Complications in Pediatric and Congenital Heart Surgery

Carl L. Backer • Constantine Mavroudis
Editors

Complications in Pediatric and Congenital Heart Surgery

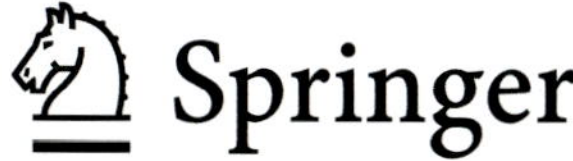

Editors
Carl L. Backer, MD
Chief, Section of Pediatric Cardiothoracic Surgery
UK Healthcare Kentucky Children's Hospital
Lexington, KY, USA

Professor, Cardiothoracic Surgery
Cincinnati Children's Hospital Medical Center
Cincinnati, OH, USA

Constantine Mavroudis, MD
Chief of Pediatric Cardiothoracic Surgery (Retired), Peyton Manning Children's Hospital
Indianapolis, IN, USA

Professor Emeritus of Surgery, Johns Hopkins University School of Medicine
Baltimore, MD, USA

ISBN 978-3-032-02660-6 ISBN 978-3-032-02661-3 (eBook)
https://doi.org/10.1007/978-3-032-02661-3

This Springer imprint is published by the registered company Springer Nature Switzerland AG
The registered company address is: Gewerbestrasse 11, 6330 Cham, Switzerland

We dedicate this book to the memory of Dr. James Tweddell, who passed away tragically at the pinnacle of his outstanding and amazingly productive career in pediatric cardiac surgery. Jim was to be the third co-editor of this textbook. His untimely passing has deprived us of his wisdom, skills, and extraordinary leadership talents.

His active participation in the creation of this book was missed. Every time that a pause would come in the writing, we would ask ourselves, "What would Jim have said?" Quite simply, it was a pleasure collaborating with him over the years. His presence and humility were rewarded by his colleagues who elected him President of the Congenital Heart Surgeons' Society and Chair of one of the most prestigious congenital heart programs in the world, Cincinnati Children's Hospital Medical Center.

As we reflect on his passing, we cannot help but feel the emotion of one who passed in the prime of his life. He was a great figure of a man, a talented surgeon, and a loyal friend. He has left a lifetime of commitment and achievement. For this, we are very much in his debt.

Preface

The raison d'etre for a book that describes perioperative complications in pediatric and congenital cardiac surgery is based on the need to define common and rare complications, offer guidelines to avoid these unwanted clinical problems, and describe solutions once these anatomic and physiologic consequences are identified. Many of these complications may seem highly unlikely until they are experienced by a given surgical team and their patient. Then the complications become reality. Emphasis will be placed on immediate diagnosis and treatment of operative mishaps, resolution of inaccurate preoperative diagnoses, and interpretation of intraoperative conditions. The book is primarily intended for practicing pediatric and adult congenital heart surgeons; however, anesthesiologists, perfusionists, supporting operating room team members, and cardiologists will find the information interesting and informative since these team members are involved in the diagnosis, evaluation, and technical resolution of the complications. The illustrations were rendered by Rachid Idriss, MFA, who illustrated our previous textbooks, atlases, and manuscripts. His artwork illustrates the problems and shows how resolution can occur in a metered manner, which plainly emphasizes the important steps of the operation. We are sad to report that shortly after the proofs for this book were completed, Rachid suddenly passed away. He was the son of the late Dr. Farouk Idriss, previous Chief of Pediatric Cardiac Surgery at Children's Memorial Hospital in Chicago. For more than 30 years we worked with Rachid on innumerable articles, book chapters, books, lectures, and presentations. Rachid was a true artist who had an amazing (gifted) understanding of human anatomy; he was able to visualize and illustrate even the most complex surgical procedures. Our publications including this one (Rachid's last book) were greatly enhanced by the illustrations that Rachid provided and we will be forever grateful for his monumental contributions. The editors also recognize the indefatigable editorial efforts by Patricia Heraty whose dedication to this publication was significant. Only experienced editors can understand the energy and patience that are required to edit chapters, secure permissions, organize prose, and communicate with the publishers. The Editors have large experience with textbooks and atlases, which have been well received. This book will likely follow previous experience. The Editors have carefully chosen contributing authors with expertise in their field that will add to the impact of the publication.

Cincinnati, OH, USA — Carl L. Backer, MD
Baltimore, MD, USA — Constantine Mavroudis, MD

In Memory of Rachid F. Idriss

Shortly after the proofs for this book were completed, our medical illustrator, Rachid F. Idriss, passed away suddenly. The editors of this book began their collaboration with Rachid when Dr. Mavroudis took over as Chief of Cardiovascular-Thoracic Surgery from Rachid's father, Dr. Farouk Idriss, at Children's Memorial Hospital in Chicago in 1989. For more than 30 years we worked with Rachid on innumerable articles, book chapters, books, lectures, and presentations. He was the principal illustrator for our textbooks, *Pediatric Cardiac Surgery, 3rd, 4th, and 5th editions*; *Atlas of Pediatric Cardiac Surgery*; *Atlas of Adult Congenital Heart Surgery*; and the present textbook, *Complications in Pediatric and Congenital Heart Surgery.*

Rachid was a true artist who had an amazing (gifted) understanding of human anatomy; he was able to visualize and illustrate even the most complex surgical procedures. The Editors have endeavored over the years to publish and lecture extensively on the procedures and techniques that we have used to repair congenital heart defects in order to educate and enlighten. Our publications were greatly enhanced by the illustrations that Rachid provided and we will be forever indebted to him.

Introduction

Perioperative complications associated with pediatric and congenital heart surgery can be challenging and potentially life-threatening if the problem is not recognized in a timely manner and rectified with appropriate measures. This book is written to heighten awareness of these unfortunate occurrences and to offer methods of diagnosis and reparative solutions. While there are many textbooks, atlases, and manuscripts dealing with pediatric and congenital heart surgery, the descriptions concentrate on the reparative parts of the operations and not so much on illustrating and resolving the complications that can occur. The narrative and the illustrations will describe how perioperative complications can occur and demonstrate how these mishaps can be resolved.

There are many examples of these unwanted complications. During an atrial septal defect closure, a prominent Eustachian flap can be misinterpreted as the inferior margin of the secundum ASD. An unaware surgeon could tunnel the flow of the inferior caval vein into the left atrium. A complicated ventricular septal defect closure associated with complex great vessel anatomy could tunnel the ventricular septal defect to an unintended great vessel. A camouflaged patent arterial duct due to thickened periductal tissue can result in an unwanted left pulmonary artery ligation. While these mishaps seem far-fetched, they have actually happened.

This book, illustrated by an experienced artist, (the late Rachid Idriss, MFA), and written by knowledgeable authors, reviews literature contributions and emphasizes how complications can occur and how to avoid them. By necessity, previously published drawings showing the important steps of the operation will be repeated in this text to contrast with new drawings highlighting the complications. The narrative will concentrate on the complications that can occur.

Contents

Complications Associated with Sternotomy, Resternotomy, and Cannulation

Constantine Mavroudis

Abstract

Complications involving sternotomy, resternotomy, and canulation procedures include uncontrolled hemorrhage, cardiac arrhythmias, and sternal fracture. Operative complications with first time sternotomy are rare; however, innominate vein injury at first time sternotomy was recently reported. Resternotomy is clearly more difficult owing to adhesions, extant hemodynamic considerations that require reoperation, and cavitary proximity to camouflaged dissection planes. Complications related to the inferior caval vein, left ventricular vent placement, and initiation of cardiopulmonary bypass are also reviewed. This chapter presents some techniques to overcome these obstacles that have been used by the editors and have been associated with excellent results and a minimal rate of unwanted cavitary reentry.

Keywords

Congenital heart disease · Surgery · Cannulation · Resternotomy · Cardioplegia

C. Mavroudis (✉)
Chief of Pediatric Cardiothoracic Surgery (Retired), Peyton Manning Children's Hospital, Indianapolis, IN, USA

Professor Emeritus of Surgery, Johns Hopkins University School of Medicine, Baltimore, MD, USA

1 Introduction

Sternotomy, resternotomy, and cannulation represent the beginning of an open-heart procedure that requires special attention to standard techniques to avoid unwanted complications. Acute operative complications with first time sternotomy are rare and only recently was innominate vein injury at first time sternotomy reported (Steely and Liu 2020). Other complications associated with first time sternotomy are more remote and centered around infections resulting in mediastinitis and sepsis (Ogus et al. 2002; Kühme et al. 2007). These infections are due to patient risk factors (Thiel and Bircks 1990), and intraoperative contamination (Webster et al. 2021).

Resternotomy is clearly more difficult owing to adhesions, extant hemodynamic considerations that require reoperation, and cavitary proximity to camouflaged dissection planes (Delius and Walters 2003). In addition, resternotomy is a predictor of operative mortality that increases with each successive mediastinal entry (Park et al. 2010). Inadvertent cavitary entry during sternal reentry can cause significant hemodynamic instability. This is especially relevant for revision operations involving Fontan conversion, right ventricular outflow tract and aortic aneurysms with substernal adherence, as well as right ventricular distention. Operative planning with preoperative computed tomography scans to determine cavitary proximity to the sternum,

C. L. Backer, C. Mavroudis (eds.), *Complications in Pediatric and Congenital Heart Surgery*,
https://doi.org/10.1007/978-3-032-02661-3_1

hemodynamic assessment to assess patient stability, and resternotomy methods are imperative before any attempts at revision operations are undertaken.

Complications of resternotomy include uncontrolled hemorrhage, cardiac arrhythmias, and sternal fracture. Any unexpected decrease in right atrial pressure due to uncontrolled hemorrhage can result in hypovolemia that unfavorably impacts the driving force (elevated central venous pressure) that controls the pulmonary circulation and cardiac output. These same hemodynamic aberrations also negatively impact patients who are undergoing ventricular-to-pulmonary conduit replacement, reoperations for tetralogy of Fallot, and tricuspid valve repairs, among others. Electrocautery dissection to separate cavitary structures from the underside of the sternum has proven to be effective and hemostatic as long as the adhesions are thin and identifiable. During this time, an electrocautery discharge on the surface of the heart can cause ventricular fibrillation requiring instant defibrillation with externally placed defibrillator pads. Under these circumstances, it is wise to continue with scissor dissection until the sternum is divided. It is for these reasons that presternotomy peripheral cannulation preparations should be considered and enacted.

2 Techniques of Safe Peripheral Cannulation to Avoid Complications

Peripheral cannulation and resternotomy techniques are principally learned and acquired during residency training, where technical expertise and confidence are nurtured. No doubt, the reader is already practicing the tenets of safe resternotomy. Collective experience reflects these principles as innovative tools for resternotomy, peripheral cannulation, and perfusion techniques that enrich the surgeon's expertise so that they are integrated into daily practice.

Figures 1, 2, 3, and 4 show the operative steps of right axillary cannulation which can be used in an emergency and also for standard arterial can-

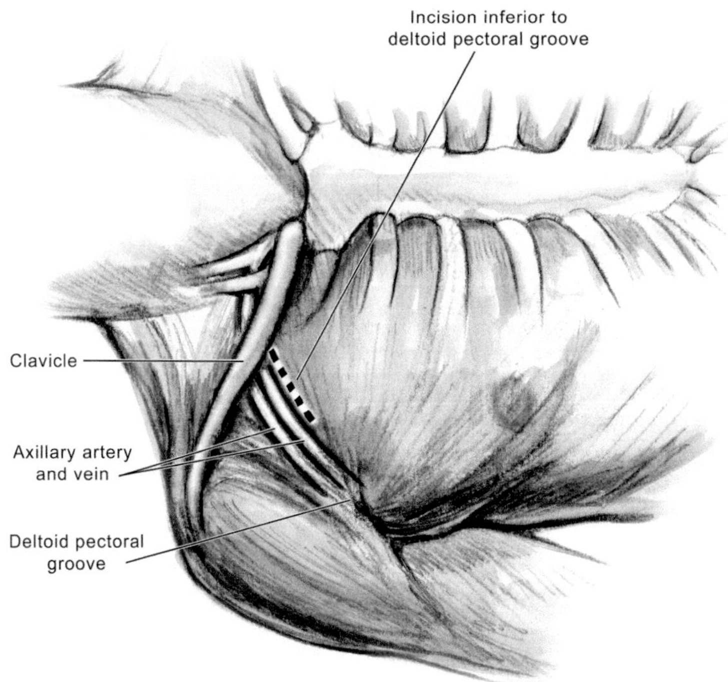

Fig. 1 Shows the topographic basic anatomy for identification and dissection of the right axillary artery in the deltopectoral groove. Axillary cannulation has the advantage of closer forward flow to the cerebral circulation, with the capability of using regional perfusion techniques in the event that arch reconstruction becomes necessary. (With permission: Mavroudis and Dearani 2020)

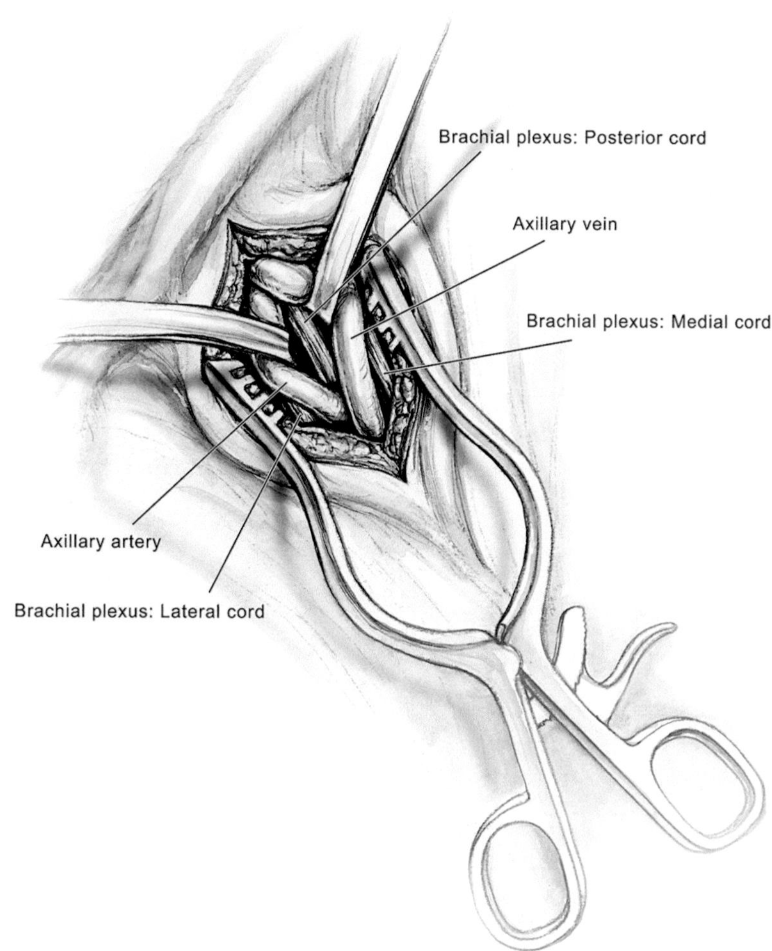

Fig. 2 Demonstrates how the dissection is performed with care to identify the axillary artery, axillary vein, and surrounding brachial plexus cords. (With permission: Mavroudis and Dearani 2020)

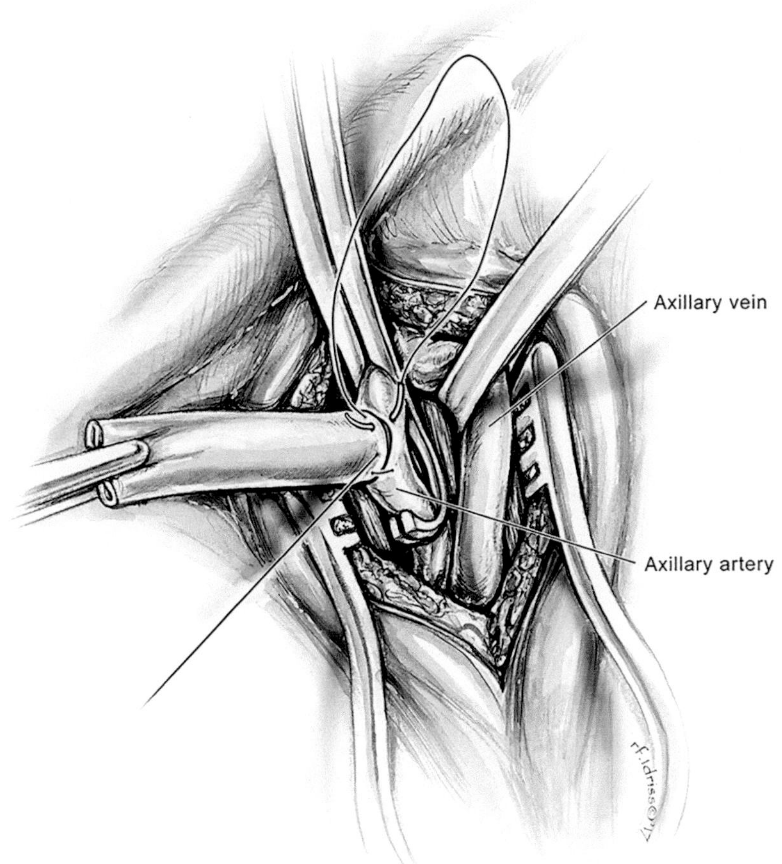

Fig. 3 The anatomic details and process of graft placement are illustrated in this figure. Once heparin is administered, the axillary artery is clamped, and an appropriately sized polytetrafluoroethylene (PTFE) graft is anastomosed end-to-side to the axillary artery. (With permission: Mavroudis and Dearani 2020)

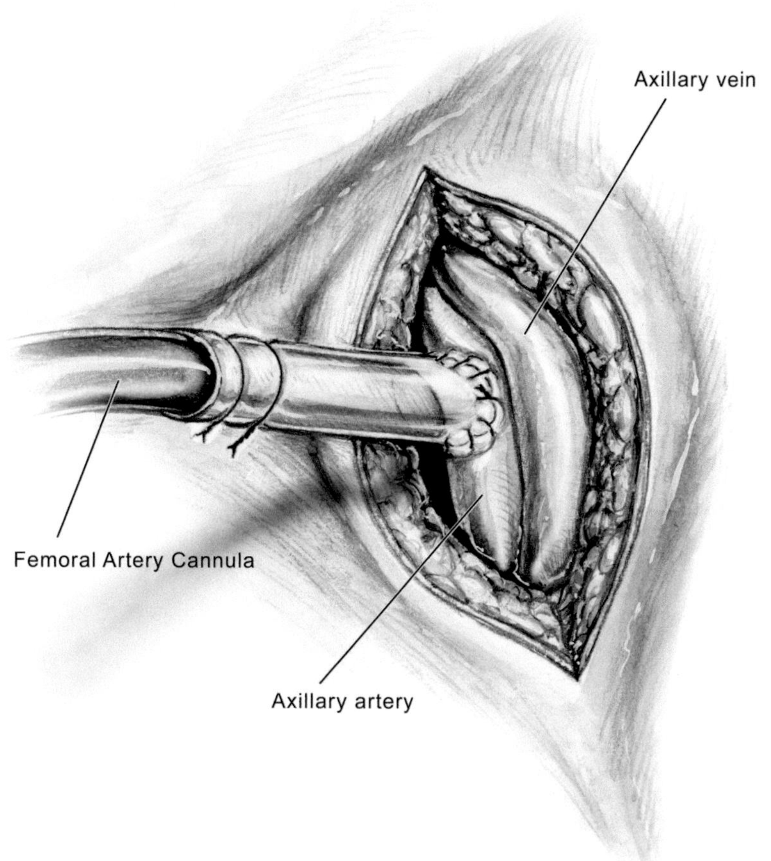

Fig. 4 Shows how the proximal graft is connected to the arterial line in preparation for cardiopulmonary bypass. Venous drainage can be instituted through the axillary vein or the femoral vein, as necessary. (With permission: Mavroudis and Dearani 2020)

nulation especially if arch reconstruction is anticipated. The steps of the operation are straightforward and well tolerated. This type of cannulation is best performed before any emergent indications since it requires an anastomosis involving a Gore-Tex graft and the axillary artery which takes time to perform. Emergent cannulation is best performed by peripheral femoral cannulation which does not routinely require graft placement. Figures 5, 6, 7, and 8 show the pro-

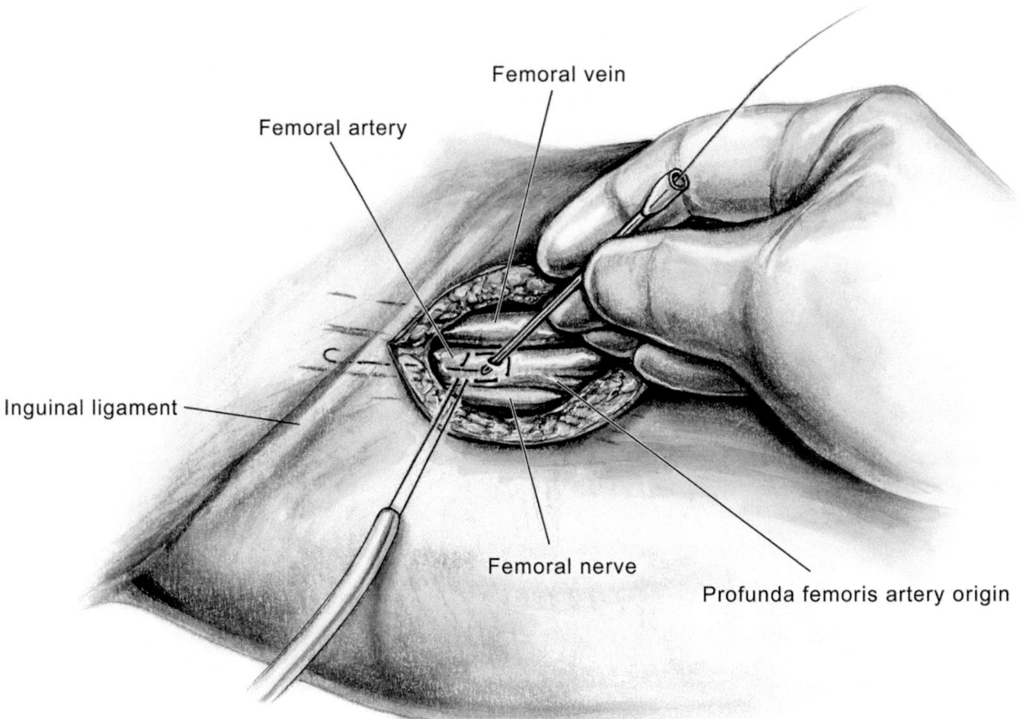

Fig. 5 The Seldinger technique of femoral arterial cannulation is depicted. Direct cannulation using this method can be accomplished without extensive dissection or subtotal femoral artery transection. Once the femoral artery is dissected and exposed, a rectangular purse string is placed in the artery. The needle and guide wire are introduced into the artery. (With permission: Mavroudis and Dearani 2020)

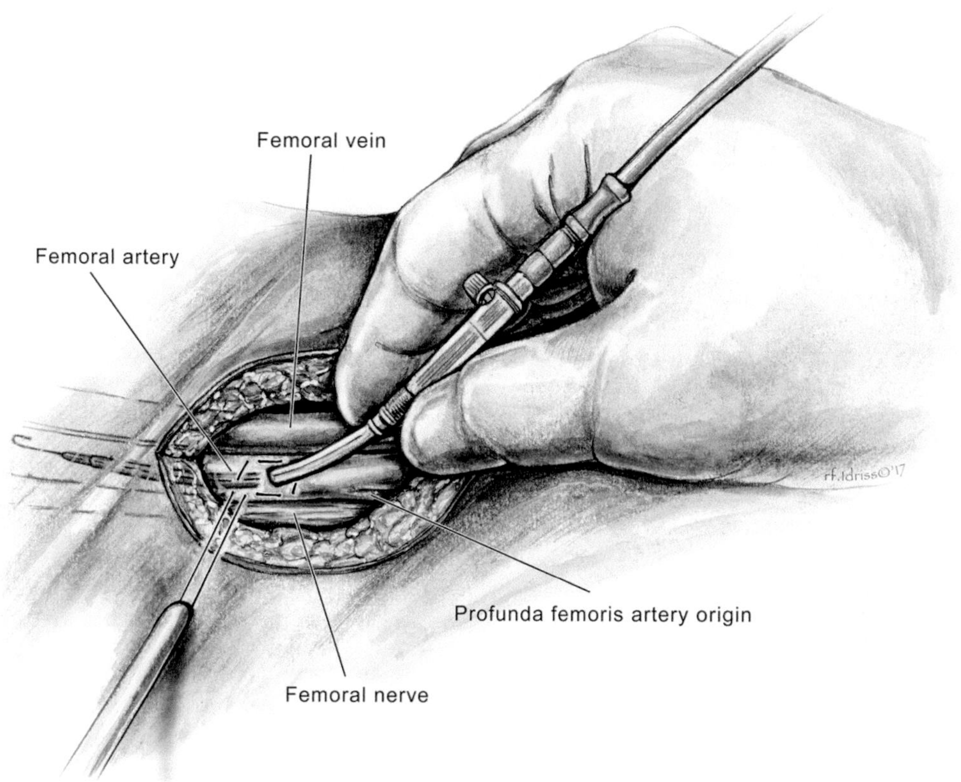

Fig. 6 Shows the result of femoral artery dilatation followed by femoral catheter placement. Often, a small incision at the wire site may be needed to facilitate the catheter placement (*not shown*). (With permission: Mavroudis and Dearani 2020)

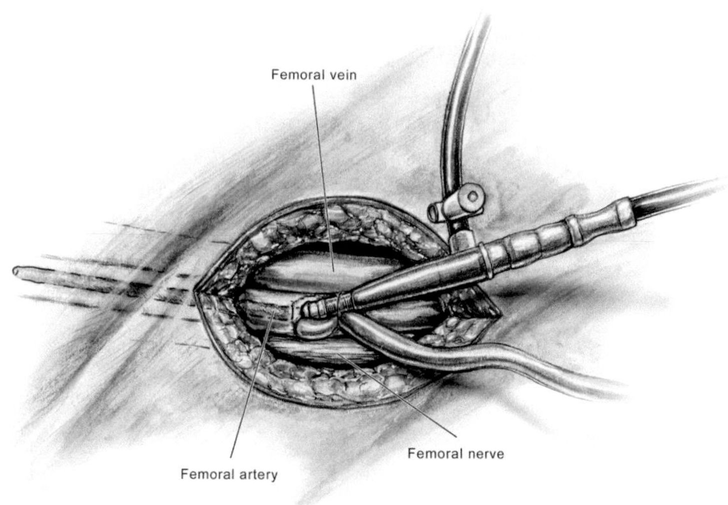

Fig. 7 The catheter is secured by a Rommel tourniquet and connected to the arterial line for immediate perfusion. (With permission: Mavroudis and Dearani 2020)

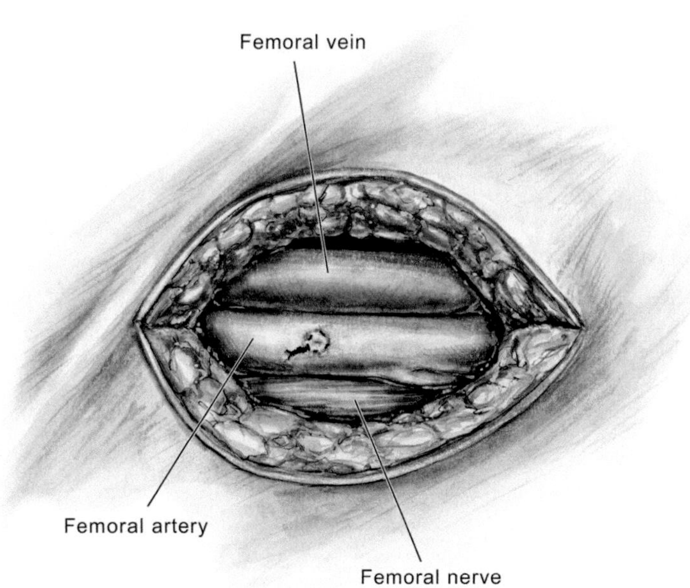

Fig. 8 Shows the repaired artery after the catheter has been removed. (With permission: Mavroudis and Dearani 2020)

cess of safe and effective cannulation and decannulation with or without minimal femoral vessel incision.

3 Resternotomy Techniques

Preparation is everything. Preoperative diagnostic computed tomography (CT) can guide the surgeon to avoid the dreaded and complicated unwanted cavitary entry. The CT scan can demonstrate the substernal relational anatomy to alert the surgeon and allow proper planning that includes peripheral cannulation, establishment of cardiopulmonary bypass (CPB), and cooling even before a mediastinal incision is performed (Ranganath et al. 2019). Transesophageal echocardiography is a less reliable tool for this purpose but can identify relational structures close to the sternum.

There are many techniques of safe resternotomy. This chapter reviews some techniques that have been used by the editors (Mavroudis and Backer 2020) and have been associated with excellent results and a minimal rate of unwanted cavitary reentry. Probably the most common approach to resternotomy uses the handheld saw (Stryker, Kalamazoo, MI), which allows the surgeon to cut the outer sternal table and allows further dissection by handheld retractors, scissor dissection, and electrocautery techniques (Bolotin et al. 2007). We have used slightly different techniques that the reader might find useful. Figures 9, 10, 11, and 12 show the progression of safe resternotomy using self-retaining mammary retractors. The particulars of the technique (Mavroudis and Backer 2020) are noted in each figure.

It is important to recognize the advantages and disadvantages of any resternotomy technique before it is attempted. Typically, electrocautery

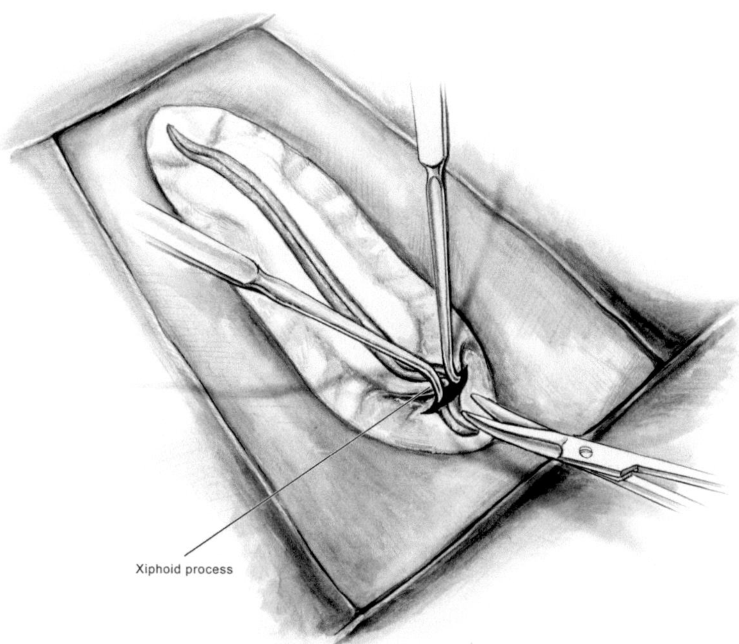

Fig. 9 These are the initial steps of a safe resternotomy. Once skin incision is performed and continued to the outer table of the sternum, the surgeon has the choice of starting the resternotomy. If the resternotomy is further challenged by dangerous adherence of vital structures to the undersurface of the sternum—which can be anticipated in patients with transposed arteries (anterior aorta), false aneurysms, central position of the right ventricular-to-pulmonary artery conduit, and gigantic right atria—peripheral cannulation is recommended for safe reentry in the event of an untoward event. Preoperative anatomic studies, the number of resternotomies, and the overall experience of the surgical team guides the use of peripheral cannulation. The resternotomy is commenced by dissecting a plane at the most inferior portion of the sternum by electrocautery or scissor dissection, assisted by handheld retractors. The motion of the heart can help to determine the safe plane between the heart and the sternum and offer a safe physical purchase for placement of the self-retaining internal mammary artery retractors. (With permission: Mavroudis and Dearani 2020)

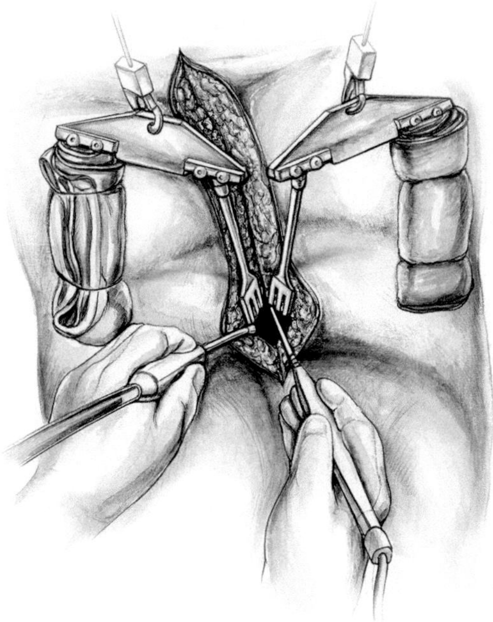

Fig. 10 Depicts the successful placement of bilateral self-retaining internal mammary artery retractors under both sides of the sternum. This maneuver allows cautious upward (anterior) retraction of the sternum away from the heart without depending on human interactions, which could be unreliable owing to normal variations of strength, attention to detail, and fatigue. Once the retraction is established, a "Delta" is created, with the superior portion of the "Delta" in the center of the undissected sternotomy. Using direct electrocautery or scissor dissection, the "Delta" is moved superiorly while the lateral planes of the underside of the sternum are enlarged and dissected into the pleural cavities, if possible. (With permission: Mavroudis and Dearani 2020)

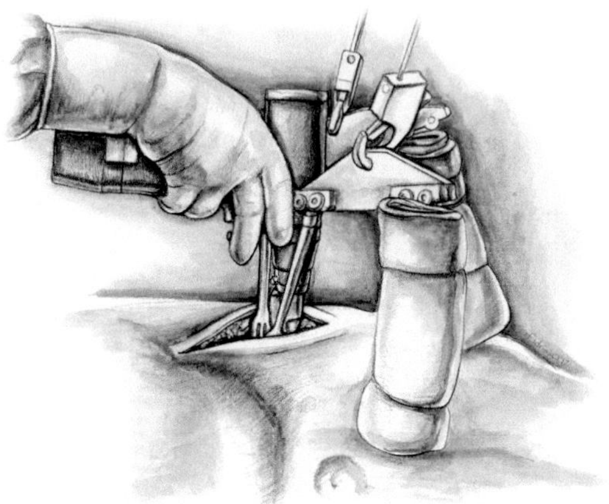

Fig. 11 The actual sternal division can be accomplished with a saw as shown in the figure, which can be used segmentally to divide the sternum up to the dissected plane that has been created. This "Delta" is then used as a dissection module to move the dissection plane superiorly until the dissection is complete. Because most self-retaining internal mammary retractors have two arms, in this application one of the arms is covered with a sterile towel to prevent unwanted injury to the surgical team. Once the sternum is opened, the second arm can be freed and used to retract each of the sternal edges for further dissection. (With permission: Mavroudis and Dearani 2020)

dissection has the advantages of creating a bloodless field during dissection and aiding in visualization of the next dissection plane. However, electrocautery can also cause cardiac arrhythmias and ventricular fibrillation requiring prompt defibrillation. Unwanted cavitary reentry can also occur with electrocautery which tends to be larger and more serious than with scissor dissection. There is no substitute for judicious application of the correct method to proceed. During sternal reentry, therefore, one can use dissection scissors to find the correct plane and then use electrocautery to continue the dissection. If arrhythmias occur with electrocautery, the surgeon may decide to switch to dissection scissors until a safer plane emerges, away from the locus of arrhythmia generation.

Furthermore, when the aorta or pulmonary artery (conduit or otherwise) has been determined by palpation to be adherent to the plane of dissection, the surgeon can continue this delicate exposure using scissors until the great vessel is safely away from the dissection plane and underside of the sternum. Awareness and attention to detail help avoid these complications. Once the resternotomy is performed, the dissection plane is extended into both thoracic cavities to facilitate eventual chest tube placement for adequate postoperative fluid and air drainage. This maneuver will allow full lung expansion and prompt extubation. This tactic is facilitated by the self-retaining internal mammary retractor that can be placed strategically to allow the surgeon increased visualization and access into both thoracic cavities as noted in Fig. 12.

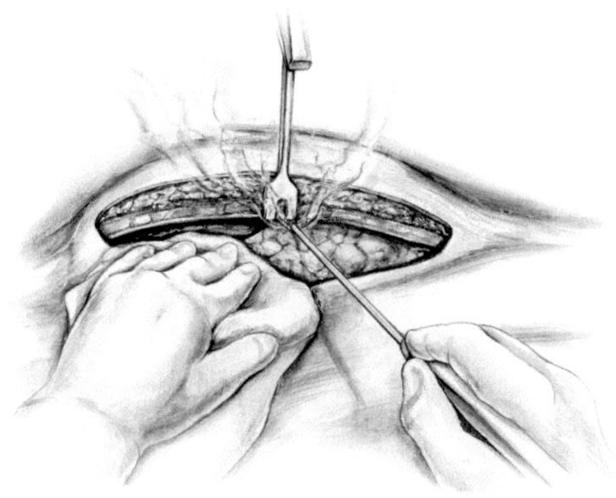

Fig. 12 Demonstrates the technique of sternal retraction using only one retractor, manual manipulation of the lung, and electrocautery dissection to lyse adhesions. (With permission: Mavroudis and Dearani 2020)

4 Unwanted Cavitary Entry

Even with the most judicious application of the aforementioned resternotomy techniques, significant bleeding can occur which can be managed as long as the proper preoperative preparations have been made. A stopgap technique to slow the bleeding and tamponade the outflow is noted in Fig. 13. The left-hand module shows the result of an extensive bleed that cannot be effectively controlled with finger digital pressure. Under these circumstances, temporary reapproximation of the dissected sternal edges as shown in the right-handed module may give the surgeon enough time to effect peripheral cannulation and commence cardiopulmonary bypass (Mavroudis and

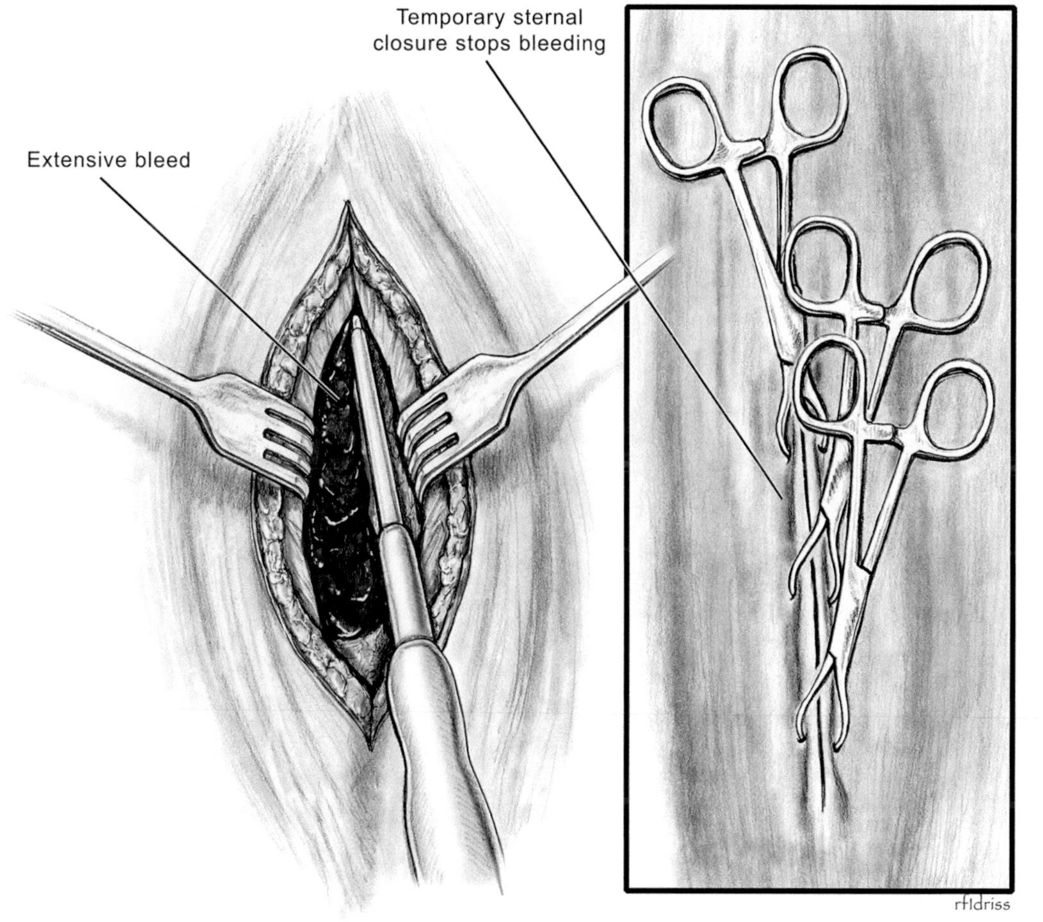

Fig. 13 (Left panel) Shows unwanted hemorrhage that can occur during resternotomy. These kinds of cavitary entry tend to occur at the apex of the sternotomy which is not convenient for digital compression and hemorrhage control. The right panel shows the judicious placement of towel clips which can reapproximate the sternal edges for temporary hemorrhage control to allow emergency peripheral cannulation for cardiopulmonary bypass

Dearani 2020). This maneuver should be considered temporary and should not be relied upon for anything except emergency measures to establish cardiopulmonary bypass.

5 Aortic Cannulation

Aortic cannulation, especially in a neonate requires special care. In general, we use only one purse string suture employing a two-needle technique as shown in Fig. 14. The site is just below and to the left of the takeoff of the common brachiocephalic artery. Figures 15, 16, 17, 18, 19, 20, 21, 22, 23, and 24 show the progression of safe aortic cannulation. In the case of an unwanted transaortic suture placement resulting in bleeding, the surgeon must assess the extent and magnitude of the bleeding. Oftentimes, but not always, a transaortic suture must be removed and replaced to prevent ongoing bleeding during the procedure, which is shown in Fig. 25a–c.

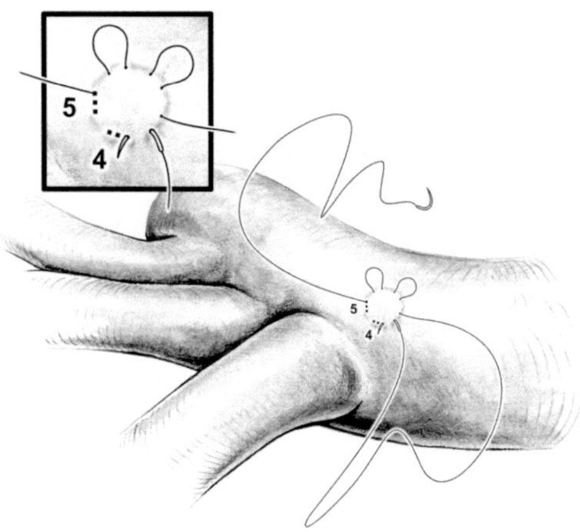

Fig. 14 Shows placement of aortic purse string using a two-needle technique for aortic cannulation The sutures are placed through the adventitia and into, but not, through the media. Transaortic sutures are avoided to prevent bleeding. (With Permission: Mavroudis 2015)

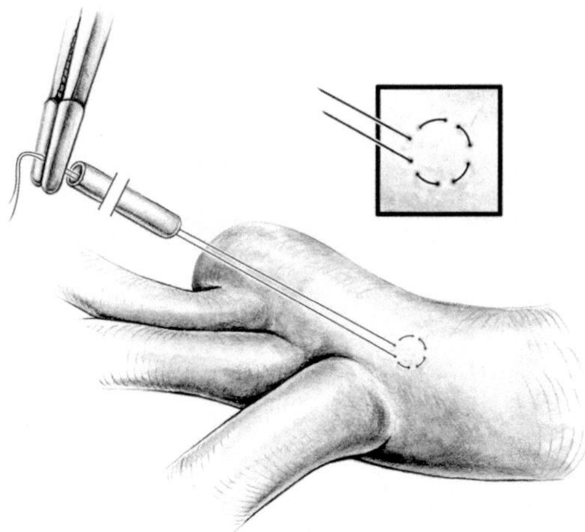

Fig. 15 Demonstrates the snugger tourniquet application after suture placement. (With Permission: Mavroudis 2015)

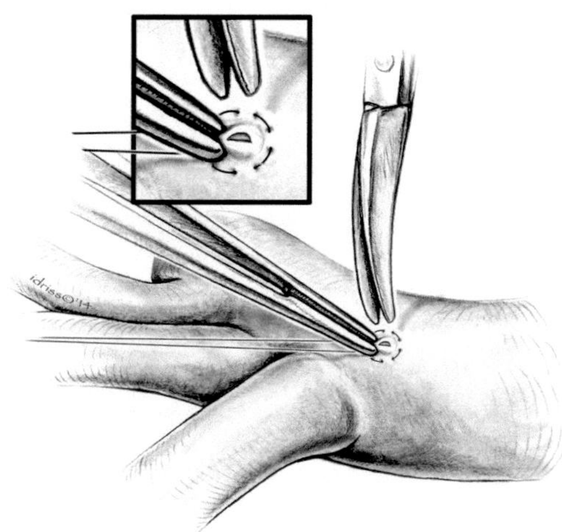

Fig. 16 The adventitia is being dissected to the media within the confines of the purse string suture line. (With Permission: Mavroudis 2015)

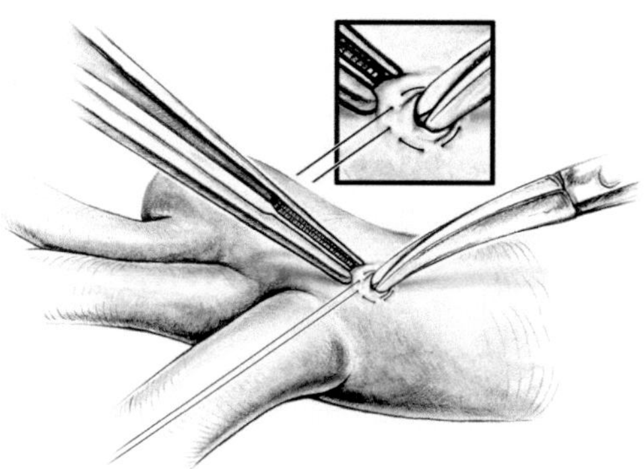

Fig. 17 The aortic cannulation site is dissected to the media to facilitate aortic cannula placement. (With Permission: Mavroudis 2015)

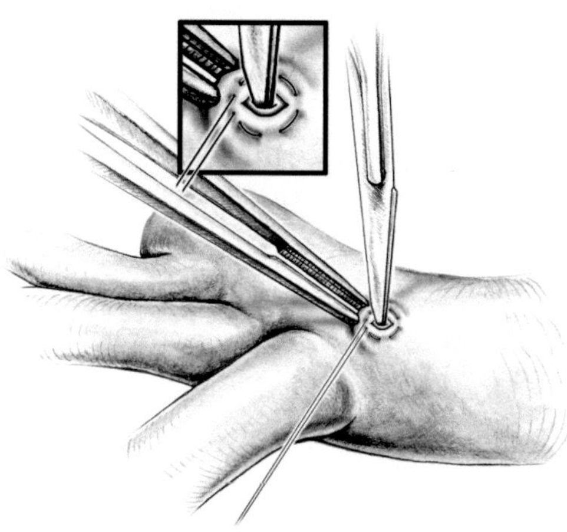

Fig. 18 With the left hand, vascular forceps firmly grip the aortic wall above (upstream to) the aortic purse string. The surgeon retracts the forceps superiorly to expose the dissected cannulation site. A #11 blade is used to perform a small horizontal aortotomy within the confines of the dissected aorta inside the suture line. As the blade is removed, downward traction is placed with the forceps thereby controlling the bleeding. (With Permission: Mavroudis 2015)

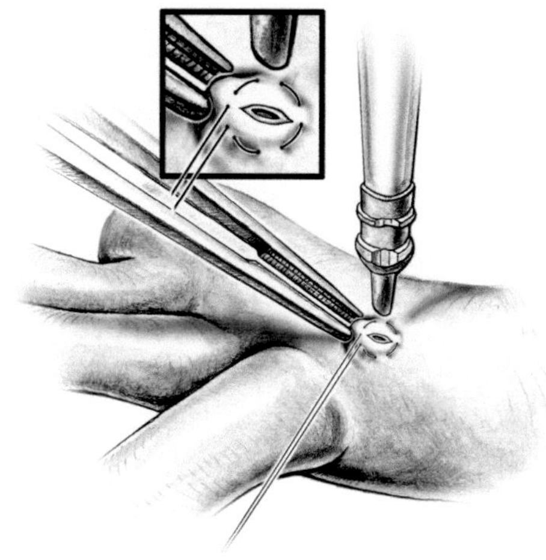

Fig. 19 In a coordinated movement, the forceps loosen the downward traction and expose the aortotomy. Sometimes the aortotomy is too small and the catheter may need to be manipulated. Other times a small, curved mosquito clamp can be inserted to dilate the opening with or without opening the clamp. (With Permission: Mavroudis 2015)

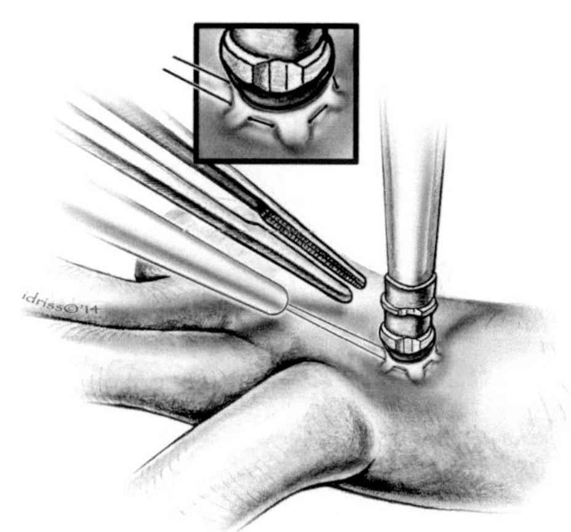

Fig. 20 Once the cannula is placed, the snugger is engaged and preparations are made to secure the cannula in place. (With Permission: Mavroudis 2015)

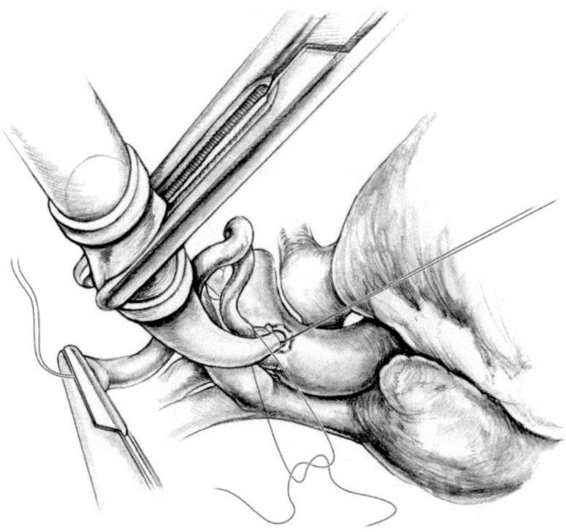

Fig. 21 Shows the placement of two separate sutures to secure the aortic cannula for successful perfusion. (With Permission: Mavroudis 2015)

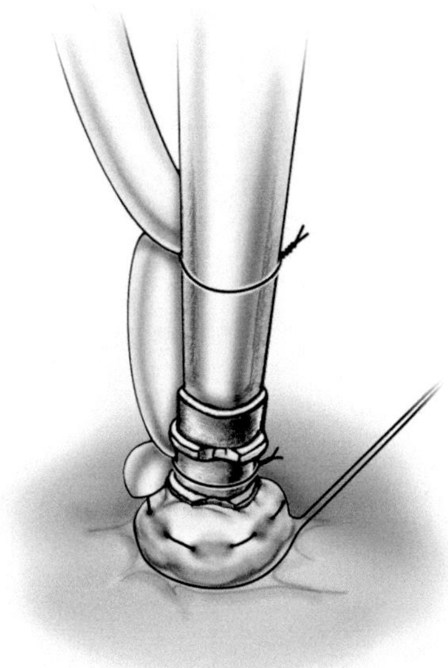

Fig. 23 This tie can act as a second suture line and generally this maneuver controls the bleeding. (With Permission: Mavroudis 2015)

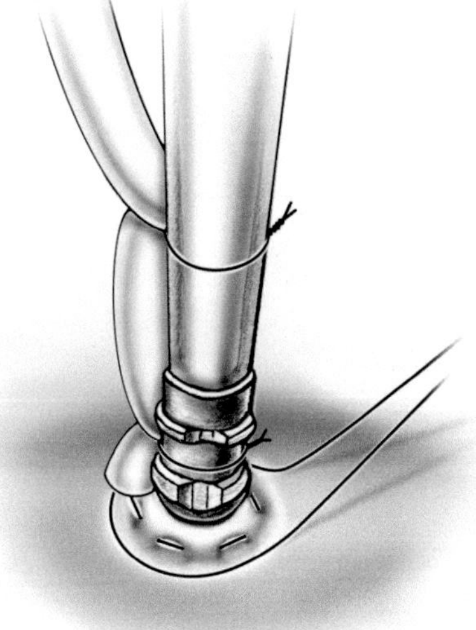

Fig. 22 If bleeding persists from the purse string suture line, a free silk tie can be placed around the base of the cannula while dragging the adventitia to the base. (With Permission: Mavroudis 2015)

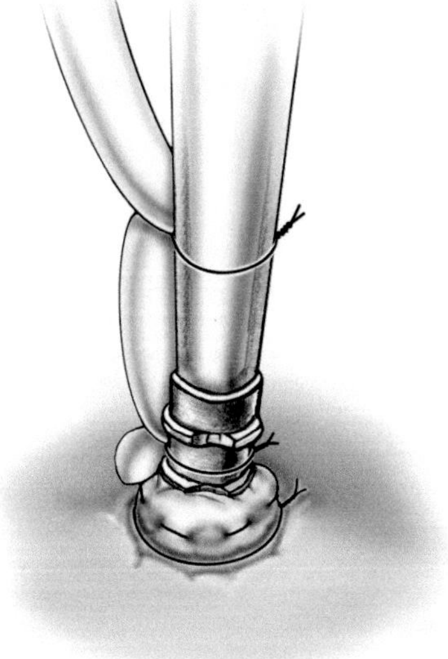

Fig. 24 Shows the completed tie around the aortic suture line resulting in hemostasis. (With Permission: Mavroudis 2015)

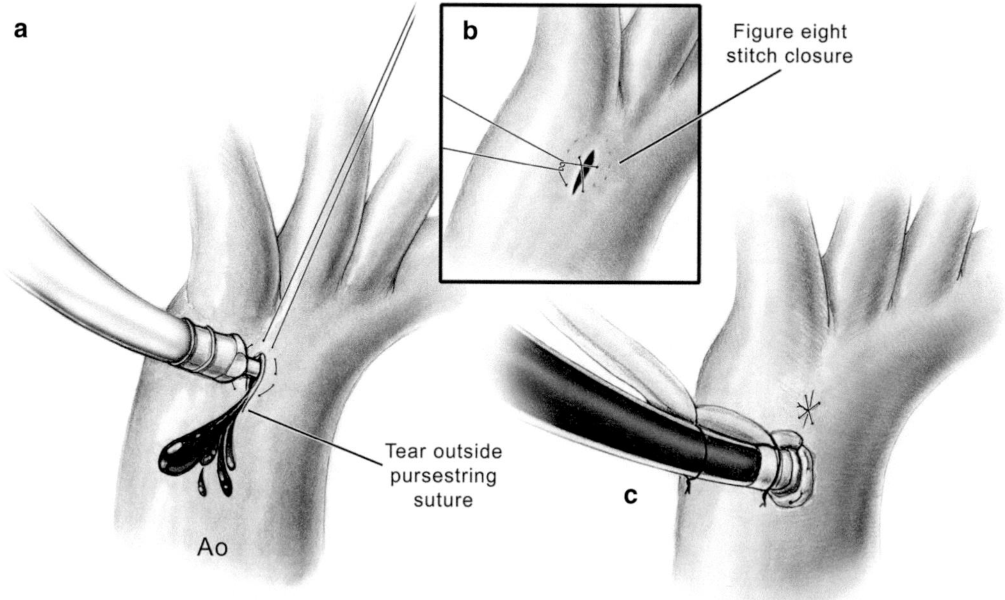

Fig. 25 This figure illustrates hemorrhage outside of the aortic suture line which is not controlled by Rommel tourniquet. This conundrum is best treated by cannula removal (**a**), aortic suture repair of the tear (**b**), and recannulation using a new aortic purse string and Rommel tourniquet (**c**). *A* aorta

6 Superior Caval Vein Cannulation

The superior caval vein (SCV) can be cannulated directly into the SCV for specific indications such as for partial anomalous pulmonary venous return, bidirectional Glenn shunt, and total cavopulmonary artery Fontan, to name but a few. Alternatively, the SCV can be cannulated via the right atrial appendage with careful advancement into the SCV. Figures 26, 27, 28, 29, 30, 31, and 32 show the proper steps of SCV cannulation using a longitudinal rectangular purse string suture and careful right angle cannula placement just downstream to the entry of the brachiocephalic vein for cardiopulmonary bypass. The azygous vein may or may not require ligation and division depending on the anatomic and physiologic circumstances.

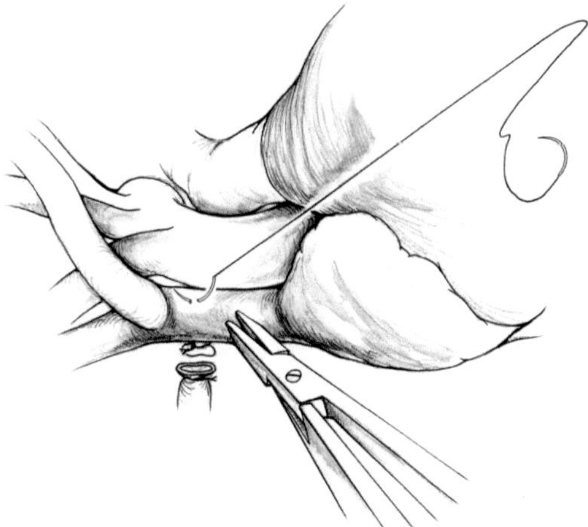

Fig. 26 These are the initial steps of superior vena cava cannulation with Prolene suture placement just downstream of the brachiocephalic vein. The azygous vein is shown ligated and divided. (With Permission: Mavroudis 2015)

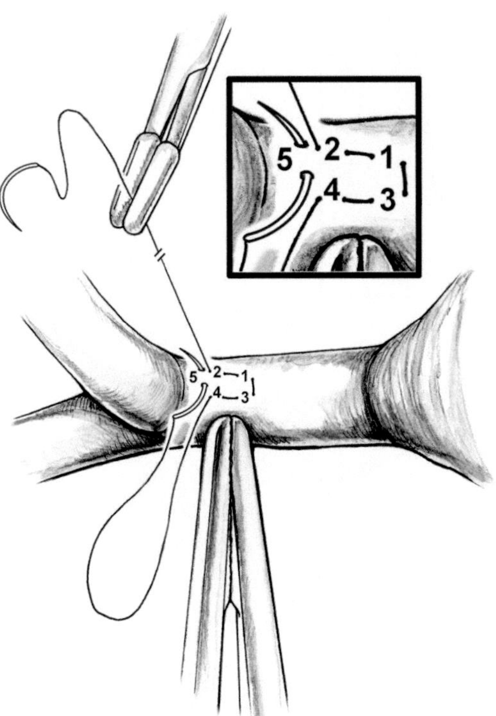

Fig. 27 Demonstrates the rectangular purse string in progress by numbered needle placement. (With Permission: Mavroudis 2015)

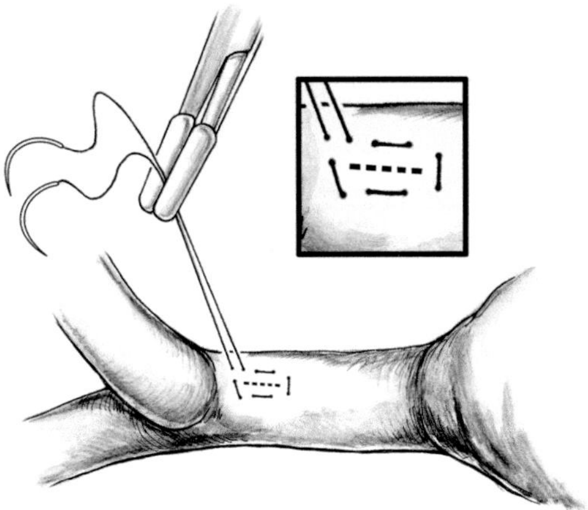

Fig. 28 Completed rectangular purse string with a dotted line to indicate the incision location for proper cannulation. (With Permission: Mavroudis 2015)

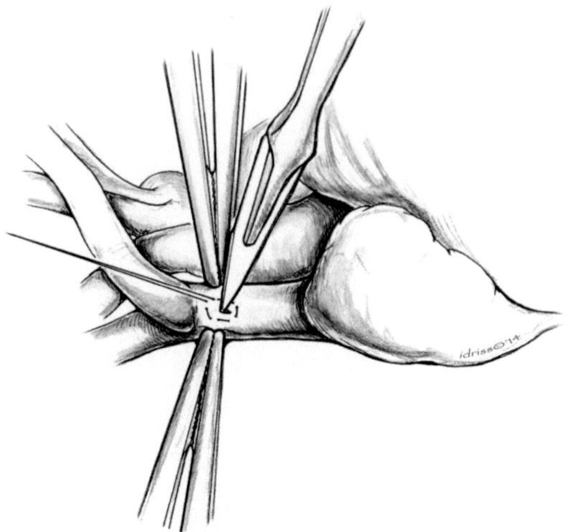

Fig. 29 This figure illustrates the surgeon and assistant gripping the medial and lateral superior vena cava walls just outside of the rectangular suture line and retracting while the surgeon performs a venotomy (#11 blade) for the length of the area within the purse string. (With Permission: Mavroudis 2015)

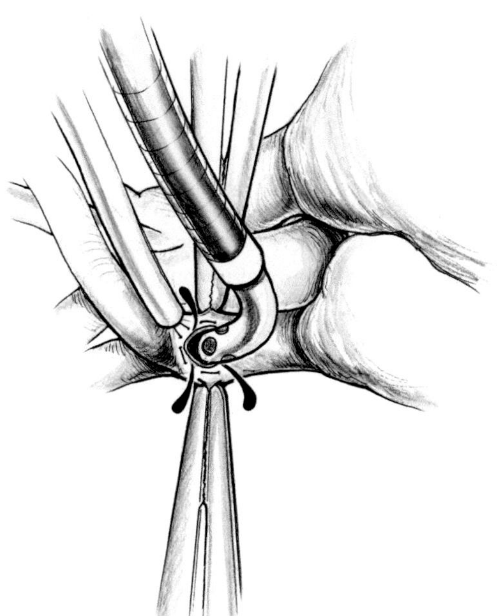

Fig. 30 Demonstrates the maneuver that the surgeons use to laterally retract the superior vena cava, open the hole, and place the right-angled catheter into the opening. (With Permission: Mavroudis 2015)

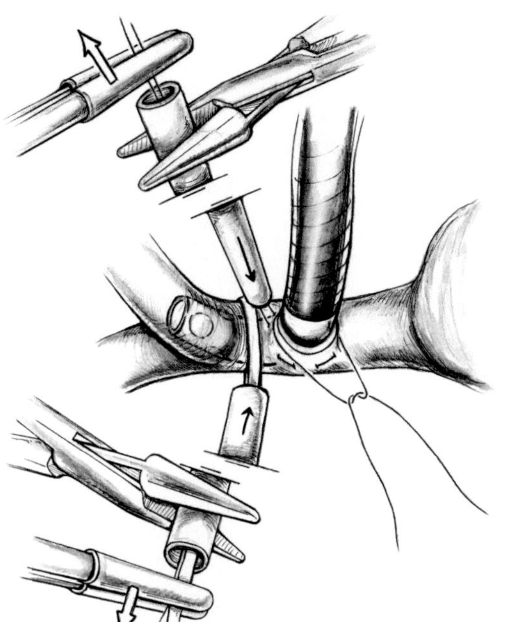

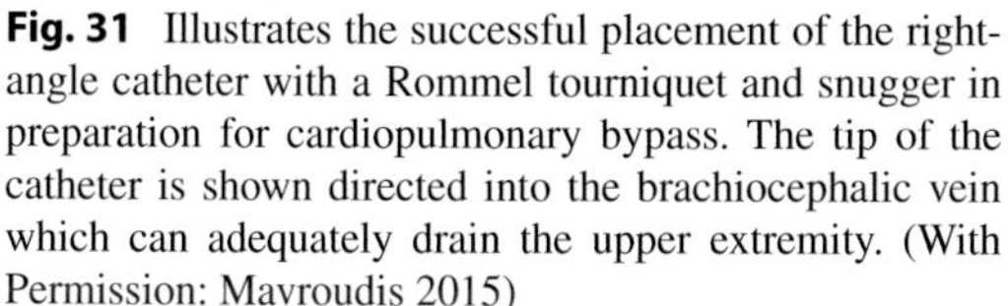

Fig. 31 Illustrates the successful placement of the right-angle catheter with a Rommel tourniquet and snugger in preparation for cardiopulmonary bypass. The tip of the catheter is shown directed into the brachiocephalic vein which can adequately drain the upper extremity. (With Permission: Mavroudis 2015)

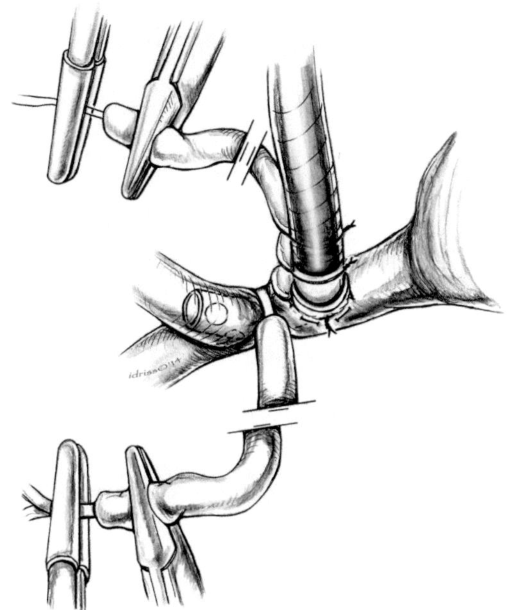

Fig. 32 After the commencement of cardiopulmonary bypass the surgeon can engage the Rommel tourniquet and proceed with the operation confident that upper extremity drainage will be unobstructed. (With Permission: Mavroudis 2015)

Occasionally, a tear may occur outside of the rectangular suture line which will require attention if proper hemostasis is to be achieved. Figure 33a shows the tear in the SCV outside of the rectangular purse-string. The initial response will generally be to place more sutures around the hole to control the bleeding. However, this may cause SCV obstruction in the long term which may not be favorable for those patients who are having an extracardiac Fontan operation, or bidirectional Glenn operation. Better to commence partial cardiopulmonary bypass with the inferior caval vein catheter, remove the SCV catheter, and perform a horizontal repair of the caval tear at the cannulation site. A horizontal repair will slightly shorten the length of the SCV but should retain the internal diameter that will facilitate upper extremity drainage without stenosis as noted in Fig. 33b. The end result should appear like the horizontally repaired SCV as noted in Fig. 33c. The patient can then be separated from cardiopulmonary bypass without concern for SCV obstruction.

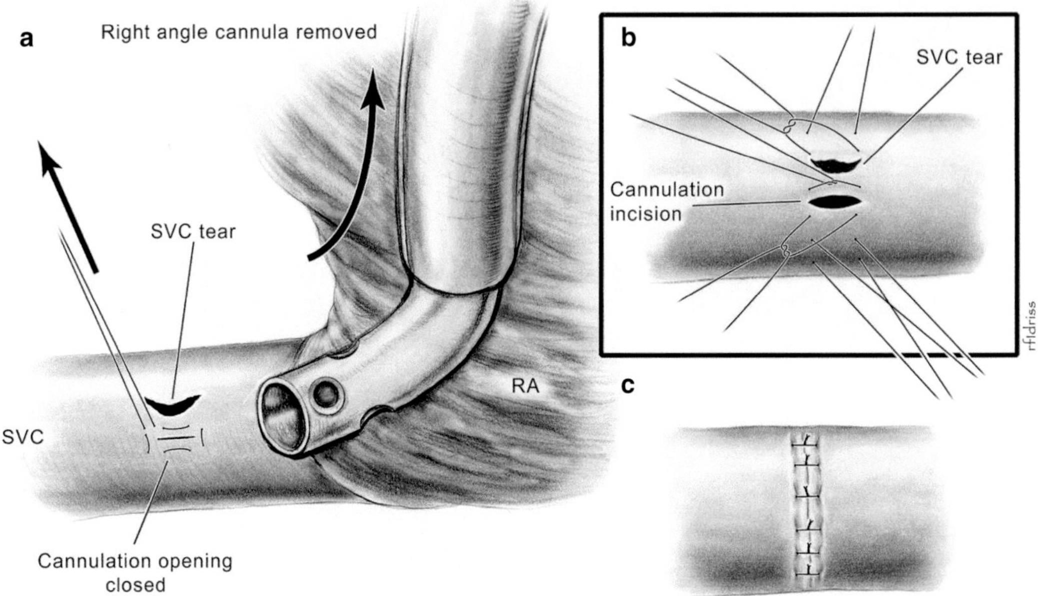

Fig. 33 (**a–c**) The completed tie around the aortic suture line resulting in hemostasis. *RA* right atrium, *SVC* superior vena cava

7 Right Atrial Appendage Cannulation

The process of right atrial appendage cannulation is straightforward and generally uncomplicated. The steps of the cannulation procedure are noted in Figs. 34, 35, 36, 37, and 38. There are some complicating factors, especially in reoperations, which should be avoided, however. Recannulation of the right atrial appendage may require additional dissection in the right atrioventricular groove where lies the course of the right coronary artery. An unwanted entry in this artery will require expedited cardiopulmonary bypass, aortic cross-clamping, and patch repair usually with a piece of pericardium or Gore-Tex patch. In addition, the redo atrial appendage purse-string may be carried more medial than appropriate and cause injury to the sinoatrial node. In general, however, these complications are rare as long as judicious awareness of the anatomy is practiced. More often than not, the surgeon will be made aware of poor venous drainage which will require catheter adjustment to enhance drainage. These complications will be discussed in the subsequent sections of this chapter.

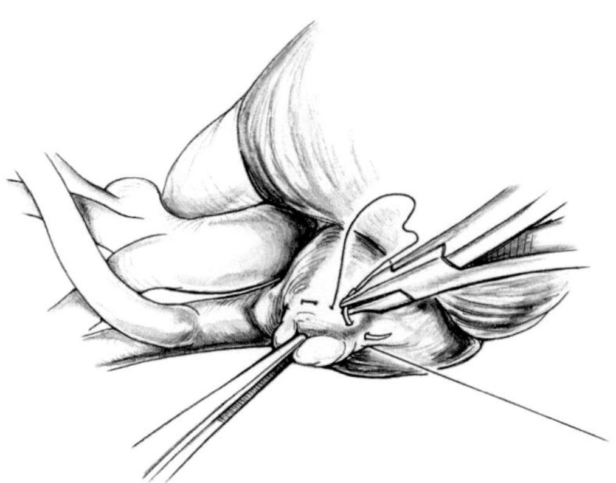

Fig. 34 A transatrial appendage cannulation can be accomplished through an atrial appendage purse string as noted. (With Permission: Mavroudis 2015)

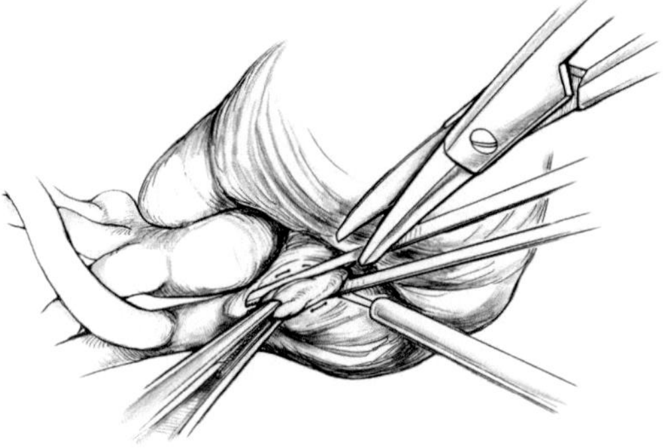

Fig. 35 The assistant surgeon holds the forceps to simulate a clamp and compresses the atrial appendage while the surgeon amputates the appendage above the purse string suture. (With Permission: Mavroudis 2015)

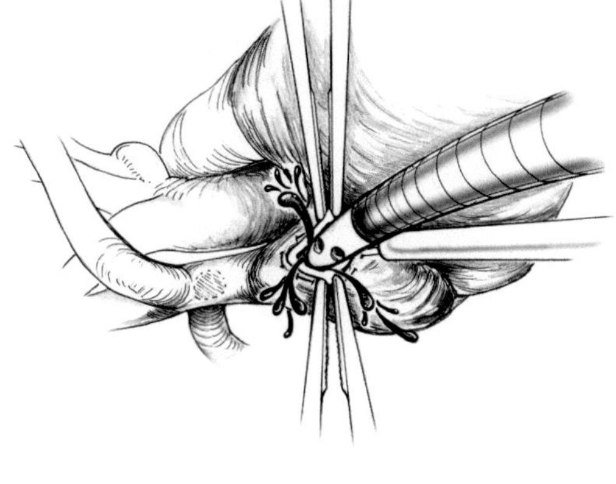

Fig. 36 Both surgeons hold the opposing ends of the cut atrial appendage and retract laterally thereby opening the hole while the surgeon inserts the catheter into the atrium, directing it to the superior vena cava. (With Permission: Mavroudis 2015)

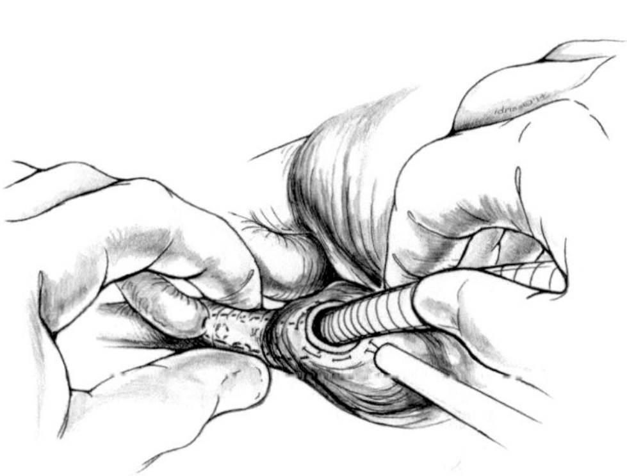

Fig. 37 The catheter is advanced, oftentimes requiring guidance with the left hand, just above the entry of the azygous vein. (With Permission: Mavroudis 2015)

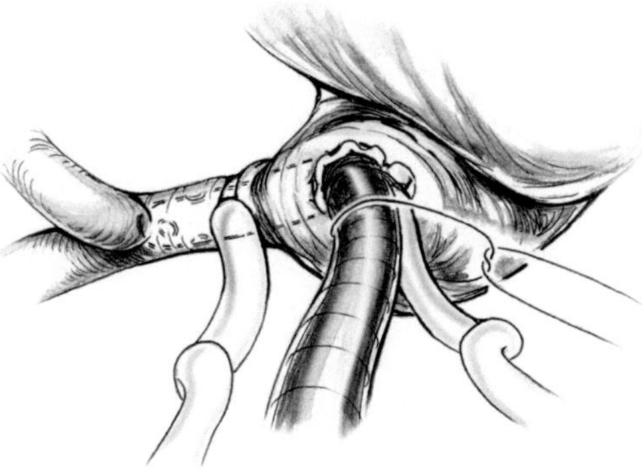

Fig. 38 The catheter is then secured by the snugger and a silk tie. When single atrial cannulation is desired by the surgeon, this transatrial appendage cannulation technique can be used to place the catheter in the atrium with the tip at the orifice of the inferior vena cava. (With Permission: Mavroudis 2015)

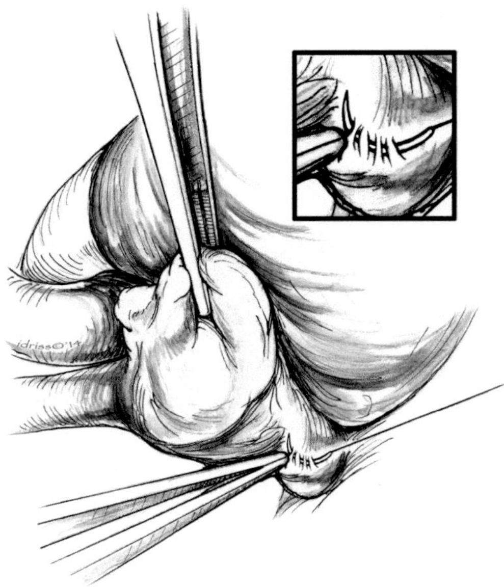

Fig. 39 The inferior vena cava (IVC) can be cannulated at its entry into the right atrium (RA). A purse string suture is placed at the IVC-RA junction or directly in the IVC depending on the operation. The assistant surgeon retracts the right atrium medially and superiorly with the right-hand using forceps while he/she and the surgeon control opposite sides of the suture line. (With Permission: Mavroudis 2015)

8 Inferior Caval Vein Cannulation

The process of safe inferior caval vein (ICV) cannulation is noted in Figs. 39, 40, 41, 42, and 43. In general, ICV cannulation should be an uncom-

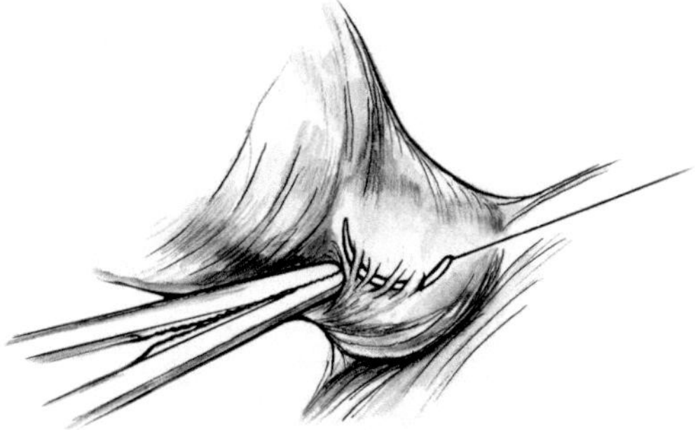

Fig. 40 Shows the first part of the purse string suture which is accomplished in a front handed fashion (assuming right handedness) inferiorly to superiorly in a clockwise fashion. (With Permission: Mavroudis 2015)

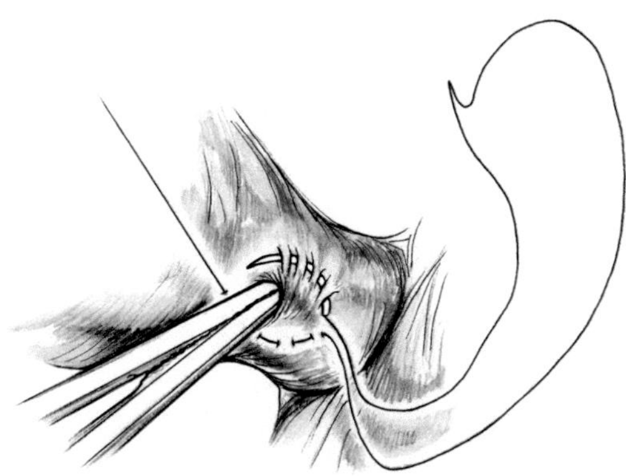

Fig. 41 This is the completion of the purse string suture which is accomplished in a back handed fashion (assuming right handedness) inferiorly to superiorly in a counter clockwise fashion. (With Permission: Mavroudis 2015)

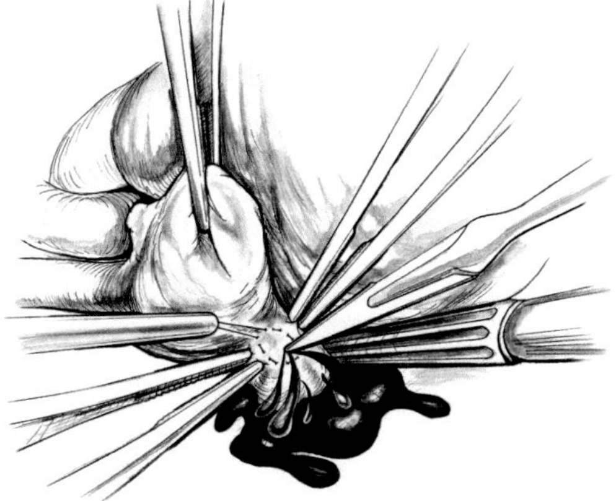

Fig. 42 A pump sucker is placed medially to the inferior vena cava. A #11 blade is used to make an incision within the suture line, after which time the surgeon and the assistant surgeon close the hole by mutual medial direct pressure. (With Permission: Mavroudis 2015)

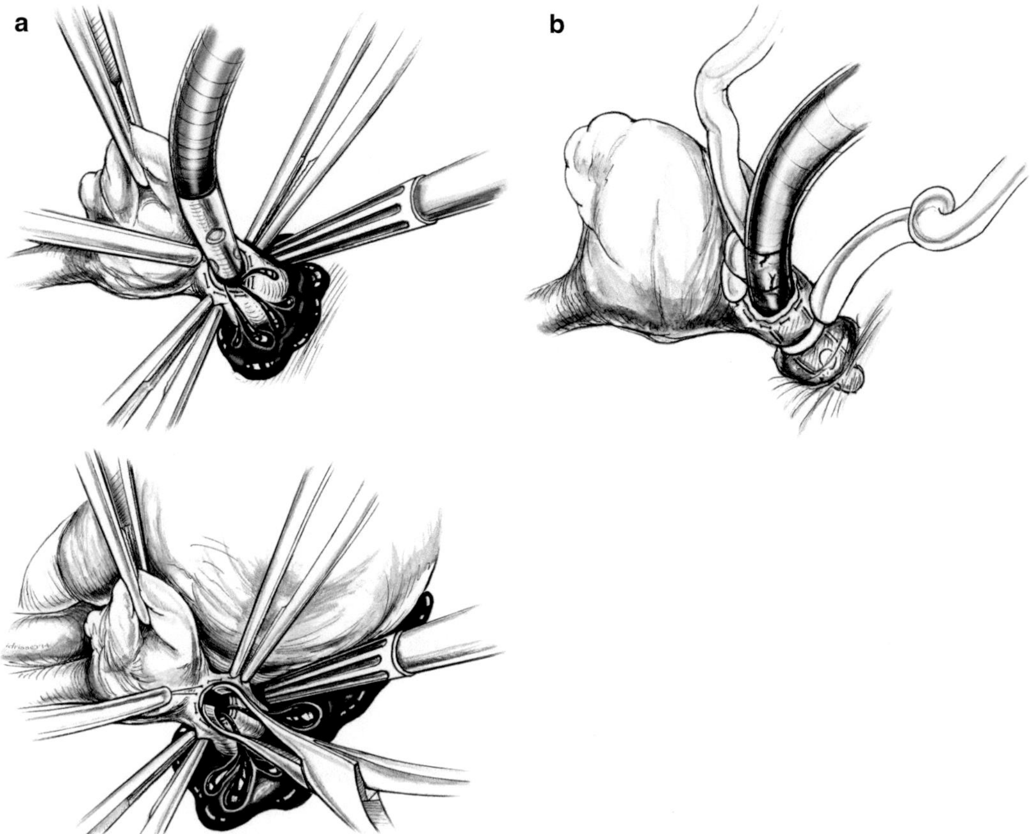

Fig. 43 The surgeon retracts laterally while a tonsil clamp is inserted into the hole for dilation followed by medial compression to control the bleeding. The processes are repeated, this time placing the catheter into the opening (Panel a) and controlling it by snugger engagement and securing ties (Panel b). (With Permission: Mavroudis 2015)

plicated part of an operation. However, there are circumstances, such as in a redo operation that placing a clamp around the ICV may result in a posterior ICV tear. This is a major complication and will need to be managed appropriately.

9 Undiagnosed Left Superior Caval Vein

Hemodynamic problems with systemic venous return at the commencement of cardiopulmonary bypass become obvious within the first 1–3 min and requires immediate attention. The most common congenital venous anomaly that challenges the safe institution of CPB is a left superior caval vein (SCV). This structure typically drains into the coronary sinus although rarely it can be associated with an unroofed coronary sinus with drainage into the left atrium. Figure 44 shows proper aortobicaval CPB with snugger application on both caval veins. The alert surgeon will recognize right atrial dilatation despite proper placement of the venous catheters and should start a search for a left SCV. The prior thymus dissection would have alerted the surgeon to such a possibility, since a left SCV is often associated with the absence of the brachiocephalic vein.

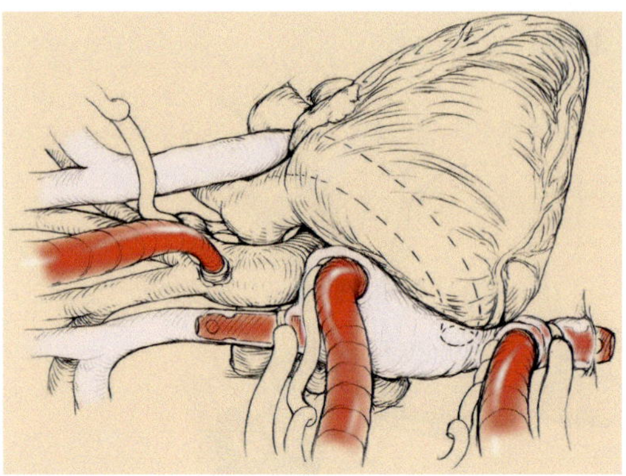

Fig. 44 Shows the undiagnosed left superior caval vein, which when not diagnosed early will result in right atrial dilatation after the commencement of cardiopulmonary bypass (With Permission: Mavroudis 2015)

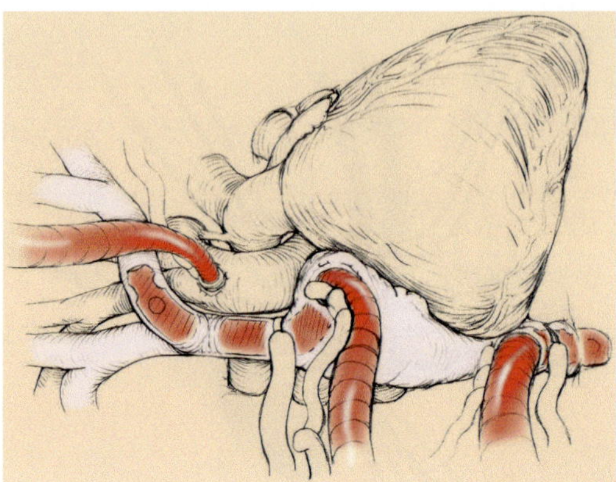

Fig. 45 Demonstrates high placement of the superior vena catheter, which preferentially drains the left innominate vein and leaves the rest of the brachiocephalic venous structures undrained. A simple adjustment of the catheter will correct this problem. (With Permission: Mavroudis 2015)

Once the diagnosis is made, the surgeon must assess the size of the left SCV and determine the need for a third drainage catheter. Catheter drainage of a large left SCV is indicated for safe and effective venous drainage. A smaller left SCV can be managed by simple snugger control during the intracardiac operation and this may be all that is needed under these condition. If the left SCV remains undiagnosed after the initiation of CPB, aortic cross-clamping, cardioplegic arrest, and right atrial entry, the condition will become obvious by venous blood filling the operative field through the coronary sinus. This situation should immediately result in a search for a left SCV, with the goal of controlling the flow by snugger application or by venous drainage if the left SCV is large.

10 Complications Associated with Venous Catheter Placement

The commencement of aortobicaval cardiopulmonary bypass is usually attended by a smooth transition from cardiopulmonary maintenance of the circulation to the heart lung machine. Within the first few minutes of cardiopulmonary bypass, there should be visual evidence of appropriate venous drainage as indicated by right atrial decompression and effective transfer of the circulation to the bypass circuit. When the right atrium is not decompressed and when there is a drainage problem as noted by the perfusionist, a thorough search for venous obstruction should result. First things first; careful inspection should ensure proper and unobstructed venous tube alignment towards the CPB pump. All effluent tubes should be inspected for unwanted kinks or inappropriate turns. The perfusionist must also ascertain that the tube clamps have been removed to institute drainage.

Assuming that there are no obvious impediments with the heart lung machine, the next course of action should confirm the proper placement of the caval vein drainage catheters. Figure 45 shows a high placement of the SCV catheter, which preferentially drains the left innominate vein leaving the rest of the brachiocephalic venous structures undrained. A simple adjustment of the catheter by the surgeon will correct this problem and should result in visual drainage and decompression of the right atrium.

A more likely cause of decreased venous drainage is the undesirable placement of the ICV catheter into one of the hepatic veins, as in Fig. 46. Figure 47 shows how the ICV snugger is released, with repositioning of the catheter to insure proper drainage. As the surgeon adjusts the catheter, improved drainage is monitored and confirmed by assessment of the right atrial volume, which will be fully decompressed upon

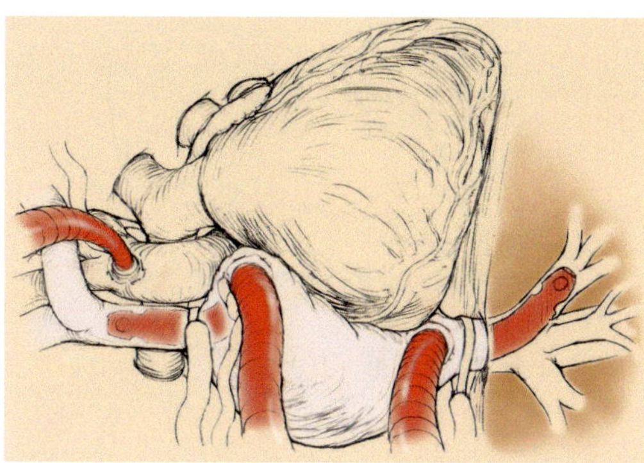

Fig. 46 This illustration shows inappropriate placement of the inferior vena cava catheter into a hepatic vein which results in poor drainage. When this condition remains undiagnosed, poor lower extremity drainage and hepatic venous congestion will ensue. (With Permission: Mavroudis 2015)

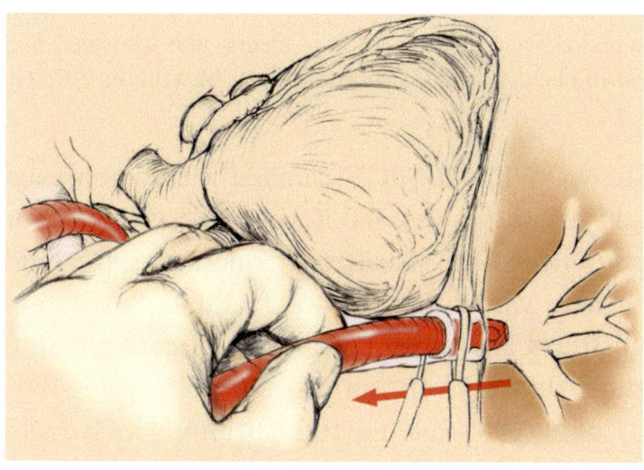

Fig. 47 Shows the gentle retraction of the inferior vena cava (IVC) while the surgeon is monitoring the visual decompression of the right atrium. This maneuver is an excellent investment of time to avoid complications during the subsequent cardiopulmonary bypass. (With Permission: Mavroudis 2015)

proper catheter placement. Failure to make these adjustments at the beginning of the operation will result in poor perfusion and multiple complications. Clearly, time is well spent on these details before continuing with the operation.

11 Management of Inferior Caval Vein Injury

Superior and inferior caval vein snuggers (tapes) to control the venous inflow can be placed around the respective venous structures either before or during the initiation of cardiopulmonary bypass. Complications associated with snugger placement especially in reoperations are not unusual and it is the rare surgeon, indeed, who has not encountered complications with this maneuver. Injury to the ICV results when a clamp is placed around the insufficiently dissected ICV for the purpose of placing the caval tape for right atrial isolation. Intense bleeding before the institution of CPB as noted in Fig. 48 or significant air in the ICV cannula after CPB indicates the injury, usually evoking dismay, embarrassment, and the recognition that the operation will become complicated and prolonged. Figures 49, 50, and 51 demonstrate maneuvers that should **not** be employed to repair this injury owing to poor exposure and possible air embolus. Embarking on epicardial repair tactics will result in frustration and continued bleeding. Figure 49 shows the result of a posterior ICV bleed with the ICV catheter in place. Bleeding under these circumstances is torrential. Adequate exposure and reparative suture placement are challenged under any circumstances. Even if the sutures are placed, tying them becomes a major consideration which likely will cause a larger tear. Such an attempt is ill advised and likely to fail.

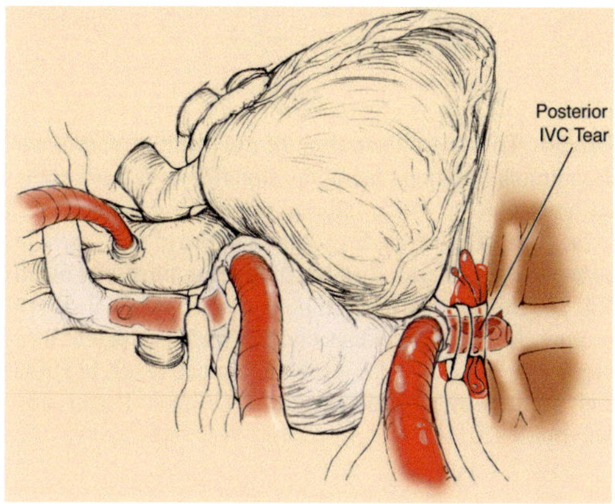

Fig. 48 Demonstrates the result of a posterior inferior caval vein injury caused by attempted passage of the caval tape around the inferior vena cava without conscientious and thorough dissection to find the proper plane. The injury tends to be directly posterior and inaccessible to uncomplicated suture repair. (With Permission: Mavroudis 2015)

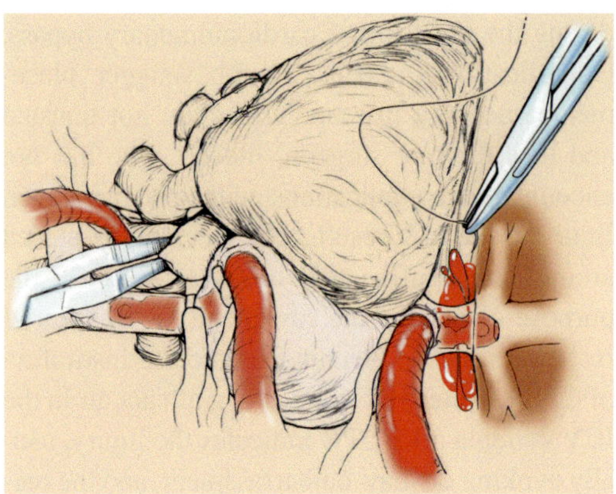

Fig. 49 Shows a posterior bleed of the inferior vena cava with the catheter in place. Bleeding in this scenario is torrential, making adequate exposure and reparative suture placement almost impossible. Even if the sutures are placed, tying them becomes a major effort. (With Permission: Mavroudis 2015)

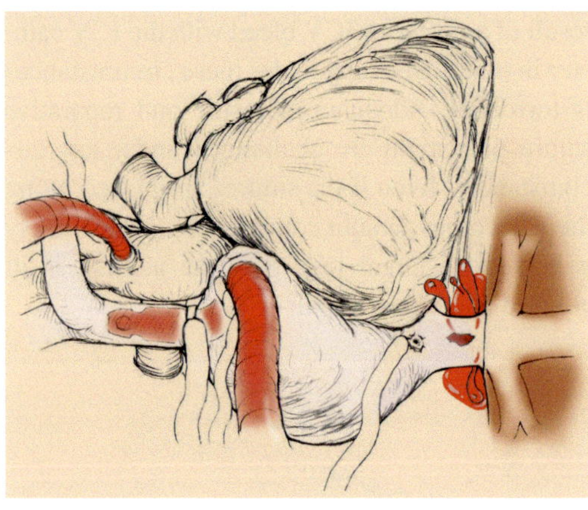

Fig. 50 This is an illustration of the result of partial cardiopulmonary bypass using the superior vena cava catheter with removal of the inferior vena cava catheter (IVC) to facilitate ICV repair. Exposure will prove to be difficult owing to the posterior location of the tear, torrential bleeding, and the danger of air embolism since the heart is still beating. Atrial air entry especially if there is a patent foramen ovale or ventricular septal defect can result in stroke and coronary insufficiency. (With Permission: Mavroudis 2015)

Figures 50 and 51 show alternative would be solutions with major drawbacks concerning control of hemorrhage and the potential for air embolus. Figure 50 shows the result of ICV cannula removal and institution of partial CPB through the SCV and a field sucker which is not

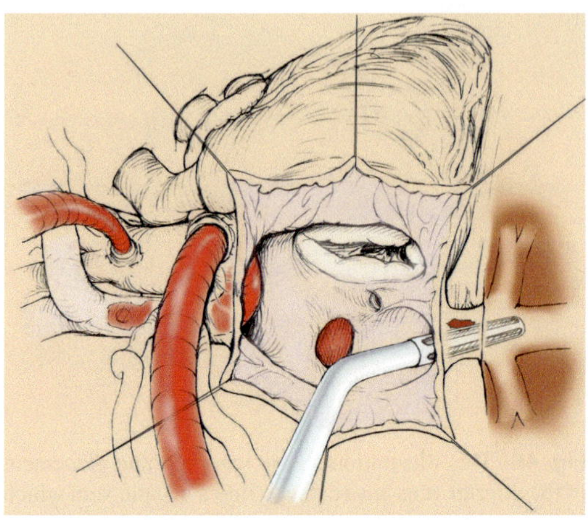

Fig. 51 Another ill-advised technique to repair the inferior vena cava tear is depicted. While the exposure for endocardial repair is appropriate, the reader will recognize that there is no cross clamp with every indication that the heart is still beating in the presence of a large atrial septal defect. This situation is clearly not indicated and should be avoided. (With Permission: Mavroudis 2015)

shown. While the ICV cannula is now removed and out of the way, the ICV tear is still posterior and difficult to visualize. Furthermore, the field sucker while placed to facilitate exposure. obstructs any effort to place an effective hemostatic suture. Even worse is the distinct possibility of air entry into the right atrium, which could embolize through patent foramen ovale or ventricular septal defect and cause irreparable harm to the brain and coronary arteries. The second misguided solution as shown in Fig. 51 which uses the recommended suture repair technique for endocardial repair of the ICV injury; namely, atrial entry, removal of the ICV cannula, and direct endocardial repair. However, the heart continues to beat, so the possibility of air embolus is compounded. The preferred technique for repair of this injury is aortic cross-clamping, cardioplegic arrest, right atrial entry, ICV cannula removal, and establishing ICV flow control by a field sucker into the orifice of the ICV as shown in Fig. 52. This exposure will allow a clear view of the tear, resulting in interrupted suture repair, replacement of the cannula, and safe application of the snugger. The operation can then be continued under more appropriate and favorable conditions.

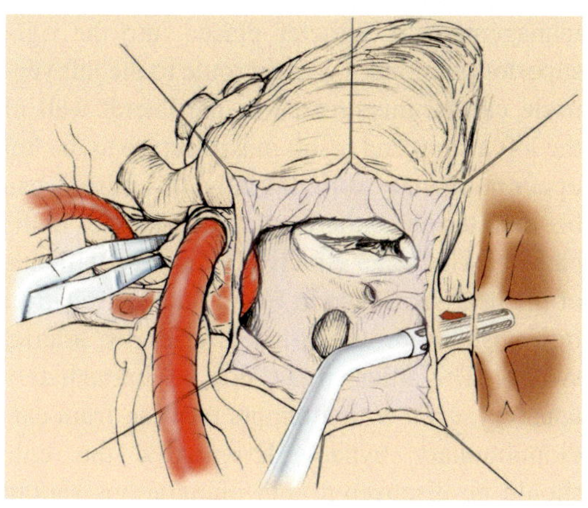

Fig. 52 Shows the proper technique for repair of a posterior tear of the inferior vena cava (IVC) using aortic cross clamping to avoid air embolus, excellent exposure for endocardial repair, and eventual IVC cannula placement with continuation of the intended operation. (With Permission: Mavroudis 2015)

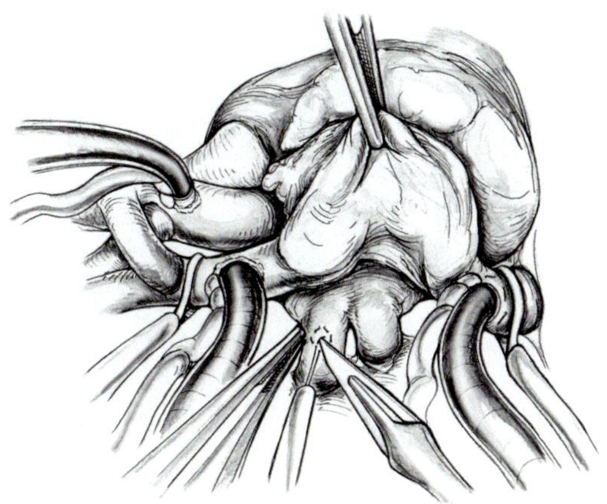

Fig. 53 Shows the exposure and purse string suture in the right superior pulmonary vein in preparation for left ventricular vent placement. A #11 blade is poised to perform a stab incision within the confines of the purse string. The heart is allowed to fill by retarding venous flow which will prevent air embolism. (With permission: Mavroudis 2015)

12 Left Ventricular Vent Placement

Many congenital heart repairs are enhanced by a left ventricular vent for ventricular decompression, enhanced exposure, and air removal at the end of the operation. Vent placement requires careful technique that will avoid instillation of air into the left side of the heart during the pre-cross-clamp stage shortly after the commencement of cardiopulmonary bypass. A purse string suture is placed at the juncture of the right superior pulmonary vein and the left atrium. The heart is allowed to fill by returning venous return to the heart lung machine which will result in positive pressure in the left atrium. In addition, vacuum assisted venous drainage, if routinely employed, should be disengaged at this time to allow the heart to fill. A #11 blade is used to puncture the right superior pulmonary vein within the confines of the purse string suture as noted in Fig. 53. The punctured site can then be dilated with a clamp if needed. Bleeding should result indicating that there is positive pressure in the left atrium. The catheter is then placed into the left atrium as shown in Fig. 54 and directed into the left ventricle via the left atrioventricular valve (Fig. 55) The Rommel tourniquet is engaged, and the catheter is tied in place. The surgeon may elect to place a finger behind the ventricle at the area of the posterior atrioventricular groove which will confirm catheter placement through the mitral valve into the left ventricle. The perfusionist can then be directed to start drainage of the left ventricle. The surgeon should be aware of the roller pump connections to ensure correct orientation

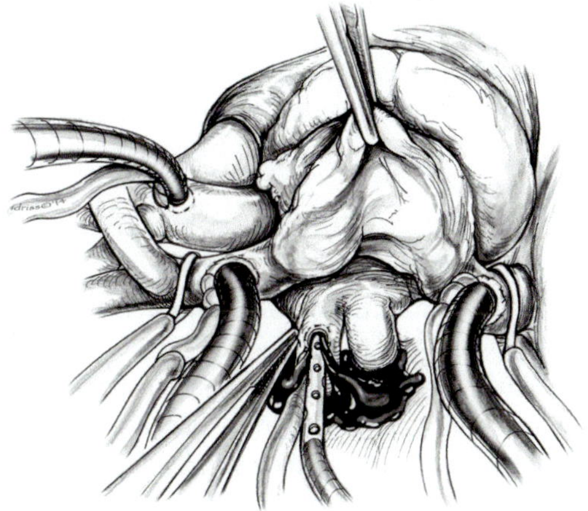

Fig. 54 The proper technique for left ventricular vent placement into the left atrium under positive left atrial pressure caused by retarding venous flow is shown. Robust bleeding as noted in the drawing ensures that air will not enter into the left side of the heart. (With permission: Mavroudis 2015)

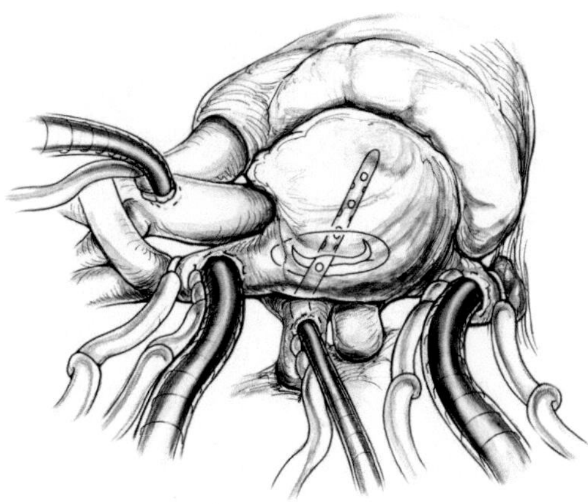

Fig. 55 The proper location of the left ventricular vent in preparation for aortic cross clamping and progression of the operation is illustrated. (With permission: Mavroudis 2015)

and effluent flow. A tubing clamp in hand will give the surgeon the option to quickly clamp the vent tubing in the unlikely event that the flow is reversed which can result in disastrous insufflation of air into the left ventricle instead of drainage.

13 Complications of Left Ventricular Vent Placement

Placement of left ventricular vents, especially in infants and young children, are not without complications, rare as they might be. As noted in other parts of this book, these complications are rare and unlikely to occur until they actually happen to the surgical team. Then, they become real and manifest which will require proper management. A catheter placed into the right superior pulmonary vein en route to the left ventricle can be misdirected to the lateral wall of the left atrium and result in a puncture to the left upper pulmonary vein. Initially, this mishap can be tolerated since there are multiple holes in the catheter which can effectively drain the left side of the heart as shown in Fig. 56 during repair of transposition of the great arteries by arterial switch. The injury may not be immediately apparent, even with attempts to wean from cardiopulmonary bypass. Eventually, the hole should be discovered, and preparations should be made to repair the damage. Figure 56a shows the actual complication with the tip of the left ventricle misdirected through the left pulmonary vein causing bleeding. The patient should be placed back on CPB with gentle ventricular retraction to visualize the tear and repair with interrupted suture technique (Fig. 56b). Gentle ventricular retraction is imperative since there are myriad suture lines associated with the arterial switch operation which should be respected to avoid unwanted further hemorrhage. Figure 56c shows the successful repair of the left pulmonary vein with interrupted suture technique.

Left ventricular vents placed through the right superior pulmonary vein into the left ventricle can also cause ventricular puncture as noted in Fig. 57a–c. This complication is less insidious and often becomes manifest shortly after separation from cardiopulmonary bypass. The best way to manage this problem is to resume CPB and place a pledgetted suture to close the hole primarily.

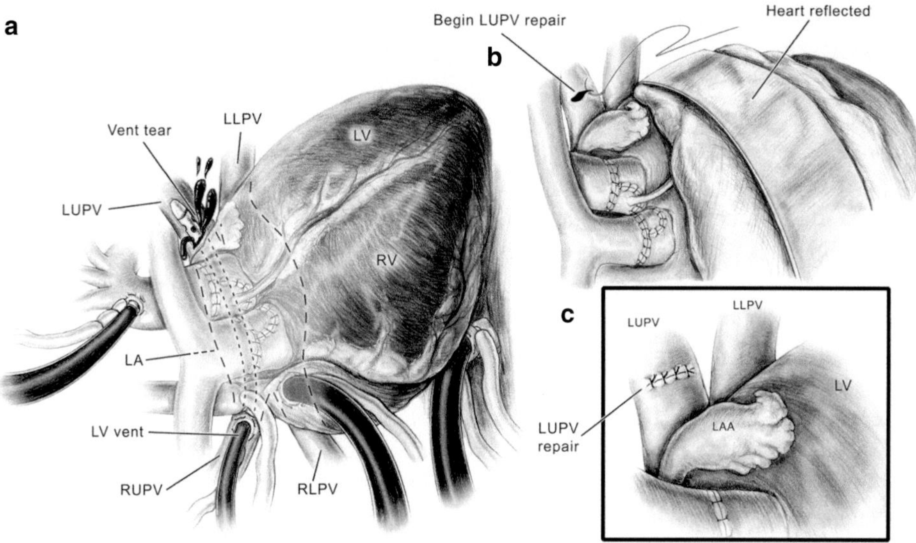

Fig. 56 This is the proper technique for repair of unwanted left pulmonary vein puncture by the left ventricular vent. Panel a shows cardiopulmonary bypass being started to avoid hypotension and arterial switch suture line disruption. Panel b shows the act of repairing the pulmonary vein with interrupted suture technique using gentle ventricular retraction. Panel c shows the completed repair en route to separation from cardiopulmonary bypass and complication resolution. *LA* left atrium, *LAA* left atrial appendage, *LLPV* left lower pulmonary vein, *LUPV* left upper pulmonary vein, *LV* left ventricle, *RLPV* right lower pulmonary vein, *RUPV* right upper pulmonary vein, *RV* right ventricle

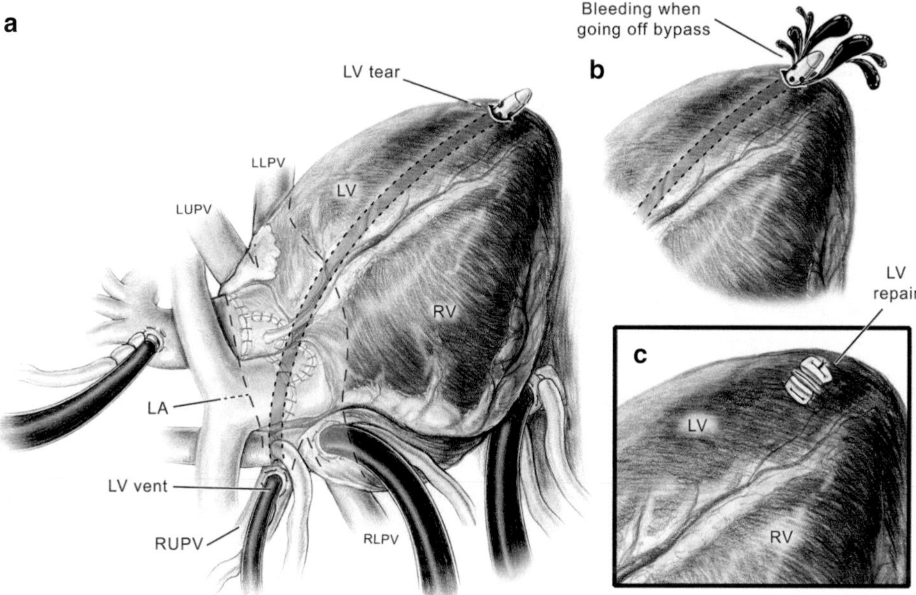

Fig. 57 shows the proper technique for repair of left ventricular puncture from a left ventricular vent as shown in Panel a. The most important issue is to quickly recognize the problem, restart cardiopulmonary bypass as noted in Panel b. Panel c demonstrates the use a pledgetted suture to repair the hole. *LA* left atrium, *LLPV* left lower pulmonary vein, *LUPV* left upper pulmonary vein, *LV* left ventricle, *RLPV* right lower pulmonary vein, *RUPV* right upper pulmonary vein, *RV* right ventricle

14 Antegrade Cardioplegia Catheter

There are various catheters and systems that can be employed for antegrade cardioplegia administration. Size appropriate catheters are used and fixed to the aorta by tourniquets. This allows for frequent cardioplegia administration as determined by the complexity of the procedure and type of cardioplegia that is employed. Furthermore, the same catheter can be used for air removal at the end of the operation.

At the time of catheter placement in the ascending aorta, care is taken not to perforate the posterior aorta by forceps stabilization during the puncture maneuver. Throughout cardioplegia administration, line pressure is measured and estimated by finger palpation of the proximal aorta (Fig. 58).

There are very few complications associated with antegrade cardioplegia. Perhaps the most insidious problem occurs when the surgeon misplaces the cross-clamp resulting in subtotal aortic occlusion. A small leak may continue undetected resulting in cardioplegia washout. As long as this problem is recognized, reapplication of an occlusive cross-clamp and reperfusion of cardioplegia can be administrated to maintain the proper state of myocardial preservation.

15 Retrograde Cardioplegia Administration

Frequently, retrograde cardioplegia is required for optimal myocardial preservation, especially for open aortic and coronary artery procedures. For infants and children, direct coronary sinus cannulation through open atriotomy is more reliable than transatrial catheter placement and distal catheter manipulation into the coronary sinus. After cannulation, a pressure monitor is used to observe the effective delivery of the cardioplegic solution as noted in Fig. 59. Occasionally, the balloon catheter slips out of the coronary sinus. Under these circumstances, a superficial purse string suture is placed around the orifice of the coronary sinus with special care not to disturb the conduction system. The catheter is then advanced into the coronary sinus, the purse string tourniquet is engaged, and the balloon is inflated as noted in Fig. 60. In the event that there is a persistent left superior caval vein draining into the coronary sinus, the left superior caval vein can be temporarily occluded at its entry into the heart to allow for retrograde cardioplegic delivery.

Interestingly, coronary sinus rupture has been reported in adults but not in infants or children. The risk factors for coronary sinus rupture in adults who have had retrograde cardioplegia include ven-

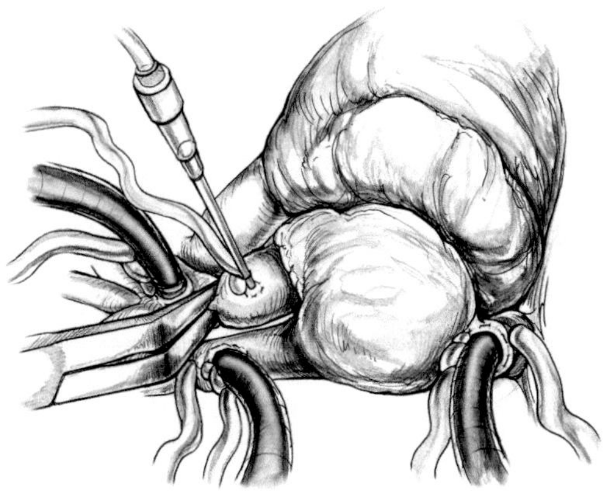

Fig. 58 Aortic cross clamping and administration of antegrade cardioplegia is demonstrated. (With permission: Mavroudis 2015)

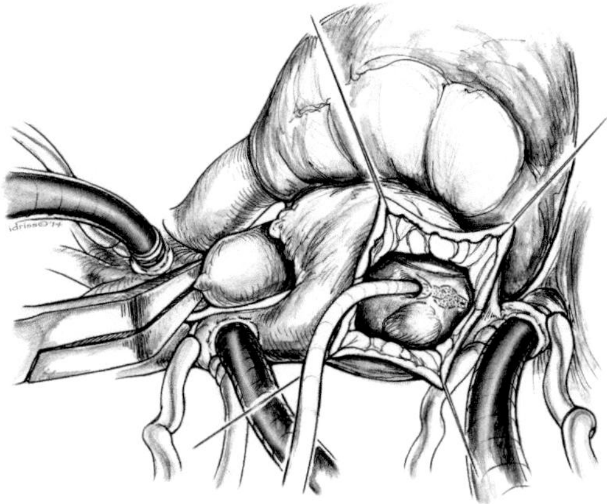

Fig. 59 shows direct transatrial placement of a retrograde cardioplegia catheter. (With permission: Mavroudis 2015)

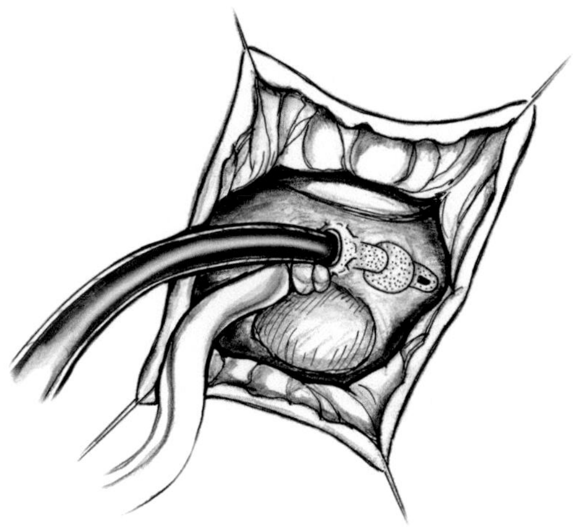

Fig. 60 shows direct transatrial placement of a retrograde cardioplegia catheter reinforced by an orifice purse string suture to keep the catheter in place during cardioplegia administration. (With permission: Mavroudis 2015)

tricular hypertrophy, advanced age, and prolonged aortic cross-clamp times (Kurusz et al. 2002). Fortunately, coronary sinus rupture associated with retrograde cardioplegia in infants and children has not been reported. Reasons are speculative. Tissue elasticity may have an important role.

16 Complications Associated with the Initiation of Cardiopulmonary Bypass

Complications associated with the initiation of cardiopulmonary bypass occur quickly and can lead to considerable complications in a matter of seconds. Arterial cannulas can be misplaced into the orifice of the innominate artery, aortic dissections can occur, catheters can be dislodged, they can be too small for the calculated flow specifications, and so on. Venous catheters can also be misplaced, resulting in poor drainage and inappropriate perfusion that can lead to acidosis, ventricular distention, and a poor outcome.

Unwanted cavitary entry at the beginning of the operation has challenges dependent on the diagnosis for which the patient is being treated. A cavitary entry into the inferior caval vein and injudicious management can lead to strokes and somatic air embolus. Unwanted entry into the innominate vein during thymus excision can lead to significant bleeding, circulatory collapse, and careless repair that can cause central venous catheter occlusion of the repair (reparative sutures placed through the venous catheter). These situations require a high degree of heightened awareness, a mature sense of equanimity, and most importantly, a thorough knowledge of the resolution techniques that will put the patient and the surgeon on the proper foundation to continue the operation.

References

Bolotin G, Buckner GD, Campbell NB, et al. Tissue-disruptive forces during median sternotomy. Heart Surg Forum. 2007;10:487–92.

Delius RE, Walters HL 3rd. Re-operative surgery in pediatric patients. Semin Thorac Cardiovasc Surg Pediatr Card Surg Annu. 2003;6:108–15.

Kühme T, Isaksson B, Dahlin LG. Wound contamination in cardiac surgery. A systematic quantitative and qualitative study of the bacterial growth in sternal wounds in cardiac surgery patients. APMIS. 2007;115:1001–7.

Kurusz M, Girouard MK, Brown PS Jr. Coronary sinus rupture with retrograde cardioplegia. Perfusion. 2002;17(1):77–80.

Mavroudis C. Cannulation techniques. In: Mavroudis C, Backer CL, editors. Atlas of pediatric cardiac surgery. London: Springer; 2015.

Mavroudis C, Dearani JA. Resternotomy and peripheral cannulation. In: Mavroudis C, Dearani JA, editors. Atlas of adult congenital heart surgery. Cham: Springer Nature; 2020. p. 1–10.

Ogus TN, Hulusi Us M, Ciçek S, Ozkan S, Yüksel Oztürk O, Isik O. Sternal cyanoacrylate gluing in mediastinitis. Effects on infection, stability and bone healing. J Cardiovasc Surg. 2002;43:741–6.

Park CB, Suri RM, Burkhart HM, et al. Identifying patients at particular risk of injury during repeat sternotomy: analysis of 2555 cardiac reoperations. J Thorac Cardiovasc Surg. 2010;140:1028–35.

Ranganath P, Singh S, Abbara S, Agarwal PP, Rajiah P. Computed tomography in adult congenital heart disease. Radiol Clin North Am. 2019;57:85–111.

Steely AM, Liu DC. Innominate vein injury secondary to first-time sternotomy. Ann Thorac Surg. 2020;110:e485–6.

Thiel R, Bircks W. Arteriovenous fistulas after median sternotomy—report of 2 cases and review of the literature. Thorac Cardiovasc Surg. 1990;38:195–7.

Webster G, Balmert LC, Patel AB, et al. Surveillance cultures and infection in 230 pacemaker and defibrillator generator changes in pediatric and adult congenital patients. World J Pediatr Congenit Heart Surg. 2021;12:331–6.

Complications Associated with Palliative Operations

Constantine Mavroudis and Carl L. Backer

Abstract

Palliative operations for neonates, infants, and children are performed in anticipation of a "complete repair" in the future. For example, pulmonary artery bands are placed to protect the pulmonary bed for a future operation or for left ventricular (LV) training in anticipation of an arterial switch operation. Systemic-to-pulmonary artery shunts are placed for cyanosis or as the sole source of pulmonary artery perfusion in anticipation of further reparative operations when anatomic and physiologic conditions are more favorable. Bidirectional Glenn shunts are placed as an interim physiologic operation en route to a Fontan operation. Complications associated with these procedures can be life-threatening and prohibitive for complete repair. For instance, a suboptimal and poorly performed systemic-to-pulmonary artery shunt can prevent a future operation such as tetralogy repair or completion Fontan procedure. Further, a poorly placed pulmonary artery band can lead to unwanted pulmonary hypertension, pulmonary artery stenosis, and pulmonary valve distortion. In this chapter we will review complications that can occur in palliative operations and offer suggestions and techniques that can rectify these missteps.

Keywords

Congenital heart surgery · Palliation · Pulmonary artery band · Modified Blalock-Taussig-Thomas shunt · Reoperation · Bidirectional Glenn

1 Introduction

Palliative operations are generally conceived and implemented to provide temporary symptomatic relief without actual correction of the main congenital or acquired defect (Joffs and Sade 2000). When applied to congenital heart surgery, the two classic palliative procedures are the aortopulmonary shunt and the pulmonary artery band (Blalock and Taussig 1945; Muller and Dammann 1952) which are generally used to increase pulmonary artery flow in the presence of cyanosis or decrease the pulmonary artery flow in the case of

C. Mavroudis (✉)
Chief of Pediatric Cardiothoracic Surgery (Retired), Peyton Manning Children's Hospital, Indianapolis, IN, USA

Professor Emeritus of Surgery, Johns Hopkins University School of Medicine, Baltimore, MD, USA

C. L. Backer
Chief, Section of Pediatric Cardiothoracic Surgery, UK Healthcare Kentucky Children's Hospital, Lexington, KY, USA

Cardiothoracic Surgery, Cincinnati Children's Hospital Medical Center, Cincinnati, OH, USA

C. L. Backer, C. Mavroudis (eds.), *Complications in Pediatric and Congenital Heart Surgery*, https://doi.org/10.1007/978-3-032-02661-3_2

pulmonary overcirculation which could lead to pulmonary hypertension.

There has been a shift away from pre-repair palliation in favor of complete neonatal/infant repair over the last half century thereby decreasing the number of palliative procedures. There are, however, important present-day indications for palliative operations which include staged univentricular repair, severe tetralogy of Fallot, Swiss-cheese ventricular septal defects (VSD), ventricular training for arterial switch operations (PA Band) and the various types of pulmonary atresia with VSD, among others. Palliative procedures therefore are important stages that lead to corrective operations and improved hemodynamic conditions (Backer et al. 2012). Complications associated with these procedures can be life-threatening in the short term and prohibitive for complete repair in the long term. For instance, a suboptimal and poorly performed systemic-to-pulmonary artery shunt can obviate a future operation such as tetralogy repair or completion Fontan procedure. Further, a poorly placed pulmonary artery band can lead to unwanted pulmonary hypertension, pulmonary artery stenosis, and pulmonary valve distortion.

It is no secret that palliative operations can be just as complicated and challenging as complete repairs. Therefore, it is imperative that these operations be performed with great attention to detail since the eventual corrective operation is highly dependent on the successful execution of the palliative procedure.

In particular, this chapter will primarily consider complications associated with pulmonary artery banding and the variant types of systemic-to-pulmonary artery shunts (Table 1). By necessity, the optimal sequence of these operations, which have been previously published (Backer and Mavroudis 2023; Mavroudis 2015), will be reproduced in order to contrast these techniques with unwanted complications that can occur. Dated systemic-to-pulmonary artery shunts (Potts, Waterston, and Cooley shunts), not used in the present era, are also reviewed herein to underscore the reality that surgeons should be cognizant of the anatomic details of these operations in order to manage the takedown procedure in association with complete repair. These situations arise when adult patients with previously performed dated palliative operations are lost to follow-up and present late for corrective surgery. Potential complications are reviewed that will be helpful in resolving mishaps should they occur.

Table 1 Aortopulmonary shunts

Shunt	Surgeon	Year
Blalock-Taussig-Thomas shunt	Alfred Blalock	1944
Potts shunt	Willis Potts	1946
Waterston shunt	David Waterston	1962
Cooley shunt	Denton Cooley	1966
Modified Blalock-Taussig-Thomas Shunt	Marc de Leval	1976

Another palliative operation is the atrial septectomy, which traditionally has been performed to increase atrial mixing in patients with transposition of the great arteries or functionally univentricular hearts and atrioventricular valve stenosis. This palliative surgical technique was first reported in 1950 by Blalock and Hanlon (1950). In the years to come, transcatheter balloon septostomy was introduced by Rashkind in 1966 and remains the accepted method (Rashkind and Miller 1966). Other more complex staged palliative operations such as the Norwood operation for hypoplastic left heart syndrome (HLHS) (Norwood et al. 1983), the Glenn procedure (Glenn 1958), and the "hybrid" approach using bilateral pulmonary artery banding in association with ductal stenting for HLHS (Gibbs et al. 1993; Galantowicz et al. 2008; Haller and Caldarone 2018) are considered in detail in Chap. 17 (Bidirectional Glenn and Fontan Operations) and Chap. 21 (Norwood operation) regarding those specific lesions.

2 Pulmonary Artery Band

Pulmonary artery banding was first reported by Muller and Dammann (1952) in 1952 for children with a large left-to-right shunt or functionally univentricular heart and excessive pulmonary blood flow. For many years, pulmonary artery banding was the preferred initial palliation for any small child with a large left-to-right shunt and increased pulmonary blood flow. Examples include ventricular septal defect, atrioventricular septal defect, and common arterial trunk. However, advances in neonatal cardiac surgical techniques have altered the indications for modern day use of the pulmonary artery band for only a few specific lesions (Backer and Mavroudis 2023). These include

1. "Swiss-cheese" muscular ventricular septal defects,
2. multiple ventricular septal defects or atrioventricular septal defect with coarctation,
3. functionally univentricular heart with increased pulmonary blood flow (i.e., tricuspid atresia type IIc) (Alsoufi et al. 2015; Lee et al. 2014)
4. to prepare and retrain the left ventricle of a patient with transposition of the great arteries for the arterial switch procedure either (a) following late presentation after 4 weeks of age (Mainwaring et al. 2018), or (b) following prior atrial repair (Mavroudis and Backer 2000)
5. to train the left ventricle in a patient with congenitally corrected transposition of the great arteries for a "double switch" (Winlaw et al. 2005; Barron and Mahendran 2019; Di Bardino et al. 2012)
6. the critically ill infant with contraindications for the use of cardiopulmonary bypass.

These previous six indications are guidelines and can be controversial depending on the surgical team. For instance, some surgeons perform a Damus-Stansel-Kaye procedure with systemic-to-pulmonary artery shunt instead of pulmonary artery band placement for a functionally univentricular heart with increased pulmonary blood flow because of the potential for subaortic obstruction under these circumstances (Franklin et al. 1990; Bradley et al. 2002).

The following sections highlight the exposure for pulmonary artery band, the operative sequence and the potential complications, which include:

1. Stenosis or distortion of one or both branch pulmonary arteries (Agasthi and Graziano 2023),
2. Alterations in the function of the pulmonary valve (Zhu et al. 2023),
3. Impingement of circumflex artery (Kawamura et al. 2012),
4. Erosion of band into the pulmonary artery (Danilowicz et al. 1990),
5. Pseudoaneurysm of pulmonary artery (Nakayama et al. 2017; Venugopal et al. 2010),
6. Hemolysis (Iannucci et al. 2013),
7. Thrombosis (Recto et al. 2013),
8. Pulmonary artery disruption (Makhija et al. 2017),
9. Unwanted unilateral pulmonary artery band (Galinanes et al. 1993).

The ensuing discussion will review how the pulmonary artery band should be performed and will consider how complications can occur by narrative and illustration.

Pulmonary artery banding in a child with normally related great vessels can be performed through a left lateral thoracotomy or a median sternotomy incision. Historically, many surgeons chose to perform left thoracotomy thinking that the future reparative operation through median sternotomy would be free of adhesions. There are, however, many advantages of mediastinal approach to pulmonary artery banding. To begin with, median sternotomy allows a safe and demonstrable display of the anatomy which can be important in unusual circumstances of pulmonary artery variations in complex defects such as heterotaxy, situs inversus, and so on. Other more subtle advantages become manifest during the banding maneuver. Tightening the band through a right thoracotomy while observing the oxygen saturation monitor may not result in an accurate hemodynamic evaluation owing to the compression of the lung. On the other hand, tightening the band through a median sternotomy does not involve lung compression thereby making the observed systemic oxygen saturation more accurate. In the longer term, the once feared problem of resternotomy has been mitigated owing to improved techniques of resternotomy (Morales et al. 2008). As a matter of technique and choice of band material, we have employed either Teflon-impregnated Dacron (infants) or a strip of polytetrafluoroethylene (PTFE) (neonates).

Figure 1 (Backer and Mavroudis 2023; Mavroudis 2015) shows the surgical exposure for a pulmonary artery banding through a median sternotomy incision. The thymus can either be divided in the midline or partially removed. To maintain ease at future resternotomy, only the superior portion of the pericardium need be opened. If a left thoracotomy is elected, the pericardium is entered anterior to the phrenic nerve with stay sutures to retract the pericardium and enhance exposure. The left atrial appendage, which can obscure the relational anatomy lies close to the pulmonary trunk. This can be retracted with stay sutures which will avoid injury and bleeding. Figures 2, 3, 4, and 5 illustrate the subtraction technique that safely facilitates proper band encirclement of the pulmonary artery trunk. As noted, the band is first placed around both the ascending aorta and the main pulmonary artery trunk. This initial maneuver serves to avoid the complication of encircling only the left pulmonary artery, which can occur with the thoracotomy approach. A plane is then developed between the aorta and the pulmonary artery with a combination of sharp dissection and electrocautery. A right-angled clamp is then passed specifically around the aorta while the free end of the band is engaged as noted in Fig. 4 (Backer and Mavroudis 2023; Mavroudis 2015). The band is pulled through the space between the aorta and pulmonary artery thereby encircling the pulmonary artery and completing the subtraction technique as noted in Fig. 5. When performed correctly,

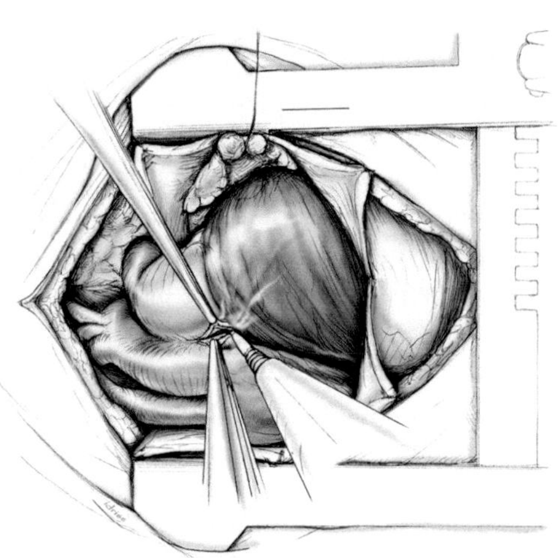

Fig. 1 Pulmonary artery band (PAB) is performed through a thoracotomy or median sternotomy, depending on the surgeon's preference. The rationale for using a thoracotomy approach has been to facilitate median sternotomy for the eventual definitive repair. Over the past 10 years, however, redo sternotomy techniques have improved, and redo is no longer a risk factor for reoperations. Most surgeons now prefer a median sternotomy approach for PAB because of the improved exposure for anatomic and physiologic manipulations. The exposure for PAB shown in this chapter, therefore, is through a median sternotomy. The figure shows electrocautery dissection between the aorta and the pulmonary artery. (With permission: Mavroudis and Dearani 2020)

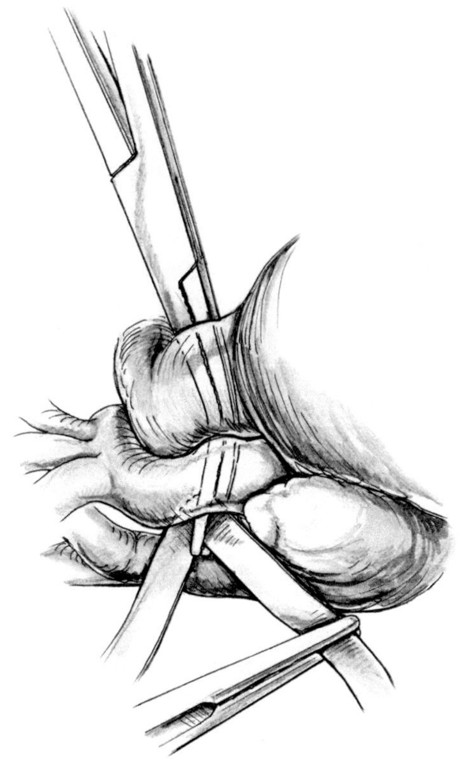

Fig. 2 Shows the initiation of the exclusion technique which is performed by a right-angle clamp being placed through the transverse sinus of the heart. The surgeon then pulls the pulmonary artery band (Teflon™) to encircle both great vessels. (With permission: Mavroudis and Dearani 2020)

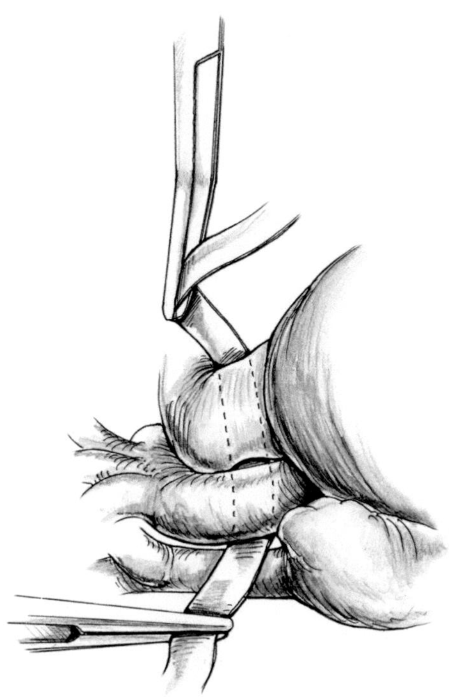

Fig. 3 Shows the completed encircled pulmonary artery band around both great vessels in preparation for the selective encircled pulmonary artery. (With permission: Mavroudis and Dearani 2020)

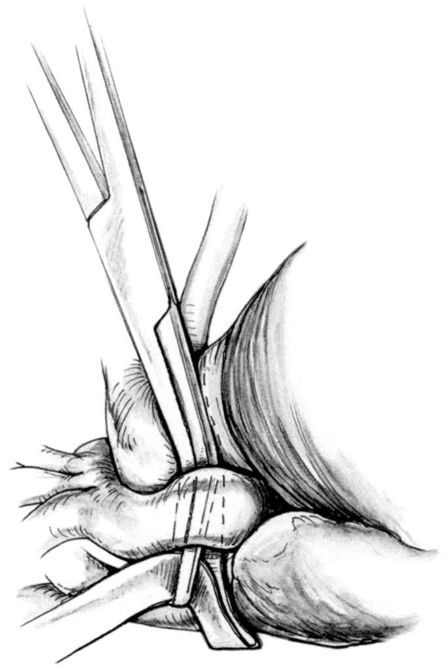

Fig. 4 Shows the right-angle clamp being placed around the aorta. The surgeon pulls the aortic end of the PAB posterior to the aorta, thereby encircling the pulmonary artery as noted in Fig. 5. (With permission: Mavroudis and Dearani 2020)

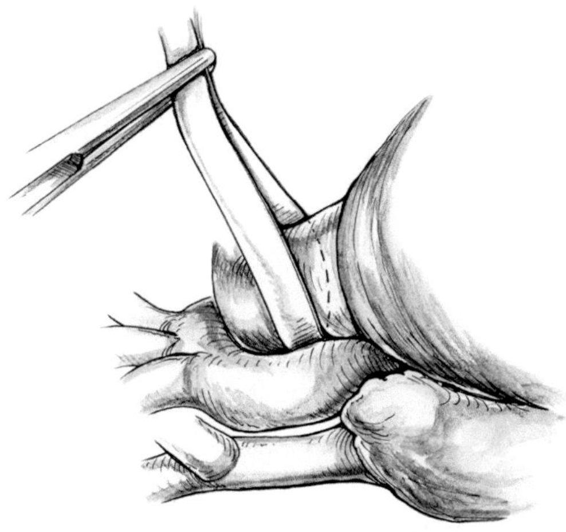

Fig. 5 Shows the completed action of encircling the pulmonary artery by the band material. This maneuver will allow the surgeon to estimate the amount of tightening for the next phase of the operation. (Pediatric Atlas). (With permission: Mavroudis and Dearani 2020)

complications can be avoided. For instance, Figs. 6, 7, and 8 show how an attempted passing of the clamp through the transverse sinus of the heart (area posterior to both the main pulmonary trunk and ascending aorta) can be misguided to emerge superior to the right pulmonary artery. The ensuing maneuvers as shown will result in a unilateral pulmonary artery band around the right pulmonary artery; the left pulmonary artery has been excluded in the band and therefore will continue to be exposed to systemic pressures which will eventually result in severe pulmonary hypertension. This condition will obviously result in a failed palliation attempt and might even preclude any chance at eventual proper complete repair. While the figures show clear and obvious anatomy, the surgeon might find unanticipated camouflaging adhesions, pulmonary artery distortion, and unusual landmarks that could result in this complication. In the case of difficult anatomy, the operating team would be wise to engage in comprehensive dissection to further define the anatomy.

Encircling a thin-walled pulmonary artery by a direct approach can be avoided by the aforementioned subtraction technique. There may be, however, situations where the surgeon elects direct main pulmonary artery encirclement. If bleeding occurs as noted in Fig. 9, consideration should be given to the institution of cardiopulmo-

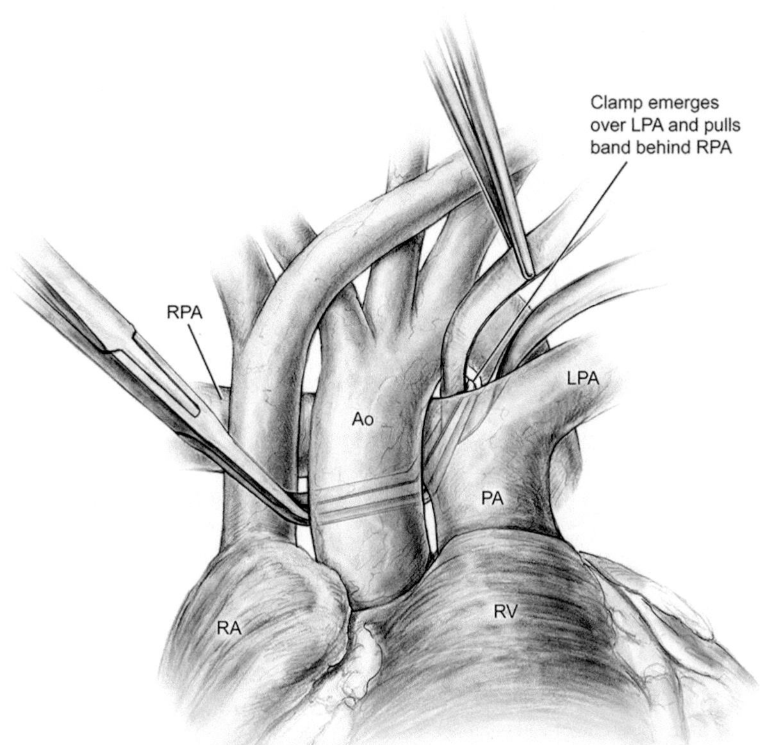

Fig. 6 Shows an angled clamp encircling the ascending aorta from the right side and misdirecting the pathway away from the transverse sinus to emerge superior to the right pulmonary artery. The pulmonary artery band is shown being clamped in an effort to encircle the intended main pulmonary artery. In this case, however, the band will mistakenly encircle the right pulmonary artery. *Ao* aorta, *LPA* left pulmonary artery, *PA* pulmonary artery, *RA* right atrium, *RPA* right pulmonary artery, *RV* right ventricle

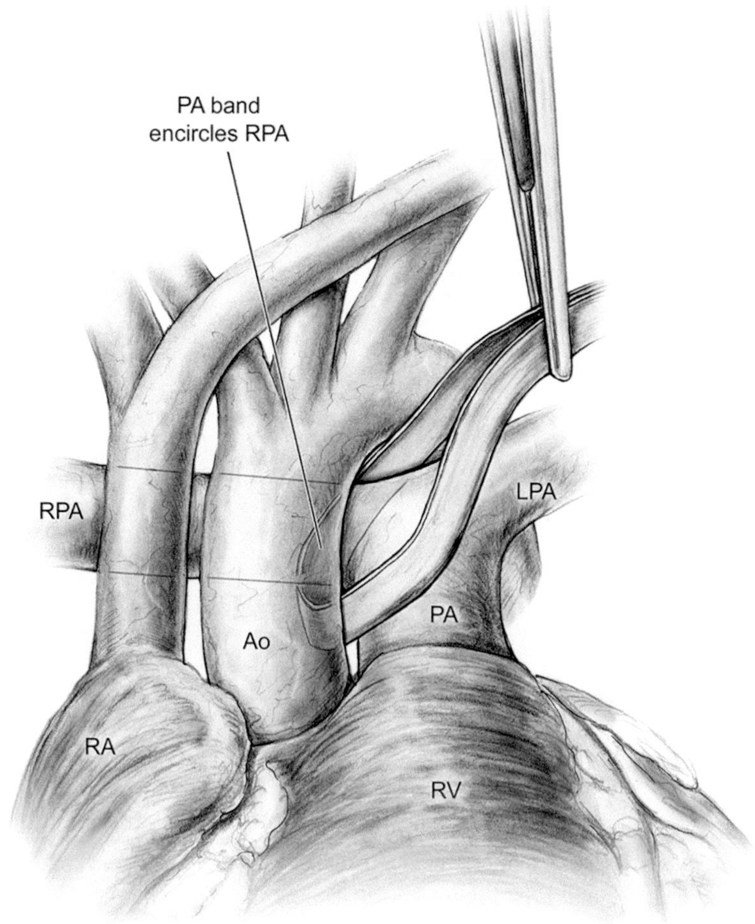

Fig. 7 Shows the completed band which has mistakenly encircled the right pulmonary artery while leaving the left pulmonary artery subjected to systemic pressures. *Ao* aorta, *LPA* left pulmonary artery, *PA* pulmonary artery, *RA* right atrium, *RPA* right pulmonary artery, *RV* right ventricle

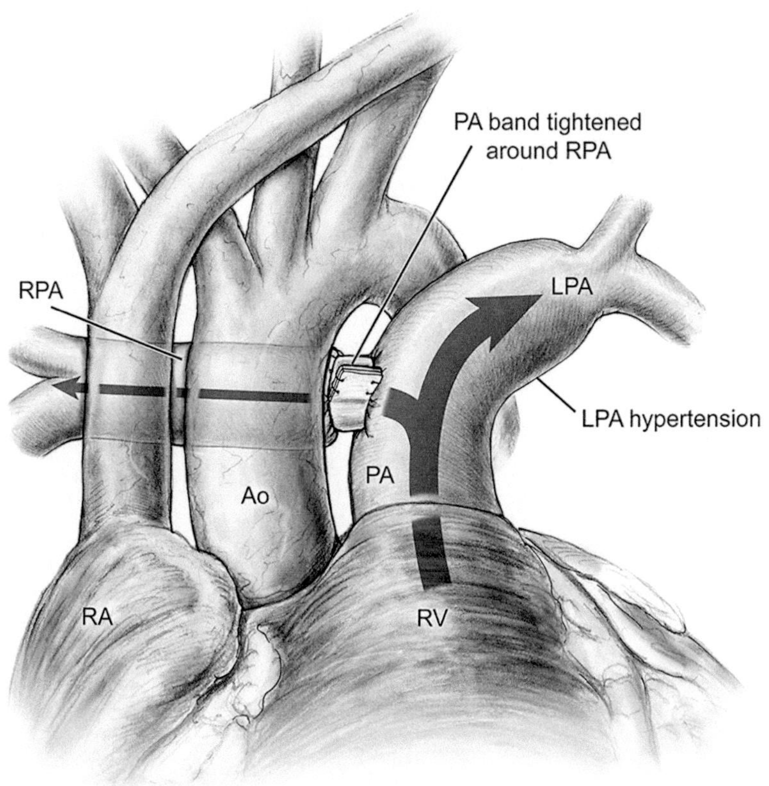

Fig. 8 Shows the completed misplaced pulmonary artery band that constricts the flow to the right pulmonary artery but leaves the left pulmonary artery unconstricted and subject to systemic pressures and eventually severe left pulmonary hypertension. *Ao* aorta, *LPA* left pulmonary artery, *PA* pulmonary artery, *RA* right atrium, *RPA* right pulmonary artery, *RV* right ventricle

nary bypass to avoid hemodynamic instability and significant blood loss. Figure 10 shows how institution of cardiopulmonary bypass and cardioplegic arrest can facilitate exposure of the injured pulmonary artery with direct suture repair or patch augmentation. Cardioplegic arrest is employed to avoid systemic air embolism in the event that there is a VSD or other left to right shunts that require repair.

The band-tightening maneuver involves a number of guidelines to help adjust the band for the most favorable hemodynamic result and anatomic location. Once the band is accurately placed to avoid pulmonary artery exclusion and bleeding, the band can be sequentially tightened by placing multiple interrupted sutures in the band, as shown in Figs. 11, 12, and 13 (Backer and Mavroudis 2023; Mavroudis 2015). Surgeons have used other techniques as well. Serial hemoclips can be used to tighten the band, each placed below the prior clip, leading to a progressively tighter band. Another technique is to grasp the two sides of the encircling band using a right-angled clamp and place sutures below the clamp to secure the band in place. This technique requires close attention to the systemic oxygen saturation and the rise in systemic pressure to gauge the adequacy of pulmonary artery banding. A more scientific way to gauge the constriction result of the banding is the Trusler formula. We have used the Trusler formula to determine the initial pulmonary artery band circumference. The original Trusler formula involved constructing the band circumference 20 mm + 1 mm for each

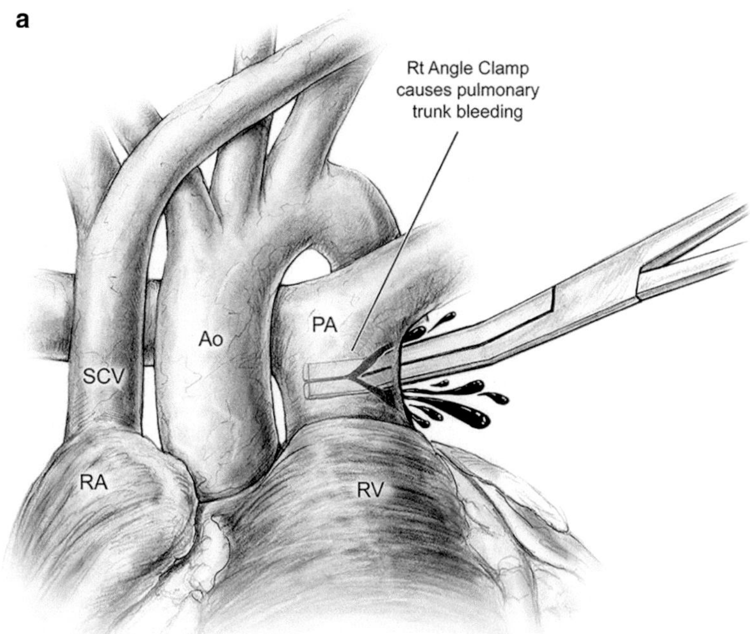

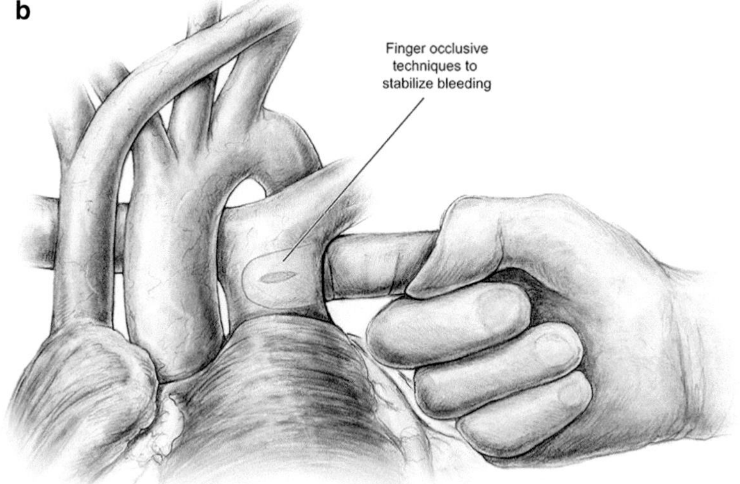

Fig. 9 Panel a shows unwanted posterior pulmonary trunk bleeding resulting from complicated direct encirclement. Panel b shows finger occlusive technique which should stabilize the situation until cardiopulmonary bypass is instituted. This will allow better exposure and more accurate repair techniques. *Ao* aorta, *PA* pulmonary artery, *RA* right atrium, *RV* right ventricle, *SCV* superior caval vein

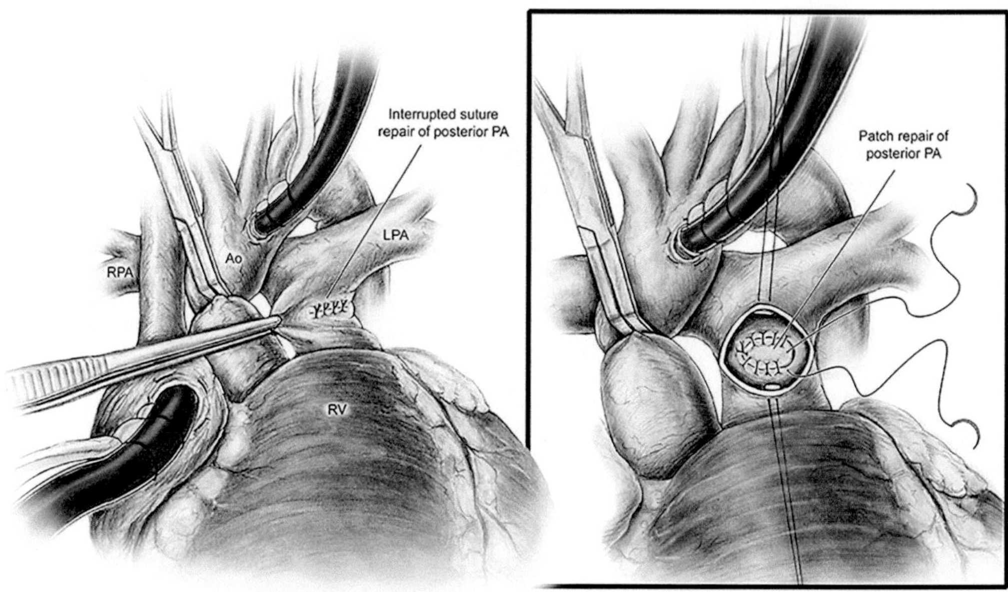

Fig. 10 Shows the completion of emergency cardiopulmonary bypass due to extensive pulmonary truck dissection to expose the injured posterior area. Cardioplegic arrest is used to prevent systemic air embolism assuming that there is a ventricular septal defect or other left to right shunt that will need repair. The left panel shows epicardial primary suture repair when appropriate. The right panel shows a transpulmonary artery incision and exposure for patch repair if the injury is large enough to require augmentation. *Ao* aorta, *LPA* left pulmonary artery, *PA* pulmonary artery, *RPA* right pulmonary artery, *RV* right ventricle

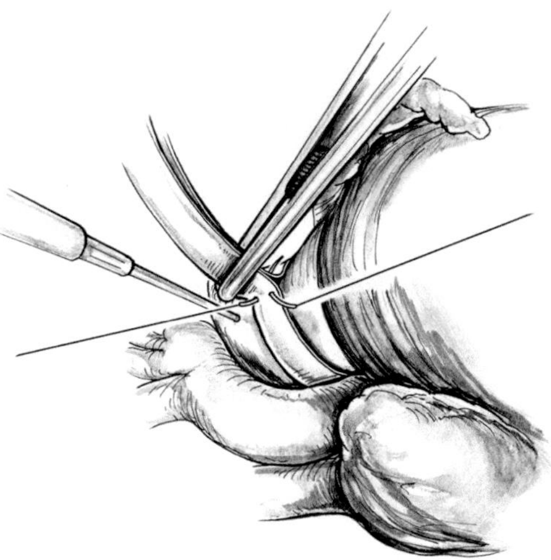

Fig. 11 The surgeon can place a distal catheter for pressure measurements and begins tightening of the PAB which is noted in the figure. (With permission: Mavroudis and Dearani 2020)

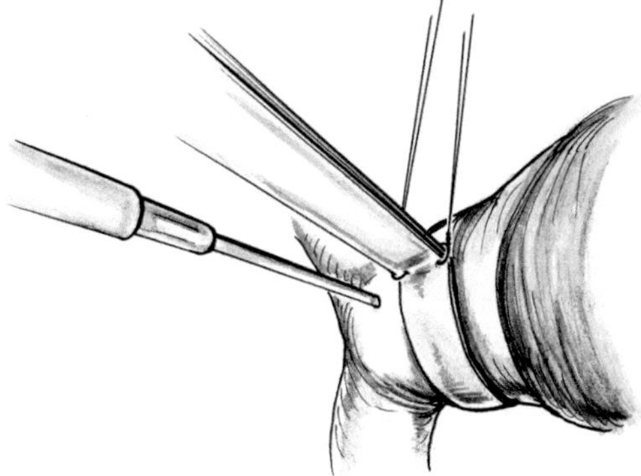

Fig. 12 Shows the initial suture that is strategically placed below the bifurcation of the main pulmonary artery and above the pulmonary valve to begin the tightening process. (With permission: Mavroudis and Dearani 2020)

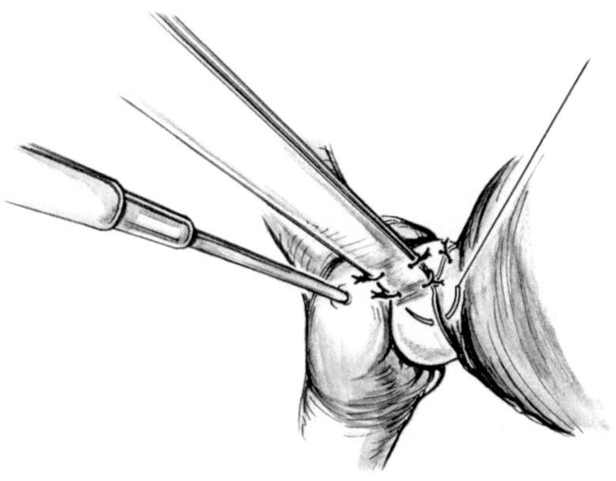

Fig. 13 In general, the PAB is tightened to achieve a distal pulmonary artery pressure that is approximately 50% of the systemic pressure as shown in the figure. (With permission: Mavroudis and Dearani 2020)

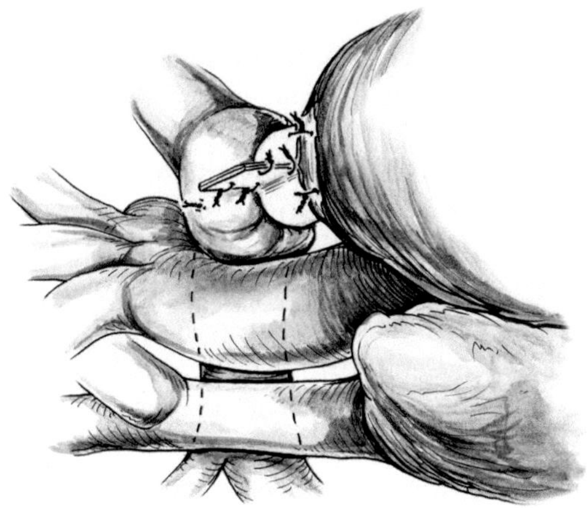

Fig. 14 It is important to suture the tightened PAB to the adventitia of the pulmonary artery in order to prevent distal migration, which can cause right or left pulmonary artery stenosis. The figure shows the completed tightening of the pulmonary artery band and tacking adventitial sutures that anchor the pulmonary artery band to the preferred location below the pulmonary artery bifurcation and above the pulmonary valve. (With permission: Mavroudis and Dearani 2020)

kg of body weight (Trusler and Mustard 1972; Albus et al. 1984). The formula has been modified by Baslaim (2009) to place a band 2.25 mm narrower in the functionally univentricular heart group. To assess band adjustment, a pressure measuring catheter can be placed in the distal pulmonary artery to compare dynamic differences with the systemic pressure as noted in Figs. 11 and 12. Alternatively, the gradient across the band can be monitored by transesophageal echocardiography. After optimal band placement, the band can be attached to the proximal pulmonary artery trunk using several interrupted polypropylene sutures which serve to prevent distal band migration and encroachment on the right pulmonary artery (Figs. 13 and 14) (Backer and Mavroudis 2023; Mavroudis 2015).

Guidelines for pulmonary artery banding generally apply to those patients who will eventually have a two-ventricle repair and those who will have a single ventricle repair (Fontan operation). The procedural recommendations for optimal results are quoted herein from our previous chapter (Backer and Mavroudis 2023). “Placement of the band should result in an elevation of the aortic systolic blood pressure by 10–20 mm Hg. For a patient who will eventually have a two-ventricle repair, the distal pulmonary artery systolic pressure should be reduced to less than 50% of the measured aortic systolic blood pressure. For a patient who is going to undergo an eventual Fontan procedure, the lowest possible distal main pulmonary artery pressure that can be achieved with acceptable oxygen saturations is desired. Oxygen saturations for a patient who is going to undergo biventricular repair should be left at 95%. For the patient who is going to undergo a Fontan operation, the oxygen saturation should preferably drop to between 80% and 85%. It should be kept in mind that as the child grows, the band will by default become “tighter” and further drop the distal pulmonary artery pressure (and saturations). One possible complication of band placement is the above-noted encroachment on the right pulmonary artery. The band can pinch off the right pulmonary artery while allowing excessive blood flow to the left pulmonary artery. This results in right pulmonary artery stenosis and left pulmonary artery hypertension. This complication can be avoided by properly anchoring the band to the proximal main pulmonary artery. Once the band has been secured in place, the pericardium is irrigated with saline, so there is less chance of intrapericardial adhesions at the time of intracardiac repair. If performed through a left thoracotomy, the pericardium is loosely approximated with several interrupted polypropylene sutures, with care being taken to avoid injury to the phrenic nerve." (Backer and Mavroudis 2023)

The idea of an externally adjustable pulmonary artery band has been proposed and discussed for many years. Only recently, however, have enough advances in this technology been established to offer guidelines for its use (Di Bardino et al. 2012; Corno 2013; EspeRare 2020; Corno et al. 2006). Talwar and associates (2016) reviewed their early experience with an adjustable pulmonary artery band and found that, "major PA distortion or stenosis was absent in the majority. One patient had pseudoaneurysm of the main pulmonary artery with sternal sinus infection and required surgical reconstruction. One patient had infective endocarditis of the pulmonary valve managed medically. Band migration was not encountered. There were two deaths after definitive repair and one after adjustable pulmonary artery band."

Large database studies have documented the continued use of pulmonary artery banding. During the period from 2015 to 2018, the Society of Thoracic Surgeons (STS) congenital database reported 2,522 pulmonary artery band procedures which comprised 2.1% of all congenital surgical procedures (STS Congenital Heart Surgery Database 2019). Corresponding data from the European Association for Cardio-thoracic Surgery (EACTS) revealed 711 cases of pulmonary artery band which comprised 2.0% of total surgical experience for the same time period. Devlin and associates reported excellent results with pulmonary artery banding in high-risk patients with complete atrioventricular septal defect (Devlin et al. 2020). Their patient population included premature infants, infants with unbalanced atrioventricular septal defect, coarctation of the aorta, and other serious comorbidities. While pulmonary artery banding for atrioventricular septal defect and aortic arch obstruction is controversial when compared with early complete repair, Shuhaiber and associates (2013) performed a multi-institutional study comparing attempted complete neonatal repair with a staged approach using pulmonary artery banding. They found that the staged approach with prior pulmonary artery banding was associated with improved survival and lower morbidity (fewer complications and unplanned reoperations). Clearly, there are proponents for pulmonary artery banding in some subsets of patients that will continue to be part of staged surgical therapy.

Pulmonary artery banding can also be performed by the "intraluminal technique" (Piluiko et al. 2005). The technique requires transpulmonary artery suture placement of an obstructive patch with a calibrated precut hole in the center into the main pulmonary artery which requires cardiopulmonary bypass. In general, this technique is reserved for patients who require cardiopulmonary bypass for other, simultaneous procedures. The hemodynamic consequences are significant reduction in pulmonary artery pressure and flow. There are, however, advantages and disadvantages of this technique. The advantages include elimination of potential band migration and pulmonary artery branch encroachment since the patch is sutured within the pulmonary artery. In addition, the band can be dilated for acquired cyanosis due to somatic growth using transcatheter techniques. The disadvantages include (1) hemolysis due to flow acceleration and jagged edges of the fenestration (Iannucci et al. 2013) and (2) the potential for pulmonary trunk distortion (Sandrio et al. 2015). These disadvantages tend to be significant and require reoperation, cardiopulmonary bypass, and reparative or palliative operative management.

Other long-term complications of pulmonary artery band not mentioned earlier in this chapter include stenosis or distortion of one or both branch pulmonary arteries (Agasthi and Graziano 2023), alterations in the function of the pulmonary valve (Zhu et al. 2023), impingement of circumflex artery (Kawamura et al. 2012), erosion of band into the pulmonary artery (Danilowicz et al. 1990), pseudoaneurysm of pulmonary artery (Nakayama et al. 2017; Venugopal et al. 2010), and thrombosis (Recto et al. 2013).

Distortion of one or both distal pulmonary arteries due to band migration is generally diagnosed by magnetic resonance imaging (MRI) or cardiac catheterization (Agasthi and Graziano 2023). Figure 15a shows the extent of branch pulmonary artery distortion. In most cases, the stenotic segment will require resection and followed by branch pulmonary artery pericardial patch augmentation and main pulmonary artery reconstruction as noted in Fig. 15b and associated inset. Proximal pulmonary artery band can cause pulmonary valve distortion (Zhu et al. 2023). Direct distortion of the pulmonary valve from proximal pulmonary artery band is shown in Fig. 16. At the time of band takedown and proximal pulmonary trunk repair, care is taken to remove the fibrosed pulmonary artery wall with incisions into the sinuses of Valsalva. This will allow appropriate enlargement that can be repaired by a series of pericardial patches before pulmonary trunk reconstruction as noted in Fig. 17. Pulmonary valve distortion due to pulmonary artery banding can also result in patients with transposition of the great arteries who undergo left ventricular training. The band causes significant pulmonary valve pressure afterload elevation which can cause neoaortic valve regurgitation after arterial switch (Mavroudis and Backer 2000). Coronary artery impingement after pulmonary artery banding can be surreptitious and difficult to diagnose (Kawamura et al. 2012). Tightening the band usually involves observation of the systemic oxygenation measurement, the systemic pressure, and the distal pulmonary artery pressure. It should also include monitoring of the electrocardiogram. Systemic pressure deterioration and electrocardiographic evidence of ischemic changes should immediately trigger a release of the band and exploration of the surface coronary artery anatomy to assess anomalous aortic origin. An adjusted pulmonary artery band location may be all that is necessary to perform an uncomplicated banding procedure. Takeyoshi and associates describe a more complicated situation and more involved solution. They wrote, "A one-month-old baby boy with a complete atrioventricular septal defect underwent pulmonary artery banding. A high take-off of the left coronary artery, overlooked on the echocardiogram, was identified. It was compressed by the right pulmonary artery that was dilated owing to pulmonary artery banding. The patient developed severe heart failure, and a Lecompte maneuver was performed. The procedure helped effectively treat this congenital heart disease with a high take-off coronary artery compressed by the right pulmonary artery (Takeyoshi et al. 2023). These situations are very rare; however, understanding the possibilities allows the surgeon to be aware and be ready to avoid the complications.

Erosion of the pulmonary artery band through the pulmonary artery wall and into the inner flow of the pulmonary artery has been described and can result in clot formation and hemolytic anemia (Danilowicz et al. 1990; Recto et al. 2013; Kutsche et al. 1985). This situation is more common when bands that have been used are made of umbilical tape or silk rather than Silastic or Teflon brands (Mahle et al. 1979). The best way to repair this problem at pulmonary artery takedown and comprehensive repair is to be mindful of the possibilities and be ready to open the pulmonary artery and remove the band and fibrous tissue by circumferential resection and reanastomosis of the pulmonary artery trunk. A careful search for associated clot formation, undiagnosed endocarditis, and camouflaged pseudoaneurysm (Shin et al. 1983) will yield the best results. Foale and associated (1984) demonstrated a large pseudoaneurysm after pulmonary artery band as noted in Fig. 18. Clear margins of the pseudoaneurysm, as shown in their report, can lead to careful intraoperative assessment and avoidance of unwanted cavitary entry during the dissection. Once the aneurysm has been dissected, standard techniques of band removal and pulmonary trunk reconstruction, as noted in the previous figures, can be implemented. While unilateral downstream pulmonary artery thrombosis after pulmonary artery band is theoretically possible, it is more likely to occur in relation to hybrid palliation and selective right and left pulmonary artery banding for hypoplastic left heart syndrome (Recto et al. 2013). We will not consider the complications of selective right and left pulmonary artery banding in this chapter.

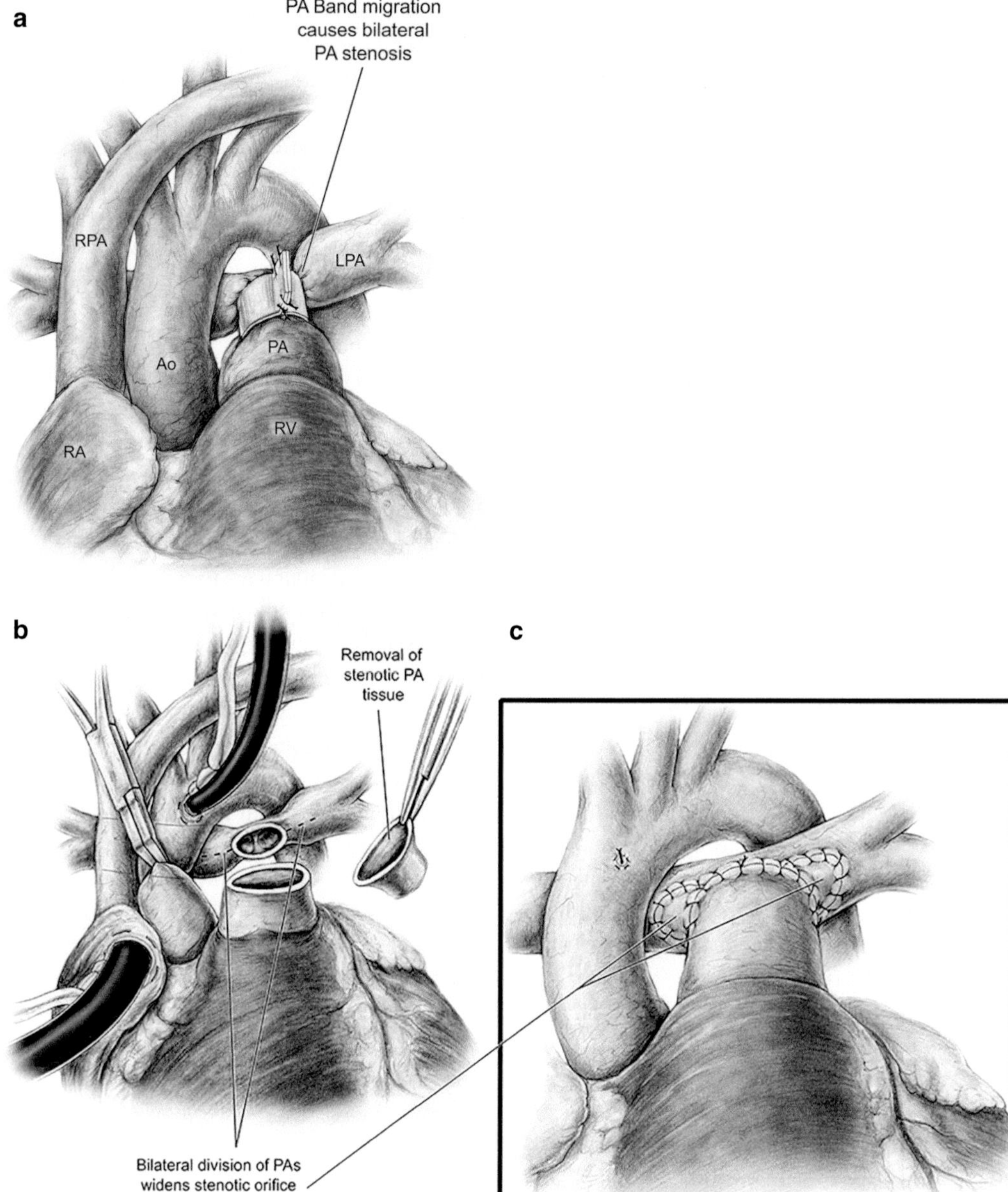

Fig. 15 (**a**) shows distal pulmonary artery distortion due to pulmonary artery band distal migration. The figure shows how the band can cause bilateral branch pulmonary artery stenosis. (**b**) shows band stenosis resection, bilateral distal pulmonary artery incisions to repair the stenosis. The inset "C" panel shows the completed repair technique using two separate pericardial patches for augmentation and main pulmonary artery reconstruction. *Ao* aorta, *LPA* left pulmonary artery, *PA* pulmonary artery, *RA* right atrium, *RPA* right pulmonary artery, *RV* right ventricle

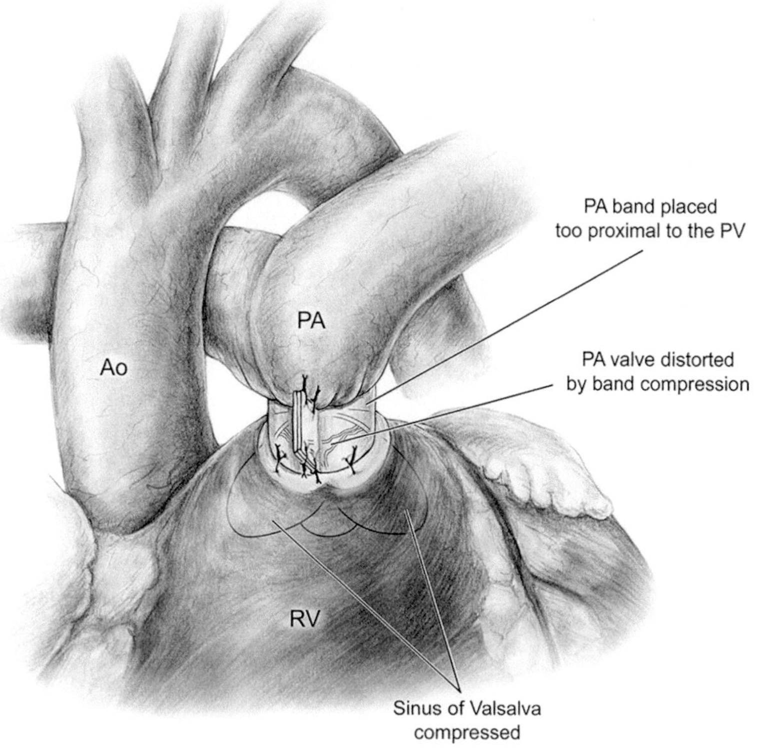

Fig. 16 Shows direct distortion of the pulmonary valve from proximal pulmonary artery banding. *Ao* aorta, *PA* pulmonary artery, *RV* right ventricle

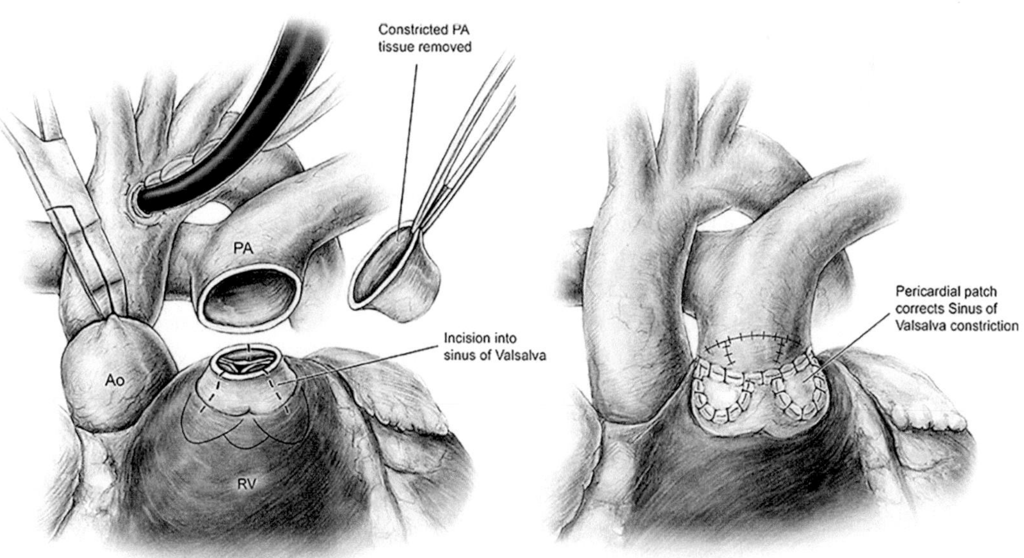

Fig. 17 Left panel shows how the supravalvar stenosis can be repaired by fibrous tissue resection and sinus of Valsalva incisions. The right panel shows sinus augmentation by pericardial patches and reconstruction. *Ao* aorta, *PA* pulmonary artery, *RV* right ventricle

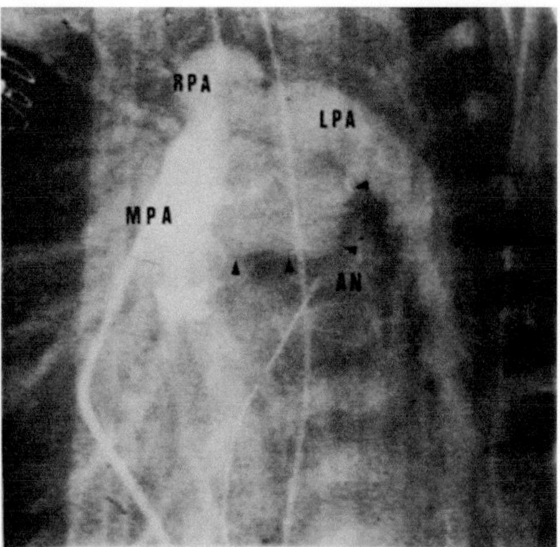

Fig. 18 Left anterior oblique projection of the angiogram demonstrating contrast medium within the main pulmonary artery (MPA) and right (RPA) and left (LPA) branches. Extrusion of contrast medium behind the main pulmonary artery delineating the pseudoaneurysm (AN) is denoted by arrowheads. (With Permission: Foale et al. 1984)

3 Pulmonary Artery Band Takedown

Pulmonary artery band takedown is performed by careful resternotomy, conscientious dissection, cardiopulmonary bypass, cardioplegic arrest in most cases, removal of the band, circumferential resection of the fibrosed segment, and pulmonary trunk reconstruction. Of those patients who have an intraluminal pulmonary artery band and who are undergoing a bidirectional Glenn shunt (single ventricle palliation), the course of the operation is slightly different. In these specific cases, pulmonary artery transection, removal of the fenestrated patch, and oversewing of the proximal pulmonary artery trunk is accomplished.

Pulmonary artery band takedown in palliated patients who are undergoing simultaneous intracardiac correction is performed through a median sternotomy. In most cases, the intracardiac repair is performed first using cardioplegic arrest. When all cardiac shunts are repaired, the pulmonary artery reconstruction can be accomplished after cross-clamp removal and while the patient is being warmed.

The specific steps of the pulmonary artery band takedown operation are reviewed in Figs. 19, 20, 21, 22, and 23. The entire pulmonary artery band should be removed to avoid posterior pulmonary wall scarring, which can cause late pulmonary artery stenosis. However, removing the band entirely is not generally sufficient to prevent residual pulmonary stenosis at the band site owing to pulmonary wall fibrosis and contraction. An exception to this rule occurs if the band is left in place for only a period of weeks, after which time, simple removal is adequate. In those cases where the band is in place for more than a few months, the area of the band must be excised as noted in Fig. 20 or patched as shown in Figs. 24, 25, 26, and 27. The excision technique as shown in Fig. 21, is followed by an end-to-end anastomosis using absorbable, fine monofilament suture as shown in Figs. 22 and 23. Care must be taken to ensure that the distal right and left pulmonary arteries are completely mobilized and that the ligamentum arteriosum is ligated and divided to allow a tension-free anastomosis.

The patch technique as illustrated in Figs. 24, 25, 26, and 27 requires patch augmentation using pericardium or polytetrafluoroethylene (PTFE) which will allow unobstructed flow to the right and left pulmonary arteries. An alternative solution to patch augmentation is the use of a "pantaloon" patch with extension into the right and left anterior sinuses of Valsalva as noted in Fig. 25. We prefer the transection and reanastomosis technique over the patch augmentation technique since the former technique virtually eliminates residual stenoses and systolic murmurs which are often seen postoperatively with the patch augmentation technique. We readily admit however, that this takedown technique is surgeon specific and can be shown to be excellent with either technique.

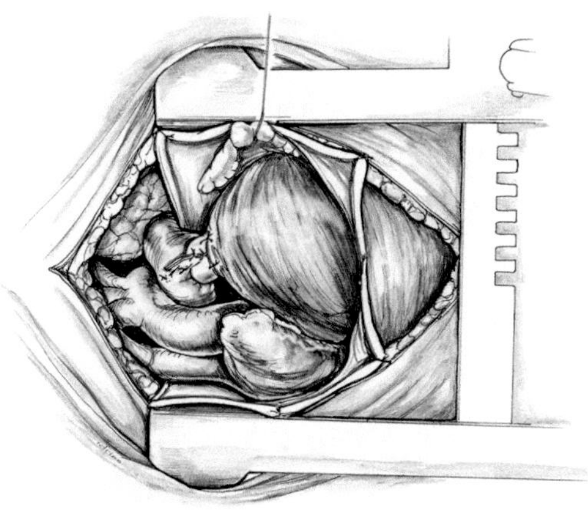

Fig. 19 Pulmonary artery banding takedown usually requires cardiopulmonary bypass, Teflon™ PAB removal, and repair by either direct anastomosis or patch technique. Each technique has its advantages and disadvantages and is illustrated. The figure shows the completed dissection of a patient with PAB in preparation for the excision and direct anastomosis technique. (With permission: Mavroudis 2015)

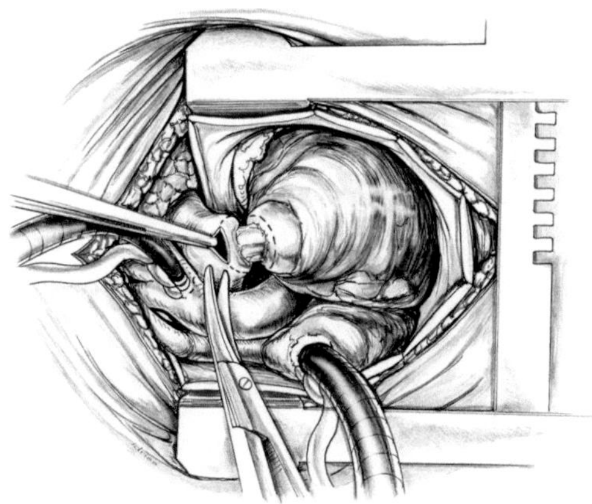

Fig. 20 After cardiopulmonary bypass, the pulmonary artery band (PAB) is removed and the surgeon is shown removing the cuff of pulmonary artery wall (*dotted lines*) that was involved in the PAB procedure. The incision is above the area of stenosis in order to create a freshened anastomotic site for the eventual repair without residual obstruction. Figures 21 and 22 do not show the application of an aortic cross-clamp and cardioplegic arrest since it is assumed that the intracardiac repair has already been performed thereby eliminating intracardiac shunts and the potential for systemic air embolism. Cardioplegic arrest is advised in those cases where an intracardiac shunt is delayed until after the pulmonary artery reconstruction procedure. The surgeon will be wise to consider all aspects of this operation before commencing. (With permission: Mavroudis 2015)

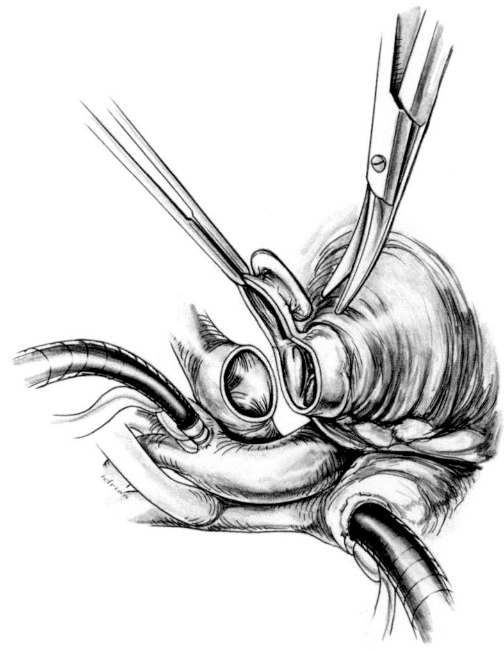

Fig. 21 Shows the completion of the banded segmental resection, leaving uninvolved native proximal and distal pulmonary artery tissue. Figures 21 and 22 do not show the application of an aortic cross-clamp and cardioplegic arrest since it is assumed that the intracardiac repair has already been performed thereby eliminating intracardiac shunts and the potential for systemic air embolism. Cardioplegic arrest is advised in those cases where an intracardiac shunt is delayed until after the pulmonary artery reconstruction procedure. The surgeon will be wise to consider all aspects of this operation before commencing. (With permission: Mavroudis 2015).

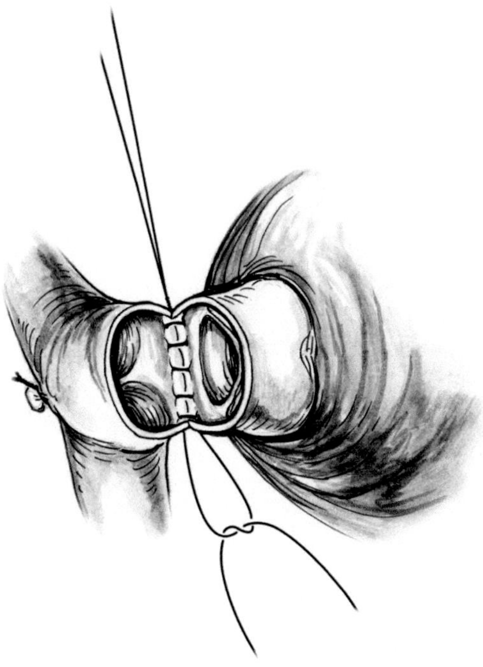

Fig. 22 The re-anastomosis is performed by interrupted suture technique, starting at the posterior wall as shown in the figure. (With permission: Mavroudis 2015)

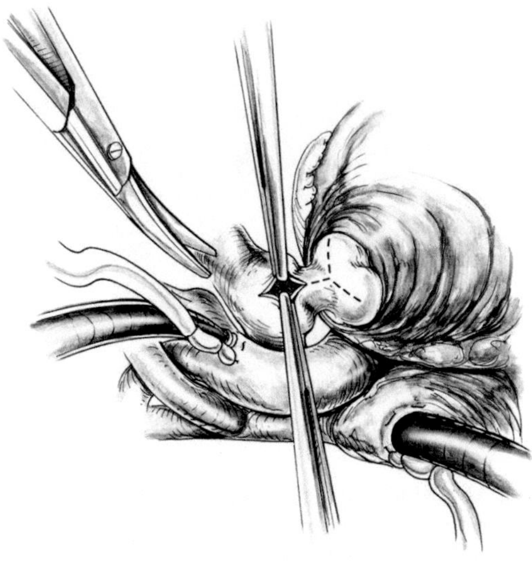

Fig. 24 Surgeons may choose to repair the pulmonary artery band (PAB) by wide incisions and placement of a biologic or synthetic patch. The figure shows a patient with the PAB removed while on cardiopulmonary bypass and aortic cross-clamp. The initial incision in the distal pulmonary artery is shown; the proposed incisions are noted by dotted lines, which extend into the anterior pulmonary artery sinuses of Valsalva. (With permission: Mavroudis 2015)

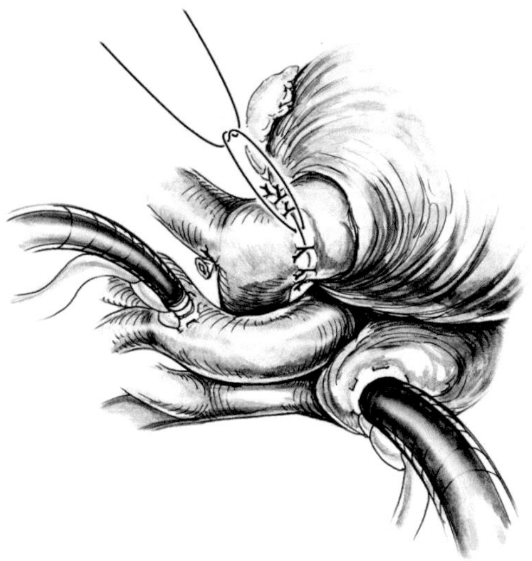

Fig. 23 Shows the completed anastomosis using interrupted suture technique. (With permission: Mavroudis 2015)

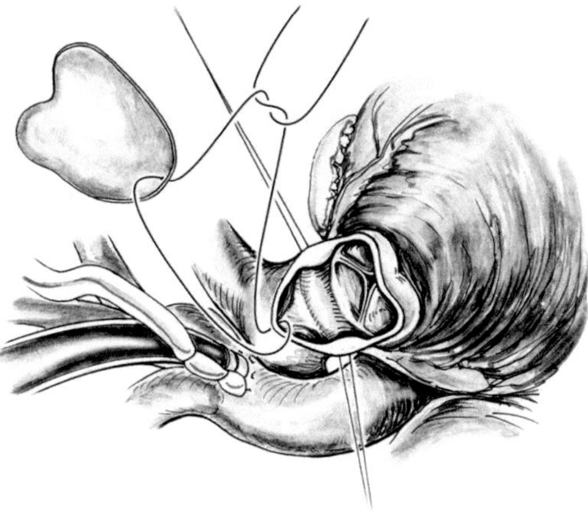

Fig. 25 The patch augmentation is performed using a pantaloon-shaped patch of autologous pericardium or prosthetic material (polytetrafluoroethylene; PTFE) as shown in the figure. The suture line can be commenced proximally or distally, depending on the circumstances. (With permission: Mavroudis 2015)

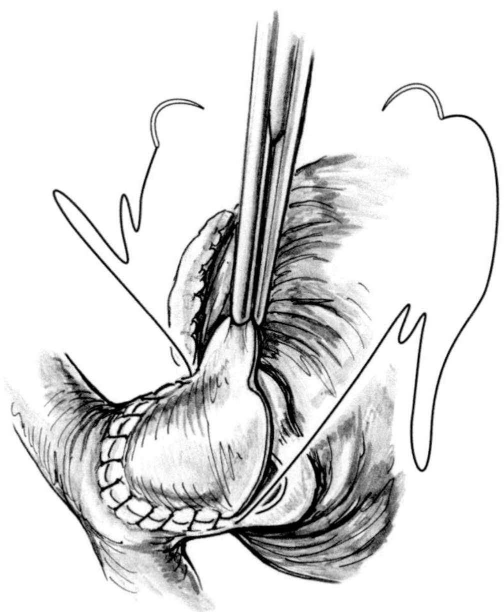

Fig. 26 Shows the placement of the pantaloon patch using running suture technique from distal to proximal sequence. (With permission: Mavroudis 2015)

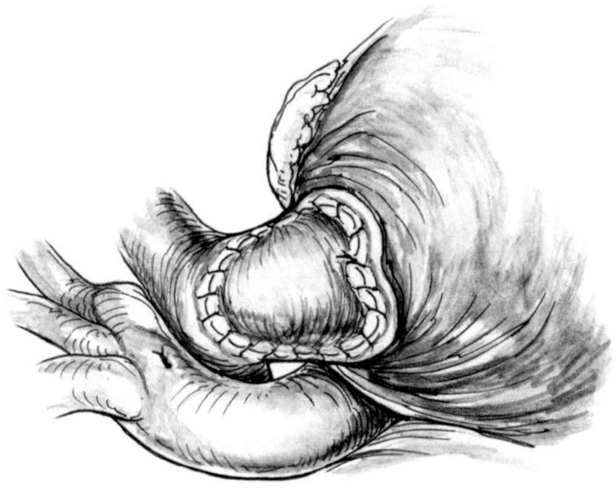

Fig. 27 Shows the completed reconstruction after separation from cardiopulmonary bypass. (With permission: Mavroudis 2015)

4 Other Indications for Pulmonary Artery Banding

During the last decade, surgeon investigators have introduced two innovative uses for pulmonary artery banding in patients. Schranz and colleagues reported their findings regarding pulmonary artery banding in infants and young children with left ventricular dilated cardiomyopathy in an effort to improve ventricular function before cardiac transplantation (Schranz et al. 2013, 2018). Banding of the pulmonary artery led to optimal ventricular interaction, improved left ventricular function, and decreased mitral regurgitation. In another group of patients, Ma and associates reported on the use of palliative pulmonary artery banding in patients with congenitally corrected transposition of the great arteries, ventricular dysfunction, and systemic (tricuspid valve) regurgitation (Ma et al. 2014). The banding procedure led to both left ventricular training and improved tricuspid regurgitation (systemic atrioventricular valve) caused by a shift in the ventricular septum towards a more midline position. While present-day surgical treatment for congenitally corrected transposition of the great arteries is tilted towards double switch procedures, the authors noted that some selected patients would benefit from prolonged palliative pulmonary artery banding over double switch.

5 Aortopulmonary Shunts

5.1 Classic Blalock-Taussig-Thomas Shunt

The Blalock-Taussig-Thomas (BTT) shunt was the first systemic-to-pulmonary shunt and ushered in the era of palliation en route to complete repair. The shunt was performed in 1944 by Alfred Blalock with the clinical encouragement of Helen Taussig and the laboratory assistance of Vivien Thomas of the Johns Hopkins University Medical Center (Blalock and Taussig 1945; Thomas 2020). As originally described, the classic BTT shunt (previously known as the Blalock-Taussig shunt) is a direct end-to-side anastomosis of the transected subclavian artery to the pulmonary artery. Alfred Blalock and Vivien Thomas used this shunt in animals in an attempt to create a model of pulmonary hypertension during their tenure at Vanderbilt University. After Blalock accepted his position at Hopkins, he persuaded

Thomas to come to Baltimore and establish the surgical research laboratory. Helen Taussig, who was the director of the pediatric cardiology program, suggested to Alfred Blalock that they apply their experimental procedure to patients who had cyanosis from insufficient pulmonary blood flow.

The first BTT operation was performed on November 28, 1944, on a 15-month-old girl with tetralogy of Fallot and severe pulmonary stenosis which proved to be a momentous moment in the progress of congenital heart surgery (Vricella et al. 2013). This tradition was highlighted by Williams and colleagues who reported on the results of 2,016 patients who had a BTT shunt between 1944 and 2006 at the Johns Hopkins Medical Center (Williams et al. 2007).

The classic BTT shunt is performed through a thoracotomy on the side opposite the aortic arch. Figure 28 (Backer and Mavroudis 2023; Mavroudis 2015) illustrates the anatomic exposure highlighting the right subclavian artery, and right pulmonary artery which are required for the BTT shunt. The figure shows ligation of the right subclavian artery branches. The carotid artery can be dissected to provide more mobility. The azygos vein is doubly ligated and divided. In preparation for the anastomosis, heparin 1 mg/kg is administered intravenously. The anastomosis is performed to connect the subclavian artery to the main pulmonary artery with vascular clamps. Great care is taken to avoid performing the anastomosis to the right upper lobe branch which will result in suboptimal hemodynamic and saturation shunt conditions The subclavian artery will then take a course in an anatomic groove posterior to the superior caval vein and the phrenic nerve. When this anastomosis is performed always in this manner, the takedown procedure is more easily approached. Therefore, takedown of the classic right BTT shunt at the time of complete correction through a median sternotomy anticipates dissection posterior to the superior caval vein. The artery can then be carefully encircled with double ligation and division.

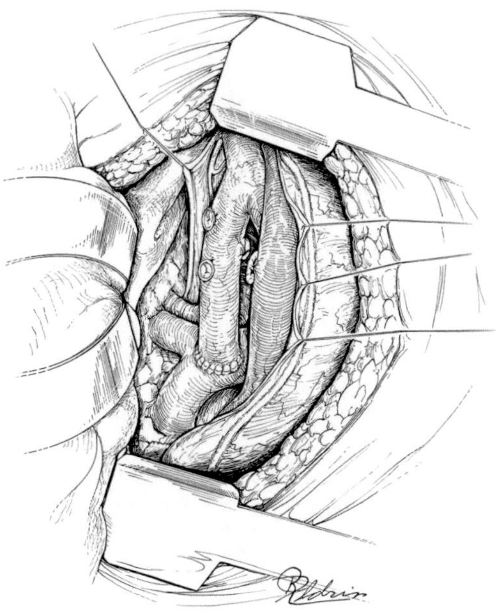

Fig. 28 For the sake of historical perspective and intellectual curiosity, The Blalock-Taussig shunt, otherwise known as the Blalock-Taussig-Thomas shunt is shown to recognize the pioneering laboratory work of Vivien Thomas at Johns Hopkins University during this golden era of heart surgery. The operation was initially developed to create an animal model of pulmonary hypertension. Its application, as seen in the figure, revolutionized the field of congenital heart surgery. (With permission: Mavroudis 2015)

The classic BTT shunt seems uniquely favorable since the pulmonary artery blood flow is limited by the orifice of the subclavian artery. Since there is no prosthetic material, the shunt grows with the patient, providing more pulmonary blood flow as the child grows. There are important negative consequences however, such as hand or arm ischemia that can occur due to the divided subclavian artery that collateral arteries do not always mitigate against (Geiss et al. 1980). The involved arm is generally shorter than the contralateral arm, cool to the touch, and pulseless. The intraoperative maneuvers to optimize the proximity between the subclavian artery and pulmonary artery include carotid artery mobilization and division of the inferior pulmonary ligament. When these actions are not enough to result in a tension free anastomosis, the short subclavian artery may cause the pulmonary artery to be "pulled" up and kink, which counteracts any of the advantages. As a result, most, if not all, centers now employ PTFE grafts for the systemic-to-pulmonary artery shunt and thereby preserve the subclavian artery.

5.2 Modified Blalock-Taussig-Thomas Shunt

A PTFE tube to create a systemic-to-pulmonary shunt was first reported by Gazzaniga and associates (1976). This experience was followed by De Leval and colleagues (1981) who termed the operation, modified Blalock-Taussig (-Thomas) shunt. Their report highlighted 99 patients operated on between 1975 and 1979 with excellent results. The advantages and disadvantages of the modified BTT shunt have been published in a previous report, "The advantages of the modified BTT shunt, which has now become the shunt of choice at most congenital heart surgery centers, include (1) preservation of the circulation to the affected arm; (2) regulation of the shunt flow by the size of the shunt; (3) guarantee of adequate shunt length; and (4) ease of shunt takedown. One disadvantage of the modified BTT shunt is the occasional leaking of serous fluid through the interstices of the fabric of the PTFE. This may result in excessive and prolonged chest tube drainage, localized seroma formation around the graft, or both (LeBlanc et al. 1984). This complication, as shown in Fig. 29 (Silva et al. 2013) occurs in less than 5% of patients. The patency rate of the modified BTT shunt has been improved by the addition of heparin coating to the PTFE graft (Ashfaq et al. 2018; Ambarsari et al. 2018)."

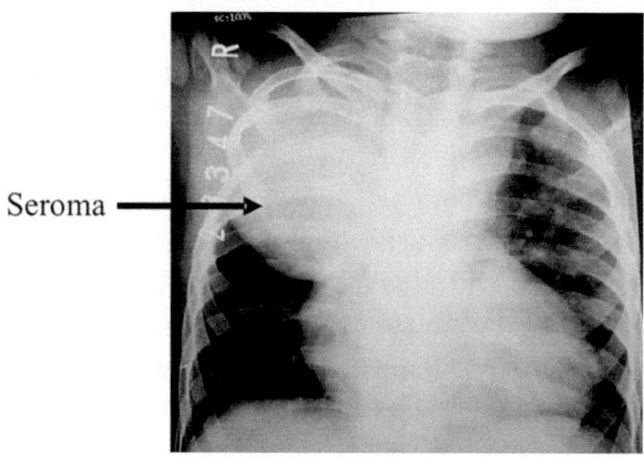

Fig. 29 Shows a chest roentgenogram which depicts a large seroma in association with the placement of a right modified Blalock-Taussig-Thomas shunt. (With permission: Silva et al. 2013)

The operative approach for the modified BTT can be performed through a left thoracotomy, a right thoracotomy or a median sternotomy. The operative exposure is dependent on the subclavian and pulmonary artery anatomy, the presence and location of a patent arterial duct, the great vessel relationship, and surgeon preference. Nowadays, most surgeons perform the modified BTT shunt through a median sternotomy. We have been using this approach for over 20 years. The sternotomy approach is technically less challenging and is associated with fewer shunt failures than the classic thoracotomy approach (Odim et al. 1995). It allows the surgeon to comfortably use cardiopulmonary bypass in the event that the patient becomes cyanotic or unstable. There are other advantages as well that decrease the incidence of complications. The median sternotomy approach renders the anatomic location of the aortic arch insignificant. The shunt can also be targeted to the main pulmonary artery (central shunt), which can be preferable in many cases. Access to the patent arterial duct for ligation for the purpose of removing a source of competitive flow is always possible. In addition, the outdated reason to avoid sternotomy to decrease adhesions has been mitigated owing to increased experience and other prophylactic measures such as PTFE pericardial substitutes (Morales et al. 2008).

The guidelines for shunt flow estimation and optimal PTFE graft size have been accurately considered in one of our previous reports and is reproduced herein (Backer and Mavroudis 2023).

"The size of the PTFE graft selected is based on the size of the patient. Importantly, the amount of flow through the shunt is determined by Poiseuille's law,

$$Q = \frac{\pi r^4 \Delta p}{8 \mu L}$$

in which Q = volumetric flow, Δp = pressure drop, r = radius of the tube, L = length, and μ = fluid viscosity. This relationship illustrates the concept that a small change in shunt diameter (radius) results in a large change in flow, relating to the diameter raised to the fourth power. If the shunt is taken from the subclavian artery, the diameter of the subclavian artery will regulate the flow. However, if the shunt is from the innominate artery (which frequently is the case with a median sternotomy approach), consideration must be given to using a smaller shunt as then the shunt size will regulate the flow. We use a 3.5-mm graft for infants weighing 2.5–4.0 kg, a 4.0-mm graft for infants 4.0–5.0 kg, and a 3.0-mm graft for infants less than 2.5 kg. Most of these children go on to second stage procedure or complete repair at 3–6 months of age and the shunt flow for that short time period is adequate and not excessive (even if the shunt comes from the innominate artery)."

In those patients for whom a right thoracotomy approach is preferred, the latissimus dorsi muscle is divided; the serratus anterior is mobilized and spared. The thorax is entered through the fourth interspace and retracted. The lung is retracted anteriorly and inferiorly. The mediastinal pleura is incised posterior to the superior caval vein and phrenic nerve. The azygos vein is doubly ligated and divided which will prevent retraction into the mediastinum and excessive bleeding. The subclavian artery is dissected and encircled with a vessel loop, with care being taken to avoid the right recurrent laryngeal nerve, which passes around the distal innominate artery at the take-off of the subclavian and common carotid arteries. The right pulmonary artery is dissected completely, with care being taken to identify the right upper lobe branch and main pulmonary artery continuation to the right lower and middle lobes. The right upper lobe and distal right pulmonary artery branches are encircled with vessel loops, which can then be occluded with small Rummel tourniquets. The patient is administered heparin 1 mg/kg intravenously.The PTFE is cut to size before the clamps are placed to accurately measure the appropriate distance between the innominate artery and right pulmonary artery. Clamps distort the distance and therefore are placed after the PTFE graft is accurately measured. The graft is generally cut to result in an implanted gentle curve. This theoretically allows for patient growth. It should not kink or distort the pulmonary artery, which can occur if the length is not accurate. We have used and prefer the "stretch" PTFE that is more forgiving regarding length estimates. The figures that describe the surgical techniques for graft construction and complications thereto are basically the same for right thoracotomy and median sternotomy. We will therefore consider the implantation techniques as viewed from the median sternotomy approach as noted in Figs. 30, 31, 32, 33, 34, 35, 36, 37, 38, 39, 40, 41, and 42.Figure 30 reviews the benefits of median sternotomy as compared with thoracotomy for systemic-to-pulmonary artery graft placement. Figure 31 illustrates the methods for azygous vein ligation and division. Surgeons are encouraged to perform double ligation and/or suture ligation to prevent unwanted suture disruption, vein retraction into the posterior mediastinum, and excessive bleeding. This can be a distressing complication since the edges of the cut end of the retracted vein are not readily visible. Focused suction and for-

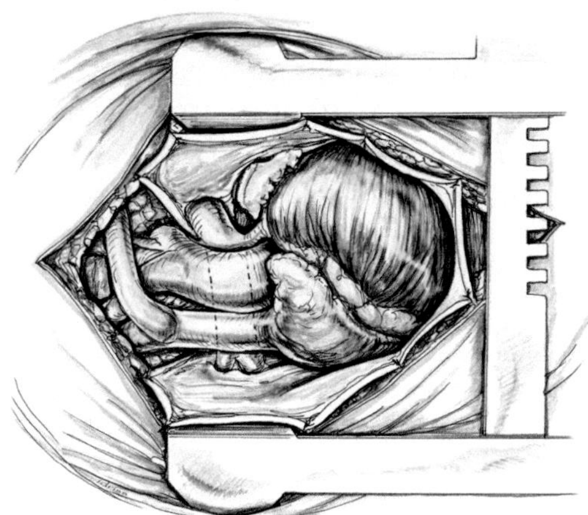

Fig. 30 Systemic-to-pulmonary artery shunts are used to palliate a number of congenital heart lesions with decreased pulmonary artery flow. The general principles are to provide enough pulmonary artery flow to relieve cyanosis but not to cause pulmonary overcirculation. In years past, surgeons preferred to perform systemic-to-pulmonary artery shunts by thoracotomy technique, thereby making a median sternotomy simpler for the eventual repair. Recently, surgeons have preferred median sternotomy, to gain better exposure and to employ cardiopulmonary bypass when deemed necessary. The figure shows a patient with tetralogy of Fallot and a tiny communication between the right ventricle and the pulmonary artery. (With permission: Mavroudis 2015)

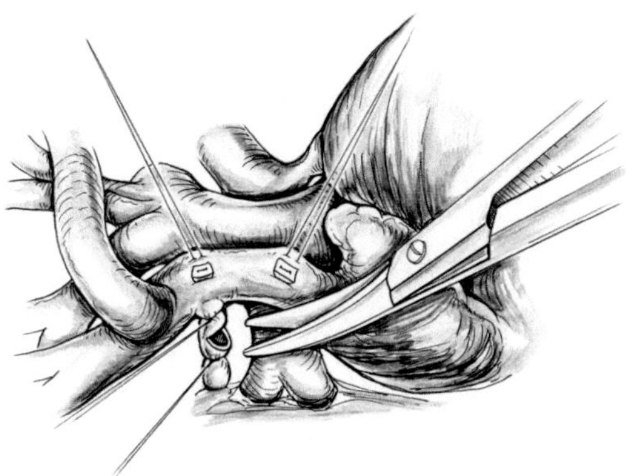

Fig. 31 In preparation for creation of a systemic-to-pulmonary artery shunt, many surgeons prefer to ligate the azygos vein, as shown in the figure, to allow identification and eventual shunt takedown easier. Pledgetted sutures are placed in the adventitia of the superior caval vein to help with exposure. (With permission: Mavroudis 2015)

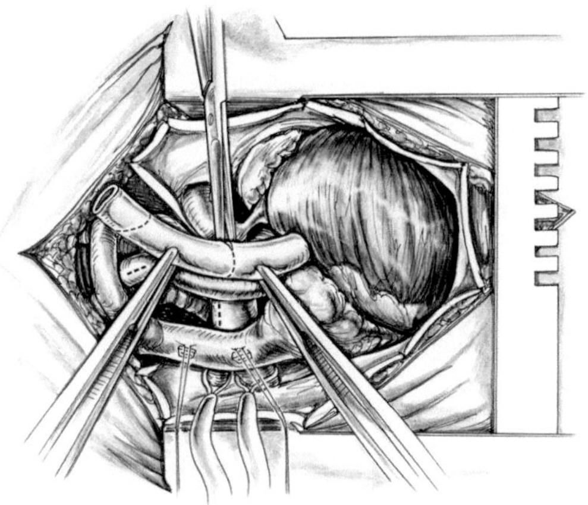

Fig. 32 Once the appropriate dissection is performed, the target shunt vessels are identified (dashed lines) and the systemic-to-pulmonary artery polytetrafluoroethylene (PTFE) graft is cut to size. In general, the innominate artery and the right pulmonary artery are the chosen vessels for shunt creation. Heparin (1 mg/kg) is administered before any clamps are applied. (With permission: Mavroudis 2015)

ceps application into the presumed area will allow the surgeon to capture the vein and elevate it into vision allowing a vascular clamp to control the vessel. Appropriate dissection and double ligation are preferrable.The PTFE graft is beveled as illustrated in Fig. 32. After heparin administration and vascular clamp placement, an arteriotomy is created in the inferior aspect of the subclavian or innominate artery as noted in Fig. 33. In most cases we use the proximal innominate artery for the anastomotic target. The length of the arteriotomy is important. The clamp placement should clasp enough artery to ensure that the edges of the arteriotomy will allow comfortable exposure to conduct the anastomosis. Not enough clasping of the artery will result in difficult conditions with the possibility of extending suture placement mistakenly from one side of the arterial incision to the other side as noted in Fig. 34. This complication will pin the opposite sides of the anastomosis and result in clotting. Better to see every stitch that is placed by ensuring proper exposure. In normal conditions and appropriate clamp placement, the PTFE graft is anastomosed to the incised innominate artery using 7-0 polypropylene suture as noted in Figs. 33, 35, 36, and 37. Another complication

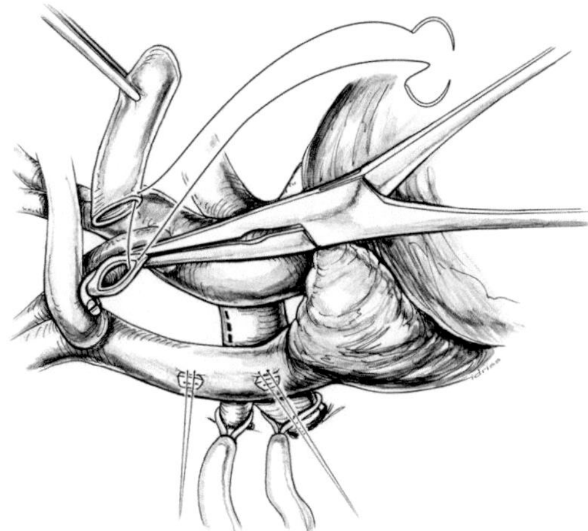

Fig. 33 Once the shunt material has been cut to size, the innominate artery is clamped in such a manner as to have the resultant anastomosis in its most inferior position. This requires placement of the clamp to isolate the inferior portion of the innominate artery and retraction anteriorly for anastomosis. A longitudinal incision is made in the isolated portion of the innominate artery to correspond with the size of the prosthetic graft. In general, the polytetrafluoroethylene (PTFE) shunt used measures of 3.5, 4.0, or 5.0 mm, depending on the patient's size. The anastomosis is then initiated using polypropylene running suture technique as shown in the figure. (With permission: Mavroudis 2015)

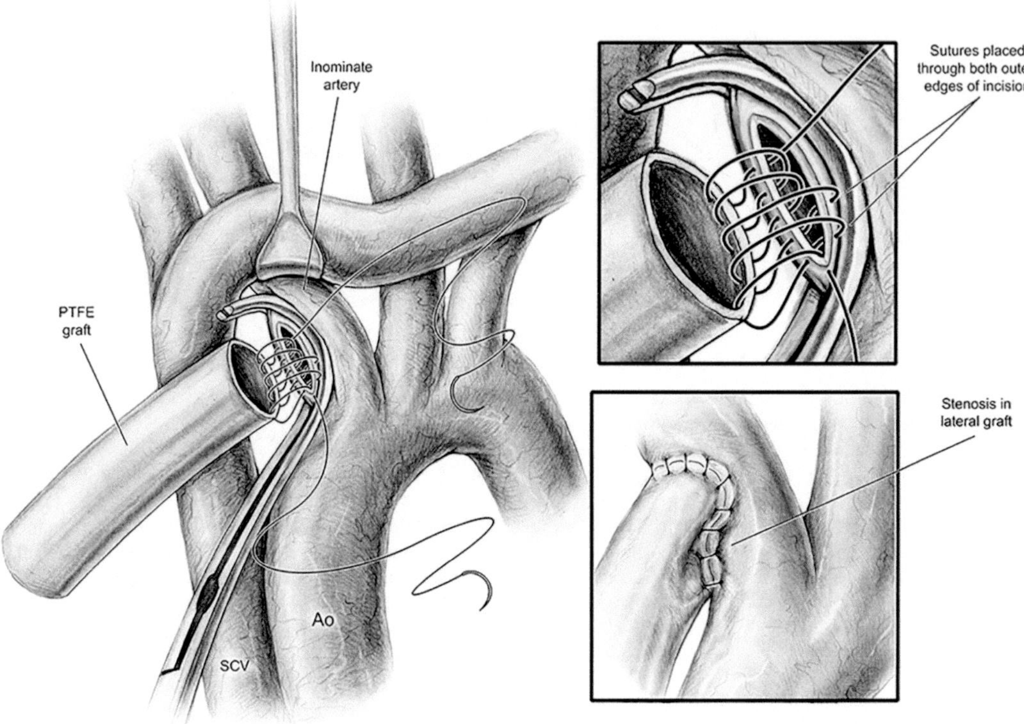

Fig. 34 Left panel shows how superficial clamp placement on the innominate artery can result in inadequate exposure of the lumen. This can result in unwanted suture placement that will connect both walls of the proposed anastomosis. The upper right inset shows a magnified view of mistaken suture placement. When not identified, the suture can coapt the edges, compress the anastomosis, and cause clotting. The right lower inset demonstrates the epicardial anatomy after the complicated anastomosis that compresses the anastomosis. An adequate placement of the vascular clamp will ensure proper luminal exposure that will avoid this complication. *Ao* aorta, *PTFE* polytetrafluoroethylene, *SCV* superior caval vein

during the arteriotomies that are required for the shunt procedure is making the incision too long either at the beginning of the proposed anastomosis or during the course of the anastomosis. Figure 38 illustrates the result of making an arterial incision too long in the innominate artery that can cause significant stenosis of the proximal graft and the distal innominate artery. The best way to deal with this complication is to take down the original anastomosis, repair the elongated incision with an augmenting patch of PTFE, and anastomose the graft to the PTFE patch as noted in Fig. 38 inset. Assuming that the proximal graft anastomosis was performed without complications, as is more often the case, attention can be given to the pulmonary artery anastomosis. The clamp on the innominate artery is left in place until the pulmonary artery anastomosis is completed. Repositioning the clamp to the PTFE graft may increase the risk of blood stasis and shunt thrombosis. The pulmonary artery is controlled with another vascular clamp as shown in Fig. 37. Rummel tourniquets are snugged on the right upper and lower distal pulmonary arteries. A longitudinal arteriotomy is created in the superior aspect of the right pulmo-

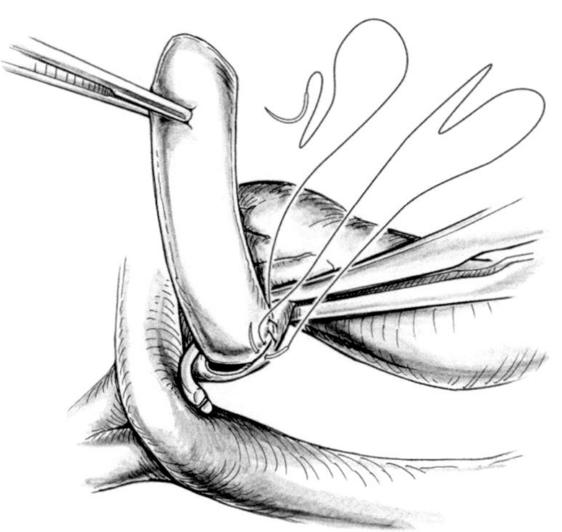

Fig. 35 Shows the performance of the posterior anastomosis, which will end near the apex of the arteriotomy. The suture sequence is outside-in on the artery and inside-out on the PTFE graft for this posterior side of the anastomosis. (With permission: Mavroudis 2015)

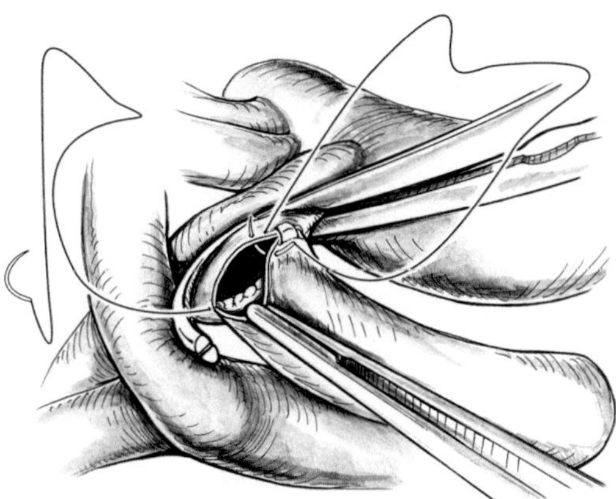

Fig. 36 Shows how the anastomosis is continued by the execution of the corresponding anterior suture line. The sequence of suturing in this case is outside-in on the PTFE graft and inside-out on the artery until the anastomosis is completed. (With permission: Mavroudis 2015)

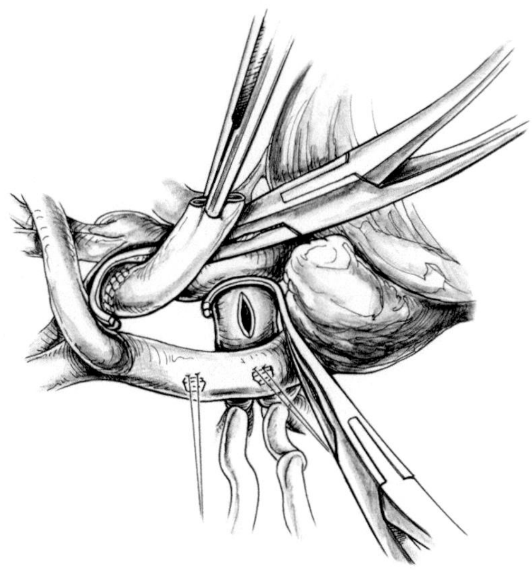

Fig. 37 Shows the completed proximal suture line. The clamp is left applied to the systemic artery because if it were removed from the artery and applied to the shunt material, an unwanted clot could form at the anastomotic site, causing shunt thrombosis. The right pulmonary artery is isolated, either with distal rubber vessel loops and a proximal clamp, as shown in the figure, or by a side-biting clamp of the right pulmonary artery (not shown). A longitudinal incision is then made as noted. Recognizing that the pulmonary artery incision tends to stretch, the surgeon is advised to make the initial incision smaller than would appear necessary, reserving the option to increase its size during the anastomosis. (With permission: Mavroudis 2015)

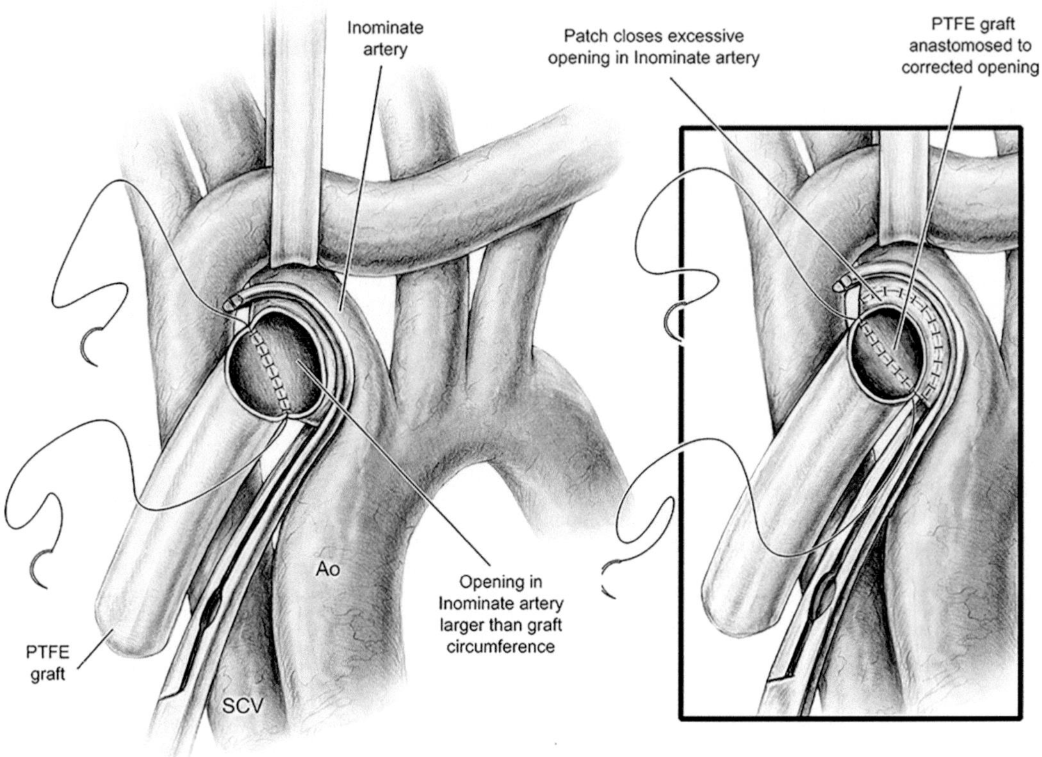

Fig. 38 Left panel shows an elongated innominate artery incision larger than the orifice of the PTFE graft. Placing more sutures to accommodate the PTFE graft could cause anastomotic disruption and stenosis. The right panel shows how a situation like this can be salvaged by a separate arterial patch repair into which the graft can be anastomosed. *Ao* aortic, *PTFE* polytetrafluoroethylene, *SCV* superior caval vein

nary artery. Using a single 7-0 polypropylene suture, the PTFE graft is anastomosed to the pulmonary artery as shown in Figs. 39 and 40.

When the clamps are simultaneously released as shown in Fig. 41, and flow established through the shunt, an instantaneous rise of 15%–20% in the patient's oxygen saturation should be expected as monitored by pulse oximetry. In addition, a thrill should be palpable in the distal pulmonary artery. To maximize the clinical effect of the systemic-to-pulmonary artery shunt, maintenance of adequate systemic perfusion pressure before, during, and after the operation is necessary to prevent early shunt thrombosis. This may require inotropic support (dopamine, epinephrine). Bleeding is controlled with Gelfoam soaked with topical thrombin. The heparin is not routinely reversed with protamine unless there is excessive bleeding from the suture lines.

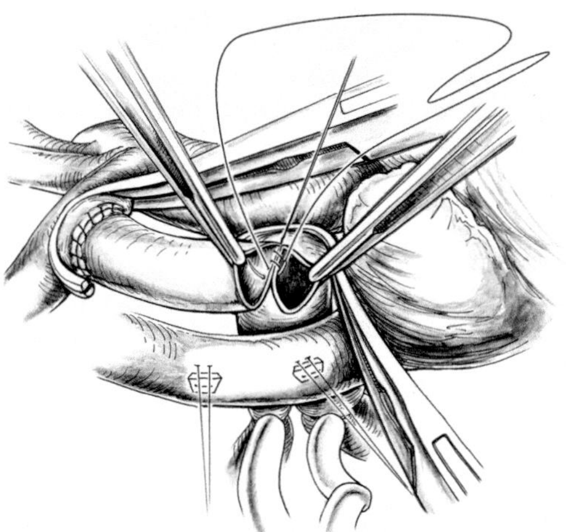

Fig. 39 The distal anastomosis is commenced by initiating the running suture line posteriorly as shown in the figure within the pulmonary artery and the PTFE shunt. Once the posterior suture line is completed, the anterior suture line can be commenced. (With permission: Mavroudis 2015)

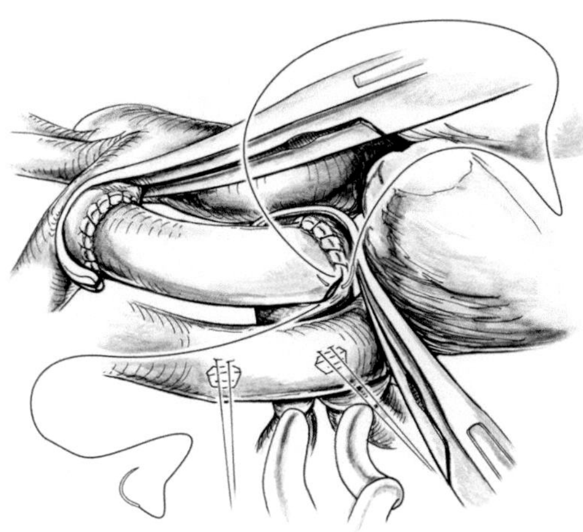

Fig. 40 The anterior suture line is performed using running suture technique, as shown in the figure. Note that both occlusive clamps are still in place. Before the last suture is placed, a heparinized solution can be instilled in the graft to remove the air and unwanted clots. (With permission: Mavroudis 2015)

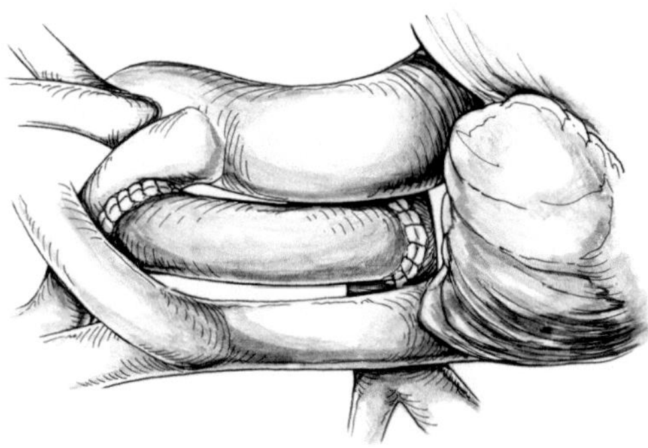

Fig. 41 The clamps are removed simultaneously and the bleeding is controlled as needed. The figure shows the completed reconstruction. (With permission: Mavroudis 2015)

There has been some controversy as to the management of a patent ductus arteriosus after completion of the shunt procedure. In other words, should the shunt be ligated or should it be left open?

The rationale of ligating the arterial duct is that this will eliminate a source of competitive pulmonary blood flow and improve the patency of the shunt. The reason not to ligate the arterial duct is that if shunt thrombosis occurs, prostaglandin E_1 can be reinitiated, providing a source of pulmonary blood flow which will give the operating team time to reoperate and repair the problem. In an analysis of the STS Congenital Heart Surgery Database by Petrucci and associates, 50% of the patent arterial ducts were ligated and 50% were left open under these circumstances, with no difference in surgical mortality (Petrucci et al. 2011). Management of the patent ductus arteriosus proves to be important, especially regarding the sequence of ligation or no ligation with regard to the shunt operation. We recommend not mobilizing the patent arterial duct until after the shunt is opened. Even minimal dissection around the patent arterial duct can result in ductal spasm or bleeding, which can lead, to an unstable clinical situation resulting in hypotension and desaturation requiring emergent initiation of cardiopulmonary bypass. Our practice has been to ligate the patent arterial duct after completing the shunt, recognizing that this operative decision is based on clinical experience.

Short- and long-term complications of systemic-to-pulmonary artery shunts are associated mostly with the original shunt construction that caused anastomotic stenosis (discussed in Figs. 34 and 38). However, these complications can be multifactorial. As noted by Sachweh and associates (1998), "pulmonary artery stenosis is not a rare event after systemic-to-pulmonary shunt operations. A patent ductus arteriosus with or without administration of Prostaglandin E1 is related to pulmonary artery stenosis on the side of the ductus arteriosus. Pulmonary artery stenosis on the side of a peripheral shunt may be caused by inappropriate surgical technique, increased intimal proliferation, or pulmonary artery kinking. Treatment depends on severity of cyanosis and on further surgical plans." Figs. 42 and 43 from Sachweh's article (Sachweh et al. 1998) are angiographic examples of these aforementioned complications. Another complication associated with the shunt procedure is pulmonary stenosis on the side of the shunt due to pulmonary artery "tenting" which occurs when the original PTFE graft proves to be too short thereby causing right and left pulmonary branch stenosis. Figure 44 shows an artist's representation of this complication with recommended resolution of

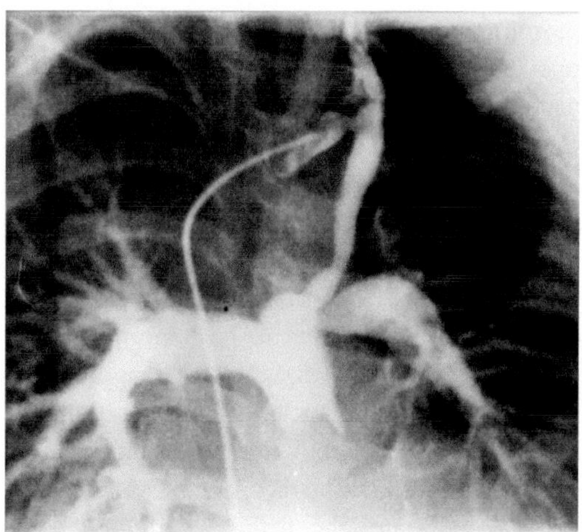

Fig. 42 Stenosis of the left pulmonary artery located ipsilaterally to the BTT shunt with an additional shunt stenosis caused by kinking due to an overlength of the graft. (With permission: Sachweh et al. 1998)

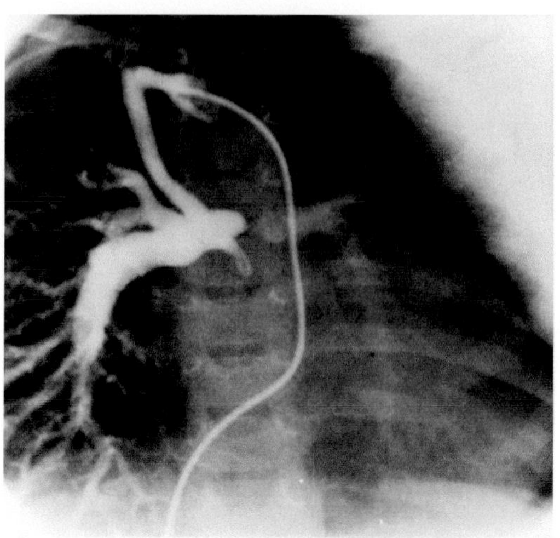

Fig. 43 Discontinuity of the left pulmonary artery at the site of the ductus arteriosus located contralaterally to the BTT shunt in a patient with a former patent ductus arteriosus and administration of PGE1. (With permission: Sachweh et al. 1998)

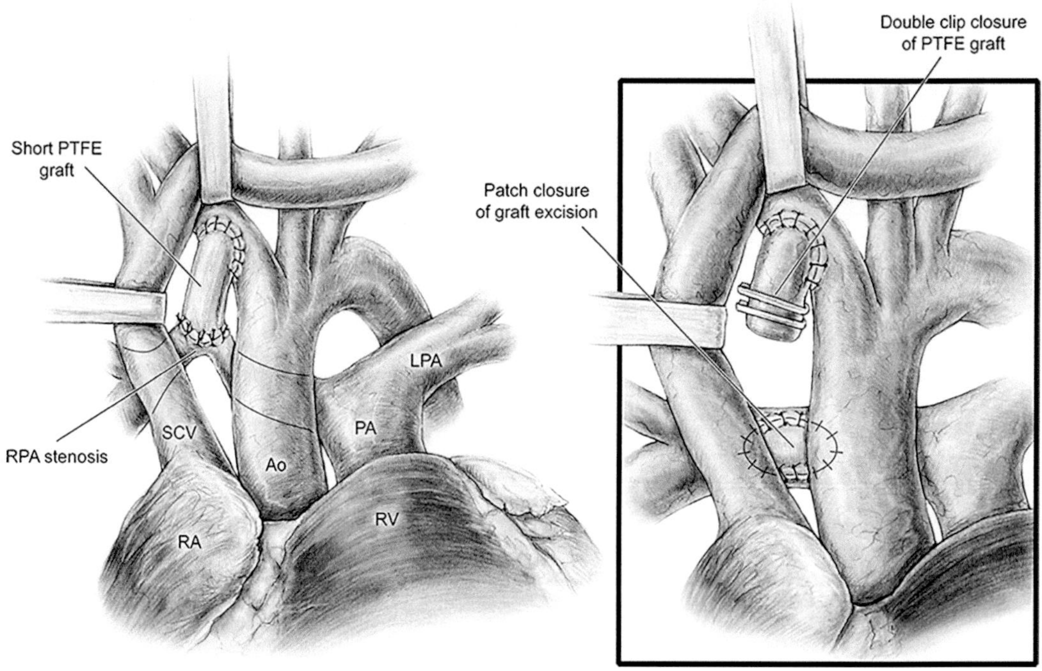

Fig. 44 Left panel illustrates the "tenting" results of a short systemic-to-pulmonary artery PTFE shunt procedure in which the shortened segment has caused distal and proximal right pulmonary artery stenosis. The inset shows how the pulmonary artery patch augmentation can be performed to mitigate this problem. *Ao* aorta, *LPA* left pulmonary artery, *PA* pulmonary artery, *PTFE* polytetrafluoroethylene, *RA* right atrium, *RPA* right pulmonary artery, *RV* right ventricle, *SCV* superior caval vein

the problem at the time of shunt takedown using an augmentation patch to restore proper unobstructed pulmonary artery anatomy.

5.3 Central Systemic-to-Pulmonary Shunt

There has been renewed interest in the central systemic-to-pulmonary artery shunt by us and others (Do et al. 2018). In the 2018 report of the STS-CHS database, central shunts accounted for 32% of recent systemic-to-pulmonary shunts (Do et al. 2018). The technique is straight forward and is especially effective when there are inadequate brachiocephalic vessels and when applied to very small neonates and infants. Our preference is to direct the shunt to the main pulmonary artery. The sequence of the systemic and pulmonary artery anastomoses is reversed for the central shunt owing to the fact that the pulmonary artery anastomosis is more difficult and allows better exposure for the aortic anastomosis once the pulmonary anastomosis is completed. Once the pulmonary artery anastomosis is completed using a side-biting clamp, another similar clamp is placed on the aorta which is followed by coronary punch creation of a suitable opening for the proximal shunt. A large, beveled opening is created on the shunt. The anastomosis to the aorta is completed and is marked with a small hemoclip to aid the cardiologists in visualizing the location of the shunt orifice at the time of eventual cardiac catheterization.

The postoperative management after a systemic-to-pulmonary artery shunt is very important and requires routine sedation and ventilation for the first 24 h postoperatively. This has been shown to be the most critical time for complications in the postoperative period. Continuing with the STS-CHS Database analysis, 33% of all shunt deaths occurred during the first 24 h postoperatively (Do et al. 2018). To optimize the success of this operation in small infants, we consistently administer an aspirin suppository (10 mg/kg) in the operating room when the shunt is completed and then 10 mg/kg daily until shunt takedown (Li et al. 2007). At the present time, we augment this regimen by the use of heparin-coated shunts. Supporting this management scheme, Ashfaq and associates reviewed 142 patients who had a modified BTT shunt. In 69 of these patients a heparin-coated shunt was used, resulting in two incidents of shunt thrombosis and two shunt-related mortalities (Ashfaq et al. 2018) which compared favorably with those patients who did not receive a heparin-coated shunt. The aforementioned STS-CHS database analysis (Do et al. 2018) showed a 7.4% shunt failure rate in 3474 infants having a modified BTT shunt. In-hospital shunt failure was related to a higher mortality rate of 32% and was associated with a lower weight at operation and preoperative hypercoagulable state. To add more granularity to this analysis, Jahangiri and associates (1999) reported 140 patients who had tetralogy of Fallot and had undergone a modified BTT shunt. All operations were performed through a thoracotomy approach. The results were favorable with no hospital deaths and equal growth of the right and left pulmonary arteries, regardless of shunt location. These outstanding results prompted them to conclude that the incidence of shunt complications is lower in patients who were palliated prior to a two-ventricle repair when compared with patients with a functionally univentricular heart (Do et al. 2018).

Takedown and division of a modified BTT shunt at the time of intracardiac repair through a median sternotomy is readily performed, especially if the shunt was placed on the right side as noted in Figs. 45, 46, 47, and 48 (Backer and Mavroudis 2023; Mavroudis 2015). As noted in Fig. 45, the shunt is identified by dissecting the medial aspect of the superior caval vein posteriorly. Locating and controlling the shunt on the left side is more difficult, which is not shown in the figures. The initial approach towards locating the shunt can be performed by (1) dissecting the left pulmonary artery, along the aorta to the shunt, or (2) by entering the pleural space and approaching the shunt laterally. There are pitfalls everywhere, however. Besides unwanted entry into the pulmonary artery and hemorrhage, the left-sided modified BTT shunt is oftentimes adjacent to the left phrenic nerve. The first encounter during the

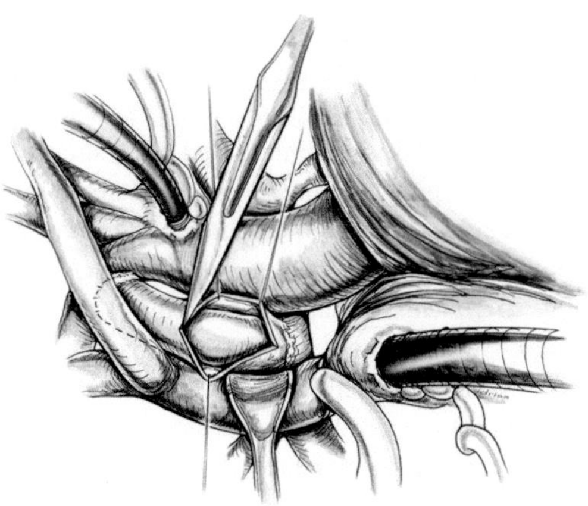

Fig. 45 Takedown of an established systemic-to-pulmonary artery shunt is a necessary part of intracardiac repair after palliation. In general, the prosthetic material needs to be identified, interrupted, and divided in order to prevent superior tenting of the pulmonary artery during subsequent somatic growth. It is therefore important to perform a comprehensive dissection in order to avoid this potential complication. The figure shows the dissection of an extant systemic-to-pulmonary artery shunt. While the patient is cannulated, cardiopulmonary bypass is not instituted until the surgeon can quickly interrupt the shunt at the beginning of bypass. The surgeon is shown dissecting the fibrous peel surrounding the shunt, which is a convenient plane to allow control of the shunt. (With permission: Mavroudis 2015)

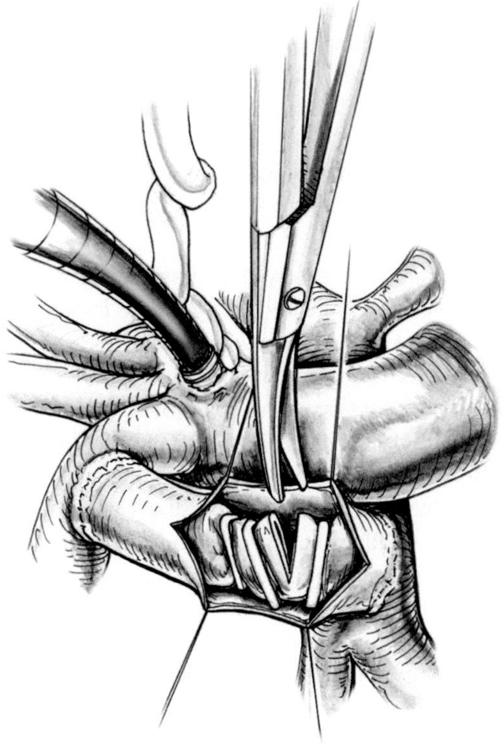

Fig. 47 Shows the transection of the systemic-to-pulmonary artery shunt after the clips have been applied. (With permission: Mavroudis 2015)

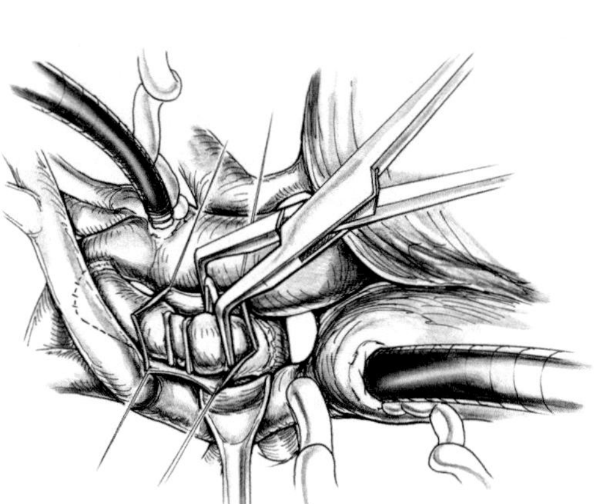

Fig. 46 Shows the commencement of cardiopulmonary bypass while two proximal clips and one distal clip are placed to interrupt the flow and prevent pulmonary over-circulation. (With permission: Mavroudis 2015)

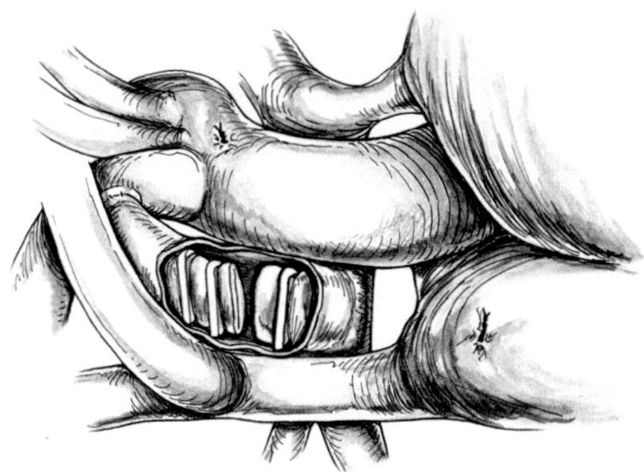

Fig. 48 Emphasizes the importance of complete dissection so that no residual connection is maintained between the shunt materials. If performed correctly, complete dissection will prevent the aforementioned tenting complication. Occasionally, the systemic-to-pulmonary artery shunt will result in a right pulmonary artery stenosis. In these circumstances, an autologous pericardial or synthetic patch will be used to perform a pulmonary arterioplasty (*not shown*). (With permission: Mavroudis 2015)

dissection will be a thick fibrous "peel," which typically forms around the PTFE graft as shown in Fig. 45. The peel surrounding the PTFE graft is entered and enough of the shunt is dissected along the peel to secure enough graft length for double hemoclip application proximally and single hemoclip application distally. Cardiopulmonary bypass is instituted before hemoclip application to prevent pulmonary overcirculation and an unwanted period of cyanosis. As noted in Figs. 46 and 47, the graft should be divided between the hemoclips and mobilized to prevent distortion of either the subclavian artery or the pulmonary artery as the patient grows and the distance between these two vessels naturally increases as emphasized in Fig. 48. No effort is made to remove the proximal portion of the graft. However, some patients will require removal of the distal graft in order to reconstruct a stenotic pulmonary artery. This is especially important if a bidirectional Glenn shunt is anticipated. If, on the other hand, the pulmonary artery is not stenosed at the site of the shunt, the distal graft can be left in place and usually does not result in residual peripheral pulmonary artery stenosis. As previously noted, preparations for cardiopulmonary bypass should be made prior to dissecting the shunt which include accessibility to the aorta and right atrium, appropriate purse string placement, and pump availability. The reason for this type of preparation is inherently clear since dissection of the shunt can lead to dislodgement, cyanosis, and hemorrhage. A rapid initiation of cardiopulmonary bypass will ameliorate the problem and allow proper management.

In the current era, transcatheter placement of a ductal stent (Bentham et al. 2018; Glatz et al. 2018) has been introduced as an alternative to surgical intervention. In properly selected patients this is rapidly becoming the procedure of choice in some centers (Benson and Van Arsdell 2018). However, early stent related complications can occur in up to 13.2%–23.1% of patents and include stent migration, stent thrombosis, in-stent restenosis, jailing of the pulmonary artery branches, and pulmonary overcirculation (Promphan and Qureshi 2021). Technical improvements have mitigated many of these complications, but some are unavoidable owing to the morphology of the ductal dependent pulmonary blood flow which is mediated and determined by ductal origin, tortuosity, and supply to the lungs (Promphan and Qureshi 2021). Reintervention for stent complications is not uncommon and includes re-dilatation, additional surgical shunt placement (Shahanavaz et al. 2021). Recent studies have shown that ductal stents for ductal dependent pulmonary circulation results in a less complicated PICU course, shorter hospital stays, but with a higher risk of vascular injury (Shaath et al. 2021; Nasser et al. 2020). While these results seem to favor ductal stenting in selected patients, there have not been any comprehensive reports citing complications associated with intraoperative takedown of the stented ductus in association with complete repair of congenital heart disease. In general, most surgeons interrupt the stented ductus by crushing techniques assisted by large hemoclips. Dissecting the stented ductus and application of hemoclips can lead to hemorrhage, recurrent laryngeal nerve injury, branch pulmonary artery stenosis, and acquired coarctation. These complications tend to be rare, but being forewarned will alert the clinician for resolution of the potential problem. As a matter of safety, when stents are being placed, precautions should be taken to have a cardiac team with cardiopulmonary bypass available to support the procedure. Inadvertent dissection of the patent arterial duct in a patient with ductal-dependent pulmonary blood flow requires emergent intervention with ECMO or initiation of cardiopulmonary bypass via emergent sternotomy.

5.4 Waterston/Cooley Shunt

Some 17 years after Blalock and associates introduced the BTT shunt, David Waterston in 1962 reported an aortopulmonary shunt that was comprised of an anastomosis between the posterior aspect of the ascending aorta and the anterior right pulmonary artery (Waterston 1962). This palliative procedure was performed through a right thoracotomy approach and posterior to the superior caval vein. Four years later, Denton Cooley (Cooley and Hallman 1966) reported the same technical and anatomic shunt with the difference being that the shunt was performed within the pericardium anterior to the superior caval vein. Initially, there were many perceived advantages for this shunt. It is relatively easy to perform; it preserves the subclavian artery; and prosthetic material is not necessary. However, as experience accrued, significant right pulmonary artery distortion occurred with corresponding difficulty in gauging the appropriate size of the shunt. The successful introduction of the modified BTT shunt largely replaced the Waterson/Cooley shunt and it is therefore rarely used in the current era.

As described earlier, there are still patients who may present with a Waterson/Cooley shunt for takedown and complete repair. For this reason, it is wise to review and consider how such a shunt can be safely taken down for the eventual repair. The technique for construction of a Waterston/Cooley shunt is shown in Figs. 49 and 50. The mobilized right pulmonary artery and ascending aorta are clamped together with a side-biting clamp while the pulmonary artery branches can be controlled with small Rummel tourniquets. As the clamp is placed, the aorta is rotated slightly anteriorly with a forceps that will allow a posterior rather than a lateral anastomosis. Figure 50 demonstrates the aligned incisions and anastomosis being performed.

A significant problem with the Waterston/Cooley shunt is that it is not as controlled a shunt as either the classic or modified BTT shunts. If the incisions in the aorta and pulmonary artery are too long and the anastomosis is too large, there will be excessive pulmonary blood flow with a risk of pulmonary vascular disease. If the incisions are too short and the opening is too small, there will be inadequate pulmonary blood flow and the patient will remain cyanotic.

Another confounding dilemma with the Waterston/Cooley anastomosis, as previously implied, is that there is considerable distortion of the right pulmonary artery as the patient grows and the aorta rotates. This situation results in

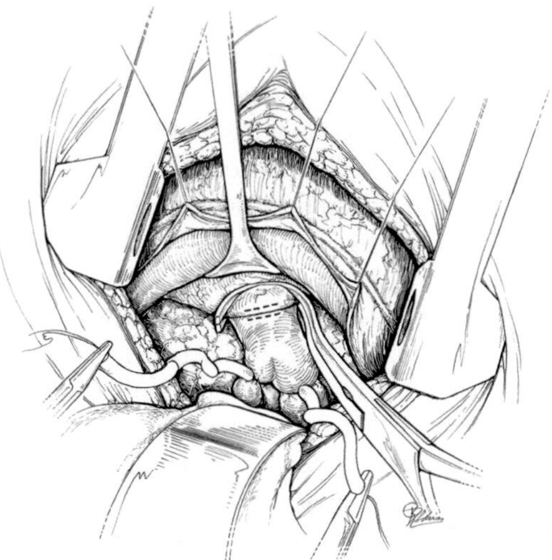

Fig. 49 The introduction of the Blalock-Taussig-Thomas shunt paved the way for the Waterston shunt, shown in the figure, that could be applied more easily to very small infants. A side-biting clamp is placed to partially occlude the ascending aorta together with the proximal right pulmonary artery while the distal pulmonary arteries are clamped separately. The dashed lines indicate the incision to be made to facilitate the side-to-side anastomosis. (With permission: Mavroudis 2015)

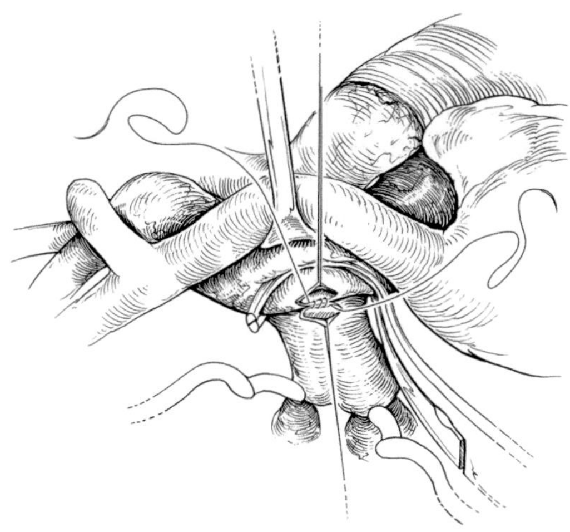

Fig. 50 Shows the side-to-side anastomosis in progress. Because this anastomosis does not involve any synthetic grafts, there is less chance of clot formation, but constructing the exact size proved to be challenging—the anastomosis often seemed either too small or too large. Moreover, constructing the anastomosis to avoid right pulmonary artery kinking was also challenging. (With permission: Mavroudis 2015)

preferential flow to one lung and significant right pulmonary artery stenosis (Wilson et al. 1981). The great majority of patients who undergo Waterston/Cooley shunt takedown in association with complete repair will require major reconstruction of the right pulmonary artery. This procedure is illustrated in Fig. 51. The preparations for performing this takedown procedure, however, are more complicated and require great attention to detail and sequence. Comprehensive dissection of the pulmonary arteries prior to cardiopulmonary bypass is advised in order to occlude the pulmonary arteries on initiation of cardiopulmonary bypass. This will prevent pulmonary overcirculation with inadequate systemic perfusion. The takedown procedure is performed on cardiopulmonary bypass with cardioplegic arrest, aortic cross-clamping distal to the shunt, and pulmonary artery occlusion to prevent cardioplegic solution runoff. The aorta and the right pulmonary artery are separated by an incision along the original anastomotic suture line. This incision is facilitated by a large aorta which can be closed primarily after the anatomic separation. The pulmonary artery will require augmentation, usually with a PTFE or pericardial patch. An alternative takedown approach for the Waterston/Cooley shunt is through the ascending aorta after safe cardioplegic arrest. This approach is characterized by aortic transection, better exposure, and comprehensive augmentation of the right pulmonary artery (Curran et al. 1997).

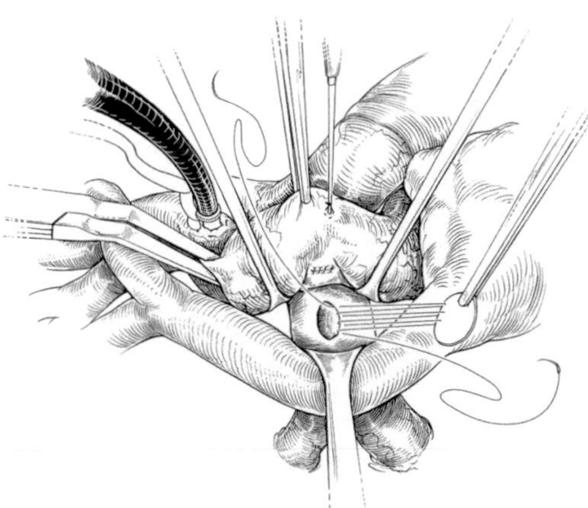

Fig. 51 Takedown of the Waterston shunt with right pulmonary artery arterioplasty is shown in the figure. The best way to accomplish this procedure is with aortobicaval cardiopulmonary bypass, aortic cross-clamping, and cardioplegic arrest. The aortic suture line can be accomplished more accurately and the right pulmonary artery can be repaired with greater precision using a synthetic or biologic patch. (With permission: Mavroudis 2015)

5.5 Potts Shunt

The Potts shunt (Fig. 52) (Backer and Mavroudis 2023; Mavroudis 2015) is a palliative operation that involves an anastomosis between the descending thoracic aorta and the left pulmonary artery that is performed through a left thoracotomy. Willis J. Potts from Children's Memorial Hospital in Chicago (Potts et al. 1946) first performed the operation on September 13, 1946. The child was 21 months of age and weighed 8.3 kg. She had been cyanotic since 3 months after birth and had multiple hypercyanotic spells.

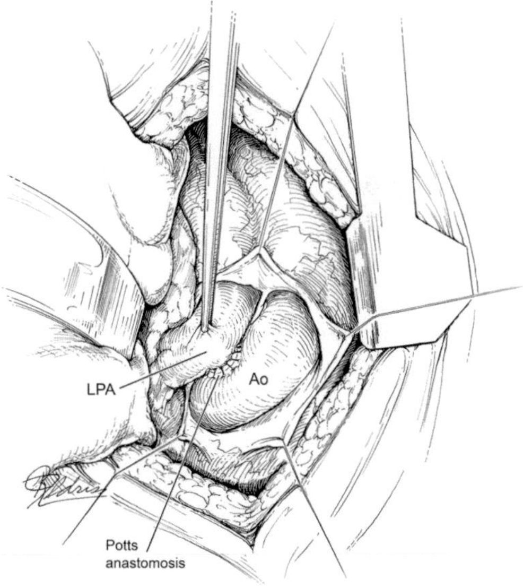

Fig. 52 Another systemic-to-pulmonary artery shunt of historical significance is the Potts shunt as noted in the figure. This exposure is through a left thoracotomy with dissection of the descending aorta (Ao) and the left pulmonary artery (LPA). The aorta and pulmonary artery are clamped together in the same manner as is used for the Waterston shunt, except that in this case it is the descending aorta and the left pulmonary artery. (With permission: Mavroudis 2015)

She was very cyanotic and had severe clubbing. To emphasize the preparatory elements that were required for this new operation, Potts performed his shunt using a special clamp that he developed that only partially occluded the descending thoracic aorta to decrease the risk of paraplegia (Baffes 1987). The proximal and distal left pulmonary artery were temporarily occluded and the anastomosis was performed between parallel 4-mm incisions created in the descending thoracic aorta and the posterior left main pulmonary artery. Historically, the first child to have had a Potts shunt survived and eventually had successful repair of tetralogy of Fallot with a conduit. She had multiple operations for conduit changes and survived to 57 years of age (Waisbren Sr. 2010).

Over the time period between 1946 and 1967, 659 Potts shunts were performed at Children's Memorial Hospital. Like the Waterston/Cooley shunt, it was technically easier to perform than the classic BTT shunt. In addition, it preserved the left subclavian artery and could be performed in neonates and infants. However, over the short and long term, several serious complications led to its abandonment. Large aneurysms of the left pulmonary artery developed as noted on the chest roentgenogram in Fig. 53 (de Hoyos et al. 2009) and proved very difficult to repair. Another complication, which was also similar to the Waterston/Cooley shunts, involved the construction of the Potts shunt which could result in either too small or too large shunt flow characteristics. The former would result in continued cyanosis; the latter would result in congestive heart failure. In addition, the Potts shunt was contraindicated in patients with a right aortic arch, even using a right thoracotomy, owing to the confounding anatomy that exists, namely that the right bronchus lies between the pulmonary artery and the aorta. Perhaps the most significant problem that awaits the surgeon is the difficulty in taking down the shunt at the time of complete correction of the existing intracardiac lesion (Kirklin and Devloo 1961). The initial attempts by simple ligation proved to be unwise and unsuccessful since there

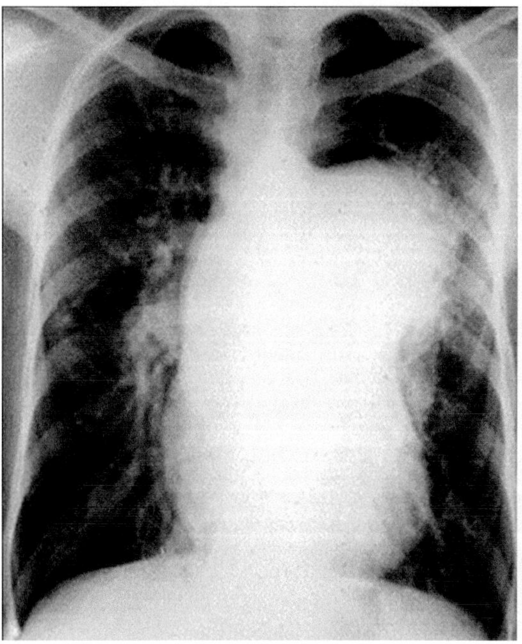

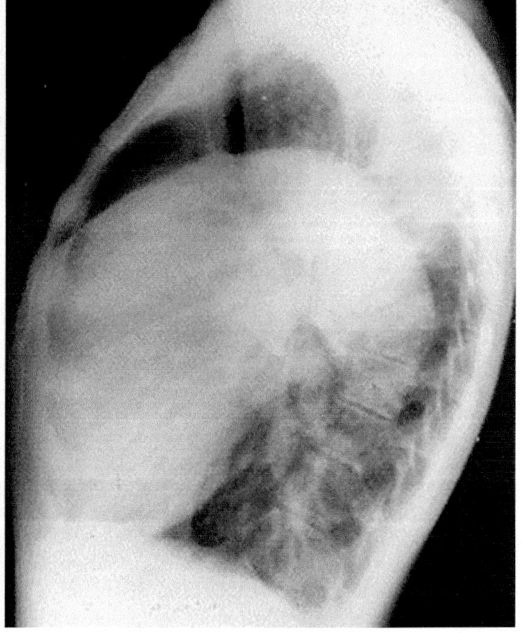

Fig. 53 Chest radiographs (posteroanterior and lateral) of a 23-year-old patient with tetralogy of Fallot 16 years after a Potts (descending aorta-to-pulmonary artery) anastomosis. The left panel shows the pulmonary artery aneurysm projecting from the mediastinum into the left chest and fills the anterior compartment shown in the right panel. (With permission: Backer and Mavroudis 2013)

was no tube-like communication between the two vessels. Invariably, this maneuver resulted in uncontrolled hemorrhage in the operating room or in the immediate postoperative period. Other methods involved shunt takedown using cardiopulmonary bypass and circulatory arrest. There was, however, a risk of stroke using this technique from air embolism if the brachiocephalic vessels were not controlled. The preferred practice now is to use deep hypothermia and circulatory arrest, with adequate precautions taken to avoid air embolism to the cerebral circulation with the descending thoracic aorta opened. A deep Trendelenburg position during the time of circulatory arrest and shunt takedown has been used in aneurysm repair patients with safe outcomes.

In particular, the sequence of Potts shunt takedown is started by median sternotomy and cardiopulmonary bypass. The aortic-pulmonary anastomosis is digitally occluded with pressure on the pulmonary artery opposite the shunt to limit the left-to-right shunt, decrease pulmonary overcirculation, and improve cooling efficiency. The brachiocephalic vessels are encircled and controlled with vessel loops. Cardioplegic arrest is induced and the brachiocephalic vessels are snared. This is followed by circulatory arrest once the target temperature (18 °C) is reached. Once these conditions are met, left pulmonary artery can be safely opened. Circulatory arrest facilitates exposure to the communication between the pulmonary artery and the aorta which allows closure with a PTFE patch which is shown in Fig. 54 (Backer and Mavroudis 2023; Mavroudis 2015). Once the communication is closed all the air maneuvers are accomplished which can lead to release of the brachiocephalic vessel snares, recommencement of cardiopulmonary bypass, and attention to the intracardiac repair for which the patient is undergoing surgical repair.

Because of the aforementioned complications of left pulmonary artery aneurysm, frequent excessive pulmonary blood flow with resultant pulmonary hypertension, and the difficulties in taking down the Potts shunt, this procedure has fallen out of favor for the purpose of a palliative systemic-to-pulmonary artery shunt in neonates, infants, and children. However, there has been a resurgence and rediscovery of the Potts shunt as an approach and strategy to palliate specific patients with severe pulmonary hypertension and suprasystemic right ventricular pressures (Blanc et al. 2004). The anastomosis allows for a right to left shunt, specifically from the pulmonary artery to aorta, in order to ameliorate sudden right ventricular failure from a pulmonary hypertensive crisis (Aggarwal et al. 2018). While the resultant pathologic physiology resulted in lower extremity desaturation, this situation did not appear to significantly affect organ function. The clinical results of this strategy helped to provide palliation to those patients in lieu of lung transplantation or while waiting for lung transplantation. Belli and associates reported on 24 patients having this procedure and concluded, "Palliative Potts shunt allows prolonged survival and dramatic, long-lasting improvement in functional capacities in children with severe, drug-refractory pulmonary arterial hypertension (PAH). The Potts shunt might be considered as a first surgical or interventional step in the management of children with severe, drug-refractory PAH, leaving

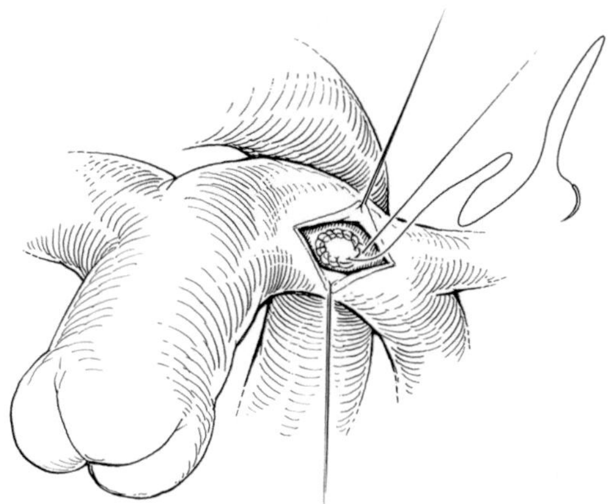

Fig. 54 Takedown of the Potts shunt is technically very demanding and may require a period of deep hypothermia and circulatory arrest while the anastomosis is approached through the pulmonary artery and the shunt is closed with a patch and running suture technique as shown in the figure. Once the shunt is closed, cardiopulmonary bypass can be reinstituted and the reparative operation can be performed. (With permission: Mavroudis 2015)

the door open for further lung transplantation, if needed." (Belli 2016; Baruteau et al. 2015) The complications, regardless of recent applications, are still operative. Proper attention to detail and the aforementioned considerations will help to prevent unwanted outcomes.

6 Conclusion

The primary and modern-day palliative operations for neonates, infants, and children with congenital heart disease are systemic-to-pulmonary artery shunts and the pulmonary artery band. As discussed in our previous publication (Backer and Mavroudis 2023) there are four keys to optimal palliation. They include: "1) a precise, complete diagnosis prior to palliation; 2) adequate, calibrated pulmonary blood flow; 3) an initial operation which addresses potential late complications; and 4) appropriately timed biventricular repair or early ventricular unloading with a bidirectional superior cavopulmonary anastomosis" (Backer et al. 2012).

The aortopulmonary shunt of choice currently is the modified BTT shunt performed with a sternotomy approach. This provides a controlled source of pulmonary blood flow, does not sacrifice the subclavian artery, and is quite easy to take down at the time of intracardiac repair. Heparin coating has improved shunt patency. Ductal stenting is now a definite alternative as initial palliation.

Pulmonary artery banding is indicated for patients with Swiss-cheese muscular ventricular septal defects, for some infants with a functionally univentricular heart and increased pulmonary blood flow, and to prepare or treat the left ventricle in select patients. It should also be considered for neonates with atrioventricular septal defect and coarctation of the aorta, and neonates who have contraindications to cardiopulmonary bypass. Hybrid techniques have led to a resurgent interest in pulmonary artery band techniques. Surgeons need to be aware of the Waterston/Cooley and Potts anastomosis, the associated complications, and the techniques required to safely take these shunts down at the time of complete repair. The Potts shunt is now being used to palliate selected patients with severe pulmonary hypertension. Palliative operatives continue to play an important role in our surgical strategies.

References

Agasthi P, Graziano JN. Pulmonary artery banding. In: StatPearls [Internet]. Treasure Island: StatPearls Publishing; 2023. PMID: 32809673.

Aggarwal M, Grady RM, Choudhry S, Anwar S, Eghtesady P, Singh GK. Potts shunt improves right ventricular function and coupling with pulmonary circulation in children with suprasystemic pulmonary arterial hypertension. Circ Cardiovasc Imaging. 2018;11(12):e007964. https://doi.org/10.1161/CIRCIMAGING.118.007964. PMID: 30558504.

Albus RA, Trusler GA, Izukawa T, Williams WG. Pulmonary artery banding. J Thorac Cardiovasc Surg. 1984;88(5 Pt 1):645–53.

Alsoufi B, Manlhiot C, Ehrlich A, et al. Results of palliation with an initial pulmonary artery band in patients with single ventricle associated with unrestricted pulmonary blood flow. J Thorac Cardiovasc Surg. 2015;149:213–20.

Ambarsari YA, Purbojo A, Blumauer R, et al. Systemic-to-pulmonary artery shunting using heparin-bonded grafts. Interact Cardiovasc Thorac Surg. 2018;27:591–7.

Ashfaq A, Soroya MS, Iyengar A, Federman M, Reemtsen BL. Heparin-coated grafts reduce mortality in pediatric patients receiving systemic-to-pulmonary shunts. Pediatr Cardiol. 2018;39:473–7.

Backer CL, Mavroudis C. Palliative operations. In: Mavroudis C, Backer CL, editors. Pediatric cardiac surgery. 4th ed. Oxford: Wiley-Blackwell; 2013.

Backer CL, Mavroudis C. Palliative operations. In: Mavroudis C, Backer CL, editors. Pediatric cardiac surgery. 5th ed. London: Wiley-Blackwell Inc; 2023.

Backer CL, Russell HM, Deal BJ. Optimal initial palliation for patients with functionally univentricular hearts. World J Pediatr Congenit Heart Surg. 2012;3:165–70.

Baffes TG. Willis J. Potts: his contributions to cardiovascular surgery. Ann Thorac Surg. 1987;44:92–6.

Barron DJ, Mahendran K. Left ventricular re-training: feasibility and effectiveness–what are the limits? Semin Thorac Cardiovasc Surg Pediatr Card Surg Annu. 2019;22:43–50.

Baruteau AE, Belli E, Boudjemline Y, et al. Palliative Potts shunt for the treatment of children with drug-refractory pulmonary arterial hypertension: updated data from the first 24 patients. Eur J Cardiothorac Surg. 2015;47:e105–10.

Baslaim G. Modification of Trusler's formula for the pulmonary artery banding. Heart Lung Circ. 2009;18:353–7.

Belli E. Invited commentary. Ann Thorac Surg. 2016;101:1543.

Benson L, Van Arsdell G. Comparisons between ductal stenting and Blalock-Taussig shunts for infants with ductal-dependent pulmonary circulation. Circulation. 2018;137:602–4.

Bentham JR, Zava NK, Harrison WJ, et al. Duct stenting versus modified Blalock-Taussig shunt in neonates with duct-dependent pulmonary blood flow: associations with clinical outcomes in a multicenter national study. Circulation. 2018;137:581–8.

Blalock A, Hanlon CR. Surgical treatment of complete transposition of the aorta and pulmonary artery. Surg Gynecol Obstet. 1950;90:1–15.

Blalock A, Taussig HB. The surgical treatment of malformations of the heart in which there is pulmonary stenosis or pulmonary atresia. JAMA. 1945;128:189–202.

Blanc J, Vouhé P, Bonnet D. Potts shunt in patients with pulmonary hypertension. N Engl J Med. 2004;350:623.

Bradley SM, Simsic JM, Atz AM, Dorman BH. The infant with single ventricle and excessive pulmonary blood flow: results of a strategy of pulmonary artery division and shunt. Ann Thorac Surg. 2002;74:805–10.

Cooley DA, Hallman GL. Intrapericardial aortic-right pulmonary arterial anastomosis. Surg Gynecol Obstet. 1966;122:1084–6.

Corno AF. FloWatch device for adjustable pulmonary artery banding. J Thorac Cardiovasc Surg. 2013;145(4):1144. [abstract].

Corno AF, Prosi M, Fridez P, Zunino P, Quarteroni A, von Segesser LK. The non-circular shape of FloWatch-PAB prevents the need for pulmonary artery reconstruction after banding. Computational fluid dynamics and clinical correlations. Eur J Cardiothorac Surg. 2006;29:93–9.

Curran RD, Mavroudis C, Backer CL. Ascending aortic extension for right pulmonary artery stenosis associated with ventricular-to-pulmonary artery conduit replacement. J Card Surg. 1997;12:372–9.

Danilowicz D, Presti S, Colvin S. The disappearing pulmonary artery band. Pediatr Cardiol. 1990;11(1):47–9.

de Hoyos A, Dodge-Khatami A, Backer CL. Vascular masses of the mediastinum. In: Shields TW, LoCicero 3rd J, Reed CE, et al., editors. General thoracic surgery, vol. 2. 7th ed. Lippincott Williams & Wilkins/ Wolters Kluwer: Philadelphia; 2009.

De Leval MR, McKay R, Jones M, et al. Modified Blalock-Taussig shunt. Use of subclavian artery orifice as flow regulator in prosthetic systemic-pulmonary artery shunts. J Thorac Cardiovasc Surg. 1981;81:112–9.

Devlin PJ, Jegatheeswaran A, McCrindle BW, et al. Pulmonary artery banding in complete atrioventricular septal defect. J Thorac Cardiovasc Surg. 2020;159:1493–503.

Di Bardino DJ, Leeman K, Bove EL. A method of transcutaneously adjustable pulmonary artery banding for staged left ventricular retraining. J Thorac Cardiovasc Surg. 2012;144:553–6.

Do N, Hill KD, Wallace AS, et al. Shunt failure–risk factors and outcomes: an analysis of the Society of Thoracic Surgeons Congenital Heart Surgery Database. Ann Thorac Surg. 2018;105:857–64.

EspeRare. FloWatch in congenital heart defects; 2020. http://www.esperare.org/en/flowatch-congenital-heart-defects. Accessed 14 Apr 2020.

Foale RA, King ME, Gordon D, Marshall JE, Weyman AE. Pseudoaneurysm of the pulmonary artery after the banding procedure: two-dimensional echocardiographic description. J Am Coll Cardiol. 1984;3(2 Pt 1):371–4.

Franklin RCG, Sullivan JD, Anderson RH, et al. Is banding of the pulmonary trunk obsolete for infants with tricuspid atresia and double inlet ventricle with a discordant ventriculoarterial connection? Role of aortic arch obstruction and subaortic stenosis. J Am Coll Cardiol. 1990;16:1455–64.

Galantowicz M, Cheatham JP, Phillips A, et al. Hybrid approach for hypoplastic left heart syndrome: intermediate results after the learning curve. Ann Thorac Surg. 2008;85:2063–70.

Galinanes M, Stanley P, Guérin R, Kratz C, Chartrand C. Pulmonary banding complicated by low origin of right pulmonary artery. Tex Heart Inst J. 1993;20(3):238–40.

Gazzaniga AB, Elliott MP, Sperling DR, et al. Microporous expanded polytetrafluoroethylene arterial prosthesis for construction of aortopulmonary shunts: experimental and clinical results. Ann Thorac Surg. 1976;21:322–7.

Geiss D, Williams WG, Lindsay WK, et al. Upper extremity gangrene: a complication of subclavian artery division. Ann Thorac Surg. 1980;30:487–9.

Gibbs JL, Wren C, Watterson KG, Hunter S, Hamilton JR. Stenting of the arterial duct combined with banding of the pulmonary arteries and atrial septectomy or septostomy: a new approach to palliation for the hypoplastic left heart syndrome. Br Heart J. 1993;69:551–5.

Glatz AC, Petit CJ, Goldstein BH, et al. Comparison between patent ductus arteriosus stent and modified Blalock-Taussig shunt as palliation for infants with ductal-dependent pulmonary blood flow. Circulation. 2018;137:589–601.

Glenn WWL. Circulatory bypass of the right side of the heart. IV. Shunt between superior vena cava and distal right pulmonary artery; report of a clinical application. N Engl J Med. 1958;259:117–20.

Haller C, Caldarone CA. The evolution of therapeutic strategies: niche apportionment for hybrid palliation. Ann Thorac Surg. 2018;106:1873–80.

Iannucci GJ, Deshpande SR, Kirshbom PM. Hemolytic anemia after placement of an intraluminal pulmonary artery band. Ann Thorac Surg. 2013;95(5):e119–20.

Jahangiri M, Lincoln C, Shinebourne EA. Does the modified Blalock-Taussig shunt cause growth of the contralateral pulmonary artery? Ann Thorac Surg. 1999;67:1397–9.

Joffs C, Sade RM. Congenital Heart Surgery Nomenclature and Database Project. Palliation, correction, or repair? Ann Thorac Surg. 2000;69:S369–72.

Kawamura A, Oshima Y, Maruo A, Matsuhisa H. Compression of an anomalous single coronary artery from pulmonary artery by banding. Eur J Cardiothorac Surg. 2012;41(4):e59–61. https://doi.org/10.1093/ejcts/ezr269. Epub 2012 Jan 13. PMID: 22246964.

Kirklin JW, Devloo RA. Hypothermic perfusion and circulatory arrest for surgical correction of tetralogy of Fallot with previously constructed Potts' anastomosis. Dis Chest. 1961;39:87–91.

Kutsche LM, Alexander JA, Van Mierop LH. Hemolytic anemia secondary to erosion of a Silastic band into the lumen of the pulmonary trunk. Am J Cardiol. 1985;55(11):1438–9.

LeBlanc J, Albus R, Williams WG, et al. Serous fluid leakage: a complication following modified Blalock-Taussig shunt. J Thorac Cardiovasc Surg. 1984;88:259–62.

Lee MGY, Brizard CP, Galati JC, et al. Outcomes of patients born with single-ventricle physiology and aortic arch obstruction: the 26-year Melbourne experience. J Thorac Cardiovasc Surg. 2014;148:194–201.

Li JS, Berezny KY, Rhodes JF, et al. Clinical outcomes of palliative surgery including a systemic-to-pulmonary artery shunt in infants with cyanotic congenital heart disease: does aspirin make a difference? Circulation. 2007;116:293–7.

Ma K, Gao H, Hua Z, et al. Palliative pulmonary artery banding versus anatomic correction for congenitally corrected transposition of the great arteries with regressed morphologic left ventricle: long-term results from a single center. J Thorac Cardiovasc Surg. 2014;148:1566–71.

Mahle S, Nicoloff DM, Knight L, Moller JH. Pulmonary artery banding: long-term results in 63 patients. Ann Thorac Surg. 1979;27(3):216–24.

Mainwaring RD, Patrick WL, Ibrahimiye AN, Watanabe N, Lui GK, Hanley FL. An analysis of left ventricular retraining in patients with dextro- and levo-transposition of the great arteries. Ann Thorac Surg. 2018;105:823–9.

Makhija N, Aggarwal S, Talwar S, Ladha S, Das D, Kiran U. Management of iatrogenic pulmonary artery injury during pulmonary artery banding. Ann Card Anaesth. 2017;20(3):379–80.

Mavroudis C. Palliation techniques. In: Mavroudis C, Backer CL, editors. Atlas of pediatric cardiac surgery. London: Springer; 2015.

Mavroudis C, Backer CL. Arterial switch after failed atrial baffle procedures for transposition of the great arteries. Ann Thorac Surg. 2000;69:851–7.

Mavroudis C, Dearani JA. Palliation techniques. In: Mavroudis C, Dearani JA, editors. Atlas of adult congenital heart surgery. Cham: Springer; 2020.

Morales D, Zafar F, Arrington K, et al. Repeat sternotomy in congenital heart surgery: no longer a risk factor. Ann Thorac Surg. 2008;86:897–902.

Muller WH Jr, Dammann JF Jr. The treatment of certain congenital malformations of the heart by creation of pulmonic stenosis to reduce pulmonary hypertension and excessive pulmonary blood flow: a preliminary report. Surg Gynecol Obstet. 1952;95:213–9.

Nakayama Y, Iwata Y, Nishimori T, Takeuchi T. Infected pulmonary aneurysm following pulmonary artery banding. Asian Cardiovasc Thorac Ann. 2017;25(9):642–4.

Nasser BA, Abdulrahman M, Qwaee AAL, Alakfash A, Mohamad T, Kabbani MS. Impact of stent of ductus arteriosus and modified Blalock-Taussig shunt on pulmonary arteries growth and second-stage surgery in infants with ductus-dependent pulmonary circulation. J Saudi Heart Assoc. 2020;32(1):86–92.

Norwood WI, Lang P, Hansen DD. Physiologic repair of aortic atresia-hypoplastic left heart syndrome. N Engl J Med. 1983;308:23–6.

Odim J, Portzky M, Zurakowski D, et al. Sternotomy approach for the modified Blalock-Taussig shunt. Circulation. 1995;92(9 Suppl):II256–61.

Petrucci O, O'Brien SM, Jacobs ML, Jacobs JP, Manning PB, Eghtesady P. Risk factors for mortality and morbidity after the neonatal Blalock-Taussig shunt procedure. Ann Thorac Surg. 2011;92:642–52.

Piluiko VV, Poynter JA, Nemeh H, et al. Efficacy of intraluminal pulmonary artery banding. J Thorac Cardiovasc Surg. 2005;129:544–50.

Potts WJ, Smith S, Gibson S. Anastomosis of aorta to pulmonary artery: certain types in congenital heart disease. JAMA J Am Med Assoc. 1946;132:627–31.

Promphan W, Qureshi SA. Technical modifications for ductal stenting in neonates with duct-dependent pulmonary circulation. Heart. 2021;2:188–201.

Rashkind WJ, Miller WW. Creation of an atrial septal defect without thoracotomy. A palliative approach to complete transposition of the great arteries. JAMA. 1966;196:991–2.

Recto MR, Doyle S, Massicotte MP, Guerra VC, Yang SG, Yeh T Jr. Right pulmonary artery thrombosis after hybrid stage 1 palliation: resolution after direct tissue plasminogen activator infusion. Pediatr Cardiol. 2013;34(1):185–8.

Sachweh J, Däbritz S, Didilis V, Vazquez-Jimenez JF, Bernuth GV, Messmer BJ. Pulmonary artery stenosis after systemic-to-pulmonary shunt operations. Eur J Cardiothorac Surg. 1998;14(3):229–34.

Sandrio S, Purbojo A, Arndt F, Toka O, Glöckler M, Dittrich S, Cesnjevar R, Rüffer A. Feasibility and related outcome of intraluminal pulmonary artery banding. Eur J Cardiothorac Surg. 2015;48(3):470–80.

Schranz D, Rupp S, Müller M, et al. Pulmonary artery banding in infants and young children with left ventricular dilated cardiomyopathy: a novel therapeutic strategy before heart transplantation. J Heart Lung Transplant. 2013;32:475–81.

Schranz D, Akintuerk H, Bailey L. Pulmonary artery banding for functional regeneration of end-stage diated cardiomyopathy in children: World Network Report. Circulation. 2018;137:1410–2.

Shaath GA, Jijeh AM, Fararjeh M, et al. Stent or shunt, what could be better for children with duct dependent pulmonary circulation? J Saudi Heart Assoc. 2021;33(4):306–12.

Shahanavaz S, Qureshi AM, Petit CJ, et al. Factors influencing reintervention following ductal artery stent implantation for ductal-dependent pulmonary blood flow: results from the Congenital Cardiac Research Collaborative. Circ Cardiovasc Interv. 2021;14(12):e010086. https://doi.org/10.1161/CIRCINTERVENTIONS.120.010086. Epub 2021 Nov 18. PMID: 34789017.

Shin MS, Ceballos R, Bini RM, Ho KJ. CT diagnosis of false aneurysm of the pulmonary artery not demonstrated by angiography. J Comput Assist Tomogr. 1983;7(3):524–6.

Shuhaiber J, Shin AY, Gossett JG, et al. Surgical management of neonatal atrioventricular septal defect with aortic arch obstruction. Ann Thorac Surg. 2013;95:2071–7.

Silva DD, et al. Perigraft seroma following Right Modified Blalock Taussig shunt in a child with complex cyanotic heart disease. Galle Med J. 2013;18(2):25–7.

STS Congenital Heart Surgery Database. Spring 2019 Harvest Report; 2019. Accessed 19 Feb 2024.

Takeyoshi D, Konuma T, Kojima A, Takeuchi T. Lecompte maneuver for compressed left coronary artery after pulmonary artery banding. Asian Cardiovasc Thorac Annu. 2023;31(9):802–4.

Talwar S, Kamat NA, Choudhary SK, Ramakrishnan S, Saxena A, Juneja R, Kothari SS, Airan B. Mid-term outcomes of patients undergoing adjustable pulmonary artery banding. Indian Heart J. 2016;68(1):72–6.

Thomas VT. Series 6. Research and laboratory materials. Vivien T. Thomas collection, The Alan Mason Chesney Medical Archives of The Johns Hopkins Medical Institutions; 2020. http://www.medicalarchives.jhmi.edu:8443/finding_aids/vivien_thomas/vivien_thomasd.html. Accessed 14 Apr 2020.

Trusler GA, Mustard WT. A method of banding the pulmonary artery for large isolated ventricular septal defect with and without transposition of the great arteries. Ann Thorac Surg. 1972;13:351–5.

Venugopal PS, Hayes N, Simpson J, Anderson D. Transection with pseudoaneurysm formation of the pulmonary trunk after placement of an adjustable pulmonary artery banding device (FloWatch-PAB) in a patient with residual muscular ventricular septal defect. J Thorac Cardiovasc Surg. 2010;139(5):e103–4.

Vricella LA, Jacobs ML, Cameron DE. The birth of a new era: the introduction of the systemic-to-pulmonary artery shunt for the treatment of cyanotic congenital heart disease. Cardiol Young. 2013;23:852–7.

Waisbren BA Sr. The other princess Diane–a story of valiant perseverance against medical odds. Victoria: Trafford Publishing; 2010.

Waterston DJ. [Treatment of Fallot's tetralogy in infants under the age of 1 year]. Rozhl Chir. 1962;41:181–3.

Williams JA, Bansal AK, Kim BJ, et al. Two thousand Blalock-Taussig shunts: a six-decade experience. Ann Thorac Surg. 2007;84:2070–5.

Wilson JM, Mack JW, Turley K, et al. Persistent stenosis and deformity of the right pulmonary artery after correction of the Waterston anastomosis. J Thorac Cardiovasc Surg. 1981;82:169–75.

Winlaw DS, McGuirk SP, Balmer C, et al. Intention-to-treat analysis of pulmonary artery banding in conditions with a morphological right ventricle in the systemic circulation with a view to anatomic biventricular repair. Circulation. 2005;111:405–11.

Zhu MZL, Fricke TA, Buratto E, Chowdhuri KR, Brizard CP, Konstantinov IE. Outcomes of neo-aortic valve and root surgery late after arterial switch operation. J Thorac Cardiovasc Surg. 2023;S0022–5223(23):00864-4. https://doi.org/10.1016/j.jtcvs.2023.09.038. Epub ahead of print. PMID: 37757970.

Complications Associated with Ligation of Patent Arterial Duct (Patent Ductus Arteriosus)

Constantine Mavroudis

Abstract

Ligation of patent ductus arteriosus (also patent arterial duct) is considered one of the simplest procedures resulting in rare morbidity and mortality. Complications that occur typically involve surgical principles and anatomic proximity to the area of closure including the laryngeal nerve, aorta, left pulmonary artery, and thoracic duct. This chapter describes complications and ways to avoid and repair unanticipated surgical errors.

Keywords

Dissection · Undiagnosed patent arterial duct · Operative exposure · Left thoracotomy · Median sternotomy · Inadvertent aortic ligation · Ductal disruption · Recurrent laryngeal nerve · Uncontrolled hemorrhage

1 Introduction

Complications associated with patent arterial duct (PAD) closure center around the choice of operative exposure (left thoracotomy vs. median sternotomy) and anatomic proximity to structures that can be injured during dissection and ligation. For those patients undergoing left thoracotomy, the most common injury involves the recurrent laryngeal nerve (Foster et al. 2021). Other reported complications are more rarely encountered and include ductal disruption and bleeding, neocoarctation at the repaired bleeding site (Qasim et al. 2017), accidental clipping of the aorta (Qasim et al. 2017), inadvertent ligation of the left pulmonary artery (Yucel and Sahin 2020; Terlemez et al. 2017; Orzel and Monaco 1986; Pontius et al. 1981), inadvertent ligation of the descending aorta (Terlemez et al. 2017), and thoracic duct injury. For those patients who undergo PAD ligation through a median sternotomy in association with other repairs, inadvertent aortic ligation, ductal disruption, and neocoarctation can occur (Qasim et al. 2017).

All of these potential complications can be avoided using established anatomic and surgical principles. However, in the event that these complications do occur, it is important to recognize them and perform reparative measures. This chapter will review the extant methods of classic PAD ligation, neighboring structures, and consequences of complications.

C. Mavroudis (✉)
Chief of Pediatric Cardiothoracic Surgery (Retired), Peyton Manning Children's Hospital, Indianapolis, IN, USA

Professor Emeritus of Surgery, Johns Hopkins University School of Medicine, Baltimore, MD, USA

C. L. Backer, C. Mavroudis (eds.), *Complications in Pediatric and Congenital Heart Surgery*, https://doi.org/10.1007/978-3-032-02661-3_3

2 Relational Anatomy

Figure 1 (Mavroudis 2015a) shows the relational anatomy of PAD highlighting the recurrent laryngeal nerve and the associated directional left-to-right shunt. The dotted lines represent the continuation of the descending aorta posterior to the left pulmonary artery (Mavroudis 2015a). The reader can appreciate the proximity of important structures that can be injured during PAD ligation. Figure 2 (Mavroudis 2015a) demonstrates operative exposure through a left thoracotomy, showing the course of the recurrent laryngeal nerve. The course of the phrenic nerve is not noted as it runs along the posterior portion of the pericardium. The visceral pleura has been incised and retracted to show the dissected PAD (Mavroudis 2015a).

There are three basic methods of PAD interruption: ligation, ligation with division, and ligation using a clip (Mavroudis 2015a). Ligation of PAD is usually approached through a limited muscle-sparing left thoracotomy (Mavroudis 2015a). The best way to ensure ductal closure is by ligation and division, but this technique is not practical when performed in the premature low-birth-weight newborn. Single ligation is preferred, either with a single ligature, a single hemoclip, or both (Mavroudis 2015a).

The important events leading to an uncomplicated ductal ligation are accurate thoracic entry (usually third or fourth interspace), careful ductal dissection to avoid injury to the recurrent laryngeal nerve, and careful ductal manipulation to avoid unwanted disruption and hemorrhage. Injury to the recurrent laryngeal nerve is likely owing to a stretch injury during dissection, and, in the end, careful assessment of anatomic structures to avoid inadvertent ligation of the left pulmonary artery (Yucel and Sahin 2020; Terlemez et al. 2017; Orzel and Monaco 1986; Pontius et al. 1981; Kim et al. 2016), inadvertent ligation of the descending aorta (Qasim et al. 2017), and inadvertent injury to the thoracic duct.

Many surgeons use electrocautery to dissect PAD to help keep the dissection free of pesky bleeding as long as the PAD, the pulmonary artery, or aorta are not entered. Skilled surgeons may use the inactivated electrocautery probe to

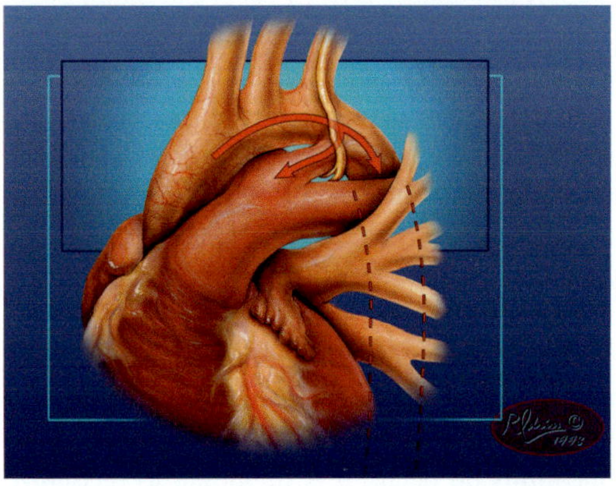

Fig. 1 Drawing shows the relational anatomy of a patient with patent arterial duct. The recurrent laryngeal nerve is highlighted in yellow; the course of the left to right shunt is shown by the red arrows, and the descending aorta is shown by the dashed red lines. The reader can appreciate the possibility of injury to the extant anatomical structures during dissection. (With permission: Mavroudis 2015c)

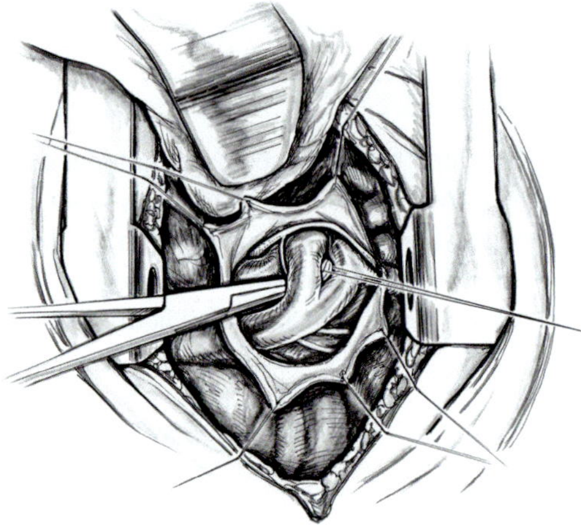

Fig. 2 Drawing demonstrates the operative exposure through a left thoracotomy showing the course of the recurrent laryngeal nerve. The course of the phrenic nerve is not noted since it runs along the posterior portion of the pericardium. A right-angle clamp is placed around the ductus from the inferior approach, underneath the patent arterial duct (PAD), and then emerging at the superior course of the PAD. This maneuver has a number of hazards such as injury to the recurrent laryngeal nerve and PAD disruption and bleeding. (With permission: Mavroudis 2015c)

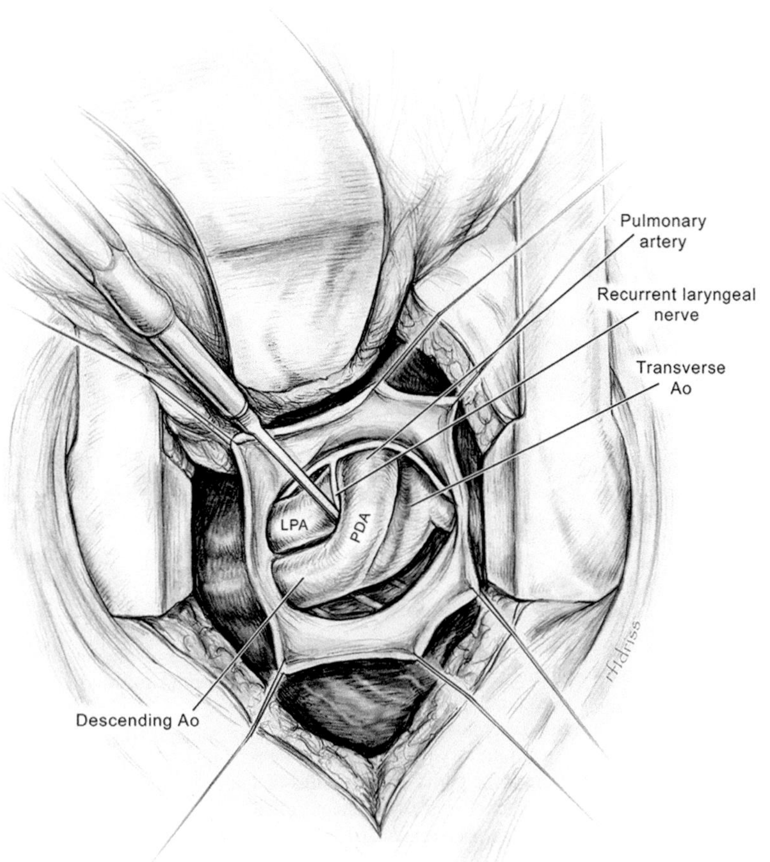

Fig. 3 Drawing shows a left thoracotomy with active dissection of the patent arterial duct using the electrocautery device. The device is shown in an inactive mode (not using the electrocautery) by the surgeon who is manually dissecting the recurrent laryngeal nerve away from the proposed site of ductal ligation. If the electrocautery device is still hot from previous use during this dissection, thermal injury can occur to the recurrent laryngeal nerve and cause temporary or long-term nerve damage. *Ao* aorta, *LPA* left pulmonary artery, *PDA* patent ductus arteriosus

dissect the ductus and push the recurrent laryngeal nerve away from the ductal dissection plane (Fig. 3). What may not be adequately appreciated is that the electrocautery dissector may still be hot despite the inactive electrocautery mode. This could cause a thermal injury and result in temporary or long-term nerve damage. It is better to use scissor dissection in this location to prevent thermal injury to the nerve. If some bleeding develops, careful and accurate electrocautery can control the situation.

When the clamp is successfully placed and sutures delivered around the PAD, it can be ligated as shown in Fig. 4 (Mavroudis 2015a). Uncontrolled bleeding can occur, and the operating team must be mindful that such a situation can be ameliorated by a well-placed suture or a hemoclip at the aortic site. Figure 5 (Mavroudis 2015a) shows successful placement of a hemoclip for standard ductal ligation. Not shown is placement under hemorrhage conditions. The maneuver is the same.

Perhaps the most consequential complications involving PAD ligation, except for uncontrolled hemorrhage, are unintentional ligation of the left pulmonary artery (Yucel and Sahin 2020; Terlemez et al. 2017; Orzel and Monaco 1986; Pontius et al. 1981; Kim et al. 2016) or descending aorta (Qasim et al. 2017; Aggarwal et al. 2013). The complication of accidental division of left pulmonary artery is more likely to occur in an infant with a large PAD and pulmonary artery hypertension (Pontius et al. 1981). Figure 6 shows a tie placed inadvertently around the left pulmonary artery and in the inset, a suture placed around the descending aorta downstream to the PAD. These unwanted consequences are generally the result of thick-

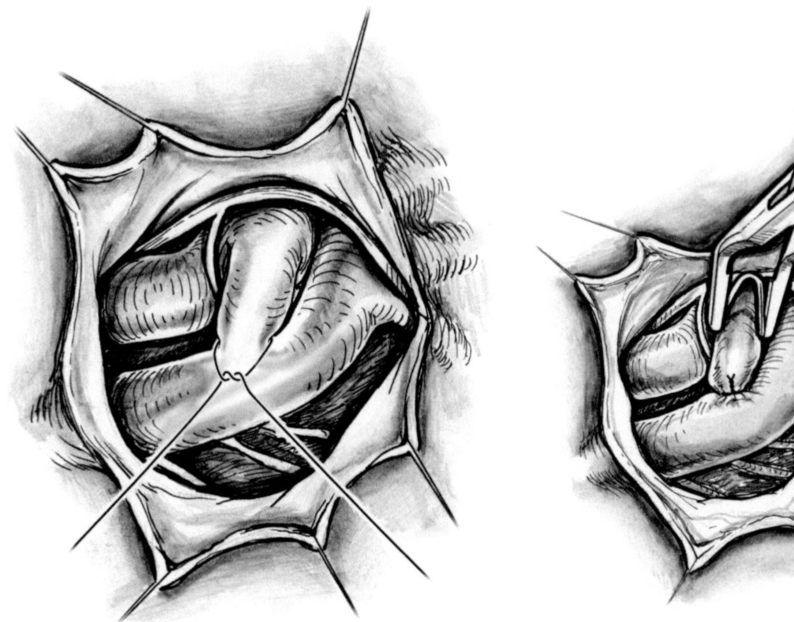

Fig. 4 Drawing shows the successful placement of the suture and ligation procedure. Note that the suture is placed closer to the aorta rather than the pulmonary artery to avoid injury to the recurrent laryngeal nerve and help control unwanted bleeding at the aortic site as sutures or a clip are easier placed under duress from uncontrolled hemorrhage. (With permission: Mavroudis 2015c)

Fig. 5 Drawing shows hemoclip ligation of the patent arterial duct under stable conditions. This method can also be used when there is uncontrolled hemorrhage owing to ductal disruption. (With permission: Mavroudis 2015c)

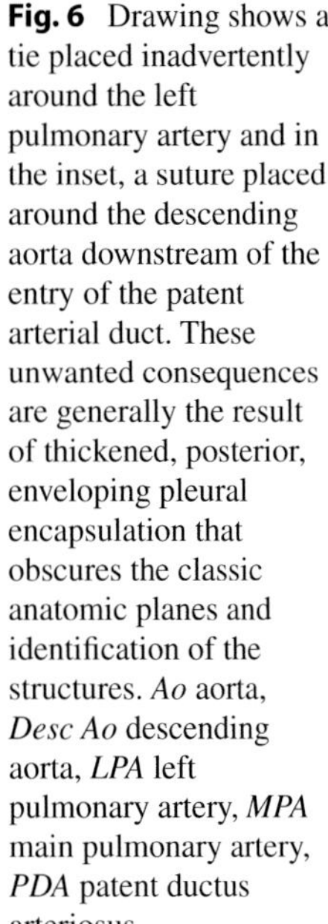

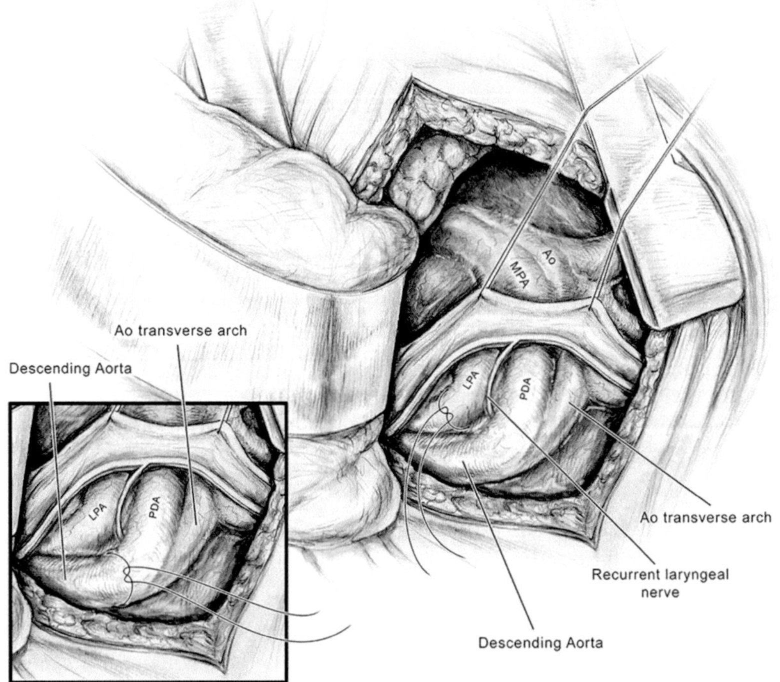

Fig. 6 Drawing shows a tie placed inadvertently around the left pulmonary artery and in the inset, a suture placed around the descending aorta downstream of the entry of the patent arterial duct. These unwanted consequences are generally the result of thickened, posterior, enveloping pleural encapsulation that obscures the classic anatomic planes and identification of the structures. *Ao* aorta, *Desc Ao* descending aorta, *LPA* left pulmonary artery, *MPA* main pulmonary artery, *PDA* patent ductus arteriosus

ened, posterior, enveloping pleural encapsulation that obscures classic anatomic planes and clear identification of the structures. When these complications occur, it is important to act immediately to avoid severe lung complications (e.g., pulmonary hypertension) and distal aortic hypoperfusion that can lead to acute organ failure and death. Ordinarily, postoperative chest roentgenograph can point to left lung hypoperfusion that can be confirmed by echocardiography. Aortic ligation can be inferred by absence of femoral pulses, poor lower extremity perfusion, and lactic acidosis.

Other complications of PAD ligation include injury to the thoracic duct and neocoarctation of the aorta (Qasim et al. 2017) in the event of ductal rupture and resultant suture repair. Thoracic duct injury can result from excessive dissection in the area of the left subclavian artery. If large amounts of clear or milky fluid are seen in the area, thoracic duct injury should be suspected, and multiple individual sutures should be placed in the area until flow has stopped.

When unwanted hemorrhage at the aortic site of the PAD leads to acquired coarctation of the aorta, the surgeon must use caution and judgment to determine whether to engage in repair. For instance, if the preexisting hemorrhage was severe and the patient suffered shock and remains acidotic, cross-clamping the aorta for such a repair may be unwarranted especially if some flow is maintained to the lower extremities. Prudence may determine when to intervene for repair of acquired coarctation.

3 Transmediastinal Patent Arterial Duct Exposure

When the PAD is approached through transmediastinal exposure (Mavroudis 2015a), care must be taken to prevent bleeding and inadvertent ligation of the transverse arch of the aorta distal to the origin of the left subclavian artery. Figure 7 shows transmediastinal exposure (left panel) of the heart with a PAD that is very close to the

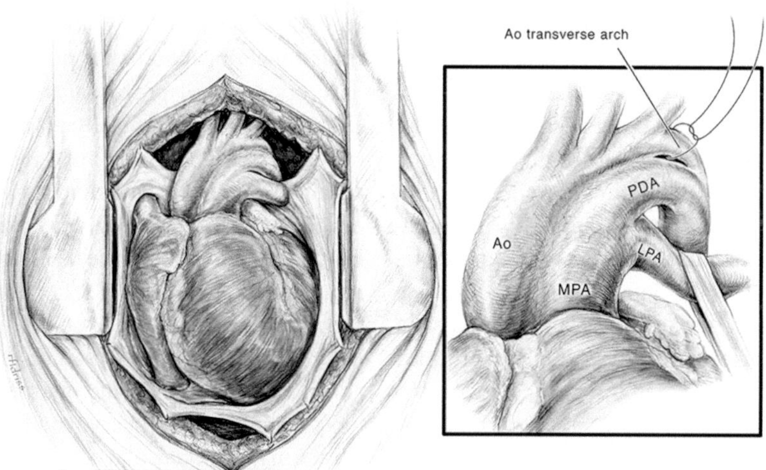

Fig. 7 Drawing shows transmediastinal exposure of the heart (left panel) with a patent arterial duct that is very close to the transverse arch. During dissection, the ductus can be injured and unwanted hemorrhage could result in recoarctation or recurrent laryngeal nerve injury. These mishaps have been discussed. Inadvertent ligation of the transverse arch can occur when mediastinal anatomy is unclear. Figure 7 inset (right panel) shows how the unwanted ligation can occur. As discussed, the condition should be identified immediately or during the early postoperative period when femoral pulses are absent with accompanying lactic acidosis. Immediate attention and repair can be lifesaving. *Ao* aorta, *LPA* left pulmonary artery, *MPA* main pulmonary artery, *PDA* patent ductus arteriosus

transverse arch. During dissection, the ductus can be injured and establish unwanted hemorrhage that may result in recoarctation or recurrent laryngeal nerve injury as discussed earlier in this chapter. It has been reported (Qasim et al. 2017; Pontius et al. 1981) that inadvertent ligation of the transverse arch can occur when the mediastinal anatomy is not clear. Figure 7 inset shows how the unwanted ligation can occur. As discussed, the condition should be recognized immediately or during the early postoperative period when femoral pulses are absent with accompanying lactic acidosis. Immediate recognition and repair can be lifesaving.

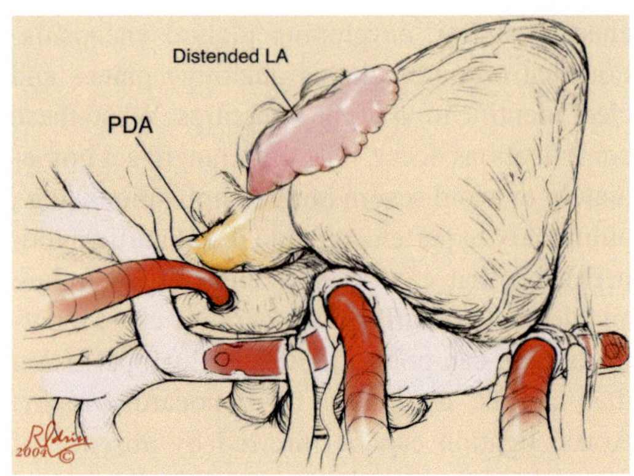

Fig. 8 Drawing shows the initial hemodynamic effects of full cardiopulmonary bypass in the presence of a large patent arterial duct. Epicardial inspection reveals supravalvar pulmonary artery trunk dilatation (yellow). If not immediately corrected, the left atrium will become distended (pink hue) indicating a large left to right shunt and ventricular overload. If the uninformed surgeon continues the search for proper crisis resolution without patent arterial duct ligation, further decompensation will occur within 30–45 s. *LA* left atrium, *PDA* patent ductus arteriosus. (With permission: Mavroudis 2015b)

4 Institution of Cardiopulmonary Bypass with Undiagnosed Patent Arterial Duct

Occasionally, the PAD may not be diagnosed preoperatively. The initiation of cardiopulmonary bypass (CPB), especially if the PAD is large, will have profound hemodynamic consequences and will require immediate attention. Figure 8 (Mavroudis 2015b) shows the initial hemodynamic effects of full CPB in the presence of a large PAD. Within 15 s of CPB commencement, the alert perfusionist should inform the surgeon that perfusion pressure is low despite full flow. Epicardial inspection reveals supravalvar pulmonary artery trunk dilatation (yellow). If not immediately resolved, the left atrium will become distended (pink) indicating a large left-to-right shunt and ventricular overload. If the uninformed surgeon continues to search for proper crisis resolution without PAD ligation, further decompensation will occur within 30–45 s. Figure 9 (Mavroudis 2015b) shows further pulmonary artery and left atrial distention. Poor coronary artery perfusion, myocardial depression, and electrocardiogram evidence of ischemia will become evident owing to the large run off of the systemic circulation into the pulmonary circulation causing misdistribution of blood flow away from the coronary arteries. The alert surgeon will recognize that a large left-to-right shunt is complicating the bypass circuit. Most likely, the cause will be a large PAD requiring immediate dissection and ligation, with special care to avoid PAD entry and injury to the recurrent laryngeal nerve. Proper identification of the right and left pulmonary arteries will prevent unwanted ligation of either vessel. A superficially placed clamp on the epicardial surface of the main pulmonary artery will help with caudal traction that will expose the distal pulmonary artery trunk and PAD. If the PAD is not identified at the usual location, search for PAD in the right or left pulmonary artery should be undertaken. Prompt ligation of the PAD will return hemodynamics to normal and allow reperfusion of the systemic structures, most notably, the coronary circulation. The operation can now proceed (Mavroudis 2015b). In the case of an undiagnosed small PAD, the left-to-right shunt might not be recognized immediately at the start of CPB. Under these circumstances, the surgeon may be confronted with unexplained blood flow accumulating in the right ventricle or right atrium alerting the surgeon to explore for the PAD and ligate, if identified. Adequacy of myocardial preservation during cardioplegic arrest will need to be assessed. The unwanted

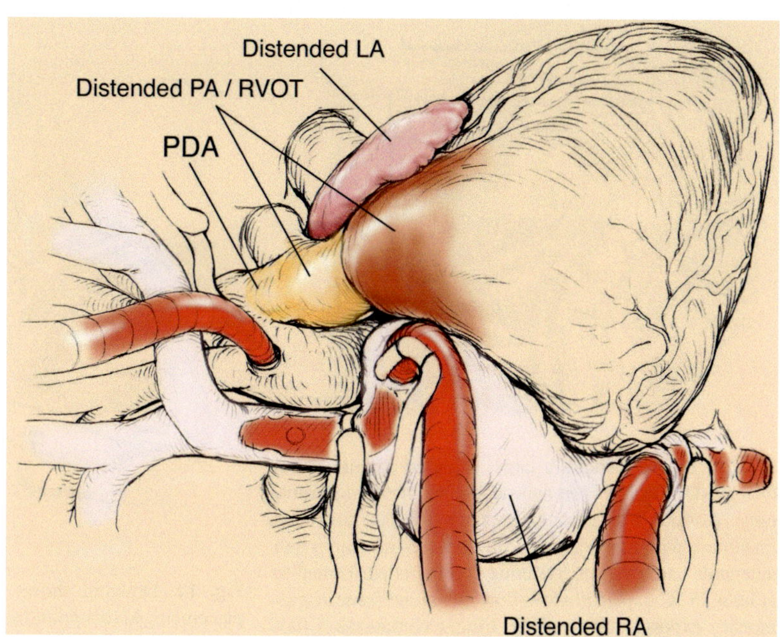

Fig. 9 Drawing shows further pulmonary artery and left atrial distention. Coronary artery malperfusion, myocardial depression, and electrocardiogram evidence of ischemia will become evident owing to the large runoff of the systemic circulation into the pulmonary circulation. *LA* left atrium, *PA* pulmonary artery, *PDA* patent ductus arteriosus, *RA* right atrium, *RVOT* right ventricular outflow tract. (With permission: Mavroudis 2015b)

PAD flow into the right ventricle and right atrium may cause endomyocardial warming. The wise surgeon may want to readminister cardioplegia to assure that myocardial preservation has been accomplished.

While not likely to be preoperatively undiagnosed, unusual causes of left-to-right runoff lesions are aortopulmonary window and hemitruncus arteriosus (anomalous takeoff of the right pulmonary artery from the aorta. These lesions have the same hemodynamic abnormalities as PAD, but resolution is much more involved than simple ligation. Separation from CPB and reassessment with intraoperative transesophageal echocardiography is the prudent course of action to be followed with the appropriate intraoperative repair.

5 PAD Ligation in the Adult with Calcified PAD

When PAD is diagnosed in the adult, calcification of the ductal wall, when present, makes ligation dangerous (Aggarwal et al. 2013) owing to uncontrolled bleeding. For this reason, the PAD can be approached through a median sternotomy and CPB to allow the surgeon to effect closure through the opened pulmonary artery, usually employing a patch technique. However, there are dangers with this approach as it can result in air embolism if the proper techniques are not used.

Figure 10 (Mavroudis 2015a) shows a large, calcified PAD that has been approached via median sternotomy. Aortobicaval CPB has been instituted with application of an aortic cross clamp and antegrade cardioplegia. Systemic cooling is performed to at least 25 °C to perform low-flow technique for transpulmonary exposure of the PAD. After conditions are acceptable, the patient is placed in the Trendelenburg position, a low-flow state established, and longitudinal pulmonary arteriotomy is performed with placement of a polytetrafluoroethylene patch at the orifice of the PAD. Figure 11 (Mavroudis 2015a) shows the placement of this patch with running suture technique. Figure 12 (Mavroudis 2015a) shows the completion of patch placement, and at this point, the CPB flow can be increased, and the patient can be rewarmed. Figure 13 (Mavroudis 2015a) shows a completed pulmonary artery arteriorrhaphy and separation from CPB.

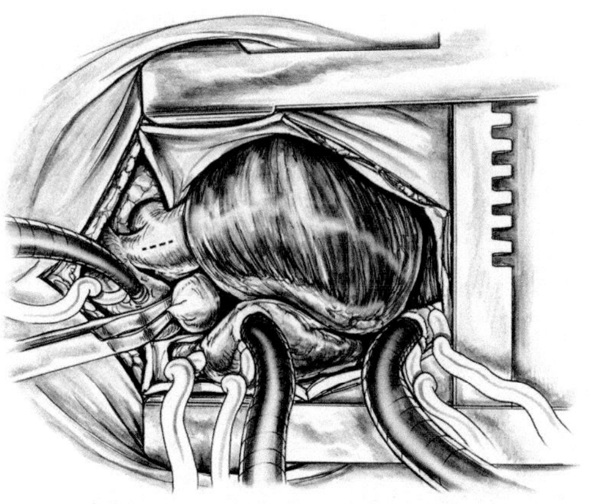

Fig. 10 Drawing shows a large, calcified patent arterial duct (PAD) that has been approached via median sternotomy. Aortobicaval cardiopulmonary bypass has been instituted, with application of an aortic cross clamp and antegrade cardioplegia. Systemic cooling is performed to at least 25 °C to perform low-flow technique for transpulmonary exposure of the PAD. Finger compression (not shown) of the PAD near the aorta is performed to avoid pulmonary overcirculation during cardiopulmonary bypass. (With permission: Mavroudis 2015c)

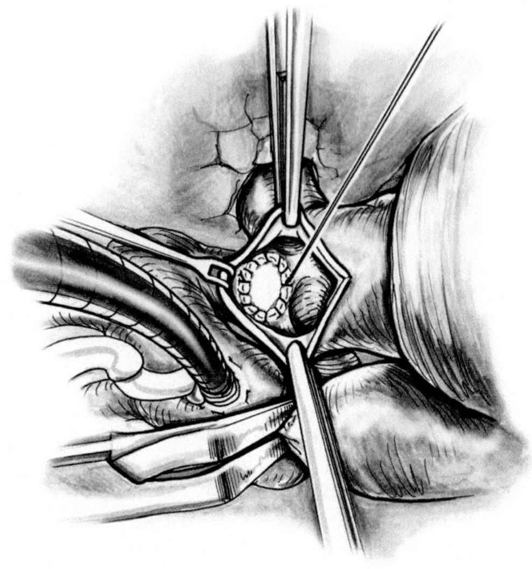

Fig. 12 Drawing shows the completion of the patch placement, At this point the cardiopulmonary bypass flow can be increased and the patient can be rewarmed. (With permission: Mavroudis 2015c)

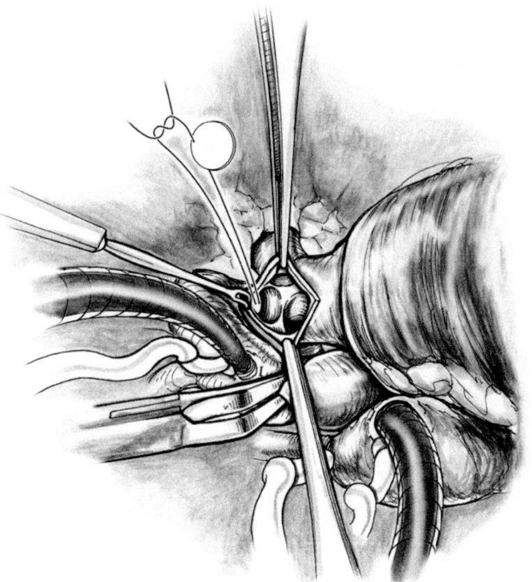

Fig. 11 Drawing shows placement of this polytetrafluoroethylene patch with running suture technique. Proper and favorable conditions for this maneuver include systemic hypothermia, Trendelenburg position, and decreased systemic flow commensurate with systemic temperature and estimated safe systemic flow at the target temperature. (With permission: Mavroudis 2015c)

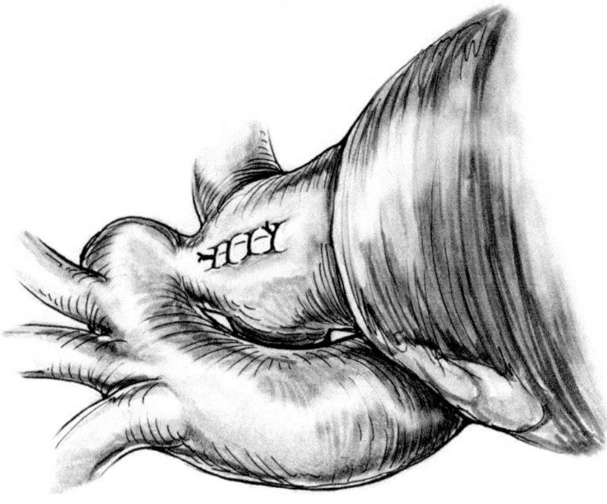

Fig. 13 Drawing shows completed arteriorrhaphy of the pulmonary artery and separation from cardiopulmonary bypass. Transesophageal echocardiography can confirm that the patent arterial duct has been closed. (With permission: Mavroudis 2015c)

6 Summary

In general, ligation of PAD is safe, effective, and simple to perform resulting in beneficial clinical results. Once the patient is weaned from the ventilator, and in essence cured of congestive heart failure, effectively free of bacterial endocarditis, the patient may continue with a normal life.

Even so and even with the most experienced of surgeons, unwanted complications can occur owing to camouflaged anatomy, poor exposure, and ineffective planning. Attention to the integrity of the recurrent laryngeal nerve, realization that the PAD can be friable and subject to hemorrhage, recognizing that anatomy can be camouflaged by surrounding tissue, and careful attention to detail and prudent dissection will assure excellent results free of complications.

References

Aggarwal S, Delius RE, Pettersen MD. Anomalous left coronary artery from the pulmonary artery with a large patent ductus arteriosus: aversion of a catastrophe. Congenit Heart Dis. 2013;8(6):E168–73.

Foster M, Mallett LH, Govande V, Vora N, Castro A, Raju M, Cantey JB. Short-term complications associated with surgical ligation of patent ductus arteriosus in ELBW infants: a 25-year cohort study. Am J Perinatol. 2021;38(5):477–81.

Kim D, Kim S, Shin H, Hong J, Lee JH, Han H. Unintended pulmonary artery ligation during PDA ligation. Heart Surg Forum. 2016;19(4):E187–8.

Mavroudis C. Atrial septal defect. In: Mavroudis C, Backer CL, editors. Atlas of pediatric surgery. London: Springer; 2015a. p. 89–98.

Mavroudis C. Complications associated with the initiation of cardiopulmonary bypass. In: Mavroudis C, Backer CL, editors. Atlas of pediatric surgery. London: Springer; 2015b. p. 401–5.

Mavroudis C. Patent ductus arteriosus ligation. In: Mavroudis C, Backer CL, editors. Atlas of pediatric cardiac surgery. London: Springer; 2015c.

Orzel JA, Monaco MP. Inadvertent ligation of the left pulmonary artery instead of patent ductus arteriosus. Noninvasive diagnosis by pulmonary perfusion imaging. Clin Nucl Med. 1986;11(9):629–31.

Pontius RG, Danielson GK, Noonan JA, Judson JP. Illusions leading to surgical closure of the distal left pulmonary artery instead of the ductus arteriosus. J Thorac Cardiovasc Surg. 1981;82(1):107–13.

Qasim A, Dasgupta S, Jain SK, Jiwani AK, Aly AM. Coarctation of the aorta as a complication of surgical ligation of patent ductus arteriosus in a premature infant. Case Rep Pediatr. 2017;2017:2647353.

Terlemez S, Işık O, Şahin S, Akcan AB, Kaynak Türkmen M. A rare complication of patent ductus arteriosus ligation: inadvertent ligation of the left pulmonary artery. Heart Surg Forum. 2017;20(6):E266–8.

Yucel SM, Sahin IO. Ligation of left pulmonary artery instead of patent ductus arteriosus. Cardiol Young. 2020;30(12):1943–5.

Complications Associated with Surgery for Vascular Rings and Pulmonary Artery Sling

Carl L. Backer

Abstract

Avoiding complications in patients with vascular rings and pulmonary artery sling is predicated on precise preoperative cross-sectional imaging to plan the optimal surgical procedure, full preoperative evaluation with echocardiogram and bronchoscopy, and careful operative technique with attention to details of vascular surgical principles.

Keywords

Double aortic arch · Right aortic arch · Vascular ring · Pulmonary artery sling · Innominate arteriopexy · Aortic Uncrossing · Kommerell diverticulum

Vascular ring operations in children can be among the most satisfying procedures that pediatric heart surgeons are entrusted with. In many cases, a child that is having difficulty breathing or issues with simply swallowing, are completely alleviated after a successful procedure. However, each of these procedures needs to be carefully managed in order to avoid potential complications or inadequate relief of the child's symptoms.

One of the key principles of avoiding complications for these children is to base the operative procedure on accurate advanced preoperative imaging. The original guidelines for vascular ring surgery were based on what we now look upon as the primitive barium swallow examination (Backer et al. 1989). Using careful interpretation of the areas of compression of the esophagus, prediction was made of what type of vascular ring would be encountered. Thankfully those days are behind us, and now every patient who undergoes a vascular ring operation should have advanced cross-sectional imaging in the preoperative evaluation. Our personal preference is for computed tomography (CT) scan with three-dimensional reconstruction (Backer et al. 2005). Alternatively, magnetic resonance imaging (MRI) can often provide nearly the same high-quality images, although may require general anesthesia. Furthermore, CT imaging provides better imaging of the trachea when compared with MRI.

In addition to the advanced cross-sectional imaging, all vascular ring patients should have a preoperative transthoracic echocardiogram to rule out associated congenital heart defects. Finally all vascular ring patients should have either a separate preoperative bronchoscopy or interoperative bronchoscopy at the time of the

C. L. Backer (✉)
Chief, Section of Pediatric Cardiothoracic Surgery, UK Healthcare Kentucky Children's Hospital, Lexington, KY, USA

Cardiothoracic Surgery, Cincinnati Children's Hospital Medical Center, Cincinnati, OH, USA
e-mail: Carl.Backer@uky.edu

C. L. Backer, C. Mavroudis (eds.), *Complications in Pediatric and Congenital Heart Surgery*,
https://doi.org/10.1007/978-3-032-02661-3_4

surgical repair to fully understand the tracheal compression, tracheal and bronchomalacia, and possible stenosis secondary to complete tracheal rings (Backer et al. 2005).

The surgical portion of the operation in general requires meticulous vascular surgical principles using vascular clamps and prolene suture for most of the procedures.

The classification of vascular rings that we have used goes back to the original STS nomenclature and database project (Backer and Mavroudis 2000). The four primary vascular rings are (1) double aortic arch, (2) right aortic arch with left ligamentum, (3) pulmonary artery sling and (4) innominate artery compression syndrome. Within each of these categories, we will now address potential complications that are to be avoided.

Children that are symptomatic with a vascular ring should undergo timely operative repair to avoid serious complications that can arise after hypoxic or apneic spells. A high index of suspicion is required. When evaluating a child with respiratory or swallowing issues delayed treatment can result in tracheobronchial damage that could have been avoided. There are reports of catastrophic erosion of the aortic arch into the trachea, or the esophagus in patients where the diagnosis was delayed (Othersen et al. 1996; Heck et al. 1993; Angelini et al. 2002). Other complications from vascular rings that had a delayed diagnosis include aortic dissection, and in particular aneurysm formation (Midulla et al. 1994). There are several reports of surgical repair of vascular rings in older adult patients, which, because of the progression of the aortic abnormalities, have a much higher incidence of complications than the operation performed in children (Saran et al. 2019; Backer 2024).

1 Double Aortic Arch

The surgical approach to a patient with an aortic arch is vitally dependent upon the preoperative three dimensional imaging. The most common anatomic configuration is where the right arch is dominant. These children are best approached through a left thoracotomy. However, if the left arch is dominant the approach should be through a right thoracotomy. This is a crucial distinction as it is difficult to divide a right arch from the left side.

If the aortic arches are balanced in nature, I would recommend a thoracotomy with division of the right aortic arch. This leaves the left arch in an essentially normal anatomic configuration. I cannot stress the importance of the preoperative imaging to select the appropriate approach.

For the typical patient with a dominant right aortic arch, the vascular ring is approached through a left fourth interspace posterolateral thoracotomy (Fig. 1). Prior to making any decisions regarding the division of the ring, careful dissection of all the essential components should be performed. The best place to start is with dividing the pleura overlying the left subclavian artery. This can then be encircled with a vessel loop. The left subclavian artery can then be traced to the origin from the left aortic arch adjacent to the origin of the left carotid artery. On the undersurface of the left aortic arch will be found the left ligamentum. The typical site of division of the left aortic arch is just distal to the origin of the left subclavian artery from the arch (Fig. 1). In more than half these cases this part of the arch will actually be atretic even though externally it appears patent.

During this dissection attention should be paid to the left recurrent laryngeal nerve (Fig. 1). Injuring the nerve, either with electrocautery or excessive traction will leave the child with a hoarse voice for a period of time. This also makes a child at risk for aspiration. Although the nerve is usually relatively easily visible anteriorly as it curls around the ligamentum, it is where the nerve ascends posterior in the tracheoesophageal groove that an injury may occur as the posterior dissection is performed.

Another structure that needs to be carefully avoided is the thoracic duct. This runs along the posterior aspect of where the dissection is performed adjacent to the spine (Fig. 1). Avoiding the thoracic duct can be achieved by making the pleural dissection slightly more anterior than posterior. Another location where the thoracic

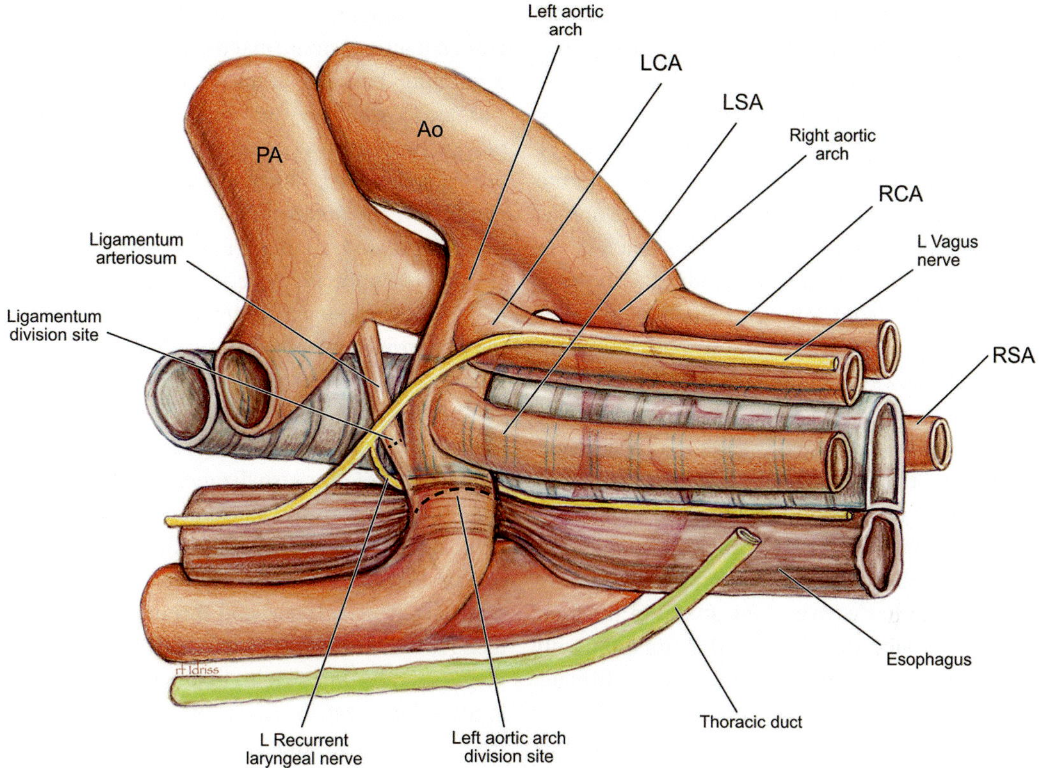

Fig. 1 Double aortic arch, right arch dominant, patent left arch. Dotted lines indicate where ligamentum and distal left arch will be divided. Note position of left recurrent laryngeal nerve and the thoracic duct. *Ao* aorta, *LCA* left carotid artery, *LSA* left subclavian artery, *PA* pulmonary artery, *RCA* right carotid artery, *RSA* right subclavian artery

duct can be injured is where the dissection on the left subclavian artery proceeds superiorly. I have seen large branches of the thoracic duct cross here and in fact have had to reoperate on patients where this was the location of a thoracic duct leak. With use of magnification and a headlamp one is often able to identify these lymphatic structures and avoid them. In some cases where the pleura is being divided at the level of the supreme intercostal vein the patient will have enlarged lymph nodes. In order to avoid a lymph leak here I have ligated and divided this lymphatic tissue along with the supreme intercostal vein. If there is a high volume of chylothorax after the procedure I recommend early repeat thoracotomy to identify and oversew the leak.

Another structure that needs to be carefully dissected is the esophagus. The esophagus, of course, has no serosa so that the dissection can inadvertently proceed into the muscular layers of the esophagus. This is particularly important If the double aortic arch is quite tight and impinging upon the esophagus. The dissection needs to remain very close to the adventitia of the vascular ring itself. I caution against using a blunt right angle to dissect beneath the ring.

I have encountered a ring that actually eroded into the esophagus. If this occurs one needs to be prepared to repair the esophagus with a standard two layer closure.

Once all of the anatomic structures have been identified temporary occlusion of the intended arch division site should be performed, assessing the left radial artery to ensure that the vascular supply to the subclavian artery is not compromised.

The actual division of the arch should be performed using vascular clamps and staged division and oversewing techniques (Fig. 2a, b). A patent arch should never be doubly ligated with a silk suture and divided. I am personally aware of cases where these sutures either cut through the arch, or came off in the postoperative care unit as the patient became hypertensive, leading to catastrophic exsanguination. Figure 2a shows a Potts ductus clamp (straight) on the proximal arch and a Castañeda clamp on the distal arch. Figure 2b shows the completed arch division.

It is important to use the staged division and oversewing techniques so if there is slippage of a clamp or accidental dislodgment, there are sutures that can be gently pulled up to replace the vascular clamp in the correct position. Simply transecting the entire arch before placing any sutures leads to the risk of the stump of the arch slipping through the clamp and a situation with catastrophic hemorrhage, which is very difficult to control. Even when the arch is atretic on CT scan I recommend division and oversewing between vascular clamps.

I recommend that the first suture line be a horizontal mattress suture and the second suture line, a running baseball stitch. Additional mattress sutures to reinforce the suture line should be placed (usually two or three). All of the suture tails are left long. When the clamp is released, they allow the suture line to be pulled up back into the clamp if there is excessive bleeding (Fig. 3). In particular, the distal end of the arch may be quite posterior in the mediastinum. When the clamp is released, the stump of the divided arch tends to retract behind the esophagus. This can be very difficult to control if the sutures are not left so long that the stump can be pulled back up into the field for visualization, possible repeat clamp placement, or placement of additional hemostatic sutures. Small bleeding points remaining after clamp release can be controlled with pieces of gelfoam and thrombin which are then removed after hemostasis has been achieved.

In patients with a right dominant aortic arch it is also important to divide the left ligamentum (Fig. 1). Should the left ligamentum not be divided you would convert the patient from a

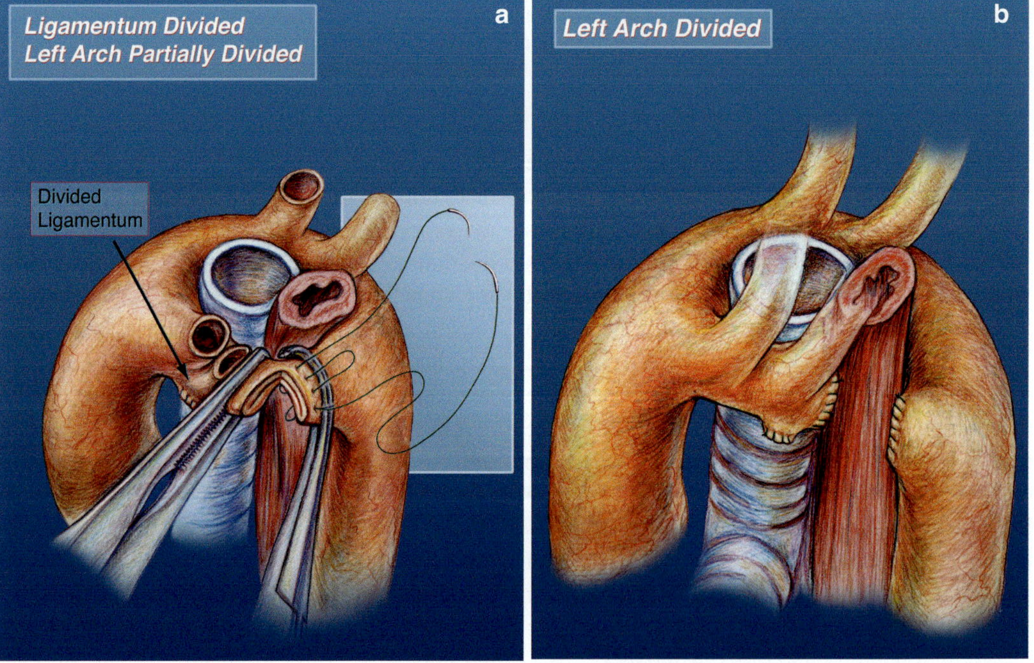

Fig. 2 (**a**, **b**) Double aortic arch, right arch dominant, patent left arch. Staged division and oversewing technique with vascular clamps is shown. The left ligamentum was divided between sutures prior to placing the clamps

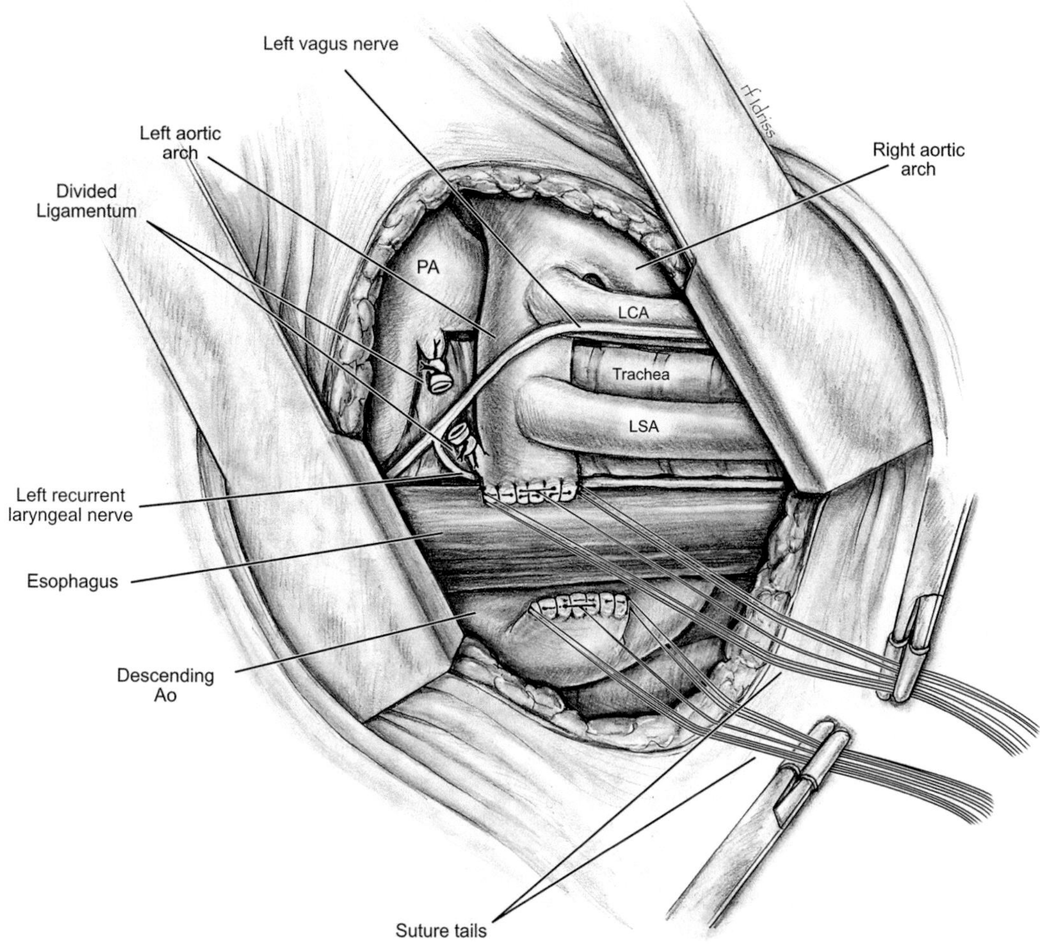

Fig. 3 Left arch has been divided. Suture tails have been kept long so divided stump can be pulled up into vascular clamp if there is excessive bleeding. Ligamentum has been ligated with silk suture and suture ligated with prolene. *LCA* left carotid artery, *LSA* left subclavian artery, *PA* pulmonary artery

double aortic arch to a right aortic arch with a left ligamentum. The ligamentum is avascular; it can be divided between silk ligatures with a reinforcing prolene suture. However, if there is any question about the patency of the ligamentum/ductus arteriosus it should be divided between vascular clamps, oversewing the stumps with prolene sutures.

Following division of the arch and ligamentum, it is important to also divide any adhesive bands that may have developed because of the chronic compression of the esophagus. These bands should be carefully divided with scissors or low level electrocautery, taking care not to enter the esophagus or injure the recurrent laryngeal nerve.

Another important part of the vascular ring division is to avoid the temptation to close the pleura. Many surgeons close the pleura after a coarctation repair. However, after a vascular ring division closure of the pleura can lead to scar tissue that can actually cause recurrence of the child's symptoms. I have had to reoperate on several patients where the pleura was closed and scar tissue developed and recurrence of symptoms occurred.

Once the procedure has been completed and hemostasis achieved the chest is closed. In our current practice, we use a Blake drain attached to a suction bulb. This allows the child to move about more easily than being attached to a pleurovac that is attached to suction. In the past 25 years, we had no complications associated with using a Blake drain instead of a chest tube and pleurovac system. The drain should be left in place for 24–48 h. The main reason for the drain is to monitor for any potential postoperative bleeding and check for lymph leaks leading to a potential for a chylothorax. We always make sure that the child eats food containing fat prior to removing the drain.

If it all possible, the child should be extubated in the operating room. Many children after a vascular ring repair will have residual tracheomalacia or bronchomalacia, and have noisy breathing. This sometimes takes weeks to months to resolve. However, the best place to extubate them is in the operating room with anesthesia standing by. You may have to spend some time observing the child in the operating room, but they will typically improve over time after the endotracheal tube has been removed.

The parents should be counseled ahead of time that it may take weeks to months for the noisy breathing and barky cough to completely disappear. It is nearly always substantially improved immediately postoperatively but may take months to completely resolve.

Some patients with a double aortic arch will have a Kommerell diverticulum (KD) that serves as the insertion site of the distal portion of the left aortic arch (Fig. 4) (Backer et al. 2019). This can also occur with an atretic distal arch, but still have a Kommerell diverticulum originating from the descending thoracic aorta. The diverticulum of course is the distal remnant of the left fourth aortic arch. This Kommerell diverticulum should be resected at the time of the double aortic arch repair. The base of the diverticulum should be clamped flush with the descending thoracic aorta (Fig. 5). Care needs to be taken not to compromise the descending thoracic aorta and create a neocoarctation. For this reason, a lower extremity

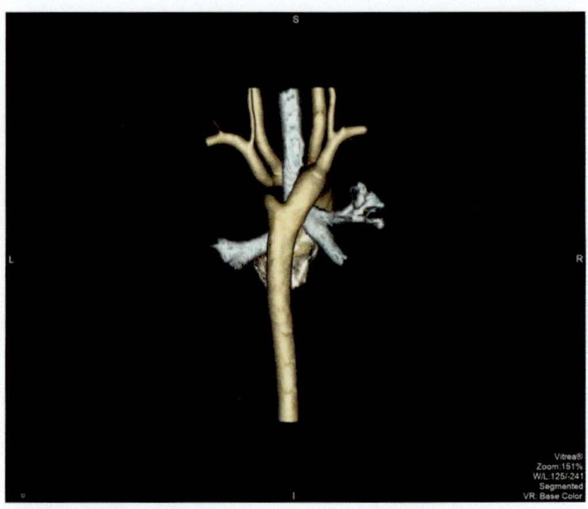

Fig. 4 Posterior view of three-dimensional reconstruction of computed tomography angiography of a 5-month-old, 7-kg child with stridor and choking episodes with feeding. Child has a double aortic arch, right arch dominant, with a Kommerell diverticulum that is a continuation of the atretic distal left aortic arch. (With permission: Backer et al. 2019)

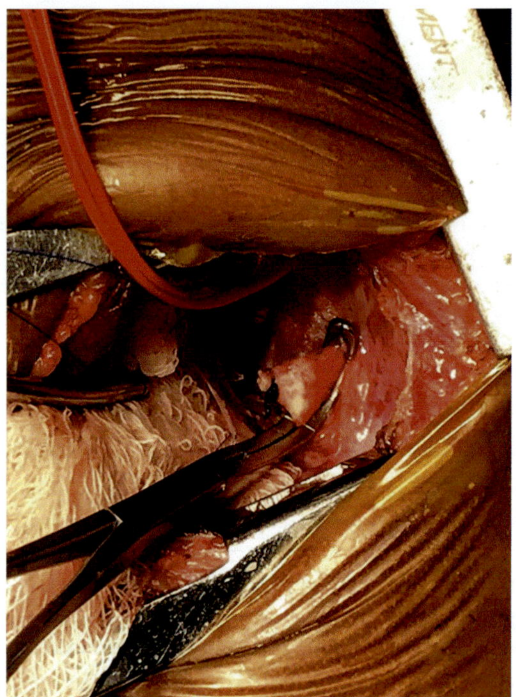

Fig. 5 The Castañeda clamp is on the Kommerell diverticulum. The stump of ligamentum remains on the diverticulum. (With permission: Backer et al. 2019)

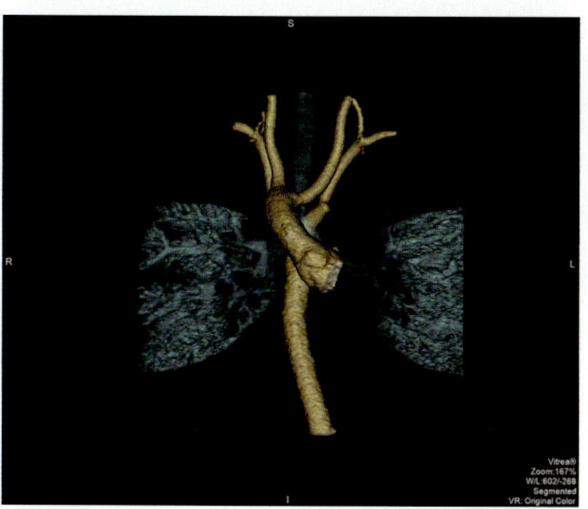

Fig. 6 Anterior view of a three-dimensional reconstruction computed tomography angiography (CTA) of a 13-month-old 8-kg child. CTA shows a double aortic arch, right arch dominant, with an atretic distal left aortic arch. The left subclavian artery originates from a Kommerell diverticulum from the descending aorta. (With permission: Backer et al. 2019)

arterial line or blood pressure cuff should be placed. The diverticulum should be resected using the same staged division and oversewing techniques as used for the division of a left aortic arch. The sutures should be placed in a similar fashion, and the prolene tails left until the clamp on the base of the diverticulum is released. We reported 10 patients in a series of 66 patients undergoing an operation for a double aortic arch that had simultaneous excision of a Kommerell diverticulum (Backer et al. 2019).

In some cases, the left aortic arch can be atretic between the left carotid artery and the Kommerell diverticulum, which is serving as the actual source of blood flow to the left subclavian artery (Fig. 6). In these cases, the atretic arch needs to be ligated and divided, the Kommerell diverticulum resected, and the left subclavian artery transferred to the left carotid artery. This is described in further detail in the section on right aortic arch.

2 Right Aortic Arch

The principles of surgical intervention for patients with a right aortic arch and left ligamentum have dramatically changed in the past 20 years. It was previously thought that simple division of the left ligamentum would offer relief for these patients. Although that was true in many cases, in other cases, particularly with the advent of advanced cross-sectional imaging we have realized that in many of these cases the vascular compression is not only from the ligamentum, completing a ring, but from a KD acting as an independent source of external compression of the trachea and esophagus. In addition, the origin of the left subclavian artery distal on the aortic arch acts to pull the right aortic arch to the left, and in many cases act as a sling, affecting particularly the esophagus. Because of this, we now recommend in the majority of cases that the diverticulum which serves as the source of blood supply to the left subclavian artery be resected, and in order to preserve the vascular supply of the arm and left hand that the left subclavian artery be transferred to the left carotid artery. This of course, is technically a more demanding procedure but with proper preparation and surgical technique is straightforward and, more importantly, more completely relieves the patient's symptoms.

Much like the double aortic arch the approach to these patients begins with advanced cross-sectional imaging. Again our preference is for CT imaging with three dimensional reconstruction but MRI imaging in many cases is also adequate. The preoperative imaging will show how the trachea and the esophagus are affected by the KD. Imaging will also show the course of the left carotid artery, and whether it will be anatomically feasible to transfer the left subclavian artery to the left carotid artery in the chest.

The approach is through a left posterolateral thoracotomy. Again the dissection begins with opening the pleura over the left subclavian artery, and then encircling the left subclavian artery with a vessel loop. The left subclavian artery is then traced to its origin from the descending thoracic aorta. Adjacent to the left subclavian artery is the usual location of the ligamentum arteriosum. There are patients who do not have a diverticulum as the source of the left subclavian artery. In these patients, I divide the left ligamentum and visualize the separation of the vascular structures, and the remaining degree of compression of the esophagus. The ligamentum can be divided with sutures on either side and reinforcing prolene sutures. However, again, if there is any question regarding patency, or if the ligamentum is extremely short, division between vascular clamps, oversewing the stumps with prolene suture is always safer (Fig. 7). In some cases, after division of the ligamentum, it will be apparent that the vascular structures have separated nicely and the esophagus is free of compression. However, in many cases, the subclavian artery remains acting as a sling that compresses the esophagus posteriorly. These patients, even if they do not have a Kommerell diverticulum will benefit from transferring the left subclavian artery to the left carotid artery.

Most frequently, the left subclavian artery will have its origin from a Kommerell diverticulum from the descending thoracic aorta. This structure can independently compress the esophagus and requires resection. In addition, the diverticulum, if not addressed, can enlarge to the point where it can actually rupture. Our specific recommendation is that if the Kommerell diverticulum is more than 1.5 times the size of the diameter of the left subclavian artery it should be resected. The conduct of this procedure requires important attention to detail. Again the recurrent laryngeal nerve needs to be carefully identified and preserved. The ligamentum is divided prior to addressing the diverticulum (Fig. 8). The left carotid artery should be dissected, and then encircled with a vessel loop prior to beginning the diverticulum resection. This often takes some time. The artery is typically in a plane posterior to the vagus nerve and anterior to the recurrent laryngeal nerve as it ascends in the tracheoesophageal groove. Dissection directly posterior from the thoracotomy incision between these two nerves will lead to the carotid artery. We monitor the cerebral NIRS, right and left side, in preparation for carotid artery clamping.

The patient should then be given a dose of heparin 100 units per kilogram prior to applying the clamps on the subclavian and carotid arteries. The base of the diverticulum is occluded with a

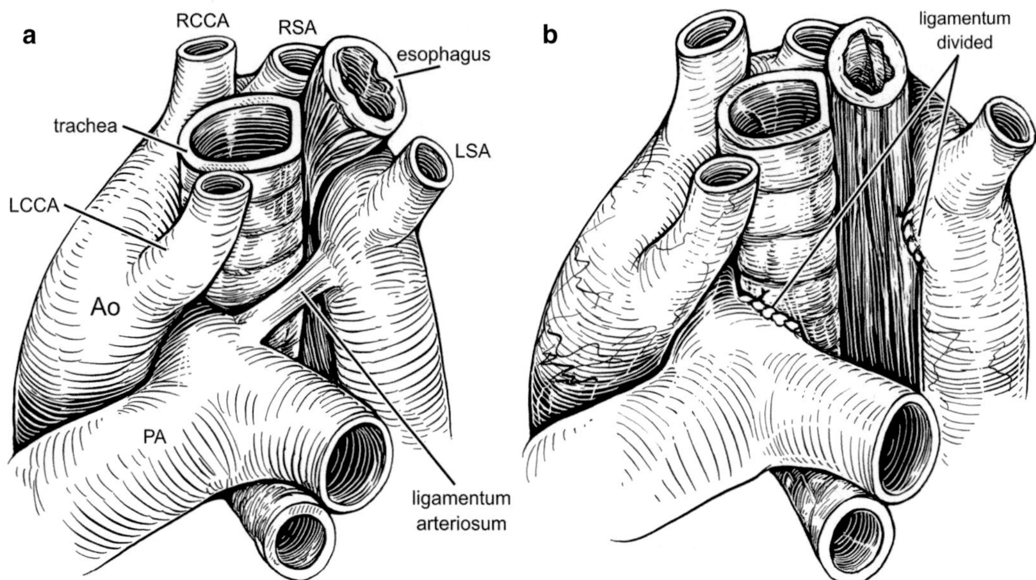

Fig. 7 (**a**) Right aortic arch, aberrant left subclavian artery, left ligamentum. (**b**) The left ligamentum has been divided and the stumps have been oversewn with running prolene suture. *Ao* aorta, *LCCA* left common carotid artery, *LSA* left subclavian artery, *PA* pulmonary artery, *RCCA* right common carotid artery, *RSA* right subclavian artery. (With permission: Backer and Mavroudis 2003)

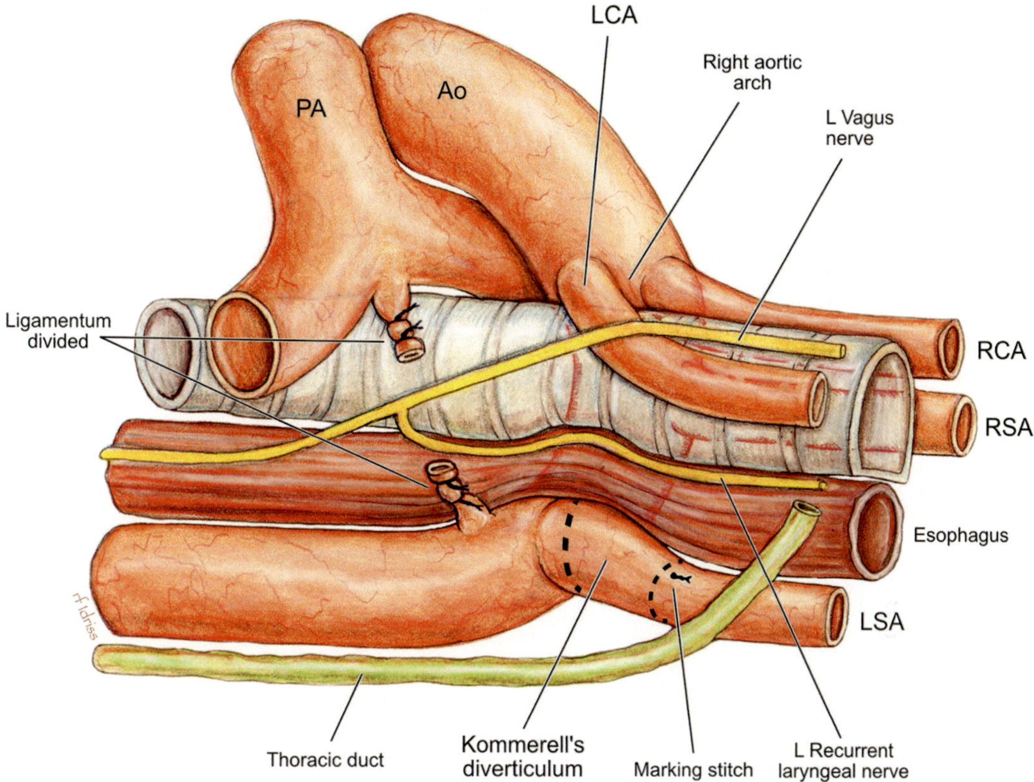

Fig. 8 This illustration shows some of the technical details of Kommerell diverticulum resection and left subclavian artery transfer. The ligamentum has been doubly ligated with silk suture and suture ligated with a prolene suture. There is still compression of the esophagus by the Kommerell diverticulum. The dotted lines indicate where the Kommerell diverticulum will be resected. A small prolene marking suture is placed on the anterior aspect of the left subclavian artery to help with orientation when the left subclavian artery is transferred to the left carotid artery. Note the location of the left carotid artery "between" the vagus nerve and the left recurrent laryngeal nerve. Also note the location of the thoracic duct. *Ao* aorta, *LCA* left carotid artery, *LSA* left subclavian artery, *PA* pulmonary artery, *RCA* right carotid artery, *RSA* right subclavian artery

vascular clamp (Fig. 9b). The subclavian artery is controlled with a small yellow vascular hemoclip. The subclavian artery is transected at a site just distal to the aneurysmal diverticulum tissue. The superior aspect of the subclavian artery should be marked with a small suture prior to the division so that the subclavian artery is not inadvertently twisted when the anastomosis is performed (Fig. 8).

The base of the diverticulum is then transected again using staged division and oversewing techniques. As the diverticulum is being excised, the suture line is advanced. It is only when the suture line is nearly completed that the diverticulum is completely removed. This prevents the suture line from slipping through the clamp. Any slippage of this clamp will result in substantial hemorrhage. Once the diverticulum has been removed and the two suture lines completed, and prior to removing the clamp I place two or three horizontal mattress sutures of prolene to reinforce the suture line. When the clamp is released, the prolene sutures are left long so that if there is substantial bleeding, the clamp can be immediately reapplied, and the suture line pulled up into the clamp (Fig. 10). Once satisfied with the hemostasis at the base of the resected diverticulum attention is directed to the anastomosis to the left carotid artery.

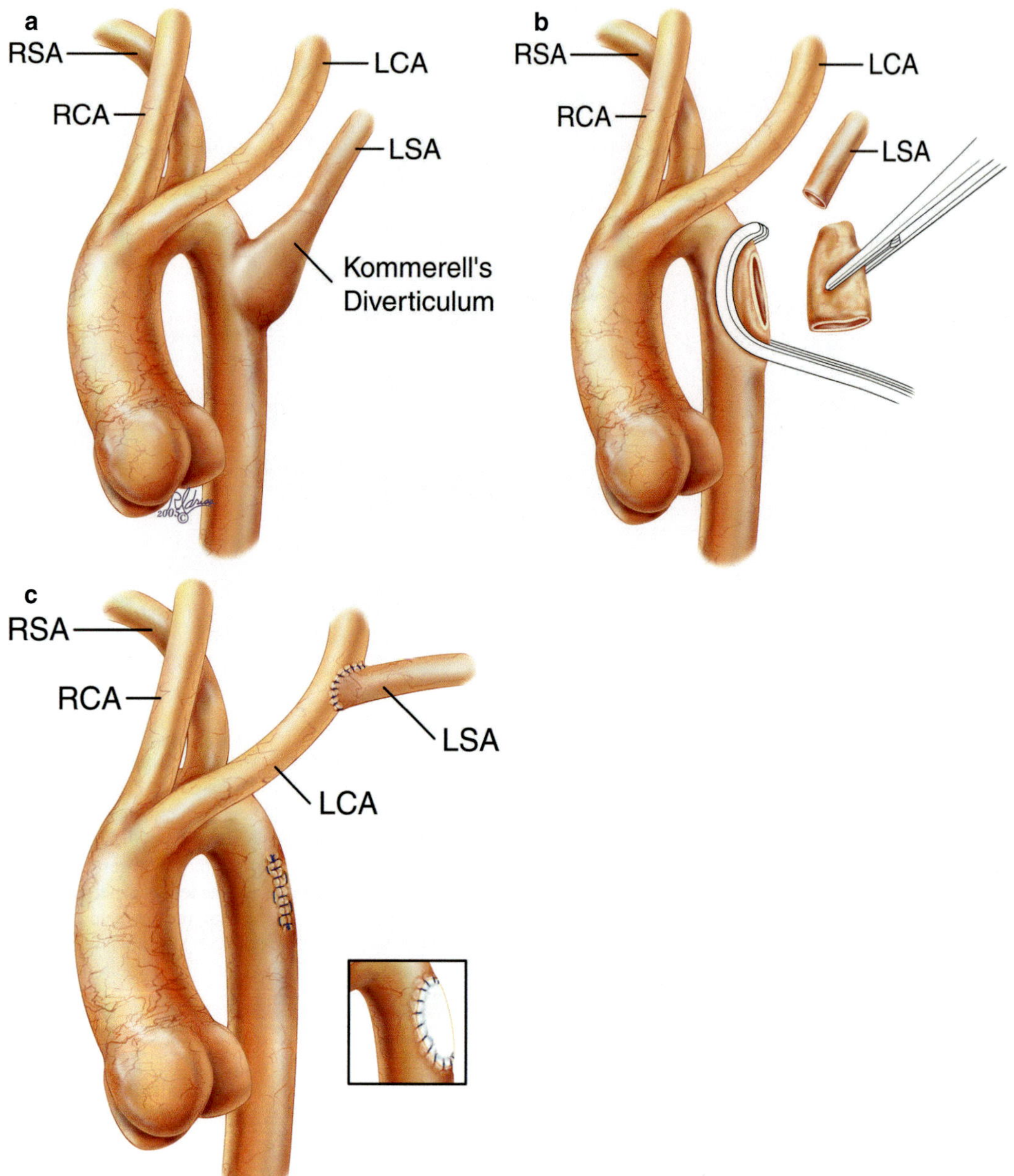

Fig. 9 Overview of Kommerell diverticulum resection (**a**) Right aortic arch with aberrant left subclavian artery and Kommerell diverticulum (ligamentum not shown). (**b**) Base of Kommerell diverticulum occluded with a vascular clamp, the Kommerell diverticulum has been resected, the left subclavian artery is controlled with a vascular clip. (**c**) Base of the Kommerell diverticulum has been oversewn and the left subclavian artery has been transferred to the left carotid artery. Inset shows a patient with a friable Kommerell diverticulum base repaired with a polytetrafluoroethylene (PTFE) patch. *LCA* left carotid artery, *LSA* left subclavian artery, *RCA* right carotid artery, *RSA* right subclavian artery. (With permission: Backer et al. 2002)

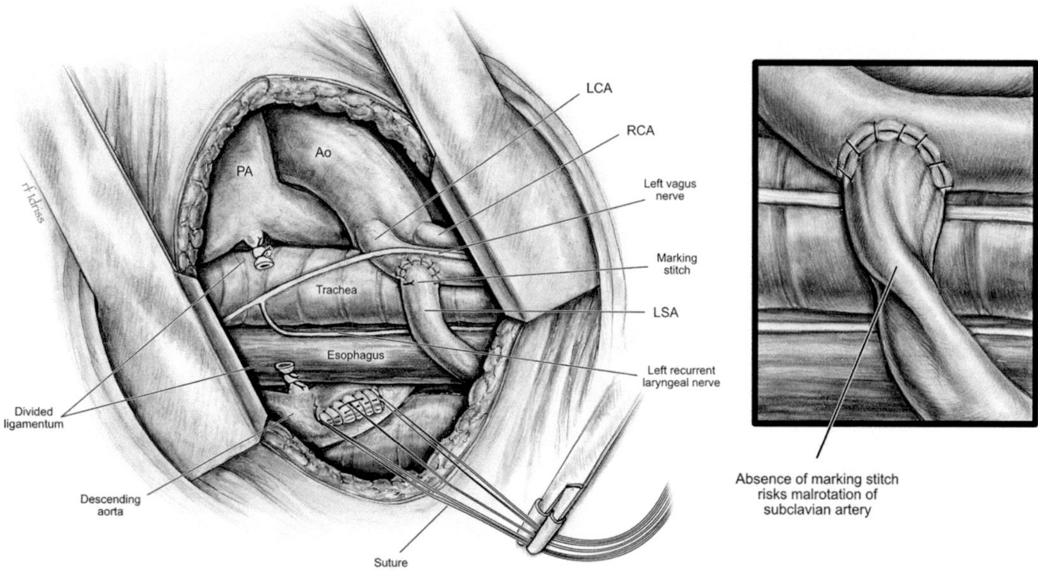

Fig. 10 The left subclavian artery has been transferred to the left carotid artery. Note the position of the marking stitch on the left subclavian artery. Suture tails on the Kommerell diverticulum have been left long in case there is bleeding necessitating pulling the stump up into the released vascular clamp. The small inset shows how the left subclavian artery can become twisted if a marking stitch is not used to maintain proper orientation. *Ao* aorta, *LCA* left carotid artery, *LSA* left subclavian artery, *PA* pulmonary artery, *RCA* right carotid artery

The carotid artery is completely occluded with a Castañeda vascular clamp. During this time the anesthesiologist should maintain a high, normal blood pressure in order to ensure adequate blood flow through the circle of Willis. We monitor the right and left cerebral NIRS and should the left cerebral NIRS begin to drop the patient's blood pressure should be increased by anesthesia. We have now performed a Kommerell diverticulum with left subclavian artery transfer in almost 100 patients with no neurologic complications.

The portion of carotid artery contained within the vascular clamp is incised with a 15 blade. This incision is extended with an angled microvascular Potts clamp to accommodate the size of the left subclavian artery. The left subclavian artery is anastomosed to this opening with 6-0 or 7-0 prolene suture. This portion of the anastomosis is facilitated by making sure that the small anterior marking suture is directed to the proximal opening of the carotid artery (Fig. 10). When the anastomosis is completed, this marking suture should be adjacent to the most proximal portion of the carotid incision. Preventing twisting of this anastomosis is critical (Fig. 10). The clamps are sequentially released by flashing the subclavian clamp, reapplying it, releasing the clamp on the carotid, and then releasing the subclavian vascular clip. There may be mediastinal tissues that impinge upon the subclavian artery as it courses "down" to the left carotid artery. These should be carefully divided with electrocautery to prevent compression/stenosis of the reimplanted left subclavian artery. A blood pressure cuff on the left arm and a pulse oximeter on the left arm should be used to assess the adequacy of the anastomosis to the carotid artery. If the pressure is low, or the waveform dampened steps should be taken to ensure that the anastomosis is not kinked or stenotic.

My experience with nearly 100 of these anastomoses is that I have only had to revise one of them because it was twisted; hence, the importance of the marking suture placed at the beginning of the procedure.

After completing the anastomosis, I typically place two interrupted prolene sutures on either side of the anastomosis to help reinforce the suture line.

Again after this procedure, the pleura is left open. The same instructions with the Blake drain are used as for the double aortic arch.

3 Circumflex Aorta

A subset of patients with a right aortic arch and left ligamentum will have a left sided descending aorta which is a distinctly different anatomic variant, called the circumflex aorta (Russell et al. 2013). This anatomic variant is now easily identified with advanced cross-sectional imaging. In these patients simple division of the ligamentum will not necessarily alleviate the patient's symptoms. Even resection of a Kommerell diverticulum if present and transfer of the left subclavian artery may not help. The problem with these patients is that the descending thoracic aorta crosses from right to left above the carina and compresses the trachea and esophagus posteriorly (Fig. 11). The circumflex aorta can also occur with a double aortic arch where the right arch is dominant (Fig. 12). These patients need to be evaluated in a slightly different manner. For some of these patients, despite the fact that there is a circumflex aorta, there is minimal compression of the trachea and operative intervention may not be required. More often though, there is posterior compression of the trachea, and they have dysphagia caused by compression of the esophagus (Fig. 13). The operation for these patients is the aortic uncrossing procedure (Backer et al. 2024). This is a major operation performed through a median sternotomy with cardiopulmonary bypass, hypothermia, and either a period of circulatory arrest or modified cerebral perfusion.

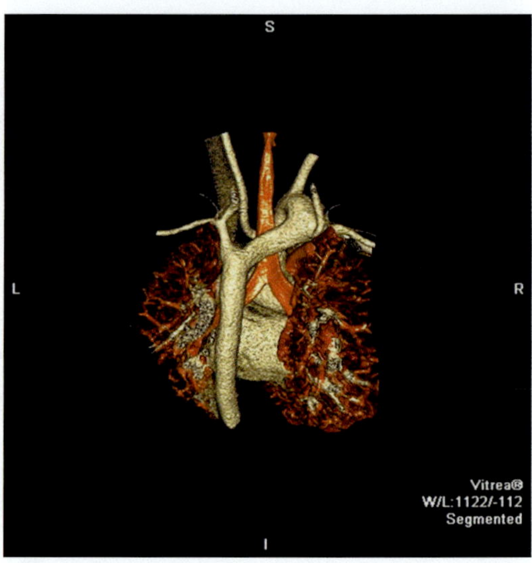

Fig. 11 This computed tomography angiogram (CTA) demonstrates the posterior view of a 4.6-year-old child with a right cervical aortic arch, left ligamentum arteriosum, and retroesophageal left subclavian artery. The descending thoracic aorta crossing right to left posterior to the trachea and superior to the carina is clearly seen on this CTA. (With permission: Russell et al. 2013)

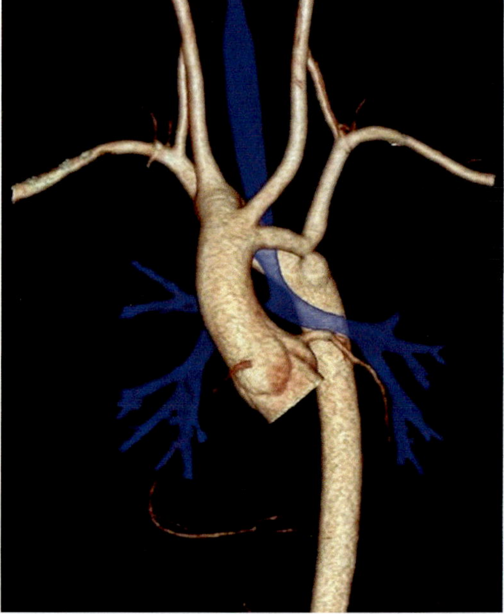

Fig. 12 Preoperative CT scan in a child with noisy breathing, harsh cough, and multiple episodes of recurrent bronchitis. There is a right dominant double aortic arch, with a circumflex aorta. The aorta crosses from right to left posterior to the trachea. (With permission: Backer et al. 2024)

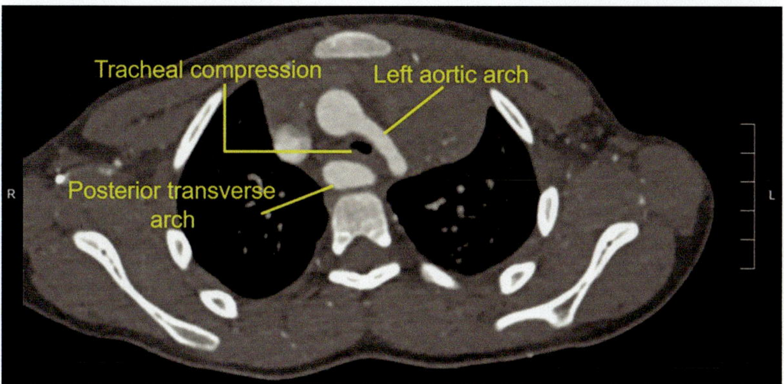

Fig. 13 Double aortic arch, right arch dominant, circumflex aorta. This axial image shows how the aorta compresses the posterior aspect of the membranous trachea. This posterior compression of the trachea by the aorta is one of the key diagnostic features that should lead the clinician to recommend an aortic uncrossing rather than simple ligamentum or left aortic arch division alone. (With permission: Backer et al. 2024)

4 Aortic Uncrossing Procedure

The aortic crossing procedure is done through a median sternotomy (Fig. 14a, b). This is in many cases, a reoperation in a patient who has had a previous ligamentum division. The usual precautions for a redo sternotomy must be taken. In addition, it is extremely important to take care when dissecting near the recurrent laryngeal nerves on both the right and left sides, and also the vagus nerve which runs in the tracheoesophageal groove (Fig. 15). These areas should be dissected either with the scissors or the electrocautery on very low settings. The operation is facilitated by complete dissection of all structures with encircling vessel loops. This includes the left carotid, right carotid, right subclavian, left subclavian, right, and left branch pulmonary arteries, and ligamentum. In our series of patients eight were operated on with deep hypothermic circulatory arrest with a mean of 34 minutes and three patients had antegrade cerebral perfusion with a median of 28 minutes. The cerebral perfusion must be performed via one of the carotid arteries, I have preferred using the left carotid artery (Fig. 15).

The aortic cross-clamp is applied and the heart arrested with cardioplegia. The ascending aorta is transected just distal to the right subclavian artery. The aortic arch is dissected under the trachea and esophagus and then transferred to the left side of the body. Care must be taken not to enter either the trachea or the esophagus during this dissection.

In order to provide an appropriate site for the reanastomosis, I place two marking sutures or use a pen to mark the side of the ascending aorta prior to placing the cross-clamp so that the aorta is full at the time of this decision process (Fig. 15). The incision in the side of the aorta may extend up onto the subclavian artery, but should be the same size as the orifice of the descending aorta. The anastomosis is performed with running prolene and the system must be carefully deaired to prevent air embolus to the brain. If the anastomosis appears to be under tension, a patch can be used to augment the anastomosis (Fig. 16). This has been the preference of

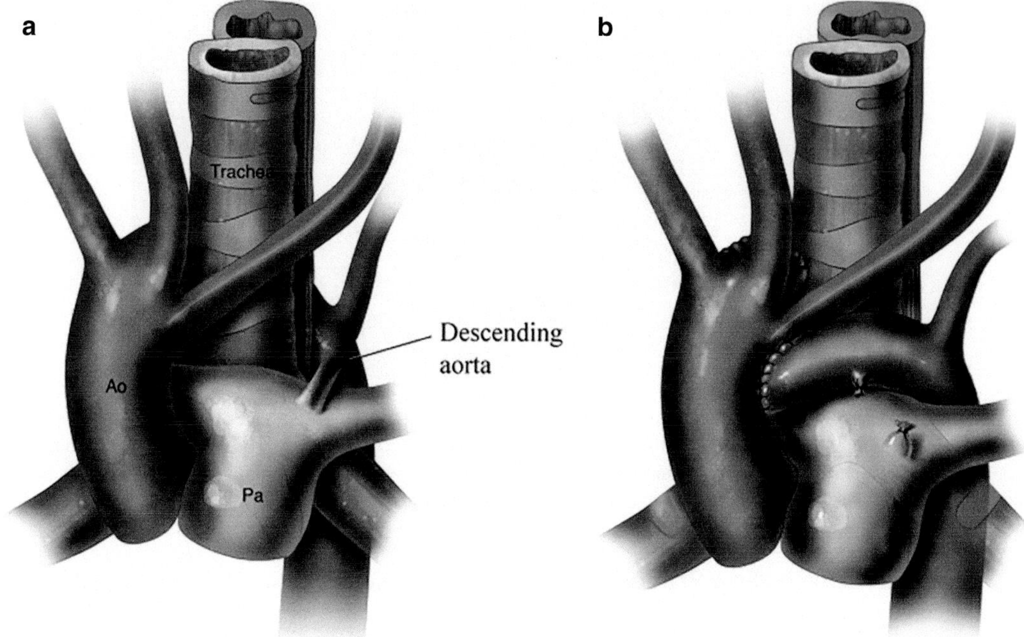

Fig. 14 (**a**) This image illustrates a patient with a circumflex aorta as exposed through a median sternotomy incision. The ascending aorta is on the right. The first brachiocephalic branch is the left carotid artery, the second branch is the right carotid artery, and the third branch is the right subclavian artery. The descending thoracic aorta crosses posterior to the trachea and esophagus and the left subclavian artery originates from the descending thoracic aorta adjacent to the ligamentum arteriosum. (**b**) The completed aortic uncrossing. The descending thoracic aorta has been brought anterior to the trachea and esophagus and anastomosed to the side of the ascending aorta. The ligamentum has been ligated and divided. The posterior compression of the trachea is now completely relieved. *Ao* aorta, *PA* pulmonary artery. (With permission: Russell et al. 2013)

the Boston Children's group (Kamran et al. 2020).

Our series has had two significant complications. The first was bilateral recurrent laryngeal nerve paresis, which required a temporary tracheostomy. Both nerves recovered over a period of months, and the tracheostomy was removed. The same patient had significant sinus tachycardia which may have reflected temporary injury to the vagus nerve. This also resolved.

Another patient who was two years old at the time of the uncrossing procedure had an ectatic

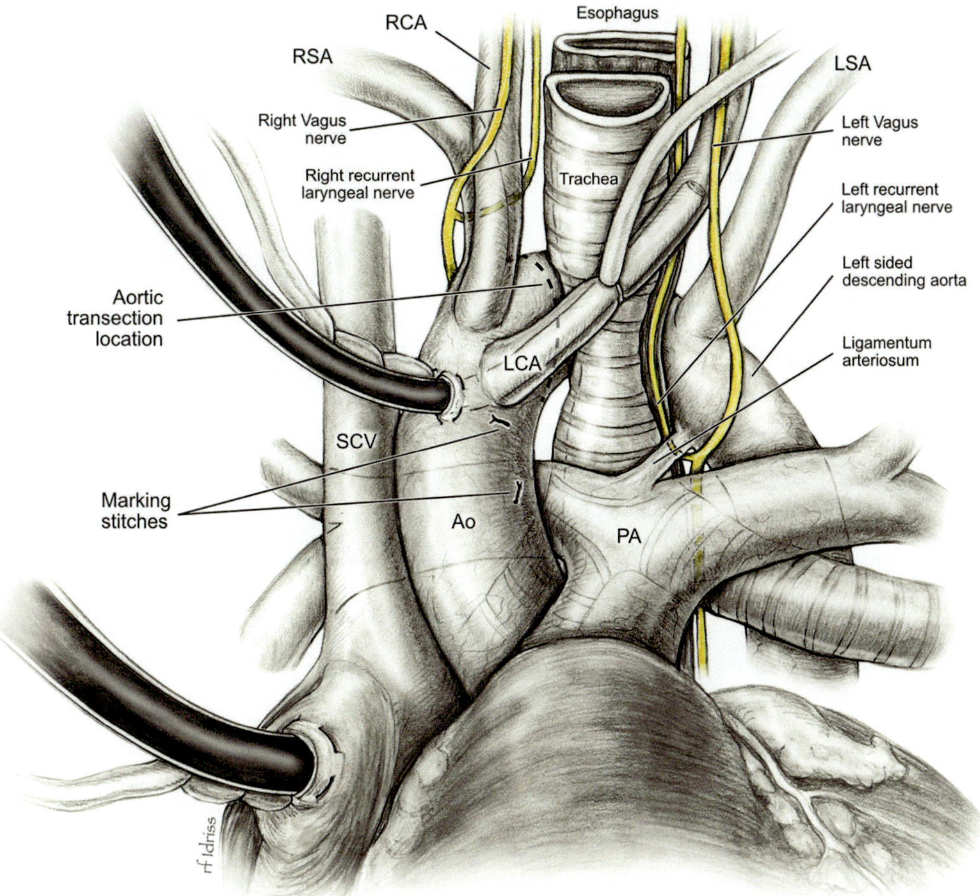

Fig. 15 This illustration demonstrates some of the finer details of the aortic uncrossing procedure. Dotted lines show the planned transverse aortic arch transection site. Marking sutures have been placed on the left side of the ascending aorta to indicate where the aortic incision will be for the aortic anastomosis. Careful attention must be paid to both the right and left recurrent laryngeal nerves. Illustration shows how the aortic cannula can be advanced into the left carotid artery for modified cerebral perfusion. *Ao* aorta, *LCA* left carotid artery, *LSA* left subclavian artery, *PA* pulmonary artery, *RCA* right carotid artery, *RSA* right subclavian artery, *SCV* superior caval vein

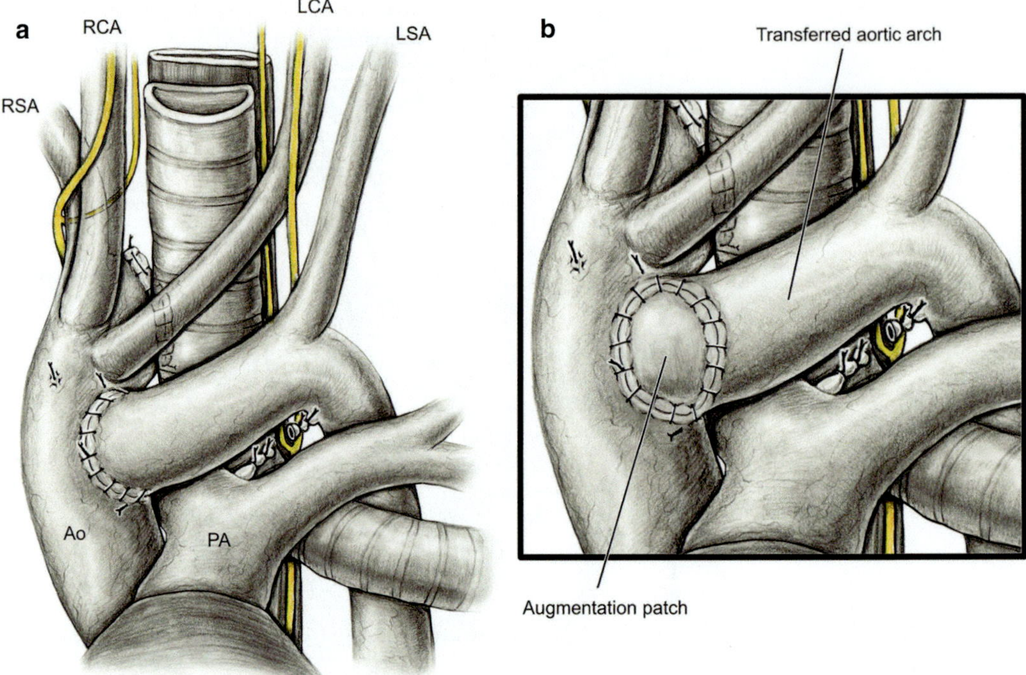

Fig. 16 This illustration shows the completed aortic uncrossing procedure. Note the carefully closed transected aortic arch with multiple reinforcing mattress sutures. The inset shows augmentation of the anastomosis with a prosthetic patch which occasionally may be required. *Ao* aorta, *LCA* left carotid artery, *LSA* left subclavian artery, *PA* pulmonary, *RCA* right carotid artery

anomalous course of the esophagus (Fig. 17a, b). Aortic uncrossing led to severe esophageal compression after the uncrossing (Fig. 18a, b). This necessitated a reoperation to open the aortopulmonary window by placing an aortic extension graft. This relieved the esophageal compression (Fig. 19), but at some point the graft will need to be upsized. It is imperative to determine the course of the esophagus prior to proceeding with the aortic uncrossing operation to avoid this complication. If recognized preoperatively, the esophagus can be mobilized and placed lateral to the translocated transverse aorta.

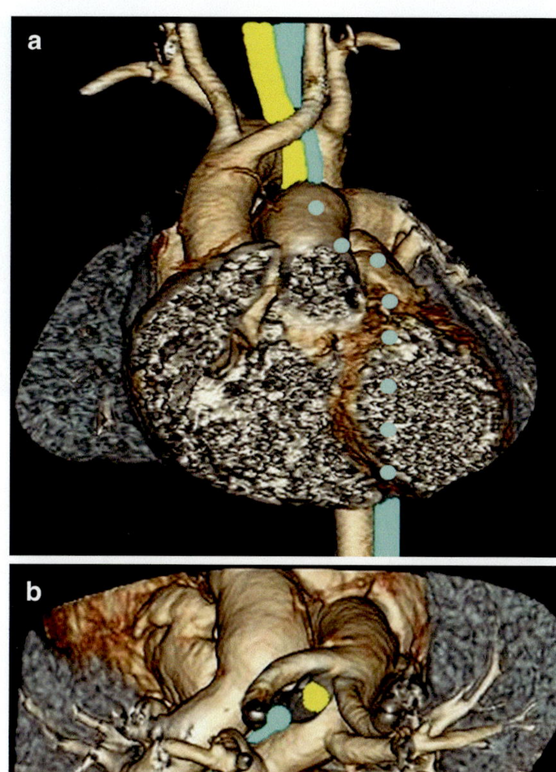

Fig. 17 (**a**). This is an anterior-posterior view of a CTA reconstruction of a 2-year-old child with a right aortic arch, aberrant left subclavian artery, and circumflex aorta. The trachea is in yellow and the esophagus is in blue. The blue dots show the course of the ectatic esophagus which was not recognized prior to the procedure. (**b**) Superior view of the preoperative anatomy. The trachea is yellow and the esophagus is blue. Note how the esophagus traverses from right to left

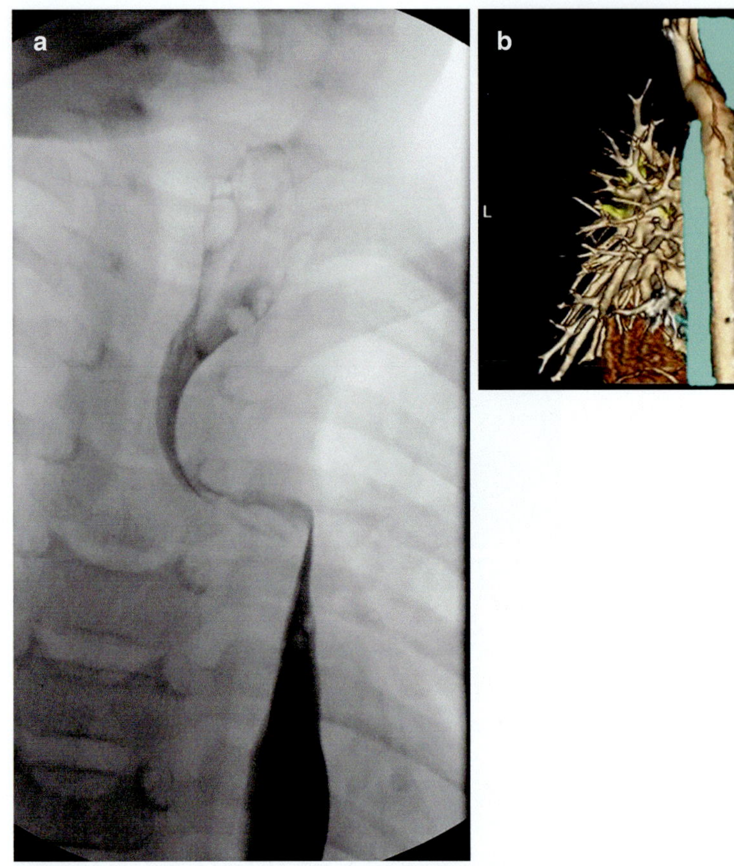

Fig. 18 (**a**) Barium swallow on PO Day #10 showed severe esophageal compression. The translocated aorta compresses the esophagus as it attempts to travel from right to left. (**b**) Posterior view of CTA showing how the esophagus is compressed as it travels under the aorta after the uncrossing as it courses from right to left

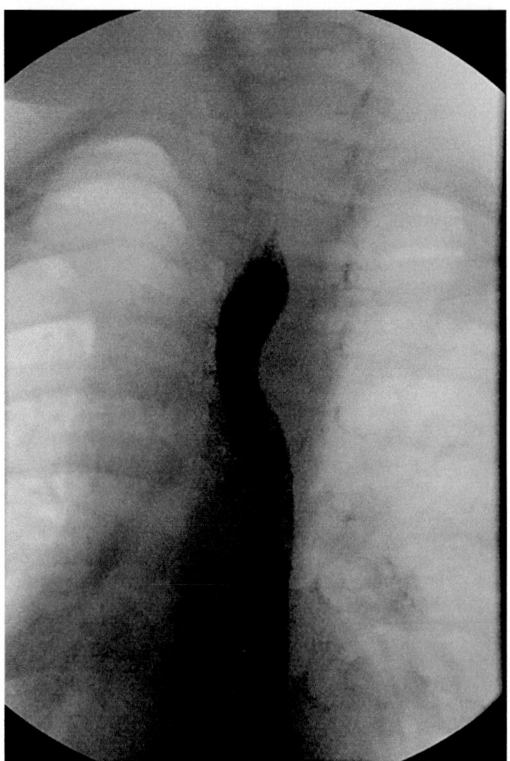

Fig. 19 Barium swallow after transverse aorta was lengthened with an extension graft

5 Pulmonary Artery Sling

Pulmonary artery sling is best repaired with a median sternotomy and cardiopulmonary bypass (Backer et al. 2012). Prior to the repair, it is extremely important to assess the patient for other cardiac anomalies, and to assess the trachea for tracheal stenosis secondary to complete tracheal rings. If there are other cardiac anomalies, in general, it is best to perform both the intracardiac repair and the pulmonary artery sling repair at the same time. In addition, if there is significant tracheal stenosis, secondary to complete tracheal rings, a slide tracheoplasty should be considered as part of the operation (Stephens et al. 2020).

Regarding the procedure itself, the operation is greatly facilitated by using cardiopulmonary bypass. Historically surgeons used a left thoracotomy but this was associated with the frequent complication of left pulmonary artery occlusion (Sade et al. 1975). Cardioplegic arrest is not usually required, unless there is an additional intracardiac issue. The initial dissection should identify the right pulmonary artery, the origin of the left pulmonary artery from the superior aspect of the right pulmonary artery, and the left ligamentum. Figure 20 shows a cutaway view with the aorta removed along with the main pulmonary artery to show the anatomic features, which is the left pulmonary artery passing beneath the trachea anterior to the esophagus en route to the left lung. Dissection of this structure needs to be carefully performed in order to not enter the trachea anteriorly or the esophagus posteriorly. We have had the occasion of having entered the trachea, which required a limited tracheal resection and end-to-end anastomosis.

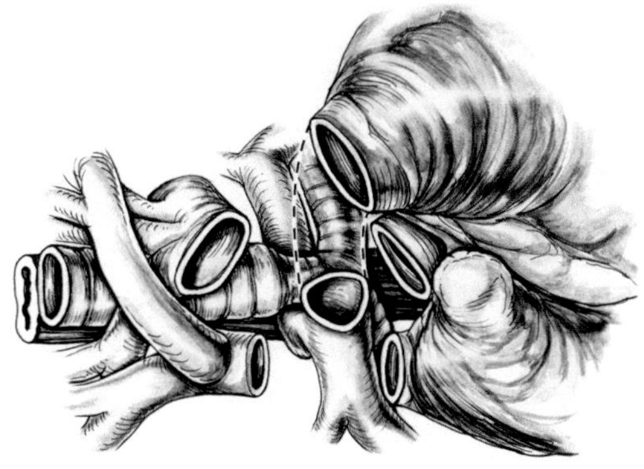

Fig. 20 Surgeon's view of a pulmonary artery sling through a median sternotomy approach. The ascending aorta and main pulmonary artery have been virtually "cut away." (With permission: Backer 2015)

Figure 21 demonstrates careful electrocautery dissection of the left pulmonary artery posterior to the trachea and anterior to the esophagus. In this illustration, the stump of the left pulmonary artery as it originates from the right pulmonary artery has been oversewn. Care should be taken when creating this stump that the right pulmonary artery is not stenosed. Because the left pulmonary artery is usually excessively long there should be no reason to not ensure an adequate stump on the right pulmonary artery.

The site of the planned anastomosis of the left pulmonary artery should be marked on the main pulmonary artery when the pulmonary artery is full prior to beginning cardiopulmonary bypass.

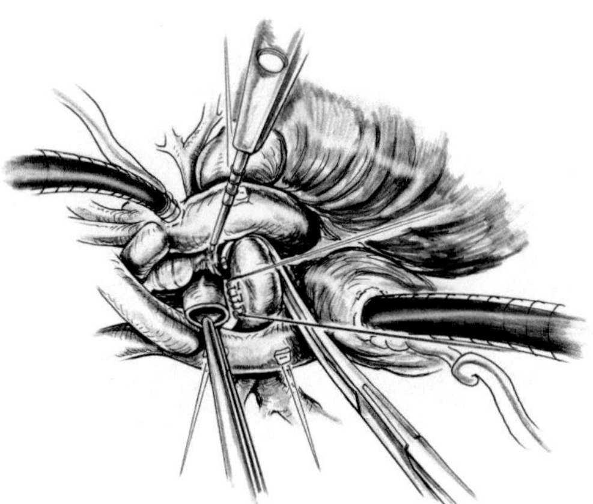

Fig. 21 Cardiopulmonary bypass canulae are in place. The stump of the left pulmonary artery on the right pulmonary artery is being oversewn. Care must be taken not to purse-string this and create right pulmonary artery stenosis. Careful electrocautery dissection is being used to free the left pulmonary artery under the trachea anterior to the esophagus. (With permission: Backer et al. 2012)

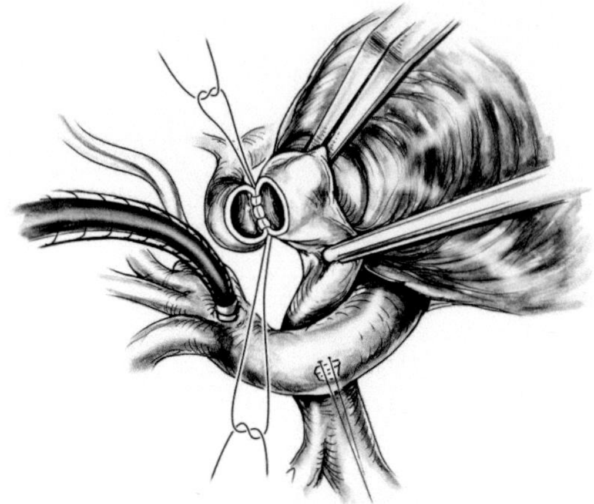

Fig. 22 The anastomosis of the left pulmonary artery to the coronary punch hole created in the main pulmonary artery. The left pulmonary artery must not be twisted, too long, or too short. This requires careful orientation and measuring. (With permission: Backer et al. 2012)

This is usually very close to the site of the left ligamentum. Great care must be taken to establish this anastomosis without kinking or twisting of the left pulmonary artery. The orifice of the left pulmonary artery can be sized with a small coronary dilator. A coronary punch is then used to create the opening in the main pulmonary artery, which has previously been marked. The anastomosis of the left artery is performed with fine, prolene suture. Early in my career I used interrupted sutures for this; currently I prefer running suture with 7-0 or sometimes 8-0 prolene suture (Fig. 22). Some surgeons have recommended beveling the left pulmonary artery to ensure an adequate orifice, I have not found this to be necessary. Other surgeons have used a pericardial patch augmentation for this orifice; again I have not found that to be necessary.

The dissection of the left pulmonary artery is close to the location of the vagus nerve on the right side, and can be close to the location of the recurrent laryngeal nerve on the left side. Both of the structures should be carefully visualized and avoided.

6 Innominate Arteriopexy

I have preferred to do this operation through a submammery right anterolateral thoracotomy (Backer et al. 1992). Through this exposure the right lobe of the thymus is exercised. Then the pericardium is opened and the innominate artery identified. Three pledgeted sutures are used to pull the artery up to the back of the sternum (Fig. 23).

The two complications which need to be carefully avoided, relate to the phrenic nerve and the right arm vascular supply. The nerve needs to be visualized and avoided carefully while the right lobe of the thymus is being removed (Fig. 24). It can also be injured when opening the pericardium from this approach. In order to not adversely affect the blood supply to the right arm it is imperative to have a pulse oximeter, and/ or an arterial line in the right radial artery. When the innominate artery is pulled up to the sternum, this pulse needs to be carefully monitored (Fig. 25). Should the pulse oximeter wave diminish or the blood pressure be diminished the suture place-

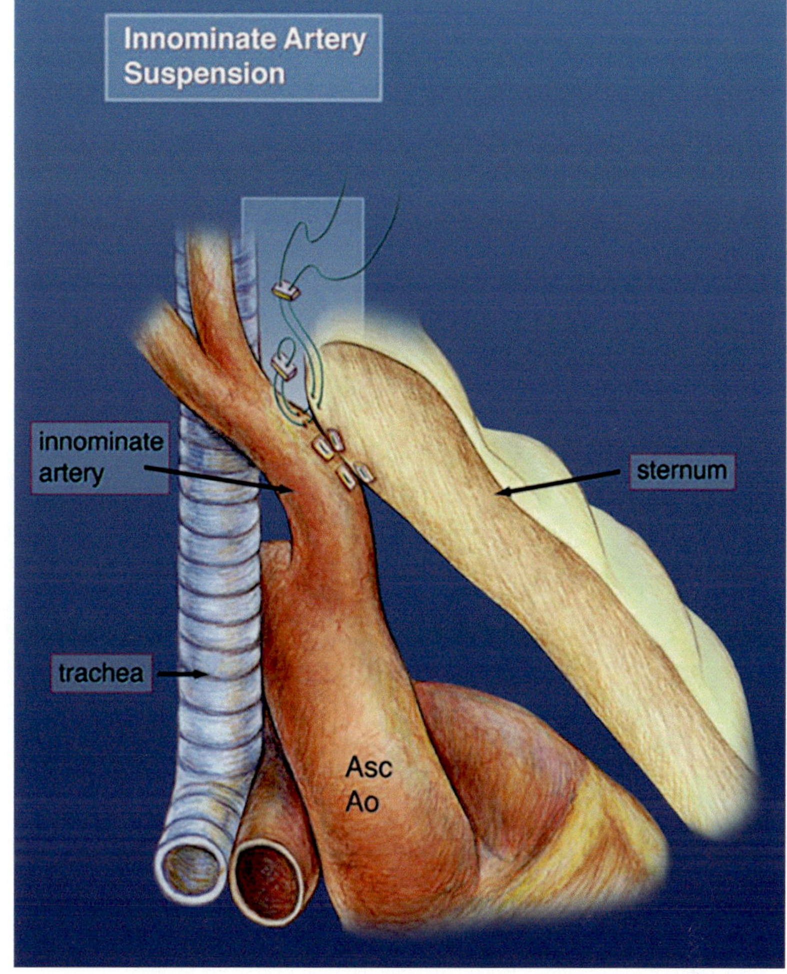

Fig. 23 Innominate arteriopexy being performed via right submammary anterolateral thoracotomy. Three pledgeted sutures are used to elevate the innominate (brachiocephalic) artery away from the trachea. *Asc Ao* ascending aorta. (With permission: Backer 2015)

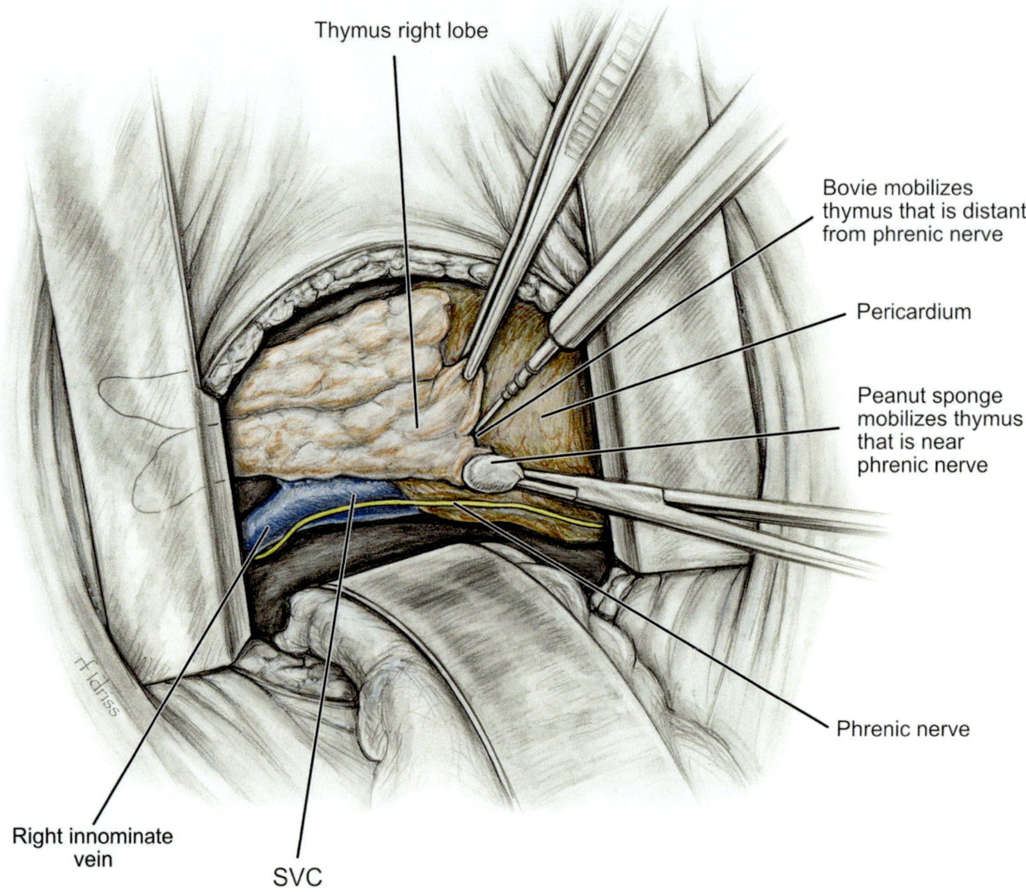

Fig. 24 Approach to the innominate artery via a right anterolateral thoracotomy. Care must be taken not to injure the phrenic nerve with the cautery when removing the right lobe of the thymus

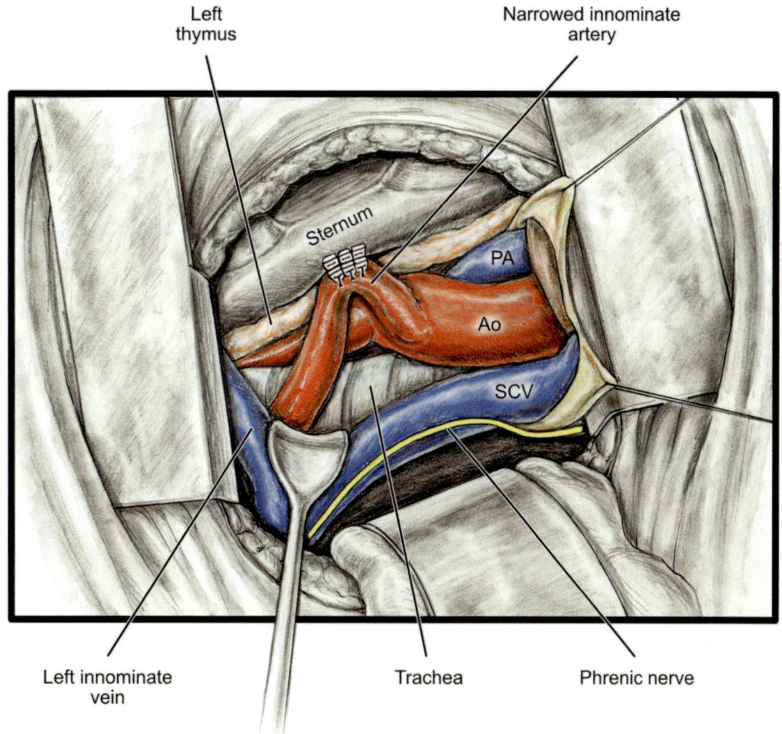

Fig. 25 Care must be taken not to kink off or narrow the innominate artery when it is sutured to the back of the sternum as is illustrated here. *Ao* aorta, *PA* pulmonary artery, *SVC* superior vena cava

ment will have to be reevaluated to prevent this from happening.

The other strategy required to prevent an inadequate postoperative result is to perform intraoperative bronchoscopy through the endotracheal tube. This allows visualization of the tracheal lumen, and the relief of compression can be assessed in real time as the pexy is being performed.

References

Angelini A, Dimopoulos K, Frescura C, Gamba P, Lo Piccolo R, Stellin G, Thiene G. Fatal aortoesophageal fistula in two cases of tight vascular ring. Cardiol Young. 2002;12(2):172–6.

Backer CL. Vascular rings, tracheoplasty, and pulmonary artery sling. In: Mavroudis C, Backer CL, editors. Atlas of pediatric cardiac surgery. Springer: London; 2015. p. 45–72.

Backer CL. Invited commentary: adults are not large children. Ann Thorac Surg. 2024;117(2):402–3.

Backer CL, Mavroudis C. Congenital Heart Surgery Nomenclature and Database Project: vascular rings, tracheal stenosis, pectus excavatum. Ann Thorac Surg. 2000;69(4 Suppl):S308–18.

Backer CL, Mavroudis C. Vascular rings and pulmonary artery sling. In: Mavroudis C, Backer CL, editors. Pediatric cardiac surgery. 3rd ed. Philadelphia: Mosby; 2003. p. 234–50.

Backer CL, Ilbawi MN, Idriss FS, DeLeon SY. Vascular anomalies causing tracheoesophageal compression. Review of experience in children. J Thorac Cardiovasc Surg. 1989;97(5):725–31.

Backer CL, Holinger LD, Mavroudis C. Innominate artery compression—division and reimplantation versus suspension. J Thorac Cardiovasc Surg. 1992;103(4):817–20.

Backer CL, Hillman N, Mavroudis C, Holinger LD. Resection of Kommerell's diverticulum and left subclavian artery transfer for recurrent symptoms after vascular ring division. Eur J Cardiothorac Surg. 2002;22(1):64–9.

Backer CL, Mavroudis C, Rigsby CK, Holinger LD. Trends in vascular ring surgery. J Thorac Cardiovasc Surg. 2005;129(6):1339–47.

Backer CL, Russell HM, Kaushal S, Rastatter JC, Rigsby CK, Holinger LD. Pulmonary artery sling: current results with cardiopulmonary bypass. J Thorac Cardiovasc Surg. 2012;143(1):144–51.

Backer CL, Bharadwaj SN, Eltayeb OM, Forbess JM, Popescu AR, Mongé MC. Double aortic arch with Kommerell diverticulum. Ann Thorac Surg. 2019;108(1):161–6.

Backer CL, Mongé MC, Wallen WJ, Eltayeb O. The aortic uncrossing procedure. J Thorac Cardiovasc Surg. 2024;167(2):413–9.

Heck HA Jr, Moore HV, Lutin WA, Leatherbury L, Truemper EJ, Steinhart CM, Pearson-Shaver AL. Esophageal-aortic erosion associated with double aortic arch and tracheomalacia. Experience with 2 infants. Tex Heart Inst J. 1993;20(2):126–9.

Kamran A, Friedman KG, Jennings RW, Baird CW. Aortic uncrossing and tracheobronchopexy corrects tracheal compression and tracheobronchomalacia associated with circumflex aortic arch. J Thorac Cardiovasc Surg. 2020;160(3):796–804.

Midulla PS, Dapunt OE, Sadeghi AM, Quintana CS, Griepp RB. Aortic dissection involving a double aortic arch with a right descending aorta. Ann Thorac Surg. 1994;58(3):874–5.

Othersen HB Jr, Khalil B, Zellner J, Sade R, Handy J, Tagge EP, Smith CD. Aortoesophageal fistula and double aortic arch: two important points in management. J Pediatr Surg. 1996;31(4):594–5.

Russell HM, Rastatter JC, Backer CL. The aortic uncrossing procedure for circumflex aorta. Oper Tech Cardiovasc Surg. 2013;18:15–31.

Sade RM, Rosenthal A, Fellows K, Castaneda AR. Pulmonary artery sling. J Thorac Cardiovasc Surg. 1975;69(3):333–46.

Saran N, Dearani J, Said S, Fatima B, Schaff H, Bower T, Pochettino A. Vascular rings in adults: outcome of surgical management. Ann Thorac Surg. 2019;108(4):1217–27.

Stephens EH, Eltayeb O, Mongé MC, Forbess JM, Rastatter JC, Rigsby CK, Backer CL. Pediatric tracheal surgery: a 25-year review of slide tracheoplasty and tracheal resection. Ann Thorac Surg. 2020;109(1):148–53.

Complications Associated with Repair of Coarctation of the Aorta

Constantine Mavroudis,
Constantine D. Mavroudis, and Richard Hallett

Abstract

Coarctation of the aorta (CoA) is a congenital heart defect where there is significant narrowing of the descending thoracic aorta. It is commonly grouped into three categories: (1) isolated coarctation, (2) coarctation and ventricular septal defect, and (3) coarctation and complex intracardiac anomalies. Complications associated with repair of CoA include paradoxical hypertension, thoracic duct injury, recurrent laryngeal nerve injury, limb ischemia, and paraplegia. This chapter will discuss the importance of preoperative evaluation to avoid errors in judgment and the proper execution of the operation to yield optimal results.

Keywords

Coarctation of the aorta · Congenital heart surgery · Extended end-to-end anastomosis · Aortoplasty

1 Introduction

The classic short-term complications associated with repair of coarctation of the aorta include paradoxical hypertension, thoracic duct injury with lymphatic leak, recurrent laryngeal nerve injury, limb ischemia if subclavian flap aortoplasty is used, residual coarctation, and paraplegia (Backer et al. 1998; Farag et al. 2019; Serfontein and Kron 2002; Amato et al. 1997). The long-term complications include sustained hypertension, aneurysm formation at the site of repair, arteriopathy leading to coronary artery disease, and femoral vascular injury in the event that balloon angioplasty is used for recurrent coarctation (Kappetein et al. 1994; Maxey et al. 2003; Venturini et al. 1978; Bromberg et al. 1989; Rheuban et al. 1985, 1986; Backer et al. 1995; Walhout et al. 2003; Waldhausen and Nahrwold 1966; Kanter et al. 2001; Midgley et al. 1978; Sousa et al. 1983; Beekman et al. 1986; Pandey et al. 2006; Barreiro et al. 2007; van Son et al. 1990; Thomson et al. 2006; Hager et al. 2009; Burch et al. 2009; Tabbutt et al. 2008; Wright et al. 2005; Kumar et al. 2011; Brown et al.

C. Mavroudis (✉)
Chief of Pediatric Cardiothoracic Surgery (Retired), Peyton Manning Children's Hospital, Indianapolis, IN, USA

Professor Emeritus of Surgery, Johns Hopkins University School of Medicine, Baltimore, MD, USA

C. D. Mavroudis
Pediatric Cardiothoracic Surgery, Children's Hospital of Philadelphia, Perelman School of Medicine, University of Pennsylvania, Philadelphia, PA, USA

R. Hallett
Department of Radiology, Stanford University School of Medicine, Stanford, CA, USA

C. L. Backer, C. Mavroudis (eds.), *Complications in Pediatric and Congenital Heart Surgery*,
https://doi.org/10.1007/978-3-032-02661-3_5

2009a, 2010; Sudarshan et al. 2006; Bassareo et al. 2009; Younoszai et al. 2002; Lock et al. 1983; Rothman et al. 2010; Fiore et al. 2005; Rodés-Cabau et al. 2007; Wong et al. 2008; Qureshi et al. 2007; Forbes et al. 2007, 2011; Clarkson et al. 1983; Shaddy et al. 1993; Franco-Paredes et al. 2002; Wilson et al. 2007).

In general, complications associated with repair of coarctation of the aorta tend to occur more often with judgment errors as opposed to technical mishaps. For instance, paraplegia is associated with (1) hyperthermia during the clamp time, (2) extended clamp time, and (3) ligating an excessive number of intercostal arteries. Furthermore, failure to assess the status of the transverse (hypoplastic transverse arch) may result in ill-advised left thoracotomy without a favorable anatomic solution (Gray et al. 2018). This situation, if recognized, should lead to left thoracotomy closure and operation through a median sternotomy with likely cardiopulmonary bypass, liberal coarctectomy and extended end-to-end anastomosis or descending aortic anastomosis to the proximal transverse arch/ascending aorta. Other complications associated with errors in judgment include using patch aortoplasty which could result in remote aneurysm formation, failure to inspect for lymphatic injury/leak, and failure to perform an arterial blood gas measurement before applying the aortic clamp. These omissions can lead to acute and chronic complications which can be ameliorated or prevented with forethought and application of basic surgical principles and judgment.

These issues will be raised as the chapter progresses through the process of coarctation definition, diagnostic methods, and procedures.

2 Coarctation of the Aorta: Definition and Associated Defects

Coarctation of the aorta, is a stenotic disease of the juxtaductal aorta, which causes upper extremity hypertension, lower extremity hypoperfusion, and various degrees of left ventricular hypertrophy or left ventricular failure depending on the tightness of the coarcted segment, the age at presentation, and associated cardiac lesions (Mavroudis 2015). Patients with coarctation of the aorta can be generally characterized into three major groups. The first group, which is the most common is isolated coarctation which can be associated with bicuspid aortic valve. The second group is comprised of patients with coarctation and ventricular septal defect. The third group are patients who have associated complex heart disease, including truncus arteriosus, transposition of the great arteries, double outlet ventricles, the various types of single ventricle, or heterotaxy syndrome. To be inclusive, a rarer form of coarctation exists in which the stenotic segment occurs in the lower thoracic and thoracoabdominal aorta. Unlike the classic form of coarctation, which is caused by ductal tissue contraction, this unusual form of coarctation is assumed to be caused by fetal vascular accidents that result in ischemic injury to the developing aortic wall. The anatomic characteristics of patients with this type of coarctation tend to have very large collateral vessels and are not amenable to extended end-to-end anastomosis. They are best treated by onlay prosthetic patches or bypass grafts if the patients are adolescents or adults (Terramani et al. 2002; Rees et al. 1990).

3 Historical Aspects and Evolution of Coarctation Repair

Coarctation repair has undergone many types of interventions and modifications. The initial procedures logically involved coarctectomy and end-to-end anastomosis (Backer et al. 1998). This operation, while successful in many cases, was complicated by restenosis caused by contraction of residual ductal tissue which was insufficiently resected. More solutions were developed and applied (Backer et al. 1998; Farag et al. 2019;

Serfontein and Kron 2002; Amato et al. 1997). Patch aortoplasty and various forms of subclavian flap aortoplasty were tried (Waldhausen and Nahrwold 1966; Kanter et al. 2001; Midgley et al. 1978; Sousa et al. 1983; Beekman et al. 1986; Pandey et al. 2006; Barreiro et al. 2007) with a certain amount of early success, but they lost popularity because of aneurysm formation (Venturini et al. 1978; Bromberg et al. 1989; Rheuban et al. 1985, 1986; Backer et al. 1995; Walhout et al. 2003), restenosis (Bromberg et al. 1989), and exercise ischemia to the left arm (van Son et al. 1990). It remained for Amato and colleagues in 1977 to introduce a new "Method of enlarging the distal transverse arch n infants with hypoplasia and coarctation of the aorta" (Amato et al. 1997). This procedure was not immediately embraced. However, once the data were analyzed (Backer et al. 1998; Farag et al. 2019; Serfontein and Kron 2002), near universal approval and application of this procedure ensued (Serfontein and Kron 2002). As a result, extended aortic arch dissection, liberal coarctectomy, and extended end-to-end anastomosis has largely replaced all of the aforementioned procedures, with excellent short-term and long-term results. For the sake of completeness, however, all of the techniques mentioned are illustrated in this chapter. Complications associated with these approaches are discussed.

4 Diagnostic Methods to Guide Operation of Choice and Operative Exposure

The initial evaluation for suspected coarctation of the aorta is blood pressure measurements in the right arm and lower extremity. Echocardiography will determine the location of the coarctation segment, the presence or absence of transverse arch hypoplasia, distance between the left common carotid artery and the left subclavian artery, associated lesions such as ventricular septal defect (VSD), and other arch abnormalities such as common brachiocephalic trunk. All of these measurements are important to determine the type of operation that will be performed, the exposure method (left thoracotomy vs. median sternotomy), and the need to perform associated procedures such as pulmonary artery band or closure of a large VSD.

In general, echocardiography is used for diagnostic purposes which should include the location of the coarcted segment and transverse arch anatomy with associated z-score measurements to assess the presence or absence of significant aortic arch hypoplasia. A long distance between the left common carotid artery and left subclavian artery should alert the diagnostician that there could be transverse arch hypoplasia (z-score less than -4 or -5-, or 4-mm transverse arch measurement in neonates and infants). Another measurement tool to determine size suitability of the transverse arch for left thoracotomy and extended end-to-end anastomosis is the number derived by the weight of the baby in kilograms plus one. If this measurement (3 kg child plus 1 = 4) is greater than the narrowest portion of the transverse arch, then the anatomy is deemed suitable (Gray et al. 2018; Ramachandran et al. 2018; Brown et al. 2009b) for repair by left thoracotomy and extended end-to-end anastomosis. If not, the operating team should consider median sternotomy, cardiopulmonary bypass using hypothermia with or without regional perfusion techniques and direct anastomosis between the ascending aorta and the descending aorta (Gray et al. 2018; Ramachandran et al. 2018; Brown et al. 2009b; Sainathan and Mulinari 2022; Tulzer et al. 2016; Anagnostopoulos 2015; Parikh et al. 2021).

Coarctation of the aorta with hypoplasia of the transverse arch, as noted, will challenge the surgeon to perform an extended end-to-end anastomosis through a left thoracotomy since the aortic clamp would need to be placed close to the origin of the innominate artery to achieve an unobstructed arch repair. Computed tomography (CT) and magnetic resonance imaging (MRI) scans, which are being used for accurate diagnosis more and more (Karaosmanoglu et al. 2015), can further delineate the anatomy. A series of CT and MRI scans are shown in Figs. 1 and 2. The scans

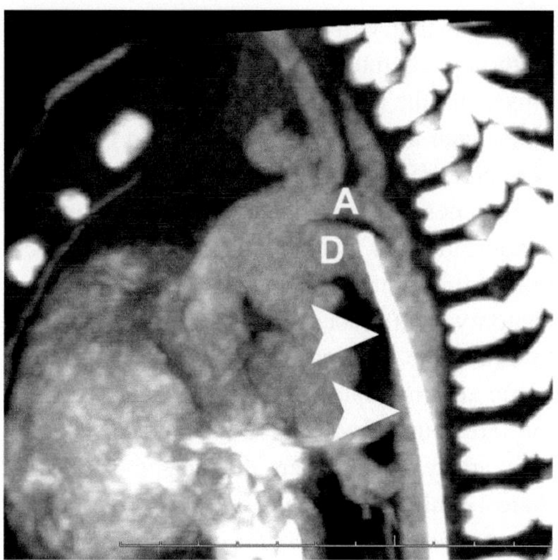

Fig. 1 Sagittal thick-slab maximum intensity projection (MIP). Note diffuse hypoplasia of the transverse thoracic aorta (A) with large patent ductus (D). An umbilical arterial line extends into the origin of the PDA (arrowheads)

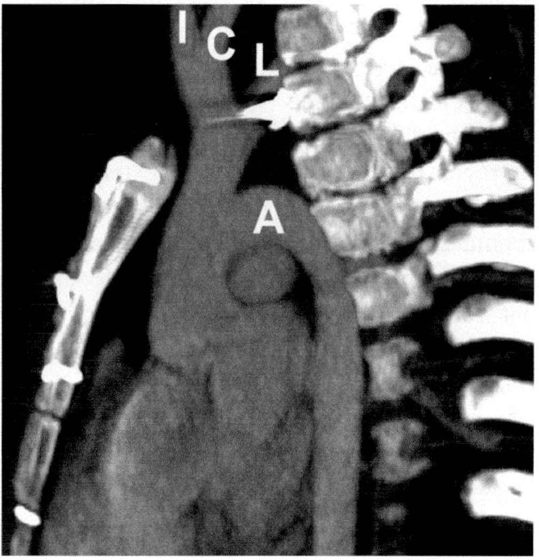

Fig. 2 Six year-old-patient status post repair of ventricular septal defect and juxta-ductal coarctation at 8 days of age, with flow acceleration in arch on surveillance echocardiogram. Thick-slab MIP reconstruction from CTA shows no significant narrowing in the postoperative arch and juxta-ductal region (A). Note a single vessel aortic arch with common trunk giving rise to the innominate (I), left common carotid (C), and left subclavian (L) arteries

show the various forms of coarctation of the aorta which can help the clinicians to determine the most advantageous exposure (left thoracotomy vs. median sternotomy) and the most appropriate operation to achieve a long-term stenosis-free outcome.

Another anatomic variant is coarctation of the aorta associated with common brachiocephalic trunk and narrow transverse arch. Approaching this anomaly through a left thoracotomy will require partial proximal placement of the cross-clamp of the common brachiocephalic trunk. This maneuver will likely cause near occlusion of the aortic arch branches owing to the common brachiocephalic trunk. To our knowledge, no published account of surgical management of this anomaly has been recorded. However, repair through a median sternotomy and cardiopulmonary bypass is highly recommended to avoid the possibilities of left ventricular outflow tract obstruction and cerebral hypoperfusion during the cross-clamp time.

5 Review of Coarctation Repair with Associated Benefits and Complications

5.1 Coarctectomy and Classic End-to-End Anastomosis Without Cardiopulmonary Bypass

The classic operative approach for the repair of coarctation of the aorta is left thoracotomy through the 4th intercostal space. Exposure and dissection for this operation is mostly confined to the area of coarctation involving the arterial duct, the left subclavian artery and the descending aorta. Figures 3, 4, and 5 show the steps of the classic coarctectomy and end-to-end anastomosis. This procedure is infrequently performed nowadays because of the success of the extended

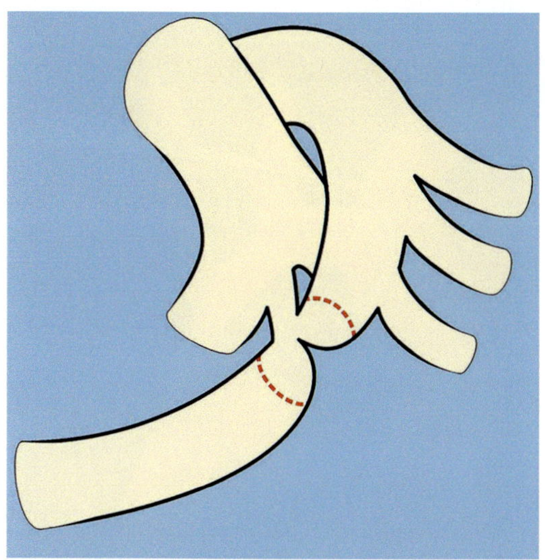

Fig. 3 This is a cartoon that demonstrates the lines of resection for the classic repair of coarctation using coarctectomy and end-to-end anastomosis. (With permission: Mavroudis 2015)

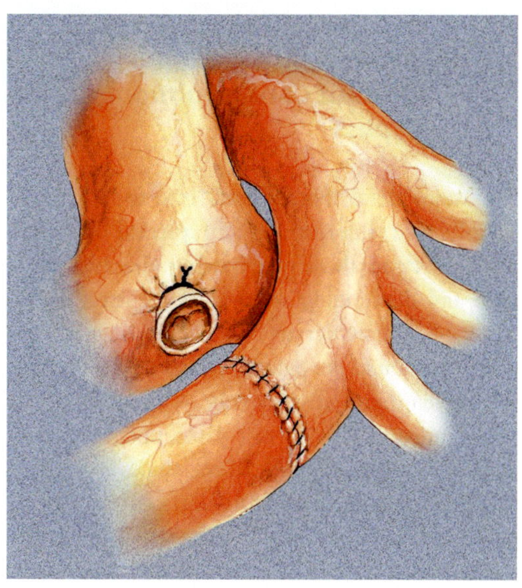

Fig. 5 Shows the completed anastomosis. (With permission: Mavroudis 2015)

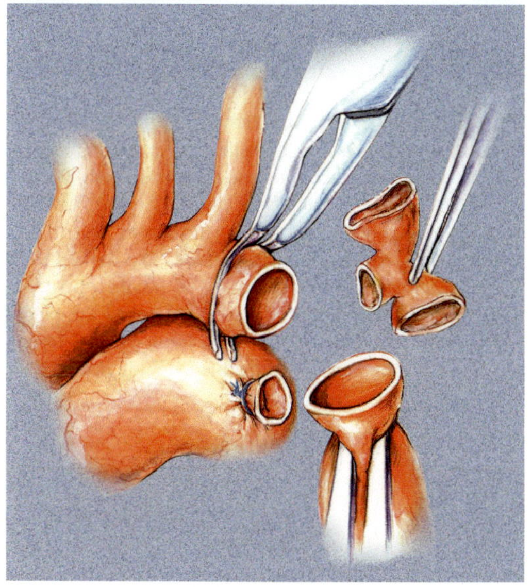

Fig. 4 Shows the clamps being applied to the transverse arch distal to the left subclavian artery and to the descending aorta downstream of the resected coarcted segment. (With permission: Mavroudis 2015)

end-to-end anastomosis. However, it can be employed in older patients with a discrete narrowing of the descending aorta away from the origin of the subclavian artery. The potential immediate surgical complications of such an approach have been noted and include injury to the recurrent laryngeal nerve, thoracic duct injury, excessive hemorrhage, and rarely, paraplegia. Long-term complications include recurrent stenosis, persistent systemic hypertension, aneurysm formation, and endocarditis.

6 Coarctectomy and Extended End-to-End Anastomosis Without Cardiopulmonary Bypass

A posterolateral thoracotomy into the 4th intercostal space is performed with pleural dissection and reflection thereby exposing the transverse arch and descending aorta. The recurrent laryngeal and phrenic nerves can usually be identified coursing around the patent arterial duct and along the pericardium, respectively. Care is taken to avoid injury due to scissor dissection or electrocautery thermal injury. The transverse arch, arterial duct, and descending aorta (with its intercostal branches) are all dissected and mobilized extensively. Anatomic mobilization is very important because a tension free extended end-to-end anastomosis is required to avoid recurrent stenosis and aneurysm formation. As previously mentioned, the transverse arch needs to be evaluated to determine anastomotic suitability. A transverse arch measurement of −4 or −5 z-score should be further evaluated by CTA to determine if the operation needs to be performed through a median sternotomy. The steps of the extended end-to-end anastomosis are shown in Figs. 6, 7, 8, and 9.

Complications associated with this operation are centered around inaccurate measurement of the aortic arch, insufficient mobilization of the aortic arch, injury to the recurrent laryngeal nerve, and injury to the thoracic duct.

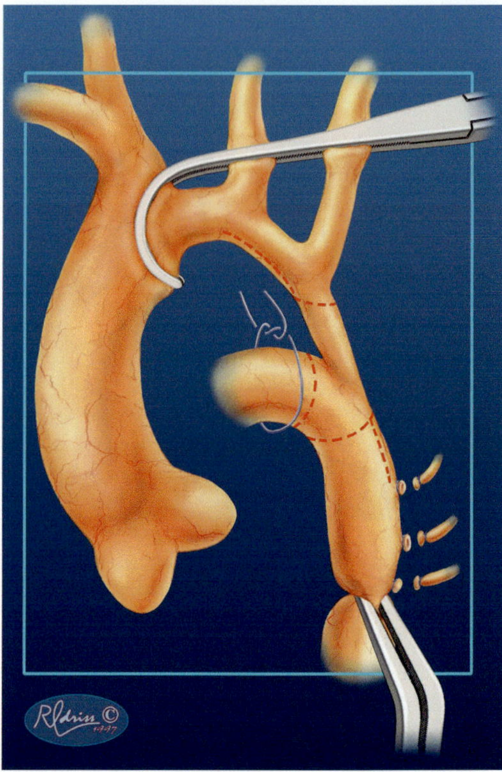

Fig. 6 Shows how the vascular clamp has been placed across the transverse arch distal to the takeoff of the innominate artery, occluding the transverse arch, the left carotid artery, and the subclavian artery. Another vascular clamp is placed on the descending aorta after several collateral arteries are ligated and divided. The dashed lines show the incision lines in preparation for the operation. Also shown in this figure is suture control of the patent ductus arteriosus. Extensive coarctectomy and end-to-end anastomosis can now be performed. (With permission: Mavroudis 2015)

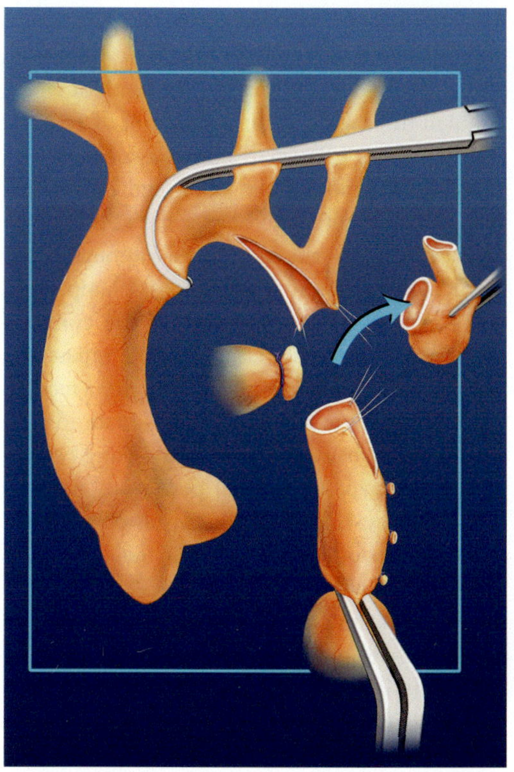

Fig. 7 Shows the removal of the coarcted segment with an incision of the undersurface of the transverse arch towards the area opposite to the orifice of the left common carotid artery. An incision is made in the descending aorta, which will correspond to the anticipated alignment for the extended end-to-end anastomosis. (With permission: Mavroudis 2015)

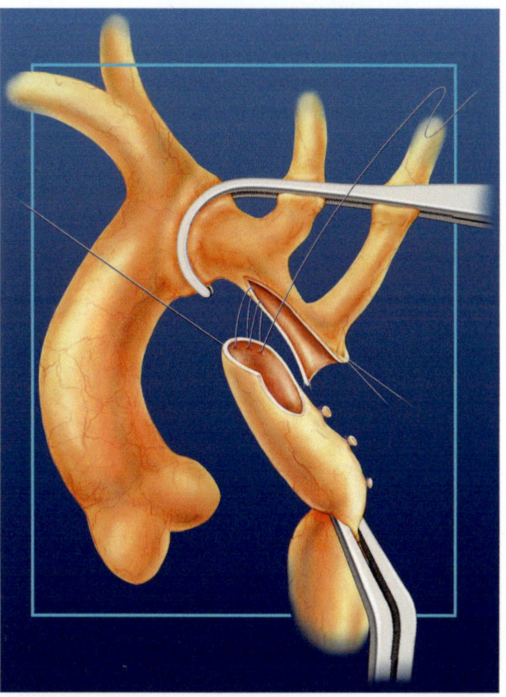

Fig. 8 Shows the extended end-to-end anastomosis in progress. The running suture line (polypropylene) is started at the apex of the transverse arch incision and is carried out posteriorly to align with the descending aorta. (With permission: Mavroudis 2015)

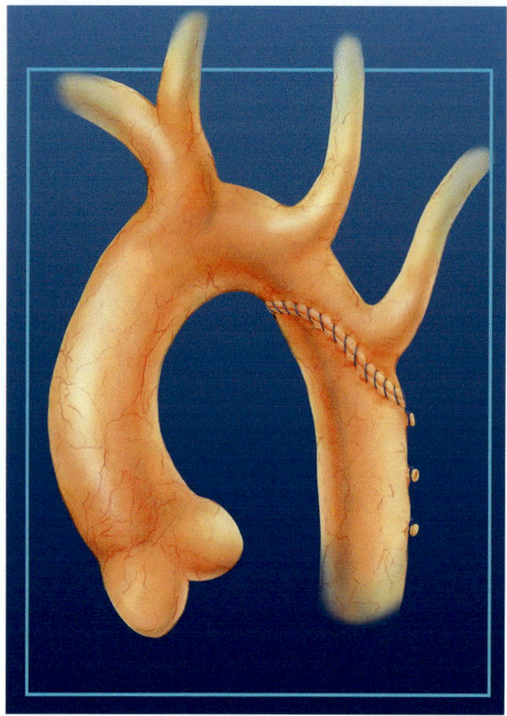

Fig. 9 Shows the completed anastomosis. (With permission: Mavroudis 2015)

Inaccurate preoperative measurement of the transverse aortic arch has been discussed and will result in an inadequate repair. Figure 10a shows the coarctation anatomy with a very narrow transverse arch which is projected to be less than a Z-score of -4. The long distance between the left carotid artery and the left subclavian artery should alert the clinician as to the possibility of a narrow arch. Figure 10b shows the transverse arch clamp placement leaving enough room for ascending aortic flow without severe left ventricular outflow tract obstruction. The trouble is that the clamp is placed across the narrow arch which will not be repaired by the proposed operation. Figure 11 shows the process of extended end-to-end anastomosis which is being performed through the left thoracic cavity. Figure 11b shows the result of an extended end-to-end anastomosis in the presence of an unresolved small aortic arch which will result in an inadequate repair and continued stenosis. This repair would have been better served by a more complete preoperative assessment of the transverse arch which could have been better approached by a median sternotomy, cardiopulmonary bypass, cardioplegic arrest, and regional perfusion, the result of which is noted in Fig. 12. A rarer variation of coarctation and small transverse arch is associated with common brachiocephalic trunk and coarctation (Fig. 13a). Figure 13b shows the result of an extended end-to-end anastomosis through a left thoracotomy. Since the aortic cross-clamp could not be safely placed upstream of the common brachiocephalic trunk, an inadequate repair was performed. Most surgeons would prefer a median sternotomy approach under these conditions to ensure an unobstructed arch repair using cardiopulmonary bypass, regional perfusion, and cardioplegic arrest. The branch vessels do not need to be reanastomosed owing to the successful unobstructed repair (Fig. 13c).

Injuries to the recurrent laryngeal nerve during thoracic surgery are not uncommon (Krasna and Forti 2006; Benouaich et al. 2012). While it is easy to state that recurrent laryngeal nerve injury should not occur, it is important to note some of the procedural steps that should decrease injury. The dissection is important. Noting the recurrent nerve as it circles the patent arterial duct will identify its course and alert the surgeon that comprehensive and careful dissection should be performed in order to allow suture closure of the duct without injuring the nerve. The dissection should be performed by scissors to avoid the inadvertent thermal injury caused by electrocautery. Electrocautery injury can be caused by unwanted direct application. It can also be caused by the unengaged electrocautery instrument for dissection, which can still be hot from previous use a few seconds prior to the new application. This is why scissors dissection is preferable. Another form of recurrent laryngeal nerve injury is placing the ductal clamp too close to the nerve during ductal division. This can be avoided by careful and thorough dissection before clamp application.

Thoracic duct injury is also uncommon during repair of coarctation. Anatomically, lymphatic vessels are thin and easily damaged during dissection. However, clinical signs are usually encountered only when disruption of the major

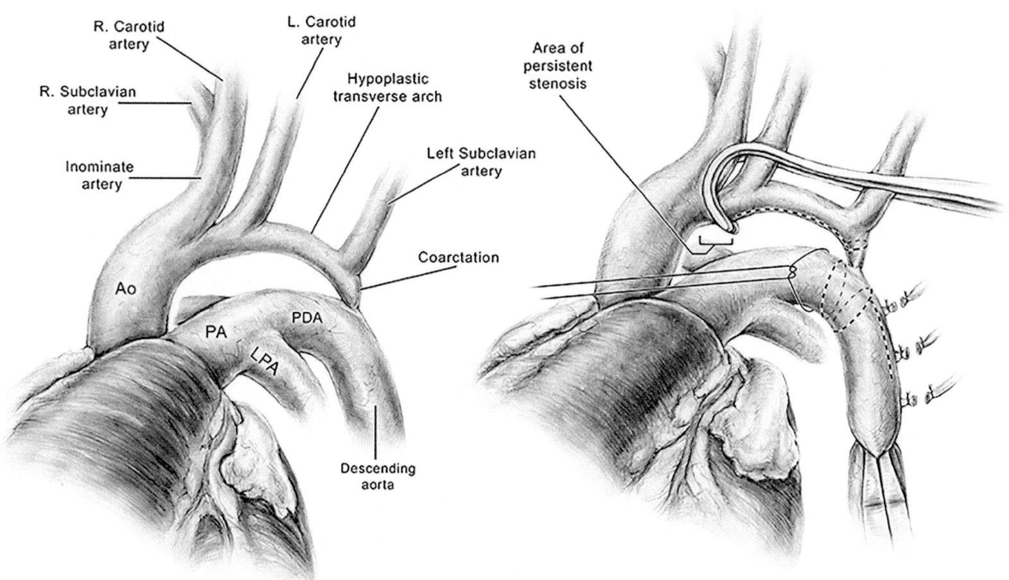

Fig. 10 (Left) depicts the narrow transverse arch which is associated with coarctation of the aorta. Note the long distance between the left carotid artery and the left subclavian artery. The transverse arch in this depiction has a Z-score of less than −4 which is associated with an insufficient repair if the narrow arch is not corrected. (Right) shows the process of attempted extended end-to-end repair. The clamp is placed across the area of aortic arch narrowing since any further upstream placement of the clamp would result in severe left ventricular outflow tract obstruction. *Ao* aorta, *LPA* left pulmonary artery, *PA* pulmonary artery

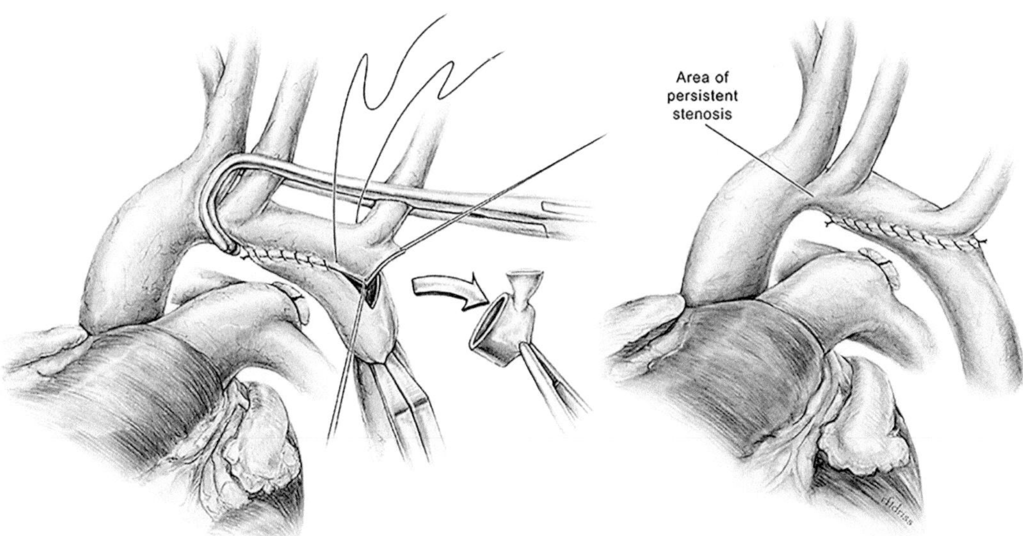

Fig. 11 (Left) shows the extended end-to-end anastomosis in process after coarctectomy and aortic mobilization. While the operation is being shown with excellent technique and good intention, the result as shown in (right) depicts the persistent narrowed aortic arch after the attempted repair. The narrowed segment could not have been addressed since any further upstream placement of the aortic clamp would have resulted in severe left ventricular outflow tract obstruction

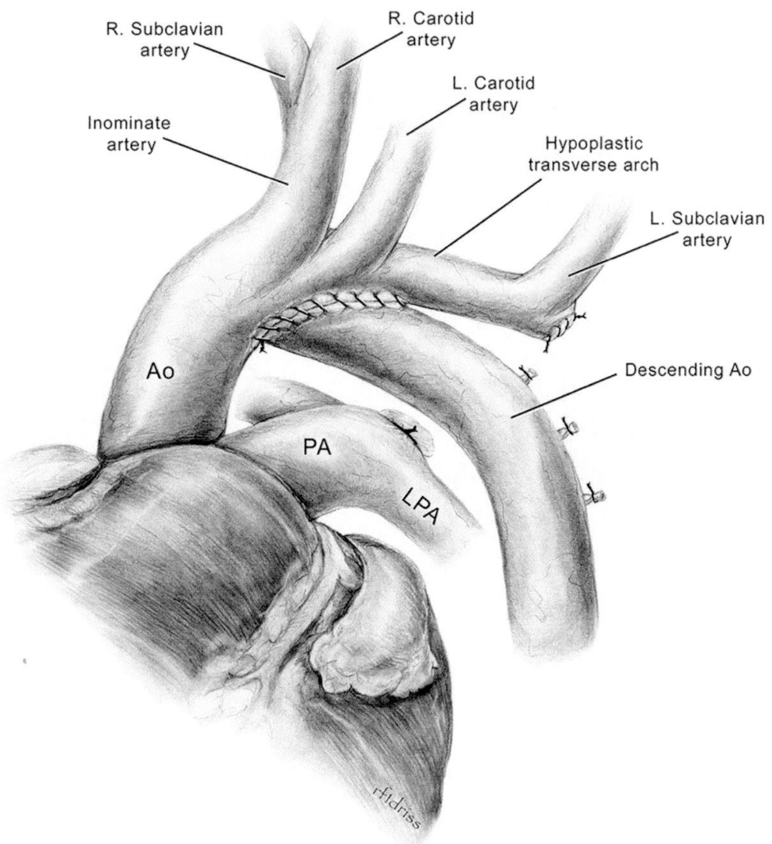

Fig. 12 Shows the ascending aortic to descending aortic anastomosis which was performed by median sternotomy, cardiopulmonary bypass, cardioplegic arrest, and regional perfusion. The transverse arch is left intact which allows adequate flow to the left carotid and left subclavian arteries. *Ao* aorta, *LPA* left pulmonary artery, *PA* pulmonary artery

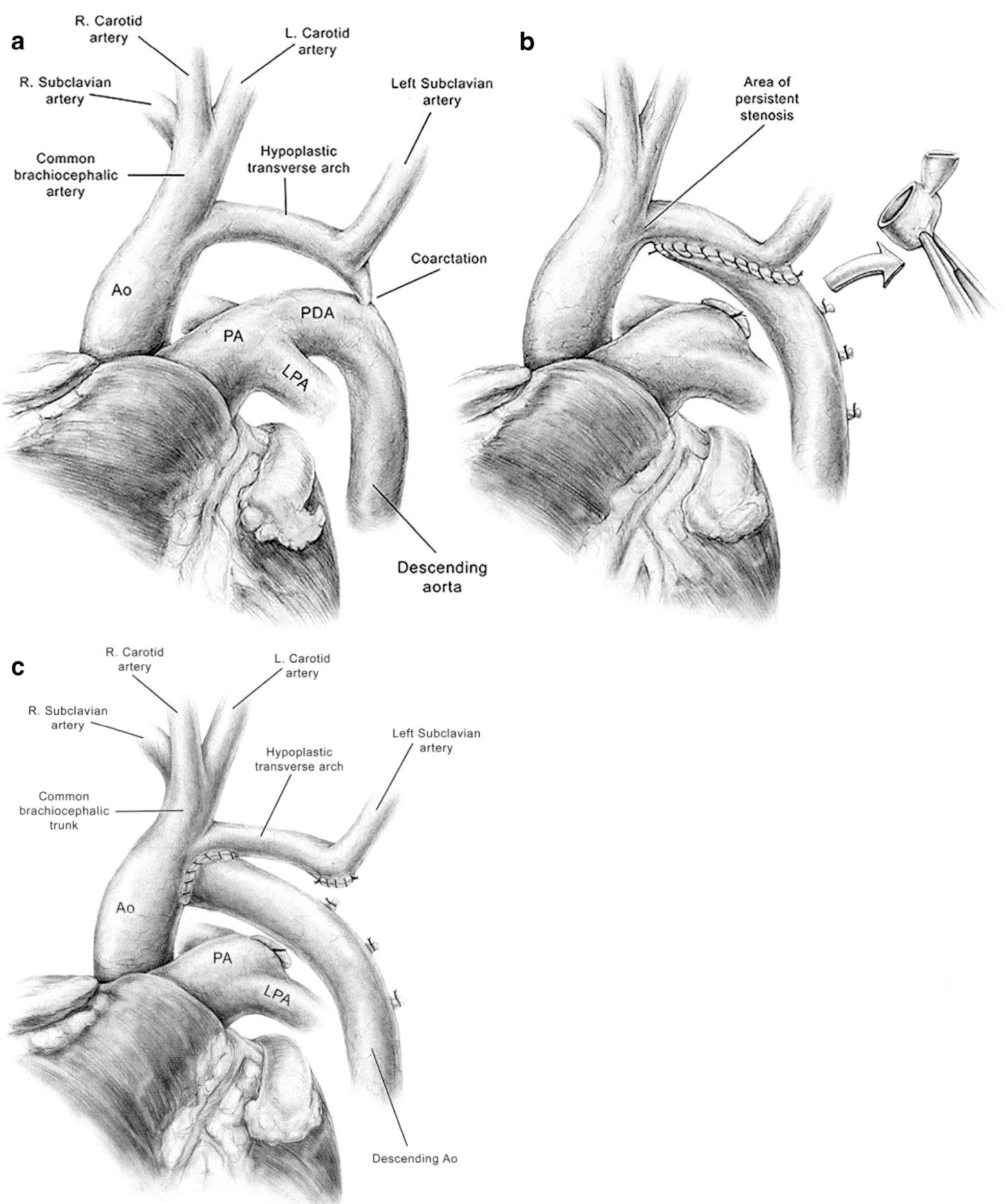

Fig. 13 (**a**) shows the surgical anatomy of a patient with coarctation of the aorta associated with common brachiocephalic trunk and narrow aortic arch. Placement of the aortic cross-clamp during attempted coarctation repair will not allow sufficient aortic exposure for an unobstructed postoperative result. (**b**) shows the inadequate repair which was approached by a left thoracotomy the results of which show a persistent aortic arch obstruction. (**c**) shows the more appropriate repair which is accomplished through a median sternotomy, cardiopulmonary bypass, cardioplegic arrest, and regional perfusion. *Ao* aorta, *LPA* left pulmonary artery, *PA* pulmonary artery, *PDA* patent ductus arteriosus

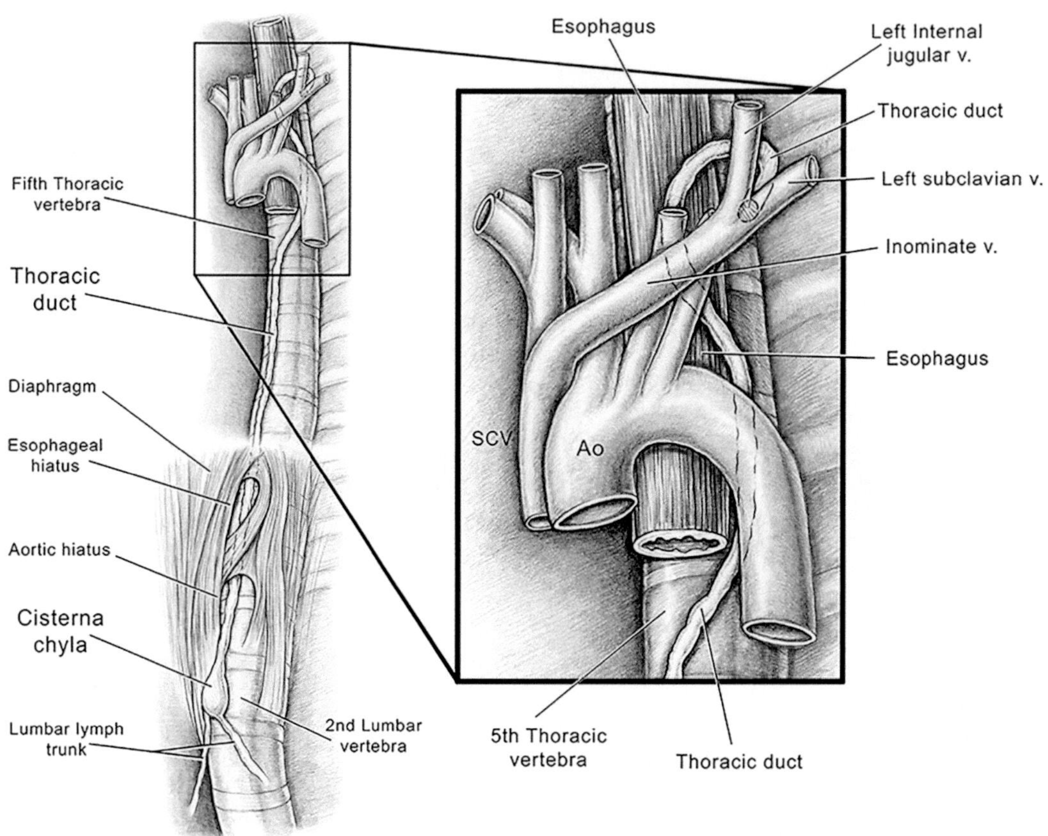

Fig. 14 Drawing of the normal thoracic duct anatomy. While the anatomy is quite variable, in general, the thoracic duct ascends from the Cisterna chyli in the abdomen through multiple channels and enters the thoracic cavity adjacent to the aorta in the right thoracic cavity. It then crosses to the left thoracic cavity at about the 5th thoracic vertebra. As the duct rises, it is protected by the spine, aorta, and mediastinum, making injury to the thoracic duct rare. *Ao* aorta, *SCV* superior caval vein

ducts occurs. This results in thoracic chylous effusions. Chylous effusions are rich in protein and immune rich fluid which when left untreated can cause malnutrition, immunosuppression, dehydration, electrolyte abnormalities, and pulmonary insufficiency due to volume compression. Before the development and introduction of total parenteral nutrition and surgical treatment of thoracic duct injuries mortality rates for thoracic duct leaks approached 50% (Said and Marey 2021; Schild et al. 2013; Cerfolio and Allen 1996; Pillay and Singh 2016; Sharkey and Rao 2012).

The thoracic duct anatomy is variable and can ascend from the Cisterna chyli in the abdomen through multiple channels. In general, however, the thoracic duct enters the thoracic cavity adjacent to the aorta in the right thoracic cavity and crosses to the left thoracic cavity at the level of the 5th thoracic vertebra (Fig. 14). Because of its location, it is protected by the spine, aorta, and mediastinum, making injury to the thoracic duct rare. Nevertheless, thoracic duct injury can occur during extensive dissection caused by unusual arterial anatomy during coarctation repair. In general, the initial pleural incision to identify the aorta and subclavian artery is accomplished directly over these structures. The anterior reflection is then developed to identify the arterial duct, recurrent laryngeal nerve, and transverse arch.

The posterior reflection is then developed to identify the lateral edge of the aorta, the intercostal arteries, and the esophagus. It is in this area between the aorta, the esophagus, the spine, and posterior mediastinum that the thoracic duct can be injured. After the extended end-to-end anastomosis is performed, the prudent surgeon will make every effort to identify a lymphatic leak which will be difficult since the baby has not eaten prior to the operation and there is no cloudy chyle emanating from the presumed injured ducts. An unusual leakage of fluid in this area should alert the surgeon to perform a longitudinal suture line to obliterate the edge of the posterior pleural reflection. Other leaking points can be addressed in the same manner.

In the event that a chylothorax is discovered postoperatively, initial management depends on volume of the leak (Said and Marey 2021). Tube thoracostomy, generally placed at the reparative operation, should be continued and must be adequate to evacuate all fluid and allow the lung to fully re-expand. All measures to reduce the volume of chyle should then be implemented which include a fat free diet enriched in medium-chain triglycerides diet or when indicated, nothing per os (NPO) and total parenteral nutrition. Some authors have used octreotide or somatostatin, which have the effect of reducing gastrointestinal secretion and absorption. This may reduce chyle production leading to resolution (Sharkey and Rao 2012; Lv et al. 2017). Electrolytes, fluids, and fat-soluble vitamins should be monitored and replaced intravenously. Those patients with low and moderately low chylothorax output generally respond well to dietary manipulation and drainage without requiring invasive interventions. Success with conservative management has been reported to be as high as 88% (Said and Marey 2021; Schild et al. 2013; Cerfolio and Allen 1996). Decreasing amounts of chylothorax output will signify successful treatment leading to resolution and implementation of appropriate diets.

What to do when there is excessive chyle leakage coming from the left tube thoracostomy? When medical therapy proves to be unsuccessful, the surgical team may decide to perform interventional therapy. Femoral cannulation of the lymphatic channel in skilled hands can offer an opportunity to deliver an occlusive coil or device to stop the chyle leak (Fig. 15) (Itkin et al. 2010). Surgical therapy can be performed by two methods The classic method is by lower right thoracotomy incision with mass ligation of the thoracic duct at the level of the diaphragm adjacent to the spine, aorta, and esophagus (Cerfolio and Allen 1996). The second method, namely, repeat left thoracotomy and exploration of the injured duct has gained acceptance recently (Bender et al. 2016). The night before the operation, cream is fed to the baby to stimulate chylous flow. Care is taken to stop the feeding at an appropriate time to avoid anesthetic complications. At re-exploration, a significant amount of chyle will be encountered in the left thoracic cavity which should help the surgical team to identify the leak and oversew the

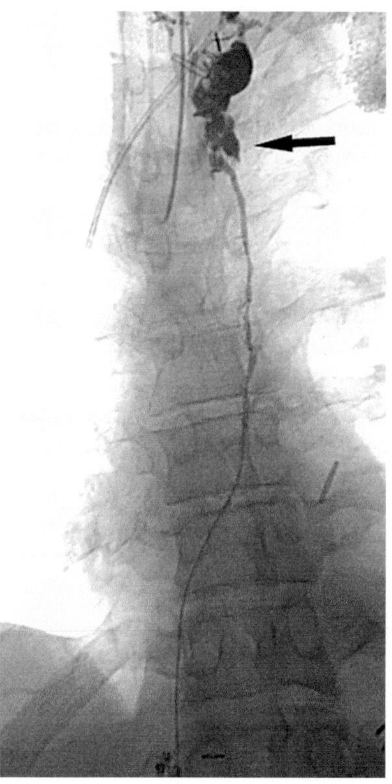

Fig. 15 Radiographic image showing extravasation of the contrast in the upper part of the thoracic duct (*arrow*), following injection of the duct with iodinated contrast through the microcatheter. (With permission: Itkin et al. 2010)

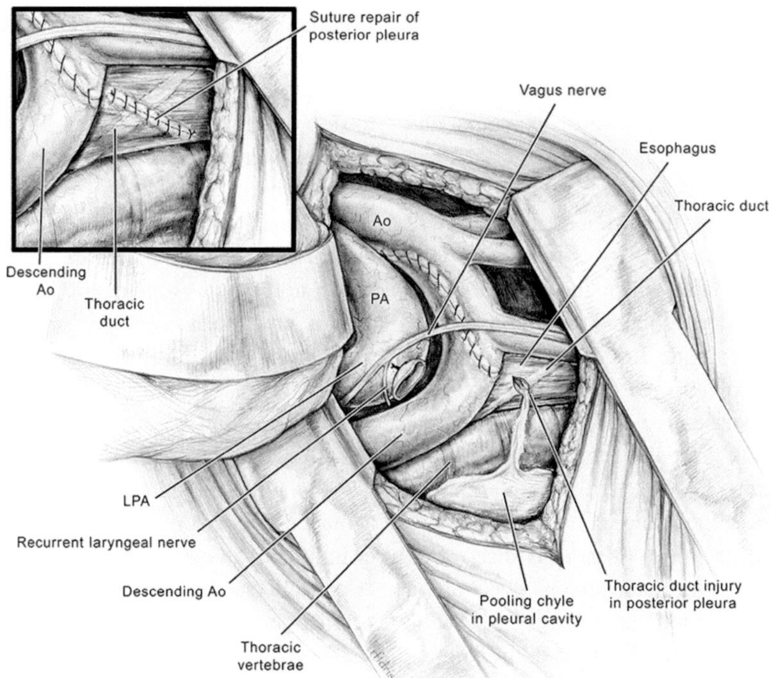

Fig. 16 Because the thoracic duct is nestled between the aorta, the esophagus, the spine, and posterior mediastinum the thoracic duct can be injured during the dissection of the posterior flap of the pleura, which is necessary to expose the anatomy. When the dissection is carried near the thoracic duct, it can be injured. The inset shows a suture line being placed at the posterior pleural flap to include the lymphatic duct injury, which resulted in cessation of lymphatic leak. An oral dose of cream facilitates the identification of the injured duct and will allow proper ligation. *Ao* aorta, *LPA* left pulmonary artery, *PA* pulmonary artery

area of leak. This technique is shown in Fig. 16. Some authors (Cerfolio and Allen 1996) have advocated using biologic pledgets to ensure tissue closure. Mechanical and/or antibiotic pleurodesis can complement the operation. These measures should be successful assuming that the proper precautions are taken.

7 Patch Aortoplasty

Patch aortoplasty is not used routinely in the present era for the management of coarctation of the aorta, but occasionally a long segment of coarcted aortic tissue may require such an approach (Fig. 17). It also can be used in patients with previous repairs who have recurrent coarctation. Figure 18 shows the application of the clamps, with an incision being made in the dotted area to expose the coarcted area for a patch aortoplasty. Figures 19, 20, 21, 22, and 23 show steps and completion of patch aortoplasty. Currently, polytetrafluoroethylene (PTFE) aortoplasty is reserved for long-segment coarctation and reoperative surgery, mainly because of the associated complications of patch aortoplasty, which include aortic aneurysm on the side opposite the PTFE graft (possibly caused by excessive resection of the posterior shelf) and false aneurysm due to suture-line disruption or infection.

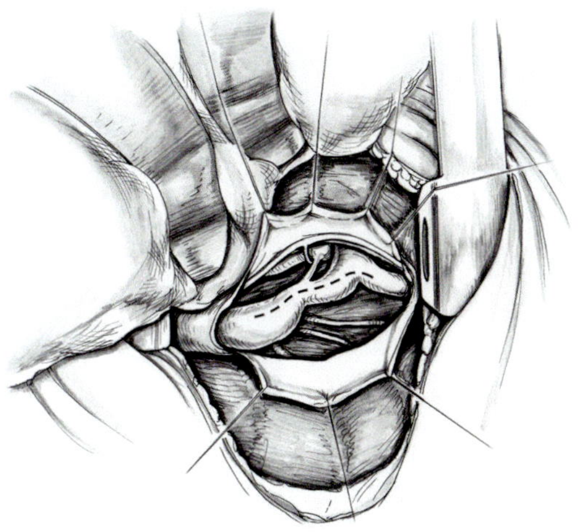

Fig. 17 Shows the dissected coarcted segment with the dotted line indicating the proposed aortic incision for patch aortoplasty once the aortic clamps are placed. (With permission: Mavroudis 2015)

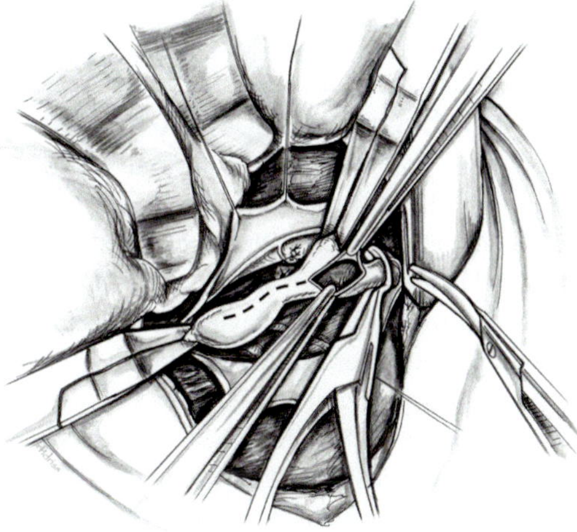

Fig. 18 Shows the application of vascular clamps, with an incision being made in the dotted area to expose the coarcted area for a patch aortoplasty. (With permission: Mavroudis 2015)

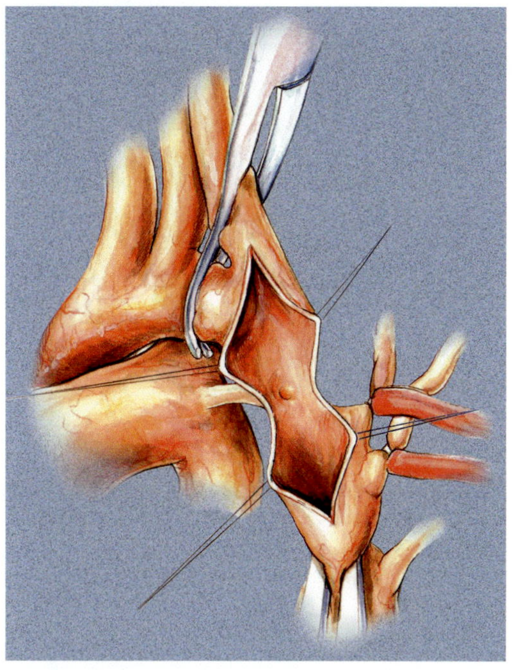

Fig. 19 Shows the application of occlusive vascular clamps, tourniquet control of intercostal arteries, and longitudinal incision across the area of coarctation. No effort is made to perform a coarctectomy, although some authors have advocated coarctectomy, posterior anastomosis, and patch aortoplasty in combination. (With permission: Mavroudis 2015)

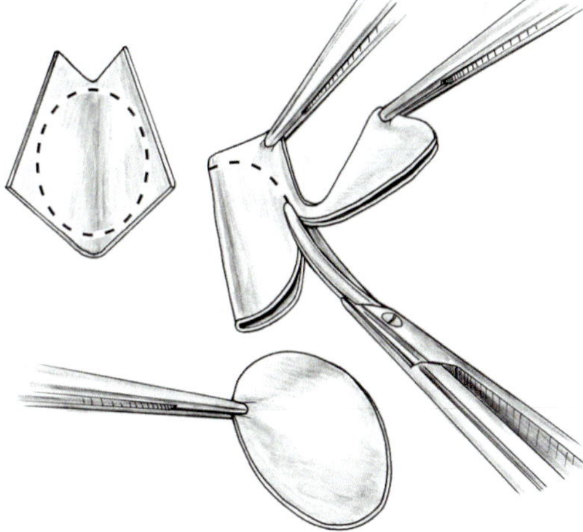

Fig. 20 Shows the method of trimming the ovoid polytetrafluoroethylene (PTFE) patch to be placed to account for growth of the surrounding aortic tissue. (With permission: Mavroudis 2015)

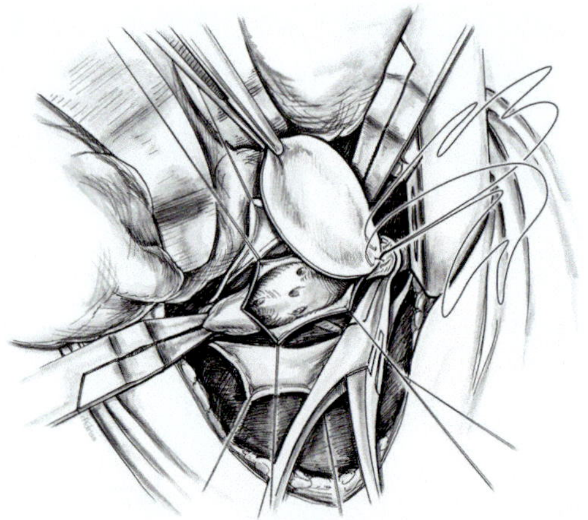

Fig. 21 Shows the beginning of PTFE aortoplasty using the running suture technique, (With permission: Mavroudis 2015)

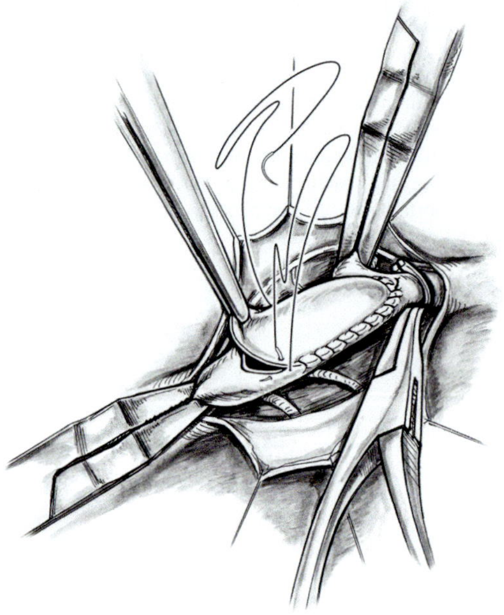

Fig. 22 Shows the application of the distal portion of the patch. (With permission: Mavroudis 2015)

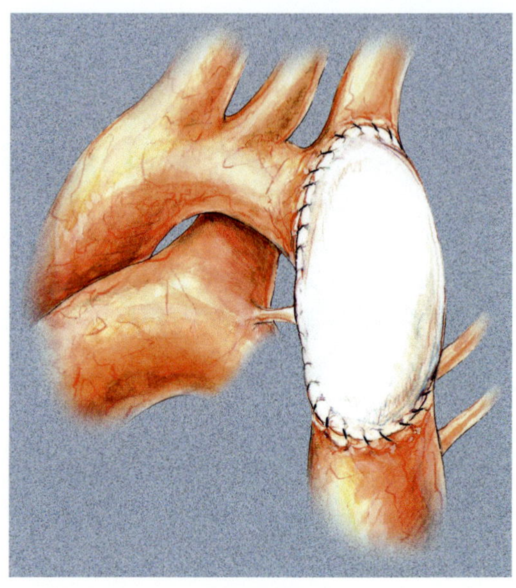

Fig. 23 Shows a completed PTFE patch aortoplasty. (With permission: Mavroudis 2015)

8 Subclavian Flap Aortoplasty

Subclavian flap aortoplasty takes its origin from the clinical experience with the classic Blalock-Taussig-Thomas (BTT) shunt, which required distal ligation of the subclavian artery and was reasonably well tolerated in the infant population on which it was practiced (Midgley et al. 1978). Besides successful repair when not associated with a narrow transverse aortic segment, the subclavian artery patch has been shown to undergo somatic growth and therefore allow continued unobstructed aortic reconstruction and avoid the problems of recurrent coarctation (Barreiro et al. 2007). Figures 24, 25, 26, and 27 show the steps of subclavian patch aortoplasty.

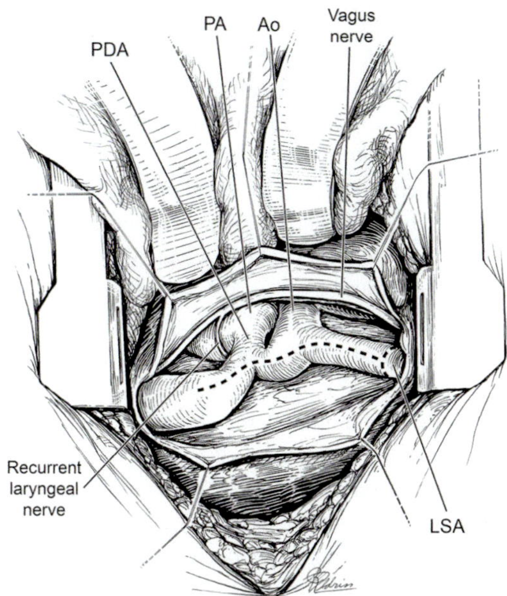

Fig. 24 Shows the relevant anatomy, highlighting the extent of the subclavian artery dissection. The dotted lines indicate the longitudinal incision required and the area of subclavian artery transection. (With permission: Mavroudis 2015). *Ao* aorta, *LSA* left subclavian artery, *PA* pulmonary artery, *PDA* patent ductus arteriosus

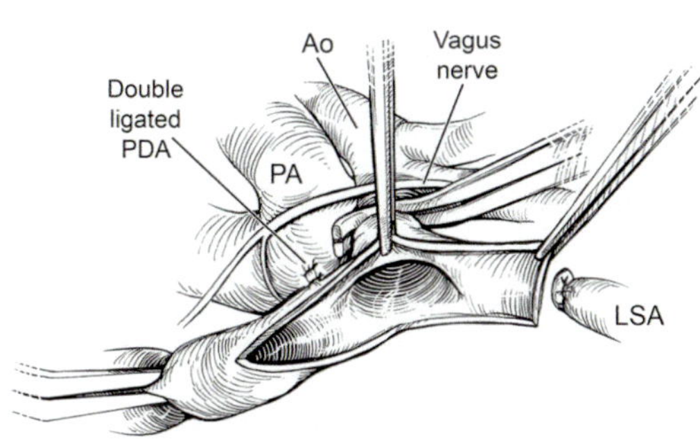

Fig. 25 Shows application of the clamps to the transverse arch and descending aorta, with the ductus arteriosus ligated and divided. The subclavian artery has been ligated and incised; it is now free to be placed onto the coarcted segment for repair. (With permission: Mavroudis 2015). *Ao* aorta, *LSA* left subclavian artery, *PA* pulmonary artery, *PDA* patent ductus arteriosus

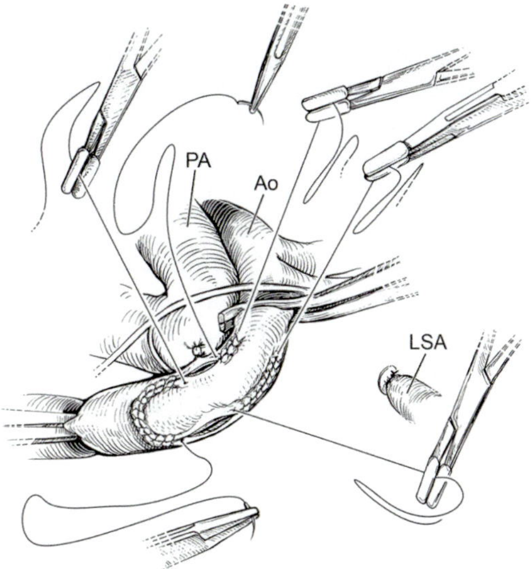

Fig. 26 Shows the subclavian flap being sutured to the edges of the aorta en route to completion. (With permission: Mavroudis 2015). *Ao* aorta, *LSA* left subclavian artery, *PA* pulmonary artery

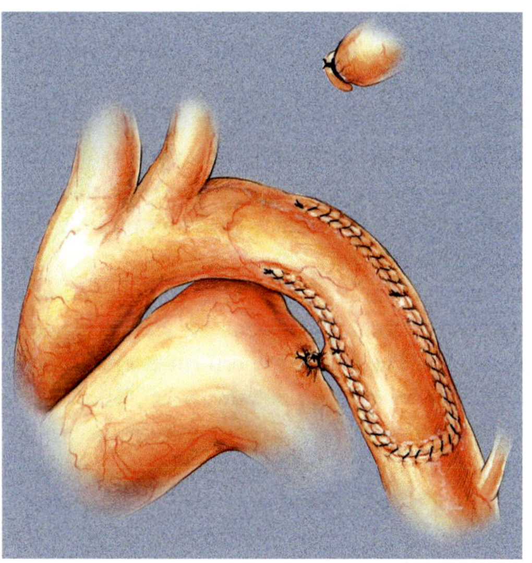

Fig. 27 Shows the completed subclavian patch aortoplasty. (With permission: Mavroudis 2015)

This operation is not generally used nowadays owing to reports of upper extremity exercise intolerance (van Son et al. 1990) despite the early experience with this operation which documented excellent upper extremity vascular tolerance in the short term (Sharma et al. 1992).

9 Transmediastinal Coarctation Repair in Association with Ventricular Septal Defect Closure

Coarctation of the aorta is often associated with a VSD, which can present the operating team with more complex difficulties in surgical management. In the case of a small VSD which may close spontaneously or can be managed medically, the surgical option is to repair the coarctation only. Clearly, this option is limited to those patients with hemodynamically insignificant VSDs. Another option reserved mostly for infants with large left-to-right shunts and severe heart failure, is coarctation repair and pulmonary artery bending through a left thoracotomy. However, most surgeons avoid pulmonary artery banding due to the association with pulmonary trunk scarring and potential right ventricular outflow tract obstruction.

Another surgical option is to concomitantly repair both lesions. This can be accomplished in two ways. The first is to perform a left thoracotomy and coarctation repair to be followed by median sternotomy and VSD closure using cardiopulmonary bypass. This method has produced excellent results (Callahan et al. 2017); however, it requires two separate operations at the same setting. Nevertheless, there are some benefits to this approach. Once the coarctation is repaired, the VSD closure through the mediastinal approach does not require deep hypothermia and regional perfusion or circulatory arrest to repair the coarctation, since it has been repaired. Furthermore, cardiopulmonary bypass can be accomplished with a more homogeneous circulatory perfusion strategy since the coarctation has been repaired. Nevertheless, most surgeons have abandoned this technique for simultaneous repair of both the VSD and coarctation through a median sternotomy.

The second option is simultaneous repair as noted. This approach has undergone improvement over the years taking advantage of perfusion techniques of deep hypothermia and circulatory arrest as well as regional perfusion (Brouwer et al. 1996; Gaynor et al. 2000; Lim et al. 2003, 2007).

While the infant is being cooled on cardiopulmonary bypass, extensive dissection of the great vessels and descending aorta permits coarctectomy and extended end-to-end anastomosis, as well as correction of hypoplasia of the transverse aortic arch. Most surgeons prefer to perform the coarctectomy and anastomosis within 15–20 min of deep circulatory arrest and then close the VSD once cardiopulmonary bypass is reestablished (Brouwer et al. 1996; Gaynor et al. 2000; Lim et al. 2003, 2007). Some surgeons use low-flow and regional perfusion techniques to limit the period of circulatory arrest as much as possible (Lim et al. 2003).

Complications regarding these techniques stem from improper use of cardiopulmonary bypass and circulatory arrest which can result in neurological injury, residual VSD, and acquired heart block (Lim et al. 2003).

10 Coarctectomy and Interposition Graft Using Partial Cardiopulmonary Bypass

While no definite cause for paraplegia has been identified in patients who undergo coarctation repair, several risk factors have been noted in the literature. They include a long cross-clamp time, hyperthermia during the cross-clamp time, and decreased distal perfusion pressure in the lower extremity. These are important considerations for the development of paraplegia and should be

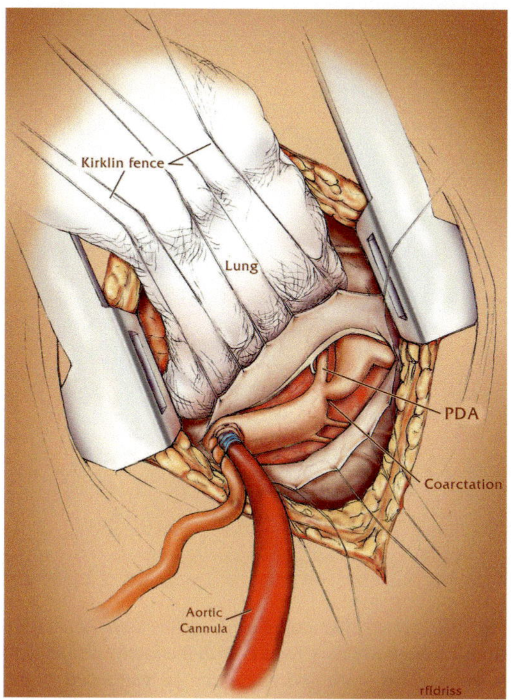

Fig. 28 Shows a completed dissection of the transverse arch, ductus arteriosus, and descending aorta in preparation for coarctectomy repair. A test clamp of the transverse arch revealed that the perfusion pressure in the lower extremity was below 30 torr. After systemic heparinization, an arterial line is placed in the descending aorta well away from the area of coarctectomy. (With permission: Mavroudis 2015)

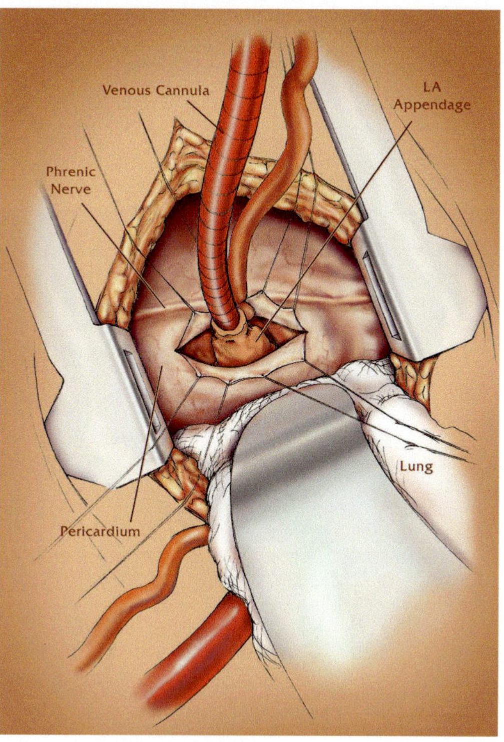

Fig. 29 Shows a transverse incision in the pericardium just posterior to the phrenic nerve for identification and isolation of the left atrial appendage. Once the left atrium is identified and controlled with a purse string suture, a venous catheter is placed making sure to avoid any air entry. Many surgeons prefer to place the left atrial cannula at the base of the left atrial appendage towards the pulmonary veins to enhance drainage and avoid coronary injury caused by atrial appendage retraction (not shown). Cardiopulmonary bypass can then be commenced in this manner by adjusting the arterial flow to approximately 40% of cardiac output and adjusting left atrial drainage to allow an upper extremity pressure in the normal range for the patient. Ventilation to the right lung is carried out during this time. (With permission: Mavroudis 2015)

avoided. Most surgeons avoid long cross-clamp times (>30 min); and prefer time periods between 15 and 20 min. The aortic cross-clamp should not be applied if the somatic temperature is above 37 °C. In those instances where the temperature is above 37 °C, iced saline can be placed in the thoracic cavity to decrease the temperature before the application of a cross-clamp. When the perfusion pressure is below 35–40 mmHg as measured by a distal arterial line, partial cardiopulmonary bypass should be strongly considered. Figures 28, 29, 30, 31, and 32 demonstrate the steps of coarctectomy and interposition graft using cardiopulmonary bypass. Important points to avoid complications are noted within the figure legends.

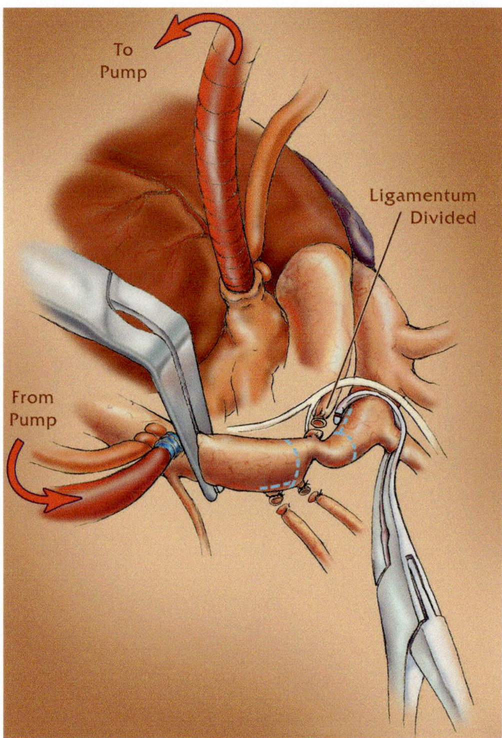

Fig. 30 Shows partial cardiopulmonary bypass in process with the bypass circuit flow annotated by the arrows. The 2 clamps are placed there by isolating the stenotic segment and the dotted lines show the anticipated resection. In this case, the patient was older and required an interposition graft to avoid anastomotic tension. (With permission: Mavroudis 2015)

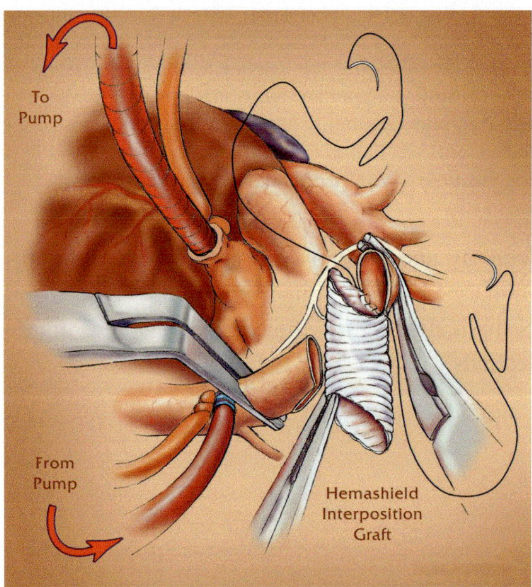

Fig. 31 Shows the proximal anastomosis in progress using a Dacron graft. Note that the recurrent laryngeal nerve is identified and preserved. (With permission: Mavroudis 2015)

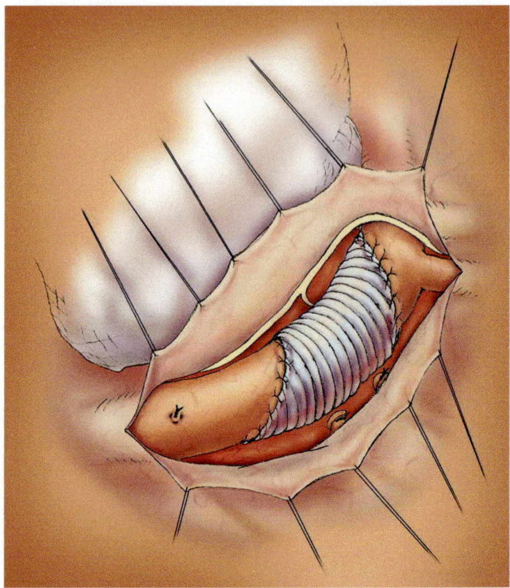

Fig. 32 Shows the completed repair after separation from cardiopulmonary bypass with the interposition graft in place. This same procedure can be employed in the event that coarctectomy and extended end-to-end anastomosis without an interposition graft could be performed. In addition, this same interposition graft can be used in older patients with limited mobilization potential without partial cardiopulmonary bypass. (With permission: Mavroudis 2015)

11 The Adult with Coarctation

Coarctation of the aorta can present during adult life during the evaluation of systemic hypertension. Physical examination usually shows differences in upper and lower extremity pulses and noninvasive blood pressure measurements. Large collateral arteries however may confound the diagnosis which will require further evaluation. There is often a history of prior coarctation repair, but some patients present with a delayed diagnosis of native coarctation, which, as noted, is usually identified during an evaluation for hypertension. Associated symptoms include exertional headaches and exercise intolerance with leg fatigue (claudication). Associated anatomic findings are bicuspid aortic valve and mitral valve abnormalities. Without treatment, significant coarctation is associated with a reduced life expectancy owing to systemic hypertension, accelerated

coronary artery disease, stroke, aortic dissection, and congestive heart failure.

The American College of Cardiology/American Heart Association (ACC/AHA) guidelines (2008) (Warnes et al. 2008) for adults with congenital heart disease (ACHD), recommend intervention for coarctation in the presence of a peak-to-peak coarctation gradient (by catheterization data) of 20 mmHg or greater, or a peak-to-peak coarctation gradient less than 20 mmHg in the presence of anatomic imaging evidence of significant coarctation (a coarctation lumen less than 50% of the aortic lumen at the diaphragm) with radiologic evidence of significant collateral flow. There are two methods of treating coarctation of the aorta: transcatheter or surgical techniques.

12 Transcatheter Methods to Repair

Transcatheter techniques to treat recoarctation and native coarctation in adults have achieved general acceptance and are the procedures of choice in many centers (Torok et al. 2015; Alkashkari et al. 2020; Qureshi 2009; Tilea et al. 2012; Kutty et al. 2008).

Transcatheter techniques for coarctation repair are usually performed by aortic dilation with stent placement. Specific noncontroversial indications for transcatheter stent positioning for either primary or recurrent coarctation include discrete, short-segment, stenosis and a favorable landing zone that does not compromise the origin of the left subclavian artery, as noted in Fig. 33. Covered stents are recommended when primary coarctation is being treated to avoid aortic wall and intimal disruption. Either uncovered or covered stents can be used for patients with recoarctation since surrounding scar tissue can prevent unwanted hemodynamically significant hemorrhage. False aneurysms however can occur which will require a covered stent (Alkashkari et al. 2020). Further to this discussion, transcatheter techniques are not always applicable especially when used to dilate a longer segment of stenotic aorta, particularly in patients with primary coarc-

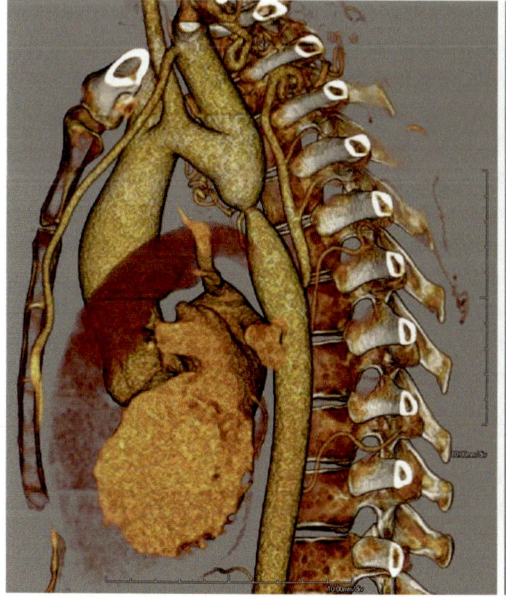

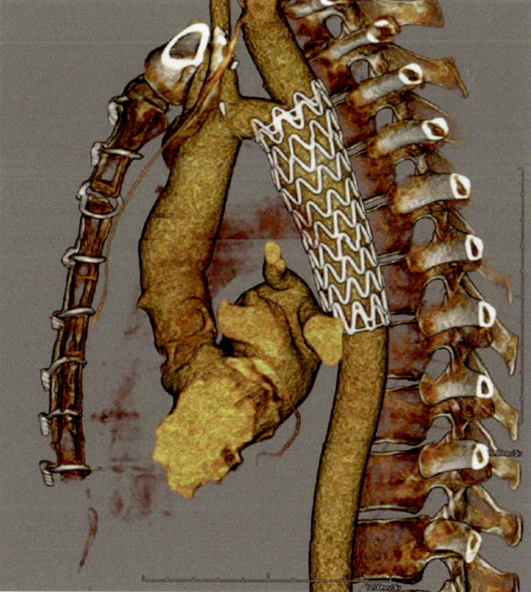

Fig. 33 Shows two MRIs showing a transcutaneous placement of a stent for recoarctation of the aorta with excellent results

tation; a tortuous, narrowed aortic isthmus; or compromise of the left subclavian artery orifice (Tilea et al. 2012; Kutty et al. 2008). When the subclavian artery is part of the aortic stenotic segment, carotid-subclavian bypass may provide an alternative solution since the stent can be deployed across the subclavian artery orifice knowing that an alternative vascular pathway can be established. These decisions regarding transcatheter versus surgical approaches are often complex and not straightforward. It is for this reason that decisions regarding the most effective and safe procedure should be made with joint interventionalist-surgeon consultation to optimize the best approach for each individual patient.

13 Surgical Methods to Repair Recoarctation or Native Coarctation in the Adult

Surgical methods to treat recoarctation or native coarctation in the adult center around creating unobstructed pulsatile flow to the lower extremity to avoid the complications noted earlier in this chapter (Mavroudis 2015; Dearani and Mavroudis 2020). This chapter presents the most commonly used methods to address aortic obstruction at the level of the aortic isthmus and/or aortic arch. The approach may be median sternotomy or left thoracotomy. Adults with undiagnosed native coarctation usually present with persistent hypertension, but rarely present with complications such as endocarditis, aneurysm, or disruption. Surgical repair of recoarctation of the aorta is a challenging procedure that requires considerable forethought and surgical planning. There are two approaches for this repair: the anatomic repair, which centers the operative procedure directly at the recoarctation segment and the extra-anatomic repair, which employs bypass graft techniques to avoid dissection at the original repair site. The surgical approach to the recoarctation site (anatomic repair) can be performed through a left thoracotomy or through a transmediastinal approach. The left thoracotomy approach is challenged by the disadvantages and problems of a redo thoracotomy, with associated blood loss, lung injury, nerve (phrenic or recurrent laryngeal) damage, and thoracic duct injury. The advantages of this approach are optimal exposure of the descending aorta, the ability to perform partial or complete cardiopulmonary bypass, and diverse options for re-repair, the interposition graft being the most common. The transmediastinal approach also has some advantages. In many cases of recoarctation, the mediastinum has not been explored, except in situations such as closure of an associated VSD earlier in life. Hemodynamic control is optimized, as it allows the surgeon the options of cardiopulmonary bypass, deep hypothermia, and circulatory arrest.

14 Left Thoracotomy Approach

This section is a narrative to iterate the important steps of these operations in adults which in turn will help to avoid complications and result in an excellent result (Dearani and Mavroudis 2020). As has been discussed, adult patients with coarctation can present for the first time (primary) or as a result of recoarctation. Left thoracotomy approach is favored for obstruction in the aortic isthmus, proximal descending aorta, and in some situations, the distal arch. In preparation for the operation the patient is placed in a right lateral decubitus position with the hips rolled out leftward to 45° to provide access to the left groin. Conscientious monitoring is accomplished by right radial and right femoral arterial cannulation. A double-lumen endotracheal tube is used to

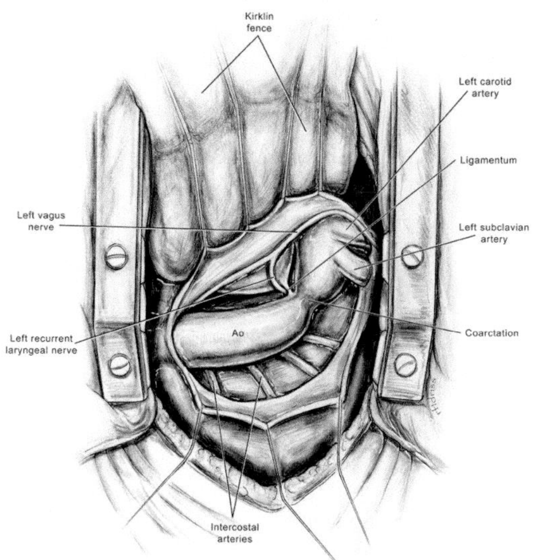

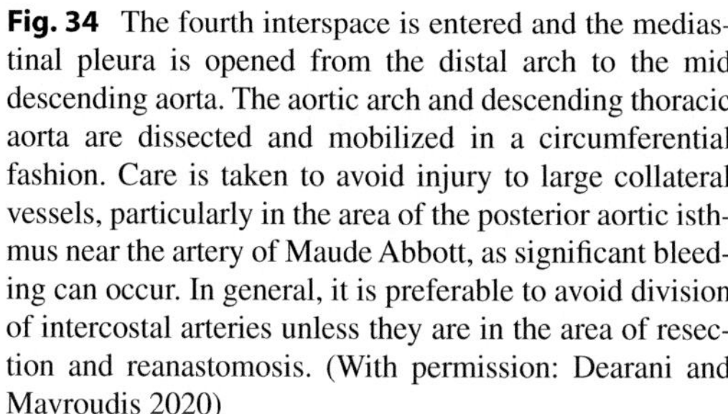
Fig. 34 The fourth interspace is entered and the mediastinal pleura is opened from the distal arch to the mid descending aorta. The aortic arch and descending thoracic aorta are dissected and mobilized in a circumferential fashion. Care is taken to avoid injury to large collateral vessels, particularly in the area of the posterior aortic isthmus near the artery of Maude Abbott, as significant bleeding can occur. In general, it is preferable to avoid division of intercostal arteries unless they are in the area of resection and reanastomosis. (With permission: Dearani and Mavroudis 2020)

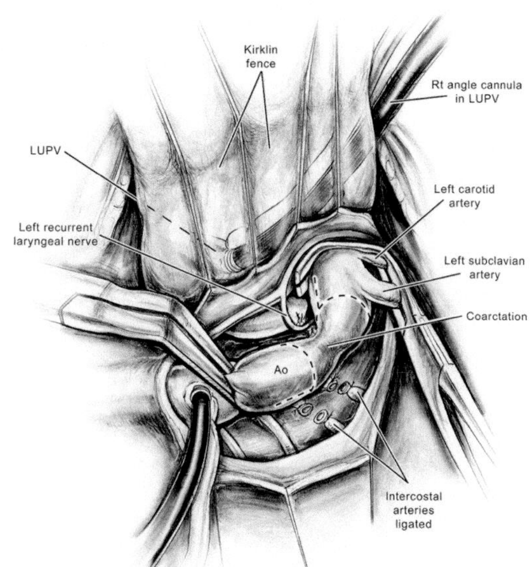

Fig. 35 Shows the preparation for the repair. An arterial line is placed in the descending aorta (if a femoral arterial line is not in place), well away from the area of coarctectomy. Partial cardiopulmonary bypass is in process. Note the hidden anatomy showing the left atrial cannula which is placed in the body of the left atrium below the atrial appendage. This position enhances outflow and prevents torsion on the left atrial appendage which could cause coronary artery injury. Two clamps are placed, isolating the stenotic segment; the *dotted lines* show the anticipated resection. In this case, an interposition graft is employed. (With permission: Dearani and Mavroudis 2020)

allow collapse of the left lung, which facilitates mediastinal dissection. Transesophageal echocardiography (TEE) is routinely used and provides pre- and postoperative evaluation. In addition, the TEE probe provides a landmark for the esophagus during the posterior mediastinal dissection. Figures 34, 35, and 36 show the important steps of the operation with special attention to avoid complications. While this series of diagrams depict partial cardiopulmonary bypass, coarctectomy and interposition graft, there are some cases where partial bypass may not be necessary. This will depend on the distal perfusion pressure after cross-clamps are placed across the aortic arch between the left subclavian and left carotid artery and the descending thoracic aorta beyond the area of anastomosis. This will allow measurement and analysis of the distal perfusion pressure. If the distal perfusion pressure is easily maintained at or above 40 mmHg, then the operating team may consider not using left heart bypass for the reconstruction. Under these circumstances, the distal perfusion pressure is more likely to be maintained in an acceptable range with primary coarctation due to significant collateralization. On the other hand, partial bypass is more often required for patients with recoarctation because of less collateralization (Dearani and Mavroudis 2020). Despite these general principles and despite the fact that an acceptable distal pressure may avert the use of left heart bypass, most surgeons will apply left heart bypass to establish predictable perfusion to avoid the need to hurry through an anastomosis in the event that the perfusion pressure falls while aortic clamps are in place.

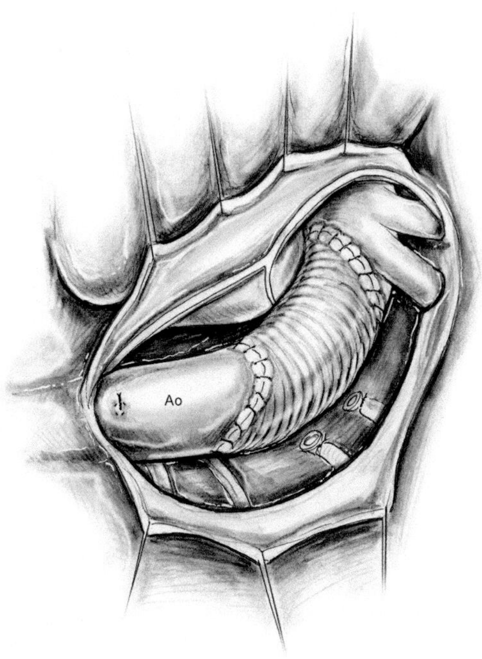

Fig. 36 Shows the completed repair after separation from cardiopulmonary bypass with the interposition graft in place; this provides an anatomic reconstruction of the descending thoracic aorta. Under these circumstances in adult patients, resection and end-to-end anastomosis is usually not feasible without undue tension at the anastomosis, so an interposition graft is used. Note that the recurrent laryngeal nerve is identified and preserved. (With permission: Dearani and Mavroudis 2020)

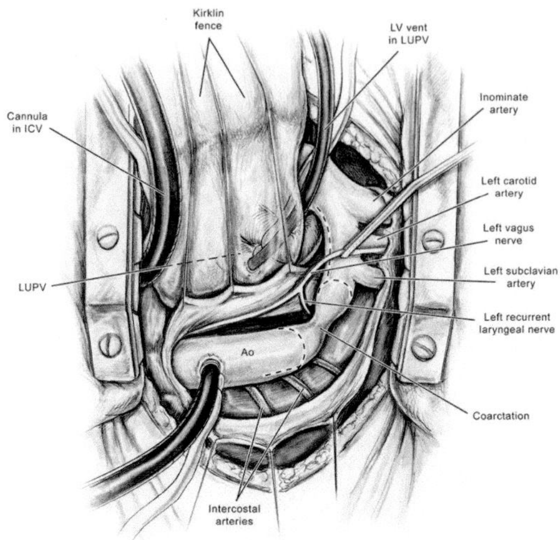

Fig. 37 Cannulation for left heart bypass is usually accomplished with either left femoral artery or descending aortic cannulation. In both situations, a flexible femoral artery cannula is used with the Seldinger technique. This is particularly helpful if the descending thoracic aorta is used in a deep-chested patient, as it avoids the need to extend the thoracotomy incision to improve exposure. The left atrium can be cannulated via the left atrial appendage or directly at the level of the left upper pulmonary vein. Preference is to cannulate the left atrium at the upper pulmonary vein with a metal-tipped right-angle cannula. This avoids manipulation of the left atrial appendage, which can be quite fragile and vulnerable to tearing. (With permission: Dearani and Mavroudis 2020)

Partial (left heart) bypass cannulation is also important and the preferred option when addressing either discrete or long-segment stenosis of the proximal descending aorta. The steps of the operation are noted in Figs. 37, 38, and 39. Distal aortic arch hypoplasia with or without descending aortic coarctation or recoarctation is better approached using complete bypass cannulation. Arterial cannulation is performed in the same manner as described. Systemic venous access is accomplished by right atrial cannulation at the inferior caval vein (ICV). The left heart is vented by catheter insertion into the left superior pulmonary vein or the left ventricular apex. This drainage technique is especially important if the patient has mild aortic regurgitation. The left ventricular catheter will avoid left ventricular dilatation during the cooling and rewarming process, when ventricular fibrillation is apt to occur. Deep hypothermia is established, with an anticipated period of circulatory arrest using retrograde total body perfusion (described below). In addition, electroencephalogram (EEG) is used routinely and helps guide the degree and effects of hypothermia.

Cooling is generally ceased when the EEG becomes isoelectric, which generally occurs at a core temperature of 18–22 °C. Ascending aortic cross-clamping with cardioplegia is not performed owing to remote proximity to the ascending aorta using this technique. Instead, myocardial protection relies on systemic deep hypothermia, which requires attention to the cooling process for optimal myocardial and tissue preservation (Dearani and Mavroudis 2020). The length of time required to perform the proximal aortic anastomosis is usually not very long (20 min or

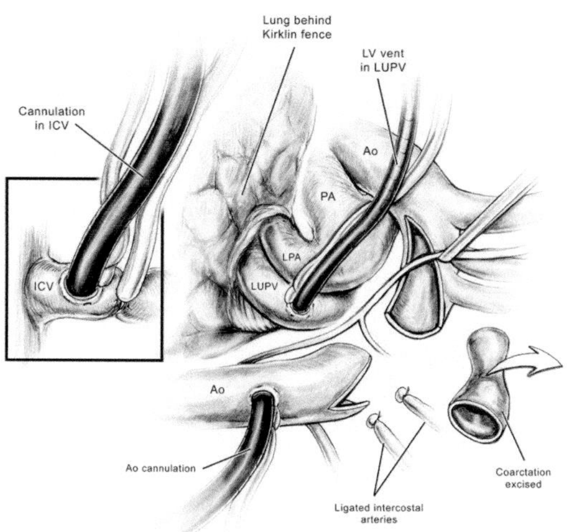

Fig. 38 The repair is accomplished by resection of the abnormal segment of thoracic aorta and placement of an interposition Dacron tube graft (Fig. 28); direct end-to-end anastomosis is usually not feasible in the adult. Post-repair analysis is achieved with both TEE imaging and examination of pressures with needles in the aorta above and below the graft. Decannulation is accomplished in the standard fashion, being sure to avoid entry of air into the left atrium with cannula removal. (With permission: Dearani and Mavroudis 2020). *Ao* aorta, *ICV* inferior caval vein, *LPA* left pulmonary artery, *LUPV* left upper pulmonary vein, *LV* left ventricle, *PA* pulmonary artery

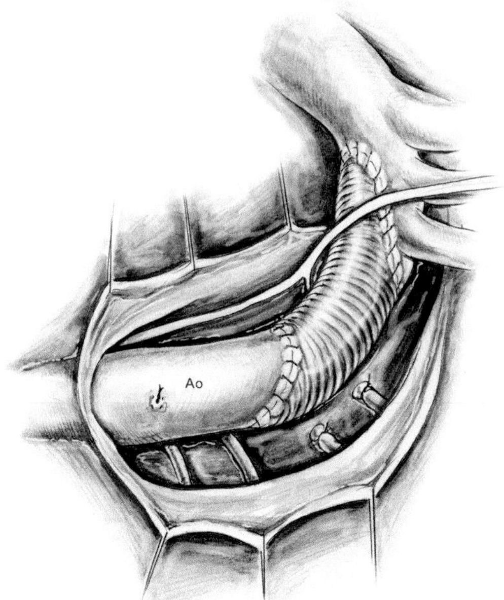

Fig. 39 Shows the completed repair which extends into the proximal transverse arch. (With permission: Dearani and Mavroudis 2020). *Ao* aorta

less), and consequently the time without myocardial perfusion is relatively short. Using this technique, normal ventricular function is usually attained at the completion of the procedure.

Other important protective technical maneuvers that are used routinely are retrograde total body perfusion through the right atrium which is accomplished by a flow rate of 800–1000 mL/min to maintain a central venous pressure <20 mmHg. Retrograde perfusion to the ICV and superior caval vein is utilized for two purposes. First, it allows perfusion to the brain and body tissues during the period of circulatory arrest. Second, the left ventricular vent is disengaged during the period of retrograde total body perfusion. As a result, the left heart and ascending aorta remain full of blood and free of air. This is extremely important since it is not possible to perform standard deairing maneuvers when the patient is in the right lateral decubitus position to deair the left heart and ascending aorta.

The full bypass strategy with deep hypothermia is used for distal arch hypoplasia or obstruction. The abnormal segment of the proximal descending aorta is excised and the underside of the distal aortic arch is incised proximally toward the brachiocephalic artery. The tube graft can be fashioned with a graft extension retained to reconstruct the underside of the distal arch. This technique is referred to as the reversed hemiarch (Dearani and Mavroudis 2020); it results in an anatomic reconstruction of the hypoplastic arch and stenotic isthmus. The distal anastomosis is performed in the usual end-to-end anastomosis with the descending aorta almost always without the need for felt Teflon strips. The repair can be analyzed using TEE and direct pressure measurements.

15 Median Sternotomy Approach

Median sternotomy is the preferred option for aortic arch hypoplasia or complex arch and proximal descending aortic obstruction. This approach is also practical if other concomitant cardiac surgical procedures are indicated, such as aortic valve repair or replacement, ascending aortic replacement, or coronary bypass grafting. As in previous pre-procedure preparations, arterial monitoring catheters in the right radial and left femoral arteries are used for pre- and postoperative analysis. A groin incision is made for femoral artery and vein access in the setting of a hazardous resternotomy.

Transesophageal echocardiography is used for pre- and postoperative repair analysis, which includes aortic flow characteristics in the descending thoracic aorta. Since deep hypothermia is established with retrograde or antegrade cerebral perfusion, the EEG is monitored and helps guide the degree of hypothermia to ensure cerebral and systemic tissue preservation. As noted, systemic cooling is ceased when the EEG becomes isoelectric, which usually occurs at a core temperature of 18–22 °C. Aortic and right atrial or bicaval cardiopulmonary bypass techniques are used, depending on the presence of associated cardiac lesions that require surgical repair. Aortic occlusion with cardioplegic arrest (antegrade and/or retrograde) techniques are used, and the left heart is vented via the right superior pulmonary vein. Figures 40 and 41 show the particulars of the operation with associated important surgical recommendations to avoid complications within the legend narration. The sequence of operative steps is dependent on the specific operation and is generally determined by the surgeon. In the majority of cases, intracardiac procedures are performed during the cooling phase of cardiopulmonary bypass, giving the operative team enough time for systemic cooling prior to arch reconstruction and circulatory arrest.

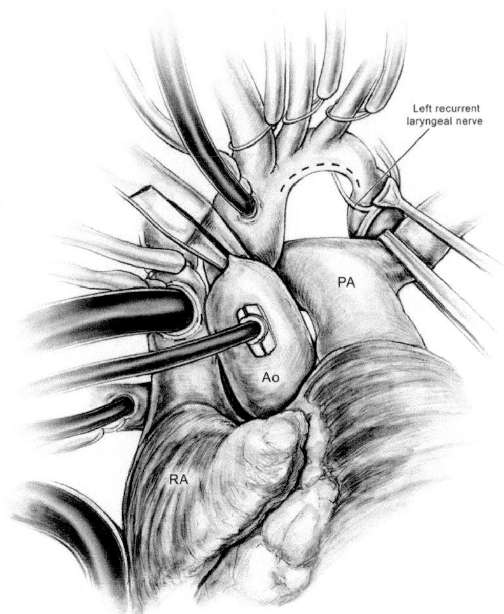

Fig. 40 Mediastinal dissection includes mobilization of the ascending aorta, arch, and arch vessels, and control of the brachiocephalic and left carotid arteries with vessel loops. Dissection is extended to the distal arch as much as safely possible prior to the institution of bypass. Identification of the ligamentum and protection of the recurrent laryngeal nerve during dissection is essential, but scar tissue from prior surgery often makes it difficult or impossible to discern the nerve. In general, the distal aortic arch up to the left subclavian artery can be safely reached from the front (i.e., sternotomy). When obstruction extends into the proximal descending thoracic aorta beyond the left subclavian artery, satisfactory exposure from the front is more difficult to achieve in an adult. When aortic obstruction extends into the proximal descending aorta, options include a clamshell incision or the use of an extra-anatomic bypass graft. (With permission: Dearani and Mavroudis 2020). *Ao* aorta, *PA* pulmonary artery, *RA* right atrium

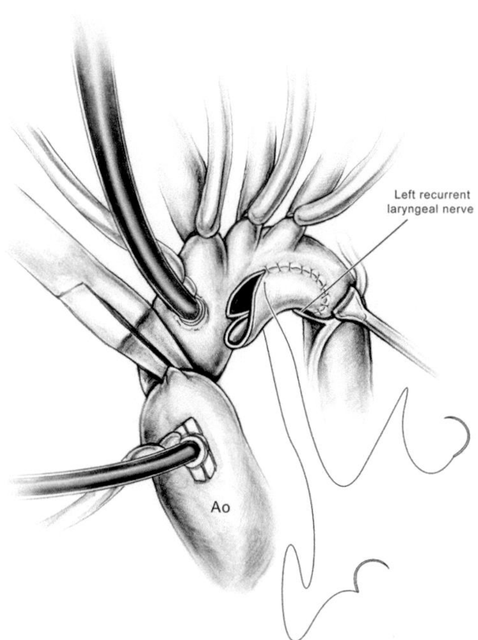

Fig. 41 Isolated aortic arch hypoplasia is best treated with patch augmentation of the underside of the arch. After satisfactory cooling with myocardial protection (antegrade and/or retrograde cardioplegia) and cerebral protection (antegrade or retrograde cerebral perfusion), the underside of the arch is incised, with the incision extended as far distally as possible, usually to the site of the left subclavian artery or slightly beyond. The incision is then extended proximally into the distal ascending aorta. An oval patch (of bovine pericardium, Dacron, or Gore-Tex) can be used, or a Dacron or Gore-Tex tube graft that is cut in half can be used to recreate the underside of the arch and provide an anatomic reconstruction. If the ascending aorta is aneurysmal and requires replacement, then a standard ascending aortic replacement with hemiarch graft extension is tailored to extend beyond the distal portion of arch hypoplasia. If concomitant aortic valve disease (stenosis, regurgitation, or both) is present, then the valve is addressed, either with valvuloplasty (valve repair or valve-sparing root replacement) or replacement of the valve, with or without root replacement, depending on the extent of root pathology. Other intracardiac procedures or coronary bypass grafting is performed as needed. (With permission: Dearani and Mavroudis 2020). *Ao* aorta

The distal arch reconstruction is then performed, followed by placement of a new arterial cannula in the graft to allow reinstitution of antegrade body perfusion (Martin and Mavroudis 2020). The remaining aortic root reconstruction or other intracardiac procedures are completed while rewarming is in progress. Additional doses of cardioplegia are administered as needed prior to cross-clamp removal to safely extend the time for additional procedures.

16 Extra-Anatomic Procedures

Extra-anatomic bypass grafting for repair of recurrent coarctation can be achieved by placement of a graft from the ascending aorta to the descending aorta. This approach has been described and used to address arch and/or proximal descending aortic obstruction (Savlania et al. 2018). The benefit to this procedure is that the native obstructive aortic abnormalities are left intact and untouched. Another benefit is that the conduct of the operation does not involve the need for deep hypothermia and circulatory arrest. In addition, it avoids dissection of the previously operated site and potential injury to the recurrent laryngeal nerve, which generally is difficult to identify. Also, it eliminates the possibility of hypoperfusion of the spinal cord because the systemic circulation is never interrupted with total aortic occlusion. The disadvantages are not insignificant. For one thing, the bypass graft is large and fills the right side of the pericardial space, which can make any future cardiac surgical procedure more difficult. In addition, the graft, if inappropriately long, can lie in the right thoracic cavity and be prone to develop a bronchial to graft fistula resulting in bleeding and or infection.

The operation is noted in Figs. 42, 43, 44, and 45. The descending thoracic aorta is best exposed and approached by aortobicaval cardiopulmonary bypass with retraction and rotation of the left ventricular apex towards the right pleural space as noted in Fig. 42. A pressure line in the femoral artery to ensure that the side-biting clamp is not completely occluding the small aorta is an important monitor. An end-to-side anastomosis is performed with continuous suture; the graft size is determined by the size of the descending aorta at the level of the diaphragm which is usually 16–20 mm. The progression of the reconstruction is continued as noted in Fig. 39.

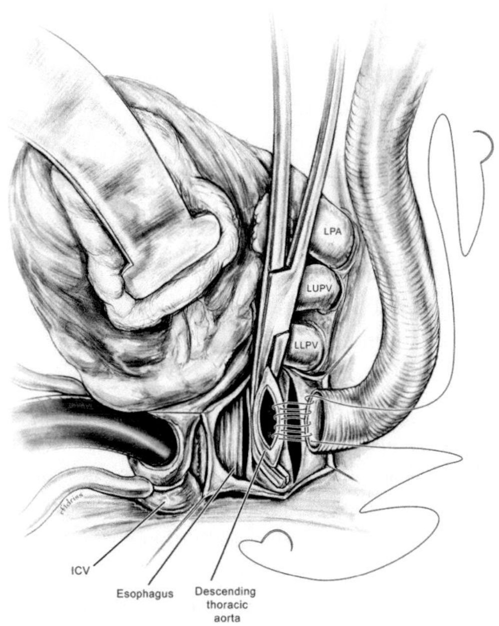

Fig. 42 Shows optimal exposure of the descending aorta for distal graft placement. Care is taken to allow enough space on the ascending aorta for graft placement. The heart is maintained beating without cardioplegic arrest. The posterior pericardium is incised longitudinally just left of the spine and over the descending thoracic aorta, which is usually small. It is important not to denude the aortic adventitia during the dissection. The esophagus will be to the right; the TEE probe is usually palpable and provides a convenient landmark to avoid inadvertent esophageal injury. A side-biting clamp is placed on the descending aorta, with the handles of the clamp directed upward toward the head, so as not to be in the way of the right arm and hand of the surgeon sewing the graft. (With permission: Dearani and Mavroudis 2020). *ICV* inferior caval vein, *LPA* left pulmonary artery, *LLPV* left lower pulmonary vein, *LUPV* left upper pulmonary vein

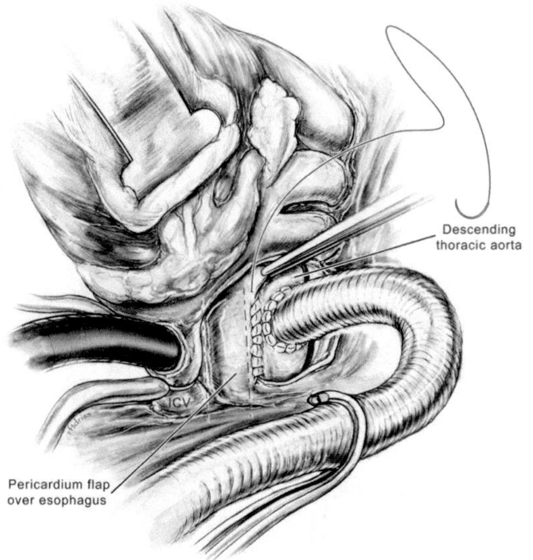

Fig. 43 After the anastomosis is completed, the side-biting clamp is removed, and hemostasis around the anastomosis is achieved with extra pledgetted mattress sutures as needed. The cut pericardial edge to the right side of the anastomosis is then sutured to the aorta just below the graft anastomosis to ensure that there is no contact between the graft and esophagus. Topical biologic sealant is applied to the anastomosis to ensure hemostasis because exposure at the end of the operation can be quite difficult without causing hemodynamic compromise once bypass has been discontinued. The graft is then placed either posterior or anterior to the inferior caval vein (ICV). In general, we prefer an anterior position, as the space between the ICV and the right inferior pulmonary vein can be a tight fit, particularly if the graft is on the larger side. The main disadvantage of the anterior position is more difficult access to the ICV for direct cannulation at a subsequent reoperation. (With permission: Dearani and Mavroudis 2020)

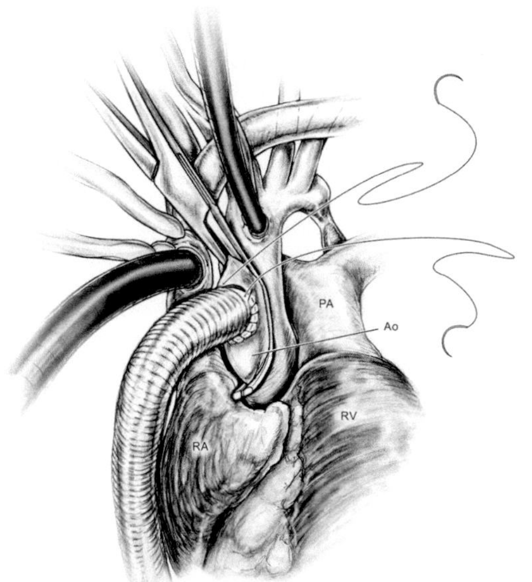

Fig. 44 The graft is brought around the right atrium and sewn end-to-side to the ascending aorta. It is preferable to place the proximal anastomosis of the extra-anatomic graft as far distal on the ascending aorta as possible (hence the reason for appropriate initial aortic arch cannulation), as some patients will need future aortic valve replacement; a more distal location allows sufficient room for an aortotomy to expose the aortic valve. The location of the graft just anterior to the ICV also allows easier access for snare or clamp placement at the time of future aortic valve replacement. When the ascending aorta is dilated and requires replacement, the extra-anatomic aortic graft is sewn end-to-side to the new ascending aortic graft. (With permission: Dearani and Mavroudis 2020). *Ao* aorta, *PA* pulmonary artery, *RA* right atrium, *RV* right ventricle

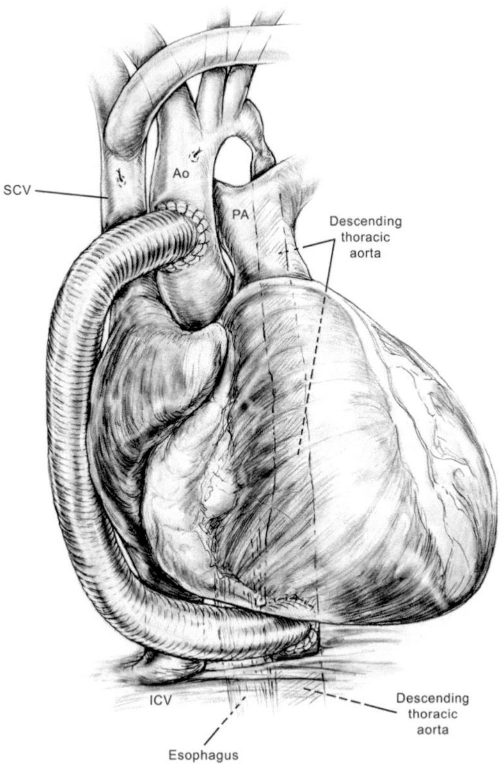

Fig. 45 Shows the completed extra-anatomic reconstruction for coarctation of the aorta. (With permission: Dearani and Mavroudis 2020). *Ao* aorta, *IVC* inferior caval vein, *PA* pulmonary artery, *SCV* superior caval vein

Protecting graft exposure to the esophagus is an important maneuver to protect against fistula formation. Figure 40 shows the proximal aortic anastomosis and the relative benefits of proper positioning. Figure 41 shows the completed reconstruction with separation from cardiopulmonary bypass.

In general, this operation is safe to perform making sure to protect the esophagus with surrounding tissue to prevent graft erosion and fistula formation. Also, there is proximity to the thoracic duct which will require vigilance to identify a leak after the completion of the operation. Long term complications include false aneurysms at the aortic anastomoses (Posacioglu and Apaydin 2004; Al-Husayni et al. 2021) and erosion of the graft into the right lung parenchyma in the event that the graft is too long and extends into the thoracic cavity (Bugge et al. 2021).

17 Summary

Coarctation of the aorta is a complex lesion with many variations which can be challenging to the surgical team. Complications such as paraplegia, thoracic duct injury, recurrent laryngeal injury, false aneurysms, endocarditis, and transverse hypoplasia have been discussed, among others. Preoperative evaluation, comprehensive and careful dissection, and appropriate conduct of the operation will yield optimal results with minimal exposure of the patient to complications.

References

Al-Husayni F, Samman A, Althobaiti M, Alghamdi A, Alkashkari W. Late complications after previous surgical repair for coarctation with extra-anatomic bypass graft: report on two cases. Cureus. 2021;13(1):e12722. https://doi.org/10.7759/cureus.12722.

Alkashkari W, Al-Husayni F, Alfouti M, Alsofyani R, Alfawaz S. Endovascular treatment for pseudoaneurysms after the surgical repair of aortic coarctation. Cureus. 2020;12:e8978. Published 2020 Jul 3. https://doi.org/10.7759/cureus.8978.

Amato J, Rheinlander H, Cleveland R. A method of enlarging the distal transverse arch in infants with hypoplasia and coarctation of the aorta. Ann Thorac Surg. 1997;23:261–3.

Anagnostopoulos PV. When to repair coarctation associated with hypoplastic aortic arch through the front; are we asking the questions that really matter? J Thorac Cardiovasc Surg. 2015;152:1475–6.

Backer C, Paape K, Zales V, Weigel T, Mavroudis C. Coarctation of the aorta. Repair with polytetrafluoroethylene patch aortoplasty. Circulation. 1995;92:II132–6.

Backer CL, Mavroudis C, Zias EA, Amin Z, Weigel TJ. Repair of coarctation with resection and extended end-to-end anastomosis. Ann Thorac Surg. 1998;66(4):1365–70; discussion 1370–1371

Barreiro CJ, Ellison TA, Williams JA, Durr ML, Cameron DE, Vricella LA. Subclavian flap aortoplasty: still a safe, reproducible, and effective treatment for infant coarctation. Eur J Cardiothorac Surg. 2007;31:649–53.

Bassareo PP, Marras AR, Manai ME, Mercuro G. The influence of different surgical approaches on arterial rigidity in children after aortic coarctation repair. Pediatr Cardiol. 2009;30:414–8.

Beekman R, Rocchini A, Behrendt D, et al. Long-term outcome after repair of coarctation in infancy: Subclavian angioplasty does not reduce the need for reoperation. J Am Coll Cardiol. 1986;8:1406–11.

Bender B, Murthy V, Chamberlain RS. The changing management of chylothorax in the modern era. Eur J Cardiothorac Surg. 2016;49:18–24.

Benouaich V, Porterie J, Bouali O, Moscovici J, Lopez R. Anatomical basis of the risk of injury to the right laryngeal recurrent nerve during thoracic surgery. Surg Radiol Anat. 2012;34:509–12.

Bromberg B, Beekman R, Rocchini A. Aortic aneurysm after patch aortoplasty repair of coarctation: a prospective analysis of prevalence, screening tests and risks. J Am Coll Cardiol. 1989;14:734–41.

Brouwer RM, Cromme-Dijkhuis AH, Erasmus ME, et al. Decision making for the surgical management of aortic coarctation associated with ventricular septal defect. J Thorac Cardiovasc Surg. 1996;111:168–75.

Brown JW, Ruzmetov M, Hoyer MH, Rodefeld MD, Turrentine MW. Recurrent coarctation: is surgical repair of recurrent coarctation of the aorta safe and effective? Ann Thorac Surg. 2009a;88:1923–30.

Brown JW, Rodefeld MD, Ruzmetov M. Transverse aortic arch obstruction: when to go from the front. Semin Thorac Cardiovasc Surg Pediatr Card Surg Annu. 2009b:66–9.

Brown ML, Burkhart HM, Connolly HM, Dearani JA, Hagler DJ, Schaff HV. Late outcomes of reintervention on the descending aorta after repair of aortic coarctation. Circulation. 2010;122(11 Suppl):S81–4.

Bugge AS, Kvitting JP, Sundset A, Birkeland S. Lung autotransplantation and extra-anatomic bypass to treat an aortobronchial fistula after previous surgery for aortic coarctation. J Card Surg. 2021;36:2924–7.

Burch PT, Cowley CG, Holubkov R, et al. Coarctation repair in neonates and young infants: is small size or low weight still a risk factor? J Thorac Cardiovasc Surg. 2009;138:547–52.

Callahan C, Saudek D, Shillingford A, et al. Single-stage repair of coarctation of the aorta and ventricular septal defect: a comparison of surgical strategies and resource utilization. World J Pediatr Congenit Heart Surg. 2017;8:559–63.

Cerfolio RJ, Allen MS. Postoperative chylothorax. J Thorac Cardiovasc Surg. 1996;112:1361–6.

Clarkson P, Nicholson M, Barratt-Boyes B, Neutze J, Whitlock R. Results after repair of coarctation of the aorta beyond infancy: a 10 to 28 year follow-up with particular reference to late systemic hypertension. Am J Cardiol. 1983;51:1481–8.

Dearani JA, Mavroudis C. Coarctation of the aorta in adulthood. In: Mavroudis C, Dearani JA, editors. Atlas of adult congenital heart surgery. Cham: Springer Nature; 2020.

Farag ES, Kluin J, de Heer F, et al. Aortic coarctation repair through left thoracotomy: results in the modern era. Eur J Cardiothorac Surg. 2019;55(2):331–7.

Fiore AC, Fischer LK, Schwartz T, et al. Comparison of angioplasty and surgery for neonatal aortic coarctation. Ann Thorac Surg. 2005;80:1659–64.

Forbes TJ, Garekar S, Amin Z, et al. Procedural results and acute complications in stenting native and recurrent coarctation of the aorta in patients over 4 years of age: a multi-institutional study. Catheter Cardiovasc Interv. 2007;70:276–85.

Forbes TJ, Kim DW, Du W, et al. Comparison of surgical, stent, and balloon angioplasty treatment of native coarctation of the aorta: an observational study by the CCISC (Congenital Cardiovascular Interventional Study Consortium). J Am Coll Cardiol. 2011;58:2664–74.

Franco-Paredes C, Workowski K, Harris M. Infective endocarditis-endarteritis complicating coarctation of the aorta. Am J Med. 2002;112:590–2.

Gaynor JW, Wernovsky G, Rychik J, Rome JJ, DeCampli WM, Spray TL. Outcome following single-stage repair of coarctation with ventricular septal defect. Eur J Cardiothorac Surg. 2000;18:62–7.

Gray WH, Wells WJ, Starnes VA, Kumar SR. Arch augmentation via median sternotomy for coarctation of aorta with proximal arch hypoplasia. Ann Thorac Surg. 2018;106:1214–9.

Hager A, Schreiber C, Nutzl S, Hess J. Mortality and restenosis rate of surgical coarctation repair in infancy: a study of 191 patients. Cardiology. 2009;112:36–41.

Itkin M, Kucharczuk JC, Kwak A, Trerotola SO, Kaiser LR. Nonoperative thoracic duct embolization for traumatic thoracic duct leak: experience in 109 patients. J Thorac Cardiovasc Surg. 2010;139:584–90.

Kanter K, Vincent R, Fyfe D. Reverse subclavian flap repair of hypoplastic transverse aorta in infancy. Ann Thorac Surg. 2001;71:1530–6.

Kappetein A, Zwinderman A, Bogers A, Rohmer J, Huysmans H. More than thirty-five years of coarctation repair. An unexpected high relapse rate. J Thorac Cardiovasc Surg. 1994;107:87–95.

Karaosmanoglu AD, Khawaja RD, Onur MR, Kalra MK. CT and MRI of aortic coarctation: pre- and postsurgical findings. AJR Am J Roentgenol. 2015;204:W224–33.

Krasna MJ, Forti G. Nerve injury: injury to the recurrent laryngeal, phrenic, vagus, long thoracic, and sympathetic nerves during thoracic surgery. Thorac Surg Clin. 2006;16:267–75.

Kumar TKS, Zurakowski D, Sharma R, Saini S, Jonas R. Prediction of recurrent coarctation by early postoperative blood pressure gradient. J Thorac Cardiovasc Surg. 2011;142:1130–6.

Kutty S, Greenberg RK, Fletcher S, Svensson LG, Latson LA. Endovascular stent grafts for large thoracic aneurysms after coarctation repair. Ann Thorac Surg. 2008;85:1332–8.

Lim C, Kim WH, Kim SC, et al. Aortic arch reconstruction using regional perfusion without circulatory arrest. Eur J Cardiothorac Surg. 2003;23:149–55.

Lim HG, Kim WH, Jang WS, et al. One-stage total repair of aortic arch anomaly using regional perfusion. Eur J Cardiothorac Surg. 2007;31:242–8.

Lock J, Bass J, Amplatz K, Fuhrman B, Castaneda-Zuniga W. Balloon dilation angioplasty of aortic coarctations in infants and children. Circulation. 1983;68:109–16.

Lv S, Wang Q, Zhao W, et al. A review of the postoperative lymphatic leakage. Oncotarget. 2017;8:69062–75.

Martin T, Mavroudis C. Congenital aortic aneurysms. In: Mavroudis C, Dearani JA, editors. Atlas of adult congenital heart surgery. Cham: Springer Nature; 2020.

Mavroudis C. Coarctation of the aorta. In: Mavroudis C, Backer CL, editors. Atlas of pediatric cardiac surgery. London: Springer; 2015.

Maxey T, Serfontein S, Reece T, Rheuban K, Kron I. Transverse arch hypoplasia may predispose patients to aneurysm formation after patch repair of aortic coarctation. Ann Thorac Surg. 2003;76:1090–3.

Midgley F, Scott L, Perry L, Shapiro S, McClenathan J. Subclavian flap aortoplasty for treatment of coarctation in early infancy. J Pediatr Surg. 1978;13:264–8.

Pandey R, Jackson M, Ajab S, Gladman G, Pozzi M. Subclavian flap repair: review of 399 patients at median follow-up of fourteen years. Ann Thorac Surg. 2006;8:1420–8.

Parikh KJ, Fundora MP, Sasaki N, Rossi AF, Burke RP, Sasaki J. Use of aortic arch measurements in evaluating significant arch hypoplasia in neonates with coarctation. Prog Pediatr Cardiol. 2021;62:101410.

Pillay TG, Singh B. A review of traumatic chylothorax. Injury. 2016;47:545–50.

Posacioglu H, Apaydin AZ. Pseudoaneurysm and aortobronchial fistula after aortic coarctation repair by patch aortoplasty. Tex Heart Inst J. 2004;31:319–21.

Qureshi SA. Use of covered stents to treat coarctation of the aorta. Korean Circ J. 2009;39:261–3.

Qureshi AM, McElhinney DB, Lock JE, Landzberg MJ, Lang P, Marshall AC. Acute and intermediate outcomes, and evaluation of injury to the aortic wall, as based on 15 years experience of implanting stents to treat aortic coarctation. Cardiol Young. 2007;17:307–18.

Ramachandran P, Khoury PR, Beekman RH, et al. Preoperative aortic arch size and late outcome after coarctation repair by lateral thoracotomy. Ann Thorac Surg. 2018;106:575–80.

Rees AH, Elbl F, Villafane J, Solinger R, Mavroudis C, Harrison H. Surgical repair of atypical coarctation of the abdominal aorta in an infant. J Ky Med Assoc. 1990;88:62–5.

Rheuban K, Carpenter M, Jedeikin R. Aortic aneurysm after patch aortoplasty for coarctation in childhood. Am J Cardiol. 1985;55:612.

Rheuban K, Gutgesell H, Carpenter M. Aortic aneurysm after patch angioplasty for aortic isthmic coarctation in childhood. Am J Cardiol. 1986;58:178–80.

Rodés-Cabau J, Miró J, Dancea A, et al. Comparison of surgical and transcatheter treatment for native coarctation of the aorta in patients > or = 1 year old. The Quebec Native Coarctation of the Aorta study. Am Heart J. 2007;154:186–92.

Rothman A, Galindo A, Evans WN, Collazos JC, Restrepo H. Effectiveness and safety of balloon dilation of native aortic coarctation in premature neonates weighing < or = 2,500 grams. Am J Cardiol. 2010;105:1176–80.

Said SM, Marey G. Successful management of postoperative chylothorax in a neonate after coarctation repair. 2021. https://doi.org/10.25373/ctsnet.14802780.

Sainathan S, Mulinari L. Coarctation of the aorta with aortic arch hypoplasia: tackle from the front or the side? J Card Surg. 2022;37:1633–4.

Savlania A, Nair HR, Pitchai S, Unnikrishnan M. Extra-anatomic ascending to descending thoracic aortic bypass for repair of adult aortic recoarctation. J Vasc Surg Cases Innov Tech. 2018;30(4):182–3.

Schild HH, Strassburg CP, Welz A, Kalff J. Treatment options in patients with chylothorax. Dtsch Arztebl Int. 2013;110(48):819–26.

Serfontein SJ, Kron IL. Complications of coarctation repair. Semin Thorac Cardiovasc Surg Pediatr Card Surg Annu. 2002;5:206–2011.

Shaddy R, Boucek M, Sturtevant J, et al. Comparison of angioplasty and surgery for unoperated coarctation of the aorta. Circulation. 1993;87:793–9.

Sharkey AJ, Rao JN. The successful use of octreotide in the treatment of traumatic chylothorax. Tex Heart Inst J. 2012;39:428–30.

Sharma BK, Calderon M, Ott DA. Coarctation repair in neonates with subclavian-sparing advancement flap. Ann Thorac Surg. 1992 Jul;54(1):137–41.

Sousa A, Bos E, Elzenga N, de Villeneuve V. Subclavian flap aortoplasty for treatment of coarctation of the aorta in infants less than 3 months of age. Thorac Cardiovasc Surg. 1983;31:160–2.

Sudarshan CD, Cochrane AD, Jun ZH, Soto R, Brizard CP. Repair of coarctation of the aorta in infants weighing less than 2 kilograms. Ann Thorac Surg. 2006;82:158–63.

Tabbutt S, Nicolson SC, Dominguez TE, et al. Perioperative course in 118 infants and children undergoing coarctation repair via a thoracotomy: a prospective, multicenter experience. J Thorac Cardiovasc Surg. 2008;136:1229–36.

Terramani TT, Salim A, Hood DB, Rowe VL, Weaver FA. Hypoplasia of the descending thoracic and abdominal aorta: a report of two cases and review of the literature. J Vasc Surg. 2002;36:844–8.

Thomson JDR, Mulpur A, Guerrero R, Nagy Z, Gibbs JL, Watterson KG. Outcome after extended arch repair for aortic coarctation. Heart. 2006;92:90–4.

Tilea I, Hadadi L, Serban RC, Tilea B. Hybrid repair of a very late, post-aortic coarctation surgery thoracic aneurysm: a case report. J Med Case Rep. 2012;30(6):255. https://doi.org/10.1186/1752-1947-6-255.

Torok RD, Campbell MJ, Fleming GA, Hill KD. Coarctation of the aorta: management from infancy to adulthood. World J Cardiol. 2015;7:765–75.

Tulzer A, Mair R, Kreutzer M, Tulzer G. Outcome of aortic arch reconstruction in infants with coarctation: importance of operative approach. J Thorac Cardiovasc Surg. 2016;152:1506–13.

van Son J, van Asten W, van Lier H, et al. Detrimental sequelae on the hemodynamics of the upper left limb after subclavian flap angioplasty in infancy. Circulation. 1990;81:996–1004.

Venturini A, Perna A, Bianchi G. Repair of coarctation of the thoracic aorta without resection. Patch graft aortoplasty. Follow-up study of 46 cases. J Cardiovasc Surg. 1978;19:49–54.

Waldhausen J, Nahrwold D. Repair of coarctation of the aorta with a subclavian flap. J Thorac Cardiovasc Surg. 1966;51:532–3.

Walhout R, Lekkerkerker J, Oron G, Hitchcock F, Meijboom E, Bennink G. Comparison of polytetrafluoroethylene patch aortoplasty and end-to-end anastomosis for coarctation of the aorta. J Thorac Cardiovasc Surg. 2003;126:521–8.

Warnes CA, Williams RG, Bashore TM, Child JS, Connolly HM, Dearani JA, et al. ACC/AHA 2008 guidelines for the management of adults with congenital heart disease: a report of the American College of Cardiology/American Heart Association task force on practice guidelines (writing committee to develop guidelines on the management of adults with congenital heart disease): developed in collaboration with the American Society of Echocardiography, Heart Rhythm Society, International Society for adult congenital heart disease, Society for Cardiovascular Angiography and Interventions, and …. Circulation. 2008;118(23):e714–833.

Wilson W, Taubert KA, Gewitz M, et al. Prevention of infective endocarditis: guidelines from the American Heart Association. Circulation. 2007;116(15):1736–54.

Wong D, Benson LN, Van Arsdell GS, Karamlou T, McCrindle BW. Balloon angioplasty is preferred to surgery for aortic coarctation. Cardiol Young. 2008;18:79–88.

Wright GE, Nowak CA, Goldberg CS, Ohye RG, Bove EL, Rocchini AP. Extended resection and end-to-end anastomosis for aortic coarctation in infants: results of a tailored surgical approach. Ann Thorac Surg. 2005;80:1453–9.

Younoszai AK, Reddy VM, Hanley FL, Brook MM. Intermediate term follow-up of the end-to-side aortic anastomosis for coarctation of the aorta. Ann Thorac Surg. 2002;74:1631–4.

Complications Associated with Repair of Interrupted Aortic Arch

Constantine Mavroudis

Abstract

Repair of interrupted aortic arch is associated with many intracardiac and extracardiac anomalies. The principles of interrupted aortic arch repair are mostly the same which include arch dissection, appropriate management of cardiopulmonary bypass and repair of the associated lesions. This chapter reviews the important steps of these operations to avoid operative complications such as cerebral ischemic injury, postoperative arch obstruction, recurrent laryngeal nerve injury, myocardial depression, and operative bleeding due to catheter disruption of the patent arterial duct.

Keywords

Congenital heart surgery · Interrupted aortic arch · Arch repair · Complications · Outcomes

C. Mavroudis (✉)
Chief of Pediatric Cardiothoracic Surgery (Retired), Peyton Manning Children's Hospital, Indianapolis, IN, USA

Professor Emeritus of Surgery, Johns Hopkins University School of Medicine, Baltimore, MD, USA

1 Introduction

Complications in association with repair of Interrupted Aortic Arch (IAA) are generally similar to operations for coarctation of the aorta (CoA) in which the operation is performed through a median sternotomy because of hypoplastic transverse aortic arch as noted in Chap. 5 "Complications Associated with Repair of Coarctation of the Aorta". For starters, the recurrent laryngeal nerve can be injured, the transverse arch reconstruction may need to be augmented, and the conduct of cardiopulmonary bypass and circulatory arrest may be mismanaged. Nevertheless, there are important distinctions regarding repair of IAA which will be explored in this chapter. This chapter on IAA will review anatomic variations, important associated lesions, conduct of the reparative operation, and the associated complications associated thereto.

Interrupted aortic arch is often associated with ventriculoseptal defect, common arterial trunk, aortopulmonary window, transposition of the great arteries, genetic syndromes, and other conotruncal abnormalities (Celoria and Patton 1959; Weisman and Kesten 1948; Hanneman et al. 2017; Collins-Nakai et al. 1976; Hartman et al. 2011; Zhang et al. 1987; Moerman et al. 1987; Paech et al. 2011; Peyvandi et al. 2013; Chen et al. 2013a; Jonas 2004). The aortic interruption can be distal to the left subclavian artery (Type A), between the left subclavian artery and

C. L. Backer, C. Mavroudis (eds.), *Complications in Pediatric and Congenital Heart Surgery*,
https://doi.org/10.1007/978-3-032-02661-3_6

the left common carotid artery (Type B), also associated with DiGeorge Syndrome and absence of the thymus, and between the innominate artery and the left common carotid artery (Type C) (Fig. 1) (Mavroudis 2015). Figures 2a–c show the anatomic variants in an anterior view as related to the patent arterial duct (patent ductus arteriosus), the ascending aorta, and the main pulmonary artery (Celoria and Patton 1959).

Historical accounts of repair of this entity involved using the brachiocephalic vessels to form the reconfigured conduit between the interrupted segments (Bamforth and Anderson 2017; Todman et al. 2013). For example, the left common carotid artery can be distally ligated while the proximal portion can be used to anastomose to the descending aorta thereby completing the continuity between the transverse arch and the descending aorta. Another report used a piece of native pulmonary artery to construct a tube connecting the interrupted arch (Lee et al. 2013; Bergoend et al. 2010). These techniques are largely historical in nature and are not used nowadays unless specific indications warrant their use.

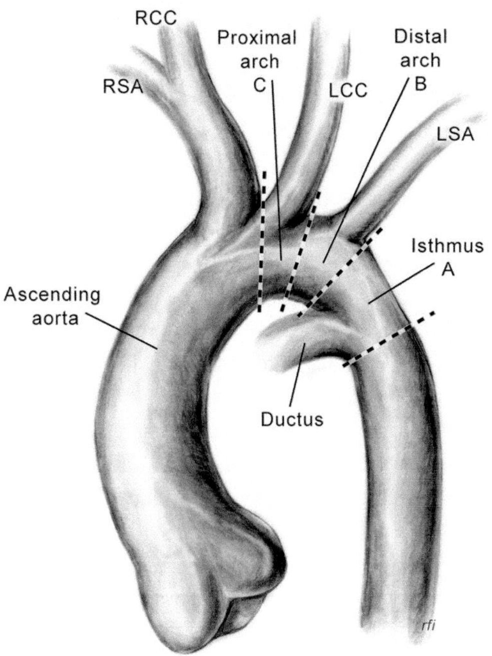

Fig. 1 Shows the aortic interruption variants with relationship to the origin of the brachiocephalic arteries. The nomenclature is counterintuitive since the A, B, C, progression is upstream to the flow and not what one would expect owing to flow related distinction. Therefore, Type A is an interruption between the left subclavian artery and the descending aorta which is also noted in the anterior view in Fig. 2a. Type B is an interruption between the subclavian artery and the left common carotid artery, which is associated with DiGeorge Syndrome and absence of the thymus. This is also shown in the anterior view in Fig. 2b. Type C interrupted aortic arch is defined as an interruption between the innominate artery and the left common carotid artery which is also shown in the anterior view in Fig. 2c. (With permission: Mavroudis 2015). *LCC* left common carotid artery, *LSA* left subclavian artery, *RCC* right common carotid artery, *RSA* right subclavian artery

The introduction of safe neonatal cardiopulmonary bypass, circulatory arrest, and regional perfusion techniques made complete repair by direct anastomosis between the ascending aorta and the descending aorta possible (Roussin et al. 2002; Sell et al. 1988; McCrindle et al. 2005; Jonas et al. 1994; Messner et al. 2002; Volpe et al. 2010; Vogel et al. 2010; Axt-Fliedner et al. 2011; Barratt-Boyes et al. 1972; Trusler and Izukawa 1975; Dillman et al. 2008; Nisli et al. 2007; Fuchigami et al. 2016; Tlaskal et al. 2010; Mery et al. 2014). The challenge was to protect the brain and the systemic organs during these operations to ensure successful outcomes and normal long-term survival. The classic one stage repair of interrupted aortic arch and ventricular septal defect has centered on simultaneous ascending aortic and descending aortic cannulation through the ductus arteriosus with deep hypothermia and circulatory arrest or the more recent application of regional perfusion techniques to preserve flow to the brachiocephalic vessels (Varghese et al. 2015; Chen et al. 2019; Morales et al. 2006; Brown et al. 2006; Joynt et al. 2009; Visconti et al. 2006; Dominguez et al. 2007; Shinkawa et al. 2012; Mainwaring and Lamberti 1997; Jegatheeswaran et al. 2010; Kalfa et al. 2007). Recent advances have supported double aortic cannulation of the innominate artery and the descending aorta at the level of the diaphragm. This technique allows moderate hypothermia, regional perfusion for the aortic reconstruction, and continuous cardiopulmonary bypass for the ventricular septal defect (VSD) closure (Serraf et al. 1996). Complications relat-

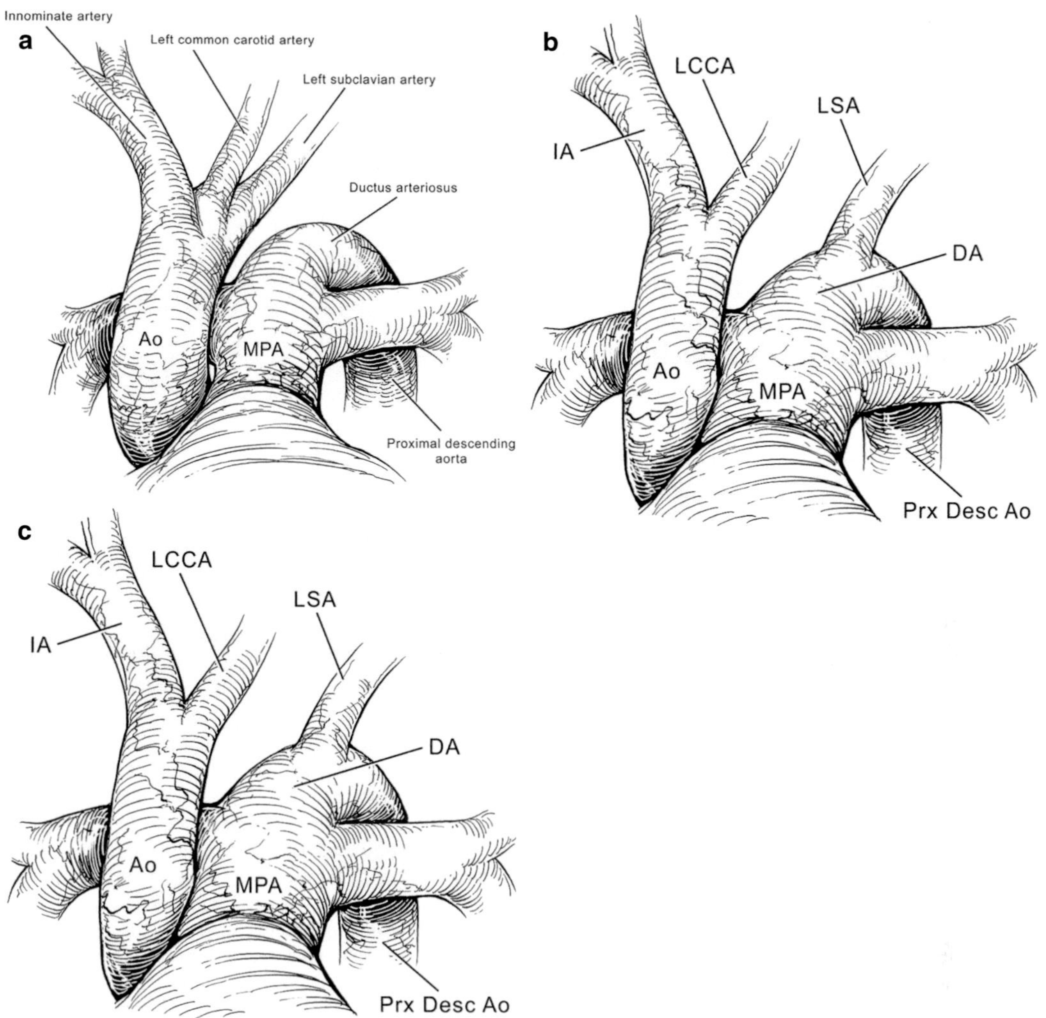

Fig. 2 (**a**) Anterior View of Type A interrupted aortic arch. (**b**) Anterior View of Type B interrupted aortic arch which is associated with DiGeorge Syndrome and absence of the thymus. (**c**) Anterior View of Type C interrupted aortic arch. (With permission: Jonas 2003). *Ao* aorta, *DA* descending aorta, *IA* innominate artery, *LCCA* left common carotid artery, *LSA* left subclavian artery, *MPA* main pulmonary artery, *Prx Desc Ao* proximal descending aorta

ing to these procedures are based on arterial cannulation, homogenous perfusion, effective whole-body cooling, management of intravascular air trapping, comprehensive cardioplegic arrest, and anastomotic alignment without tension.

2 Interrupted Aortic Arch: Cannulation for Repair Using Circulatory Arrest Technique

In the era before the introduction of double aortic and regional perfusion techniques, (Varghese et al. 2015; Chen et al. 2019; Morales et al. 2006; Brown et al. 2006; Joynt et al. 2009; Visconti et al. 2006; Dominguez et al. 2007; Shinkawa et al. 2012; Mainwaring and Lamberti 1997; Jegatheeswaran et al. 2010; Kalfa et al. 2007; Serraf et al. 1996) the accepted cardiopulmonary bypass system to achieve homogeneous somatic cooling and organ preservation was accomplished by double arterial cannulation: namely, one arterial catheter perfusing the ascending aorta and the other in the main pulmonary artery with bilateral proximal pulmonary artery occlusion as an in-parallel circuit that ensured continuous and simultaneous flow to the upper and lower extremities, respectively, as shown in Fig. 3. Care is taken to avoid direct patent arterial duct cannulation for the inferior circulation since the ductus is thin- walled and subject to tearing and bleeding when cannulated. Figure 4 shows how a direct patent arterial duct cannulation can result in bleeding and unstable circulatory circumstances. The best way to resolve this complication is to remove the ductal cannula, tie the purse string, if possible, and establish sucker bypass using the ascending aortic cannula as the transfusion method while the ductal tear is repaired using pericardial pledgets to avoid further tearing. Once this calamity is resolved a new purse string can be placed in the more suitable distal main pulmonary artery which can hold sutures better. Recannulation at this site (Fig. 4 inset) can be accomplished with commencement of cardiopulmonary bypass as shown in Fig. 5. The other complications as noted above will require vigilance to identify and resolve in the event that they occur. For instance, arterial and venous cannulation problems have been reviewed in Chap. 1 “Complications Associated with Sternotomy, Resternotomy, and Cannulation”, which will serve as the basis for crisis resolution in these circumstances as well. Furthermore, accurate cerebral and systemic temperature measurements will allow confidence that systemic cooling is occurring. Cardioplegic arrest will be assessed by prompt cardiac arrest, topical cooling, and optimal coronary perfusion pressure as measured by the perfusionist. Clearing intravascular and intra-

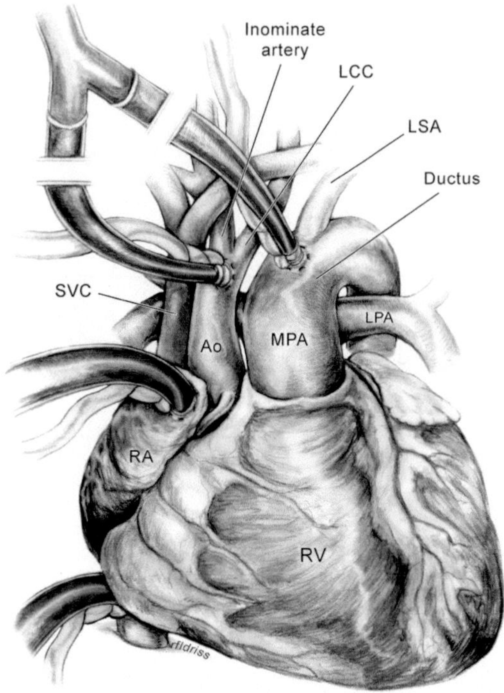

Fig. 3 Shows the cannulation technique before the era of double aortic and regional perfusion techniques, the accepted cardiopulmonary bypass system to achieve homogeneous somatic cooling and organ preservation. It is performed by double arterial cannulation: one arterial catheter perfusing the ascending aorta and the other in the main pulmonary artery perfusing the inferior circulation. Bilateral proximal pulmonary artery occlusion is accomplished to avoid pulmonary artery run-off and overcirculation (not shown in the drawing). Bicaval venous cannulation is established for VSD closure as needed. (With permission: Mavroudis 2015). *Ao* aorta, *LCC* left common carotid artery, *LPA* left pulmonary artery, *LSA* left subclavian artery, *MPA* main pulmonary artery, *RA* right atrium, *RV* right ventricle, *SVC* superior vena cava

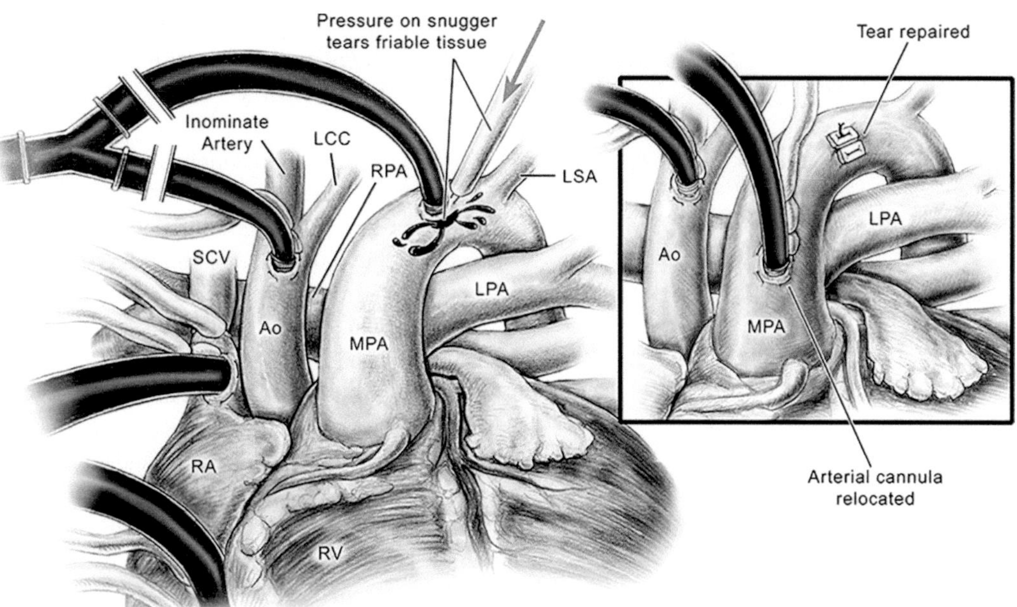

Fig. 4 Shows arterial duct disruption caused by purse string suture tearing through the thin-walled arterial duct. This problem can be resolved by catheter removal, closure of the ductal tear with pledgetted sutures and recannulation in a location closer to the body of the distal pulmonary trunk. In the event that uncontrolled hemorrhage occurs, sucker bypass can be established with infusion of lost blood into the ascending aortic cannula. The inset shows the successful closure of the ductal tear and recannulation at the distal pulmonary trunk. *Ao* aorta, *LCC* left common carotid artery, *LPA* left pulmonary artery, *LSA* left subclavian artery, *MPA* main pulmonary artery, *RA* right atrium, *RV* right ventricle, *SVC* superior vena cava

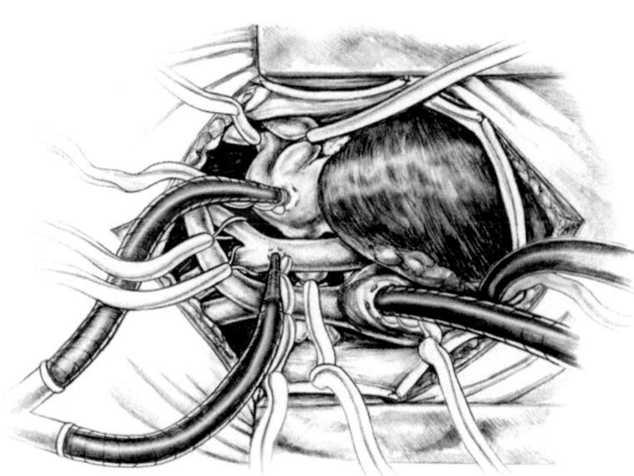

Fig. 5 Shows biarterial cannulation; one in the ascending aorta and the other in the pulmonary artery. The commencement of cardiopulmonary bypass requires right and left proximal snugger occlusion so that the pulmonary artery catheter can direct flow through the patent arterial duct en route to the lower extremity, the result of which is total body perfusion during the cooling phase of the operation. (With permission: Mavroudis 2015)

cardiac trapped air can be performed by a number of methods. The most important part of this procedure is to choose a tried-and-true method and make sure that it is performed accurately and conscientiously. Further to the diagnosis in Fig. 5, the drawing shows an anatomic display of the brachiocephalic arteries which show a type B interrupted aortic arch with left subclavian artery arising from the descending aorta. The figure also shows initiation of cardiopulmonary bypass with right and left proximal pulmonary artery temporary occlusion and snugger placement without occlusion of the brachiocephalic vessels. This perfusion method provides flow to the brachiocephalic vessels and descending aorta through the patent arterial duct. Bicaval cannulation is noted for eventual VSD closure during

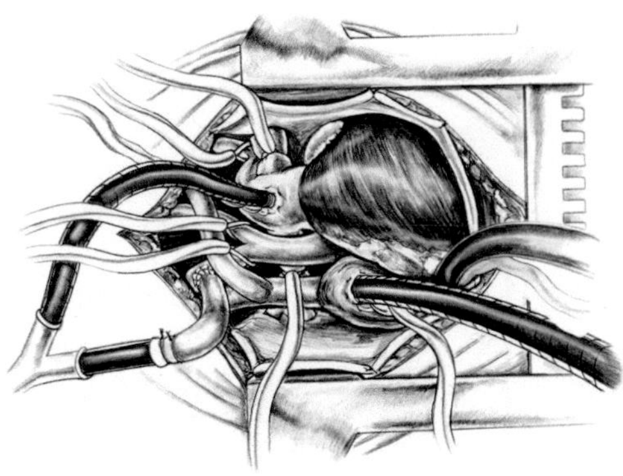

Fig. 6 Shows the double arterial perfusion technique established by anastomosing a PTFE graft to the innominate artery through which upper extremity arterial cannulation can be accomplished. The lower extremity perfusion technique is driven by a pulmonary artery catheter with proximal pulmonary artery control by snuggers. (With permission: Mavroudis 2015)

cardiopulmonary bypass after the IAA repair is completed. This perfusion technique will ensure careful and conscientious cooling that will protect the brain during the period of safe circulatory arrest which has been estimated to be 35–45 min or less. As noted, and as reviewed in Chap. 5 "Complications Associated with Repair of Coarctation of the Aorta", newer techniques of brain preservation using regional perfusion methods require arterial cannulation of the innominate artery with an interposition graft. Regional flow can then be established during the arch repair as shown in Fig. 6. These techniques have challenged the long-held maxim that circulatory arrest is the preferred technique for repair of IAA-VSD (Kreuzer et al. 2018); however, no prospective controlled study has confirmed the superiority of regional perfusion. Consequently, many congenital heart programs continue to employ the circulatory arrest technique based on excellent clinical results and laboratory findings (Myung et al. 2004). The principles of the operation however as shown in these drawings are similar whether regional perfusion or circulatory arrest is used.

3 Repair of Interrupted Aortic Arch by Regional Perfusion Techniques

As noted in the aforementioned paragraph, Fig. 6 shows the double arterial perfusion technique by anastomosing a polytetrafluoroethylene (PTFE) graft to the innominate artery through which upper extremity arterial cannulation can be implemented. Care should be taken to perform a leakproof and obstruction proof anastomosis as much as possible. Unwanted anastomotic bleeding can cause continuous visual exposure problems which can cause frustration and impediments to the flow of the operation. An obstructive PTFE to innominate anastomosis can cause poor systemic perfusion and counterbalance the beneficial effects of regional perfusion. The careful construction of this anastomosis cannot be emphasized enough.

Figure 7 demonstrates biarterial perfusion after systemic cooling to 18 °C. Also noted is removal of the descending arterial cannula, regional perfusion techniques by brachiocephalic tourniquet occlusion, descending aorta clamping and maintaining arterial flow to the brachiocephalic artery using low-flow techniques. Figure 7 also shows the act of removal of the ductus arteriosus, mobilization of the ascending and descending aorta, preservation of the origin of the left subclavian artery from the descending aorta, and preparation for the aortic arch reconstruction. Care must be taken to avoid recurrent laryngeal nerve injury during the descending aortic clamp placement. In general, the recurrent laryngeal nerve can be identified in its location around the patent arterial duct. There is enough mobility of the nerve to retract it inferiorly while the clamp is placed. This is noted and explained in Chap. 3 "Complications Associated with Ligation of Patent Arterial Duct (Patent Ductus Arteriosus)" where special attention to the nerve is emphasized by avoiding nearby use of electrocautery which can cause injury during the dissec-

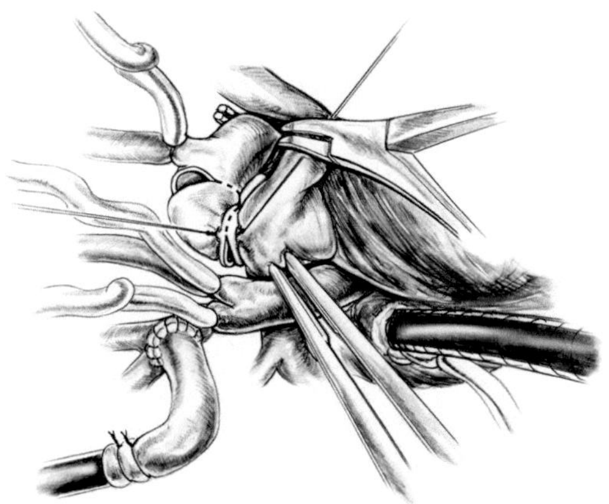

Fig. 7 Shows the later stages of cardiopulmonary bypass after systemic cooling to 18 °C, removal of the descending arterial cannula, establishing regional perfusion techniques by brachiocephalic tourniquet occlusion, descending aorta clamping and maintaining arterial flow to the brachiocephalic artery using low-flow techniques. Also shown is the removal of the ductus arteriosus, mobilization of the ascending and descending aorta, preservation of the origin of the left subclavian artery from the descending aorta, and preparation for the aortic arch reconstruction. (With permission: Mavroudis 2015)

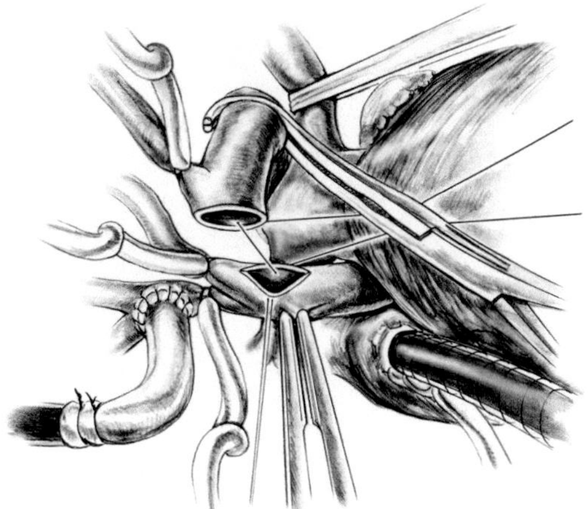

Fig. 8 Shows aortic reconstruction in progress by extensive arch mobilization and end-to-side anastomosis of the descending aorta to the ascending aorta. Notice that flow can be continued using regional perfusion through the innominate artery by way of the PTFE graft. (With permission: Mavroudis 2015)

tion with or without electrocautery engagement owing to the continued heat of the instrument during dissection. Better to use sharp or blunt dissection in this area and only usc clectrocautery when the nerve is clearly away from the bleeding site. Figures 8 and 9 show the aortic reconstruction in progress using regional perfusion techniques. The anastomotic union can be performed using polypropylene suture which is continued to the anterior suture line. After the aortic anastomosis is completed, the tourniquets can be released, air maneuvers can be accomplished, and full cardiopulmonary bypass can be established with systemic rewarming. During the performance of the air maneuvers, many surgeons place the patient in a deep Trendelenburg position to facilitate air removal from the os of the brachiocephalic vessels. Figure 10 shows the completed operation after separation from cardiopulmonary bypass. Note that 2 clips are placed on the residual stump of the PTFE graft which, when removed, can be used for emergent recannulation for arterial perfusion and extracardiac membrane oxygenation.

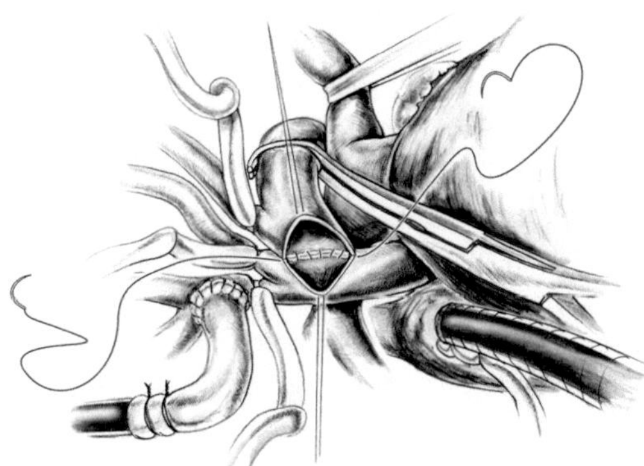

Fig. 9 Shows the posterior suture line completed with the anterior suture line in progress. (With permission: Mavroudis 2015)

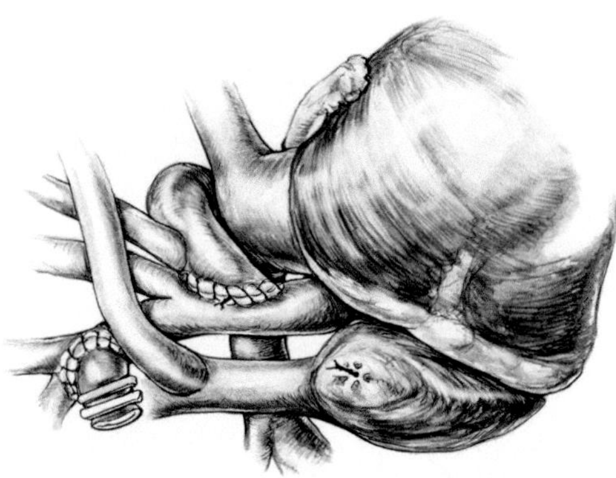

Fig. 10 Demonstrates the completed interrupted aortic arch reconstruction. Notice that the atump of the innominate artery PTFE graft is preserved by two hemoclips in the event that arterial cannulation and rapid institution of postoperative extracorporeal membrane oxygenation should be necessary. (With permission: Mavroudis 2015)

There are some anatomic variants, such as Type B interrupted aortic arch which may require left subclavian artery ligation and division to allow an unobstructive arch reconstruction free from ductal tissue, free from the potential for eventual constriction, and free from restenosis.

Figures 11, 12, and 13 show the important steps of repair of Type B interrupted aortic arch using deep hypothermia, circulatory arrest, and subclavian artery ligation/division. Once the arch repair is completed, systemic cardiopulmonary bypass and rewarming can proceed while the VSD is repaired. Conal VSDs can be repaired

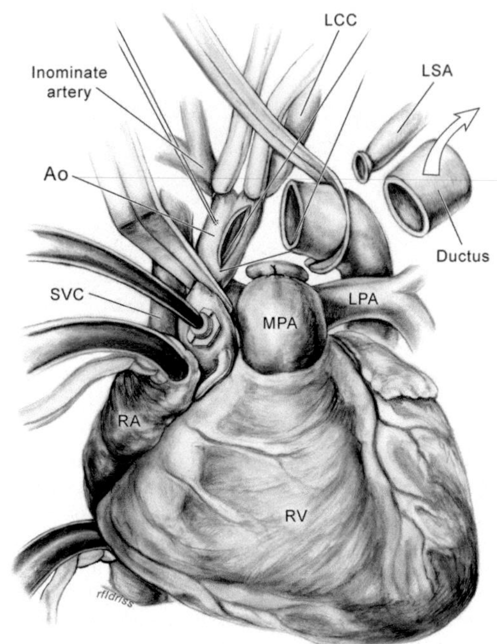

Fig. 11 Shows cannulation techniques for circulatory arrest, subclavian artery ligation, extensive arch mobilization, and end-to-side aortic anastomosis. The aortic cross-clamp was used for antegrade cardioplegia before the initiation of deep hypothermic circulatory arrest. Once the neoaortic reconstruction is completed, cardiopulmonary bypass can be resumed, and attention can be shifted to the ventricular septal defect. (With permission: Mavroudis 2015). *Ao* aorta, *LCC* left common carotid artery, *LPA* left pulmonary artery, *LSA* left subclavian artery, *MPA* main pulmonary artery, *RA* right atrium, *RV* right ventricle, *SVC* superior vena cava

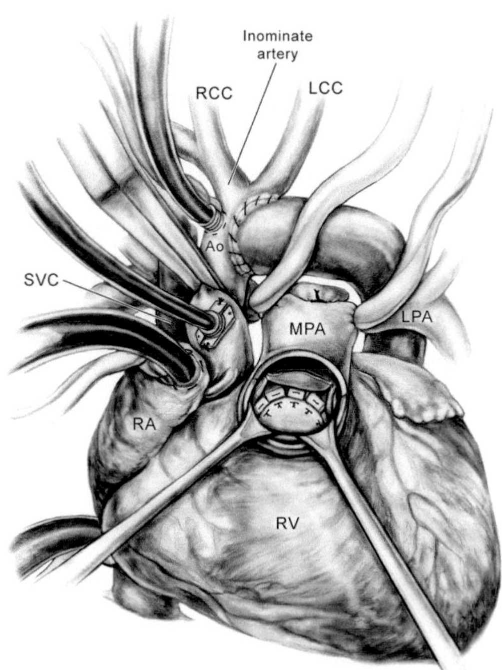

Fig. 12 Shows complete closure of a conal ventricular septal defect through a transpulmonary artery exposure. Perimembranous ventricular septal defects are better approached through the right atrium as noted in Chapter "Complications Associated with Ventricular Septal Defect Closure". (With permission: Mavroudis 2015). *Ao* aorta, *LCC* left common carotid artery, *LPA* left pulmonary artery, *MPA* main pulmonary artery, *RA* right atrium, *RV* right ventricle, *SVC* superior vena cava

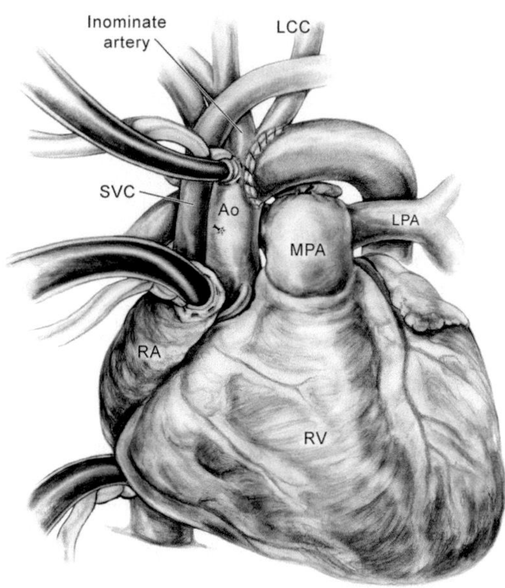

Fig. 13 Demonstrates the completed repair in preparation for separation from cardiopulmonary bypass. (With permission: Mavroudis 2015). *Ao* aorta, *LCC* left common carotid artery, *LPA* left pulmonary artery, *MPA* main pulmonary artery, *RA* right atrium, *RV* right ventricle, *SVC* superior vena cava

through the pulmonary artery while perimembranous VSDs are better approached through the right atrium as noted in Chap. 8 "Complications Associated with Ventricular Septal Defect Closure".

Repair of interrupted aortic arch is associated with many intracardiac and extracardiac anomalies. The principles of IAA repair are mostly the same which include arch dissection, appropriate management of cardiopulmonary bypass, and repair of the associated lesions. This chapter reviews the important steps of these operations to avoid operative complications such as cerebral ischemic injury, postoperative arch obstruction, recurrent laryngeal nerve injury, myocardial depression, and operative bleeding due to catheter disruption of the patent arterial duct. Careful attention to detail will prevent these complications and result in excellent clinical outcomes (Kellermann et al. 2018; Chen et al. 2013b; Hirata et al. 2010; Alsoufi et al. 2016; Backer 2016; Oosterhof et al. 2004; Miyamoto et al. 2013; Karimi et al. 2010; Patel et al. 2016; Rauch et al. 1998; McDonald et al. 2013; Simsic et al. 2009; Mahle et al. 2003; O'Byrne et al. 2014b; O'Byrne et al. 2014a).

References

Alsoufi B, Schlosser B, McCracken C, et al. Selective management strategy of interrupted aortic arch mitigates left ventricular outflow tract obstruction risk. J Thorac Cardiovasc Surg. 2016;151:412–20.

Axt-Fliedner R, Kawecki A, Enzensberger C, et al. Fetal and neonatal diagnosis of interrupted aortic arch: associations and outcomes. Fetal Diagn Ther. 2011;30:299–305.

Backer CL. Interrupted aortic arch: measure twice, cut once. J Thorac Cardiovasc Surg. 2016;151:422–3.

Bamforth SD, Anderson RH. Understanding the morphogenesis of the left-sided arterial duct in the setting of a right-sided aortic arch. Cardiol Young. 2017;27:369–72.

Barratt-Boyes BG, Nicholls TT, Brandt PW, Neutze JM. Aortic arch interruption associated with patent ductus arteriosus, ventricular septal defect, and total anomalous pulmonary venous connection. Total correction in an 8-day-old infant by means of profound hypothermia and limited cardiopulmonary bypass. J Thorac Cardiovasc Surg. 1972;63:367–73.

Bergoend E, Bouissou A, Paoli F, Roullet-Renoleau N, Duchalais A, Neville P. A new technique for interrupted aortic arch repair: the Neville tube. Ann Thorac Surg. 2010;90:1375–6.

Brown JW, Ruzmetov M, Okada Y, Vijay P, Rodefeld MD, Turrentine MW. Outcomes in patients with interrupted aortic arch and associated anomalies: a 20-year experience. Eur J Cardiothorac Surg. 2006;29:666–74.

Celoria GC, Patton RB. Congenital absence of the aortic arch. Am Heart J. 1959;58:407–13.

Chen CP, Huang MC, Chen YY, et al. Prenatal diagnosis of de novo interstitial deletions involving 5q23.1-q23.3 and 18q12.1-q12.3 by array CGH using uncultured amniocytes in a pregnancy with fetal interrupted aortic arch and atrial septal defect. Gene. 2013a;531:496–501.

Chen PC, Cubberley AT, Reyes K, et al. Predictors of reintervention after repair of interrupted aortic arch with ventricular septal defect. Ann Thorac Surg. 2013b;96:621–8.

Chen Q, Caputo M, Stoica S, Lansdowne W, Parry AJ. Direct arterial cannulation allows easy and safe continuous selective cerebral perfusion during repair of interrupted aortic arch even for low birth weight neonates. World J Pediatr Congenit Heart Surg. 2019;10(4):464–8.

Collins-Nakai RL, Dick M, Parisi-Buckley L, Fyler DC, Castaneda AR. Interrupted aortic arch in infancy. J Pediatr. 1976;88:959–62.

Dillman JR, Yarram SG, D'Amico AR, Hernandez RJ. Interrupted aortic arch: spectrum of MRI findings. AJR Am J Roentgenol. 2008;190:1467–74.

Dominguez TE, Wernovsky G, Gaynor JW. Cause and prevention of central nervous system injury in neonates undergoing cardiac surgery. Semin Thorac Cardiovasc Surg. 2007;19:269–77.

Fuchigami T, Nagata N, Nishioka M, Akashige T, Takahashi K. Repair of vascular ring with right-sided interrupted aortic arch and right-sided descending aorta. Ann Thorac Surg. 2016;101:e41–3.

Hanneman K, Newman B, Chan F. Congenital variants and anomalies of the aortic arch. Radiographics. 2017;37(1):32–51.

Hartman RJ, Rasmussen SA, Botto LD, et al. The contribution of chromosomal abnormalities to congenital heart defects: a population-based study. Pediatr Cardiol. 2011;32:1147–57.

Hirata Y, Quaegebeur JM, Mosca RS, Takayama H, Chen JM. Impact of aortic annular size on rate of reoperation for left ventricular outflow tract obstruction after repair of interrupted aortic arch and ventricular septal defect. Ann Thorac Surg. 2010;90:588–92.

Jegatheeswaran A, McCrindle BW, Blackstone EH, et al. Persistent risk of subsequent procedures and mortality in patients after interrupted aortic arch repair: a Congenital Heart Surgeons' Society study. J Thorac Cardiovasc Surg. 2010;140:1059–75.

Jonas RA. Comprehensive surgical management of congenital heart disease. London: Hodder Arnold; 2004.

Jonas RA. Interrupted aortic arch. In: Mavroudis C, Backer CL, editors. Pediatric cardiac surgery. Philadelphia: Mosby; 2003.

Jonas RA, Quaegebeur JM, Kirklin JW, Blackstone EH, Daicoff G. Outcomes in patients with interrupted aortic arch and ventricular septal defect. A multi-institutional study. Congenital Heart Surgeons' Society. J Thorac Cardiovasc Surg. 1994;107:1099–113.

Joynt CA, Robertson CM, Cheung PY, et al. Two-year neurodevelopmental outcomes of infants undergoing neonatal cardiac surgery for interrupted aortic arch: a descriptive analysis. J Thorac Cardiovasc Surg. 2009;138:924–32.

Kalfa D, Ghez O, Kreitmann B, Metras D. Secondary subaortic stenosis in heart defects without any initial subaortic obstruction: a multifactorial postoperative event. Eur J Cardiothorac Surg. 2007;32:582–7.

Karimi M, Farouk A, Golden A, Gilkeson R. Hybrid palliation of interrupted aortic arch in a high-risk neonate. Ann Pediatr Cardiol. 2010;3:74–6.

Kellermann S, Janssen C, Münch F, et al. Deep hypothermic circulatory arrest or tepid regional cerebral perfusion: impact on haemodynamics and myocardial integrity in a randomized experimental trial. Interact Cardiovasc Thorac Surg. 2018;26(4):667–72. Erratum in: Interact Cardiovasc Thorac Surg. 26(4):715. PMID: 29272381

Kreuzer M, Sames-Dolzer E, Schausberger L, et al. Double-arterial cannulation: a strategy for whole body perfusion during aortic arch reconstruction. Interact Cardiovasc Thorac Surg. 2018;27(5):742–8.

Lee MG, Brizard CP, d'Udekem Y. Limitations in the use of left carotid artery turndown for interrupted aortic arch repair. J Thorac Cardiovasc Surg. 2013;146:1307–8.

Mahle WT, Crisalli J, Coleman K, et al. Deletion of chromosome 22q11.2 and outcome in patients with pulmonary atresia and ventricular septal defect. Ann Thorac Surg. 2003;76:567–71.

Mainwaring RD, Lamberti JJ. Mid- to long-term results of the two-stage approach for type B interrupted aortic arch and ventricular septal defect. Ann Thorac Surg. 1997;64:1782–6.

Mavroudis C. Interrupted aortic arch. In: Mavroudis C, Backer CL, editors. Atlas of pediatric cardiac surgery. London: Springer; 2015.

McCrindle BW, Tchervenkov CI, Konstantinov IE, et al. Risk factors associated with mortality and interventions in 472 neonates with interrupted aortic arch: a Congenital Heart Surgeons' Society study. J Thorac Cardiovasc Surg. 2005;129:343–50.

McDonald R, Dodgen A, Goyal S, et al. Impact of 22q11.2 deletion on the postoperative course of children after cardiac surgery. Pediatr Cardiol. 2013;34:341–7.

Mery CM, Guzmán-Pruneda FA, Carberry KE, et al. Aortic arch advancement for aortic coarctation and hypoplastic aortic arch in neonates and infants. Ann Thorac Surg. 2014;98:625–33.

Messner G, Reul GJ, Flamm SD, Gregoric ID, Opfermann UT. Interrupted aortic arch in an adult single-stage extra-anatomic repair. Tex Heart Inst J. 2002;29:118–21.

Miyamoto T, Yoshii T, Inui A, Ozaki S. Staged repair for aortic arch reconstruction and intracardiac repair following bilateral pulmonary artery banding in 3 critical patients. Interact Cardiovasc Thorac Surg. 2013;16:892–4.

Moerman P, et al. Interrupted right aortic arch in DiGeorge syndrome. Br Heart J. 1987;58:274–8.

Morales DL, Scully PT, Braud BE, et al. Interrupted aortic arch repair: aortic arch advancement without a patch minimizes arch reinterventions. Ann Thorac Surg. 2006;82:1577–84.

Myung RJ, Petko M, Judkins AR, et al. Regional low-flow perfusion improves neurologic outcome compared with deep hypothermic circulatory arrest in neonatal piglets. J Thorac Cardiovasc Surg. 2004;127(4):1051–7.

Nisli K, Aydogan U, Tansel T. Left-sided aortic arch, right-sided descending aorta, and right-sided arterial duct associated with interruption of the aortic arch and presence of Abbott's artery. Cardiol Young. 2007;17:445–7.

O'Byrne ML, Mercer-Rosa L, Zhao H, et al. Morbidity in children and adolescents after surgical correction of interrupted aortic arch. Pediatr Cardiol. 2014a;35:386–92.

O'Byrne ML, Yang W, Mercer-Rosa L, et al. 22q11.2 Deletion syndrome is associated with increased perioperative events and more complicated postoperative course in infants undergoing infant operative correction of truncus arteriosus communis or interrupted aortic arch. J Thorac Cardiovasc Surg. 2014b;148:1597–605.

Oosterhof T, Azakie A, Freedom RM, Williams WG, McCrindle BW. Associated factors and trends in outcomes of interrupted aortic arch. Ann Thorac Surg. 2004;78:1696–702.

Paech C, Kostelka M, Grothoff M. First report of right sided interrupted aortic arch type A in combination with atrioventricular septal defect and microdeletion 22q11. Int J Cardiol. 2011;152:397–8.

Patel A, Costello JM, Backer CL, et al. Prevalence of noncardiac and genetic abnormalities in neonates undergoing cardiac operations: analysis of The Society of Thoracic Surgeons Congenital Heart Surgery Database. Ann Thorac Surg. 2016;102:1607–14.

Peyvandi S, et al. 22q11.2 deletions in patients with conotruncal defects: data from 1,610 consecutive cases. Pediatr Cardiol. 2013;34:1687–94.

Rauch A, Hofbeck M, Leipold G, et al. Incidence and significance of 22q11.2 hemizygosity in patients with interrupted aortic arch. Am J Med Genet. 1998;78:322–31.

Roussin R, Belli E, Lacour-Gayet F, et al. Aortic arch reconstruction with pulmonary autograft patch aortoplasty. J Thorac Cardiovasc Surg. 2002;123:443–50.

Sell JE, Jonas RA, Mayer JE, Blackstone EH, Kirklin JW, Castañeda AR. The results of a surgical program for interrupted aortic arch. J Thorac Cardiovasc Surg. 1988;96:864–77.

Serraf A, Lacour-Gayet F, Robotin M, et al. Repair of interrupted aortic arch: a ten-year experience. J Thorac Cardiovasc Surg. 1996;112:1150–60.

Shinkawa T, Jaquiss RD, Imamura M. Single institutional experience of interrupted aortic arch repair over 28 years. Interact Cardiovasc Thorac Surg. 2012;14:551–5.

Simsic JM, Coleman K, Maher KO, Cuadrado A, Kirshbom PM. Do neonates with genetic abnormalities have an increased morbidity and mortality following cardiac surgery? Congenit Heart Dis. 2009;4:160–5.

Tlaskal T, Vojtovic P, Reich O, Hucin B, Gebauer R, Kucera V. Improved results after the primary repair of interrupted aortic arch: impact of a new management protocol with isolated cerebral perfusion. Eur J Cardiothorac Surg. 2010;38:52–8.

Todman SH, Eltayeb O, Ruzmetov M, et al. Outcomes of interrupted aortic arch repair using the carotid artery turndown procedure. J Thorac Cardiovasc Surg. 2013;145:176–82.

Trusler GA, Izukawa T. Interrupted aortic arch and ventricular septal defect. Direct repair through a median sternotomy incision in a 13-day-old infant. J Thorac Cardiovasc Surg. 1975;69:126–31.

Varghese R, Saheed SB, Omoregbee B, Ninan B, Pavithran S, Kothandam S. Surgical repair of interrupted aortic arch and interrupted pulmonary artery. Ann Thorac Surg. 2015;100:e139–40.

Visconti KJ, Rimmer D, Gauvreau K, et al. Regional low-flow perfusion versus circulatory arrest in neonates: one-year neurodevelopmental outcome. Ann Thorac Surg. 2006;82:2207–13.

Vogel M, Vernon MM, McElhinney DB, Brown DW, Colan SD, Tworetzky W. Fetal diagnosis of interrupted aortic arch. Am J Cardiol. 2010;105:727–34.

Volpe P, Tuo G, De Robertis V, et al. Fetal interrupted aortic arch: 2D-4D echocardiography, associations and outcome. Ultrasound Obstet Gynecol. 2010;35:302–9.

Weisman D, Kesten HD. Absence of transverse aortic arch with defects of cardiac septums; report of a case simulating acute abdominal disease in a newborn infant. Am J Dis Child. 1948;76(3):326–30.

Zhang Z, Huynh T, Baldini A. Mesodermal expression of Tbx1 is necessary and sufficient for pharyngeal arch and cardiac outflow tract development. Development. 1987;133:3587–95.

Complications Associated with Atrial Septal Defect, Partial Anomalous Pulmonary Venous Return, and Scimitar Syndrome Repairs

Constantine Mavroudis

Abstract

Early challenges of atrial septal defect closure have decreased as repair techniques and modern era innovations developed, including the heart lung machine, myocardial protection techniques, and the intensive care unit. Today, complications are rarely encountered. However, occasionally, complications of embolism, stroke, and coronary insufficiency can occur if proper methods of deairing are not employed. Operative complications owing to unexpected anatomic variances can cause flow aberrations that can result in cyanosis, pathway obstruction, and arrythmias. A redundant Eustachian valve can complicate repair and cause inappropriate flow from the inferior caval vein to the left atrium, or in rare cases, occlusion of the inferior caval vein. Other documented complications involve superior caval vein syndrome caused by an expanding pericardial hematoma near the superior caval vein, impediments to flow owing to stenotic baffle construction, and overcoming the atrial anatomic characteristics that may require complex baffle preparation and implementation to avoid early and late atrial obstruction. This chapter reviews techniques to resolve possible complications experienced during repair.

Keywords

Pericardial effusion · Eustachian valve · Hemodynamic compromise · Superior caval vein syndrome · Limbus resection · Multipatch repair · Intra-atrial baffle · ASD devices · Transcatheter septal occluders

1 Introduction

Closure of atrial septal defects (ASDs) has a storied history in developmental repair techniques that were devised to ensure circulatory integrity, avoid cerebral air embolism, and accomplish complete defect closure. Early challenges of atrial appendage inversion (Murray 1948; Mavroudis et al. 2022), systemic hypothermia and inflow occlusion (Bigelow et al. 1950, 1954; Lewis and Taufic 1953), and atrial well techniques (Gross et al. 1952; Barratt-Boyes et al. 1956), proved to be unsatisfactory owing to incomplete closure, inaccurate diagnoses, and high mortality.

Gibbon performed the first successful closure of an ASD using a heart lung machine that he developed (Gibbon 1954). Kirklin improved the heart lung machine and applied this technology to care for patients with a variety of congenital

C. Mavroudis (✉)
Chief of Pediatric Cardiothoracic Surgery (Retired), Peyton Manning Children's Hospital, Indianapolis, IN, USA

Professor Emeritus of Surgery, Johns Hopkins University School of Medicine, Baltimore, MD, USA

C. L. Backer, C. Mavroudis (eds.), *Complications in Pediatric and Congenital Heart Surgery*,
https://doi.org/10.1007/978-3-032-02661-3_7

heart defects (Kirklin et al. 1955; Dushane et al. 1956).

The modern era saw further development of the heart lung machine, myocardial protection techniques, and the institution of the intensive care unit (Warden et al. 1954, 1955; Lillehei et al. 1955a, b, c, 1956; DeWall et al. 1957; Lillehei 1955, 1994; Melrose et al. 1955; Kolff et al. 1956; Effler et al. 1956; Gibbon 1937, 1939, 1978; Dennis et al. 1951; Reisner-Sénélar 2011). Closure of ASDs were thought to be low risk-high benefit operations. Complications are rare with the exception of undiagnosed postoperative pericardial effusions or persistent pulmonary hypertension in the unusual adult patient with increased preoperative pulmonary vascular resistance (Beghetti and Tissot 2009; Lindberg et al. 2002; Adrichem et al. 2019; Baskett et al. 2003). Anatomic complications are rarely encountered. However, they can occur and can be quite consequential if not recognized.

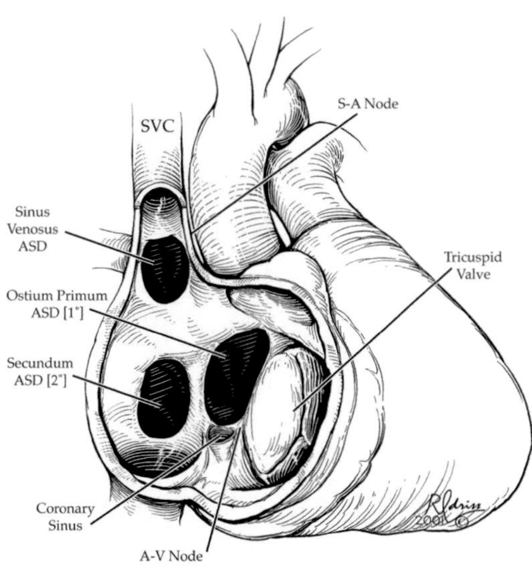

Fig. 1 A composite view of the most common types of atrial septal defect (*ASD*), including ostium primum ASD (partial atrioventricular [*AV*] canal), without the zone of apposition in the anterior leaflet of the left AV valve. A single atrium has no remnant of atrial septal tissue and is generally thought to be a partial AV canal with absence of the septum primum and septum secundum. *A-V* atrioventricular, *S-A* sinoatrial, *SVC* superior caval vein. (Reproduced with permission from: Mavroudis 2015)

2 Basic Anatomy

In our *Atlas of Pediatric Cardiac Surgery* (Mavroudis 2015), we defined an ASD as

> "a hole in the atrial septum that allows blood flow to shunt between the left and right atria. Atrial septal defects are characterized as (1) secundum type (hole in the septum primum), (2) sinus venosus type (hole in the atrial septum associated with the superior caval vein/inferior caval vein and accompanying anomalous pulmonary venous return), (3) ostium primum ASD that is better defined as partial atrioventricular (AV) canal because it is generally associated with a cleft or zone of apposition in the anterior left leaflet, and (4) single atrium with no remnant of atrial septal tissue and generally thought to be a partial AV canal with absence of the septum primum and septum secundum.
>
> To complete the classification, a patent foramen ovale, or a stretched patent foramen ovale, generally have small interatrial communications. The difference between a patent foramen ovale and a secundum ASD is determined by the amount of residual septum primum and its relationship to the septum secundum, which is superiorly located. These two septa are located in different planes in a flap-like configuration. The septum secundum is superior and slightly lateral while the septum primum is inferior and slightly medial in location. If the planes of the septa are superimposed and if there is enough tissue in the septum primum to effectively cause closure of the defect, then the hole is a patent foramen ovale. If there is a deficit of septum primum that will not effectively close the hole, then the hole is a secundum ASD." (Mavroudis 2015)

Figure 1 (Mavroudis 2015; Backer and Mavroudis 2013) shows a composite view of the most common types of ASD including ostium primum ASD (partial AV canal), although the zone of apposition in the anterior leaflet of the left AV valve is not shown (Mavroudis 2015).

In addition, there are several anatomic variants of the atrial septa and associated structures that may confound the interpretation of the margins of the ASD. For instance, multiple septal fenestrations and a prominent Eustachian valve can temporarily confuse the surgeon and cause unwanted complications, leading to undesirable baffle pathway reconstructions, baffle stenoses, caval vein stenoses and obstructions, among other complications (Mavroudis 2015).

3 Closure Techniques for Secundum Atrial Septal Defects

Over the years, many methods have been used to close ASDs, typically influenced by surgical training and settled practice. While not often used nowadays, some surgical teams have used induction of ventricular fibrillation and bicaval venous cannulation (Kugelberg 1976). While this method was successful in the past, there is always the danger that unwanted defibrillation may occur owing to wire dislodgment or hardware failure. This can result in systemic air embolism, stroke, and coronary insufficiency. Since the advent of routine use of cardioplegic arrest it became safe and efficient to employ this system having the aorta clamped, and threat of unwanted defibrillation is no longer possible.

4 Complications Resulting with Ostium Secundum Atrial Septal Defect Closure

Figure 2 shows the relevant anatomy before closure of an ostium secundum ASD. Notice the location of the Eustachian valve at the inferior margin of the atrium located near the coronary sinus (Mavroudis 2015).

Yavuz and associates (2002) described Eustachian valve development in utero as "directing oxygen-rich blood from the inferior caval vein toward the foramen ovale and away from the tricuspid valve. Once the foramen ovale is closed, there is no specific function, and in echocardiographic examination, the valve may appear as a thin flap originating from the orifice of the inferior caval vein or may be totally absent. Sometimes it may appear as a rigid, elongated structure in the inferior portion of the right atrium or as a membranous, undulating, echogenic mass within the right atrial cavity (Yavuz et al. 2002)." The Eustachian valve may be large enough to extend from the orifice of the inferior caval vein to the interatrial septum. The anatomic appearance may mask as a septal structure dividing the right atrium into two chambers (Yavuz et al. 2002).

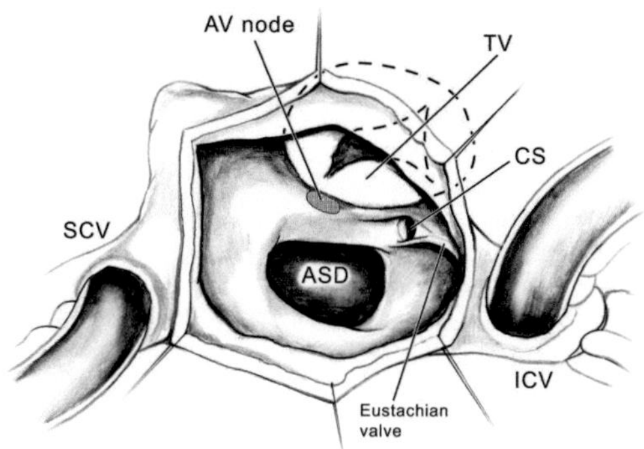

Fig. 2 A large secundum atrial septal defect (*ASD*) is shown with the important anatomic structures that should be noted and respected to avoid complications. The atrioventricular (*AV*) node is depicted as is the coronary sinus (*CS*), inferior caval vein (*ICV*), and superior caval vein (*SCV*). *TV* tricuspid valve. (Reproduced with permission from: Mavroudis 2015)

A redundant Eustachian valve may complicate the repair of an ASD by recreating the fetal blood flow course of the inferior caval vein to the left atrium. Figure 3 shows proximity of the prominent Eustachian valve to the inferior rim of the ASD, which in some cases may be missing and thereby camouflage appropriate closing techniques even further. The Eustachian valve is anterior to the os of the inferior caval vein, and the rim of the ASD or the right atrial-left atrial junction is posterior to the os of the inferior caval vein, leaving the flow of the inferior caval vein to course between these structures. Figure 4 depicts ASD patch placement en route to ASD closure. The suture line is started at the most superior location within the atrium. Notice the proximity of the Eustachian valve with the patch. Figure 5 shows the suture line being carried inferiorly as the surgeon mistakenly includes the redundant Eustachian valve as the inferior margin of the ASD. The suture line is then sutured toward the lateral portion of the ASD engaging eventually

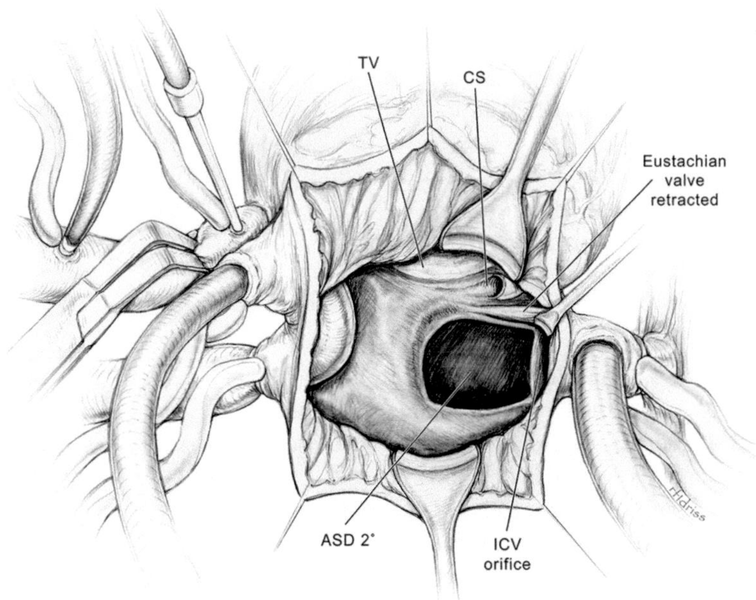

Fig. 3 The illustration shows proximity of the prominent Eustachian valve to the inferior rim of the atrial septal defect (*ASD*) that in some cases may be missing and may camouflage the accurate closing technique even further. The Eustachian valve is anterior to the os of the inferior caval vein (ICV). The rim of the ASD or the right atrial-left atrial junction is posterior to the os of the inferior caval vein. The flow of the ICV therefore courses between these structures. *CS* coronary sinus, *TV* tricuspid valve

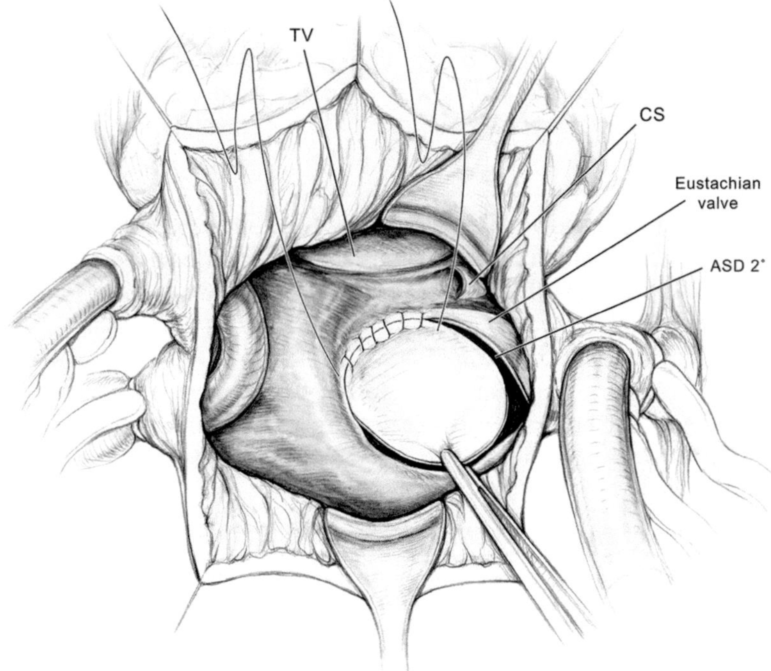

Fig. 4 Placement of the atrial septal defect (*ASD*) patch en route to ASD closure is depicted. The suture line is started at the most superior location within the atrium. Notice the proximity of the Eustachian valve with the patch. *TV* tricuspid valve, *CS* coronary sinus

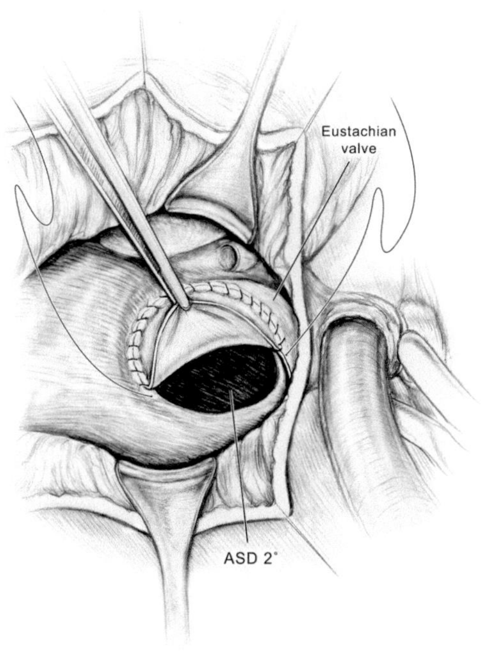

Fig. 5 The illustration shows the suture line being carried inferiorly as the surgeon mistakenly includes the redundant Eustachian valve as the inferior margin of the atrial septal defect (*ASD*). The suture line is then sutured toward the lateral portion of the ASD engaging eventually with the true ASD margin

with the true ASD margin. Figure 6a (inset) shows how the Eustachian valve is sutured to the patch. Figure 6b further depicts with arrows the resultant flow from the inferior caval vein to the left atrium and the superior caval vein to the tricuspid valve causing cyanosis owing to the atrial level right-to-left shunt. This mishap occurs more than is reported and can be misdiagnosed for many years (Thiruchelvam et al. 2021; Hallali et al. 1988; Munet et al. 1997; Aliter et al. 2011; Bjork et al. 1958; Mustard 1964; Shuntoh et al. 1997; Desnick et al. 1976; Effler and Groves 1961; Ross and Johnson 1972). A variation of this complication is the unwanted suturing of the Eustachian valve and the posterior orifice of the inferior caval vein to the patch. This anatomic configuration results in occlusion of the inferior caval vein with attendant hemodynamic compromise (Patel et al. 2021). Figure 7a, b shows how this anatomic mishap can occur if the surgeon is not alert to anatomic findings. Clearly, this is a very rare occurrence, but it has been reported in the literature (Patel et al. 2021). One can only imagine other unpublished mishaps that have occurred. Nowadays, these complications can be avoided by careful assessment and location of the os of the inferior caval vein, starting the suture line inferiorly at the os of the inferior caval vein if no ridge is present, and carrying the suture line superiorly all the time making sure that the structures are identified and respected. This includes the atrioventricular node, the sinoatrial node, the tricuspid valve, and the crista terminalis laterally. The postoperative measurement of oxygen saturation and the transesophageal echocardiogram alert the team to inappropriate flow of the inferior caval vein into the left atrium. Like many complications in this textbook, readers may express doubt that this complication can happen, until it actually does happen. The intraoperative adjustment once discovered, can be rectified by reinstitution of cardiopulmonary bypass, cardioplegic arrest, baffle takedown, and revised anatomically correct ASD closure.

Another report documents superior caval vein syndrome after ASD closure. The complication does not involve ASD closure per se, but the detection of an expanding pericardial hematoma over time near the superior caval vein leading to occlusion (Saboe et al. 2021). Mediastinal re-exploration revealed a large pericardial hematoma with residual topical hemostatic material. Although the patient did well after the operation, this complication begs the question of whether it is wise to remove topical hemostatic material once the bleeding has been controlled. These intraoperative decisions are generally personal in nature and are the result of specific training. Clearly, removing topical hemostatic agents that might cause cardiac or great vessel obstruction is imperative. However, should one remove topical hemostatic agents after bleeding is controlled? The case for removal is to eliminate any problems relating to a mass effect; the case for leaving the hemostatic agents is to control bleeding that can arise from an area that is difficult to control with sutures.

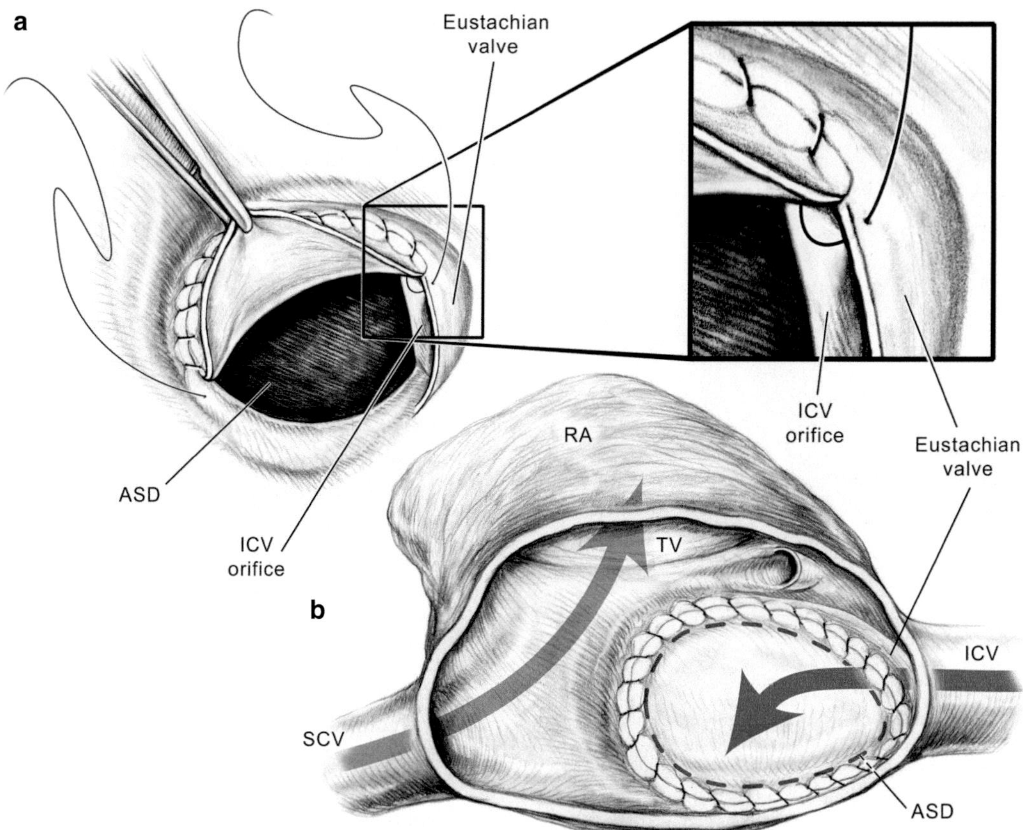

Fig. 6 (**a**, **b**) The illustration (*inset*) shows how the Eustachian valve is sutured to the patch (**a**) and (**b**) depicts with arrows the resultant flow from the inferior caval vein (*IVC*) to the left atrium and the superior caval vein (*SVC*) to the tricuspid valve (*TV*) causing cyanosis owing to atrial right-to-left shunt. *ASD* atrial septal defect, *RA* right atrium

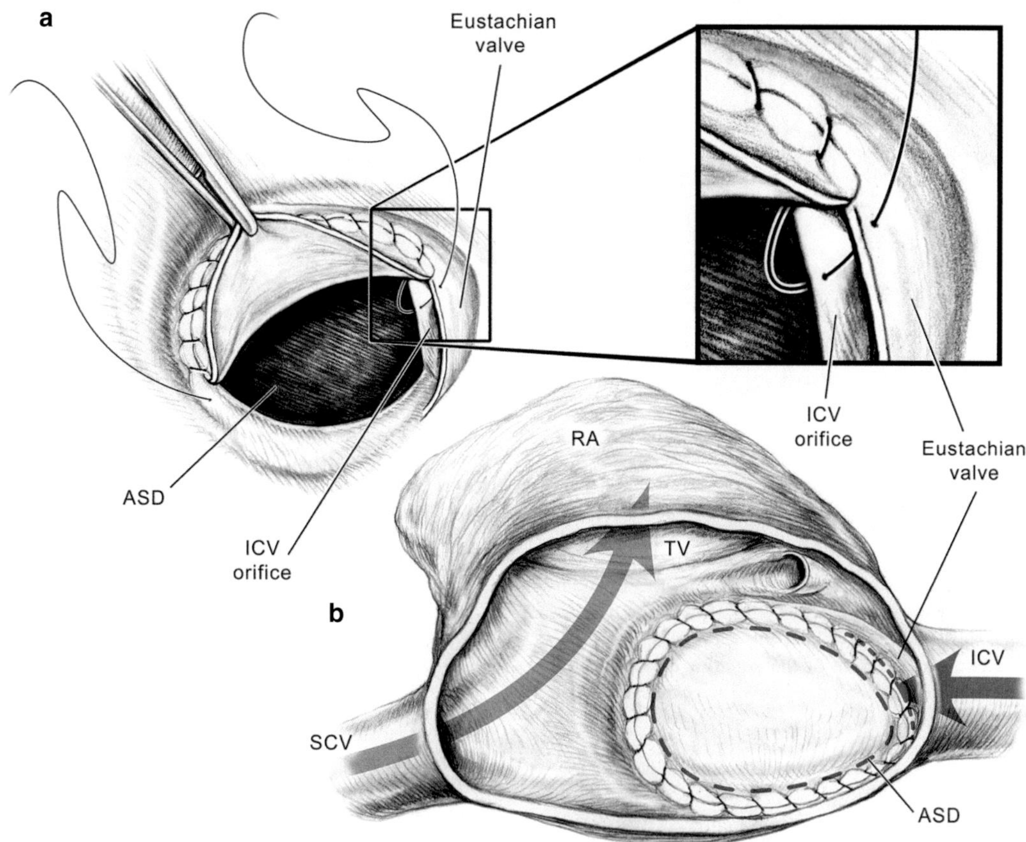

Fig. 7 (**a**, **b**) The illustration depicts a variation of the complication shown in Fig. 6. The unwanted suturing of the Eustachian valve and the posterior orifice of the inferior caval vein (*ICV*) to the patch (**A**) results in an anatomic configuration that causes occlusion of the ICV with the attendant hemodynamic compromise (**B**). *ASD* atrial septal defect, RA right atrium, *SCV* superior caval vein, *TV* tricuspid valve

5 Complications Resulting with Repair of Partial Anomalous Pulmonary Return and Sinus Venosus Atrial Septal Defect

> "Closure of a superior caval vein sinus stenosis ASD centers around the entrance point of the right anomalous pulmonary venous return into the superior caval vein. The more superior the entry of the anomalous pulmonary veins into the superior caval vein, the more difficult the operation and the higher incidence of atrial arrhythmias due to potential injury to the sinoatrial node. (Mavroudis 2015)

Figure 8 (Mavroudis 2015) demonstrates the operative exposure (median sternotomy) in a patient with sinus venosus ASD and anomalous pulmonary venous return. The right pleural cavity is exposed to note the height and the number of anomalous pulmonary veins in relationship to the phrenic nerve which must be preserved. In this case, the entry of the veins is at the juncture of the superior caval vein-right atrial junction. Figure 9 (Mavroudis 2015) after cardioplegic arrest, the atrial incision is performed respecting the distance from the sinoatrial node to avoid injury and preserve normal sinus rhythm. The illustration clearly shows the large sinus venosus ASD with entry of the right upper and right middle pulmonary veins into the right atrium. Figure 10 (Mavroudis 2015)

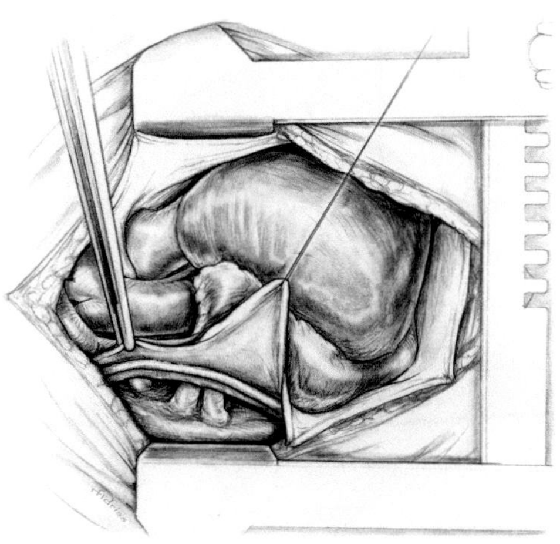

Fig. 8 The illustration demonstrates the operative exposure in a patient with sinus venosus atrial septal defect and anomalous pulmonary venous return. The right pleural cavity is exposed to note the height and number of anomalous pulmonary veins in relationship to the phrenic nerve which must be preserved. In this case, the entry of the veins is at the juncture of the superior caval vein-right atrial junction. (Reproduced with permission from: Mavroudis 2015)

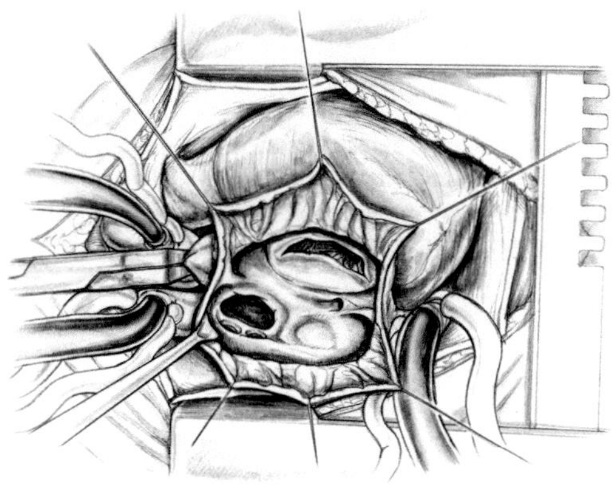

Fig. 9 The figure shows cardioplegic arrest and the atrial incision performed respecting the distance from the sinoatrial node to avoid injury and preserve normal sinus rhythm. The illustration clearly shows the large sinus venosus atrial septal defect with entry of the right upper and right middle pulmonary veins into the right atrium. (Reproduced with permission from: Mavroudis 2015)

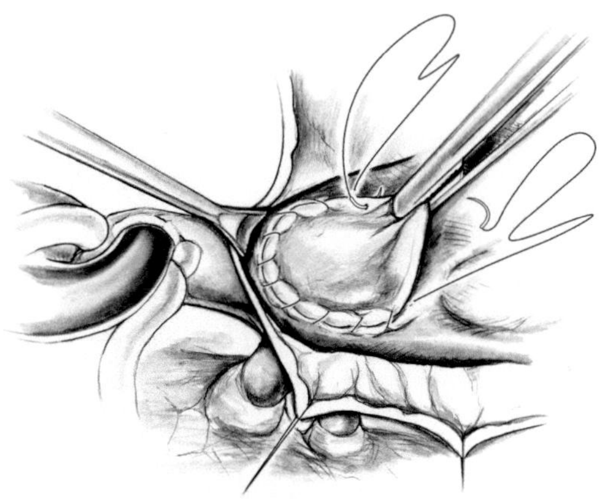

Fig. 10 Placement of a pericardial patch, with the suture line commencing at the superior edge of the atrial septal defect allowing tunneling of the pulmonary veins into the left atrium and concomitant flow from the superior caval vein into the right atrium without obstruction to either pathway. A slightly redundant pericardial patch avoids pulmonary venous obstruction without causing superior caval vein stenosis. (Reproduced with permission from: Mavroudis 2015)

> shows placement of a pericardial patch with the suture line commencing at the superior edge of the ASD that allows tunneling of the pulmonary veins into the left atrium and concomitantly flow from the superior caval vein into the right atrium without obstruction to either pathway. A slightly redundant pericardial patch will avoid pulmonary venous obstruction without causing superior caval vein stenosis as noted in Fig. 11." (Mavroudis 2015)

In some cases, the partial anomalous pulmonary veins are associated with a secundum ASD that is located further into the atrium than the sinus venosus ASD. Under these circumstances, there are significant potential impediments to flow and possible injury to the sinoatrial node. Figure 12 shows the location of the anomalous pulmonary veins and secundum ASD with a prominent limbus and location of the sinoatrial node that can be injured during repair. The surgeon may be tempted to perform a local limbus resection to avoid possible limbus obstruction during repair. As far as

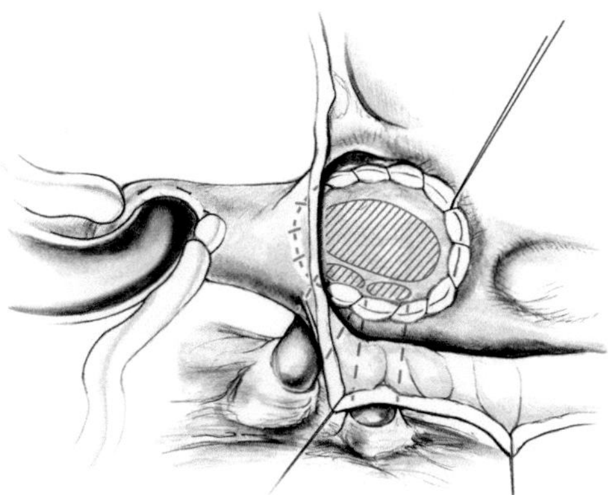

Fig. 11 The completed patch is shown with ghost views of the pulmonary veins under the pericardial patch with resultant unobstructed flow. (Reproduced with permission from: Mavroudis 2015)

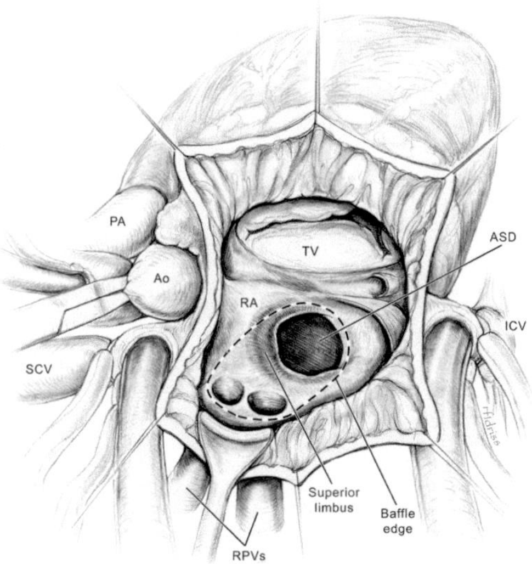

Fig. 12 The figure shows the length between the anomalous pulmonary veins and the secundum atrial septal defect (*ASD*), existent or otherwise created. The prominent superior limbus (septum secundum) represents a potential flow impediment that must be overcome by patch augmentation during the baffle creation. *Ao* aorta, *ICV* inferior caval vein, *PA* pulmonary artery, *RA* right atrium, *RPVs* right pulmonary veins, *SCV* superior caval vein, *TV* tricuspid valve

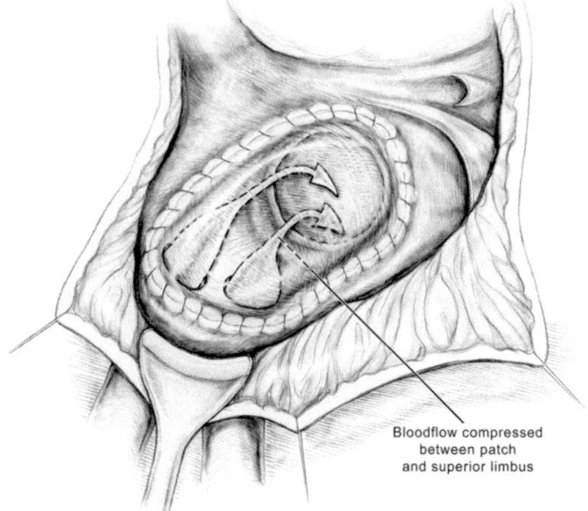

Fig. 13 The result of a pericardial baffle causes obstruction at the site of the septum secundum. The arrows represent the flow characteristics of the resultant reconstruction. The arrows are wide at the orifices of the pulmonary veins to signify excellent flow. The arrows become narrower over the septum secundum and into the left atrium signifying obstruction. When transesophageal echocardiography shows this type of flow with turbulence, the surgeon is duty bound to repair the defect as shown in Fig. 14

we know, limbus resection has been reported only by Geggel et al. (2020) to repair complex scimitar syndrome. Limbus resection to repair partial anomalous pulmonary veins and secundum ASD is not recommended. The shape and size of the reparative pericardial patch must consider the limbus that could cause a focal obstruction. Too large of a baffle may result in superior caval vein stenosis; too small of a baffle may result in pulmonary venous obstruction. Figure 13 shows a pericardial baffle that can cause obstruction at the site of the septum secundum. The arrows represent the flow characteristics of the resultant reconstruction. The arrows are wide at the orifices of the pulmonary veins to signify excellent flow. The arrows become narrower over the septum secundum indicating obstruction at the site of the septum secundum. Figure 14 shows revision of the intra-atrial baffle to enlarge the pathway. This can be managed by placing a measured probe into the partially repaired baffle. The pathway should be 1–2 mm larger than the confluence of the anomalous pulmonary veins en route to the secundum ASD. At the superior suture line, care must be taken to respect the location of the sinoatrial node. These potential conditions can be evaluated and identified by a transesophageal echocardiogram and can guide the surgical team to appropriately adjust baffle size during an immediate reoperation.

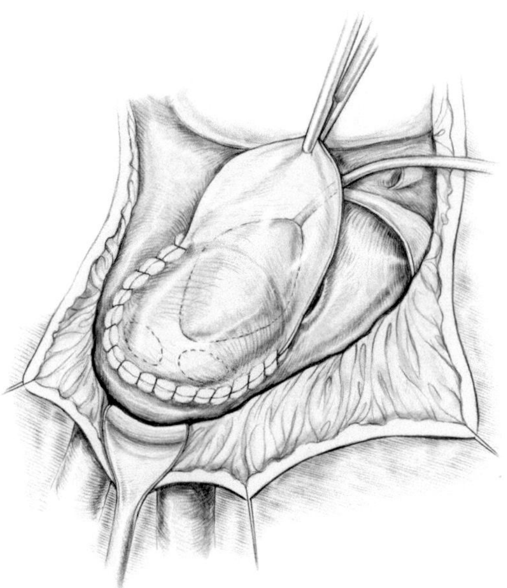

Fig. 14 The figure shows the creation of the pericardial baffle using a measured dilator to guide the ample baffle reconstruction

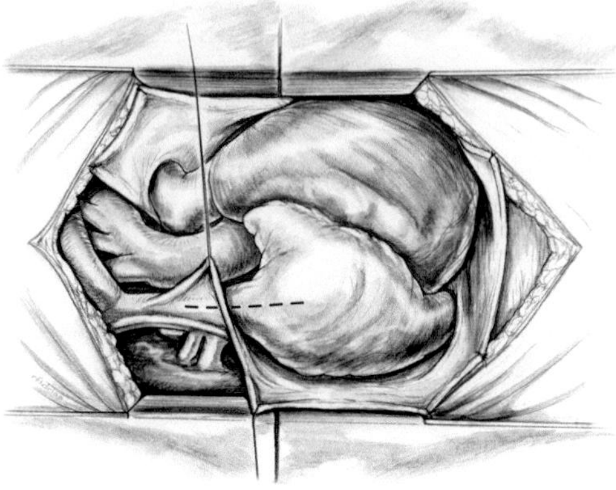

Fig. 15 In cases where the right anomalous pulmonary veins drain high in the superior caval vein as noted in this drawing, pericardial tunneling is challenged by potential obstruction of both the pulmonary venous and superior caval vein pathways. Adequate differential unobstructed flow into the right and left atria cannot be accomplished using only one patch. The classic resolution to this problem is the two-patch technique. The drawing shows the course of the phrenic nerve; the dashed line represents the incision made in the right atrium and extended to the superior caval vein. (Reproduced with permission from: Mavroudis 2015)

6 Two-Patch Technique for Sinus Venosus Atrial Septal Defect Closure for High Superior Caval Vein Entry of the Anomalous Pulmonary Veins

"In cases where the right anomalous pulmonary veins drain high in the superior caval vein, pericardial tunneling is challenged by potential obstruction of both the pulmonary venous and superior caval vein pathways. Adequate differential unobstructed flow into the right and left atria cannot be accomplished using only one patch. The classic resolution to this problem is the two-patch technique as depicted in Figs. 15, 16, 17, 18, 19, 20, and 21 (Mavroudis 2015) The operative exposure shows the sinus venosus ASD and high entry of the pulmonary veins into the superior caval vein. The atrial incision is extended into the superior caval vein opposite the entry of the anomalous pulmonary veins, The figures show the placement of the first patch which directs the pulmonary veins into the left atrium, while the second patch shows the augmentation of the distal superior caval vein to ensure adequate systemic venous flow into the right atrium. (Mavroudis 2015)

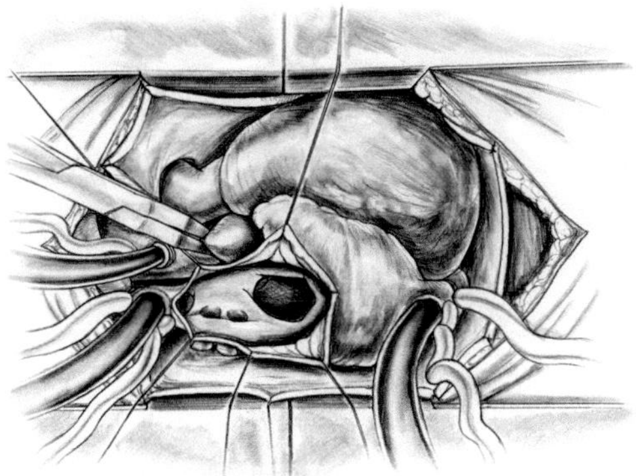

Fig. 16 The illustration demonstrates the operative exposure in a patient with sinus stenosis atrial septal defect and high superior caval vein inflow of the anomalous pulmonary venous return. An incision has been made into the os of the superior caval vein to adjust for differential pulmonary and systemic venous flow pathways. (Reproduced with permission from: Mavroudis 2015)

Complications associated with this repair are superior caval vein stenosis, anomalous pulmonary vein stenosis, and atrial arrhythmias caused by suture proximity to the sinoatrial node. Careful and

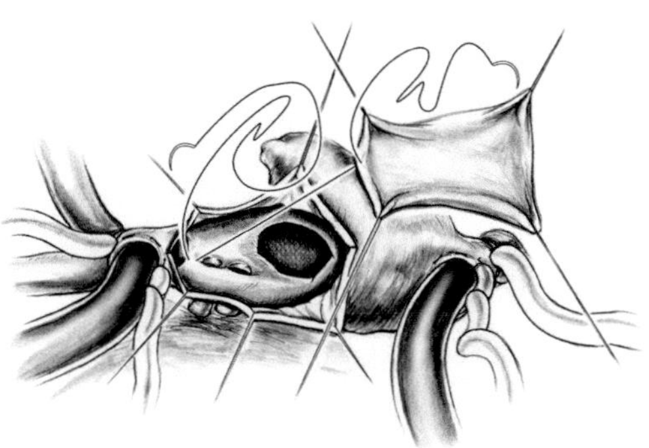

Fig. 17 Placement of the pericardial patch to baffle the anomalouos pulmonary veins to the sinus venosus atrial septal defect. The suture line is started from the posterior os of the superior caval vein. (Reproduced with permission from: Mavroudis 2015)

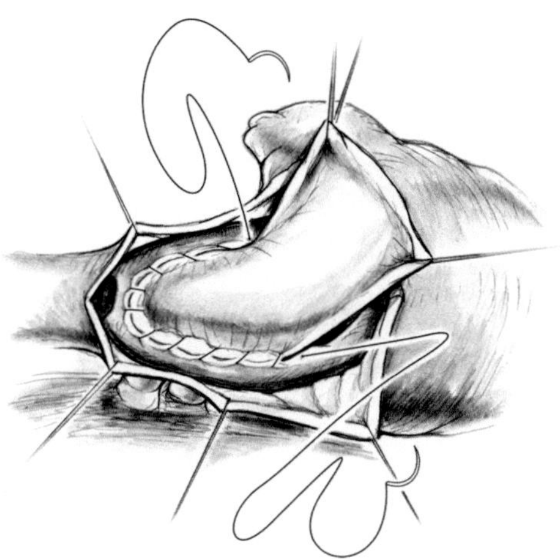

Fig. 18 The suture line is developed with special care to avoid the sinus node. The baffle is constructed to establish unobstructed flow from the pulmonary veins to the atrial septal defect. (Reproduced with permission from: Mavroudis 2015)

> comprehensive intraoperative transesophageal echocardiography can identify turbulence within both venous pathways if there is iatrogenic stenosis of the baffles." (Mavroudis 2015)

Figure 22 shows the stenosed pulmonary venous and superior caval vein pathways by differential arrow positioning. The surgical team must respond to these findings as any attempt at postoperative stenting of the superior caval pathway will certainly cause obstruction of the underlying pulmonary venous pathway. In the event that the pulmonary venous pathway is obstructed, access to the affected site will be challenged by

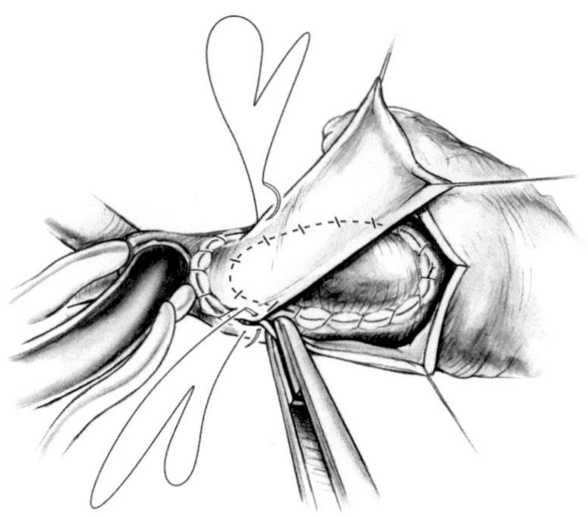

Fig. 19 Once the tunneling of the pulmonary veins into the atrial septal defect is complete and thereby the atrial septal defect closed, a second pericardial patch is placed to augment the flow of the superior caval vein into the body of the right atrium without causing obstruction to either the systemic or pulmonary venous return. This is done with special care to avoid any injury to the sinoatrial node that can cause unwanted atrial arrhythmias. (Reproduced with permission from: Mavroudis 2015)

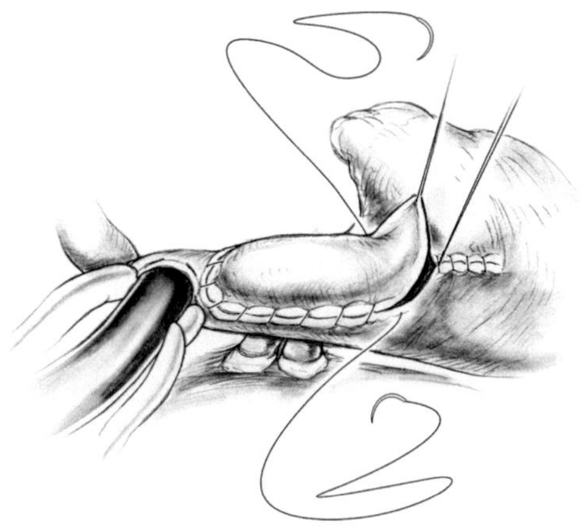

Fig. 20 The illustration shows completion of the augmented superior caval vein pathway. Oftentimes the patch comes into contact with the atriorrhaphy that was used to expose the atrial structures. (Reproduced with permission from: Mavroudis 2015)

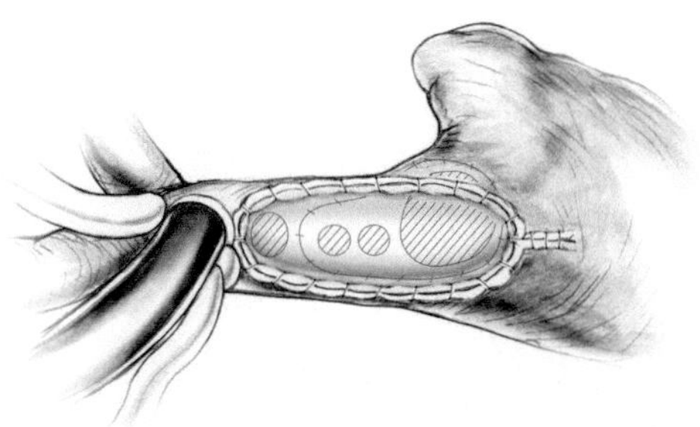

Fig. 21 The completed two classic two-patch repair with ghost views showing the differential venous pathways. (Reproduced with permission from: Mavroudis 2015)

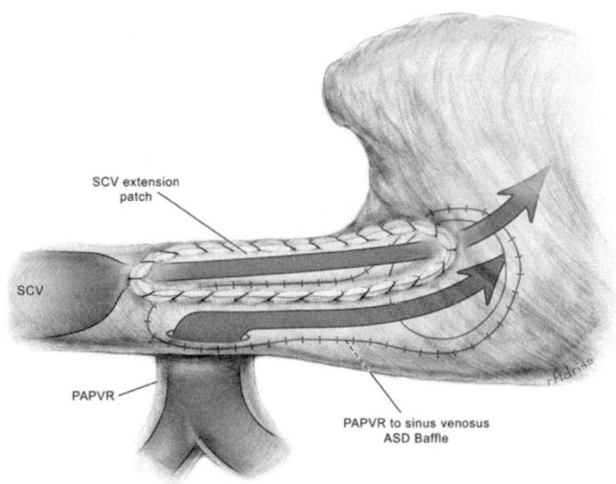

Fig. 22 The illustration shows how the two-patch repair can cause resultant pulmonary and systemic venous pathway obstruction. The arrows signify turbulence noted on transesophageal echocardiography. The demonstrated larger width of the arrow at the superior portion of the superior caval vein (*SCV*) and the upstream portion of the pulmonary veins represents normal flow. The narrow extension of both arrows represents decreased flow caused by the pathway stenosis, requiring immediate reoperation and pericardial augmentation of the stenotic pathways. *ASD* atrial septal defect, *PAPVR* partial anomalous pulmonary venous return

difficult access through the systemic venous pathway. The better option is to recommence cardiopulmonary bypass, cardioplegic arrest, take down the repair, and perform larger pericardial baffles that alleviate any hemodynamic obstructions as shown in Fig. 23.

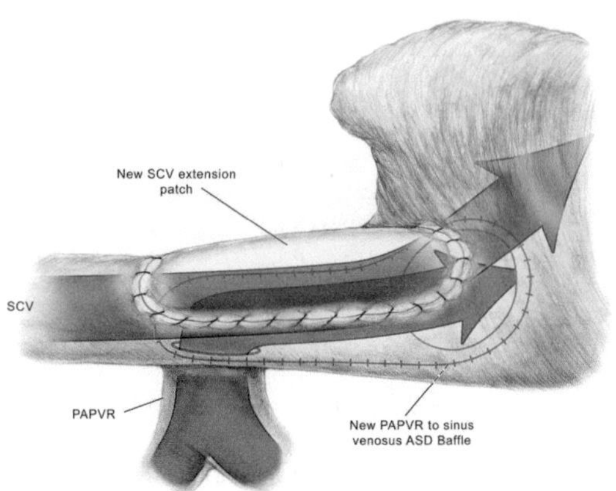

Fig. 23 The re-repair of the two-patch technique is necessary when pathway obstruction is noted by transesophageal echocardiography. The pathways have been repaired with enlarged patches that result in absence of pathway stenosis as noted by the differential arrows. The width of the arrows is the same in both pathways signifying normal flow. *ASD* atrial septal defect, *PAPVR* partial anomalous pulmonary venous return, *SCV* superior caval vein

Avoidance of atrial arrhythmias using the two-patch technique has been advocated by some (Elzein et al. 2020) suggesting a lateral superior caval vein incision away from the sinoatrial node. Others embraced the Warden procedure to avoid atrial arrhythmias and venous pathway obstructions (Stewart et al. 2007; Warden et al. 1984; Stephens et al. 2021).

7 Warden Procedure for Sinus Venosus Atrial Septal Defect Closure for High Superior Caval Vein Entry of the Anomalous Pulmonary Veins

"Some authors (Mavroudis 2015; Stewart et al. 2007; Stephens et al. 2021) have noted that the two-patch technique was attended by a high incidence of sinus node dysfunction and nodal rhythm, which led to an ingenious surgical solution as described by Warden and his colleagues

(Mavroudis 2015; Warden et al. 1984). The concept is to transect the superior caval vein and direct the flow of the anomalous pulmonary veins through the vena cava into the left atrium by a pericardial patch. This leaves the right atrial appendage to be anastomosed end-to-end to the transected superior caval vein. In theory and practically, the sinus node is preserved while the systemic venous return is maintained by unobstructed flow from the superior caval vein into the right atrial appendage. Figures 24, 25, 26, 27, 28, 29, 30, and 31 (Mavroudis 2015; Stewart et al. 2007) show the procedural progression of the Warden procedure. The potential complications of this operation are centered around the pulmonary venous baffle when a secundum ASD is encountered and the superior caval vein anastomosis to the right atrial appendage or the body of the right atrium." (Mavroudis 2015)

The pulmonary venous to left atrium baffle is relatively easy when there is a sinus venosus ASD. When there is a secundum defect or if an ASD must be created in the fossa ovalis, the baffle is more challenging owing to the limbus (septum secundum) which can act as an "anatomic hill" over which the baffled pulmonary venous flow must pass. "Eyeballing" or estimating the size of the baffle is one way of creating this baffle. Another preferable way is to start the baffle at the orifice of the pulmonary veins and use a suitably sized dilator to guide the size and width of the baffle for an unobstructed pathway.

In young patients who are undergoing a Warden procedure (Warden et al. 1984), it is not uncommon that the superior caval vein anastomosis to the right atrial appendage could be stenotic despite careful resection of the appendage trabeculations and use of interrupted suture technique. Any indication of anastomotic stenosis either by visual epicardial inspection or transesophageal demonstration of turbulence should be attended by recommencement of cardiopulmonary bypass and

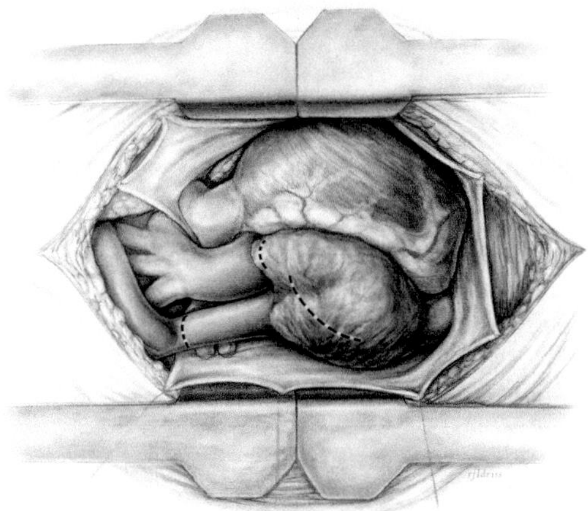

Fig. 24 The illustration shows operative exposure through a median sternotomy in a patient with sinus venosus atrial septal defect and high entry of the anomalous pulmonary veins. The dotted lines show the area of superior caval vein transection, the area of right atrial appendage incision, and the right atrial incision for exposure and repair of the defect. (Reproduced with permission from: Mavroudis 2015)

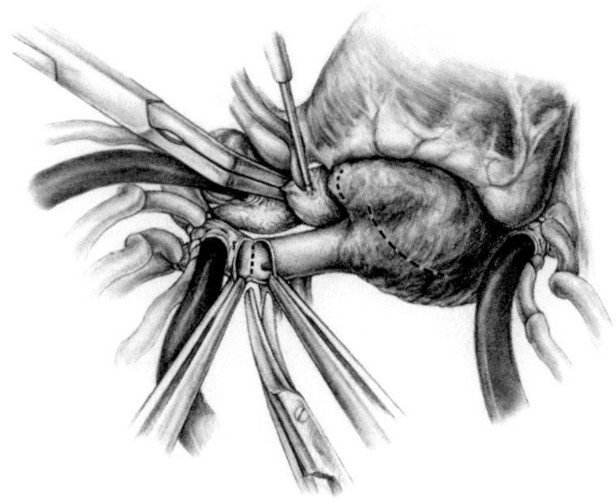

Fig. 25 The illustration shows aortobicaval cardiopulmonary bypass and cardioplegic arrest. Transection of the high superior caval vein is shown while preserving the entry of the pulmonary veins into the body of the cardiac portion of the superior caval vein. (Reproduced with permission from: Mavroudis 2015)

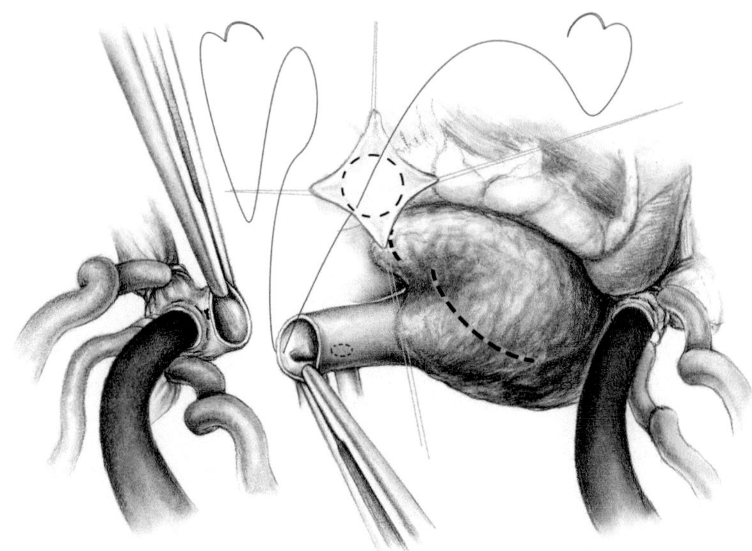

Fig. 26 The area of the sinoatrial node is shown intact. Pericardial patch closure of the cardiac end of the superior caval vein is performed to ensure unobstructed flow of the pulmonary veins into this segment. This is a very important maneuver since linear closure may obstruct one or both of the anomalous pulmonary veins. (Reproduced with permission from: Mavroudis 2015)

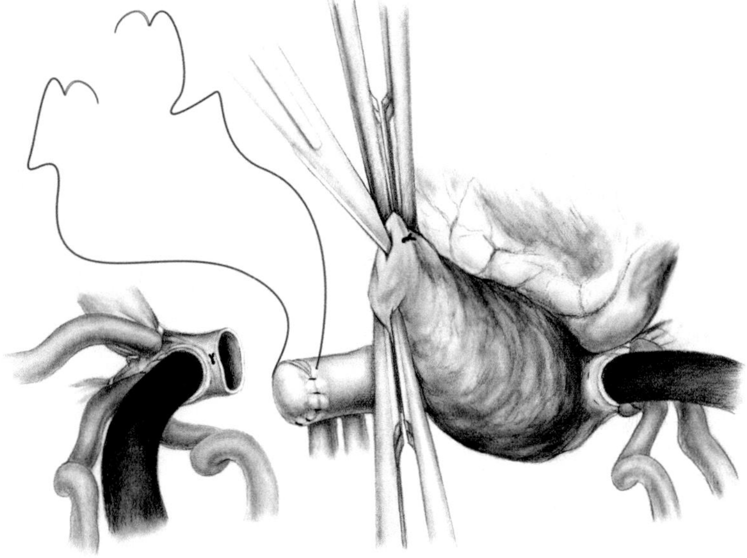

Fig. 27 This drawing shows the completion of the pericardial patch on the superior caval vein and incision of the right atrial appendage. This is done very carefully to ensure length for the eventual end-to-end anastomosis with the superior caval vein. (Reproduced with permission from: Mavroudis 2015)

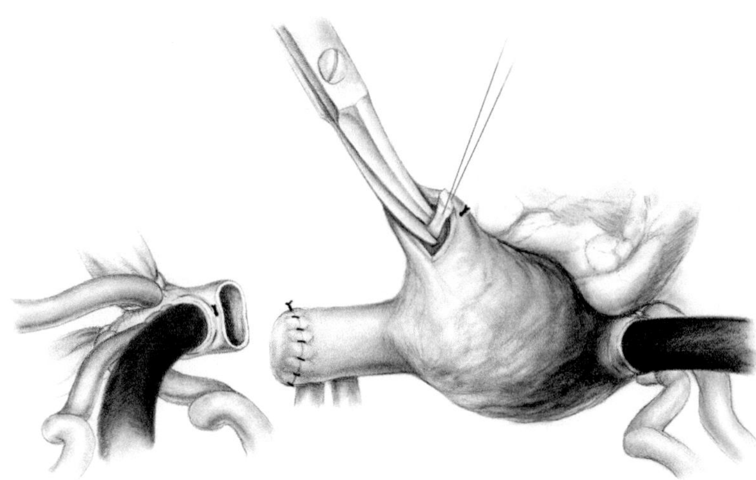

Fig. 28 Resection of the trabeculated portion of the right atrial appendage to ensure unobstructed flow during the end-to-end anastomosis with the superior caval vein. Care must be taken to avoid unwanted perforations of the atrial appendage during this delicate part of the operation. (Reproduced with permission from: Stewart et al. 2007)

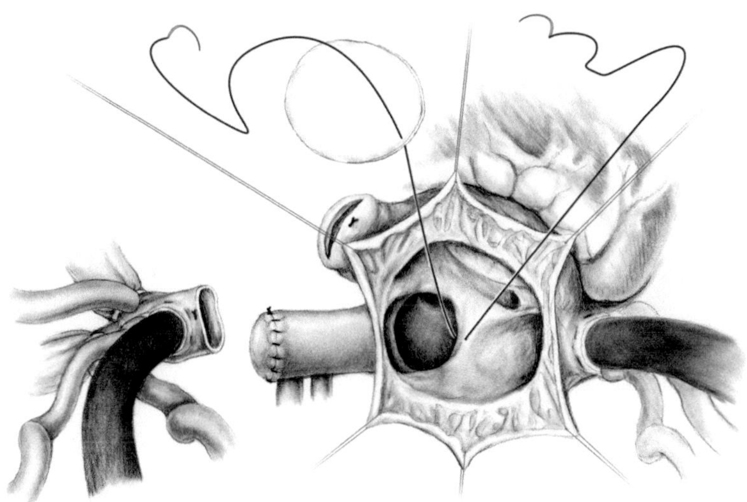

Fig. 29 Suture placement is shown at the inferior rim of the atrial septal defect in preparation for patch closure. (Reproduced with permission from Mavroudis 2015)

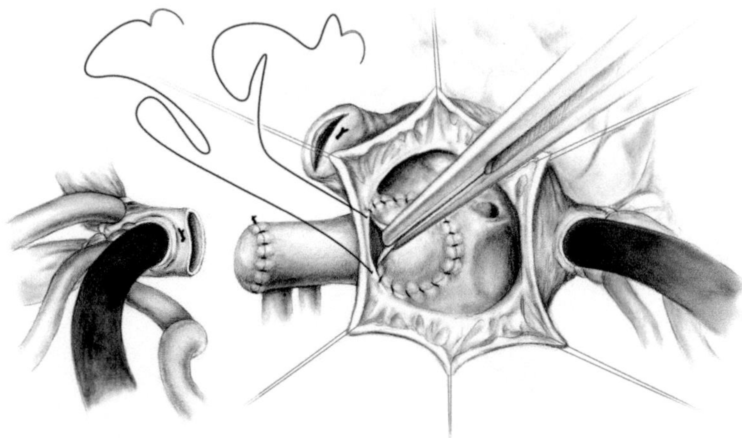

Fig. 30 Closure of the atrial septal defect is shown with a separate pericardial patch in such a way as to direct the entire orifice of the superior caval vein into the left atrium. This is clearly different from the previously described atrial septal defect closure that directed superior caval vein flow into the right atrium. In this situation, the superior caval vein that is connected to the pulmonary veins is now draining oxygenated blood into the left atrium. (Reproduced with permission from: Stewart et al. 2007)

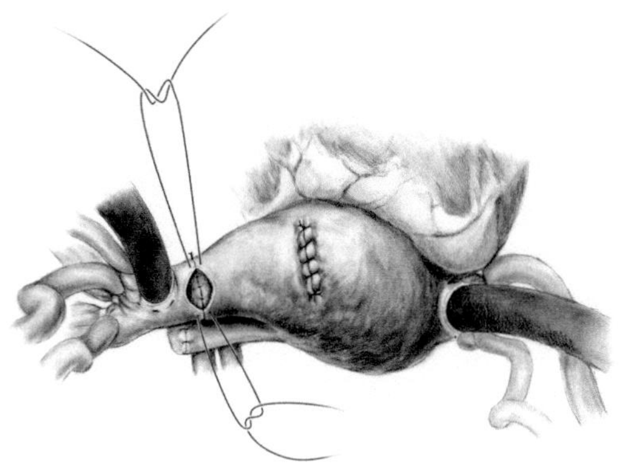

Fig. 31 Once the atrial suture line is completed as shown, the end-to-end anastomosis using interrupted suture technique is performed between the superior caval vein and the right atrial appendage. This maneuver divides the venous flow patterns without obstruction. (Reproduced with permission from: Stewart et al. 2007)

pericardial patch anastomotic augmentation as noted in Fig. 32. Counting on future subsequent balloon dilation and stent placement is not favorable in the long term. Anastomotic problems, therefore, should be addressed at the time of the initial operation.

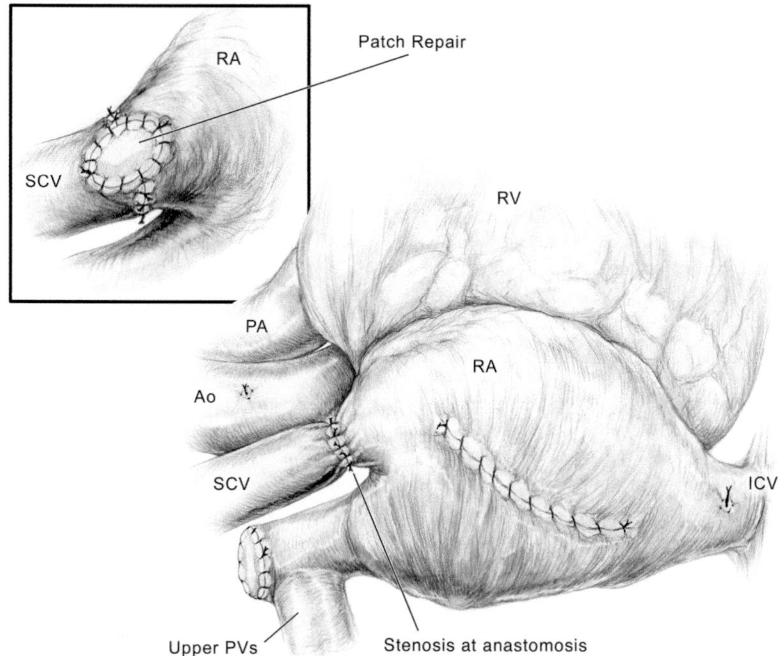

Fig. 32 In young patients who are undergoing a Warden procedure, it is not uncommon that the superior caval vein (*SVC*) anastomosis to the right atrial appendage could be stenotic despite careful resection of the appendage trabeculations and use of interrupted suture technique. Any indication of anastomotic stenosis either by visual epicardial inspection or transesophageal demonstration of turbulence should be attended by recommencement of cardiopulmonary bypass and pericardial patch anastomotic augmentation as noted. *Ao* aorta, *IVC* inferior caval vein, *PA* pulmonary artery, *PVs* pulmonary veins, *RA* right atrium

8 Complications Associated with Scimitar Syndrome

As noted in our *Atlas of Adult Congenital Cardiac Surgery* (Mavroudis and Dearani 2020),

> "Scimitar syndrome is a rare combination of anomalies that includes total or partial anomalous pulmonary venous connection of the right lung to the inferior caval vein, dextroposition of the heart, hypoplasia of the right lung and right pulmonary artery, and an anomalous systemic artery to the right lung from the abdominal aorta that penetrates the diaphragm. The cardiac silhouette on chest radiograph reveals the curved vertical shape of this vein that resembles a curved Turkish sword or scimitar—hence the nomenclature. Other frequently associated cardiac anomalies occur in up to 70% of patients with scimitar syndrome, with the most common being ASD. The degree of left-to-right shunt caused by the anomalous vein determines the severity of symptoms. Pulmonary hypertension, parenchymal lung disease, and associated intracardiac lesions can further complicate the clinical presentation. Affected patients tend to present with two separate clinical profiles. Infants present in the first few months of life with failure to thrive, cyanosis, respiratory distress, and congestive heart failure often with severe pulmonary hypertension. When inflammatory parenchymal changes are extensive or if the patient has persistent hemoptysis or marked hypoplasia of the right lung, pulmonary resection or pneumonectomy should be considered because resection eliminates the left-to-right shunt as well as lung infection. (Mavroudis and Dearani 2020)

Adult patients present with only mild symptoms of exertional dyspnea and recurrent respiratory infections. The diagnosis in adults is generally made by echocardiography that identifies associated intracardiac lesions and locates the anomalous vein regarding proximity to the cardiac chambers. Cardiac catheterization and angiography are diagnostic and can be partially therapeutic, as the anomalous systemic artery from the descending aorta that penetrates the diaphragm and supplies blood to the right lower lobe can be embolized,

> thereby facilitating the subsequent operative repair. In general, results depend primarily on the degree of preoperative pulmonary hypertension and associated cardiac lesions. Older patients with minimal symptoms have an excellent prognosis. (Mavroudis and Dearani 2020)
>
> Most approaches to repair of this anomaly center on ligation of the systemic arterial supply to the lung (for all cases) and redirection of the anomalous pulmonary vein to the left atrium. The systemic artery generally perforates the diaphragm and can be found as it courses within the inferior pulmonary ligament to the lung, where it can be readily ligated. The scimitar pulmonary vein is another matter; the surgical solution to this problem is individualized on the basis of symptomatic assessment and clinical findings at cardiac catheterization. (Mavroudis and Dearani 2020)
>
> In the recent past, surgeons have used pericardial patches to tunnel the extant orifice of the anomalous pulmonary vein at its entry into the inferior caval vein to the left atrium through an extant ASD or a surgically created pathway through the interatrial septum. This anatomic solution is fraught with complications leading to both pulmonary vein and inferior caval vein stenoses." (Mavroudis and Dearani 2020)

Najm and associates (1996) reported 32 patients with scimitar syndrome operated over a 20-year time period. Nineteen were diagnosed in the first year of life. The anomalous vein was baffled to the left atrium in 17 patients. Over a 9 year follow-up, no deaths occurred although 8 patients that included all 6 infants had postoperative evidence of pulmonary vein stenosis (Najm et al. 1996).

Alternative strategies have included polytetrafluoroethylene grafts that are anastomosed to the scimitar pulmonary vein and can be directed either through the right atrium en route to the left atrium through the ASD or directly into the left atrium (Munet et al. 1997; Guerra et al. 2016; Casha et al. 2003; Tsuchida et al. 1987; Brown et al. 2003). While these surgical techniques are ingenious in creativity and scope, stenosis (Geggel et al. 2020) as well as thrombosis (Pelletier and Spray 2001) have been reported.

More recent strategies have emphasized direct anastomosis of the anomalous pulmonary vein to the left atrium (Mavroudis and Dearani 2020). Brown and colleagues have treated 18 patients (mean age, 5.8 years) undergoing right thoracotomy with direct anastomosis of the scimitar vein to the left atrium, without use of cardiopulmonary bypass, and with no mortalities or reinterventions (Brown et al. 2003; Herrmann and Brown 2020). Other reports have enhanced the idea of direct anastomosis of the scimitar pulmonary vein to the left atrium (Mavroudis and Dearani 2020). The steps of the operation seem clear and complication proof (Figs. 33, 34, 35, and 36) (Mavroudis and Dearani 2020); however, mobilization of the scimitar vein can be challenging and result in anastomotic tension with the left atrium requiring a well-placed pericardial patch or an interposition graft to affect long-term repair.

A standard protocol for repair of the anomalous pulmonary scimitar vein is not altogether agreed upon. Geggel et al compared early scimitar vein surgery with a new operation based on multiple atrial patches with a total of 22 patients; 11 underwent baffling or reimplantation and 11 underwent the new operation that included resection of the atrial septum and removal of the

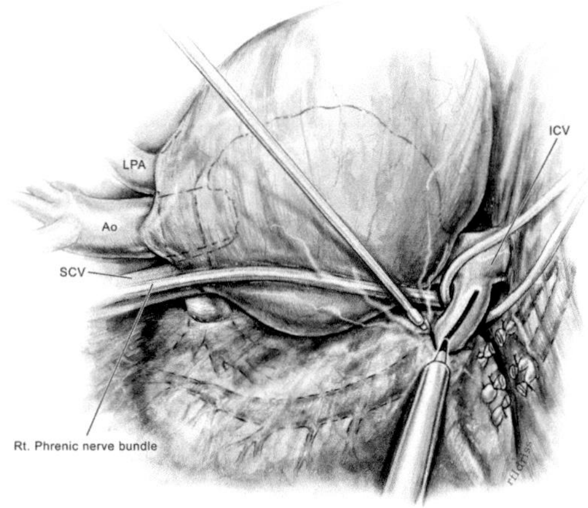

Fig. 33 The epicardial dissection of the scimitar pulmonary vein is shown at its entry to the inferior caval vein. Because anastomotic orientation can be challenging after the scimitar vein is transected, it is prudent to use a marker (*shown*) to avoid unwanted twisting during the repair. Aortobicaval cardiopulmonary bypass is instituted with aortic cross-clamping and cardioplegic arrest. This is followed by scimitar vein transection and orifice enlargement to better align the anastomosis to the left atrium. (Reproduced with permission from: Mavroudis and Dearani 2020)

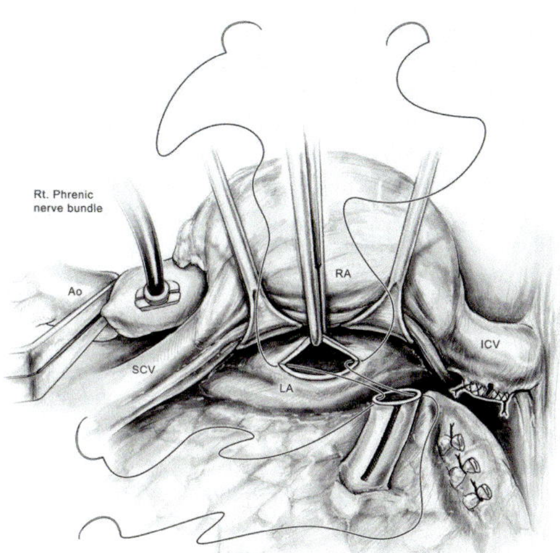

Fig. 34 The entry point to the inferior caval vein (*ICV*) is sutured closed as noted in the drawing. The previously placed mark on the scimitar vein helps to orient the anastomosis after an appropriate incision is made in the left atrium. Two sutures are placed to align the subsequent running suture technique. *Ao* aorta, *LA* left atrium, *RA* right atrium, *SCV* superior caval vein. (Reproduced with permission from: Mavroudis and Dearani 2020)

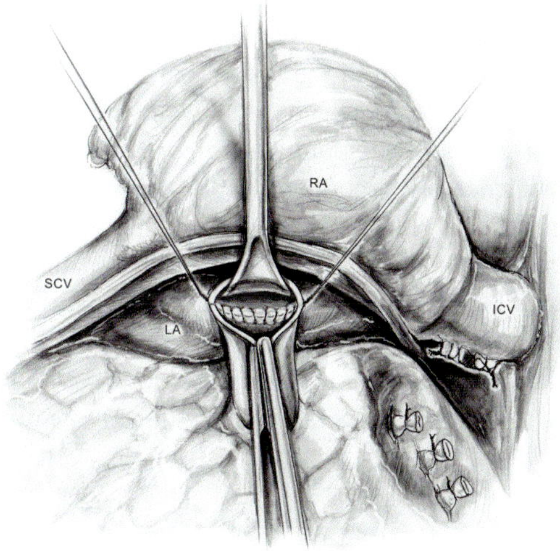

Fig. 35 The posterior anastomotic suture line is depicted. *ICV* inferior caval vein, *LA* left atrium, *RA* right atrium, *SCV* superior caval vein. (Reproduced with permission from: Mavroudis and Dearani 2020)

muscular limbus (Geggel et al. 2020). Of the 11 patients who underwent baffling or reimplantation, 5 developed pulmonary vein obstruction associated with baffle thrombosis or tension on

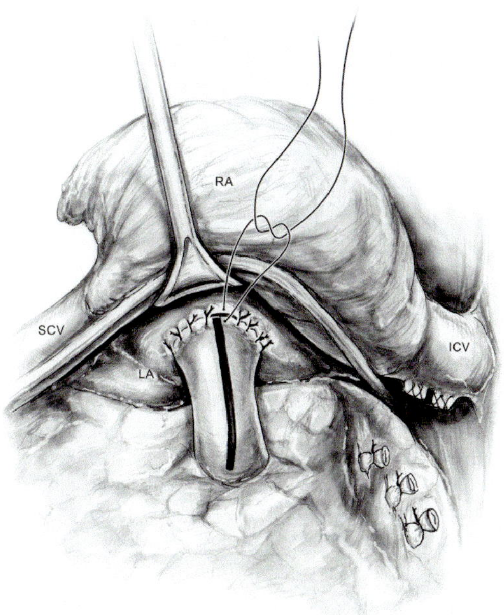

Fig. 36 The completed direct anastomosis of the scimitar vein and the left atrium are shown. *ICV* inferior caval vein, *LA* left atrium, *RA* right atrium, *SCV* superior caval vein. (Reproduced with permission from: Mavroudis and Dearani 2020)

the pulmonary vein between 45 days and 9.5 months after surgery. None of the 11 patients who underwent the new multipatch procedure developed pulmonary vein obstruction in the short- to intermediate-term of postoperative monitoring up to 3.6 years.

The multipatch procedure created an unobstructed and tension-free pathway from the scimitar vein into the left atrium and was described as follows (Geggel et al. 2020):

> "The novel surgical technique incorporated a double- or triple-patch repair depending on the distance between the scimitar vein and atrial tissue (Figs. 37 and 38; (Geggel et al. 2020)). Autologous pericardium was harvested, fixed for 2 minutes in 0.6% glutaraldehyde, and rinsed. The scimitar vein was dissected free. Cardiopulmonary bypass was established, cardioplegia administered, and diastolic arrest achieved. If the scimitar vein was near the right atrial–inferior caval vein junction, an inferior caval vein cannula was placed inferiorly in a typical position; if the scimitar vein entered at or below the diaphragm, an open-drop suction catheter was used. A right atriotomy was performed. The atrial septum was fully resected critically

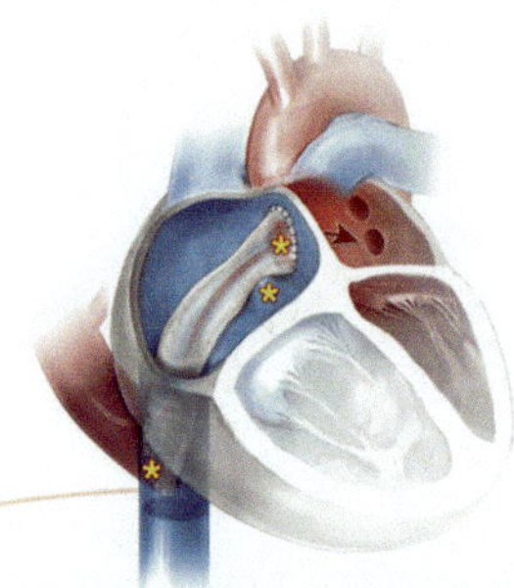

Fig. 37 Sites of obstruction associated with traditional baffle repair of scimitar syndrome are shown as is the depiction of traditional baffle repair. The stars depict sites of potential obstruction associated with the long angulated course of the scimitar vein baffle pathway, including at the proximal segment of the scimitar vein baffle pathway, superior limbic band, and atrial septal defect. (Reproduced with permission from: Geggel et al. 2020)

removing the area of the muscular limbus (Fig. 38b, c). This resection included the back wall of the left atrium to that the heart was exited posteriorly. The back wall of the left atrium was pulled rightward and downward toward the inferior caval vein to shorten the distance from the scimitar vein (Fig. 38c, insert) and run together with interlocking polypropylene suture. A right lateral atriotomy in the posterior part of the right atrium was made and opened down at a right angle into the scimitar vein creating a V-shaped incision (Fig. 38d). This space was patch augmented with a thin pulmonary homograft with running polypropylene suture in an L-shaped fashion effectively enlarging the left atrium, taking any tension or torsion off the scimitar vein so as not to pull it too tightly to the left atrium, and shortening the scimitar pulmonary venous pathway. A pulmonary homograft patch was chosen rather than a pericardial patch since it is more likely to conform to angles and not kink. If the scimitar vein coursed adjacent to the left or right atrium, a V-shaped incision was made in the vein and the atrium was pulled down into this region and directly connected to the scimitar vein with running polypropylene suture without kinking or tension. The scimitar vein was not detached from the inferior caval vein to not change the angulation of the scimitar vein. This avoids acute angle changes in the scimitar vein where it meets the lung parenchyma, where a fulcrum effect could lead to obstruction. Atrial septation was accomplished with a second patch of autologous pericardium that was sewn between the inferior caval vein and patched scimitar vein and carried up onto the superior limbus with running polypropylene suture completely closing the atrial septal defect and separating the inferior caval vein from the left atrium (Fig. 38e). The inferior caval vein was opened anteriorly down to the diaphragm and a third patch of autologous pericardium with running polypropylene suture was used to augment the inferior caval vein area where the atrial septation baffle patch had been placed (Fig. 38f). The right atriotomy was closed, heart deaired, aortic cross clamp removed, patient warmed, and weaned from cardiopulmonary bypass." (Geggel et al. 2020)

It is clear from the current literature that multiple variations have been introduced to prevent baffle or reimplantation stenosis as well as resultant thrombosis. So, whatever operation is elected for repair, care must be taken to insure an adequate and tension-free pathway from pulmonary vein to left atrium. If an intra-atrial baffle is elected, the surgical team must be attentive to the postoperative echocardiogram and respond to areas of turbulence as recorded. Under these circumstances, an enlarged baffle or an inferior caval vein patch may be necessary. Either pathway could be affected. Whichever turbulent pathway, the pulmonary vein or inferior caval vein, reoperation and correction is advisable to prevent the risk of a future reoperation that will be more difficult to perform.

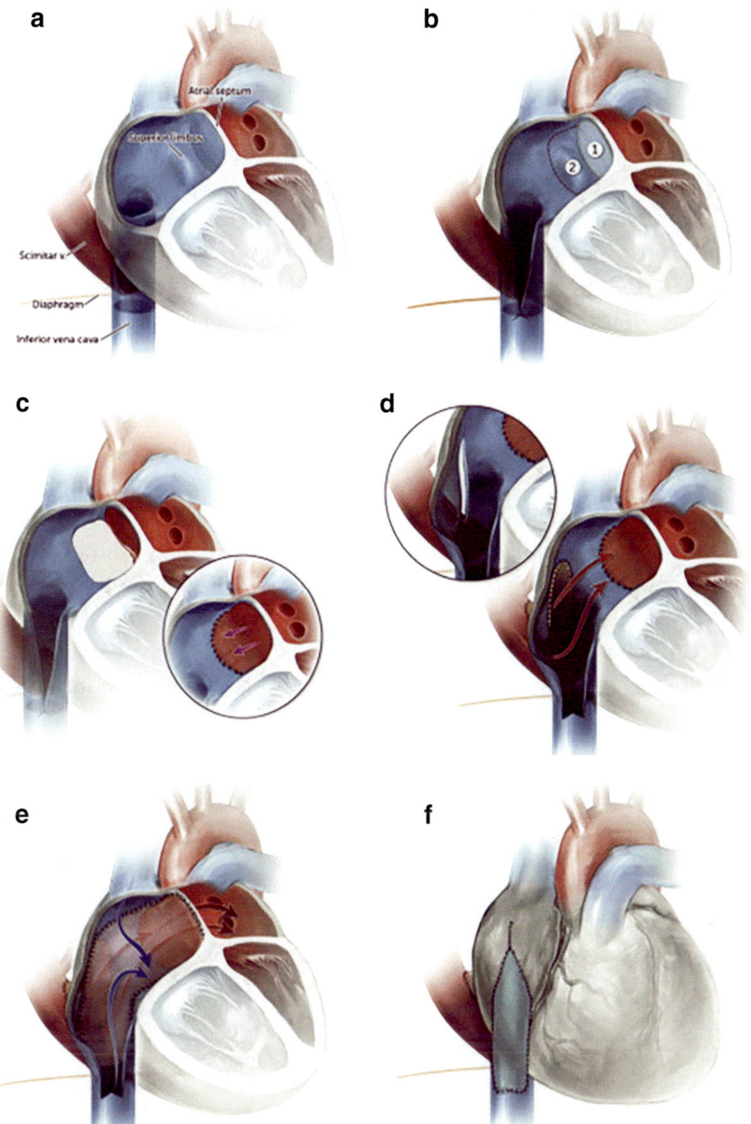

Fig. 38 Triple patch operative technique is shown to repair scimitar syndrome. (**a**) The baseline anatomy showing the scimitar vein connected to the inferior caval vein superior to the diaphragm and intact atrial septum. (**b**), Incision in the right atrium and inferior caval vein to determine the origin of the scimitar vein (The atrial septum [**1**] and superior limbic band [**2**] are noted). (**c**), Resection of the atrial septum and superior limbic band; the left atrium is pulled downward and anastomosed to the right atrial tissue bringing the left atrium closer to the scimitar vein. (**d**), V-shaped incision made in the atrium and scimitar vein and the space filled in with a thin pulmonary homograft. (**e**), An autologous pericardial patch is placed to divide the scimitar vein from the inferior caval vein and direct flow from the scimitar vein via baffle to the left atrium (red arrows) effectively closing the atrial septal defect. The caval vein flow courses anterior to this patch (blue arrows). (**f**), A pericardial patch is placed in the inferior caval vein in the region where the baffle patch was placed to raise the roof and augment the caliber of this region. (Reproduced with permission from: Geggel et al. 2020)

9 Rescue Techniques After Complicated Atrial Septal Defect Device Closure

Atrial septal defect closure devices have been developed and introduced to clinical practice with great success in patients with favorable anatomic landing sites. These anatomic conditions include well-formed ASD fibrous rims, absence of unroofed coronary sinus, absence of sinus venosus ASD, absence of ostium primum ASD (partial atrioventricular canal) with anterior leaflet atrioventricular valve cleft (Butera et al. 2008; Akagi 2015).

During the early experience complications from ASD device closures included embolization, malposition, erosion, arrhythmias, endocarditis, and thromboembolic events (Levi and Moore 2004; DiBardino et al. 2009; Abaci et al. 2013; Johnson et al. 2011; Nyboe et al. 2015; Szkutnik et al. 2008; Gatzoulis et al. 1999; Mantovan et al. 2003; Krumsdorf et al. 2004; Jalal et al. 2016; Tamura et al. 2021). In particular, device embolization and device erosion into nearby structures such as the aortic annulus have been the focus of potential surgical intervention (Crawford et al. 2012; Preventza et al. 2004; Trepels et al. 2003; Moore et al. 2013). Device erosion into nearby structures usually occurs days to weeks after device placement and can cause catastrophic conditions especially if the erosion occurs into the base of the aorta. Figure 39 demonstrates a modified coronal view of the heart depicting a transverse section of the aortic root, the left and right coronary arteries, and the proximity of the implanted device to the aortic annulus. The right and left atria are divided by the ASD device that is shown eroding through the left atrial wall and abutting the aortic annulus. The inset shows erosion of the aortic root owing to the local pressure of the implanted closure device. This can result in intrapericardial hemor-

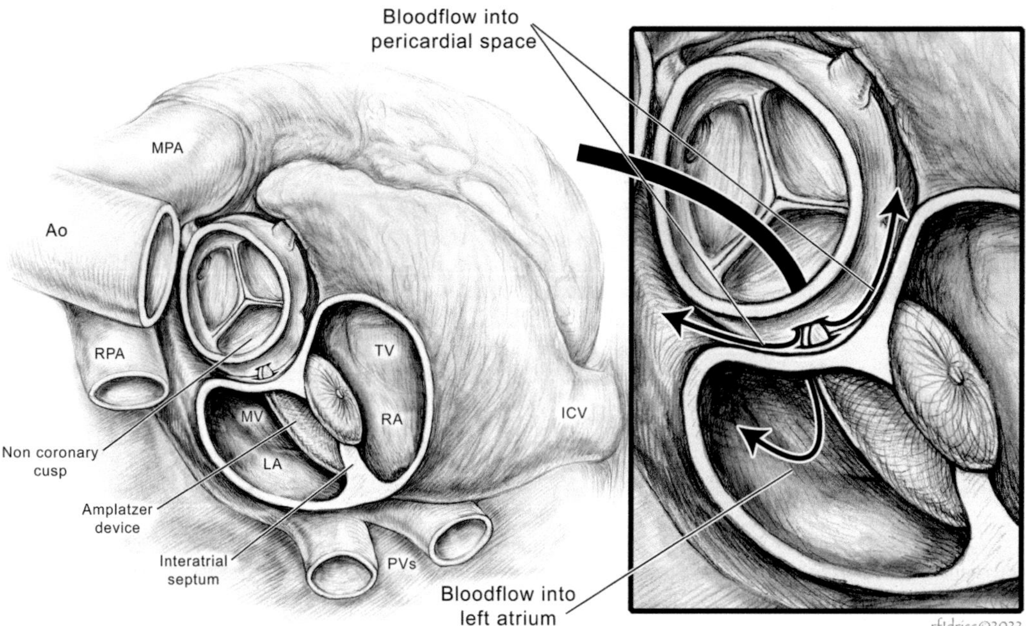

Fig. 39 A modified coronal view of the heart showing a transverse section of the aortic root, the left and right coronary arteries, and the proximity of the implanted device to the aortic annulus. The right and left atria are divided by the atrial septal defect device which is depicted as eroding through the left atrial (*LA*) wall and abutting the aortic annulus. The inset shows erosion of the aortic root by the implanted closure device resulting in intrapericardial hemorrhage and tamponade. This situation is life threatening and requires immediate operative intervention for survival. *Ao* aorta, *ICV* inferior caval vein, *MPA* main pulmonary artery, *MV* mitral valve, *PVs* pulmonary veins, *RA* right atrium, *RPA* right pulmonary artery, *TV* tricuspid valve

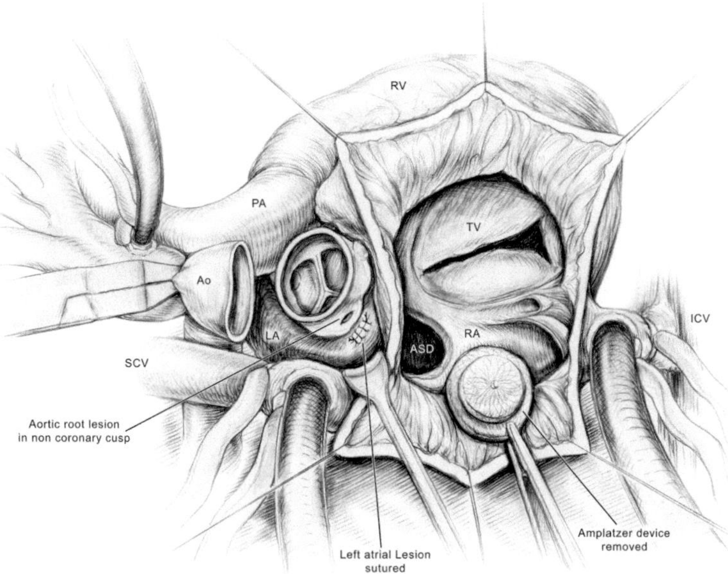

Fig. 40 The illustration shows operative exposure for repair of device erosion in the base of the aorta. Aortobicaval cardiopulmonary bypass, cardioplegic arrest, aortic transection, right atriotomy, and removal of the atrial septal defect (*ASD*) device are clearly shown. The ominous proximity of the ASD device to the aortic annulus can be appreciated. *Ao* aorta, *ICV* inferior caval vein, *LA* left atrium, *PA* pulmonary artery, *RA* right atrium, *RV* right ventricle, *SCV* superior caval vein, *TV* tricuspid valve

rhage and tamponade and is life threatening and requires immediate operative intervention for survival. Figure 40 shows operative exposure for repair of device erosion into the base of the aorta. Aortobicaval cardiopulmonary bypass, cardioplegic arrest, aortic transection, right atriotomy, and removal of the ASD device are clearly shown. One can appreciate the dangerous proximity of the ASD device to the aortic annulus when proper anatomic principles are not considered at the time of device closure. Repair can be accomplished by judicious placement of a pericardial patch from within the aorta to effect closure while respecting the important neighboring structures such as coronary arteries and aortic leaflets. Figure 41 (*left inset*) shows the accurate closure of the eroded aortic annulus from within the aorta using pericardium. Figure 41 (*right inset*) demonstrates pericardial patch closure of the original secundum ASD using the running suture technique. The aorta is reanastomosed, the right atrium is closed, the heart is deaired, and the cross-clamp is removed. After rewarming, the patient can be weaned from cardiopulmonary bypass.

Kamla and associates (2021) presented 2 patients with aortic erosion between the left atrium and aortic root following Amplatzer™ atrial septal occluder device (Abbott, Chicago, IL) with hemopericardium occurring within 72 h following implantation. Perforation or rupture owing to atrial septum occluders varies between 0.1% and 4% in the US (Kamla et al. 2021), and erosion from the Amplatzer septal occluder, specifically, occurs in 1–3 of every 1000 implantations (Kamla et al. 2021; United States Food and Drug Administration 2010). Clearly, atrio-aortic erosion owing to septal occluders is a surgical emergency that should be attended to immediately. Fortunately, with time, incidence of transcatheter septal occlusion of ASD has declined (Moore et al. 2013; Turner et al. 2017), although it remains a serious complication, and therefore, it is important to be vigilant and prepared for such an occurrence.

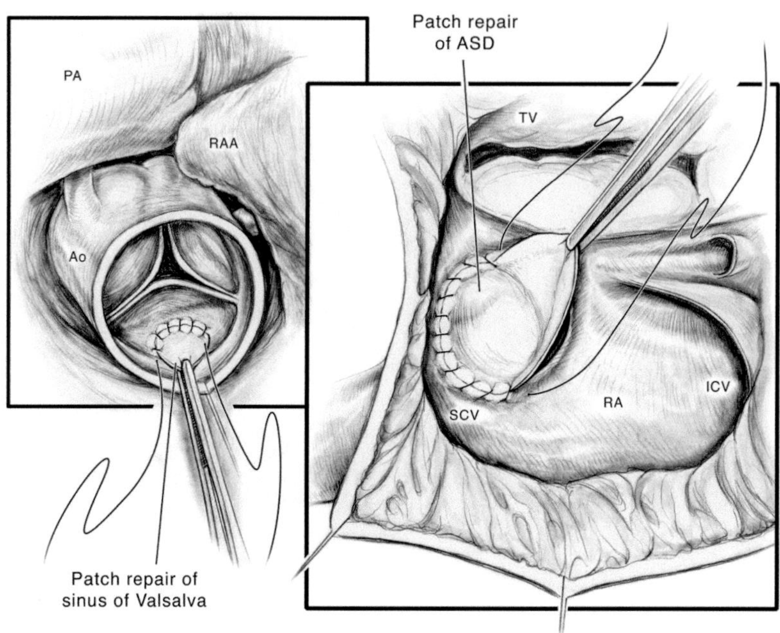

Fig. 41 The figure (*left inset*) shows the accurate closure of the eroded aortic annulus from within the aorta (*Ao*) using pericardium, with demonstrated (*right inset*) pericardial patch closure of the original secundum atrial septal defect (*ASD*) using running suture technique. Once the Ao is reanastomosed and the right atrium (*RA*) is closed, the patient can be weaned from cardiopulmonary bypass. *IVC* inferior caval vein, *PA* pulmonary artery, *RAA* right atrial appendage, *SVC* superior caval vein, *TV* tricuspid valve

Occasionally, transcatheter septal occluders can embolize owing to device ASD mismatch (Kamla et al. 2021; Fraise et al. 2018). In general, these potential complications can be avoided at the initial procedure since the occluder device is still attached to the transcutaneous catheter and can be immediately retrieved if necessary. The problem arises when the device is placed and seems to result in an excellent outcome and later results in device embolization. Most anatomic sites of embolization are the main pulmonary artery and left ventricular outflow tract (Hierlmeier et al. 2020; Cho et al. 2015; Nath and Pandit 2017; Her et al. 2018; Fernando et al. 2012; Goel et al. 2013), and occasionally, transcatheter techniques can be employed to retrieve the embolized devices. Occasionally, surgery will be required (Moore et al. 2013) to retrieve the device and close the ASD using standard techniques. Figure 42 is a modified coronal view showing transected structures while emphasizing the left atrial view, the mitral valve, and the pulmonary veins. The embolized occluder device is

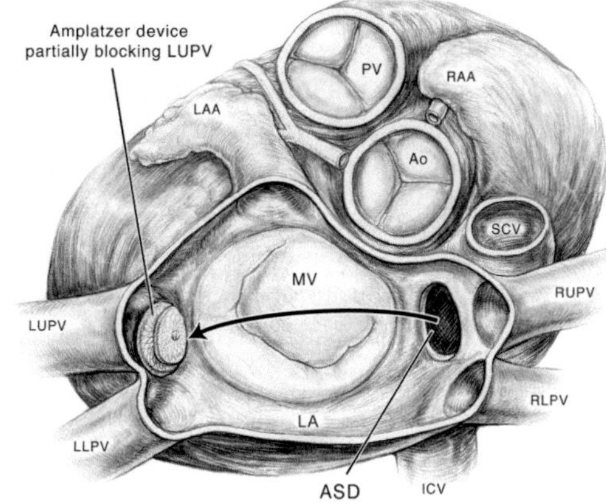

Fig. 42 A modified coronal view is shown with transected structures emphasizing the left atrial (*LA*) view, the mitral valve (*MV*), and the pulmonary veins (*PVs*). The embolized occluder device is shown in the orifice of the left upper pulmonary vein (*LUPV*). Transcatheter techniques can usually retrieve this device. When necessary, surgical retrieval can be performed through the atrial septal defect (*ASD*) attended by closure using standard techniques. *Ao* aorta, *IVC* inferior caval vein, *LAA* left atrial appendage, *LLPV* left lower pulmonary vein, *RAA* right atrial appendage, *RPA* right pulmonary artery, *RLPV* right lower pulmonary vein, *RUPV* right upper pulmonary vein, *SVC* superior caval vein

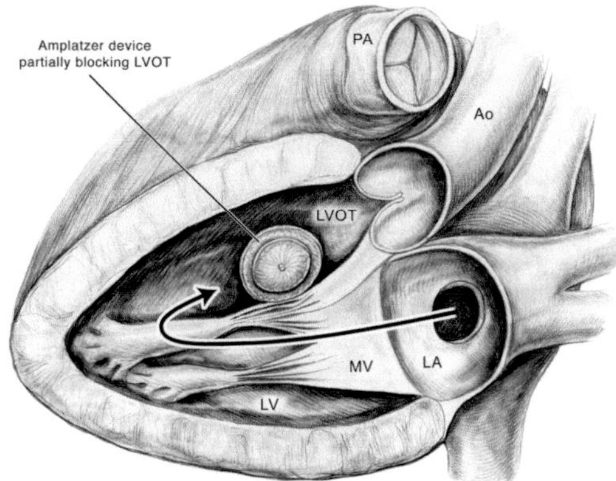

Fig. 43 Rarely, the device can embolize to the left ventricular outflow tract (*LVOT*) as shown. Transcatheter retrieval can occur through the aortic valve and successful transcatheter device closure of the atrial septal defect using a larger device. Alternatively, the surgical approach can start with transaortic exposure and augmented by transatrial-transseptal defect exposure if needed. *Ao* aorta, *LA* left atrium, *LV* left ventricle, *MV* mitral valve, *PA* pulmonary artery

shown in the orifice of the left upper pulmonary vein. As noted, transcatheter techniques can usually retrieve this device. When necessary, surgical retrieval can be performed through the ASD attended by closure using standard techniques. Rarely, the device can embolize to the left ventricular outflow tract as noted in Fig. 43. A recent report demonstrated transcatheter retrieval through the aortic valve and successful transcatheter device closure of the ASD using a larger device (Hierlmeier et al. 2020). Alternatively, the surgical approach can start with transaortic exposure and augmented by transatrial-trans-ASD exposure if needed.

As noted, transcatheter ASD device closure has evolved into a safe procedure with rare complications. The aforementioned conditions should be recognized by the surgical team and provide guidelines for resolution of the problem.

10 Summary

Complications associated with ASD, partial anomalous pulmonary venous return, and scimitar syndrome repairs can occasionally challenge the surgical team. Attention to detail, anatomic considerations, and transesophageal echocardiography can help to identify problems during the operation and allow the team to institute reparative techniques to arrive at an excellent outcome.

References

Abaci A, Unlu S, Alsancak Y, Kaya U, Sezenoz B. Short and long term complications of device closure of atrial septal defect and patent foramen ovale: meta-analysis of 28,142 patients from 203 studies. Catheter Cardiovasc Interv. 2013;82(7):1123–38.

Adrichem R, Le Cessie S, Hazekamp MG, Van Dam NAM, Blom NA, Rammeloo LAJ, et al. Risk of clinically relevant pericardial effusion after pediatric cardiac surgery. Pediatr Cardiol. 2019;40:585–94.

Akagi T. Current concept of transcatheter closure of atrial septal defect in adults. J Cardiol. 2015;65(1):17–25.

Aliter H, El-Haddad A, Gallo R, Al-Halees Z. Atrial septal defect with drainage of the inferior vena cava into the left atrium. Eur J Cardiothorac Surg. 2011;40:1256–7.

Backer CL, Mavroudis C. Atrial septal defect, partial anomalous pulmonary venous connection, and scimitar syndrome. In: Mavroudis C, Backer C, editors. Pediatric cardiac surgery. 4th ed. Hoboken: Wiley Blackwell; 2013. p. 295–310.

Barratt-Boyes BG, Ellis FH Jr, Kirklin JW. Technique for repair of atrial septal defect using the atrial well. Surg Gynecol Obstet. 1956;103:646–9.

Baskett RJF, Tancock E, Ross DB. The gold standard for atrial septal defect closure: current surgical results, with an emphasis on morbidity. Pediatr Cardiol. 2003;24:444–7.

Beghetti M, Tissot C. Pulmonary arterial hypertension in congenital heart diseases. Semin Respir Crit Care Med. 2009;30:421–8.

Bigelow WG, Callaghan JC, Hopps JA. General hypothermia for experimental intracardiac surgery; the use of electrophrenic respirations, an artificial pacemaker for cardiac standstill and radio-frequency rewarming in general hypothermia. Ann Surg. 1950;132:531–9.

Bigelow WG, Mustard WT, Evans JG. Some physiologic concepts of hypothermia and their applications to cardiac surgery. J Thorac Surg. 1954;28:463–80.

Bjork VO, Johansson L, Jonsson B, Norlander O, Nordenstrom B. The operation and management of a case after diversion of the inferior vena into the left atrium after the open repair of an atrial septal defect. Thorax. 1958;13:261–6.

Brown JW, Ruzmetov M, Minnich DJ, et al. Surgical management of scimitar syndrome: an alternative approach. J Thorac Cardiovasc Surg. 2003;125(2):238–45.

Butera G, Romagnoli E, Carminati M, et al. Treatment of isolated secundum atrial septal defects: impact of age and defect morphology in 1,013 consecutive patients. Am Heart J. 2008;156(4):706–12.

Casha AR, Sulaiman M, Cale AJR. Repair of adult Scimitar syndrome with an intra-atrial conduit. Inter CardioVasc Thorac Sur. 2003;2(2):128–30.

Cho JY, Kim KH, Yoon HJ, et al. Percutaneous retrieval of embolized Amplatzer septal occluder after treatment of double atrial septal defect: a case report. J Korean Med Sci. 2015;30(9):1361–6.

Crawford GB, Brindis RG, Krucoff MW, Mansalis BP, Carroll JD. Percutaneous atrial septal occluder devices and cardiac erosion: a review of the literature. Catheter Cardiovasc Interv. 2012;80(2):157–67.

Dennis C, Spreng DS Jr, Nelson GE, Karlson KE, Nelson RM, Thomas JV, et al. Development of a pump-oxygenator to replace the heart and lungs: an apparatus applicable to human patients and application to one case. Ann Surg. 1951;134:709–21.

Desnick SJ, Neal WA, Nicoloff DM, Moller JH. Residual right-to-left shunt following repair of atrial septal defect. Ann Thorac Surg. 1976;21:291–5.

DeWall RA, Warden HE, Varco RL, Lillehei CW. The helix reservoir pump-oxygenator. Surg Gynecol Obstet. 1957;104:699–710.

DiBardino DJ, McElhinney DB, Kaza AK, Mayer JE Jr. Analysis of the US Food and Drug Administration manufacturer and user facility device experience database for adverse events involving Amplatzer septal occluder devices and comparison with the Society of Thoracic Surgery Congenital Cardiac Surgery database. J Thorac Cardiovasc Surg. 2009;137(6):1334–41.

Dushane JW, Kirklin JW, Patrick RT, Donald DE, Terry HR Jr, Burchell HB, et al. Ventricular septal defects with pulmonary hypertension; surgical treatment by means of a mechanical pump-oxygenator. JAMA J Am Med Assoc. 1956;160:950–3.

Effler DB, Groves LK. Pitfalls in the surgical closure of atrial septal defect. Based on experience with one hundred and fifteen cases. Cleve Clin Q. 1961;28:166–75.

Effler DB, Groves LK, Sones FM, Kolff WJ. Elective cardiac arrest in open-heart surgery; report of three cases. Cleve Clin Q. 1956;23:105–14.

Elzein C, Abdulkarim M, Abbas U, Vricella L, Ilbawi M. Repair of superior sinus venosus atrial septal defect using a modified two-patch technique. Ann Thorac Surg. 2020;109:583–7.

Fernando RR, Koranne KP, Barker CM. AMPLATZER septal occluder failure resulting in paradoxical cerebral embolism. Tex Heart Inst J. 2012;39(5):647–52.

Fraise A, Latchman M, Sharma SR, et al. Atrial septal defect closure: indications and contra-indications. J Thorac Dis. 2018;10(Suppl 24):S2874–81.

Gatzoulis MA, Freeman MA, Siu SC, et al. Atrial arrhythmia after surgical closure of atrial septal defects in adults. N Engl J Med. 1999;340(11):839–46.

Geggel RL, Gauvreau K, Callahan R, Feins EN, Baird CW. Scimitar syndrome: A new multipatch technique and incidence of postoperative pulmonary vein obstruction. JTCVS Tech. 2020;4:208–16.

Gibbon JH Jr. Artificial maintenance of the circulation during experimental occlusion of the pulmonary artery. Arch Surg. 1937;34:1105–31.

Gibbon JH Jr. The maintenance of life during experimental occlusion of the pulmonary artery followed by survival. Surg Gynecol Obstet. 1939;69:602–14.

Gibbon JH Jr. Application of a mechanical heart and lung apparatus to cardiac surgery. Minn Med. 1954;37:171–85.

Gibbon JH Jr. The development of the heart-lung apparatus. Am J Surg. 1978;135:608–19.

Goel SS, Aksoy O, Tuzcu EM, Krasuski RA, Kapadia SR. Embolization of patent foramen ovale closure devices: incidence, role of imaging in identification, potential causes, and management. Tex Heart Inst J. 2013;40(4):439–44.

Gross RE, Pomeranz AA, Watkins E Jr, Goldsmith EI. Surgical closure of defects of the interauricular septum by use of an atrial well. N Engl J Med. 1952;247:455–60.

Guerra NC, Pernot M, Nesseris G, et al. Scimitar syndrome repair in adults: intermediate-term results using an extracardiac conduit. Ann Thorac Surg. 2016;102(6):2070–6.

Hallali P, Tcheng P, Davido A, Leriche H, Corone P. [Atrial septal defect and cyanosis. Apropos of 6 cases related to abnormal drainage of the inferior vena cava into the left atrium]. Arch Mal Coeur Vaiss.1988;81:783–6.

Her AY, Lim KH, Shin ES. Transcatheter retrieval of embolized atrial septal defect occluder device by waist capture technique. Int Heart J. 2018;59(1):226–8.

Herrmann JL, Brown JW. Commentary: Scimitar syndrome: cutting through the details. JTCVS Tech. 2020;1(C):81. https://doi.org/10.1016/j.xjtc.2019.12.009.

Hierlmeier BJ, Ostrovsky G, Zarth M. Embolization of an atrial septal defect occluder device into the left ventricle. Cureus. 2020;12(11):e11417. https://doi.org/10.7759/cureus.11417.

Jalal Z, Hascoet S, Baruteau AE, et al. Long-term complications after transcatheter atrial septal defect closure: a review of the medical literature. Can J Cardiol. 2016;32(11):1315.e11–8.

Johnson JN, Marquardt ML, Ackerman MJ, et al. Electrocardiographic changes and arrhythmias following percutaneous atrial septal defect and patent foramen ovale device closure. Catheter Cardiovasc Interv. 2011;78(2):254–61.

Kamla CE, Buech J, Doldi PM, Hagl C, Juchem G, Dashkevich A. Atrio-aortic erosion caused by Amplatzer atrial septal occluder—a case report. J Cardiothorac Surg. 2021;16(1):36. https://doi.org/10.1186/s13019-021-01411-3.

Kirklin JW, Dushane JW, Patrick RT, Donald DE, Hetzel PS, Harshbarger HG, et al. Intracardiac surgery with the aid of a mechanical pump-oxygenator system (Gibbon type): report of eight cases. Proc Staff Meet Mayo Clinic. 1955;30:201–6.

Kolff WJ, Effler DB, Groves LK, Peereboom G, Moraca PP. Disposable membrane oxygenator (heart-lung machine) and its use in experimental surgery. Cleve Clin Q. 1956;23:69–97.

Krumsdorf U, Ostermayer S, Billinger K, et al. Incidence and clinical course of thrombus formation on atrial septal defect and patent foramen ovale closure devices in 1,000 consecutive patients. J Am Coll Cardiol. 2004;43(2):302–9.

Kugelberg J. Electrical induction of ventricular fibrillation in the human heart. A study of excitability levels with alternating current of different frequencies. Scand J Thorac Cardiovasc Surg. 1976;10:237–40.

Levi DS, Moore JW. Embolization and retrieval of the Amplatzer septal occluder. Catheter Cardiovasc Interv. 2004;61(4):543–7.

Lewis FJ, Taufic M. Closure of atrial septal defects with the aid of hypothermia; experimental accomplishments and the report of one successful case. Surgery. 1953;33:52–9.

Lillehei CW. Controlled cross circulation for direct-vision intracardiac surgery: correction of ventricular septal defects, atrioventricularis communis, and tetralogy of Fallot. Postgrad Med. 1955;17:388–96.

Lillehei C. Section III: cardiopulmonary bypass and myocardial protection. In: Stephenson LW, Ruggero R, editors. Heart surgery classics. Boston: Adams Publishing Group; 1994. p. 126–8.

Lillehei CW, Cohen M, Warden HE, Varco RL. The direct vision intracardiac correction of congenital anomalies by controlled cross circulation: results in 32 patients with ventricular septal defects, tetralogy of Fallot, and atrioventricular communis defects. Surgery. 1955a;38:11–29.

Lillehei CW, Cohen M, Warden HE, Read RC, Aust JB, DeWall RA, et al. Direct vision intracardiac surgical correction of the tetralogy of Fallot, pentalogy of Fallot, and pulmonary atresia defects: report of first ten cases. Ann Surg. 1955b;142:418–42.

Lillehei CW, Cohen M, Warden HE, Ziegler NR, Varco RL. The results of direct vision closure of ventricular septal defects in eight patients by means of controlled cross-circulation. Surg Gynecol Obstet. 1955c;101:446–66.

Lillehei CW, DeWall RA, Read RC, Warden HE, Varco RL. Direct vision intracardiac surgery in man using a simple, disposable artificial oxygenator. Ds Chest. 1956;29:1–8.

Lindberg L, Olsson AK, Jögi P, Jonmarker C. How common is severe pulmonary hypertension after pediatric cardiac surgery? J Thorac Cardiovasc Surg. 2002;123:1155–63.

Mantovan R, Gatzoulis MA, Pedrocco A, et al. Supraventricular arrhythmia before and after surgical closure of atrial septal defects: spectrum, prognosis and management. Europace. 2003;5(2):133–8.

Mavroudis C. Atrial septal defect. In: Mavroudis C, Backer CL, editors. Atlas of pediatric surgery. London: Springer; 2015. p. 89–98.

Mavroudis C, Dearani JA. Atrial septal defect; partial pulmonary venous return; Scimitar syndrome; robotic closure of atrial septal defect. In: Mavroudis C, Dearani JA, editors. Atlas of adult congenital cardiac surgery. Philadelphia: Springer; 2020. p. 79–90.

Mavroudis C, Ong CS, Vricella LA, Gott VL, Cameron DE. Milestones in congenital cardiac surgery. In: Yuh DD, Vricella LA, Yang S, Doty JR, editors. Johns Hopkins medicine textbook of cardiothoracic surgery. 3rd ed. New York: McGraw-Hill Education; 2022.

Melrose DG, Dreyer B, Bentall HH, Baker JB. Elective cardiac arrest. Lancet (London). 1955;269(6879):21–2.

Moore J, Hegde S, El-Said H, ACC IMPACT Steering Committee, et al. Transcatheter device closure of atrial septal defects: a safety review. JACC Cardiovasc Interv. 2013;6(5):433–42.

Munet M, Gayet C, Buttard P, Ninet J, Chapon P, Tremeau G et al. [Late discovery of inferior vena cava draining into the left atrium after surgical closure of atrial septal defect]. Arch Mal Coeur Vaiss. 1997;90:991–4.

Murray G. Closure of defects in cardiac septa. Ann Surg. 1948;128:843–52.

Mustard WT. Diversion of the venae cavae into the left atrium during closure of atrial septal defects. J Thorac Cardiovasc Surg. 1964;47:317–24.

Najm HK, Williams WG, Coles JG, Rebeyka IM, Freedom RM. Scimitar syndrome: twenty years' experience and results of repair. J Thorac Cardiovasc Surg. 1996;112(5):1161–9.

Nath RK, Pandit N. Asymptomatic late embolization of Amplatzer septal occluder device. Indian Heart J. 2017;69(3):338–40.

Nyboe C, Olsen MS, Nielsen-Kudsk JE, Hjortdal VE. Atrial fibrillation and stroke in adult patients with atrial septal defect and the long-term effect of closure. Heart. 2015;101(9):706–11.

Patel P, Lee A, Zaid J, Tenuto J, Waldman B, Rosenbloom M, et al. Inferior vena cava obstruction following surgical repair of a secundum atrial septal defect. JACC Case Rep. 2021;3:82–6.

Pelletier GJ, Spray TL. Repair of Scimitar syndrome. Op Tech Thor Cardiovasc Surg. 2001;6(1):32–49.

Preventza O, Sampath-Kumar S, Wasnick J, Gold JP. Late cardiac perforation following transcatheter atrial septal defect closure. Ann Thorac Surg. 2004;77(4):1435–7.

Reisner-Sénélar L. The birth of intensive care medicine: Björn Ibsen's records. Intensive Care Med. 2011;37:1084–6.

Ross JK, Johnson DC. Complications following closure of atrial septal defects of the inferior vena caval type. Thorax. 1972;27:754–8.

Saboe A, Pramanda AN, Hasan M, Kusumawardhani NY, Maryani E, Ruhimat U, et al. Superior vena cava syndrome due to pericardial hematoma: a case report and mini-review of literature. SAGE Open Med Case Rep. 2021;9:2050313X211057700. https://doi.org/10.1177/2050313X211057700.

Shuntoh K, Wada Y, Kawai T, Oka T. [Diversion of the inferior vena cava into the left atrium after repair of atrial septal defect with partial anomalous pulmonary venous drainage]. Kyobu Geka. 1997;50:740–2.

Stephens EH, Mongé MC, Eltayeb O, et al. Evolution and current results of a unified strategy for sinus venosus surgery. Ann Thorac Surg. 2021;111(3):980–6.

Stewart RD, Bailliard F, Kelle AM, Backer CL, Young L, Mavroudis C. Evolving surgical strategy for sinus venosus atrial septal defect: effect on sinus node function and late venous obstruction. Ann Thorac Surg. 2007;84:1651–5.

Szkutnik M, Lenarczyk A, Kusa J, Bialkowski J. Symptomatic tachy- and bradyarrhythmias after transcatheter closure of interatrial communications with Amplatzer devices. Cardiol J. 2008;15(6):510–6. PMID:19039754

Tamura Y, Yonehara Y, Horibata Y, Uesugi H, Sawamura T, Sakamoto T. The first described case of late infective endocarditis after implantation of Figulla Flex IIASD occluder. J Cardiol Cases. 2021;23(5):214–7.

Thiruchelvam A, Haranal M, Abdul-Aziz KA, Sivalingam S. Iatrogenic closure of coronary sinus: an unforseen complication of surgical atrial septal defect closure. Indian J Thorac Cardiovasc Surg. 2021;37:688–90.

Trepels T, Zeplin H, Sievert H, et al. Cardiac perforation following transcatheter PFO closure. Catheter Cardiovasc Interv. 2003;58(1):111–3.

Tsuchida K, Anzai N, Hashimoto A, Fukushima Y, Yamada M. Intraatrial conduit repair in Scimitar syndrome. Chest. 1987;92(6):1120–2.

Turner DR, Owada CY, Sang CJ Jr, Khan M, Lim DS. Closure of secundum atrial septal defects with the AMPLATZER septal occlude: a prospective, multicenter, post-approval study. Circ Cardiovasc Interv. 2017;10(8):e004212. https://doi.org/10.1161/CIRCINTERVENTIONS.116.004212.

United States Food and Drug Administration. Rare and serious erosion events associated with St. Jude Amplatzer atrial septal occluder (ASO); 2010. https://citoday.com/news/fda-issues-alert-regarding-rare-erosion-events-with-st-jude-medicals-amplatzer-atrial-septal-occluder.

Warden HE, Cohen M, Read RC, Lillehei CW. Controlled cross circulation for open intracardiac surgery; physiologic studies and results of creation and closure of ventricular septal defects. J Thorac Surg. 1954;28:331–43.

Warden HE, Cohen M, DeWall RA, Schultz EA, Buckley JJ, Read RC, et al. Experimental closure of intraventricular septal defects and further physiological studies on controlled cross circulation. Surg Forum. 1955;5:22–8.

Warden HE, Gustafson RA, Tarnay TJ, Neal WA. An alternative method for repair of partial anomalous pulmonary venous connection to the superior vena cava. Ann Thorac Surg. 1984;38(6):601–5.

Yavuz T, Nazli C, Kinay O, Kutsal A. Giant Eustachian valve with echocardiographic appearance of divided right atrium. Tex Heart Inst J. 2002;29:336–8.

Complications Associated with Ventricular Septal Defect Closure

Constantine Mavroudis and Robert H. Anderson

Abstract

Ventricular septal defect closure is important for patients with congenital heart disease, as it occurs in association with many cardiac anomalies. Although common complications can occur and result in postoperative arrhythmias, heart block, residual ventricular septal defect, infection, and injury to the aortic, tricuspid, or pulmonary valves. Various forms of closure techniques, choice of patch material, and type of suture technique can impact resultant complications. Possible complications are noted herein, with intentions to avoid injury to anatomic structures and prevent complications while achieving successful and uncomplicated closure.

Keywords

Conal VSD · Doubly committed VSD · Supracristal VSD · Perimembranous VSD · Conoventricular VSD · Central VSD · Inlet defect · Atrioventricular canal VSD · Muscular defect VSD · Closure · Transatrial closure · Tricuspid valve retraction · Residual VSD

1 Introduction

Complications associated with ventricular septal defect (VSD) closure are centered around postoperative arrhythmias, including heart block; residual defects, aortic, tricuspid, and pulmonary valvar injury; and infection (Mavroudis 2015; Mavroudis et al. 2013, 2020, 2023; Kelle et al. 2012; Mavroudis and Backer 2002, 2010; Schipper et al. 2017; Menting et al. 2015; Gaynor et al. 2001; Kazmi et al. 2009; Chaudhry et al. 2011; Pedersen et al. 2008; Vaksmann et al. 1989; Andersen et al. 2006; Karonis et al. 2016; Jortveit et al. 2016; Russell et al. 2011; Dodge-Khatami et al. 2014). The incidence of such complications varies between centers. In general, closure is performed using aortobicaval cardiopulmonary bypass, left ventricular venting, and cardioplegic arrest. Various techniques are used for closure, including the choice of patch material, such as pericardium, polytetrafluoroethylene, or Dacron, and either use of a running suture, or interrupted pledgetted sutures (Mavroudis et al. 2013, 2020, 2023; Mavroudis 2015; Kelle et al. 2012; Mavroudis and Backer 2010; Schipper et al. 2017).

C. Mavroudis (✉)
Chief of Pediatric Cardiothoracic Surgery (Retired), Peyton Manning Children's Hospital, Indianapolis, IN, USA

Professor Emeritus of Surgery, Johns Hopkins University School of Medicine, Baltimore, MD, USA

R. H. Anderson
Biosciences Division, Newcastle University, Newcastle-upon-Tyne, UK

C. L. Backer, C. Mavroudis (eds.), *Complications in Pediatric and Congenital Heart Surgery*,
https://doi.org/10.1007/978-3-032-02661-3_8

To contemplate complications of closure, it is advantageous to review historical perspectives, assess classification, and recognize interrelated anatomic structures (Mavroudis et al. 2013, 2020, 2023; Mavroudis 2015; Kelle et al. 2012; Mavroudis and Backer 2010; Schipper et al. 2017; International Society for Nomenclature of Paediatric and Congenital Heart Disease 2024). Without a functioning knowledge of these principles, the operating surgeon would be hard pressed to identify the conduction system, anatomic borders of the defects, and hidden cardiac leaflets and cords. The strategy is to avoid injury to these important structures en route to a successful and uncomplicated closure.

2 Historical Insights

Closure of ventricular septal defects is an important procedure in all aspects of congenital heart surgery simply because the ventricular septum is deficient in association with many cardiac anomalies. The surgical exposure utilized for closure has evolved over time. Initially, extended ventriculotomies were performed to visualize the entire defect to achieve accurate closure (Lillehei et al. 1955; Kirklin and Dushane 1961; Kirklin et al. 1980; Serraf et al. 1992), although this resulted in right ventricular arrhythmias and various degrees of right ventricular dysfunction. This led surgeons to develop a right atrial approach that is used almost exclusively today (Vaksmann et al. 1989; Jortveit et al. 2016; Lam and Friedman 2011). In this text, surgical repair is shown by the interrupted, pledgetted suture technique using a synthetic patch. Many surgeons employ the running suture technique, and in certain circumstances insert devices to achieve closure under direct vision, especially with muscular defects (Mavroudis et al. 2013, 2023; Kitagawa et al. 1998). We selectively employ running suture technique in small babies when closure is associated with the arterial switch, interruption of the aortic arch, and other very complex procedures where preservation of cross-clamp time is a consideration. Our bias to use the interrupted, pledgetted suture technique stems from our published series showing a very low incidence of residual defects (Mavroudis et al. 2013, 2020, 2023; Mavroudis 2015; Mavroudis and Backer 2002, 2010). We feel that the slightly extra cross-clamp time associated with this technique is time well spent to assure accurate suture placement and optimal patch position. Caution and judgment concerning extended ischemic arrest times dictate the type of closure technique that is best suited to patient and surgeon.

3 Anatomy and Nomenclature

Anatomic characterization of hearts with deficient ventricular septation has been considered and published by many congenital heart specialists, but no consensus has emerged to unify various systems (Mavroudis et al. 2013, 2020, 2023; Spicer et al. 2014; Soto et al. 1980; Van Praagh et al. 1989; Becu et al. 1956; Capelli et al. 1983). The multiple systems, collectively, have failed to provide consistent guidance for interpretation of the anatomic features and location of the defects that are imperative for optimal surgical closure. Underscoring these difficulties is the fact that the holes between the ventricles, even when seen in isolation, can show baffling variation in morphology. One well-respected classification, favored for some time by the surgical community, accounts for four types of defect in numeric fashion, as shown in Fig. 1 (Mavroudis et al. 2013). One of us, with his colleagues (Mavroudis et al. 2013, 2020, 2023; Mavroudis 2015), has offered a simplified version of this scheme that depends on highlighting the phenotypic variability according to the nature of anatomic borders of the defects. This approach permits the recognition of three, rather than four, categories. The system, importantly, does not ignore the equally important feature of location of the defect relative to landmarks of the right ventricle, nor the presence of septal malalignment. The three classes are those defects that, when viewed from the right ventricle, are directly juxtapulmonary, are perimembranous, or those with exclusively muscular borders (Mavroudis et al. 2013, 2023). The specificity provided by concentration on these pheno-

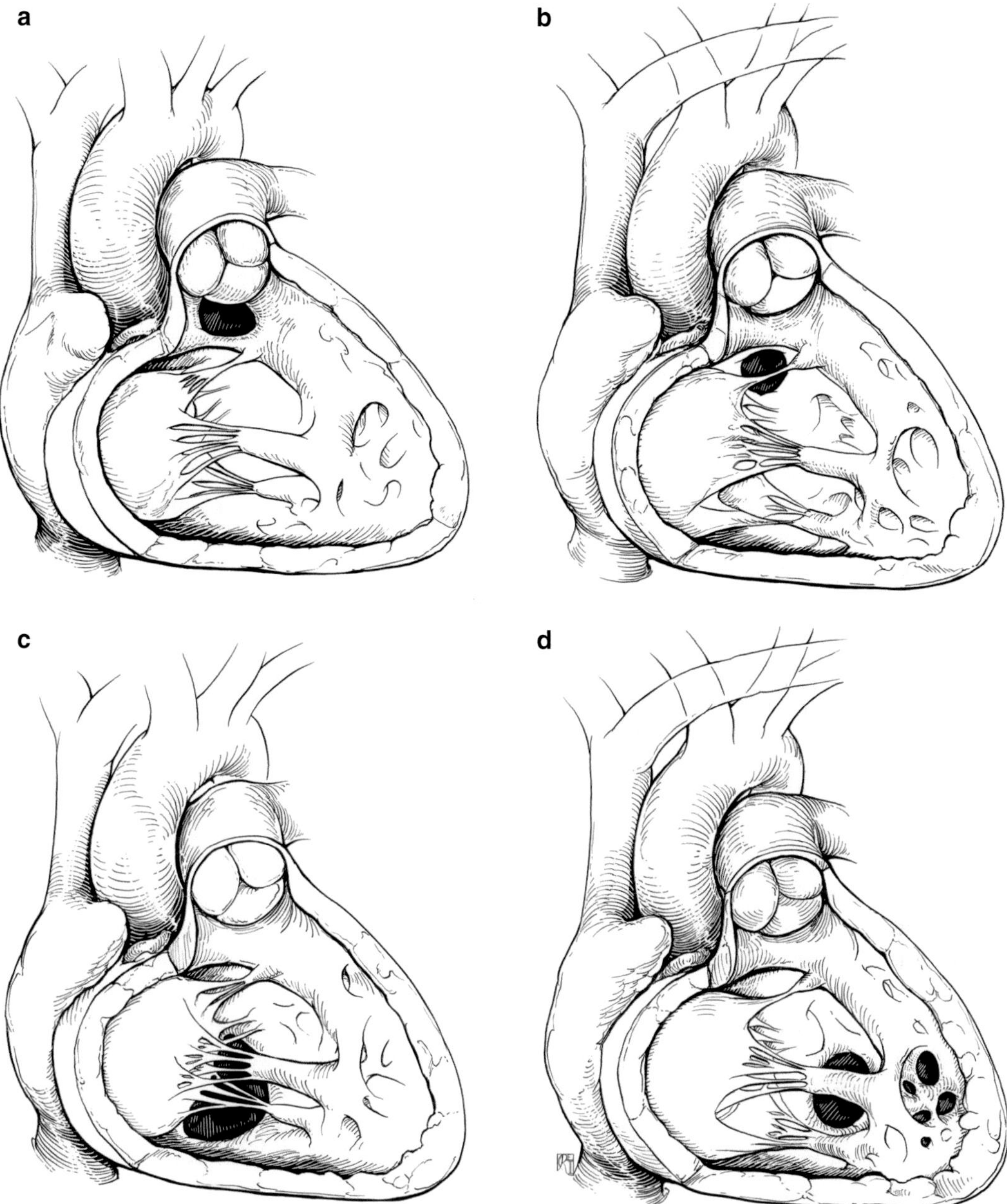

Fig. 1 Shows a well-respected classification favored for some time by the surgical community that accounts for four types of defects in numeric fashion. **Panel A** shows the so-called Type I defect, which is directly adjacent cranially to the leaflets of the pulmonary valve. The Type II defect, **panel B**, opens centrally to the right ventricle at the base of the ventricular mass. The Type III defect, **panel c**, is a large defect opening to the inlet of the right ventricle and extending across the full width of the orifice of the tricuspid valve. **Panel d** shows several of the so-called Type IV defects. The defects open apically and are surrounded by the musculature of the ventricular septum. (With permission: Mavroudis et al. 2020)

typic features with regard to the likely location of the conduction tissues reinforces the simplicity of the approach (Mavroudis et al. 2013, 2023).

This simplified anatomic approach also serves as the basis for exploring how complications can occur, how they can be recognized, and how they can be repaired. For instance, placing sutures through the tricuspid valve can result in injury to the aortic valve, or one of the leaflets of the tricuspid valve itself. Similarly, sutures placed in the pulmonary root can result in injury to the pulmonary leaflets and/or the aortic leaflets. In addition, knowing the variable anatomy of the conduction system can help surgeons avoid heart block. In the discussion that follows, we will consider the anatomic details of each type, course of the conduction system, and potential anatomic risk factors that can lead to complications.

3.1 The Juxta-Arterial Defects, Previously Known as Type I Defect, Conal VSD, Doubly Committed VSD, Supracristal VSD, and Others

The juxta-arterial defect, as noted in Fig. 1 (panel a) (Mavroudis et al. 2013) opens to the outlet of the right ventricle immediately beneath the pulmonary valve (Mavroudis et al. 2013, 2023). Its phenotypic feature is fibrous continuity between the leaflets of the aortic and pulmonary valves in the roof of the defect, owing to failure of muscularization of the subpulmonary infundibulum. For this reason, the defect is considered by some to represent conal hypoplasia (Mavroudis et al. 2013, 2023; Van Praagh et al. 1989). Indeed, it is frequently possible to recognize a fibrous raphe in fibrous continuity between the arterial valves. This is the hypoplastic outlet septum, which is fibrous rather than myocardial. The vestigial septum can be malaligned in either a cranial direction, potentially obstructing the subpulmonary outflow tract, or a caudal direction, potentially obstructing the subaortic outflow tract (Mavroudis et al. 2013, 2023). Because of failure of formation of the subpulmonary infundibular sleeve, the defect opens to the right ventricle between the limbs of the septal band (Mavroudis et al. 2013, 2023). In Fig. 2 (Mavroudis et al. 2020; International Society for Nomenclature of Paediatric and Congenital Heart Disease 2024), the phenotypic feature of the defect is shown.

Some considered the defect to be supracristal (Mavroudis et al. 2013, 2023; Becu et al. 1956; Capelli et al. 1983) as it opens into the right ventricle between the limbs of the septomarginal trabeculation, or septal band. Those naming the defect as supracristal are choosing the septal band to represent the crista. But the so-called infracristal defect also opens between the limbs of the septal band. In the latter defect, it is the outlet septum that is taken to represent the crista. Thus, in this system of classification, it was the structure taken to represent the crista that had changed, rather than the location of the defect itself (Mavroudis et al. 2013, 2023). The defect is better described as being juxta-arterial. As such, it is also doubly committed. In most cases, its posteroinferior rim is muscular, formed by fusion between the caudal limb of the septal band and the ventriculo-infundibular fold. The muscle bar thus formed protects the atrioventricular conduction axis. In a minority of cases, the defect can extend to the central area of the ventricular base. It is then bordered posteroinferiorly by an area of fibrous continuity between the leaflets of the aortic and tricuspid valves. This is the phenotypic feature of the perimembranous defect. In the numeric classification, this lesion represents the Type II defect (Fig. 1, panel b) (Mavroudis et al. 2013). Recognition of the extent of the defect to become perimembranous is of major surgical significance, as the conduction axis is at greater risk when the defect extends to reach the area of mitral-to-tricuspid fibrous continuity (Mavroudis et al. 2013, 2023).

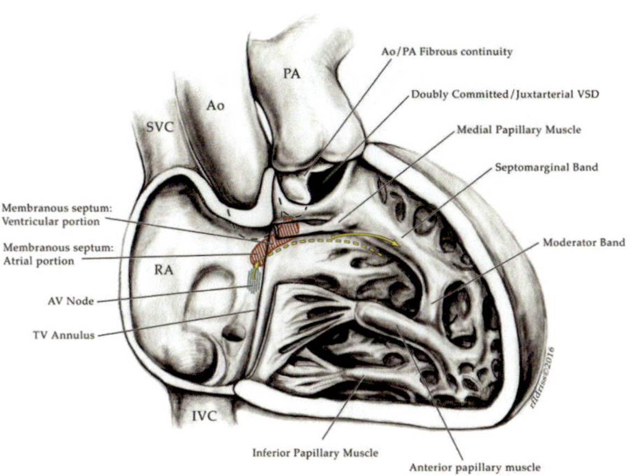

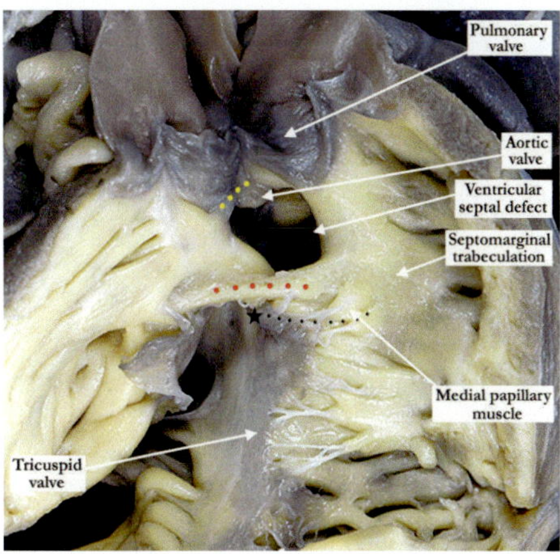

Fig. 2 The **left panel** shows the phenotypic feature of the so-called Type I VSD. It is directly juxtapulmonary but also doubly committed because of the fibrous continuity between the leaflets of the aortic and pulmonary valves. This feature reflects the failure of formation of the free-standing subpulmonary infundibular sleeve. In most instances, as shown in this figure, the defect has a muscular posteroinferior rim. The **right panel** shows how the muscular rim protects the atrioventricular conduction axis. In some instances, however, the defect can extend so as to open centrally when it is also perimembranous. (With permission: Mavroudis et al. 2020). *Ao* aorta, *AV* atrioventricular, *IVC* inferior caval vein, *PA* pulmonary artery, *RA* right atrium, *SVC* superior caval vein, *TV* tricuspid valve, *VSD* ventricular septal defect

3.2 The Perimembranous, Type II, Conoventricular, or Central VSD

The most common defect that is encountered during cardiac surgery is perimembranous (Mavroudis et al. 2013, 2023). It exists because the tertiary embryonic interventricular communication failed to close and opens to the right ventricle at the center of the cardiac base (Mavroudis et al. 2013, 2023). The central location of the defect is critical to understanding its phenotypic feature, which is fibrous continuity postero-inferiorly between the leaflets of mitral and tricuspid valves (Figs. 3 and 4) (Mavroudis et al. 2020; International Society for Nomenclature of Paediatric and Congenital Heart Disease 2024). The proximity of the defect to the tricuspid valve, the aortic valve, and the conduction system alerts the cautious surgeon to avoid unwanted complications of valvar injury and heart block. Although always incorporating a deficiency at the central part of the base of the right ventricle, these perimembranous defects can extend so as to open to either the outlet or the inlet of the right ventricle. On occasion, they can extend in both directions. Such large perimembranous defects can then be described as being confluent. Outlet defects are associated with some degree of malalignment of the muscular outlet septum. As with the fibrous outlet septum, such malalignment can be cranial or caudal (Mavroudis et al. 2020). Cranial malalignment is most frequent, is associated with overriding of the aortic root, and produces the lesion known as the Eisenmenger defect (Fig. 5) (Mavroudis et al. 2020; International Society for Nomenclature of Paediatric and Congenital Heart Disease 2024). The feature of all perimembranous defects is the postero-inferior location of the ventricular conduction tissues.

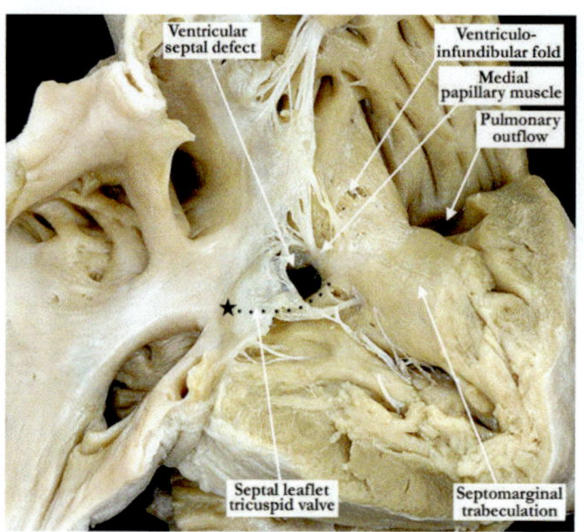

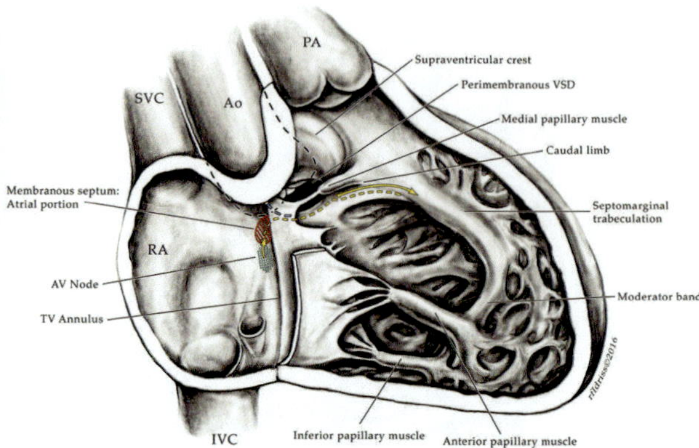

Fig. 3 (**left panel**) shows a defect opening centrally at the base of the right ventricle. As shown in the **right panel**, its phenotypic feature is fibrous continuity at its posteroinferior margin between the leaflets of the mitral and tricuspid valves. It opens inferior and posterior to the caudal limb of the septomarginal trabeculation, and behind the septal leaflet of the tricuspid valve, with the supraventricular crest inserted in normal fashion between the limbs of the trabeculation. As shown, the atrioventricular conduction axis runs posteroinferior to the defect, but is at risk in this corner. The atrioventricular component of the membranous septum is incorporated within this fibrous border, as seen in the **right panel**. The defect was initially interpreted on the basis of failure of formation of the membranous septum, so it was considered a membranous defect. A remnant of the interventricular part of the membranous septum, known as the membranous flap, is frequently found reinforcing the posteroinferior margin of the defect. The defect does not exist because the membranous septum is absent but rather because its muscular margins are deficient. For this reason, it was subsequently described as being perimembranous. Depending on the deficiency of its muscular borders, the central defect can also extend to open more to the inlet of the right ventricle, rather than being beneath the septal leaflet of the tricuspid valve. It can also open to the right ventricular outlet, or if large can be described as being confluent. (With permission: Mavroudis et al. 2020). *Ao* aorta, *AV* atrioventricular, *IVC* inferior caval vein, *PA* pulmonary artery, *RA* right atrium, *SVC* superior caval vein, *TV* tricuspid valve, *VSD* ventricular septal defect

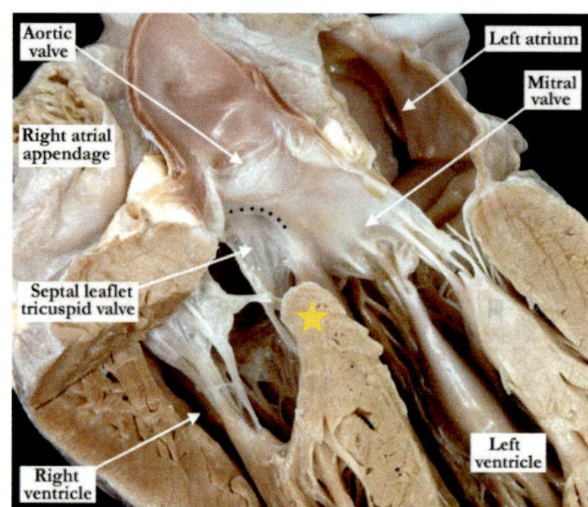

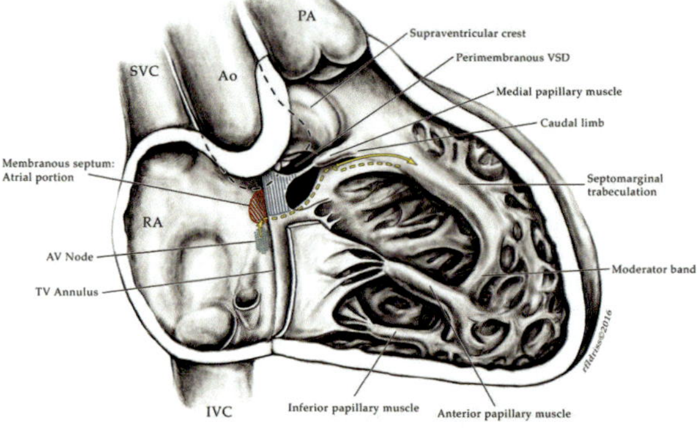

Fig. 4 (**Left panel**) shows a right ventricular section through a heart with a defect located centrally within the ventricular base, but extending inferiorly so as to open to the inlet of the right ventricle, being shielded by the septal leaflet of the tricuspid valve. Because the defect retains the phenotypic feature of fibrous continuity between the leaflets of the mitral and tricuspid valves, the conduction axis continues to run posteroinferiorly, relative to the defect when viewed from the right ventricle (**right panel**). (With permission: Mavroudis et al. 2020). *Ao* aorta, *AV* atrioventricular, *IVC* inferior caval vein, *PA* pulmonary artery, *RA* right atrium, *SVC* superior caval vein, *TV* tricuspid valve, *VSD* ventricular septal defect

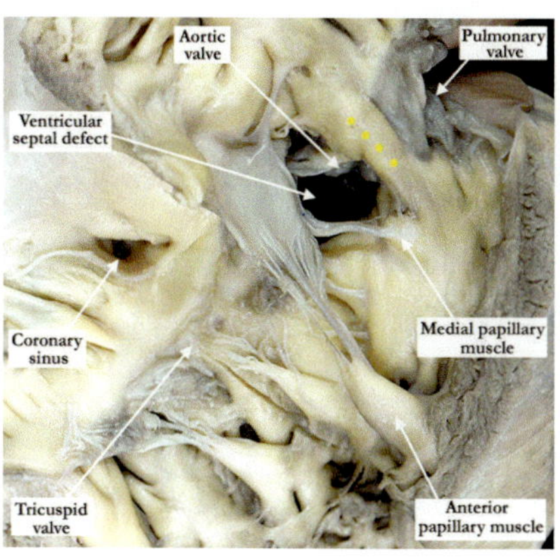

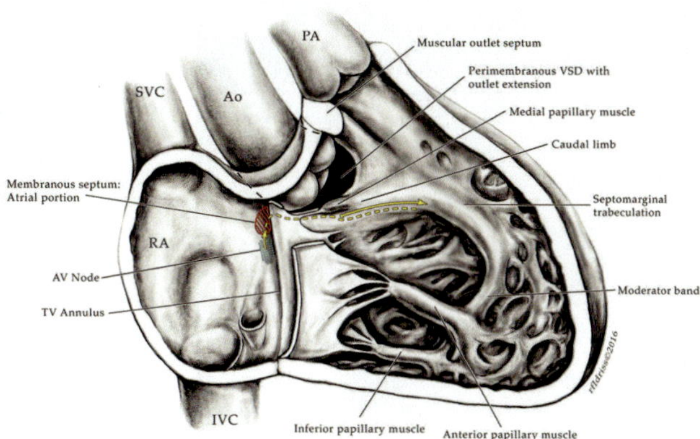

Fig. 5 The **left panel** shows a defect with malalignment of the muscular outlet septum and associated overriding of the aortic root. It extends centrally to become perimembranous (the so-called Eisenmenger defect). As shown in the **right panel**, because the defect extends to become perimembranous, the conduction axis continues to extend posteroinferiorly relative to the margins of the defect. It is in this setting that the muscular outlet septum becomes recognizable as forming the cranial margin of the defect. This defect is described by some as being conoventricular. Its right ventricular opening, like the juxtapulmonary or Type I defect, is cradled between the limbs of the septal band. In terms of its physical location, it is an outlet defect, and hence might be classified as a Type I defect by those using the initial surgical classification. Like the central defect, nonetheless, and also the central defect extending to open to the inlet of the right ventricle, the defect extending to open to the right ventricular outlet shares the feature of fibrous continuity between the leaflets of the mitral and tricuspid valves; hence, it is perimembranous *Ao* aorta. (With permission: Mavroudis et al. 2020). *AV* atrioventricular, *IVC* inferior caval vein, *PA* pulmonary artery, *RA* right atrium, *SVC* superior caval vein, *TV* tricuspid valve, *VSD* ventricular septal defect

3.3 The Perimembranous Inlet Defect with Atrioventricular Septal Malalignment, also Known as Type III Defect, Inlet Defect, or Atrioventricular Canal Type

This defect, as emphasized above, has many synonyms. It exists because of incomplete expansion of the atrioventricular canal during embryonic development (Mavroudis et al. 2020). Because of this feature, there is straddling and overriding of the tricuspid valve. The phenotypic feature is malalignment between the atrial septum and the apical ventricular septum (Fig. 6) (Mavroudis et al. 2013, 2020; Kelle et al. 2012; Andersen et al. 2006, 2011, 2014; International Society for Nomenclature of Paediatric and Congenital Heart Disease 2024; Spicer et al. 2014). Because there is still fibrous continuity between the leaflets of the mitral and tricuspid valves, the defect remains perimembranous. But, because of the malalignment, the ventricular conduction axis is unable to take origin from the regular atrioventricular node (Mavroudis et al. 2020). Instead, an anomalous node is formed at the site of union between the malaligned ventricular septum and the inferior atrioventricular junction (Mavroudis et al. 2020; International Society for Nomenclature of Paediatric and Congenital Heart Disease 2024). Another feature of the defect with straddling tricuspid valve is the presence of separate right and left atrioventricular junctions. In a minority of patients having an atrioventricular septal defect in the setting of an unequivocal common atrioventricular junction, it is possible for shunting across the defect to be confined at the ventricular level because the bridging leaflets of the common valve are attached to the leading edge of the atrial septum (Mavroudis et al. 2020), as shown in Fig. 7 (Mavroudis et al. 2013). These are the true ventricular defects of atrioventricular canal type. As might be expected, the atrioventricular conduction axis is then found as anticipated for the majority of atrioventricular septal defects (Fig. 7) (Mavroudis et al. 2013). Defects with exclusively muscular borders can also open to the inlet of the right ventricle (Fig. 8, left panel) (Mavroudis

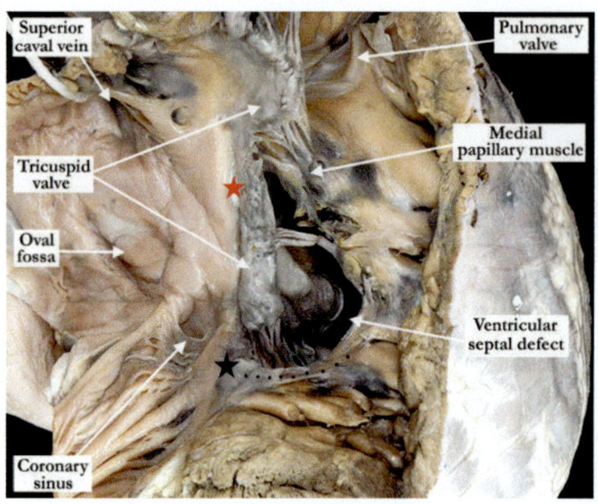

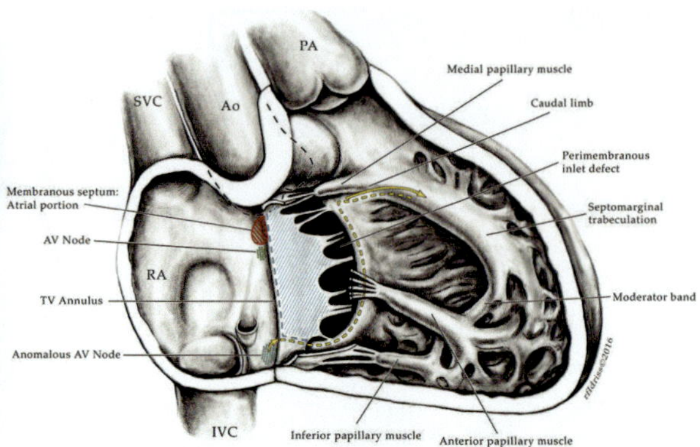

Fig. 6 The Type III defect in the initial surgical classification is considered to represent an inlet defect. It is described in this fashion because of its location relative to the landmarks of the right ventricle. As seen in Fig. 4, however, the phenotypic feature of the Type III defect is malalignment between the apical muscular septum and the atrial septum, as shown in the **left panel** of this figure. This image shows a defect unequivocally opening to the inlet of the right ventricle. Its phenotypic feature, however, results in straddling and overriding of the tricuspid valve. As is shown in the **right panel**, because of the malalignment of the muscular septum, which carries the atrioventricular conduction axis, the axis arises from an anomalous atrioventricular node formed at the point where the malaligned ventricular septum meets the inferior component of the atrioventricular junction. The regular atrioventricular node is hypoplastic, but it remains in its expected position within the triangle of Koch. (With permission: Mavroudis et al. 2020). *Ao* aorta, *AV* atrioventricular, *IVC* inferior caval vein, *PA* pulmonary artery, *RA* right atrium, *SVC* superior caval vein, *TV* tricuspid valve, *VSD* ventricular septal defect

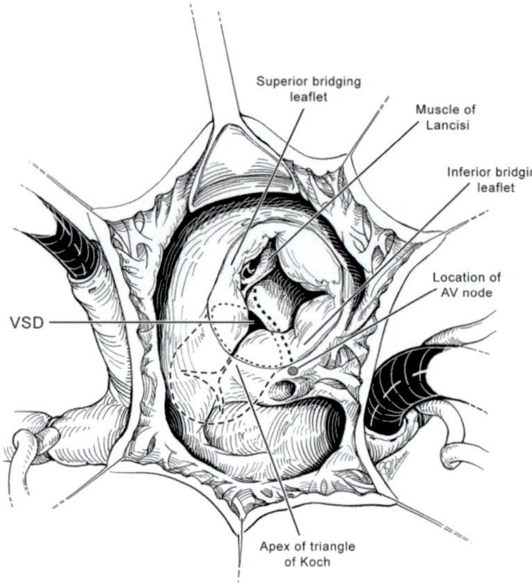

Fig. 7 Shows the features of an atrioventricular septal defect with exclusively ventricular shunting, by virtue of the attachment of the bridging leaflets of the common valve to the leading edge of the atrial septum. In this setting, the conduction axis arises from an anomalous node located at the cardiac crux, rather than at the apex of the triangle of Koch. (With permission: Mavroudis et al. 2013). *AV* atrioventricular, *VSD* ventricular septal defect

et al. 2020; International Society for Nomenclature of Paediatric and Congenital Heart Disease 2024). When a defect opening to the right ventricular inlet has exclusively muscular anatomic borders, the conduction axis is at risk anterosuperiorly, or to the left of the surgeon operating through the tricuspid valve (Fig. 8, right panel) (Mavroudis et al. 2013, 2020).

The course of the conduction system is obviously very important, as it is crucial to locate the conduction system during VSD closure. If the inlet VSD has exclusively muscular anatomic borders, the conduction system follows the course as noted in Fig. 8 (Mavroudis et al. 2013, 2020; International Society for Nomenclature of Paediatric and Congenital Heart Disease 2024). This conduction system still follows the anatomic configuration of the other lesions, namely that it courses on the left ventricular side of the septum and can be avoided if sutures are placed superficially enough to avoid heart block.

It should of course, be remembered that the perimembranous defect without atrioventricular

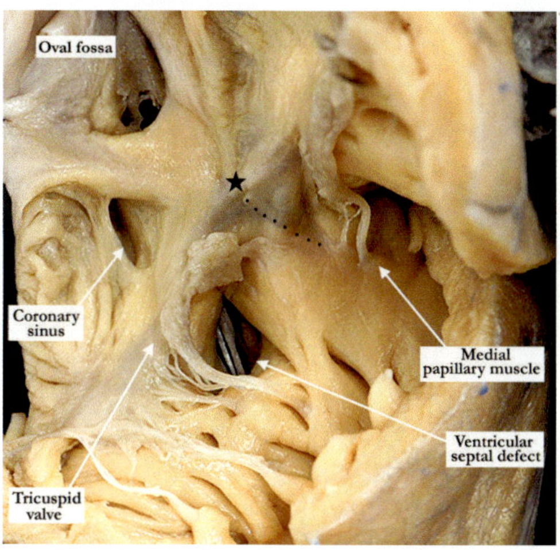

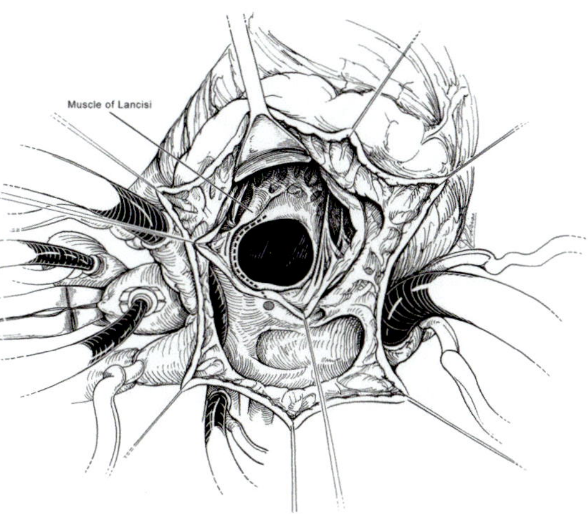

Fig. 8 (**Left panel**) shows a coronal section through a heart with a defect located centrally within the ventricular base but extending inferiorly so as to open to the inlet of the right ventricle, being shielded by the septal leaflet of the tricuspid valve. Because the defect retains the phenotypic feature of fibrous continuity between the leaflets of the mitral and tricuspid valves, the conduction axis continues to run posteroinferiorly, relative to the defect when viewed from the right ventricle. (With permission: Mavroudis et al. 2020). The **right panel** shows the defect with exclusively muscular borders that open to the inlet of the right ventricle. Although correctly classified as muscular, because of its position and exclusively muscular borders, it has a different relationship to the atrioventricular conduction axis. (With permission: Mavroudis et al. 2013). *AV* atrioventricular, *VSD* ventricular septal defect

septal malalignment, as discussed before, can extend inferiorly. In this setting, the defect can also be characterized as an inlet defect (Fig. 9, left panel) (Mavroudis et al. 2013, 2023). With this variant, however, unlike the perimembranous defect found with straddling tricuspid valve (Fig. 9, right panel) (Mavroudis et al. 2013, 2023), the atrioventricular conduction axis retains its anticipated origin from the atrioventricular node located at the apex of the triangle of Koch, although both triangle and node are deviated inferiorly within the right atrium (Mavroudis et al. 2013, 2023).

3.4 Muscular, or Type IV, Defects

These defects are characterized as holes in the ventricular septum with exclusively muscular borders (Fig. 10) (Mavroudis et al. 2020; Jacobs and Jacobs 2010). Some defects opening to the outlet of the right ventricle might be considered to be juxta-arterial. If, however, they have a muscular outlet septum, then they would not be juxta-arterial, although still opening between the limbs of the septal band (Fig. 11) (Mavroudis et al. 2020; International Society for Nomenclature of Paediatric and Congenital Heart Disease 2024). In terms of classification, they are correctly described as muscular outlet defects. If the muscular outlet septum is particularly hypoplastic, the defects will also be doubly committed.

Muscular defects can also be observed in all locations within the basal, middle, or apical part of the muscular ventricular septum. They can be further characterized as being anterior or posterior relative to the septal band (Fig. 10) (Mavroudis et al. 2013,2020, 2023). All these muscular defects exist because of incomplete compaction of the developing apical part of the septum (Anderson et al. 2011, 2014). If large, the defects can be crossed by right ventricular trabeculations, so that a defect that appears solitary when viewed from the left ventricular aspect, but seemingly has multiple orifices when viewed from the right ventricle (Mavroudis et al. 2013, 2023). Such defects can be quite challenging to close effectively, and closure may result in

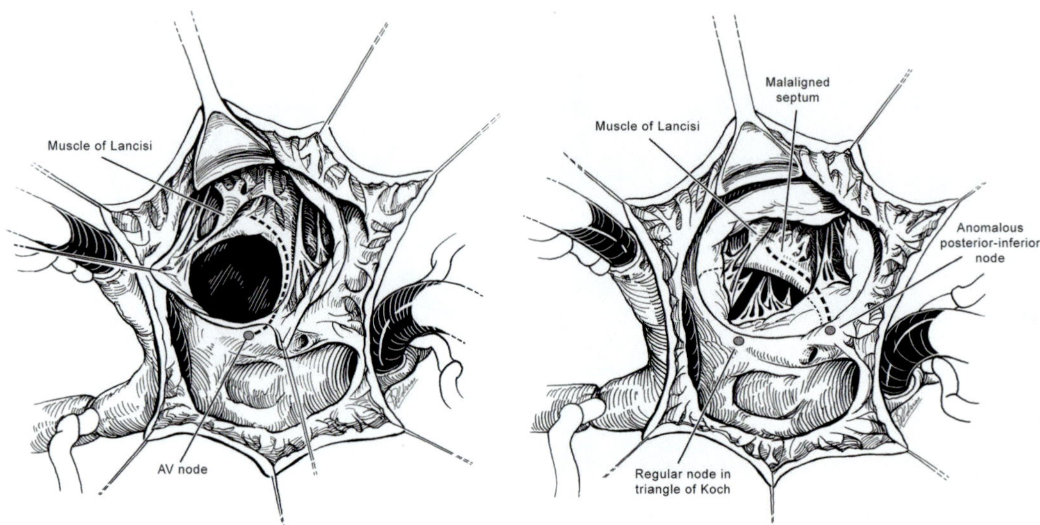

Fig. 9 Drawings show the location of the conduction axis in the setting of defects extending inferiorly from the central perimembranous area so as to open primarily to the inlet of the right ventricle, but in the settings of atrioventricular septal alignment (**left panel**) and atrioventricular septal malalignment (**right panel**). When the septal components are aligned, as in the left panel, the atrioventricular node remains located at the apex of the triangle of Koch, but the triangle and the node are displaced inferiorly, although they are not located at the cardiac crux as is the case for the atrioventricular septal defect with exclusive ventricular shunting (compare with Fig. 7 (Mavroudis et al. 2013)). When there is septal malalignment, in contrast, the conduction axis arises from an anomalous atrioventricular node (right panel). Because the defect found with straddling and overriding of the tricuspid valve is also associated with fibrous continuity between the leaflets of the mitral and tricuspid valves, it remains a perimembranous defect, but with the additional essential feature of malalignment between the atrial septum and the muscular ventricular septum. (With permission: Mavroudis et al. 2013). *AV* atrioventricular, *VSD* ventricular septal defect

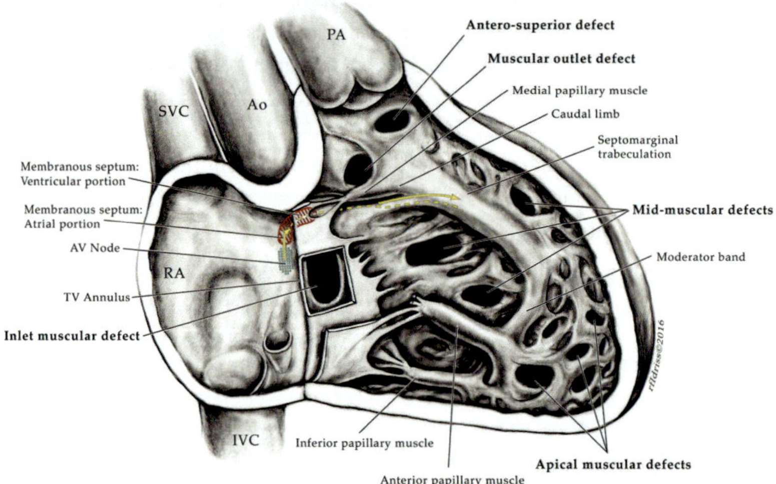

Fig. 10 Shows how defects with exclusively muscular borders, defined as Type IV in the initial surgical classification, can open to any part of the morphologically right ventricle, so that they vary with regard to their relationship to the atrioventricular conduction axis. They can show marked variability in terms of their physical location. As already described, some open to the inlet of the right ventricle (Fig. 8), which may justify their classification as Type III defects. (With permission: Mavroudis et al. 2020). *Ao* aorta, *AV* atrioventricular, *IVC* inferior caval vein, *PA* pulmonary artery, *RA* right atrium, *SVC* superior caval vein, *TV* tricuspid valve, *VSD* ventricular septal defect

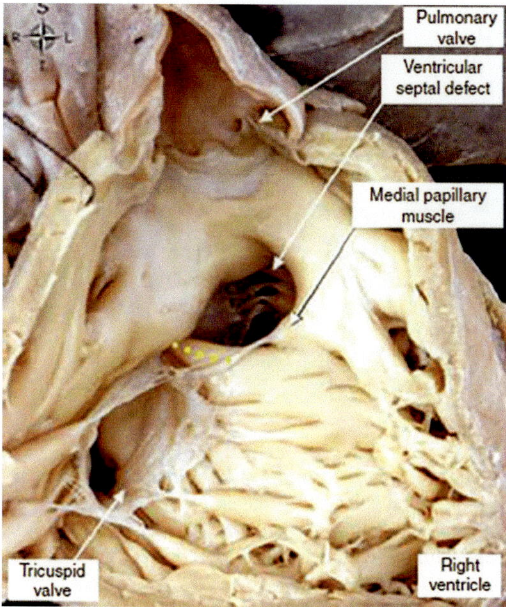

Fig. 11 Shows the location of a muscular defect opening to the outlet of the right ventricle. It exists because of separation between the subpulmonary infundibular sleeve and the crest of the muscular ventricular septum. The posteroinferior muscular rim of the defect protects the atrioventricular conduction axis (dotted line). The muscular outlet defects exist because of separation between the muscular septum and the subpulmonary infundibulum, so they can also be considered. (With permission: Mavroudis et al. 2020)

chordal entrapment, or even left ventricular dysfunction if the patch used is too large (Yoshimura et al. 2016; Hofmeyr et al. 2013). Other muscular defects have been characterized in terms of the Swiss-cheese septum (Mavroudis et al. 2013, 2023). These multiple small defects usually occur within the apical septum (Yoshimura et al. 2016; Hofmeyr et al. 2013). Any of the muscular defects, including the Swiss-cheese septum, can coexist with perimembranous defects (Mavroudis et al. 2013, 2023). If the muscular defect in such a combination opens to the inlet of the right ventricle, the conduction axis runs within the muscular bar interposing between the defects (Mavroudis et al. 2013, 2023). This myocardial entity can be very thin, making it difficult to close the defects independently without producing atrioventricular block (Mavroudis et al. 2013, 2023).

Not included in the original numeric classification is the so-called Gerbode defect (Fig. 12) (Kelle et al. 2012; Yuan 2014). This defect, which in essence is a left ventricular-to-right atrial shunt, can take two forms. The more common form is a communication first through a perimembranous defect, and then through the tricuspid valve at the area of the junction between the septal and anterosuperior leaflets (Fig. 12, left panel) (Kelle et al. 2012). The much rarer variant (Fig. 12, right panel) (Kelle et al. 2012) is characterized by a congenital deficiency of the atrioventricular component of the membranous septum.

Associated Lesions

As we have noted in previous publications, all types of defect can be associated with additional lesions (Mavroudis et al. 2013, 2023). The most important are obstruction of the ventricular outflow tracts, and prolapse of the aortic valvar leaflets. Aortic valvar prolapse can lead to valvar regurgitation. It is found usually with either the juxta-arterial defects, or with malalignment outlet defects, with or without perimembranous extension. Outflow tract obstruction is most usually associated with malalignment of the outlet septum, be it muscular or fibrous. Anterocephalad malalignment is the main feature of tetralogy of Fallot. Posterocaudal malalignment, in contrast, is associated with subaortic obstruction, which is typically associated with either severe aortic coarctation or interruption of the aortic arch. The suggested unifying approach for categorization and description of defects presented herein combines the features of location of the defect relative to the landmarks of the right ventricle, its phenotype defined on the basis of the anatomic nature of its borders, and the presence of septal malalignment (Mavroudis et al. 2013, 2023).

As we have shown, our preferred system shows but minimal departures from the initial numerical surgical classification. The major feature of our preferred classification is to use the borders of the defect as seen during surgical closure as the first step in the hierarchical classification. A hierarchy is required in any categorization, especially if potential risk factors are to be identi-

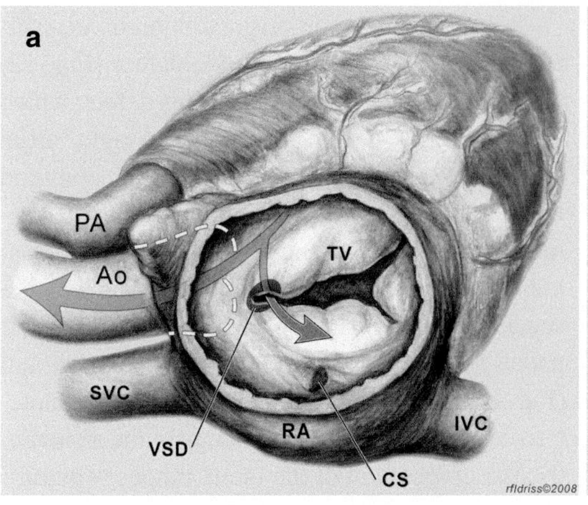

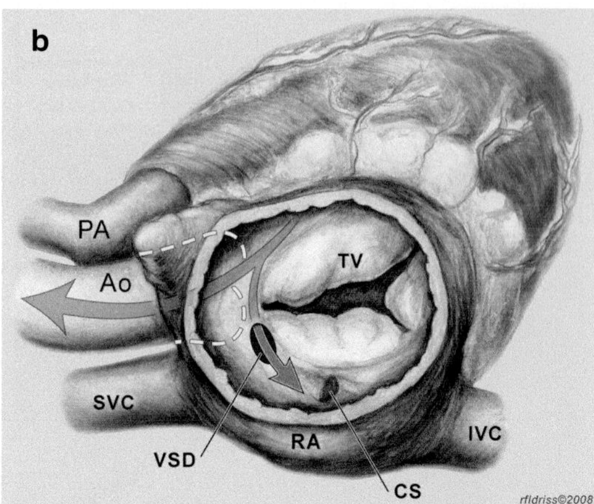

Fig. 12 **Left and right panels** show the Gerbode defects, which were not included in the initial numeric classification. They provide direct communication between the cavities of the left ventricle and the right atrium. They can take two forms. In most cases, the ventriculo-atrial shunting is through a central perimembranous defect, but with deficiency of the septal leaflet of the tricuspid valve (**left panel**) Much more rarely, the lesion represents a congenital deficiency of the atrioventricular component of the membranous septum (**right panel**). These defects are considered here for the sake of completeness, but they could also be placed in the chapter devoted to atrioventricular septal defects. It is the absence of tricuspid regurgitation that distinguishes the true Gerbode defect (**right panel**) from the indirect forms (**left panel**). Spontaneous closure is very rare in either instance, so surgical closure is recommended and is associated with excellent results. (With permission: Kelle et al. 2012). *Ao* aorta, *AV* atrioventricular, *CS* coronary sinus, *IVC* inferior caval vein, *PA* pulmonary artery, *RA* right atrium, *SVC* superior caval vein, *TV* tricuspid valve, *VSD* ventricular septal defect

fied by those who report their results to databases such as those maintained by the Society of Thoracic Surgeons and the Congenital Heart Surgeons' Society. By concentrating on the borders, the surgeon will automatically be directed to structures that will require identification and preservation if complications are to be avoided. For comparison and analysis of surgical results, it is our belief that the hierarchy based on anatomic borders will have the most utility, especially as our modification includes all the information regarding physical presentation and septal malalignment (Mavroudis et al. 2013, 2023).

4 Techniques of VSD Closure, Identification of Potential Pitfalls, and Resolution

This chapter has established the complex characteristics of VSD anatomy, the various courses of the conduction system, and the VSD borders that provide the anatomic classification system that alerts the surgeon to the possible variants and adjacent important structures. We now explore the operative techniques for VSD closure and the possible complications that could attend the operation. Where appropriate, illustrative repair techniques are offered.

4.1 Closure of the Juxta-Arterial Defects

Closure of these defects is best achieved by cardioplegic arrest and transpulmonary artery exposure (Mavroudis et al. 2013, 2020, 2023). Occasionally, as noted in Fig. 11 (Mavroudis et al. 2020; International Society for Nomenclature of Paediatric and Congenital Heart Disease 2024), a limited right ventriculotomy may be required to close a large subpulmonic muscular defect that is similarly doubly committed. The exposure techniques are noted in Fig. 13 (Mavroudis 2015) and explained in the legend. The conduct of the operation is shown in Fig. 14 (Mavroudis 2015). The parts of the operation that

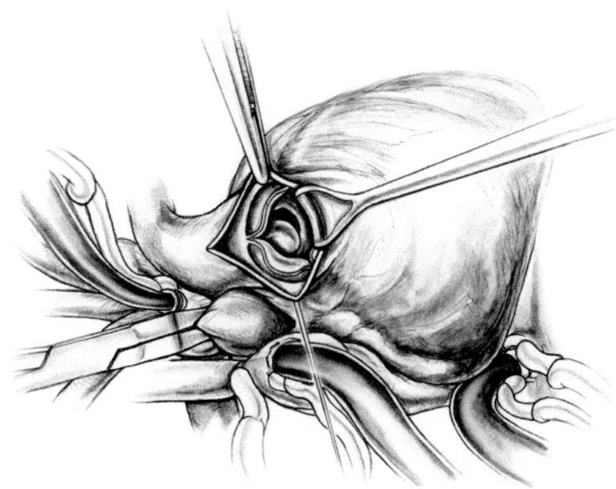

Fig. 13 Shows the cannulation technique and application of an aortic cross-clamp with cardioplegic arrest in preparation for transpulmonary arterial patch closure of a doubly committed and juxtapulmonary defect. A longitudinal pulmonary arteriotomy has been performed for exposure. The illustration demonstrates retraction of the anterior pulmonary leaflet, which exposes the defect just below the leaflets of the pulmonary valve. The right coronary aortic leaflet often can be seen prolapsing through the defect, as noted in the drawing. (With permission: Mavroudis 2015). *Ao* aorta, *AV* atrioventricular, *CS* coronary sinus, *IVC* inferior caval vein, *PA* pulmonary artery, *RA* right atrium, *SVC* superior caval vein, *TV* tricuspid valve, *VSD* ventricular septal defect

are potentially harmful are (1) manipulation of the pulmonary leaflets that can cause damage, (2) deep suturing through the pulmonary root that can cause aortic valve disruption, and (3) residual defects that can occur near their medial portion, where the muscular borders meet the pulmonary root.

Owing to the morphology of the fibrous pulmonary valve leaflets, gentle handling of the tissue with forceps is critical (Devlin et al. 2014). Figure 15 (left panel) illustrates the manner in which manipulation of the forceps can cause leaflet disruption. When this is recognized, leaflet repair (Fig. 15, right panel) can be accomplished with the careful interrupted suture technique with fine sutures. This is best done after the defect is closed using patch material as described in Fig. 14 (Mavroudis 2015).

As noted, deep suturing through the pulmonary root can disrupt the aortic valve. Figure 16 (left panel) shows accurate placement of transpulmonary sutures to close the defect. Figure 16 (right panel) inset shows the magnified view of the repair highlighting the area of the pulmonary root, and the base of the neighboring aortic root. The anchoring suture is placed in such a way as to avoid any distortion of the aortic valvar orifice. Figure 17 (left panel) shows a deep anchoring suture placed in the pulmonary root that has traversed the tissue plane and encompassed and trapped the aortic leaflet. This situation can cause valvar disruption, as well as valvar distortion, both of which can cause significant aortic regurgitation, as shown by the arrow in the right panel. The inset shows a magnified view of the unwanted suture placement that causes aortic valvar distortion, and resultant aortic valvar regurgitation. The best way to manage this complication is to recognize the problem, recommence cardiopulmonary bypass, apply aortic cross-clamping, and prepare to revise the repair, exploring the aortic valve through an aortotomy. The revision can be accomplished with suture takedown and accurate replacement to avoid the aortic valve leaflets. The aortic valve should be inspected and repaired, if needed, with the interrupted suture technique. Rarely will a patch be necessary.

4.2 Transatrial Closure of Central Perimembranous Ventricular Septal Defect by Tricuspid Valve Retraction for Exposure

As previously noted, transatrial closure of the central perimembranous defect is a common procedure, both as isolated closure and in association with other lesions. The potential complications of closure include residual shunting, heart block, tricuspid valvar entrapment, and aortic valvar injury (Mavroudis et al. 2013, 2020, 2023; Mavroudis 2015; Kelle et al. 2012; Mavroudis and Backer 2010; Schipper et al. 2017; Menting et al. 2015).

Perhaps, residual shunting is the most common complication, but not necessarily clinically relevant, as postoperative residual shunts tend to close with time (Schipper et al. 2017; Menting et al. 2015; Deng et al. 2020; Dodge-Khatami et al. 2007; Bol-Raap et al. 2003, 2007). Deng and associates (2020) have reported that residual

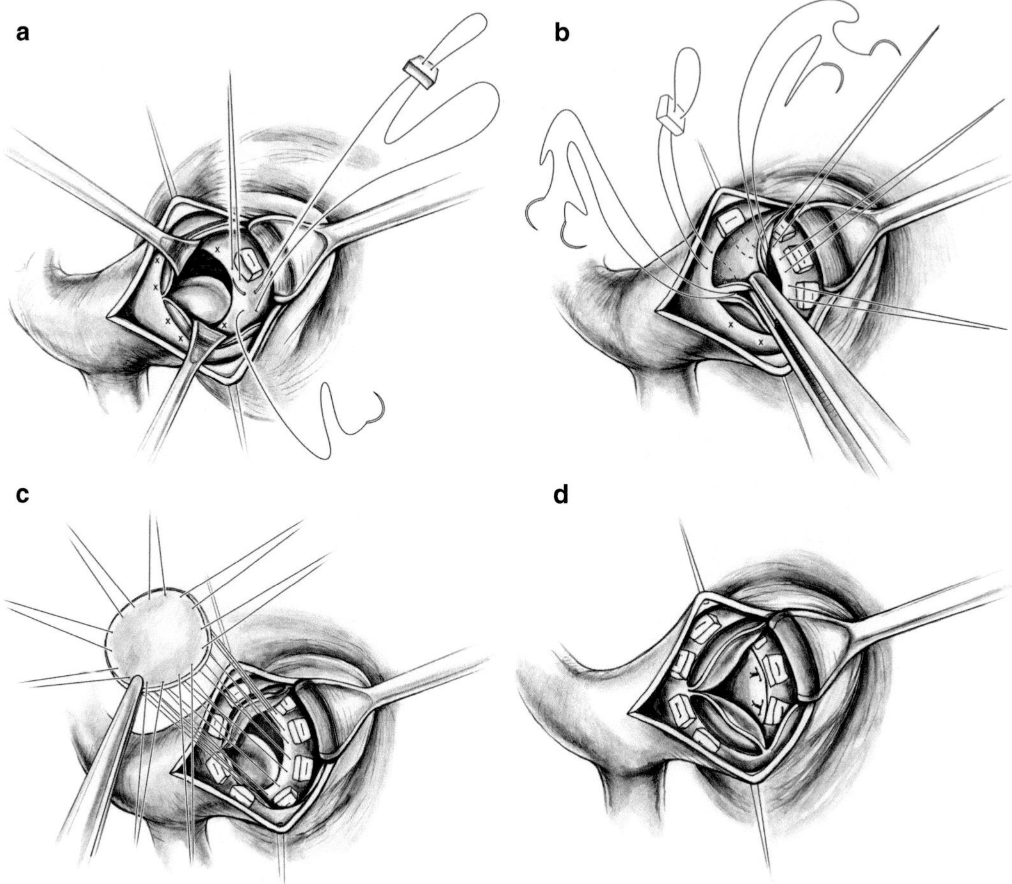

Fig. 14 Closure is commenced (**Panel a**) by placing superficial interrupted, pledgetted sutures at the crest of the septum. The sutures should be placed approximately 2 to 4 mm from the edge of the septum, with no deeper than 50% penetration into the muscular septum. Although the conduction system is anatomically remote from the suture placement, deeper bites are unnecessary and potentially could injure the atrioventricular node in the case of an anomalous course of the node. **Panel b** highlights suture placement in the pulmonary valvar sinus, emerging on the ventricular side to facilitate patch attachment. The lateral sutures are placed in the pulmonary root, and the medial sutures are placed in the shared pulmonary and aortic roots. This part of the operation has the potential for leaflet disruption or aortic valve injury if the sutures are not placed well or if the leaflets are roughly handled. **Panel c** shows the sutures being placed through a synthetic patch before the patch is lowered into the defect for closure that we generally use because the edges do not fray; this feature allows more uniform apposition to the muscle and fibrous tissues, ensuring a more secure closure. **Panel d** demonstrates the completed repair with the pulmonary leaflets partially closed to emphasize the differential placement of the pledgetted sutures (some in the valvar sinus and some in the right ventricle at the crest of the septum). (With permission: Mavroudis 2015)

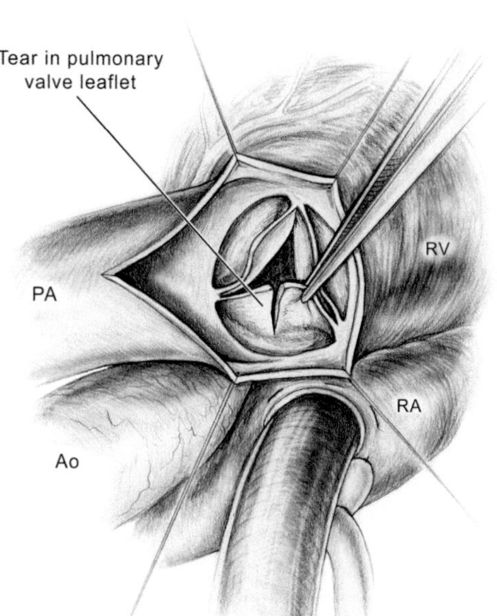

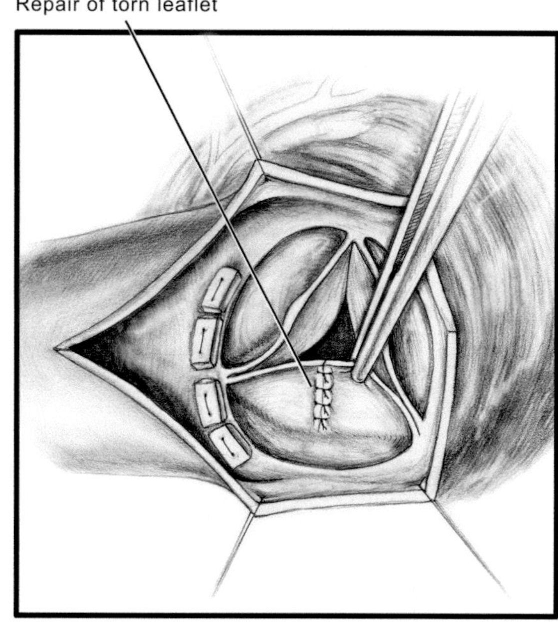

Fig. 15 (**Left panel**) shows how rough forceps manipulation of the pulmonary valve can cause leaflet disruption and potential pulmonary valvar regurgitation. This injury can be repaired by interrupted fine suture technique **(right panel**). Closure of the defect should be performed before approaching repair of the pulmonary leaflet. *Ao* aorta, *PA* pulmonary artery, *RA* right atrium, *RV* right ventricle, *VSD* ventricular septal defect

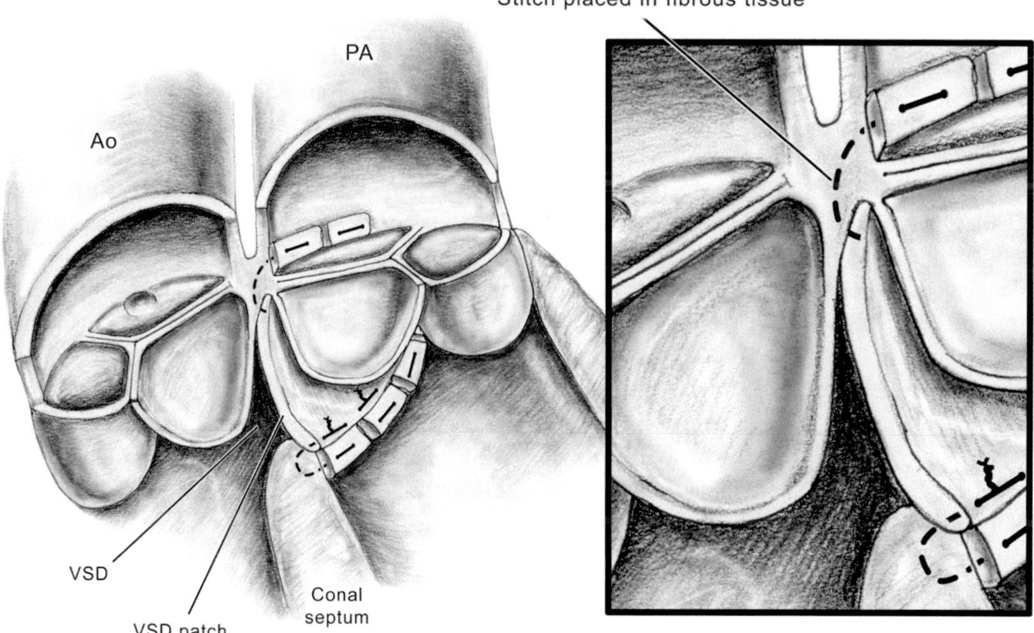

Fig. 16 Shows a coronal view of patch placement and the anchoring sutures with reference to the surrounding structures. Note that sutures are placed in the fibrous support of the valvar leaflets, and that ventricular sutures are placed superficially in the right ventricular crest. The inset shows a magnified view of the repair highlighting the area of the conjoined pulmonary and aortic roots. The anchoring suture is placed in such a way as to avoid any distortion of the aortic valvar fibrous support. *Ao* aorta, *PA* pulmonary artery, *VSD* ventricular septal defect

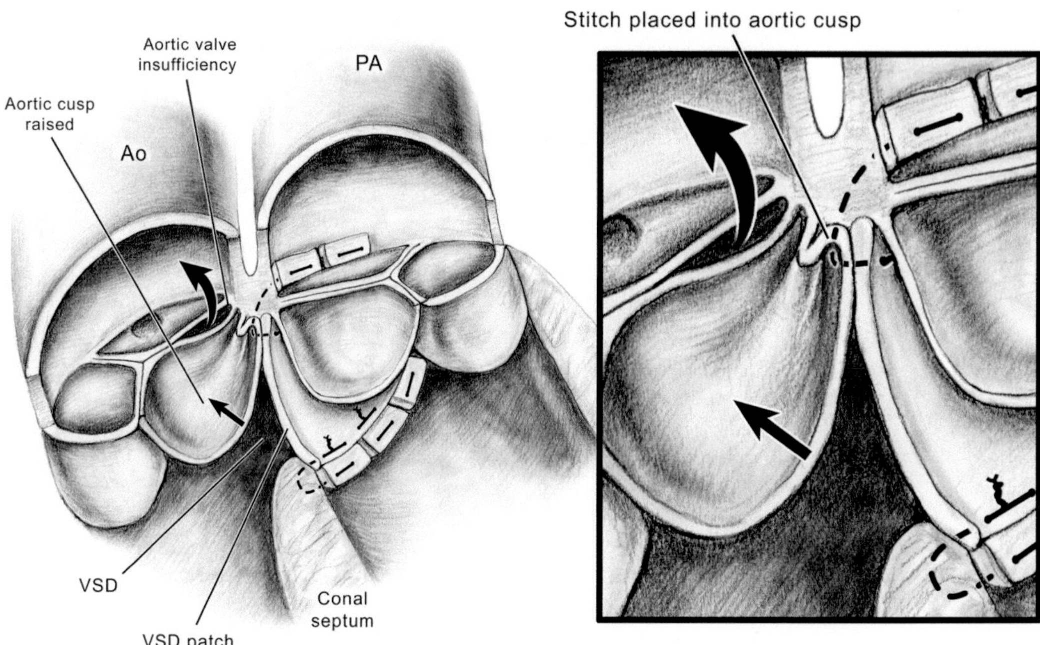

Fig. 17 Shows a deep anchoring suture placed in the pulmonary root that has traversed the tissue plane and encompassed and trapped the aortic leaflet. This situation can cause valvar disruption as well as valvar distortion, both of which can cause significant aortic regurgitation, noted by the arrow. The inset shows a magnified view of the unwanted suture placement that causes distortion and resultant aortic valvar regurgitation. *Ao* aorta, *PA* pulmonary artery, *VSD* ventricular septal defect

defects measuring less than 1.25 mm at discharge echocardiography tend to undergo spontaneous closure within 6 months. Residual defects larger than 1.25 mm had a lower short-term closure rate, but seemed not to differ from smaller shunts beyond 300 days postoperatively (Deng et al. 2020). Other reports have noted similar findings with slightly different sizes and time periods for spontaneous closure of residual defects (Dodge-Khatami et al. 2007; Bol-Raap et al. 2003, 2007).

Cao and associates (2020) have undertaken a more aggressive policy. They advocate for immediate reoperation for residual defects larger than 2 mm, using beating heart surgery to identify the defect and render complete closure more accurately. They found this strategy safe and effective without air-related complications.

It appears that 2 mm is the size of the residual defect that results in the most problems concerning long-term prophylactic antibiotic therapy and overcirculation (Cao et al. 2020). Achievement of complete closure at the primary operation, therefore, is paramount. This requires adequate exposure, accurate suture placement, and proper cardioplegic administration. This is why we advocate for interrupted pledgetted suture technique where possible. Notable exceptions to this management scheme include neonatal operations, such as for transposition with VSD, common arterial trunk, and interrupted aortic arch with VSD. These procedures require a prolonged cardioplegic arrest time. Under these circumstances, it is reasonable to perform closure using careful and deliberate running suture technique.

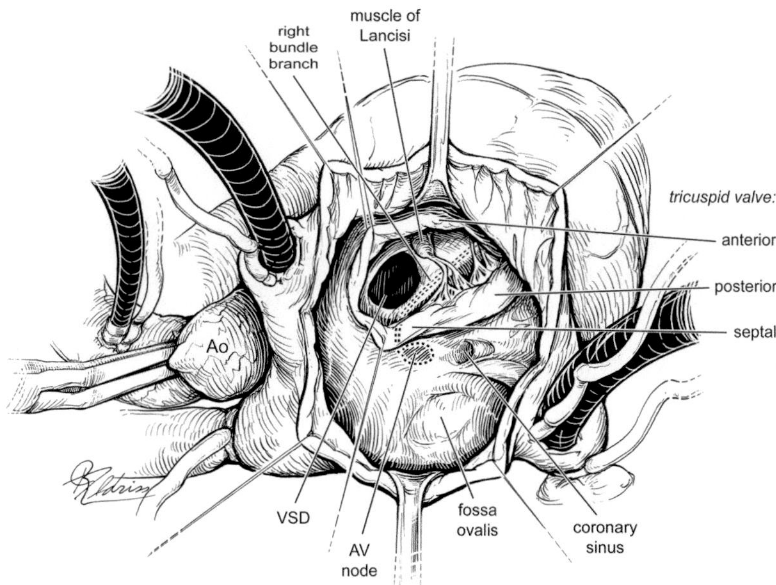

Fig. 18 Shows right atrial exposure after aortobicaval cardiopulmonary bypass and cardioplegic arrest for central perimembranous defect closure. The defect is exposed by retraction of the tricuspid valvar leaflets, and the important surrounding structures are noted. Interrupted pledgetted sutures can be placed on the right ventricular surface of the septum, aortic root, and tricuspid annulus while avoiding injury to these structures. (With permission: Mavroudis et al. 2013). *Ao* aorta, *AV* atrioventricular, *VSD* ventricular septal defect

Figure 18 (Mavroudis et al. 2013) shows right atrial exposure and structure identification after aortobicaval cardiopulmonary bypass and cardioplegic arrest for closure of the central perimembranous defect. The VSD is exposed by retraction of the tricuspid valvar leaflets. Interrupted pledgetted sutures can be placed on the right ventricular surface of the septum in such a manner as to avoid injury to the aortic and tricuspid valves, along with the conduction pathway, which is represented by the double dotted lines traversing on the left ventricular side of the septum.

Figure 19 (Mavroudis 2015) panels show the organized closure steps of a central perimembranous VSD using tricuspid leaflet retraction and interrupted pledgetted suture technique. Suture placement is deliberate to avoid residual leaks, valve injury, and heart block. Despite these well-intentioned techniques, complications can still occur.

Figure 20 is a good example of careful suture technique to avoid injury to the conduction system The sutures are place on the right ventricular side of the septum, being placed no deeper than

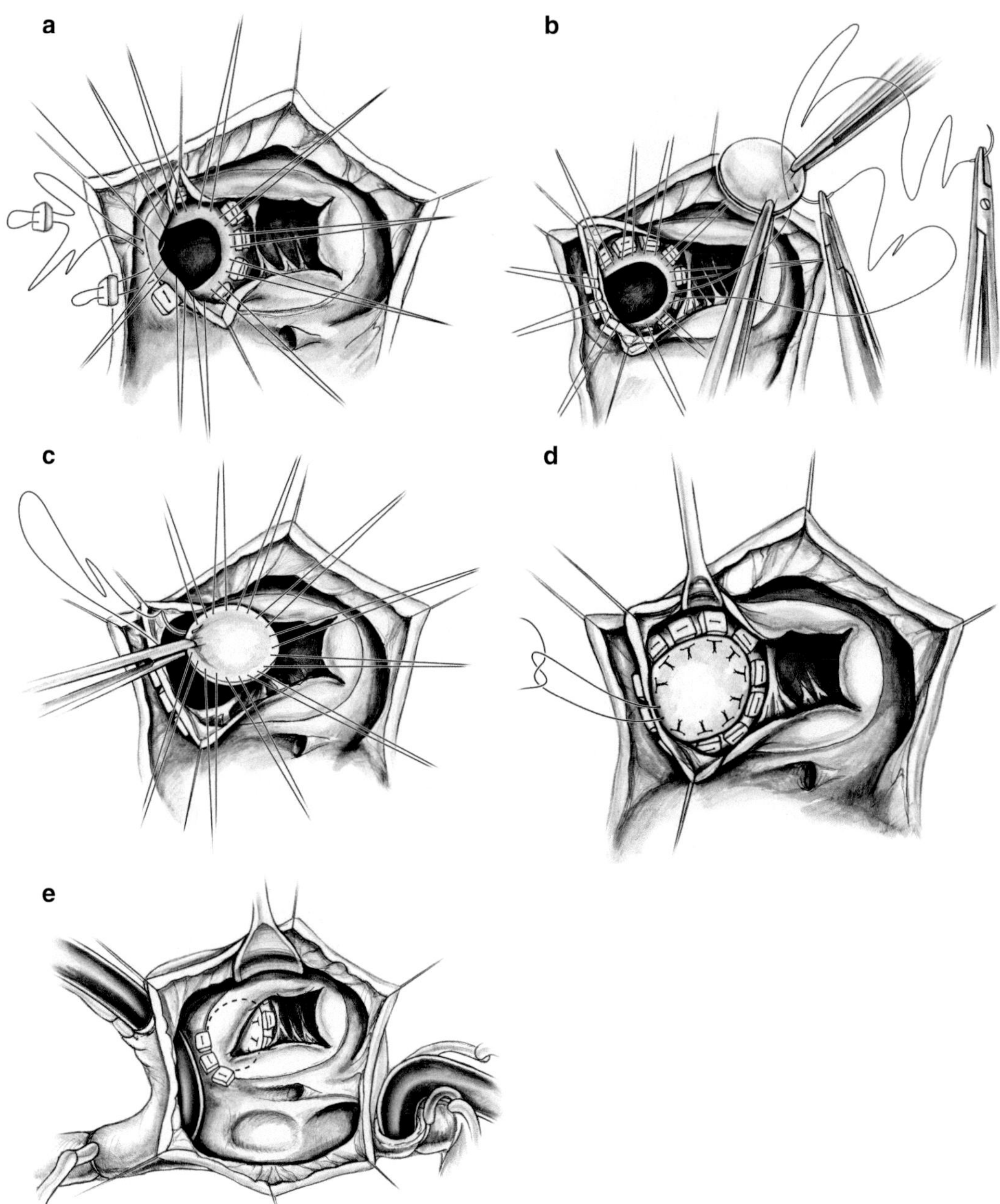

Fig. 19 **Panel a** shows pledgetted sutures placed on the crest of the right ventricular septum, annulus of the tricuspid valve, and aortic root with its fibrous support as the anatomy accords. The sutures are placed with special care to avoid injury to the aforementioned structures and, in particular, the conduction system that lies on the left ventricular surface. **Panel b** shows the proper manner to place the pledget without twists on the crest of the septum, superiorly near the aortic valve, and on the right atrial side of the tricuspid annulus to avoid muscle tearing, valve disruption, and injury. **Panel c** demonstrates sutures placed through the edges of a synthetic patch to ensure proper coaptation of the patch to the myocardium. The patch is lowered onto the defect in **Panel d** and the sutures are individually tied. **Panel e** shows the patch in place under the tricuspid valve, which is allowed to assume its normal place. A bulb syringe can be used to test the tricuspid valve for competency. (With permission: Mavroudis 2015)

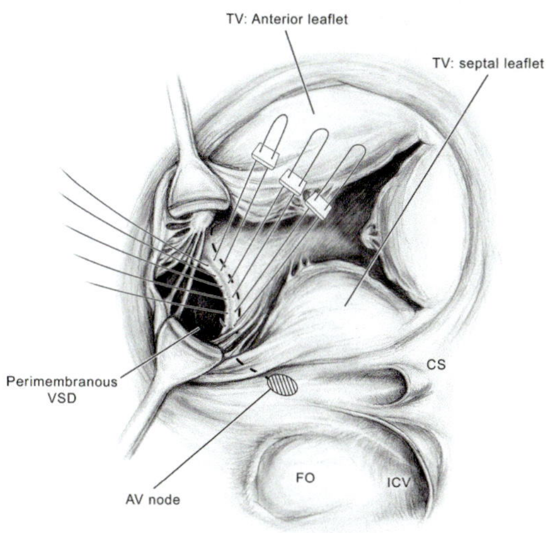

Fig. 20 Shows the execution of the careful suturing technique to ensure firm septal muscle engagement for snug patch apposition and proper closure. The conduction system and surrounding structures are noted for identification and relative visualization. The sutures are placed on the right ventricular side of the muscular ventricular septum, no deeper than 50% of its thickness. *AV* atrioventricular, *CS* coronary sinus, *ICV* inferior caval vein, *FO* fossa ovalis, *TV* tricuspid valve, *VSD* ventricular septal defect

50% of the thickness of the muscular septum. The important structures are shown to enhance the exposure for proper identification and accurate suture placement. On the other hand, Fig. 21 shows how departure of the aforementioned technique can result in conduction system injury and heart block. The three sutures shown visually at approximately 3 to 5 o'clock have been placed transeptally. They are dangerously close to the conduction system, which runs on the left ventricular side of the muscular septum. For this reason, it is imperative to keep the anchoring sutures on the right ventricular side deep enough to provide a secure anchor, but sufficiently superficial not to traverse the septum so as to cause heart block.

Another complication that can occur during closure is the unwanted entrapment of chordal structures that can cause tricuspid regurgitation (Yoshimura et al. 2016; Hofmeyr et al. 2013). Figure 22 shows two panels involving the unfortunate execution of chordal entrapment. The left panel demonstrates the well placed interrupted sutures in the proper location of the muscular septum, except that the pledgetted suture at 12 o'clock has entrapped the chordal attachment to the tricuspid valve. The right panel shows a detailed view of the 12 o'clock suture that can easily happen without proper attention to the repair technique. Once the sutures are tied, and the defect is closed, the surgeon can determine if there is a problem by using a saline bulb syringe to test for tricuspid regurgitation. The resolution to this problem can usually be performed through takedown of the flawed suture and replacement with another pledgetted suture anchored in such a way as to free the cord while still effectively closing the defect. If the chordal entrapment is not appreciated, and if the problem is found at a subsequent time, the repair technique requires a different solution, as the patch and entrapped cord are ensconced in fibrous tissue that does not allow freeing of the entangled cord. The solution to this problem is tricuspid valvuloplasty as noted in Fig. 23. The left panel shows tricuspid regurgitation (arrow) and the entrapped cord of the hidden anatomy behind the anterior leaflet. The right panel shows the classic solution using tricuspid valvoplasty by partial bicuspidization of the tricuspid valve at the area of the commissure between the anterosuperior and septal leaflets (Russell et al. 2011; Dodge-Khatami et al. 2007, 2014). In almost all cases, suturing these leaflets will repair the tricuspid regurgitation without causing stenosis.

The tricuspid valve can also be entrapped during repair by ill-fated sutures that were destined to be placed in the tricuspid annulus during closure, as noted in Fig. 19e (Mavroudis 2015). These sutures are generally safe to place and serve as a secure anchor. Sometimes, however, sutures are inappropriately placed in the body of the anterosuperior leaflet away from the annulus toward the free leaflet into the right ventricle. Figure 24 demonstrates this problem in a sectional view of the right atrium, right ventricle, and left ventricle. In the left panel, the properly placed anchoring pledgetted sutures in the tricus-

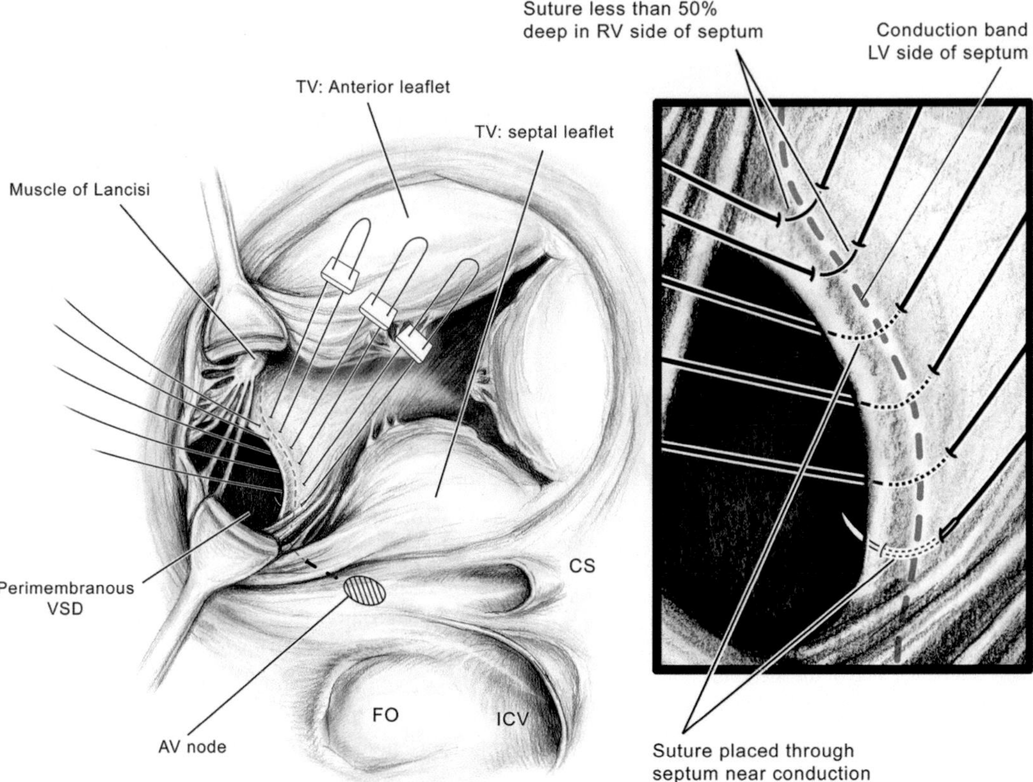

Fig. 21 Shows how the ill-advised suture technique that transverses the muscular septum can cause heart block. The three sutures shown diagrammatically at approximately 3 to 5 o'clock have been place transeptally, very close to the conduction system that traverses on the left ventricular side of the muscular septum. Avoiding this maneuver is critical to keep the anchoring sutures on the right ventricular side deep enough to provide a secure anchor and superficial enough not to traverse the septum and cause heart block. This principle should be followed whether interrupted suture technique or running suture technique is employed. *AV* atrioventricular, *CS* coronary sinus, *ICV* inferior caval vein, *FO* fossa ovalis, *TV* tricuspid valve, *VSD* ventricular septal defect

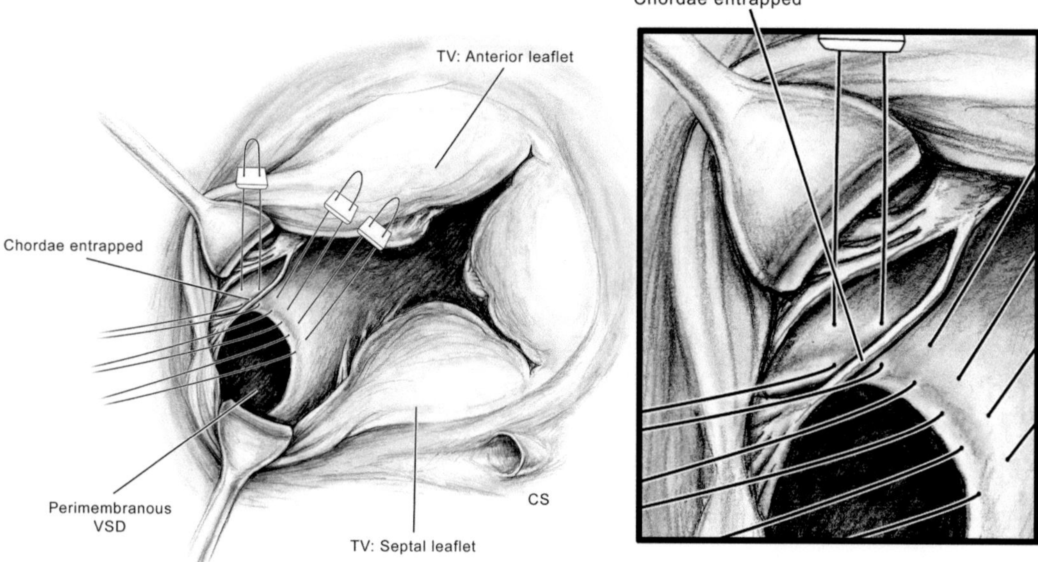

Fig. 22 The left panel demonstrates the well-placed interrupted sutures in the proper location of the muscular septum, except that the pledgetted suture at 12 o'clock has entrapped the chordal attachment to the tricuspid valve. The inset shows a detailed view of the 12 o'clock suture that can easily occur without proper attention being given to the repair technique. Once the sutures are tied and the defect is closed, the surgeon can identify the problem with a saline bulb syringe to test for tricuspid regurgitation. If found, a conscientious exploration can identify the anatomic problem. The resolution to this problem can usually be performed by takedown of the offending suture and replacement with another pledgetted suture anchored in such a way as to free the cord while still effectively closing the defect. If the chordal entrapment is not appreciated and the problem is found at a subsequent time, the repair technique requires a different solution as the patch and entrapped cord are incorporated in fibrous tissue. *CS* coronary sinus, *TV* tricuspid valve, *VSD* ventricular septal defect

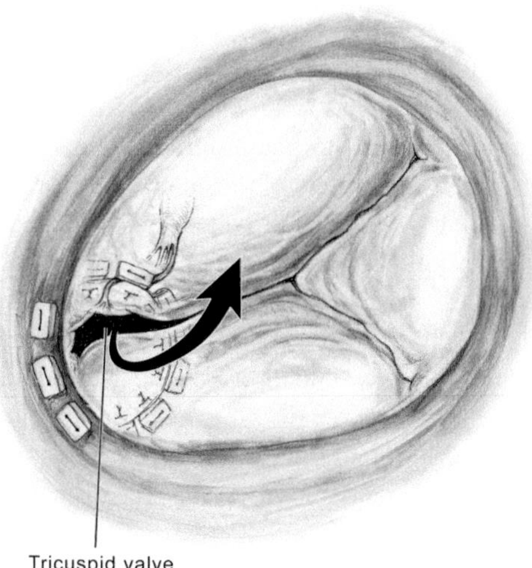

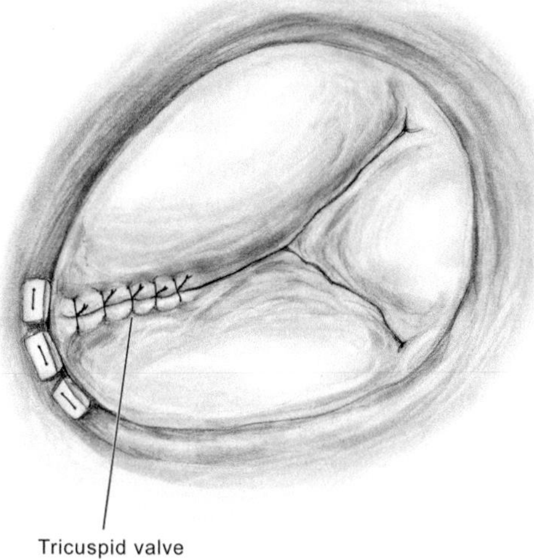

Fig. 23 The left panel shows tricuspid regurgitation (arrow) at the commissure between the anterosuperior and septal leaflets of the tricuspid valve. The hidden anatomy behind the anterosuperior leaflet demonstrates the entrapped cord. The right panel shows tricuspid valvuloplasty by partial bicuspidization of the tricuspid valve at the area of the commissure. Suturing these aspects of the leaflets using an interrupted suture technique repairs the tricuspid regurgitation without causing stenosis

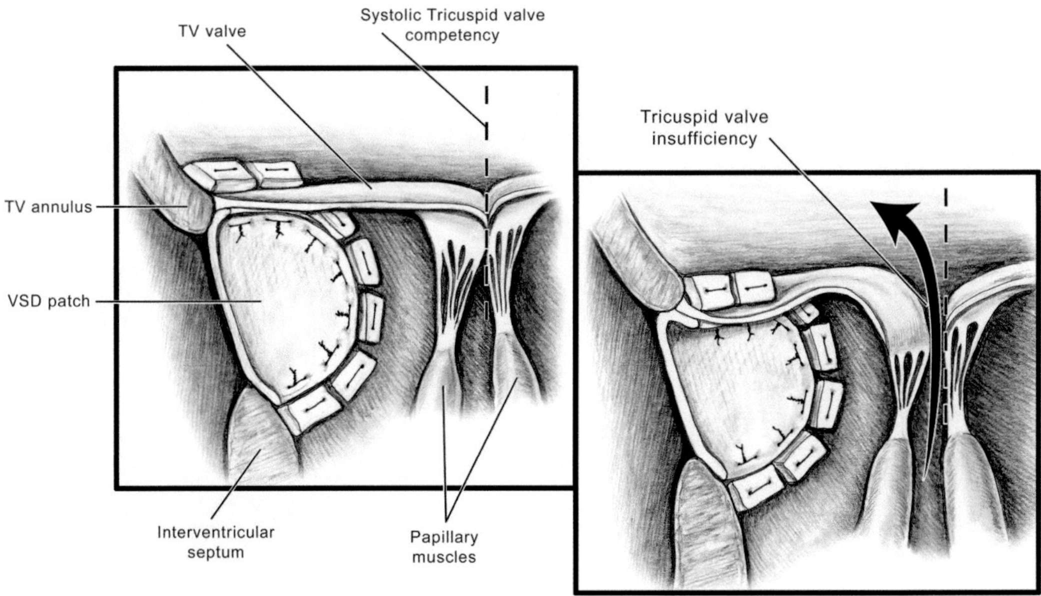

Fig. 24 Demonstrates how a misplaced suture in the body of the anterosuperior leaflet en route to central perimembranous defect closure can cause important tricuspid regurgitation. This potential problem can be viewed in cross-sectional display of the right atrium, right ventricle, and left ventricle. The left panel shows the properly placed anchoring pledgetted sutures in the tricuspid annulus, which are connected to the patch that lies comfortably under the leaflet. This maneuver results in secure closure of the defect without tricuspid injury. The right panel shows the ill-fated sutures placed through the anterosuperior leaflet body instead of the annulus. When the sutures are tied, the leaflet is tethered and fails to align closely with the remaining leaflets. This causes unwanted tricuspid regurgitation. This may also be associated with a residual defect because of poor placement of the sutures. *TV* tricuspid valve, *VSD* ventricular septal defect

pid annulus of the anterior leaflet are connected to the patch that lies comfortably under the leaflet, demonstrating a secure closure of the defect without tricuspid injury. In the right panel, the ill-fated sutures have been placed through the anterior leaflet body instead of the annulus. When the sutures are tied, the leaflet is tethered and fails to align closely with the remaining leaflets causing unwanted tricuspid regurgitation. This may also be associated with residual shunting because of the poor placement of the sutures (Kelle et al. 2012; Mavroudis and Backer 2002; Varghese et al. 2016; Saker et al. 2017). If this situation is recognized, immediate reoperation is warranted, with patch revision and freeing of the leaflet. More often than not, this situation is not well recognized, or is thought to be insignificant. This could be true; however, continued tricuspid regurgitation may require reoperation.

Figure 25 shows the result of tricuspid valve entrapment owing to inappropriate suture placement through the body of the anterosuperior leaflet. The arrow in the left panel notes the area of regurgitation. The right panel shows tricuspid valvoplasty using the partial bicuspidization technique as noted in Figure 23 right panel. Oftentimes, this situation is associated with remote tetralogy repair, where the combination of pulmonary regurgitation and tricuspid regurgitation lead to reoperation. Tricuspid repair using this technique is efficient and will allow the time required for pulmonary valve implant.

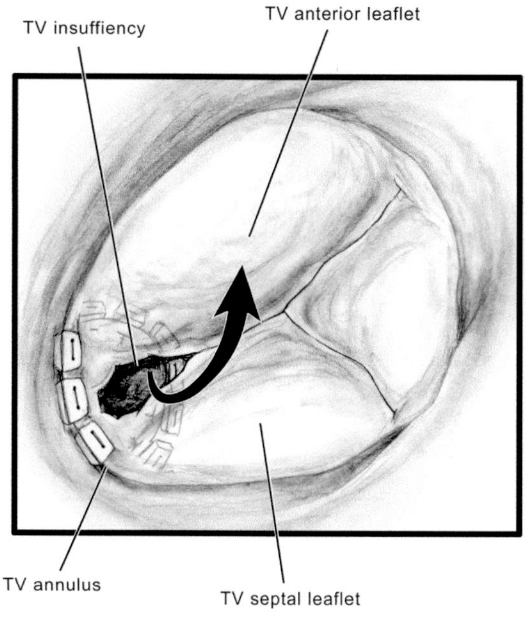

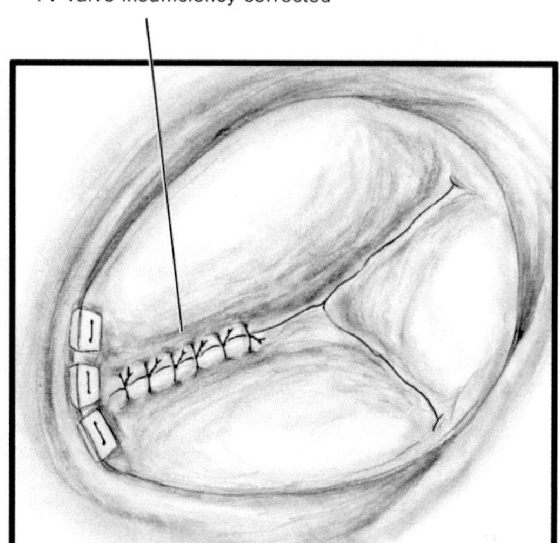

Fig. 25 Shows the result of tricuspid valvar entrapment owing to inappropriate suture placement through the body of the anterosuperior leaflet. The arrow shows the area of regurgitation. The right panel shows tricuspid valvoplasty using the partial bicuspidization technique as noted in Fig. 23 (**right panel**). This situation can be associated with remote tetralogy repair where the combination of pulmonary regurgitation and tricuspid regurgitation lead to reoperation. *TV* tricuspid valve, *VSD* ventricular septal defect. (With permission: Mavroudis et al. 2013)

4.3 Transatrial Closure of Central Perimembranous Ventricular Septal Defect by Radial Tricuspid Valve Incision for Exposure

In the majority of cases, these defects close naturally because of accessory fibrous tricuspid valve tissue and septal hypertrophy (Deng et al. 2020; Dodge-Khatami et al. 2007; Ben Farhat et al. 2020). Some, however, persist despite this natural closing process, and often present in older children. The anatomy under these circumstances can be confusing because, during the natural closing mechanism, a so-called tricuspid valve pouch can develop, which can obstruct the exposure of the defect during repair (Mavroudis et al. 2013, 2023; Mavroudis 2015; Mavroudis and Backer 2010; Feigl et al. 1986; Idriss et al. 1992; Nakamura et al. 2022). Importantly, the tricuspid pouch obstructs the underlying larger defect, and may be responsible for multiple escape routes or jets. Primary closure of an apparent solitary fibrous hole may not consider the other escape routes, which then become manifest after primary closure. The true defect beneath the tricuspid valve needs to be exposed for proper patch closure, aortic support, and tricuspid valvar integrity (Mavroudis et al. 2013, 2023; Mavroudis 2015; Mavroudis and Backer 2010; Russell et al. 2011; Dodge-Khatami et al. 2014; Idriss et al. 1992; Nakamura et al. 2022). Figure 26 (Mavroudis et al. 2013) shows right atrial exposure after aortobicaval cardiopulmonary bypass and cardioplegic arrest. The tricuspid valve pouch is noted with the important surrounding structures. The tricuspid pouch is being retracted by forceps, and the dotted line demonstrates the area that can be incised with a scalpel to fully expose the limits of the defect. Care must be taken to avoid injury to the aortic valve, which can lie in close proximity to the tricuspid pouch. Complications associated with this maneuver will be discussed further. If any doubt as to the

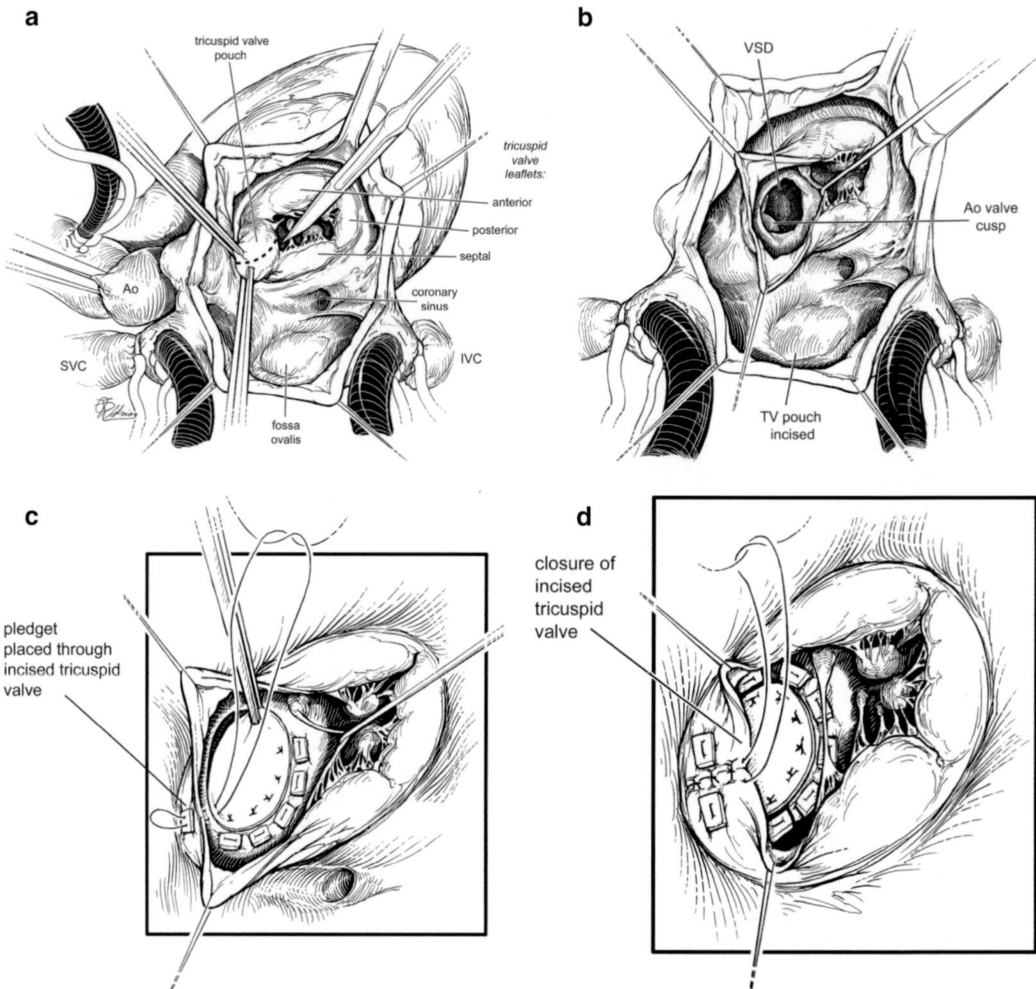

Fig. 26 **Panel a** shows right atrial exposure after aortobicaval cardiopulmonary bypass and cardioplegic arrest for closure in the presence of a tricuspid valvar pouch, as noted together with important surrounding structures. The dotted line with forceps retraction shows the area that can be incised with a scalpel. Great care is taken to avoid injury to the aortic valve, which can lie very close to the tricuspid pouch. When in doubt, administration of antegrade cardioplegia can help to define the anatomic extent of the aortic leaflets, which can help to define and direct the tricuspid pouch incision. **Panel b** shows exposure after the tricuspid valve pouch is radially incised to identify the extent of the defect and aortic valvar leaflets. Once the anatomic landmarks are identified, interrupted pledgetted sutures can be placed on the septal crest. The tricuspid annulus, and portions of the aortic root to effectively close the defect with a synthetic patch, as noted in **Panel c**. The tricuspid valve can then be repaired using interrupted sutures, as shown in **Panel d**. The resultant repaired tricuspid valve can be tested by the bulb syringe technique to guide further suture placement as necessary. (With permission: Mavroudis et al. 2013). *Ao* aorta, *CS* coronary sinus, *IVC* inferior caval vein, *SVC* superior caval vein, *TV* tricuspid valve, *VSD* ventricular septal defect

location of the aortic valve arises, administration of antegrade cardioplegia can help to define the anatomic extent of the aortic leaflets. This will help to define and address the tricuspid pouch incision. Figure 26b–d (Mavroudis et al. 2013) demonstrate the important steps of patch closure without aortic valve injury, preserving the integrity of the conduction system, and insured tricuspid valve competence using proper repair techniques.

Complications associated with exposure by radial incision of the tricuspid valve can occur, especially if there is aortic valvar prolapse (Mavroudis et al. 2013; Idriss et al. 1992). Radial incision, if not performed carefully, can result in aortic leaflet injury (Mavroudis et al. 2013; Idriss et al. 1992). Figure 27 shows the process of aortic valve leaflet injury during radial tricuspid valvar incision. To avoid this complication, the incision should be performed in stages, each incremental incision being evaluated for its proximity to the aortic valve leaflet (Mavroudis et al. 2013). The incision should be stopped when the tricuspid valve annulus is defined, with continued integrity of the aortic valve leaflet. In the unlikely event that the valve is injured, the operation should be reevaluated with the idea that the original repair will be longer and more complex owing to the aortic valve injury. The valve can be repaired

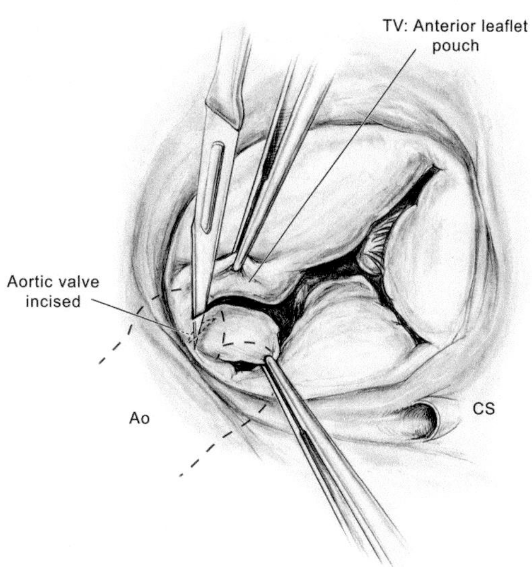

Fig. 27 Shows how the aortic valvar leaflet can be injured by radial tricuspid valvar incision for exposure of the defect. While this complication is rare, methods to avoid aortic valvar injury should be practiced in every case. The incision in the tricuspid valve should be performed in linear stages, each time evaluating the distance from the last incision to the aortic leaflet and tricuspid annulus. The incision can be stopped when the tricuspid valve annulus is identified with clear integrity of the aortic leaflet. The illustration shows how an unwanted scalpel incision can injure the aortic leaflet. The aortic valve should always be identified and inspected for such a complication. A short administration of antegrade cardioplegia can evaluate the valve for potential regurgitation. *Ao* aorta, *CS* coronary sinus, *TV* tricuspid valve, *VSD* ventricular septal defect

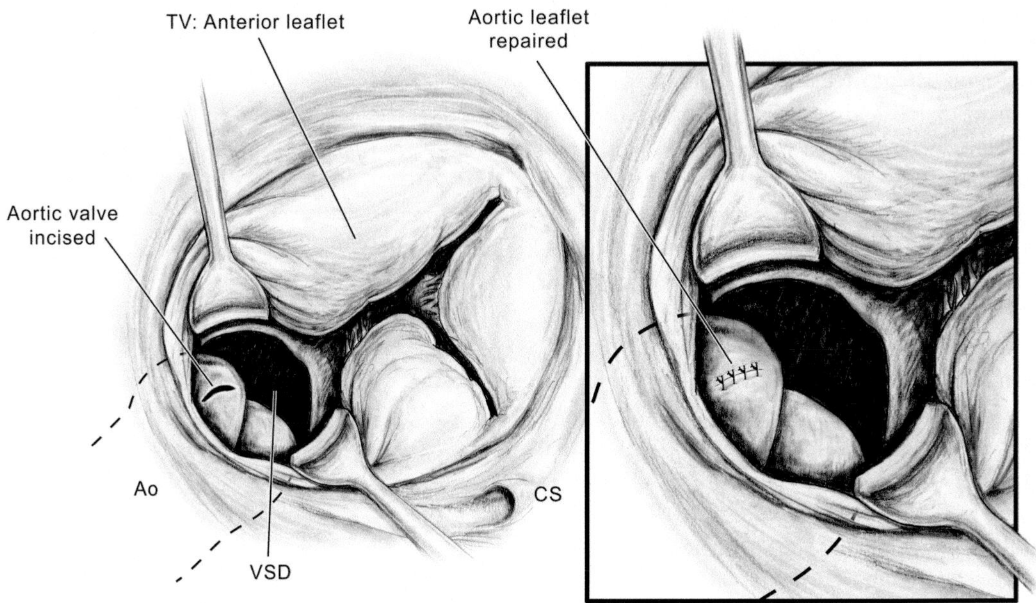

Fig. 28 Demonstrates injury to an aortic leaflet as a result of radial incision for the purpose of exposing the underlying septal defect (**left panel**). The result of valve repair using interrupted suture technique is that the defect can then be repaired by patch closure and tricuspid valve repair (**right panel**). *Ao* aorta, *CS* coronary sinus, *TV* tricuspid valve, *VSD* ventricular septal defect

through the defect, or by aortotomy. Figure 28 (left panel) shows the result of unintended aortic leaflet injury. The right panel shows the valve being repaired via the unrepaired defect using interrupted suture technique. Patch closure (not shown) can be performed in the event that the leaflet injury is very large. The defect can then be repaired by patch closure and tricuspid valve repair.

5 Complications Associated with Transatrial Closure of Central Perimembranous Ventricular Septal Defect Via Tricuspid Valve Circumferential Incision

In some cases, the commissure between the tricuspid valve anterior leaflet and septal leaflet obscures the underlying defect with many obstructive cords that are necessary for tricuspid valve function but challenging for adequate exposure for closure (Russell et al. 2011; Dodge-Khatami et al. 2014). A radial incision for exposure of the underlying defect may not prove to be sufficient. Alternatively, a circumferential incision can be performed, thereby exposing the entire circumference of the underlying defect (Mavroudis et al. 2013; Mavroudis and Backer 2010). Figure 29 (Mavroudis and Backer 2010) shows optimal exposure and closure for this type of camouflaged defect and associated closure techniques.

As with the tricuspid radial incision for exposure, the circumferential incision exposes the aortic valve leaflet to incisional injury during the operation, especially if a severely prolapsed leaflet is not detected (Mavroudis and Backer 2010; Gaynor et al. 2001).

Figure 30 (left panel) shows how a deep incision without regard to the hidden aortic valve leaflet anatomy can cause aortic valve injury. The precautionary steps of this kind of exposure

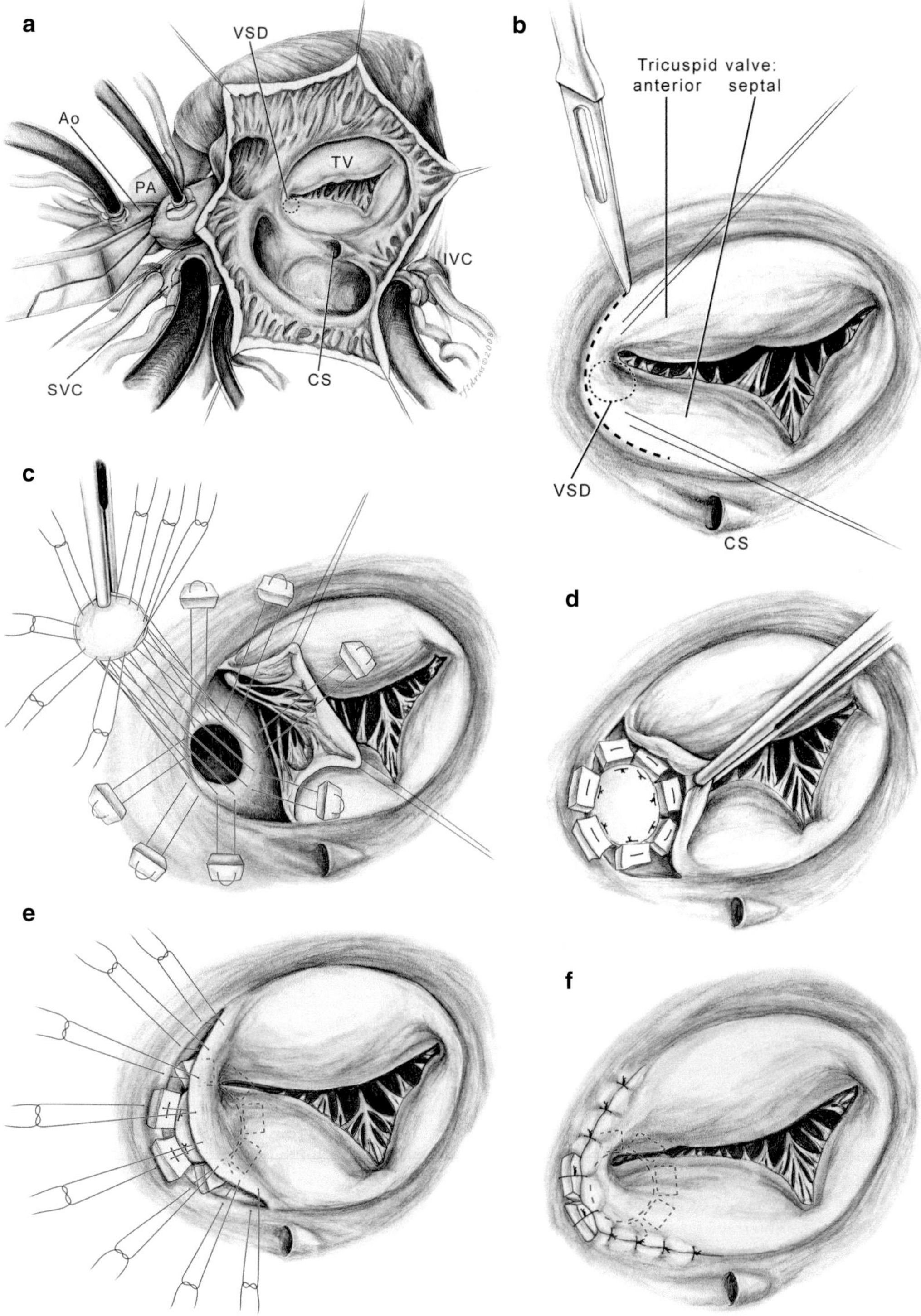

Fig. 29 (continued)

Fig. 29 **Panel a** shows right atrial exposure after aortobicaval cardiopulmonary bypass and cardioplegic arrest, with the noted important surrounding structures. The defect is covered by portions of the septal and anterosuperior leaflets, which have numerous obstructing chordal attachments. Under these circumstances, a circumferential incision with partial takedown of the tricuspid valve affords optimal exposure. In **Panel b**, the dotted circle on the tricuspid valve depicts the location of the defect, and the larger dotted line indicates the incision in the tricuspid valve planned for valvar takedown and exposure of the defect. The aortic valve is at risk when such an incision is performed. This figure also shows the incision commencing at the anterosuperior leaflet. When such an incision is planned, it is wise to place a traction suture in the leaflet of the valve for retraction. Alternatively, one could start the incision in the middle of the septal leaflet and extend it superiorly while inspecting for and identifying the aortic leaflets. An injury to the aortic valve under these circumstances would prove to be problematic. With the valve retracted, the defect is easily viewed, and pledgetted sutures can be placed around the perimeter in such a way as to avoid any injury to the aortic valvar leaflets and the conduction system. The sutures can then be placed into a polytetrafluoroethylene patch, as noted on **Panel c,** The completed closure is shown in **Panel d** with forceps retraction of the tricuspid valve. **Panel e** shows reattachment of the tricuspid valve to the annulus using interrupted suture technique, thereby reconstructing the integrity of the valve. **Panel f** shows the completed closure and reattachment of the tricuspid valve, which can be tested for competency with a bulge syringe. (With permission: Mavroudis and Backer 2010). *Ao* aorta, *CS* coronary sinus, *IVC* inferior caval vein, *SVC* superior caval vein, *TV* tricuspid valve, *VSD* ventricular septal defect

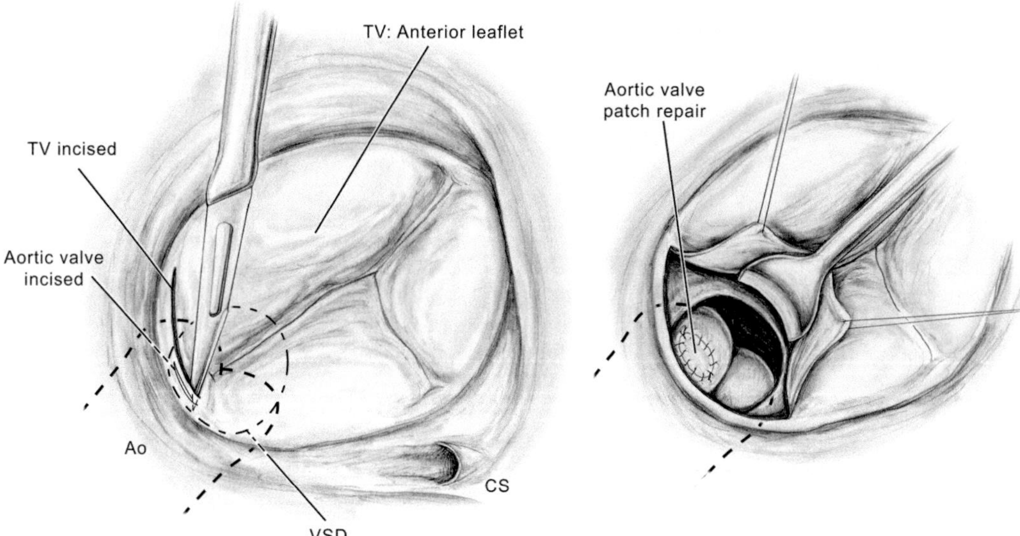

Fig. 30 Left panel shows how a deep circumferential incision to expose the underlying defect can cause injury to the aortic valve, especially if there is significant aortic leaflet prolapse. Aortic valvar injury can be close to the aortic root or in the body of the leaflet. The repair techniques can be either interrupted suture technique or patch repair as shown in the right panel. Prudence determines the proper method to use to enhance long-term function and avoid future aortic valve replacement/repair. *Ao* aorta, *CS* coronary sinus, *TV* tricuspid valve, *VSD* ventricular septal defect

have been delineated in Fig. 29 (Mavroudis and Backer 2010) and should be used. As noted previously, the operation will take a different tone with reassessment of myocardial preservation techniques to safely approach the injured aortic valve and apply repair techniques as in Fig. 30 (right panel).

6 Closure of a Central Perimembranous Ventricular Septal Defect with Inlet Extension

As discussed earlier, there are many anatomic variations of defects opening to the inlet of the right ventricle (Figs. 6, 7, 8, and 9) (Mavroudis et al. 2013, 2020; International Society for Nomenclature of Paediatric and Congenital Heart Disease 2024). They are referenced again in this section because there is a higher incidence of heart block associated with their repair, reflecting the different patterns that govern the course of the conduction system (Mavroudis et al. 2020). We do not illustrate here the closure of these defects, as the principles are the same as discussed previously (Figs. 18 and 19) (Mavroudis et al. 2013, 2020; Mavroudis 2015; Andersen et al. 2006, 2014; International Society for Nomenclature of Paediatric and Congenital Heart Disease 2024). The underlying principle is to be aware of the conduction system, understand the variations, and make every effort to avoid injury to the conduction system.

7 Complications Associated with Closure of Muscular Defects

In general, muscular defects are approached and closed through the right atrium and tricuspid valve (Mavroudis et al. 2013, 2020, 2023; Mavroudis and Backer 2010; Russell et al. 2011; Dodge-Khatami et al. 2014). These defects are often challenging to identify owing to the muscular trabeculations at the apex of the right ventricle, which are rarely in one plane (Mavroudis and Backer 2002; Jacobs and Jacobs 2010; Feigl et al. 1986; Nakamura et al. 2022). Under these circumstances, suture placement may be inaccurate, leaving residual defects after repair. Some authors (Mavroudis et al. 2020, 2023; Kitagawa et al. 1998) have advocated primary closure of such defects using pledgetted sutures without synthetic patches. We (Mavroudis and Backer 2002) have excised the trabeculations for better visualization and more accurate suture placement. Still others have used transventricular device techniques, which can be deployed without the need for cardiopulmonary bypass (Holzer et al. 2004; Jameel et al. 2006; Lim et al. 2007; Vasilyev et al. 2008). Ventriculotomy is rarely required. Under some conditions, nonetheless, a large apical defect can be closed through a very limited apical left ventriculotomy, which more easily identifies the defect because of few trabeculations in this area, as noted in Fig. 31 (Mavroudis et al. 2013). Complications with closure depend in large part on the location of the defect (Kitagawa et al. 1998). Important anatomic considerations include proximity to the conduction system, as in inlet muscular defects, proximity of the defect to the tricuspid cords, and its size, which will ensure the need for large patches and probability of postoperative ventricular dysfunction (Yoshimura et al. 2016; Hofmeyr et al. 2013). All of these potential complications can be avoided as long as the aforementioned principles and techniques are followed and implemented.

Hybrid techniques using device closure now can be used effectively in many circumstances when the patient is very small, when the muscular defect is large, and when tricuspid cords are not complicating factors. Echocardiographic guidance allows the surgeon to insert a perventricular catheter through the right ventricular free wall with advancement through the defect into the left ventricle, as noted in Fig. 32. The successful partial device deployment is noted in Fig. 32, inset. When followed by complete deployment in the right ventricle, the defect is closed as noted in Fig. 33. The inset shows the sectional view of the successful deployment with

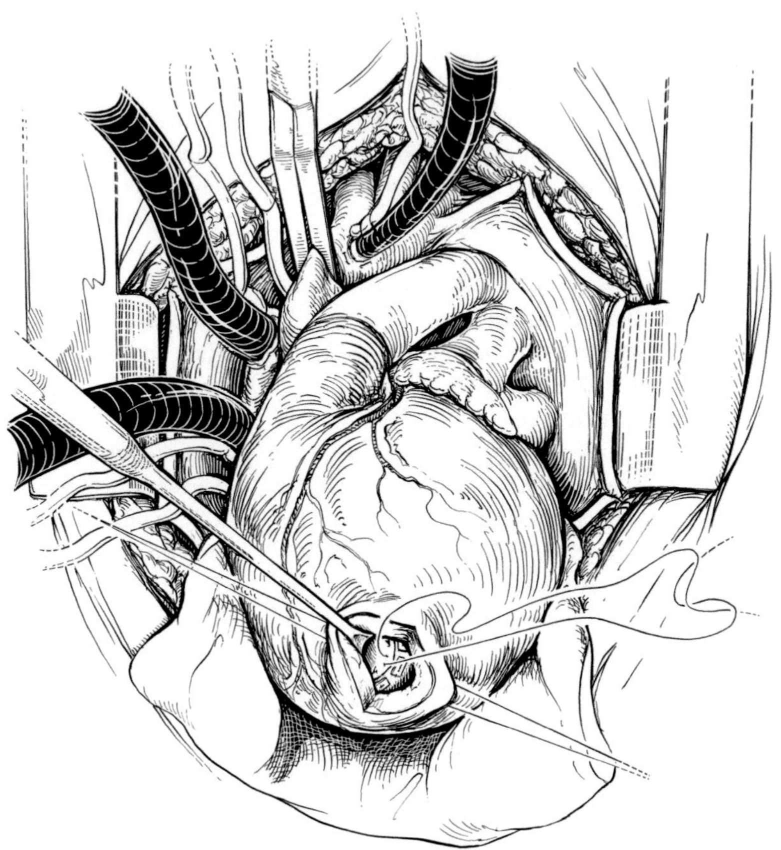

Fig. 31 Shows the exposure by left ventricular apical incision for repair of apical muscular defect. This exposure reduces trabeculations that can make apical closure through the right atrium/right ventricle difficult and insecure. This method however exposes the patient to left ventricular dysfunction in the long-term owing to left ventricular incision and is not used often in the present era. (With permission: Mavroudis et al. 2013)

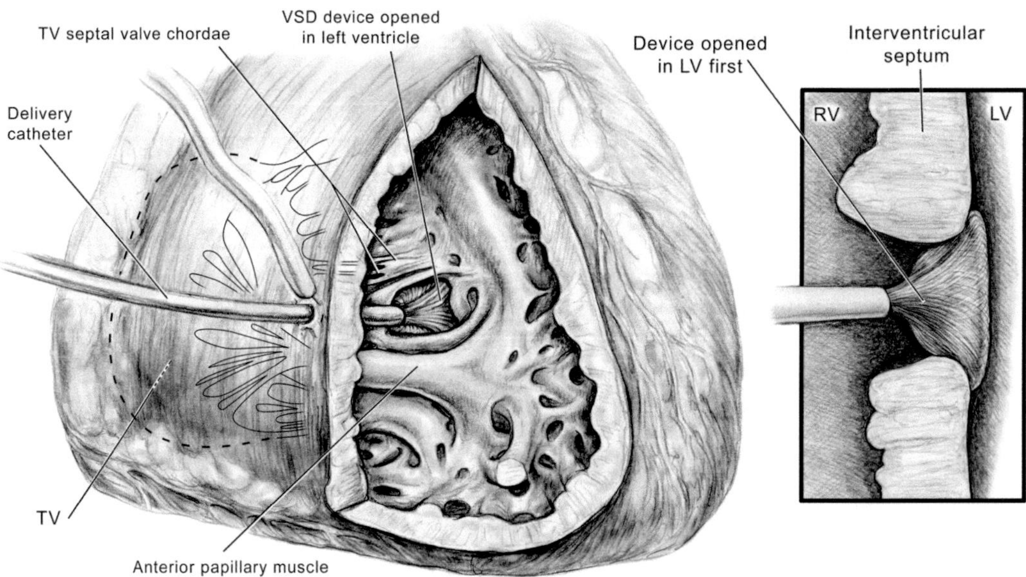

Fig. 32 Shows perventricular advancement of catheter with partial opening of device in the left ventricle. The inset depicts a modified coronal view of device placement in the left ventricular cavity. The device is then fully deployed by opening it in the right ventricular portion of the defect. *LV* left ventricle, *RV* right ventricle, *TV* tricuspid valve, *VSD* ventricular septal defect

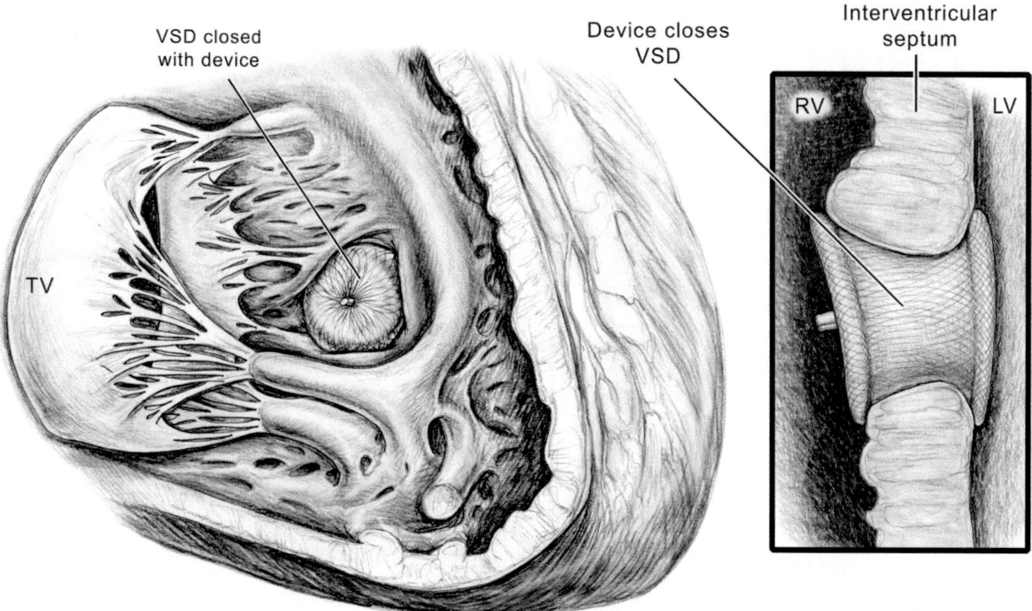

Fig. 33 It is a coronal view of the right ventricle showing the successful device deployment and closure. The inset demonstrates a sectional view of the device secured on the edges of the defect. *LV* left ventricle, *RV* right ventricle, *TV* tricuspid valve, *VSD* ventricular septal defect

appropriate closure. Care is taken to make sure that no tricuspid cords are entrapped, and excellent apposition of the device is accomplished before the device is disconnected from the retrieval mechanism. At this point, there is high probability of achieving closure without the risk of heart block, which can complicate device closure for perimembranous defects. The appeal and benefit of this approach for closure of muscular defects is that the procedure can be performed without cardiopulmonary bypass. There are, nonetheless, potential complications of injury to the tricuspid valve and/or papillary muscles as well as embolization in the event that ventricular apposition is not accomplished. Figure 34 (left panel) shows unwanted dislodgement and embolization of the device into the right ventricular cavity owing to higher left ventricular pressure that can propel the device away from the defect if device apposition is not optimal. Figure 34 (right panel) shows how device deployment can cause tricuspid chordal entrapment and regurgitation, and can be avoided if proper device deployment is confirmed by intraoperative transesophageal echocardiography before device retrieval and disengagement. There are occasions, however, that embolization can occur after confirmed deployment and may require open heart surgery, device retrieval, and subsequent closure.

8 Residual Ventricular Septal Defects in Anatomically Challenging Locations

As noted earlier, residual defects after surgical closure generally close over time if the defect is 1.25 mm or less in size (Deng et al. 2020; Dodge-Khatami et al. 2007; Bol Raap et al. 2007, 2003). When the residual defect is 2.0 mm or more, authors have advocated repeat operation at the time of initial surgery (Deng et al. 2020; Dodge-Khatami et al. 2007). In the long-term, when the defect continues to require decongestive therapy, residual defects are associated with and identified by the characteristic disruption of the previously placed patch. The typical anatomic aberration of a residual defect shows disruption of the previ-

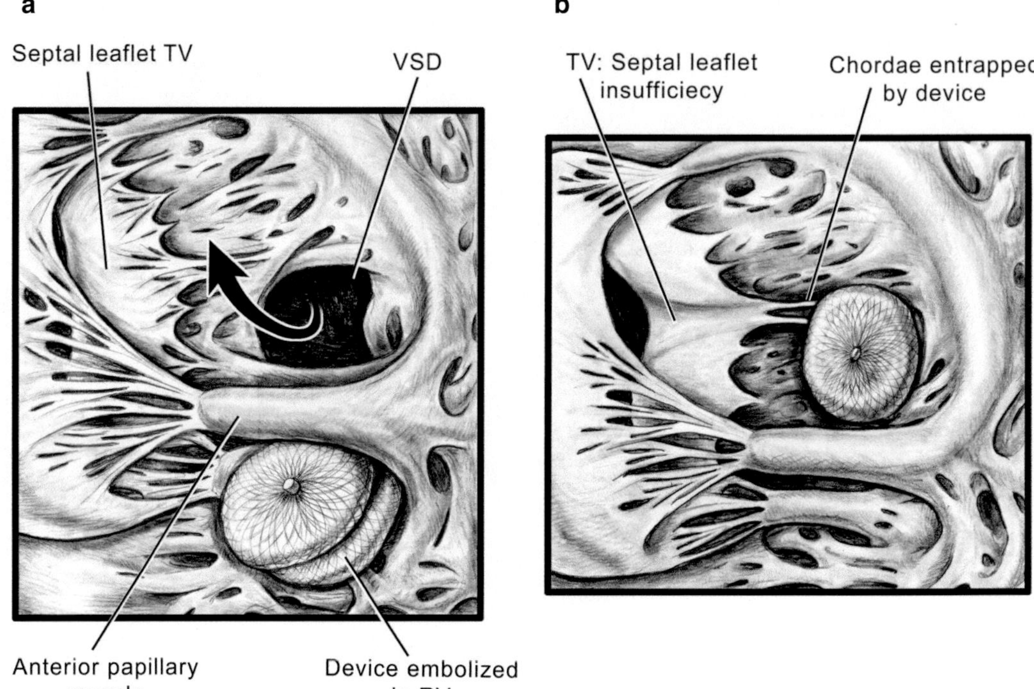

Fig. 34 Shows embolization of the device to the right ventricle (**left panel**). Device deployment appears around the cords and can cause tricuspid regurgitation (**right panel**). *RV* right ventricle, *TV* tricuspid valve, *VSD* ventricular septal defect

ously placed patch away from the surrounding tissues, which include the ventricular muscular ridge, the tricuspid annulus, and the aortic root. The literature to document the best way to close these defects is sparse; however, practical wisdom has determined that a separate patch should be employed to close the residual defect. Primary suture closure is not recommended as it could result in pulling away of the patch, resulting in yet another residual defect. The most recognizable residual defect can be found in the right ventricular inlet and is readily amenable to patch closure without much risk of heart block or injury to the tricuspid valve. Other residual defects are more difficult to visualize. The complexity of repair is increased owing to camouflaging effects of the tricuspid valve. This situation may require radial or circumferential tricuspid incision/detachment for adequate exposure and effective closure. Even more difficult is the residual defect located in the subaortic region. This defect is hidden by muscular attachments, the tricuspid valve, and anatomic complexity created by redo operation. If the borders of these residual defects cannot be readily identified, transaortic exposure allows the surgeon better access to the residual borders for suture placement and patch closure. Care must be taken while applying anchoring sutures to avoid injury to the conduction system and the aortic valve leaflets during patch closure.

9 Summary

This chapter has considered the complications associated with the phenotypic variability underscoring different courses of the conduction system, configuration of the borders of the defects, and techniques that emphasize adequate exposure that will affect secure and lasting closure. A comprehensive analysis of the different anatomic characteristics of the defects has allowed for a clear-cut understanding of pitfalls that can complicate the operation.

References

Andersen HØ, de Leval MR, Tsang VT, Elliott MJ, Anderson RH, Cook AC. Is complete heart block after surgical closure of ventricular septum defects still an issue? Ann Thorac Surg. 2006;82(3):948–56.

Anderson RH, Mohun TJ, Moorman AF. What is a ventricle? Cardiol Young. 2011;21(Suppl 2):14–22.

Anderson RH, Spicer DE, Brown NA, Mohun TJ. The development of septation in the four-chambered heart. Anat Rec (Hoboken). 2014;297(8):1414–29.

Becu LM, Burchell HB, Dushane JW, Edwards JE, Fontana RS, Kirklin JW. Anatomic and pathologic studies in ventricular septal defect. Circulation. 1956;14(3):349–64.

Ben Farhat S, Slim M, ElHraiech A, et al. Prevalence and factors associated with spontaneous closure of congenital ventricular septal defects. Tunis Med. 2020;98(12):980–5.

Bol Raap G, Meijboom FJ, Kappetein AP, Galema TW, Yap SC, Bogers AJ. Long-term follow-up and quality of life after closure of ventricular septal defect in adults. Eur J Cardiothorac Surg. 2007;32(2):215–9.

Bol-Raap G, Weerheim J, Kappetein AP, Witsenburg M, Bogers AJ. Follow-up after surgical closure of congenital ventricular septal defect. Eur J Cardiothorac Surg. 2003;24(4):511–5.

Cao Z, Chai Y, Liu J, et al. Revising ventricular septal defect residual shunts without aortic re-cross-clamping: a safe and effective surgical procedure. Ann Transl Med. 2020;8(18):1134.

Capelli H, Andrade JL, Somerville J. Classification of the site of ventricular septal defect by 2-dimensional echocardiography. Am J Cardiol. 1983;51(9):1474–80.

Chaudhry TA, Younas M, Baig A. Ventricular septal defect and associated complications. J Pak Med Assoc. 2011;61(10):1001–4.

Deng X, Huang P, Luo J, et al. Residual shunts following isolated surgical ventricular septal defect closure: risk factors and spontaneous closure. Pediatr Cardiol. 2020;41(1):38–45.

Devlin PJ, Russell HM, Monge MC, et al. Doubly committed and juxtaarterial ventricular septal defect: outcomes of the aortic and pulmonary valves. Ann Thorac Surg. 2014;97(6):2134–40.

Dodge-Khatami A, Knirsch W, Tomaske M, et al. Spontaneous closure of small residual ventricular septal defects after surgical repair. Ann Thorac Surg. 2007;83(3):902–5.

Dodge-Khatami A, Mavroudis CD, Frost J, Jacobs JP, Mavroudis C. Repairing the tricuspid valve in congenital heart diseases other than Ebstein's. Cardiol Young. 2014;24(6):1077–87.

Feigl D, Feigl A, Sweetman KM, Lobo FV, Moller JH, Edwards JE. Accessory tissue of the tricuspid valve protruding into the left ventricle through a septal defect. Arch Pathol Lab Med. 1986;110(2):144–7.

Gaynor JW, O'Brien JE Jr, Rychik J, et al. Outcome following tricuspid valve detachment for ventricular septal defects closure. Eur J Cardiothorac Surg. 2001;19(3):279–82.

Hofmeyr L, Pohlner P, Radford D. Long-term complications following surgical patch closure of multiple muscular ventricular septal defects. Congenit Heart Dis. 2013;8(6):541–9.

Holzer R, Balzer D, Cao Q-L, Lock K, Hijazi ZM, Amplatzer Muscular Ventricular Septal Defect Investigators. Device closure of muscular ventricular septal defects using the Amplatzer muscular ventricular septal defect occluder: immediate and mid-term results of a U.S. registry. J Am Coll Cardiol. 2004;43(7):1257–63.

Idriss FS, Muster AJ, Paul MH, et al. Ventricular septal defect with tricuspid pouch with and without transposition Anatomic and surgical considerations. J Thorac Cardiovasc Surg. 1992;103(1):52–9.

International Society for Nomenclature of Paediatric and Congenital Heart Disease. Archiving Working Group; 2024. http://ipccc-awg.net. Accessed 13 Feb 2024.

Jacobs ML, Jacobs JP. Operative techniques for repair of muscular ventricular septal defects. Op Tech Thor Cardiovasc Surg. 2010;15(1):2–10.

Jameel AA, Arfi AM, Arif H, Amjad K, Omar GM. Retrograde approach for device closure of muscular ventricular septal defects in children and adolescents, using the Amplatzer muscular ventricular septal defect occluder. Pediatr Cardiol. 2006;27(6):720–8.

Jortveit J, Leirgul E, Eskedal L, et al. Mortality and complications in 3495 children with isolated ventricular septal defects. Arch Dis Child. 2016;101(9):808–13.

Karonis T, Scognamiglio G, Babu-Narayan SV, et al. Clinical course and potential complications of small ventricular septal defects in adulthood: late development of left ventricular dysfunction justifies lifelong care. Int J Cardiol. 2016;208:102–6.

Kazmi U, Sadiq M, Hyder SN. Pattern of ventricular septal defects and associated complications. J Coll Physicians Surg Pak. 2009;19(6):342–5.

Kelle AM, Kaushal S, Anderson R, Backer C. The Gerbode defect: a ventriculo-atrial defect. CTSNet; 2012. https://www.ctsnet.org/article/gerbode-defect-ventriculo-atrial-defect. Accessed 11 Feb 2024.

Kirklin JW, Dushane JW. Repair of ventricular septal defect in infancy. Pediatrics. 1961;27:961–6.

Kirklin JK, Castaneda AR, Keane JF, Fellows KE, Norwood WI. Surgical management of multiple ventricular septal defects. J Thorac Cardiovasc Surg. 1980;80(4):485–93.

Kitagawa T, Durham LA 3rd, Mosca RS, Bove EL. Techniques and results in the management of multiple ventricular septal defects. J Thorac Cardiovasc Surg. 1998;115(4):848–56.

Lam W, Friedman RA. Electrophysiology issues in adult congenital heart disease. Methodist DeBakey Cardiovasc J. 2011;7(2):13–7.

Lillehei CW, Cohen M, Warden HE, Ziegler NR, Varco RL. The results of direct vision closure of ventricular septal defects in eight patients by means of controlled cross circulation. Surg Gynecol Obstet. 1955;101(4):446–66.

Lim DS, Forbes TJ, Rothman A, Lock JE, Landzberg MJ. Transcatheter closure of high-risk muscular ventricular septal defects with the CardioSEAL occluder: initial report from the CardioSEAL VSD registry. Catheter Cardiovasc Interv. 2007;70(5):740–4.

Mavroudis C. Ventricular septal defect. In: Mavroudis C, Backer CL, editors. Atlas of pediatric cardiac surgery. London: Springer; 2015. p. 99–116.

Mavroudis C, Backer CL. Closure of ventricular septal defect. Op Tech Thorac Cardiovasc Surg. 2002;7(1):11–21.

Mavroudis C, Backer CL. Technical tips for three congenital heart operations: modified Ross-Konno procedure, optimal ventricular septal defect exposure by tricuspid valve incision, coronary unroofing and endarterectomy for anomalous aortic origin of the coronary artery. Oper Tech Thorac Cardiovasc Surg. 2010;15(1):18–40.

Mavroudis C, Backer CL, Jacobs JP, Anderson RH. Ventricular septal defect. In: Mavroudis C, Backer CL, editors. Pediatric cardiac surgery. 4th ed. Hoboken: Wiley; 2013. p. 311–41.

Mavroudis C, Dearani JA, Anderson RH. Ventricular septal defect. In: Mavroudis C, Dearani JA, editors. Atlas of adult congenital cardiac surgery. Cham: Springer Nature; 2020. p. 91–116.

Mavroudis C, Backer CL, Anderson RH. Ventricular septal defect. In: Mavroudis C, Backer CL, editors. Pediatric cardiac surgery. 5th ed. Oxford: Wiley; 2023. p. 317–60.

Menting ME, Cuypers JAAE, Opic P, et al. The unnatural history of the ventricular septal defect: outcome up to 40 years after surgical closure. J Am Coll Cardiol. 2015;65(18):1941–51.

Nakamura Y, Kumada Y, Mori A, Kawai N, Ishida N, Kasugai T. [Huge tricuspid pouch with heart failure: report of a case]. Kyobu Geka. 2022;75(5):392–5.

Pedersen TA, Andersen NH, Knudsen MR, Christensen TD, Sørensen KE, Hjortdal VE. The effects of surgically induced right bundle branch block on left ventricular function after closure of the ventricular septal defect. Cardiol Young. 2008;18(4):430–6.

Russell HM, Forsberg K, Backer CL, Wurlitzer KC, Kaushal S, Mavroudis C. Outcomes of radial incision of the tricuspid valve for ventricular septal defect closure. Ann Thorac Surg. 2011;92(2):685–90.

Saker E, Bahri GN, Montalbano MJ, et al. Gerbode defect: a comprehensive review of its history, anatomy, embryology, pathophysiology, diagnosis, and treatment. J Saudi Heart Assoc. 2017;29(4):283–92.

Schipper M, Slieker MG, Schoof PH, Breur JMPJ. Surgical repair of ventricular septal defect; contemporary results and risk factors for a complicated course. Pediatr Cardiol. 2017;38(2):264–70.

Serraf A, Lacour-Gayet F, Bruniaux J, et al. Surgical management of isolated multiple ventricular septal defects: logical approach in 130 cases. J Thorac Cardiovasc Surg. 1992;103(3):437–43.

Soto B, Becker AE, Moulaert AJ, Lie JT, Anderson RH. Classification of ventricular septal defects. Br Heart J. 1980;43(3):332–43.

Spicer DE, Hsu HH, Co-Vu J, Anderson RH, Fricker FJ. Ventricular septal defect. Orphanet J Rare Dis. 2014;9:144.

Vaksmann G, Fournier A, Chartrand C, Stanley P, Davignon A. [Arrhythmia disorders after repair of ventricular septal defects. Comparison of atrial and ventricular approaches]. Arch Mal Coeur Vaiss. 1989;82(5):731–5.

Van Praagh R, Geva T, Kreutzer J. Ventricular septal defects: how shall we describe, name and classify them? J Am Coll Cardiol. 1989;14(5):1298–9.

Varghese R, Saheed S, Ravi AK, Sherrif EA, Agarwal R, Kothandam S. The "excluding" suture technique for surgical closure of ventricular septal defects: a retrospective study comparing the standard technique. Ann Pediatr Cardiol. 2016;9(3):229–35.

Vasilyev NV, Melnychenko I, Kitahori K, et al. Beating-heart patch closure of muscular ventricular septal defects under real-time three-dimensional echocardiographic guidance: a preclinical study. J Thorac Cardiovasc Surg. 2008;135(3):603–9.

Yoshimura N, Fukahara K, Yamashita A, et al. Current topics in surgery for multiple ventricular septal defects. Surg Today. 2016;46(4):393–7.

Yuan S. Left ventricular to right atrial shunt (Gerbode defect): congenital versus acquired. Postepy Kardiol Interwencyjne J. 2014;10(3):185–94.

Complications Associated with Repair of Atrioventricular Septal Defect

Carl L. Backer

Abstract

The primary complications to be avoided with atrioventricular septal defect (AVSD) repairs are: left AV valve insufficiency or stenosis, residual atrial or ventricular level shunts, injury to the AV node, right AV valve insufficiency or stenosis, and left ventricular outflow tract obstruction. Pulmonary hypertension is avoided by appropriate surgical timing.

Keywords

Atrioventricular septal defect · Atrioventricular canal · Mitral valve cleft · Atrioventricular valve insufficiency · Pulmonary hypertension · Trisomy 21

The repair of children with atrioventricular (AV) canal defects, also referred to as atrioventricular septal defects (AVSD) has the opportunity for many different complications. There are also many steps that can be taken to avoid or correct these complications when they occur.

The first step to avoiding complications in this group is to operate on these patients at the correct age. For complete atrioventricular septal defects we recommend surgery at 4–6 months of age (Jacobs et al. 2010). This is after the neonatal period when tissues are very friable, but before they develop pulmonary hypertension that is difficult to deal with. For partial AVSD we recommend surgery at 18–24 months of age (Devlin et al. 2016). This is at a point where the valve tissue has excellent integrity but the child has not developed progressive valvular insufficiency secondary to the chronic volume overload. I also recommend pulmonary artery banding for very small, premature infants that are in congestive heart failure (Devlin et al. 2020). Embarking upon a complete repair in these children with their friable AV valve tissue is fraught with potential complications.

1 Partial AVSD

For partial AVSD the operation has two primary components (Fig. 1). First is closure of the atrial septal defect for which I prefer an autologous non-glutaraldehyde treated pericardial patch. The

C. L. Backer (✉)
Chief, Section of Pediatric Cardiothoracic Surgery, UK Healthcare Kentucky Children's Hospital, Lexington, KY, USA

Cardiothoracic Surgery, Cincinnati Children's Hospital Medical Center, Cincinnati, OH, USA
e-mail: carl.backer@uky.edu

C. L. Backer, C. Mavroudis (eds.), *Complications in Pediatric and Congenital Heart Surgery*,
https://doi.org/10.1007/978-3-032-02661-3_9

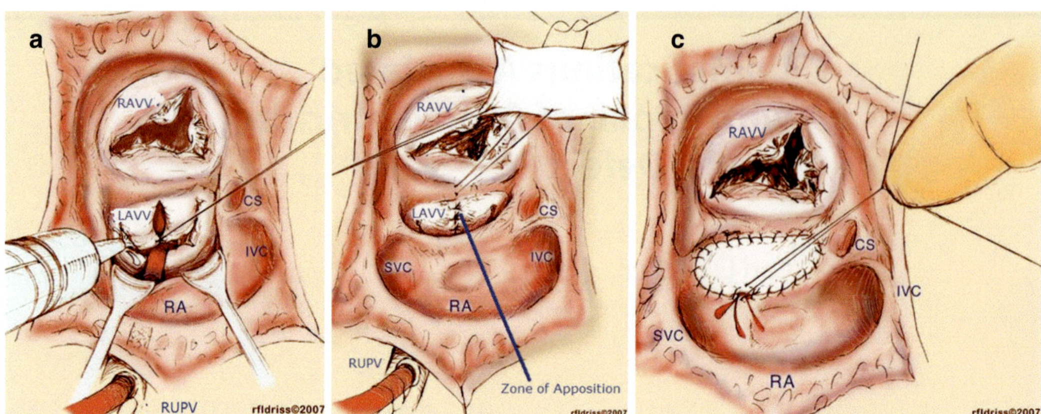

Fig. 1 Operative technique for partial AVSD. (**a**) Saline insufflation is used to assess left atrioventricular (AV) valve and plan closure of zone of apposition. (**b**) Pericardial patch is sutured in place to close atrial component of defect. This shows completed closure of zone of apposition. (**c**) Air is removed from left side of heart through suture line before tying knot. Coronary sinus remains draining to right atrium. Abbreviations: *CS* coronary sinus, *IVC* inferior vena cava, *LAVV* left atrioventricular valve, *RA* right atrium, *RAVV* right atrioventricular valve, *RUPV* right upper pulmonary vein, *SVC* superior vena cava. (With permission: Devlin et al. 2016)

second component is closure of the left AV valve "cleft," or zone of apposition. The primary complications to be avoided are complete heart block and residual AV valve regurgitation or stenosis. There are two separate surgical strategies to avoid AV block. My preference is to take superficial bites of atrium in the region between the coronary sinus orifice and the AV valve junction (Fig. 1). Other surgeons have deviated the suture line in such a fashion that the coronary sinus is committed to the left atrium rather than the right atrium (Nicholson et al. 1999). The comparison studies between these two strategies have equipoise and both result in a very low incidence of heart block. I prefer to leave the coronary sinus draining into the right atrium (normal physiology). My experience with this technique of taking careful shallow bites in the region of the conducting system has led to an extremely low incidence of postoperative heart block (Devlin et al. 2016). If operative AV block occurs I place temporary atrial and ventricular pacing wires, and then observe the patient for 7–10 days. The chances of the heart block recovering after 10 days is very low (Weindling et al. 1998).

To ensure the best possible left AV valve function, I carry the sutures of the AV valve cleft closure all the way to the insertion of the chordae tendineae on the superior and inferior left AV valve leaflets. To analyze residual left AV valve insufficiency the postoperative transesophageal echo is extremely important. If this shows that there is still insufficiency through the AV valve cleft and if the insufficiency is more than moderate, I would resume cardiopulmonary bypass and place additional sutures in the cleft. If the AV valve insufficiency is not related to the cleft, then I would consider placing annuloplasty sutures in the annulus of the left valve at the commissures (Fig. 2).

In decision making between left AV valve insufficiency and left AV valve stenosis, it has been shown that mild stenosis with mild regurgitation is better than no stenosis with moderate regurgitation (Alghamdi et al. 2011). I am always struck by the fact that a valve that by measurement seems as if it will be too stenotic is often adequate with less stenosis by ECHO than one would predict.

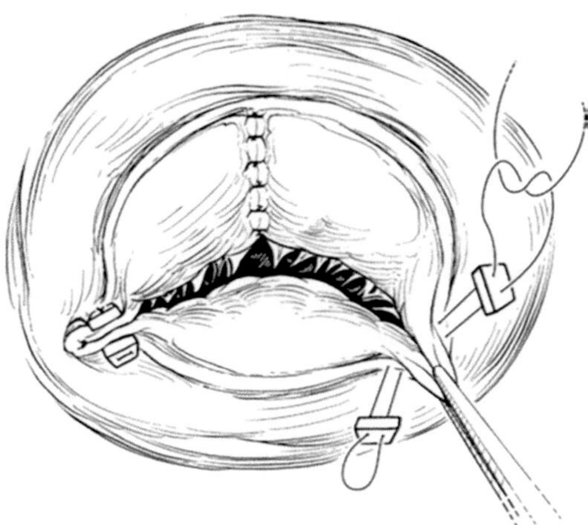

Fig. 2 Annuloplasty sutures placed at the commissures after left AV valve cleft closure. It is best to use mattress sutures reinforced with a biologic pledget for repair, as simple suturing technique tends to rip through the tissue, resulting in early repair failure. Pericardial pledgets are optimal for this maneuver. Commissural annuloplasty sutures can downsize the annulus and therefore treat central coaptation problems. (With permission: Mavroudis and Dearani 2020)

In some cases inflow to the left AV valve is impeded by closely spaced papillary muscles. This can be corrected by carefully cutting the attached trabecular muscle bundles.

2 Complete AVSD

For patients with a complete AVSD there have been two strategies for repair that are employed by the majority of surgeons. These are the modified single patch repair and the two patch repair. In the current era a large multicenter report from Australia demonstrated essentially no difference in outcomes between the two repairs (Fong et al. 2020; Backer 2020). Most surgeons who learn a certain technique are more comfortable with that technique and continue using that technique after their training.

Our preference is to use the modified single-patch technique for smaller babies, and for situations where the ventricular septal defect component is shallow in nature, less than 12 mm in depth (Backer et al. 2015a; Stephens and Backer 2022). The double-patch technique is in our experience indicated when the patient has a large VSD or the combination of tetralogy of Fallot with atrioventricular septal defect (Prifti et al. 2004).

Some principles apply to both techniques and are important to avoid complications. At the beginning of the case, a considerable amount of time should be spent looking at the transesophageal echocardiogram with the pediatric cardiologist (Cohen and Stevenson 2007). Careful attention should be paid to the AV valve and the VSD location. When the procedure is being performed on cardiopulmonary bypass the exposure of the valves and septal defect is extremely important. This is facilitated by carrying the atrial incision between the inferior vena cava (IVC) and the ventricular mass. The heart is in effect rotated out of the pericardium to allow full access and visualization of the intracardiac anatomy.

Another principal is to now carefully evaluate the intracardiac anatomy. At times this can take even as long as 10–15 min. Floating the AV valves with saline and identifying the valve leaflets and how they appose and mentally trying to reconstruct how this will be accomplished is extremely important. I have preferred to place a small marking suture on the superior and inferior bridging leaflets at what is called the "kissing point" when the valves are insufflated with saline (Fig. 3).

Whether the technique is a modified single-patch or double-patch technique, it is important that the sutures used for the ventricular component be pledgeted to ensure that they do not pull through the muscle (Figs. 4 and 5).

Also important is that when the left AV valve cleft is closed, the sutures must approximate the

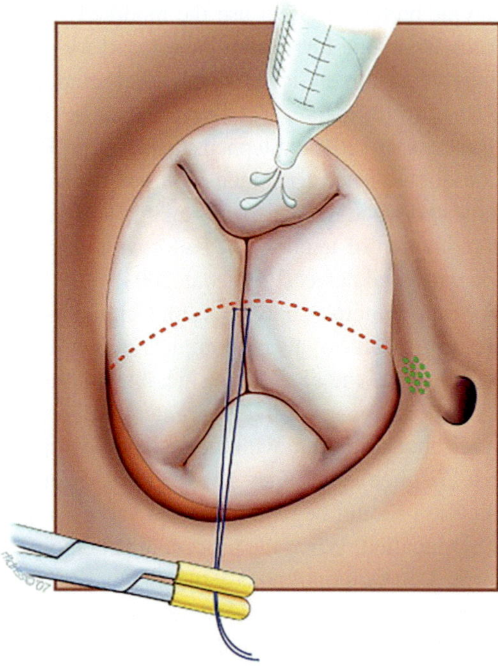

Fig. 3 For both a two-patch or modified single-patch repair insufflation of the atrioventricular valve with saline to evaluate the valve is very important. A single loose suture has been placed to mark the predicted demarcation between right and left atrioventricular valve components (dotted lines). The cluster of green dots indicates the location of the AV node. (With permission: Backer et al. 2007)

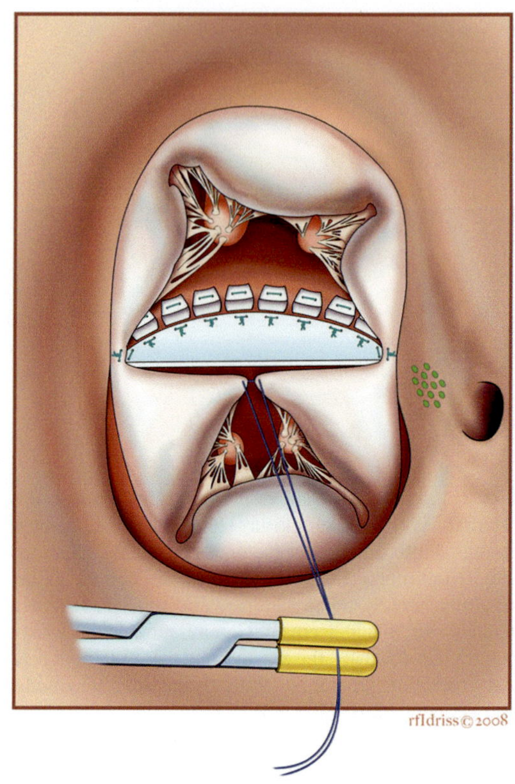

Fig. 4 This illustration demonstrates a polytetrafluoroethylene (PTFE) patch in place anchored by pledgeted sutures for a two-patch repair. (With permission: Backer et al. 1995)

tissue without crushing it. This is an extremely important part of the operation and a great deal of time and care should be taken with these knots (Fig. 6).

Potential complications of complete atrioventricular septal defect repair are as follows: (1) left AV valve insufficiency, (2) left AV valves stenosis, (3) residual ventricular or atrial septal defect, (4) AV conduction injury, (5) right AV valve insufficiency, (6) right AV valve stenosis, (7) left ventricular outflow tract obstruction, and (8) pulmonary hypertension.

Most of these potential complications can be avoided by careful surgical planning and intraoperative technique.

One recommendation to avoid complications is to avoid cutting the AV valve leaflets. This was actually part of the classic teaching for the classic single patch technique. However, cutting AV valve tissue and then reapproximating it leads to some loss of the actual valve leaflet length. It also makes the patient susceptible to potential dehiscence of the valve where it has been cut, and then reapproximated. In my career I have rarely had to cut the AV valves to perform the repair.

For very small premature infants, I prefer preliminary pulmonary artery banding rather than complete repair. Although for many years, surgeons were afraid that this would increase AV valve insufficiency, several recent studies have shown that this is not the case (Devlin et al. 2020, 2024; Kobayashi et al. 2024). In several series, the outcomes of preliminary pulmonary artery banding have been either equivalent or better than primary repair. I have had experience with AV valve tissue essentially falling apart during attempted repair in very small babies. Because

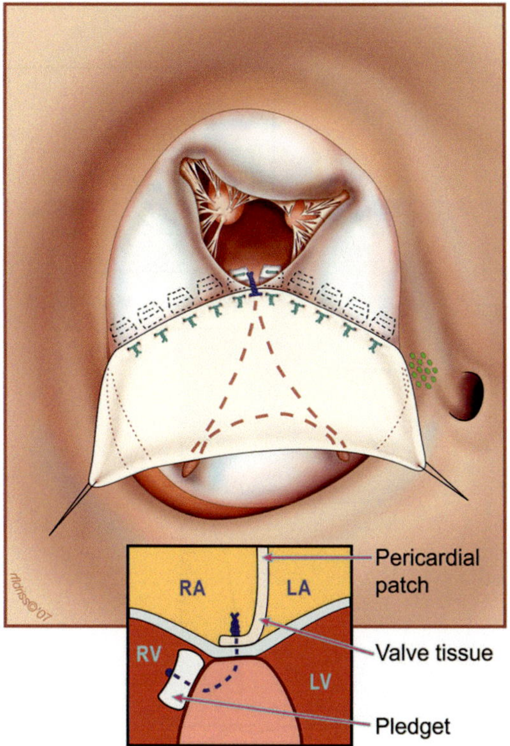

Fig. 5 This illustration demonstrates the pledgets for a modified single-patch repair. Note that the AV valve is "sandwiched" between the pericardium and the pledget. (With permission: Backer et al. 2007)

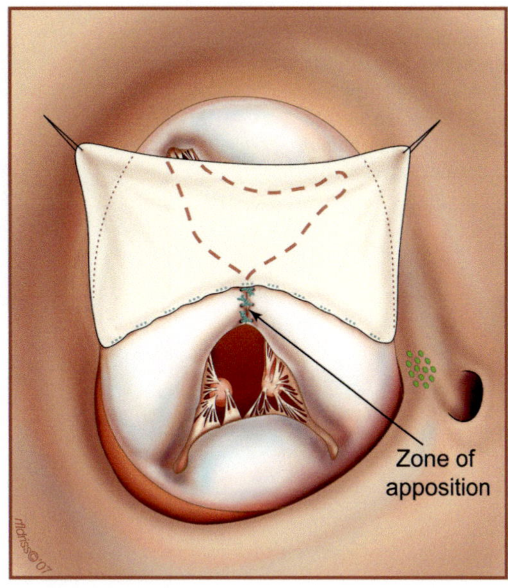

Fig. 6 The zone of apposition (or "cleft") of the left atrioventricular valve is closed with interrupted prolene sutures to the point where the chordae tendineae insert on the free edge of the leaflets. These knots need to be carefully tied and approximated but not crush the valve tissue. (With permission: Backer et al. 2007)

there is not a good bail out this is a very concerning situation, which can be avoided by appropriate use of pulmonary artery banding. However, should a complete repair be contemplated in a smaller baby, the modified single-patch technique is much easier and more applicable than a two-patch technique (Stephens and Backer 2022; Stephens et al. 2015).

In contrast, for the patient with a large ventricular septal component, greater than 12 mm as measured from the AV valve to the crest of the ventricular septum during diastole, I would recommend use of a two-patch technique (Backer et al. 1995). I have used Gore-Tex for the ventricular patch. The superior portion of the Gore-Tex patch is attached to the AV valves and is reinforced by using the pericardial patch that will be used to close the atrial component as a pledget for all of the sutures. This helps prevent dehiscence of the AV valves (Fig. 7) (Katz et al. 1981).

The closure of the cleft or zone of apposition is similar to the partial AVSD repair. An autologous pericardial patch is now used to close the atrial component. The operation will have the same potential AV conduction issues as with partial AVSD closure. In Figs. 3, 4, 5, 6, and 7 the cluster of small green dots shows the location of the AV node. It is in this area that careful superficial suture bites should be taken.

Although there was concern that the modified single-patch technique would increase the incidence of left ventricular outflow tract obstruction from subaortic stenosis, long-term follow-up of these patients have not shown this to be the case (Backer et al. 2015b). If patients develop subaortic stenosis, it is usually a fibromuscular ring beneath the aortic valve, which is unrelated to the previous repair. If the patient develops this sub-

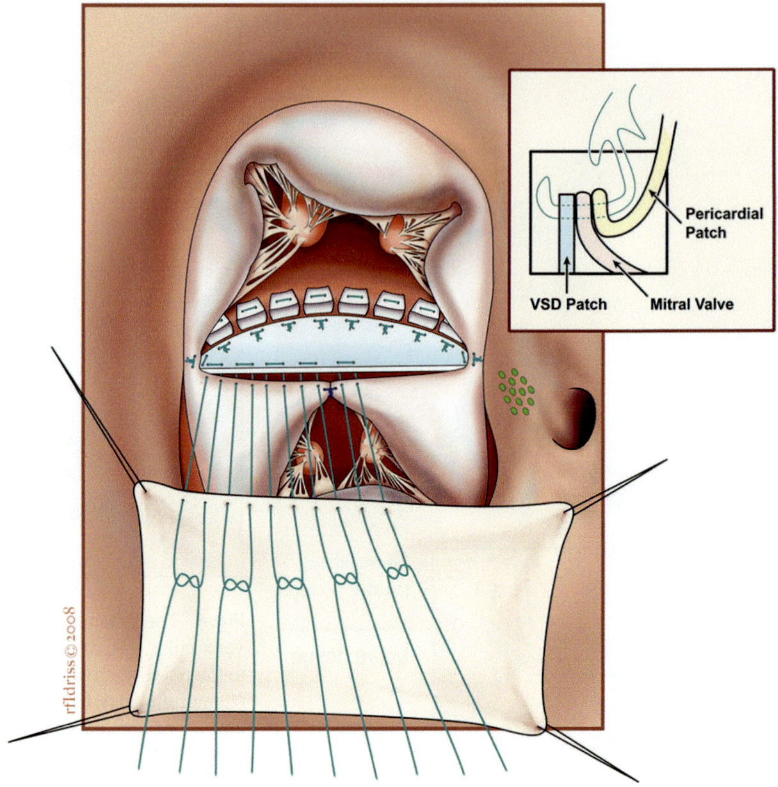

Fig. 7 In the two-patch technique the left atrioventricular valve is "sandwiched" between the PTFE patch and the pericardial patch helping to prevent valve dehiscence

aortic stenosis, it is usually years later, after the initial AV septal defect repair (Pontailler et al. 2015). It is typically approached through an aortic incision and involves resection of the fibromuscular ring. Occasionally, there are redundant chords to the left AV valve, crowding the left ventricular outflow tract. These must be carefully resected (Perez et al. 2023).

After the procedure, the post repair transesophageal echocardiogram assessment is very important. The echo should be used to assess the right and left AV valves for stenosis or regurgitation. It is quite rare that there is AV valve stenosis, especially if the valve orifice is sized with a dilator and kept within the normal range for weight. If there is AV valve regurgitation, then it is extremely important to find the location, the severity, and the mechanism. These can all lead to potential solutions if the AV valve sufficiency is moderate or greater.

When attempting to decide whether one should leave stenosis or regurgitation, a classic article from Toronto demonstrated that residual, mild mitral valve stenosis, was associated with less hazard than mild to moderate regurgitation (Alghamdi et al. 2011).

If there is an atrial or ventricular level shunt then a postop QP:QS assessment can be done by measuring the saturation in the pulmonary artery (PA), the right atrium (RA), and the aorta (Ao). The following equation can then be used to determine the QP:QS:

$$\frac{\text{Ao Sat} - \text{RA Sat}}{\text{Ao Sat} - \text{PA Sat}}$$

If the QP:QS is greater than 1.5:1.0 then I would resume cardiopulmonary bypass and close the residual defect. Another helpful parameter is the size of the color jet Doppler. If it is more than 3–4 mm that is an indication that the patient probably needs a reoperation to close the residual VSD (Dodge-Khatami et al. 2007).

If the patient has severe left AV valve regurgitation and attempted repairs are ineffective then consideration should be given to mitral valve

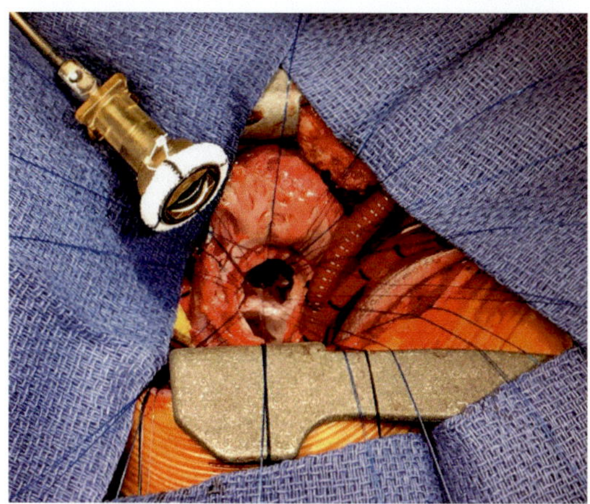

Fig. 8 Mitral valve (left atrioventricular valve) replacement in a 9-month-old child weighing 7.0 kg. The valve is anchored with interrupted 5-0 prolene sutures without pledgets

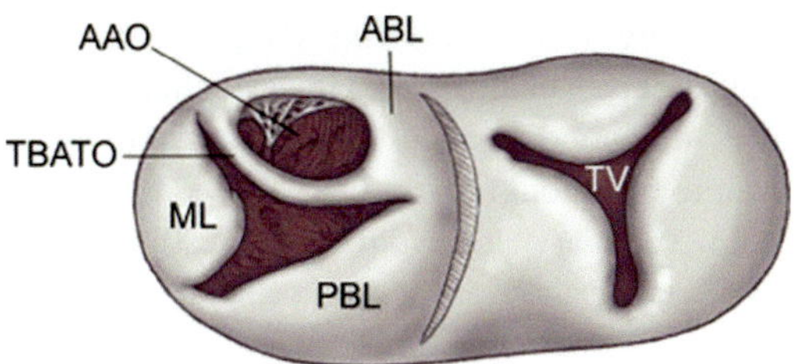

Fig. 9 Schematic example of a double orifice left atrioventricular valve. Abbreviations: AAo, anterior accessory orifice; ABL, anterior bridging leaflet; ML, mural leaflet; PBL, posterior bridging leaflet; TBATO, tissue bridge between accessory and true orifices. (With permission: Sharma et al. 2012)

replacement (Fig. 8). In the current era there is a 15 mm mechanical mitral valve available, which we have used in patients as small as 5 kg (Eltayeb et al. 2019). Another alternative is to place a Melody valve, typically used as a transcatheter valve, but this can be placed into the left AV valve orifice, balloon dilated, and sutured in place (Freud et al. 2017; Dranseika et al. 2021).

A specific AV valve issue that must be carefully dealt with is the double orifice left AV valve (Sharma et al. 2012) (Fig. 9). The principle here is to not cut the bridge between the two orifices as this will lead to severe AV valve insufficiency. In many of these cases one orifice, which is smaller and leaking, may need closure with a patch.

If there is a parachute left AV valve, the zone of apposition (or cleft) may need to be left partially open (Sharma et al. 2013). Some of these patients have essentially no mural leaflet. In those cases, partial cleft closure, or no cleft closure may be required. Consideration should be given to papillary muscle splitting to enlarge the inflow to the ventricle.

Treatment of residual left AV valve insufficiency may require as mentioned for partial AVSD, annuloplasty sutures placed at the commissures (Fig. 2). This appears to work best by placing the pledgeted sutures at the commissures. This reduces the size of the AV valve orifice and aids with approximation of the leaflets.

Another alternative for valve repair if there is significant regurgitation is use of an Alfieri stitch where the anterior and posterior AV valves leaflets are sutured together in the midline creating a double orifice valve (Alfieri et al. 2001). If there is a perforation of a leaflet, this can be closed. If there is stenosis of the valve it may require papillary muscle splitting. In some cases, the valve may benefit from being lengthened by placing a pericardial patch (Mitchell et al. 2007).

Children with a complete AVSD operated on later in life, meaning over 6–9 months of age, may have difficulty with postoperative pulmonary hypertension (Talwar et al. 2010). If this is a concern, then the pulmonary artery pressure should be monitored in the operating room with a PA line. This can be effectively treated by keeping the patient paralyzed and ventilated for 24–72 h after the operation. The patient should be maintained on milrinone infusion with mild hyper ventilation. Finally, in extreme cases inhaled nitric oxide can be used which would be converted to oral sildenafil therapy. If a PA line is used it should be placed in the right ventricular outflow tract via a pledgeted suture so that it does not bleed when it is removed.

When we were performing cardiac catheterization on all patients with a complete AVSD the pulmonary vascular resistance (PVR) at 0–3 months was a mean of 2.1 Wood units. At 4–6 months of age the mean PVR was 4.0 Wood units. At 7–12 months of age, the mean PVR was 5.7. Wood units (Backer et al. 1995). In all cases, the pulmonary vascular resistance dropped with pulmonary vasodilators like oxygen and nitric oxide (Curran et al. 1995). However, this emphasizes the importance of performing the repair prior to 6–9 months of age.

In summary to avoid complications with AVSD repair there are several principles:

1. careful evaluation of the pre-and postoperative echocardiogram;
2. adequate exposure and careful evaluation of the AV valves by floating them with saline prior to the procedure;
3. avoid cutting AV valve leaflets;
4. appropriate use of technique; modified single patch for smaller patients with shallow VSDs, and a two patch technique for patients with a large ventricular septal defect or AV canal with tetralogy of Fallot;
5. the zone of apposition should be closed completely;
6. if there is a double orifice, mitral valve, do not cut the bridge between the two orifices;
7. mitral valve replacement for moderate plus AV valve regurgitation that cannot be repaired; and
8. preemptive treatment of pulmonary hypertension.

References

Alfieri O, Maisano F, De Bonis M, Stefano PL, Torracca L, Oppizzi M, La Canna G. The double-orifice technique in mitral valve repair: a simple solution for complex problems. J Thorac Cardiovasc Surg. 2001;122(4):674–81.

Alghamdi AA, Yanagawa B, Singh SK, Horton A, Al-Radi OO, Caldarone CA. Balancing stenosis and regurgitation during mitral valve surgery in pediatric patients. Ann Thorac Surg. 2011;92(2):680–4.

Backer CL. Commentary: this case is closed. J Thorac Cardiovasc Surg. 2020;159(3):1028.

Backer CL, Mavroudis C, Alboliras ET, Zales VR. Repair of complete atrioventricular canal defects: results with the two-patch technique. Ann Thorac Surg. 1995;60(3):530–7.

Backer CL, Stewart RD, Mavroudis C. What is the best technique for repair of complete atrioventricular canal? Semin Thorac Cardiovasc Surg. 2007;19(3):249–57.

Backer CL, Eltayeb O, Mongé MC, Costello JM. No ventricular septal defect patch atrioventricular septal defect repair. Oper Tech Cardiovasc Sug. 2015a;20(3):279–92.

Backer CL, Eltayeb O, Mongé MC, Wurlitzer KC, Hack MA, Boles LH, Sarwark AE, Costello JM, Robinson JD. Modified single patch: are we still worried about subaortic stenosis? Ann Thorac Surg. 2015b;99(5):1671–5.

Cohen GA, Stevenson JG. Intraoperative echocardiography for atrioventricular canal: decision-making for surgeons. Semin Thorac Cardiovasc Surg Pediatr Card Surg Annu. 2007;10:47–50.

Curran RD, Mavroudis C, Backer CL, Sautel M, Zales VR, Wessel DL. Inhaled nitric oxide for children with congenital heart disease and pulmonary hypertension. Ann Thorac Surg. 1995;60(6):1765–71.

Devlin PJ, Backer CL, Eltayeb O, Mongé MC, Hauck AL, Costello JM. Repair of partial atrioventricular septal defect: age and outcomes. Ann Thorac Surg. 2016;102(1):170–7.

Devlin PJ, Jegatheeswaran A, McCrindle BW, Karamlou T, Blackstone EH, Williams WG, DeCampli WM, Mertens L, Fackoury CT, Eghtesady P, Jacobs JP, Baffa JM, Fleishman CE, Dodge-Khatami A, Pizarro C, Pourmoghadam K, Cohen MS, Meyer DB, Overman DM. Pulmonary artery banding in complete atrioventricular septal defect. J Thorac Cardiovasc Surg. 2020;159(4):1493–503.

Devlin PJ, Argo M, Habib RH, McCrindle BW, Jegatheeswaran A, Jacobs ML, Jacobs JP, Backer CL, Overman DM, Karamlou T. Contemporary applications and outcomes of pulmonary artery banding: an analysis of The Society of Thoracic Surgeons Congenital Heart Surgery Database. Ann Thorac Surg. 2024;117(1):128–35.

Dodge-Khatami A, Knirsch W, Tomaske M, Prêtre R, Bettex D, Rousson V, Bauersfeld U. Spontaneous closure of small residual ventricular septal defects after surgical repair. Ann Thorac Surg. 2007;83(3):902–5.

Dranseika V, Pretre R, Kretschmar O, Dave H. Melody valve to replace the mitral valve in small children: lessons learned. Ann Pediatr Cardiol. 2021;14(1):35–41.

Eltayeb OM, Readdy WJ, Mongé MC, Sarwark AE, Patel A, Backer CL. Mitral valve replacement in infants using a 15-mm mechanical valve. Ann Thorac Surg. 2019;108(2):552–7.

Fong LS, Betts K, Bell D, Konstantinov IE, Nicholson IA, Winlaw DS, Orr Y, Australian CAVSD Study Group. Complete atrioventricular septal defect repair in Australia: results over 25 years. J Thorac Cardiovasc Surg. 2020;159(3):1014–25.

Freud LR, Marx GR, Marshall AC, Tworetzky W, Emani SM. Assessment of the Melody valve in the mitral position in young children by echocardiography. J Thorac Cardiovasc Surg. 2017;153(1):153–60.

Jacobs JP, Jacobs ML, Mavroudis C, Chai PJ, Tchervenkov CI, Lacour-Gayet FG, Walters H 3rd, Quintessenza JA. Atrioventricular septal defects: lessons learned about patterns of practice and outcomes from the congenital heart surgery database of the society of thoracic surgeons. World J Pediatr Congenit Heart Surg. 2010;1(1):68–77.

Katz NM, Blackstone EH, Kirklin JW, Bradley EL, Lemons JE. Suture techniques for atrioventricular valves: experimental study. J Thorac Cardiovasc Surg. 1981;81(4):528–36.

Kobayashi Y, Kasahara S, Sano S, Suzuki H, Suzuki E, Yorifuji T, Kotani Y. Staged repair for complete atrioventricular septal defect in patients weighing less than 4.0 kg. J Thorac Cardiovasc Surg. 2024;167(3):1136–44.

Mavroudis C, Dearani JA. Atrioventricular septal defects. In: Mavroudis C, Dearani JA, editors. Atlas of adult congenital heart surgery. Cham: Springer Nature; 2020. p. 117–38.

Mitchell ME, Litwin SB, Tweddell JS. Complex atrioventricular canal. Semin Thorac Cardiovasc Surg Pediatr Card Surg Annu. 2007:32–41.

Nicholson IA, Nunn GR, Sholler GF, Hawker RE, Cooper SG, Lau KC, Cohn SL. Simplified single patch technique for the repair of atrioventricular septal defect. J Thorac Cardiovasc Surg. 1999;118(4):642–6.

Perez Y, Dearani JA, Miranda WR, Stephens EH. Subaortic stenosis in adult patients with atrioventricular septal defect. Ann Thorac Surg. 2023;115(2):479–84.

Pontailler M, Capderou A, Lebret E, Vergnat M, Ly M, Roussin R, Belli E. Subaortic area at risk for development of obstruction after surgical repair of atrioventricular septal defect: myth or reality? World J Pediatr Congenit Heart Surg. 2015;6(3):407–12.

Prifti E, Bonacchi M, Bernabei M, Leacche M, Bartolozzi F, Murzi B, Battaglia F, Nadia NS, Vanini V. Repair of complete atrioventricular septal defect with tetralogy of fallot: our experience and literature review. J Card Surg. 2004;19(2):175–83.

Sharma V, Burkhart HM, Schaff HV, Cabalka AK, Grogan MA, Dearani JA. Double-orifice left atrioventricular valve in patients with atrioventricular septal defects: surgical strategies and outcome. Ann Thorac Surg. 2012;93(6):2017–20.

Sharma V, Burkhart HM, Schaff HV, Cetta F, Cabalka A, Dearani JA. Management of zone of apposition in parachute left atrioventricular valve in atrioventricular septal defect. Ann Thorac Surg. 2013;95(5):1665–9.

Stephens EH, Backer CL. Teaching the modified single-patch technique for complete atrioventricular septal defect. World J Pediatr Congenit Heart Surg. 2022;13(3):371–5.

Stephens EH, Ibrahimiye AN, Yerebakan H, Yilmaz B, Chelliah A, Levasseur S, Mosca RS, Chen JM, Chai P, Quaegebeur J, Bacha EA. Early complete atrioventricular canal repair yields outcomes equivalent to late repair. Ann Thorac Surg. 2015;99(6):2109–16.

Talwar S, Singh V, Chandra N, Marwah A, Sharma R. Challenges in delayed repair of atrioventricular septal defects. World J Pediatr Congenit Heart Surg. 2010;1(1):87–90.

Weindling SN, Saul JP, Gamble WJ, Mayer JE, Wessel D, Walsh EP. Duration of complete atrioventricular block after congenital heart disease surgery. Am J Cardiol. 1998;82(4):525–7.

Complications Associated with Repair of Common Arterial Trunk

Constantine Mavroudis
and Constantine D. Mavroudis

Abstract

Common arterial trunk (CAT), also called truncus arteriosus, is a congenital heart defect that is characterized by a single arterial trunk arising from the heart. The arterial trunk overrides the interventricular septum and gives rise to the systemic, pulmonary, and coronary circulations. The nomenclature for CAT has undergone significant revisions owing to the recognition of varying pulmonary artery origins, interrupted aortic arch, and relative sizes of the aortic and pulmonary trunks, leading to a more generalized categorization based on aortic or pulmonary trunk dominance. This chapter will review the operative steps for repair of common arterial trunk and the complications that might arise during the conduct of the operation.

Keywords

Congenital heart surgery · Truncus arteriosus · Truncal regurgitation · Truncus with interrupted aortic arch

1 Anatomy and Classification

Common Arterial Trunk, also known as Truncus Arteriosus, is a congenital heart defect that is defined by a single arterial trunk arising from the heart, overrides the interventricular septum and gives rise to the systemic, pulmonary, and coronary circulations (Calder et al. 1976; Fyler 1992; Rowe et al. 1981; Schaff et al. 1985; Anderson et al. 2012; Van Mierop et al. 1978; Radford et al. 1988; Collett and Edwards 1949; Butto et al.

C. Mavroudis (✉)
Chief of Pediatric Cardiothoracic Surgery (Retired), Peyton Manning Children's Hospital, Indianapolis, IN, USA

Professor Emeritus of Surgery, Johns Hopkins University School of Medicine, Baltimore, MD, USA

C. D. Mavroudis
Pediatric Cardiothoracic Surgery, Children's Hospital of Philadelphia, Perelman School of Medicine, University of Pennsylvania, Philadelphia, PA, USA

C. L. Backer, C. Mavroudis (eds.), *Complications in Pediatric and Congenital Heart Surgery*,
https://doi.org/10.1007/978-3-032-02661-3_10

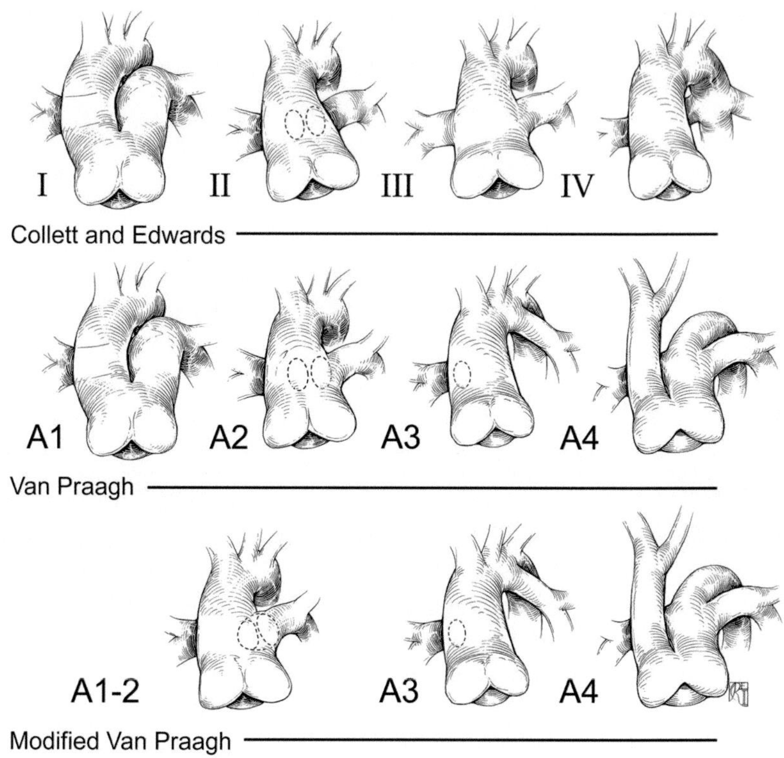

Fig. 1 Shows the similarities between the Collett and Edwards, Van Praagh, and modified Van Praagh classifications. This nomenclature has undergone significant revisions owing to the recognition of varying pulmonary artery origins, interrupted aortic arch, and relative sizes of the aortic and pulmonary trunks. This has led to a more generalized categorization based on aortic or pulmonary trunk dominance. (With permission: Mavroudis and Backer 2003)

1986; Van Praagh and Van Praagh 1965; Russell et al. 2011; Jacobs 2000; Jacobs and Anderson 2012; Lenox et al. 1992; Oddens et al. 1994). Common Arterial Trunk (CAT) can be distinguished from the severe forms of tetralogy of Fallot since there are no pulmonary valve remnants in common arterial trunk (Van Praagh and Van Praagh 1965). The basic anatomy and classification criteria are noted in Fig. 1. Figure 2 (left and right panels) shows a recent classification of truncus arteriosus as a common arterial trunk associated with either predominantly aortic (Fig. 2, left panel) or pulmonary artery (Fig. 2, right panel) characteristics (Russell et al. 2011). This definition is more inclusive and allows for categorization of all the anatomic variations, including interrupted aortic arch, pulmonary artery variations, and coronary anomalies, which are associated with this entity. An inclusive hierarchical nomenclature database structure can therefore be established. Consequently, this classification scheme can catalogue all of the variations for data analysis and comprehensive review (Jacobs 2000; Jacobs and Anderson 2012).

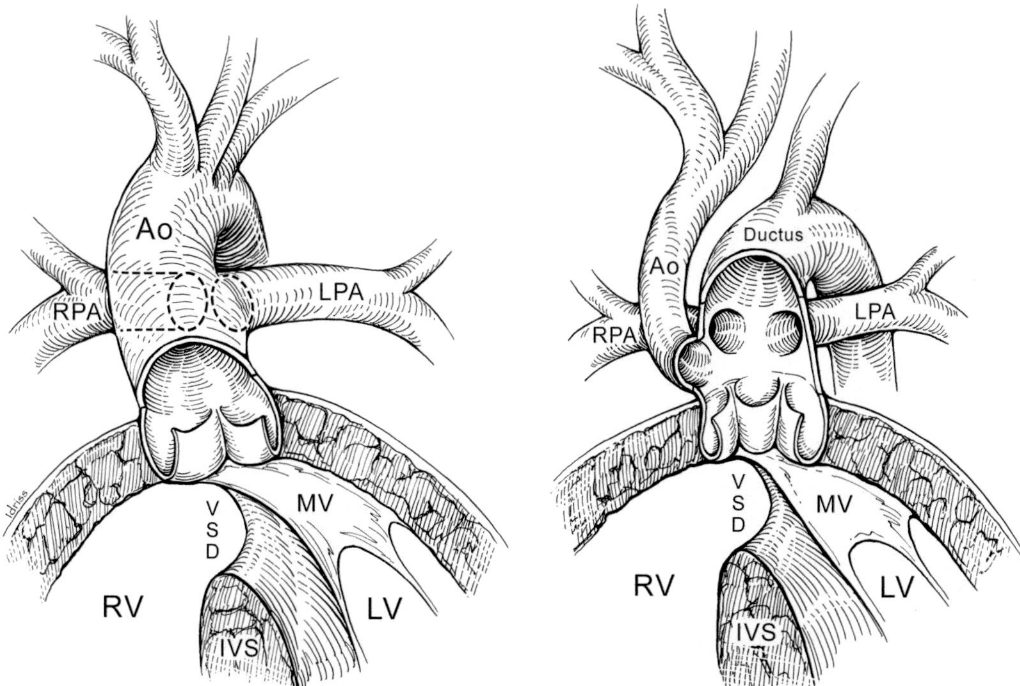

Fig. 2 (Left panel) shows anatomic categorization of the more common type of Common Arterial Trunk (Truncus Arteriosus), namely, Aortic Type. This type of Common Arterial Trunk is generally not associated with interrupted aortic arch. The pulmonary artery origins however can be variable and can differ between a complete separate pulmonary trunk arising from the common trunk to posterior pulmonary arteries arising separately. (Right panel) shows anatomic categorization of the less common type of Common Arterial Trunk (Truncus Arteriosus), namely, Pulmonary Artery Type. This type of Common Arterial Trunk is generally associated with interrupted aortic arch. The pulmonary artery origins generally arise posteriorly from the common arterial trunk. (With permission: Mavroudis 2015). *Ao* aorta, *IVS* interventricular septum, *LPA* left pulmonary artery, *LV* left ventricle, *MV* mitral valve, *RPA* right pulmonary artery, *RV* right ventricle, *VSD* ventricular septal defect

Figure 3 shows the two main types of ventricular septal defect (VSD) that are associated with Common Arterial Trunk. The more common one is the outlet type which is oriented below the overriding common trunk very much like a doubly committed VSD. A rare variant occurs when the crest of the VSD fuses with the base of the overriding common trunk thereby dividing the right and left ventricle with parallel outlets to the common trunk. This is generally noted as

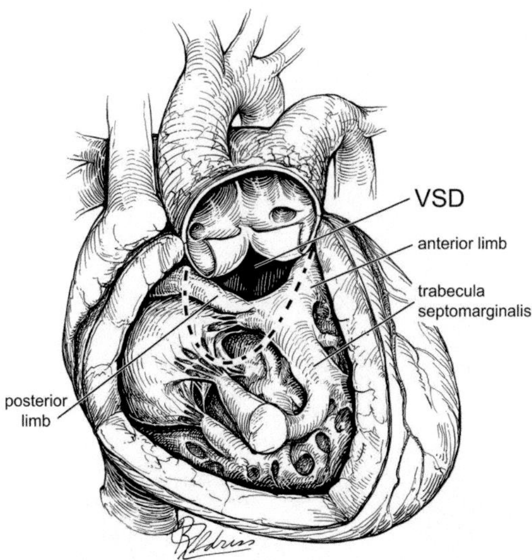

Fig. 3 Shows the two main types of ventricular septal defect (VSD) associated with Common Arterial Trunk. The first and the more common is the outlet type which is shown in the figure as VSD. The conduction system is generally far from the interventricular septum and is not associated with heart block. The second type is the perimembranous type. The neighboring structures of this VSD are the tricuspid annulus, interventricular septum and common trunk annulus. This type of VSD is larger and more difficult to close owing to the surrounding structures and proximity to the conduction system which can subject the patient to heart block. (With permission: Mavroudis and Backer 2003)

Common Arterial Trunk without VSD (Fig. 4). Intuitively, this type of Common Arterial Trunk does not make sense. How can the left or right ventricle empty into the common arterial trunk if neither one of them is not connected directly? The answer lies in the anatomic reality that the interventricular septum is attached to overriding dysplastic valve tissue that abuts to the opposing valve leaflets of the right ventricular and left ventricular outflow tract (Fig. 4a). So, the left ventricular outflow in this depiction has two leaflets which oppose together with the overriding dysplastic leaflet that is centrally attached to the interventricular septum in order to maintain valvar sufficiency. In the same manner, the right ventricular outflow in this depiction shows one leaflet that opposes the dysplastic central leaflet that is attached to the interventricular septum. McElhinney, Reddy, Brook, and Hanley (McElhinney et al. 1997) offered a unique and ingenious method to repair this entity as shown in redrawn depictions in Figs. 4 and 5. Figure 5a shows the repair technique which recreates the left ventricular outflow by attaching the right ventricular valve leaflet to the corresponding overriding dysplastic leaflet of the right side of the interventricular septum. This maneuver closes the right ventricular outflow tract while allowing only left ventricular outflow to the neoaorta without ventricular mixing as shown in Fig. 5b. The subvalvar hypertrophied left ventricular outflow tract can be resected as needed and determined by the operating team. Right ventricular continuity with the pulmonary artery is then accomplished with a right ventricular-to-pulmonary artery valved conduit.

The second type of ventricular septal defect (VSD) is the perimembranous type, shown in Fig. 3 which is generally larger and more difficult to close due to the tricuspid attachments and proximity to the conduction system. Recognizing the type of VSD will alert the surgeon to the potential risk associated with these VSD variations.

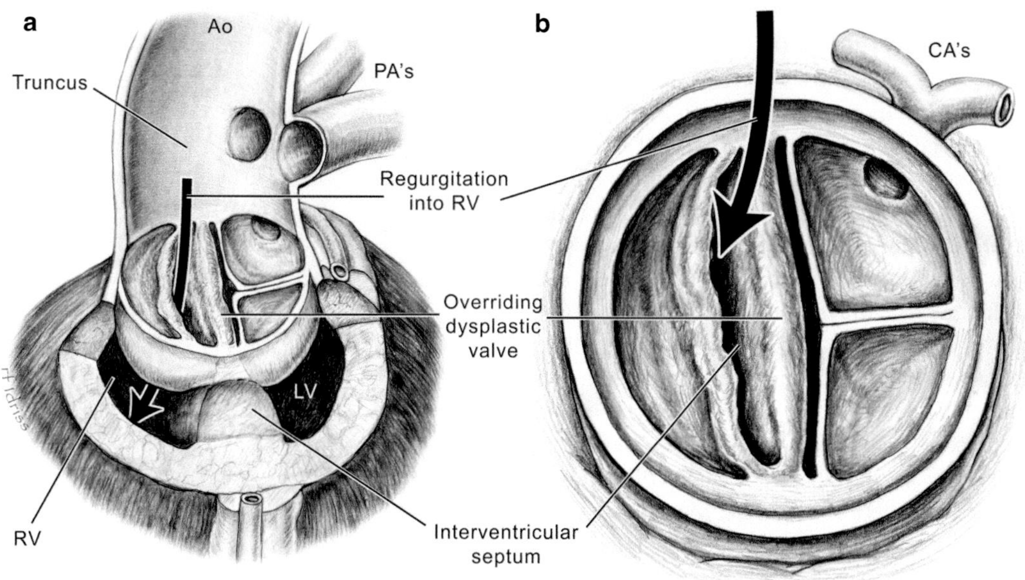

Fig. 4 (**a**, **b**) shows the anatomic variant of Common Arterial Trunk without ventricular septal defect (VSD). Note that the interventricular septum is attached to an overriding dysplastic valve running the length of the septum which serves as the abutting leaflet to the two leaflets of the left ventricular outflow tract and the one leaflet of the right ventricular outflow tract, respectively. The drawing also shows hypertrophied subvalvar muscle below the two outflow tracts. The arrow depicts the area of valvar regurgitation which was confined to the right ventricular outflow tract. *Ao* aorta, *CA* coronary artery, *LV* left ventricle, *PA* pulmonary artery, *RV* right ventricle

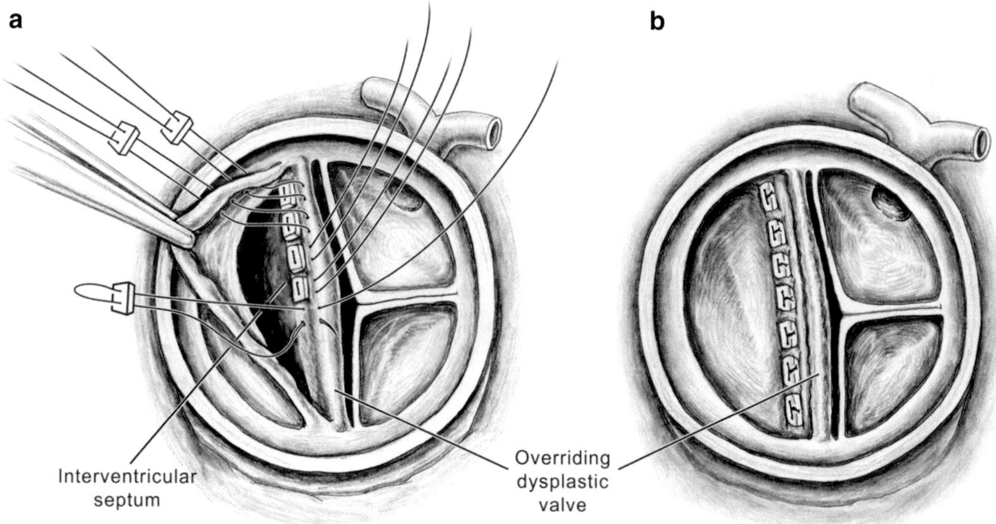

Fig. 5 Shows the attachment of the right sided valve leaflet to the overriding dysplastic valve in process. The pledgetted sutures which are placed in the overriding dysplastic valve are anchored on the ventricular side while the continuation of the sutures are brought through the corresponding leaflet from the ventricular side to the neoaortic side. This is the reason why only one side of the pledgets are noted from the neoaortic view. This maneuver will close the right ventricular outflow tract which will prevent biventricular mixing and allow only left ventricular outflow into the neoaorta. A right ventricular-to-pulmonary artery conduit (not shown) will establish continuity between the right ventricle and the pulmonary artery

2 Surgical Repair of Common Arterial Trunk

Repair of common arterial trunk (truncus arteriosus) depends on the particular type of CAT and the associated anatomic features that have been noted in the preceding paragraphs (Mavroudis et al. 2015; Wilson 1798; Buchanan 1864; Victoria et al. 1969; Shapiro 1930; Lev and Saphir 1943; Mavroudis and Backer 2013; Mavroudis and Backer 2003; Armer et al. 1961; Heilbrunn et al. 1964; Smith et al. 1964; Behrendt et al. 1974; McGoon et al. 1968; Squarcia and Squarcia 2007; Wallace et al. 1969; Rastelli et al. 1967; Bowman et al. 1973; Ebert 1976; Ebert et al. 1984; Ebert 1981, 1989; Mosca and Bove 1996; Bove et al. 1989, 1993; Jahangiri et al. 2000; Rajasinghe et al. 1997; Brizard et al. 1997; Raisky et al. 2009; Brown et al. 2001; Urban et al. 1998; Imamura et al. 1999; Mavroudis and Backer 2001; Espinola-Zavaleta et al. 2008; Marcelletti et al. 1976, 1977; Castaneda 1989; Hanley et al. 1993; Pearl et al. 1992; Pearl et al. 1991; Heinemann et al. 1993; Lacour-Gayet et al. 1996; Losay et al. 1991; Slavik et al. 1994; Laudito et al. 2006; Nemoto et al. 2011; Alfieris et al. 2010; Curi-Curi et al. 2010; Ramirez-Marroquin et al. 2017). Figures 6, 7, 8, 9, 10, 11, and 12 show the important steps of repair of CAT, aortic type. Figure 6 outlines the important issues of commencing cardiopulmonary bypass in relation to the complicating factors of truncal regurgitation and coronary artery anomalies. Figure 7 reviews the essential steps of pulmonary trunk separation, right ventriculotomy, and patch aortoplasty. Obstruction of a high origin of the left main coronary artery can prove to be a significant complication if not identified and corrected (Russell et al. 2011; Jacobs 2000). The first part of pulmonary trunk separation is to make a transverse truncal incision starting at the midpoint of the ascending trunk well away from the truncal valve as shown in Fig. 8. A pause in the action with a comprehensive internal truncal exploration will allow identification and preservation of the left main coronary artery orifice. Figure 8 also shows a high origin of the left main coronary artery which is very close to the anterior

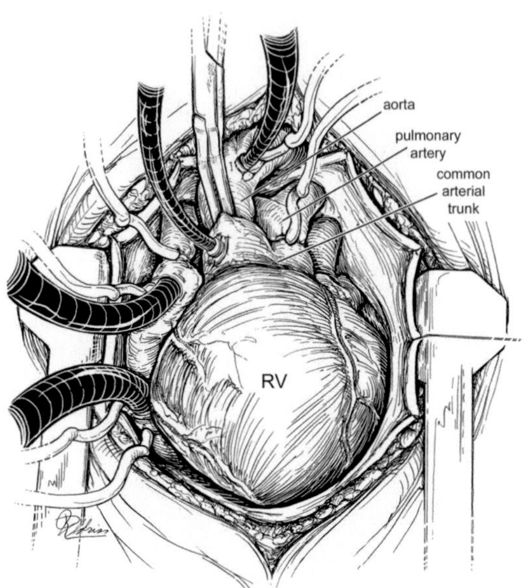

Fig. 6 Shows aortobicaval cardiopulmonary bypass, left ventricular venting, and pulmonary artery trunk constriction to prevent pulmonary overcirculation and systemic hypoperfusion. The aortic clamp is applied and antegrade cardioplegia is administered. In the event that significant truncal valve insufficiency is present, alternative administration techniques must be initiated such as direct coronary infusion or retrograde cardioplegia. (With permission: Mavroudis and Backer 2003). *RV* right ventricle

incision and may be injured during the separation of the pulmonary artery trunk. This situation is fraught with danger and should be recognized in order to perform a coronary artery augmentation if necessary. Figure 9b shows the careful and deliberate suturing technique to respect the boundary of the coronary artery orifice edge with autologous pericardium. In this case, the orifice of the coronary artery is not injured, and the pericardial patch will be sufficient to insure coronary flow. The pericardial patch extends to the edges of dissected neoaorta wherefrom emerged the pulmonary artery trunk. In the event that the orifice of the coronary artery is unwantedly breached, a more complex resolution will be necessary. Figure 10 shows an unwanted coronary artery entry during the removal of the common pulmonary artery trunk. The edges of the injury are freshened to allow for repair by coronary artery pericardial patch arterioplasty which extends into the orifice and vessel integrity of the

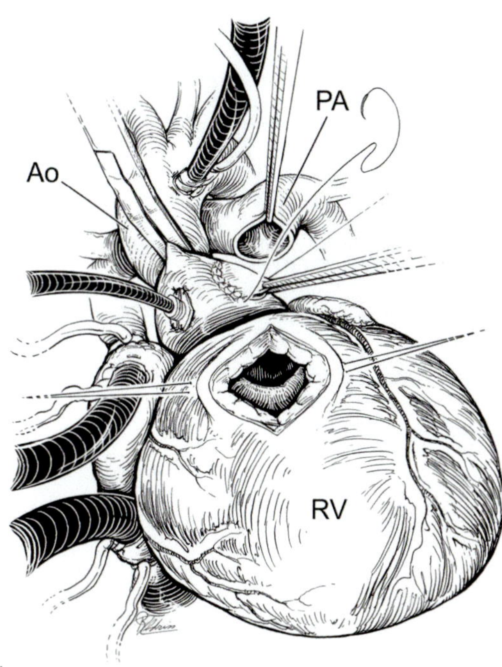

Fig. 7 Shows the next stage of the operation, namely, pulmonary trunk separation, right ventriculotomy, and patch aortoplasty of the common trunk which is to become the aorta or neoaorta depending on one's preference for nomenclature. Not shown is separation of the pulmonary trunk from the common trunk. Common arterial trunk has numerous coronary anomalies including high takeoff of the left main coronary artery. During separation of the pulmonary trunk from the common trunk, careful attention must be paid to the origin of all coronary arteries to prevent unwanted injury. This is the reason why it is best to repair the moiety of the common trunk with a biologic or prosthetic patch which will maintain neoaortic configuration and guard against coronary artery obstruction from suture line distortion. (With permission: Mavroudis and Backer 2003). *Ao* aorta, *PA* pulmonary artery, *RV* right ventricle

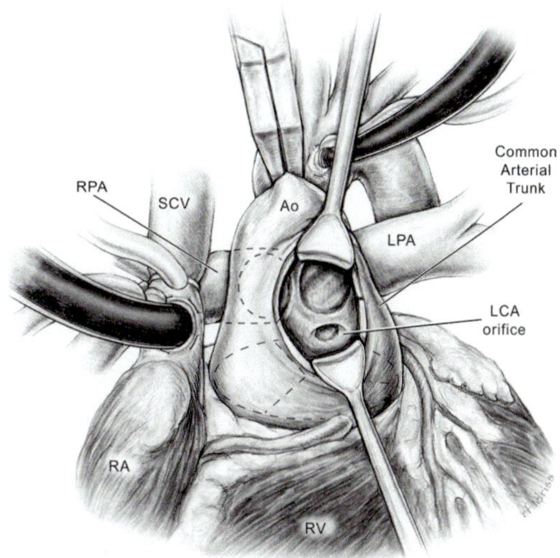

Fig. 8 Shows an anterior transverse incision upstream to the truncal valve with a pause in the action to allow the surgeon to identify the origin of the left main coronary artery which is very close to the pulmonary trunk separation incision. *Ao* aorta, *LCA* left coronary artery, *LPA* left pulmonary artery, *RPA* right pulmonary artery, *RA* right atrium, *RV* right ventricle, *SCV* superior caval vein

left main coronary artery which is shown in the inset. This repair must be accomplished by fine suture technique much like what is required for coronary artery bypass surgery. Once the coronary artery arterioplasty is performed, another tissue patch is used to augment the moiety that was created after the pulmonary artery trunk removal for the eventual repair as noted by the completed repair in Fig. 11. The inset shows the completed neoaortic reconstruction from the posterior view with emphasis on the coronary arterioplasty and truncal aortoplasty to augment the

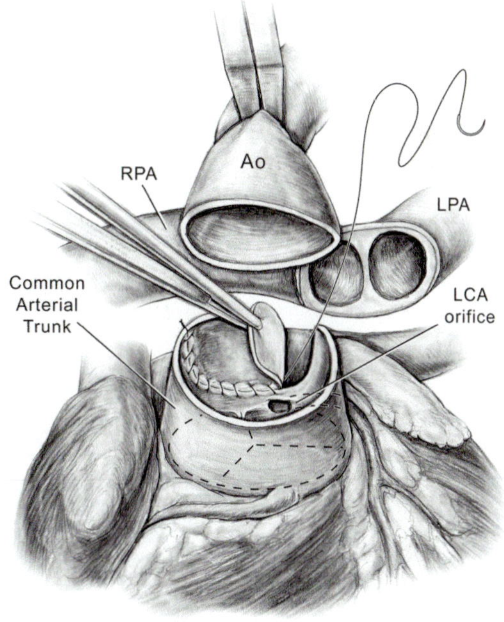

Fig. 9 Shows the careful suturing technique to insure coronary artery flow after truncal transection and coronary artery identification. *Ao* aorta, *LCA* left coronary artery, *LPA* left pulmonary artery, *RPA* right pulmonary artery

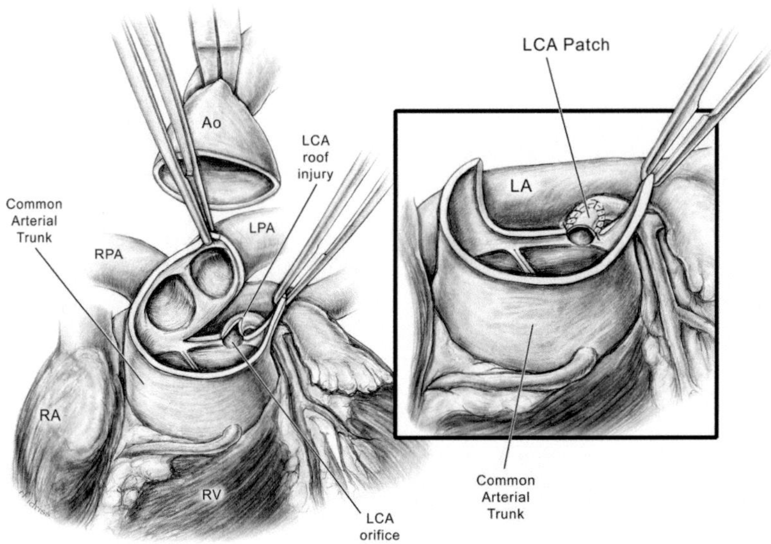

Fig. 10 If an unwanted coronary incision progresses too close or into the orifice, an autologous pericardial patch will be helpful to create an open anastomosis in preparation for the completion aortoplasty. The figure shows an unwanted coronary entry with a freshened incision to enlarge the orifice of the coronary artery. The repair as noted in the inset is performed by coronary artery pericardial patch arterioplasty which extends into the orifice and vessel integrity of the left main coronary artery. Fine suture technique much like what is used for coronary bypass will ensure anastomotic integrity and prevent the use of repair sutures in a very difficult to expose posterior location. *Ao* aorta, *LCA* left coronary artery, *LPA* left pulmonary artery, *RA* right atrium, *RPA* right pulmonary artery, *RV* right ventricle

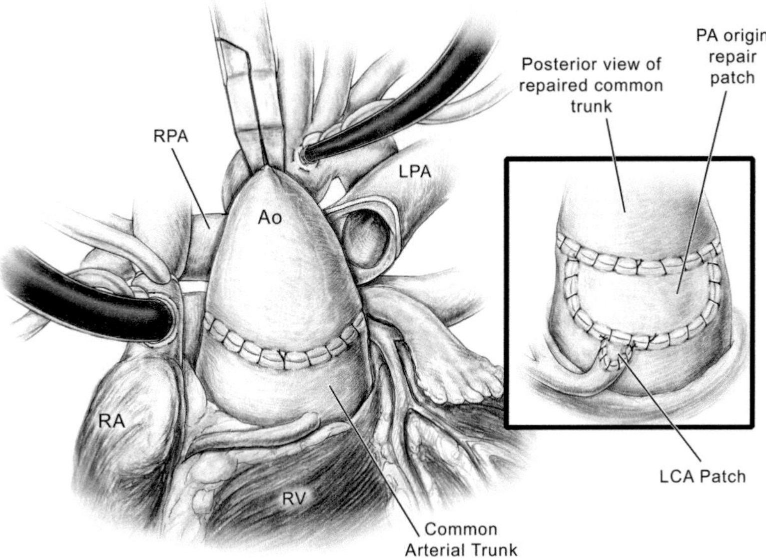

Fig. 11 Shows the completed repair of the neoaorta. Shown using hidden anatomy technique is the coronary artery patch augmentation and truncal root aortoplasty to fill out the dissected neoaortic area wherefrom arose the pulmonary artery trunk. The inset shows a posterior view to better delineate the pericardial patch augmentation of the coronary artery as well as the tissue patch to repair the moiety that was created by the removal of the pulmonary artery root. *Ao* aorta, *LCA* left coronary artery, *LPA* left pulmonary artery, *PA* pulmonary artery, *RA* right atrium, *RPA* right pulmonary artery, *RV* right ventricle

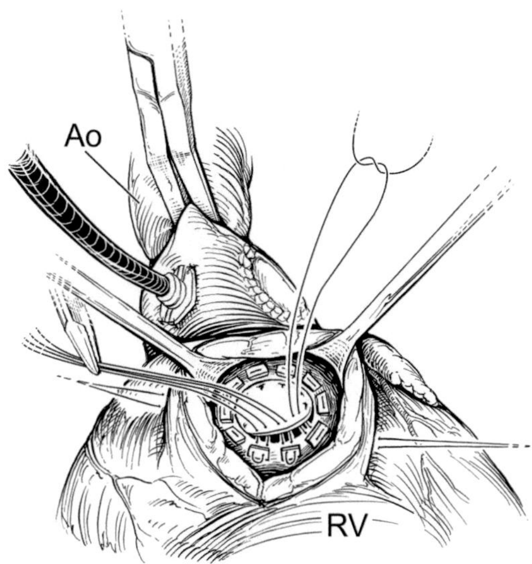

Fig. 12 Shows the technique of ventricular septal defect (VSD) closure using interrupted suture technique for an outlet VSD (more common type) through a ventriculotomy. Many surgeons use running suture technique for this patch placement. Others use the interrupted technique as shown herein. Once the VSD is closed, the aortic cross-clamp can be removed, and systemic warming can begin. This maneuver is mildly controversial since the patent foramen ovale was not closed and it is likely that the heart will recover to sinus rhythm before the ventriculotomy is closed. This problem can be managed by leaving the left ventricular vent on suction and discontinuing the assisted suction venous drainage in the right atrium. This will allow a reservoir of right atrial volume and decrease the possibility of air shifts to the left atrial and left ventricular cavities. Alternatively, the cross-clamp can be left in place until the proximal conduit connection has been completed. (With permission: Mavroudis and Backer 2003). *Ao* aorta, *RV* right ventricle

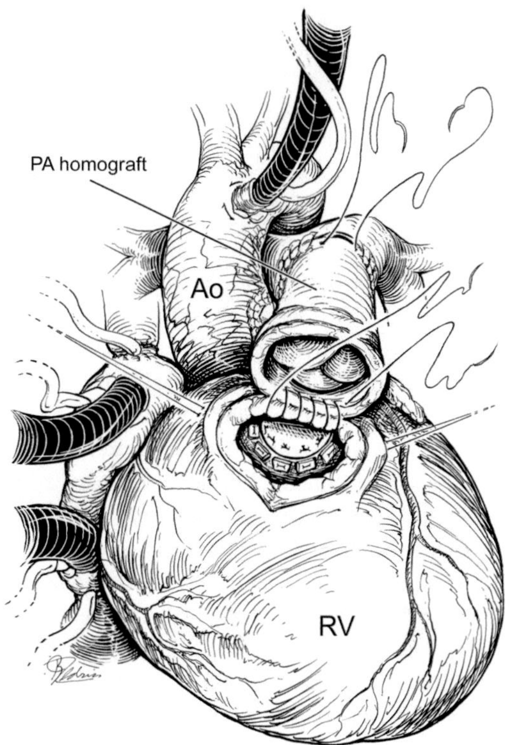

Fig. 13 Shows the right ventricular-to-pulmonary artery reconstruction using a pulmonary homograft. The distal anastomosis is performed first after careful measurement to ensure an optimal length which will prevent pulmonary artery compression in the event that the graft is too long or prevent coronary obstruction and conduit stenosis in the event that the graft is too short. (With permission: Mavroudis and Backer 2003). *Ao* aorta, *PA* pulmonary artery, *RV* right ventricle

dissected arterial wall wherefrom arose the pulmonary artery trunk.

For those patients who undergo pulmonary artery removal and aortoplasty without complication, Fig. 12 shows the particulars of the ventriculotomy, VSD closure, and protective features that will allow a shorter cross-clamp time while preventing unwanted air embolism during the proximal conduit reconstruction.

Most surgeons prefer to establish right ventricular-to-pulmonary artery continuity using a valved conduit as shown in Fig. 13 (Appelbaum et al. 1976; Parenzan et al. 1980; Stark et al. 1978; Ebert 1983; Kalavrouziotis et al. 2006; Thompson et al. 2001; Ullmann et al. 2003; Tlaskal et al. 2010; Vohra et al. 2010; Hawkins et al. 2010; Arslan et al. 2014; Chen et al. 2016; Naimo et al. 2016; Asagai et al. 2016). There are several methods that can be used to complete this portion of the operation. Pulmonary or aortic homografts can be applied by using a proximal hood technique to complete the right ventricle to pulmonary artery connection. Contegra grafts (Bovine Internal Jugular vein grafts) have been used (Brown et al. 2011; Gober et al. 2005; Kocher et al. 2006; Meyns et al. 2004; Tiete et al. 2004; Hickey et al. 2008; Beckerman et al. 2018; Mery et al. 2016); the traditional porcine Dacron valved conduit can be used; and in addition, some surgeons prefer direct pulmonary artery to right ventricle anastomosis without a valve (Agarwal et al. 1981, 1982; Berger et al. 1972; Bisset et al. 1981; Bull et al. 1987; Edwards et al. 1983; Fontan et al. 1984; Fry et al. 1964; Haverich et al. 1984; Hoots and Watson Jr. 1989; Jonas et al. 1985; Jonas et al. 1987; Kay and Ross 1985; Kirklin et al. 1987; McGoon et al. 1982; Naito et al. 1980; Ross and Somerville 1966; Schaff et al. 1984; Wesolowski 1965; Boyce et al. 1988; Angelini et al. 1989; Kobayashi et al. 1993; Reddy et al. 1995; Weipert et al. 1995; Chan et al. 1994; Chen et al. 2005; Danton et al. 2001; Derby et al. 2008; Sodian et al. 2000; Stock et al. 2000). As noted, however, most surgeons prefer some kind of valved conduit, although there have not been any prospective studies on this issue (Appelbaum et al. 1976; Parenzan et al. 1980; Stark et al. 1978; Ebert 1983; Kalavrouziotis et al. 2006; Thompson et al. 2001; Ullmann et al. 2003; Tlaskal et al. 2010; Vohra et al. 2010; Hawkins et al. 2010; Arslan et al. 2014; Chen et al. 2016; Naimo et al. 2016; Asagai et al. 2016; Brown et al. 2011; Gober et al. 2005; Kocher et al. 2006; Meyns et al. 2004; Tiete et al. 2004; Hickey et al. 2008; Beckerman et al. 2018; Mery et al. 2016; Agarwal et al. 1981; Agarwal et al. 1982; Berger et al. 1972; Bisset et al. 1981; Bull et al. 1987; Edwards et al. 1983; Fontan et al. 1984; Fry et al. 1964; Haverich et al. 1984; Hoots and Watson Jr. 1989; Jonas et al. 1985; Jonas et al. 1987; Kay and Ross 1985; Kirklin et al. 1987; McGoon et al. 1982; Naito et al. 1980; Ross and Somerville 1966; Schaff et al. 1984; Wesolowski 1965; Boyce et al. 1988; Angelini et al. 1989; Kobayashi et al. 1993). Figure 14 shows the distal pulmonary artery anastomosis and the proximal ventricular anastomosis being performed using the hood technique (Mavroudis and Backer 2003). The distal pulmonary anastomosis is performed with running suture technique as an end-to-end configuration. In cases where

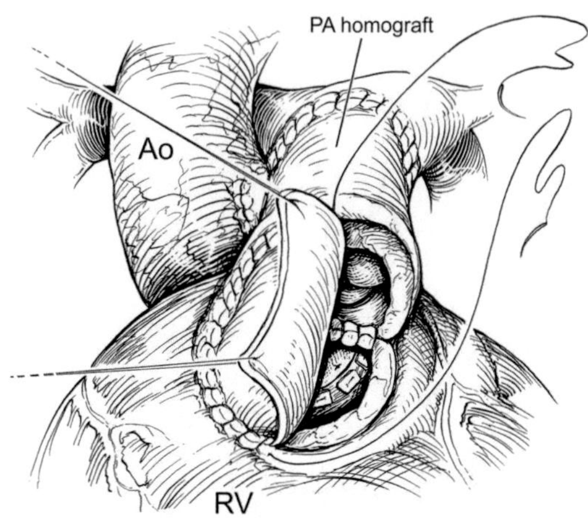

Fig. 14 Depicts the distal pulmonary artery anastomosis and the proximal ventricular anastomosis being performed using the hood technique. The distal pulmonary anastomosis is performed with running suture technique as an end-to-end configuration. In situations of an oversized conduit, a left and or right pulmonary artery incision is made to accommodate the anatomic discrepancy. The proximal portion of the conduit is anastomosed to the superior portion of the ventriculotomy for about 30% of the conduit circumference. The right ventricular outflow tract completion is shown using the patch hood technique. (With permission: Mavroudis and Backer 2003). *Ao* aorta, *PA* pulmonary artery, *RV* right ventricle

the conduit proves to be oversized, a left or right pulmonary artery incision is made to accommodate the anatomic discrepancy. The proximal conduit to ventricle reconstruction is performed by direct anastomosis of the conduit to the superior portion of the ventriculotomy for approximately one-third of the circumference in preparation for right ventricular outflow tract completion using the patch hood technique (Fig. 13) that will align the conduit for an appropriate positioning that will prevent sternal compression. The optimal position for the conduit is towards the left thoracic cavity away from the central anterior mediastinum; in other words, not under the sternal midline. The hood technique is

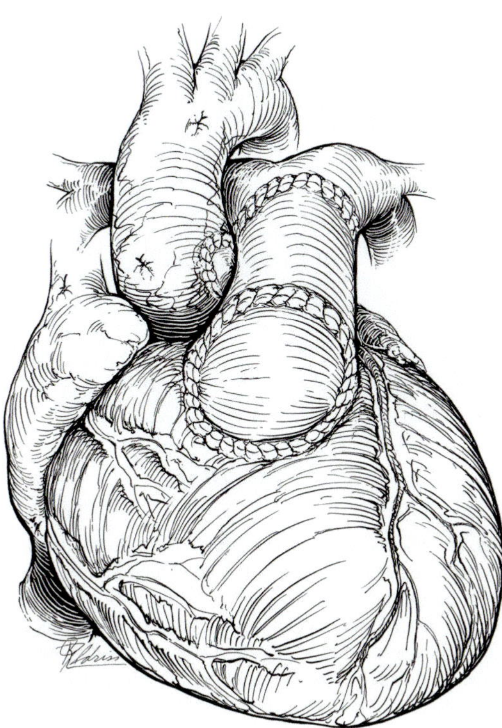

Fig. 15 Shows the completed right ventricular-to-pulmonary artery reconstruction using a pulmonary homograft and hood technique for the proximal connection. (With permission: Mavroudis and Backer 2003)

not necessary if a Contegra or Dacron valved graft is employed since the distal conduit can be cut on a bevel which will result in the same orientation as the homograft-hood technique. The ventricular anastomosis for the homograft-hood technique and the Contegra graft does not generally require Dacron felt strips for reinforced suturing. On the other hand, the porcine Dacron valved conduit is stiff and suturing to the friable ventricular edge almost always requires Dacron felt to reinforce the anastomosis, especially in young infants who are undergoing first time repair. The completed truncus repair using the hood technique is shown in Fig. 15.

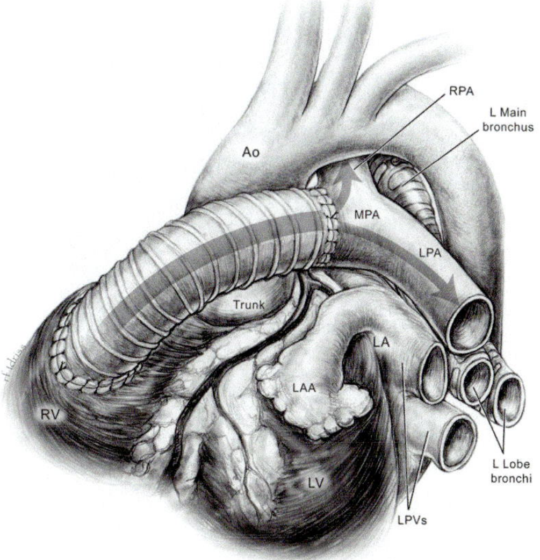

Fig. 16 Shows a left anterior oblique drawing of a completed repair of common arterial trunk. In particular, the conduit is depicted as a prosthetic externally supported graft connecting the right ventricle and the main pulmonary artery trunk which was disconnected from the common arterial trunk en route to this complete repair. Notice that there is equal flow to the pulmonary arteries as shown by the arrows which indicate, by their width, the equal separation of flow to the right and left pulmonary arteries. Also notice that there is no compression of the pulmonary arteries and there is no compression of the left main coronary artery posterior to the graft, The position of the left main coronary artery is variable and can be situated posteriorly away from the conduit or very close to the conduit as shown in this drawing. *Ao* aorta, *LA* left atrium, *LAA* left atrial appendage, *LPA* left pulmonary artery, *LPV* left pulmonary vein, *LV* left ventricle, *MPA* main pulmonary artery, *RPA* right pulmonary artery, *RV* right ventricle

3 Complications Associated With Pulmonary Artery Conduit Orientation

Pulmonary artery conduits that are used for right ventricular-to-pulmonary artery continuity require proper attention to conduit length and orientation. Figure 16 shows a left anterior oblique

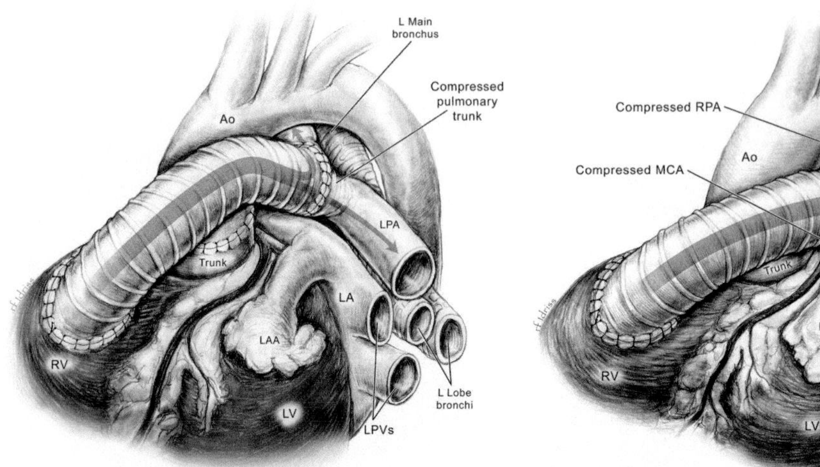

Fig. 17 Shows how a long right ventricular-to-pulmonary conduit can cause distal bifurcation pulmonary artery compression, poor pulmonary artery flow, cyanosis, and hemodynamic compromise. A telltale sign that a conduit that is too long can be appreciated by anterior conduit kinking as shown in the drawing. This anatomic configuration can cause upstream compression of the pulmonary artery connection and result in stenosis and hemodynamic instability. The arrows depicting the flow pattern shows a wide pre-anastomotic flow pattern with much narrower arrows which depicts decreased upstream flow. *Ao* aorta, *LA* left atrium, *LAA* left atrial appendage, *LPA* left pulmonary artery, *LPV* left pulmonary vein, *LV* left ventricle, *RV* right ventricle

Fig. 18 Shows how a short length of the right ventricular-to-pulmonary artery conduit reconstruction can cause pressure on the muscular portion of the right ventricular outflow tract that could cause coronary compression and right pulmonary artery proximal stenosis. Notice how a short conduit can cause right pulmonary artery stenosis by downstream traction resulting in obstructed flow from the conduit to the distal right pulmonary artery. The arrow shows normal flow within the conduit with decreased flow, depicted by a narrow arrow, into the distal right pulmonary artery. In addition to this hemodynamic problem is the possibility of the conduit causing left main coronary artery compression which can cause coronary hypoperfusion, ventricular dysfunction and failure to wean from cardiopulmonary bypass. *Ao* aorta, *LA* left atrium, *LAA* left atrial appendage, *LPA* left pulmonary artery, *LPV* left pulmonary vein, *LV* left ventricle, *MCA* main coronary artery, *MPA* main pulmonary artery, *RPA* right pulmonary artery, *RV* right ventricle

drawing of the completed repair of common arterial trunk. This drawing will serve as a proper view for complication descriptions to follow. Most surgeons prefer to establish the conduit orientation to occupy a position towards the left chest cavity to avoid a position directly underneath the sternal midline. This position will prevent sternal compression and acute conduit stenosis in the short term and easier re-entry for a future operation. Consequently, it is better to orient the conduit away from the sternal midline. However, constructing a conduit to occupy a position in the left chest may result in a long conduit which could potentially cause compression of the right and left pulmonary arteries at the distal anastomosis as noted in Fig. 17. This may cause obstruction to flow, cyanosis, and hemodynamic compromise requiring reinstitution of cardiopulmonary bypass. On the other end of the spectrum is constructing the conduit in a manner that is too short. Figure 18 shows how a short length of the right ventricular to pulmonary artery conduit can cause coronary artery compression posteriorly and right pulmonary artery proximal stenosis anteriorly (Daskalopoulos et al. 1983). Careful attention to appropriate length of the conduit will avoid these complications and allow an excellent hemodynamic result until the patient outgrows the conduit size which will require reoperation and upsized conduit replacement (Daskalopoulos et al. 1983).

4 Surgical Repair of Common Arterial Trunk When the Pulmonary Artery Trunk Is Posterior

During the early to mid-1970s and before the introduction of more comprehensive and inclusive nomenclature anatomic schemes, surgeons frequently noted that the origin of the pulmonary artery trunk was somewhat between the Collett and Edwards Type I and the Collett and Edwards Type II. Consequently, the anatomic continuum between these two subtypes was noted to occupy an area halfway between each type resulting in another informal type characterized as Type 1½. With further analysis, this type proved to be more common than either of the Collet and Edwards types. The differences notwithstanding, this discovery turns out to have important surgical considerations that are explained in the next series of drawings.

Figures 19, 20, 21, 22, 23, 24, 25, 26, 27, 28, and 29 show the important steps of the operation which include management of the so-called Truncus Arteriosus type 1½ which has proved to be a common anatomic variant of Common Arterial Trunk (Truncus Arteriosus). Figure 19 identifies, using hidden anatomy, the courses of the posterior pulmonary artery segments, the proximity of the left main coronary artery, and the truncal valve leaflets. The most important issue is not so much the common arterial trunk type, but the conduct of the operation that will emphasize a more accurate pulmonary trunk excision, coronary artery preservation, and proximal arterial trunk reconstruction. These are the considerations that could lead to coronary artery injury, pulmonary artery malposition, and injury to the truncal valve leaflets. Figure 20 shows the detailed anatomy of the exposed common arterial trunk after cardiopulmonary bypass, aortic cross-clamping and cardioplegic arrest. The anterior incision has been made to identify the important anatomic considerations. In this case it is obvious that in order to make an adequate pulmonary artery cuff, aortic transection will have to be performed. The dashed lines indicate the incision points for the pulmonary artery excision with special attention to the adjacent structures. Figure 21 reviews the important steps of the operation which are designed to avoid orifice coronary artery stenosis, truncal regurgitation or both. If the surgeon notices that the pulmonary root excision occurred too close to the orifice of the left main coronary artery, consideration should

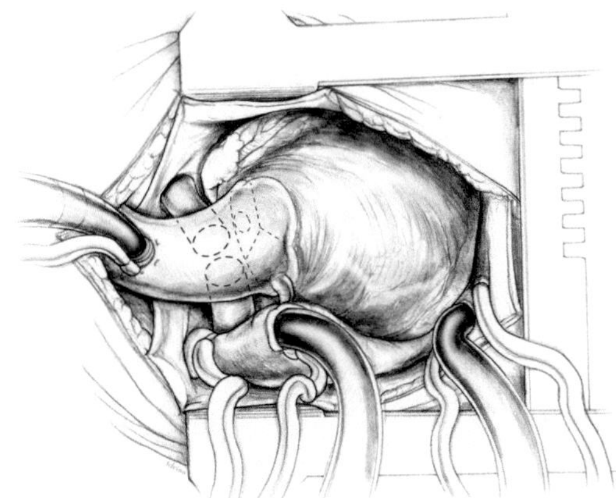

Fig. 19 Shows aortobicaval cardiopulmonary bypass preparations in a patient with Truncus Arteriosus Type 1½ or Type II depending on one's subjective analysis. The hidden anatomy depicts the origin of both pulmonary arteries, the proximity of the left main coronary artery, and the leaflets of the truncal valve. (With permission: Mavroudis 2015)

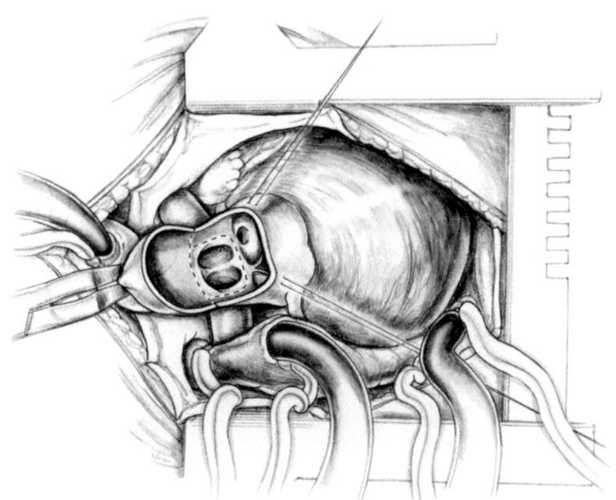

Fig. 20 Shows aortic cross-clamp and clear exposure of the common trunk before the pulmonary artery trunk is excised. Note that the left main coronary artery is very close to the orifice of the pulmonary artery trunk. Also note that removal of the pulmonary artery trunk without truncal transection can be associated with suboptimal exposure which will place the coronary artery orifice in jeopardy. (With permission: Mavroudis 2015)

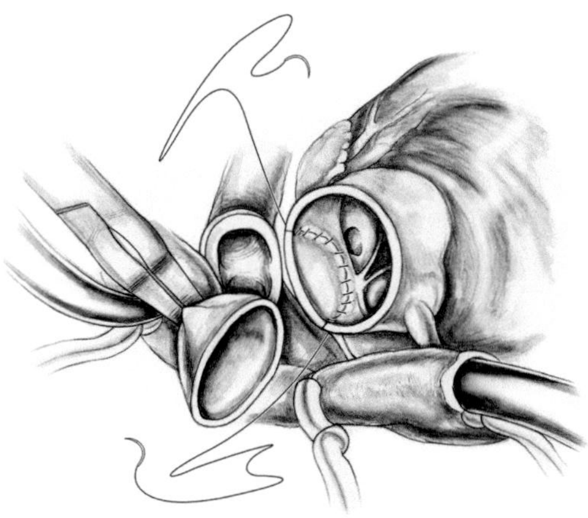

Fig. 21 Shows the excised pulmonary trunk under direct vision which allows for proximal truncal reconstruction with a prosthetic/biological patch all the while respecting the orifice of the coronary artery. Also shown is the neoaortic arterioplasty to reconstruct the neoaortic wall wherefrom came the left main coronary artery. This arterioplasty is performed with great attention to the course of the left main coronary artery and the leaflets of the truncal valve. Sutures taken too close to the coronary artery and the truncal valve could cause coronary artery insufficiency and truncal valve regurgitation, respectively. (With permission: Mavroudis 2015)

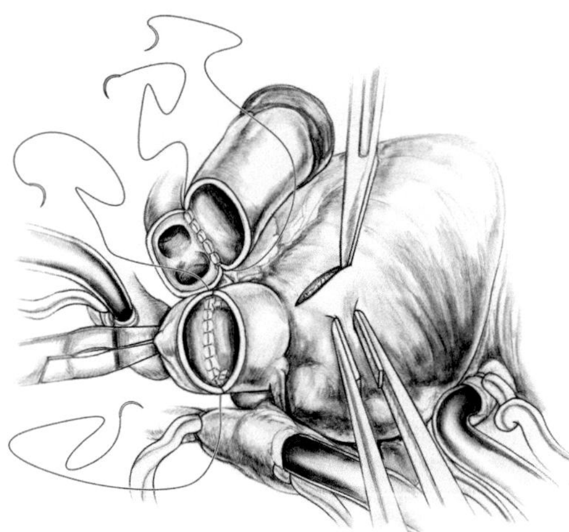

Fig. 22 Shows the progression of the operation which is performed in separate stages. The pulmonary artery homograft is being sutured end-to-end into the confluence of the pulmonary arteries; the aorta is being reconstructed using an end-to-end technique to ensure accurate suturing; and a right ventriculotomy is being performed for the eventual ventricular septal defect closure and proximal attachment of the pulmonary conduit. (With permission: Mavroudis 2015)

be given to augment the orifice of the coronary artery with a pericardial patch and fine suture technique as described in Figs. 8, 9, 10, and 11. If necessary, a coronary artery arterioplasty will allow a better arterial cuff for the pulmonary artery arterioplasty to fill out the truncal wall moiety wherefrom originated the pulmonary artery trunk. Despite this coronary artery reconstruction, the surgeon will be advised that there is the potential for a coronary artery problem when separating from cardiopulmonary bypass. Significant ST changes and poor ventricular function on transesophageal echocardiogram should result in re-exploration of the coronary artery reconstruction.

Figure 22 shows the progression of the operation which involves neoaortic reanastomosis, distal pulmonary artery to conduit anastomosis, and right ventriculotomy en route to ventricular septal defect closure and proximal outlet for the pulmonary artery conduit. Figure 23 shows the characteristics of VSD closure using interrupted suture technique. The sutures are being placed at the crest of the interventricular septum which is relatively far away from the conduction system since most patients with common arterial trunk have an outlet ventricular defect as noted early in this chapter. The suture placement for the VSD repair is being completed as shown in Fig. 24. Residual VSDs can be avoided if careful attention is given to proper exposure and accurate

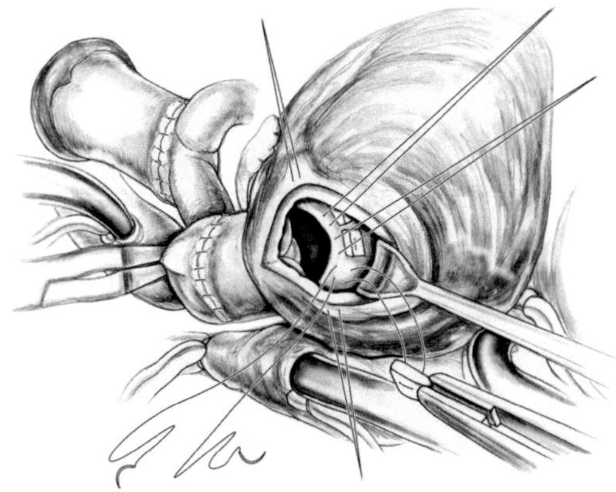

Fig. 23 Shows the pledgetted sutures being placed on the crest of the ventricular septal defect. (With permission: Mavroudis 2015)

placement of the sutures. The completed VSD closure with a Gore-Tex patch is shown in Fig. 25. Many surgeons remove the cross-clamp after the VSD closure; others wait until the proximal conduit reconstruction is completed owing to the possibility of air embolus through the patent foramen ovale which is generally left open. A careful adjustment of avoiding venous drainage suctioning should allow enough blood in the right atrium to avoid this complication. Figure 26 shows the hood technique being started with either autologous or bovine pericardium. The pericardial hood can be trimmed during the placement to create an appropriate length and width as shown in Fig. 27 which demonstrates the completion of the right ventricular to pulmonary artery reconstruction. Separation from cardiopulmonary bypass requires careful attention to the possibility of coronary artery compression and conduit malposition as noted earlier in this chapter.

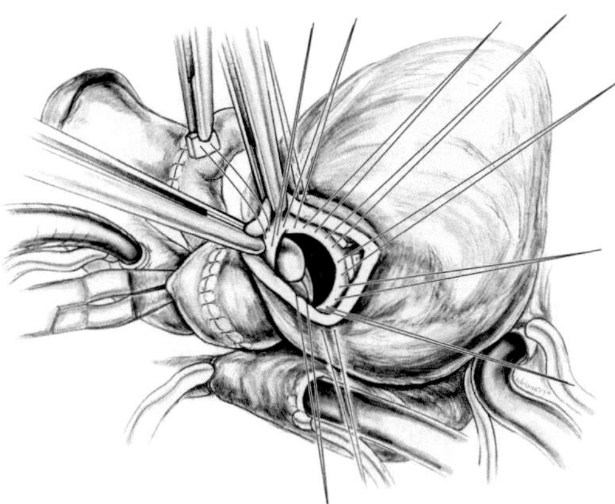

Fig. 24 Emphasizes the retraction that is often necessary to place the superior sutures near the truncal annulus for an accurate and secure attachment point that will avoid unwanted residual ventricular septal defects. (With permission: Mavroudis 2015)

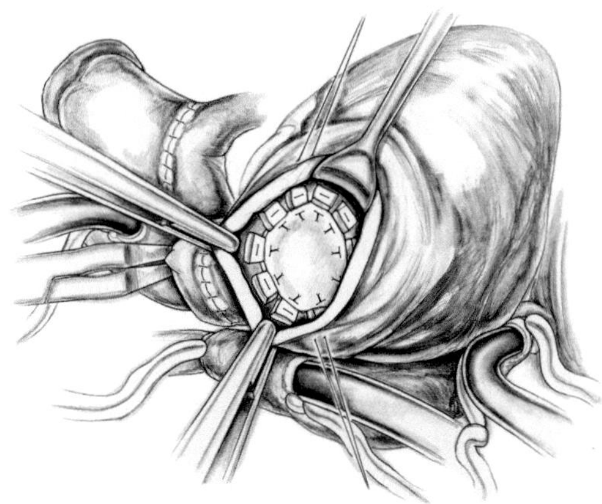

Fig. 25 Demonstrates the completed ventricular septal defect closure. The cross-clamp can now be removed, and pulmonary conduit can be sutured to the ventricular edges. (With permission: Mavroudis 2015)

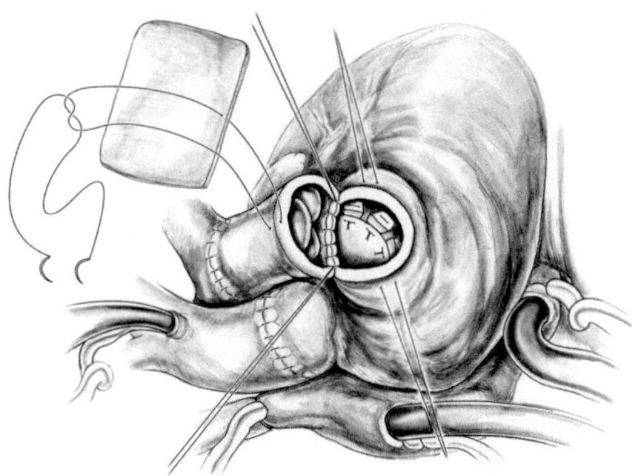

Fig. 26 Shows the placement of autologous or bovine pericardium en route to form a hood that will complete the right ventricular-to-pulmonary artery conduit. (With permission: Mavroudis 2015)

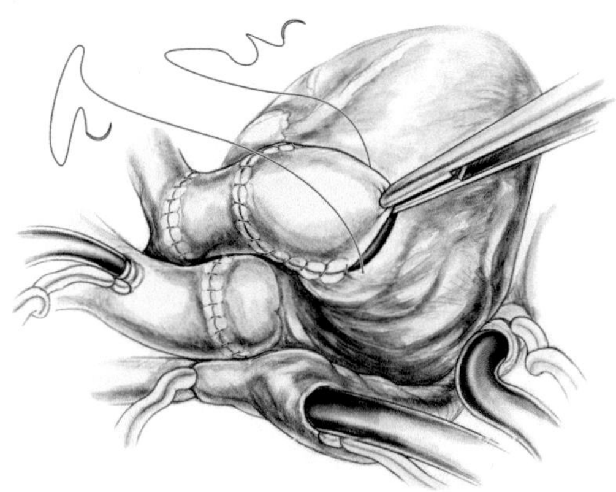

Fig. 27 The hood technique completes the ventricular-to-pulmonary artery continuity. (With permission: Mavroudis 2015)

5 Surgical Repair of Common Arterial Trunk (Truncus Arteriosus) with Interrupted Aortic Arch

Surgical repair of common arterial trunk with interrupted aortic arch is a very demanding operation that requires comprehensive management of cardiopulmonary bypass, myocardial preservation, and attention to technique (Nakae et al. 1995; Pretre et al. 1996; Rao et al. 1995; McKay et al. 1989; Berdjis et al. 1996; Cohen 1995; Haydar 1996; Lacour-Gayet et al. 1997; Mohamed and Ott 1993; Tlaskal et al. 2005; Brown et al. 2006; Chen et al. 2006; Konstantinov et al. 2006; Konstantinov 2006; de Siena et al. 2011; Bohuta et al. 2011; Yokoyama et al. 2013). Figure 28 demonstrates the cannulation technique for the initiation of cardiopulmonary bypass. If there is any advantage to cardiopulmonary bypass in CAT patients it is that a single aortic cannulation site is sufficient, unlike other patients with interrupted aortic arch who require dual cannulation, namely one in the ascending aorta and the other in the patent arterial duct to perfuse the lower extremity during the cooling phase of the operation. The patient with CAT and interrupted aortic arch requires only one aortic cannula since the descending aortic perfusion is accomplished by flow in the common arch which when the pulmonary arteries are clamped allows for flow to the descending aorta unobstructed through the patent arterial duct (Mavroudis and Backer 2003). Not shown in Fig. 28 is another option for arterial perfusion, namely, to anastomose a PTFE graft to the innominate artery which can also be used for regional perfusion during the aortic arch reconstruction. This system can avoid circulatory arrest especially if the surgeon perceives that the reconstruction will be complex and take more time to accomplish. This system requires right and left pulmonary artery snugging to prevent pulmonary overcirculation and systemic hypoperfusion. In addition, a left ventricular vent is placed through the right superior pulmonary vein. The potential complications involving this cannulation technique include malposition of the aortic cannula which can interfere with the neoaortic reconstruction, recurrent nerve injury, and left ventricular vent placement which could cause left atrial and left ventricular perforation (see chapter on Cannulation).

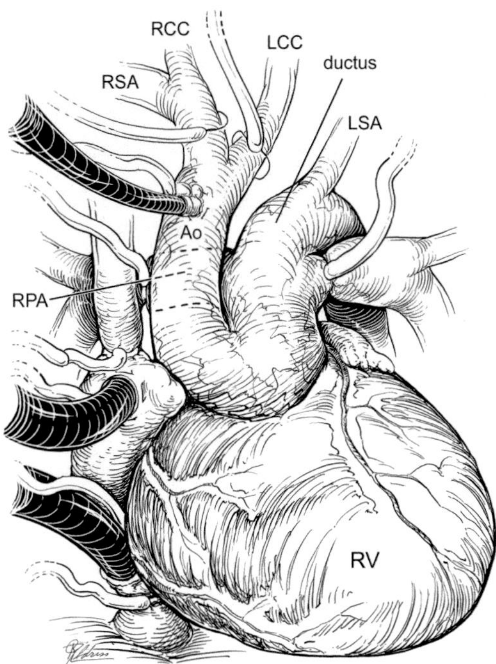

Fig. 28 Shows the cannulation technique for commencement of cardiopulmonary bypass for a patient with Common Arterial Trunk and Interrupted Aortic Arch. (With permission: Mavroudis and Backer 2003). *Ao* aorta, *LCC* left carotid artery, *LSA* left subclavian artery, *RCC* right carotid artery, *RPA* right pulmonary artery, *RSA* right subclavian artery, *RV* right ventricle

Once aortobicaval cardiopulmonary bypass is established, the patient is then cooled to 18 C° and circulatory arrest or regional perfusion is established. Antegrade and/or retrograde cardioplegia is then administered. The pulmonary artery snuggers are released, the patent arterial duct is ligated and divided, and the pulmonary artery trunk is removed with special care not to injure the left coronary artery and the truncal valve. The proximal truncal moiety wherefrom arose the pulmonary artery trunk is generally closed with a prosthetic/biological patch. Once this part of the operation is performed, exposure for the aortic reconstruction can take place. The descending aorta is then mobilized and brought into apposition with the distal ascending aorta. To complete this reconstruction, a longitudinal incision is made in the distal aorta and extended to the left common carotid artery if needed. A wide anastomosis can then be performed (Fig. 29). When the ascending to descending aortic anastomosis signals undue tension an anterior patch to augment the aortic reconstruction can be performed to ensure a large reconstruction free of any potential stenosis (Fig. 30)

After the aortic reconstruction is completed, the midproximal ascending aorta is transected in order to perform the maneuver of Lecompte resulting in translocation of the pulmonary artery anterior to the aortic arch. The aorta is then reanastomosed and cardiopulmonary bypass is restarted. The aortic cross-clamp is maintained while continued cardioplegic administration is performed. Slow systemic warming can be started while a right ventriculotomy is performed for the purpose of closing the VSD with interrupted suture technique with either a PTFE or biologic patch. Once the VSD is securely closed, air maneuvers are performed, and the aortic cross-clamp can be removed. The proximal portion of the conduit is anastomosed to the right ventriculotomy to establish right ventricular-to-pulmonary artery continuity in the same manner as noted in the previous section (Mavroudis and Backer 2003).

The important complications during the repair of common arterial trunk and interrupted aortic arch are failure to construct an adequate and tension free aortic arch repair, oversizing of the pulmonary conduit, and an extended cross-clamp

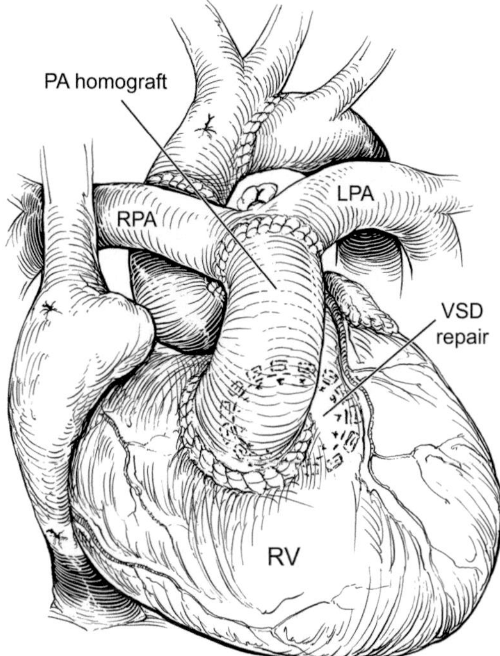

Fig. 29 Shows the completed reconstruction for a patient with Common Arterial Trunk and Interrupted Aortic Arch. The ventricular septal defect closure using pledgetted sutures is shown as hidden anatomy located in the right ventricular outflow tract just below the origin of the pulmonary artery conduit. The repair for the interrupted aortic arch is shown by a direct anastomosis between the distal ascending aorta and the mobilized descending aorta. In this case, the surgeon preferred to perform the Lecompte Maneuver by anterior translocation of the right pulmonary artery. This was accomplished by mid-ascending aortic transection pulmonary artery translocation and reanastomosis of the ascending aorta (pictured just superior to the course of the right pulmonary artery. (With permission: Mavroudis and Backer 2003). *LPA* left pulmonary artery, *PA* pulmonary artery, *RPA* right pulmonary artery, *RV* right ventricle, *VSD* ventricular septal defect

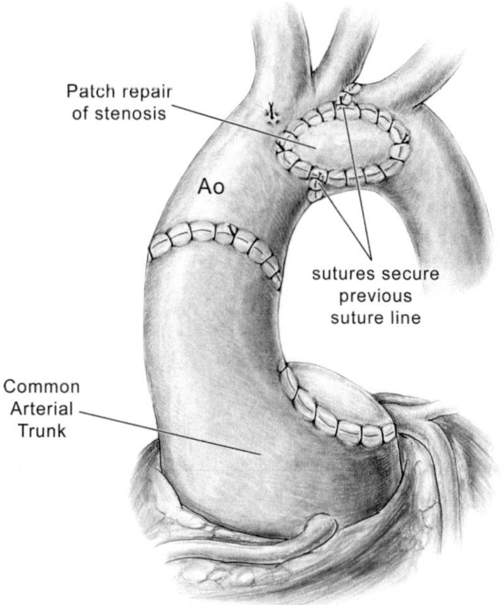

Fig. 30 Anterior autologous pericardial patch augmentation of the ascending aorta-to-descending aortic anastomosis. This patch can help to secure a tension free anastomosis and avoid stenosis and false aneurysms. *Ao* aorta

time. Anastomotic bleeding, residual VSD, heart block, and unexpected truncal valve regurgitation all have an adverse effect on hemodynamic outcome. Diligence, precise suture placement, and careful geometric orientation will optimize the clinical result (Mavroudis and Backer 2003).

6 Truncal Valve Repair for Truncal Regurgitation

In some instances, patients will present with common arterial trunk regurgitation. Mild or moderate truncal regurgitation is well tolerated in infant repair and most surgeons caution against truncal repair unless the regurgitation is rated as moderate-severe or sever truncal regurgitation. Some authors recommend repair as a primary procedure at the initial reparative operation or at subsequent operations in association with conduit replacement (Black et al. 1998; Elami et al. 1994; McElhinney et al. 1998; De Leval et al. 1974; Henaine et al. 2008; Bahrami et al. 2009; Kaza et al. 2010; Russell et al. 2012a, b; Myers et al. 2013; Perri et al. 2013; Patrick et al. 2016; Elkins et al. 1990). Truncal valve anatomy can serve as an important guide to repair of truncal regurgitation which can be associated with a quadricuspid truncal valve. The quadricuspid valve often has a prolapsing small leaflet in association with three other normally formed leaflets as noted in Fig. 31. This anomaly can be approached using a leaflet and cusp resection, reduction annuloplasty and re-suspension of the remaining leaflets to reconstruct a tricuspid truncal valve. This technique is well illustrated in Figs. 32, 33, 34, and 35. Procedure notes indicate the careful suturing techniques to avoid complications such as suture line disruption and insecure leaflet apposition.

In some cases, the surgeon may elect to perform truncal valve valvuloplasty by suturing the prolapsed valve leaflets to the adjoining leaflets in order to support the prolapsing valve and create valvar sufficiency. This technique converts the quadricuspid valve into an effective bicuspid valve as shown in Fig. 36. This technique while seemingly attractive because of its simplicity

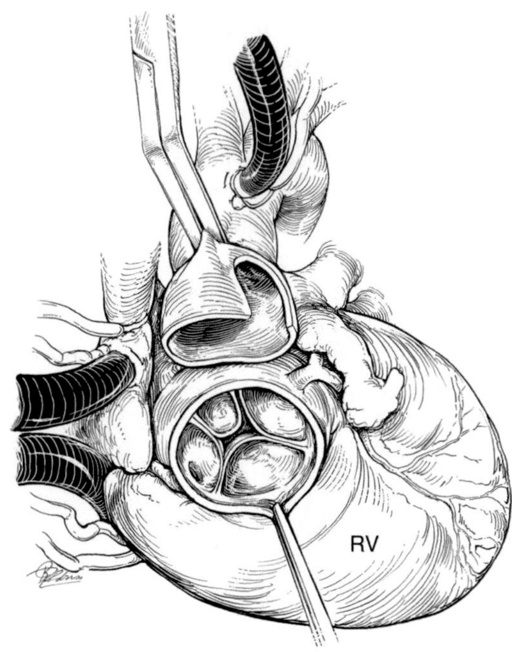

Fig. 31 The exposure is by aortobicaval cardiopulmonary bypass and aortic transection. Proper evaluation of the truncal valve, the leaflet orientation, and the coronary arteries can then be accomplished. Oftentimes it is the smallest leaflet of the quadricuspid truncal valve that is prolapsed and the cause of the regurgitation. (With permission: Mavroudis and Backer 2003). *RV* right ventricle

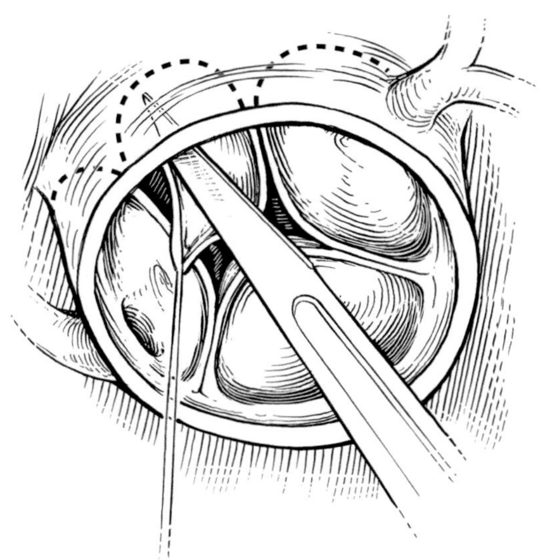

Fig. 32 Shows the resection of the small, prolapsed leaflet leaving enough leaflet tissue to close the moiety in order to form the trileaflet valve. (With permission: Mavroudis and Backer 2003)

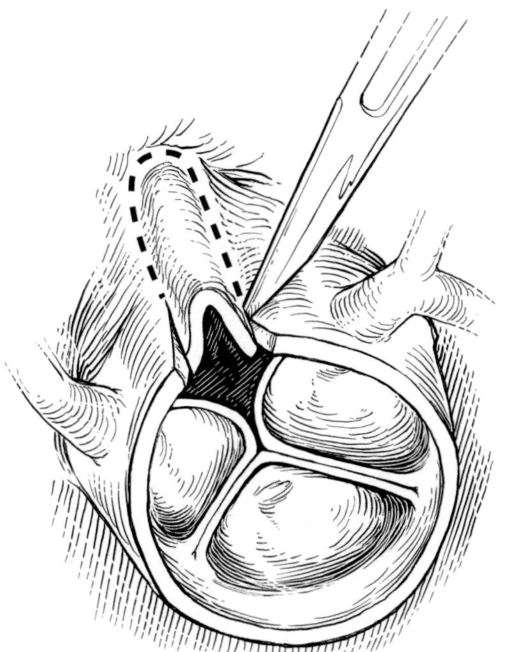

Fig. 33 A localized truncal wall resection in the area of the resected prolapsed valve down to the annulus is performed en route to annular reduction and resuspension of the truncal leaflets. (With permission: Mavroudis and Backer 2003)

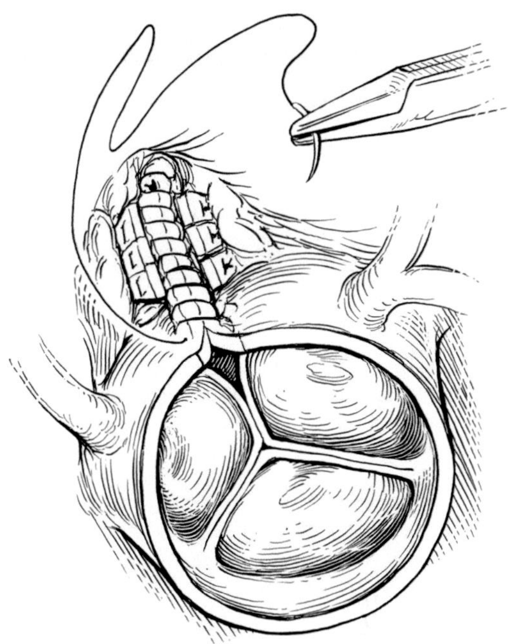

Fig. 34 A linear reanastomosis of the resected aortic segment is performed using pledgetted sutures for the reduction annular reconstruction. Once this is done, the edges of the remaining leaflet are sutured together to form the new commissure (not shown). Also shown are two suture lines. The first is demonstrated by the pledget supported sutures that have been placed to perform the annular reduction portion of this reconstruction. After this, the edges of the remaining aortic wall are reapproximated with running suture technique all the while recognizing that this suture line will form the basis of the new commissure. (With permission: Mavroudis and Backer 2003)

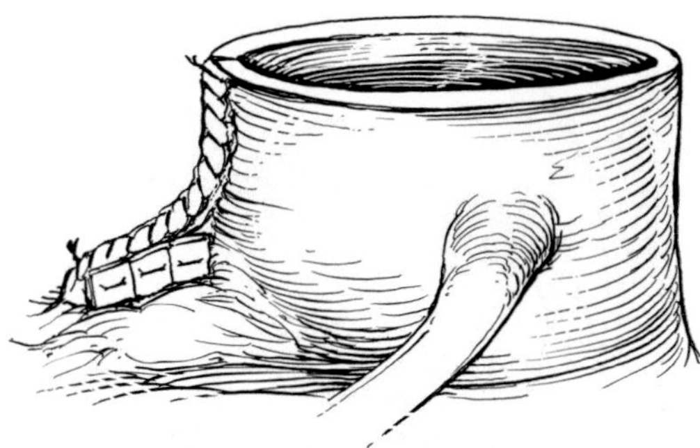

Fig. 35 Shows the reconstructed truncal reduction annuloplasty and the newly created commissure as noted from the exterior. (With permission: Mavroudis and Backer 2003)

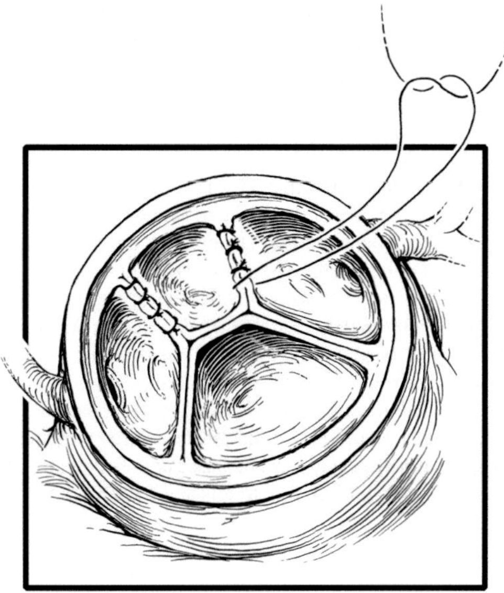

Fig. 36 Shows truncal valve repair by truncal valve valvuloplasty performed by suture apposition of the prolapsed valve leaflets to the adjoining leaflets which can support the prolapsing valve and create a normally functional valve. This maneuver converts the quadricuspid valve into an effective bicuspid valve. Care must be exercised for this procedure since the leaflets in a neonate are flimsy and do not always hold sutures well. Therefore, this technique should not be the first choice for truncal repair in our opinion. It could however help to provide an improvement in truncal valve function in difficult situations where cross-clamp time is important. (With permission: Mavroudis and Backer 2003)

must be used infrequently due to the flimsy and thin characteristics of the neonatal truncal valve which may not hold sutures well.

7 Truncal Valve Repair in the Presence of Coronary Artery Anatomy Concerns

In very rare circumstances, a coronary artery can originate from the diminutive coronary cusp which is associated with a prolapsing valve that is selected for resection. This can be managed by coronary artery transfer much the same way that is used for the arterial switch operation. Figure 37 shows the careful dissection and mobilization of the coronary artery button from the affected sinus of Valsalva, in the same manner that is used to accomplish coronary artery mobilization for the arterial switch operation. In addition, the same drawing shows the prolapsed leaflet being sharply dissected away from the sinus of Valsalva in

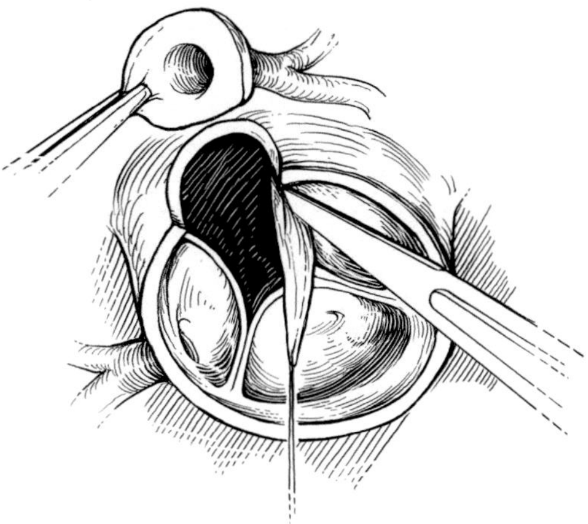

Fig. 37 Shows coronary artery button removal from the sinus of Valsalva that supports the prolapsing valve of this quadricuspid valve. The figure also shows the removal of the prolapsing valve by sharp dissection making sure to avoid any injury to the adjacent normal leaflets which will eventually be aligned to form a normal truncal valve. (With permission: Mavroudis and Backer 2003)

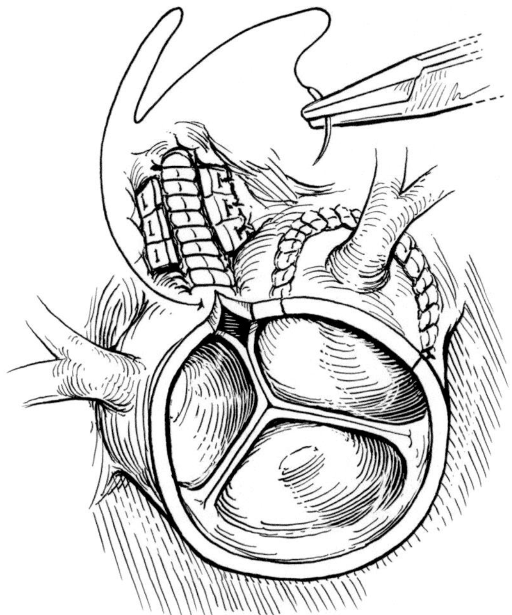

Fig. 38 Shows the reduction annuloplasty and recreation of the commissure with the coronary button already anastomosed to the adjacent sinus of Valsalva. The coronary artery button must be carefully and extensively mobilized onto the ventricular surface in order to avoid kinking and obstruction to flow. (With permission: Mavroudis and Backer 2003)

preparation for the reduction annuloplasty and commissural reconstruction. Figure 38 shows the completed repair with coronary transfer to an adjacent sinus of Valsalva, reduction annuloplasty, and recreation of the valvar commissure to insure valvar competency and unobstructed coronary artery perfusion.

References

Agarwal KC, Edwards WD, Feldt RH, Danielson GK, Puga FJ, McGoon DC. Clinicopathological correlates of obstructed right-sided porcine-valved extracardiac conduits. J Thorac Cardiovasc Surg. 1981;81(4):591–601.

Agarwal KC, Edwards WD, Feldt RH, Danielson GK, Puga FJ, McGoon DC. Pathogenesis of nonobstructive fibrous peels in right-sided porcine-valved extracardiac conduits. J Thorac Cardiovasc Surg. 1982;83(4):584–9.

Alfieris GM, Gangemi JJ, Schiralli MP, Swartz MF, Cholette JM. Modified repair of truncus arteriosus to maintain pulmonary artery architecture. Ann Thorac Surg. 2010;90(3):1038–9.

Anderson RH, Chaudhry B, Mohun TJ, Bamforth SD, Hoyland D, Phillips HM, Webb S, Moorman AF, Brown NA, Henderson DJ. Normal and abnormal development of the intrapericardial arterial trunks in humans and mice. Cardiovasc Res. 2012;95:108–15.

Angelini GD, Witsenburg M, Ten Kate FJ, Hiddema PA, Quaebebeur JM. Severe stenotic scar contracture of the Microvel Hemashield right-sided extracardiac conduit. Ann Thorac Surg. 1989;48(5):714–6.

Appelbaum A, Bargeron LM Jr, Pacifico AD, Kirklin JW. Surgical treatment of truncus arteriosus, with emphasis on infants and small children. J Thorac Cardiovasc Surg. 1976;71(3):436–40.

Armer RM, De Oliveira PF, Lurie PR. True truncus arteriosus: review of 17 cases and report of surgery in 7 patients (abstr). Circulation. 1961;24:878.

Arslan AH, Ugurlucan M, Yildiz Y, Ay S, Bahceci F, Besikci R, Cicek S. Surgical treatment of common arterial trunk in patients beyond the first year of life. World J Pediatr Congenit Heart Surg. 2014;5(2):211–5.

Asagai S, Inai K, Shinohara T, Tomimatsu H, Ishii T, Sugiyama H, Park IS, Nagashima M, Nakanishi T. Long-term Outcomes after truncus arteriosus repair: a single-center experience for more than 40 years. Congenit Heart Dis. 2016;11:672–7.

Bahrami S, Mitropoulos F, Leong F, Levi DS, Laks H, Plunkett MD. Truncal valve repair in neonates using pericardial leaflet extension. Congenit Heart Dis. 2009;4(4):281–3.

Beckerman Z, DeLeon LE, Sea-Vera Rm Mery CM, Fraser. High incidence of late infective endocarditis in bovine jugular vein valved conduits. J Thorac Cardiovasc Surg. 2018;156:728–34.

Behrendt DM, Kirsh MM, Stern A, Sigmann J, Perry B, Sloan H. The surgical therapy for pulmonary artery–right ventricular discontinuity. Ann Thorac Surg. 1974;18:122–37.

Berdjis F, Wells WJ, Starnes VA. Truncus arteriosus with total anomalous pulmonary venous return and interrupted arch. Ann Thorac Surg. 1996;61(1):220–2.

Berger K, Sauvage LR, Rao AM, Wood SJ. Healing of arterial prostheses in man: its incompleteness. Ann Surg. 1972;175(1):118–27.

Bisset GS 3rd, Schwartz DC, Benzing G 3rd, Helmsworth J, Schreiber JT, Kaplan S. Late results of reconstruction of the right ventricular outflow tract with porcine xenografts in children. Ann Thorac Surg. 1981;31(5):437–43.

Black MD, Adatia I, Freedom RM. Truncal valve repair: initial experience in neonates. Ann Thorac Surg. 1998;65(6):1737–40.

Bohuta L, Hussein A, Fricke TA, d'Udekem Y, Bennett M, Brizard C, Konstantinov IE. Surgical repair of truncus arteriosus associated with interrupted aortic arch: long-term outcomes. Ann Thorac Surg. 2011;91(5):1473–7.

Bove EL, Beekman RH, Snider AR, et al. Repair of truncus arteriosus in the neonate and young infant. Ann Thorac Surg. 1989;47:499–505.

Bove EL, Lupinetti FM, Pridjian AK, et al. Results of a policy of primary repair of truncus arteriosus in the neonate. J Thorac Cardiovasc Surg. 1993;105:1057–65.

Bowman FO, Hancock WD, Malm JR. A valve-containing Dacron prosthesis: its use in restoring pulmonary artery-right ventricular continuity. Arch Surg. 1973;107:724–8.

Boyce SW, Turley K, Yee ES, Verrier ED, Ebert PA. The fate of the 12 mm porcine valved conduit from the right ventricle to the pulmonary artery. A ten-year experience. J Thorac Cardiovasc Surg. 1988;95(2):201–7.

Brizard CP, Cochrane A, Austin C, Nomura F, Karl TR. Management strategy and long-term outcome for truncus arteriosus. Eur J Cardiothorac Surg. 1997;11:687–96.

Brown JW, Ruzmetov M, Okada Y, Vijay P, Turrentine MW. Truncus arteriosus repair: outcomes, risk factors, re-operation and management. Eur J Cardiothorac Surg. 2001;20:221–7.

Brown JW, Ruzmetov M, Okada Y, Vijay P, Rodefeld MD, Turrentine MW. Outcomes in patients with interrupted aortic arch and associated anomalies: a 20-year experience. Eur J Cardiothorac Surg. 2006;29(5):666–6734.

Brown JW, Ruzmetov M, Rodefeld MD, Eltayeb O, Yurdakok O, Turrentine MW. Contegra versus pulmonary homografts for right ventricular outflow tract reconstruction: a ten-year single-institution comparison. World J Pediatr Congenit Heart Surg. 2011;2:541–9.

Buchanan A. Malformation of the heart. Undivided truncus arteriosus. Heart otherwise double. Trans Pathol Soc Lond. 1864;15:89.

Bull C, Macartney FJ, Horvath P, Almeida R, Merrill W, Douglas J, et al. Evaluation of long-term results of homograft and heterograft valves in extracardiac conduits. J Thorac Cardiovasc Surg. 1987;94(1):12–9.

Butto F, Lucas RV Jr, Edwards JE. Persistent truncus arteriosus: pathologic anatomy in 54 cases. Pediatr Cardiol. 1986;7:95–101.

Calder L, Van Praagh R, Van Praagh S, Sears WP, Corwin R, Levy A, et al. Truncus arteriosus communis. Clinical, angiocardiographic, and pathologic findings in 100 patients. Am Heart J. 1976;92(1):23–38.

Castaneda AR. Truncus arteriosus. Ann Thorac Surg. 1989;47(4):491–2.

Chan KC, Fyfe DA, McKay CA, Sade RM, Crawford FA. Right ventricular outflow reconstruction with cryopreserved homografts in pediatric patients: intermediate-term follow-up with serial echocardiographic assessment. J Am Coll Cardiol. 1994;24(2):483–9.

Chen JM, Glickstein JS, Davies RR, Mercando ML, Hellenbrand WE, Mosca RS, et al. The effect of repair technique on postoperative right-sided obstruction in patients with truncus arteriosus. J Thorac Cardiovasc Surg. 2005;129(3):559–68.

Chen Q, Modi P, Caputo M, Pawade A. Truncus arteriosus with interrupted aortic arch: successful repair using modified cardiopulmonary bypass and surgical techniques. Ann Thorac Surg. 2006;82(5):1884–6.

Chen Q, Gao H, Hua Z, Yang K, Yan J, Zhang H, Ma K, Zhang S, Qi L, Li S. Outcomes of Surgical repair for persistent truncus arteriosus from neonates to adults: a single center's experience. PLoS One. 2016;11(1):e0146800. https://doi.org/10.1371/journal.pone.0146800.

Cohen DM. Lecompte maneuver for truncus arteriosus with type B arch interruption: is this a panacea? Ann Thorac Surg. 1995;60(1):229.

Collett RW, Edwards JE. Persistent truncus arteriosus; a classification according to anatomic types. Surg Clin North Am. 1949;29:1245–70.

Curi-Curi P, Cervantes J, Soulé M, Erdmenger J, Calderón-Colmenero J, Ramírez S. Early and midterm results of an alternative procedure to homografts in primary repair of truncus arteriosus communis. Congenit Heart Dis. 2010;5(3):262–70.

Danton MH, Barron DJ, Stumper O, Wright JG, De Giovannni J, Silove ED, et al. Repair of truncus arteriosus: a considered approach to right ventricular outflow tract reconstruction. Eur J Cardiothorac Surg. 2001;20(1):95–104.

Daskalopoulos DA, Edwards WD, Driscoll DJ, Danielson GK, Puga FJ. Coronary artery compression with fatal myocardial ischemia. A rare complication of valved extracardiac conduits in children with congenital heart disease. J Thorac Cardiovasc Surg. 1983;85(4):546–51.

De Leval MR, McGoon DC, Wallace RB, Danielson GK, Mair DD. Management of truncal valvular regurgitation. Ann Surg. 1974;180(4):427–32.

de Siena P, Rajakaruna C, Parry AJ, Caputo M. Reverse subclavian flap and aorto-pulmonary window technique for repair of interrupted aortic arch and truncus arteriosus. Interact Cardiovasc Thorac Surg. 2011;13(3):354–5.

Derby CD, Kolcz J, Gidding S, Pizarro C. Outcomes following non-valved autologous reconstruction of the right ventricular outflow tract in neonates and infants. Eur J Cardiothorac Surg. 2008;34(4):726–31.

Ebert PA. Pulmonary artery conduits in infants younger than six months of age. J Thorac Cardiovasc Surg. 1976;72:351–6.

Ebert P. Management of patients with right ventricle to pulmonary artery discontinuity. Cardiovasc Clin. 1981;11:337–42.

Ebert PA. Truncus arteriosus. In: Glenn WWL, Baue AE, Geha AS, editors. Thoracic and cardiovascular surgery. 4th ed. Norwalk: Appleton-Century-Crofts; 1983.

Ebert PA. Atlas of congenital cardiac surgery. New York: Churchill Livingstone Inc; 1989.

Ebert PA, Turley K, Stanger P, Hoffman JIE, Heymann MA, Rudolph AM. Surgical treatment of truncus arteriosus in the first 6 months of life. Ann Surg. 1984;200:451–6.

Edwards WD, Agarwal KC, Feldt RH, Danielson GK, Puga FJ. Surgical pathology of obstructed, right-sided, porcine-valved extracardiac conduits. Arch Pathol Lab Med. 1983;107(8):400–5.

Elami A, Laks H, Pearl JM. Truncal valve repair: initial experience with infants and children. Ann Thorac Surg. 1994;57(2):397–402.

Elkins RC, Steinberg JB, Razook JD, Ward KE, Overholt ED, Thompson WM Jr. Correction of truncus arteriosus with truncal valvar stenosis or insufficiency using two homografts. Ann Thorac Surg. 1990;50(5):728–33.

Espinola-Zavaleta N, Munoz-Castellanos L, Gonzalez-Flores R, Kuri-Nivon M. [Common truncus arteriosus in adults]. Arch Cardiol Mex. 2008;78(2):210–6.

Fontan F, Choussat A, Deville C, Doutremepuich C, Coupillaud J, Vosa C. Aortic valve homografts in the surgical treatment of complex cardiac malformations. J Thorac Cardiovasc Surg. 1984;87(5):649–57.

Fry WJ, Deweese MS, Kraft RO, Ernst CB. Importance of porosity in arterial prostheses. Arch Surg. 1964;88:836–42.

Fyler DC. Truncus arteriosus. In: Fyler DC, editor. Nadas; pediatric cardiology. Philadelphia: Hanley & Belfus; 1992.

Gober V, Berdat P, Pavlovic M, Pfammatter JP, Carrel TP. Adverse mid-term outcome following RVOT reconstruction using the Contegra valved bovine jugular vein. Ann Thorac Surg. 2005;79(2):625–31.

Hanley FL, Heinemann MK, Jonas RA, Mayer JE Jr, Cook NR, Wessel DL, et al. Repair of truncus arteriosus in the neonate. J Thorac Cardiovasc Surg. 1993;105(6):1047–56.

Haverich A, Oelert H, Maatz W, Borst HG. Histopathological evaluation of woven and knitted Dacron grafts for right ventricular conduits: a comparative experimental study. Ann Thorac Surg. 1984;37(5):404–11.

Hawkins JA, Kaza AK, Burch PT, Lambert LM, Holubkov R, Witte MK. Simple versus complex truncus arteriosus: neutralization of risk but with increased resource utilization. World J Pediatr Congenit Heart Surg. 2010;1(3):285–91.

Haydar S. Lecompte maneuver in truncus arteriosus repair: potential risks! Ann Thorac Surg. 1996;62(4):1241.

Heilbrunn A, Kittle CF, Diehl AM. Pulmonary arterial banding in the treatment of truncus arteriosus. Circulation. 1964;29:102–7.

Heinemann MK, Hanley FL, Fenton KN, Jonas RA, Mayer JE, Castaneda AR. Fate of small homograft conduits after early repair of truncus arteriosus. Ann Thorac Srg. 1993;55(6):1409–12.

Henaine R, Azarnoush K, Belli E, Capderou A, Roussin R, Planché C, Serraf A. Fate of the truncal valve in truncus arteriosus. Ann Thorac Surg. 2008;85(1):172–8.

Hickey EJ, McCrindle BW, Blackstone EH, Yeh T Jr, Pigula F, Clarke D, et al. Jugular venous valved conduit (Contegra) matches allograft performance in infant truncus arteriosus repair. Eur J Cardiothorac Surg. 2008;33(5):890–8.

Hoots AV, Watson DC Jr. Construction of an aortic homograft conduit for right ventricle to pulmonary artery continuity. Ann Thorac Surg. 1989;48(5):731–2.

Imamura M, Drummond-Webb JI, Sarris GE, Mee RBB. Improving early and intermediate results of truncus arteriosus repair: a new technique of truncal valve repair. Ann Thorac Surg. 1999;67:1142–6.

Jacobs ML. Congenital Heart Surgery Nomenclature and Database Project: truncus arteriosus. Ann Thorac Surg. 2000;69(4 Suppl):S50–5.

Jacobs ML, Anderson RH. Rationalising the nomenclature of common arterial trunk. Cardiol Young. 2012;22:639–46.

Jahangiri M, Zurakowski D, Mayer JE, del Nido PJ, Jonas RA. Repair of the truncal valve and associated interrupted arch in neonates with truncus arteriosus. J Thorac Cardiovasc Surg. 2000;119:508–14.

Jonas RA, Freed MD, Mayer JE Jr, Castaneda AR. Long-term follow-up of patients with synthetic right heart conduits. Circulation. 1985;72(3 Pt 2):II77–83.

Jonas RA, Schoen FJ, Ziemer G, Britton L, Castaneda AR. Biological sealants and knitted Dacron conduits: comparison of collagen and fibrin glue pretreatments in circulatory models. Ann Thorac Surg. 1987;44(3):283–90.

Kalavrouziotis G, Purohit M, Ciotti G, Corno AF, Pozzi M. Truncus arteriosus communis: early and midterm results of early primary repair. Ann Thorac Surg. 2006;82(6):2200–6.

Kay PH, Ross DN. Fifteen years' experience with the aortic homograft: the conduit of choice for right ventricular outflow tract reconstruction. Ann Thorac Surg. 1985;40(4):360–4.

Kaza AK, Burch PT, Pinto N, Minich LL, Tani LY, Hawkins JA. Durability of truncal valve repair. Ann Thorac Surg. 2010;90(4):1307–12.

Kirklin JW, Blackstone EH, Maehara T, Pacifico AD, Kirklin JK, Pollock S, et al. Intermediate-term fate of cryopreserved allograft and xenograft valved conduits. Ann Thorac Surg. 1987;44(6):598–606.

Kobayashi J, Backer CL, Zales VR, Crawford SE, Muster AJ, Mavroudis C. Failure of the Hemashield extension in right ventricle-to-pulmonary artery conduits. Ann Thorac Surg. 1993;56(2):277–81.

Kocher TZ, Pestaner JP, Koutlas TC. Early complication after repair of truncus arteriosus with Contegra conduit. Ann Thorac Surg. 2006;82(5):1949.

Konstantinov IE. Repair of persistent truncus arteriosus with interrupted aortic arch: what did we learn? Eur J Cardiothorac Surg. 2006;29(4):635–6; author reply 6–7

Konstantinov IE, Karamlou T, Blackstone EH, Mosca RS, Lofland GK, Caldarone CA, Williams WG, Mackie AS, McCrindle BW. Truncus arteriosus associated with interrupted aortic arch in 50 neonates: a Congenital Heart Surgeons Society Study. Ann Thorac Surg. 2006;81(1):214–22.

Lacour-Gayet F, Serraf A, Komiya T, Sousa-Uva M, Bruniaux J, Touchot A, et al. Truncus arteriosus repair: influence of techniques of right ventricular outflow tract reconstruction. J Thorac Cardiovasc Surg. 1996;111(4):849–56.

Lacour-Gayet F, Serraf A, Galletti L, Bruniaux J, Belli E, Piot D, et al. Biventricular repair of conotruncal anomalies associated with aortic arch obstruction: 103 patients. Circulation. 1997;96(9 Suppl):II-328–34.

Laudito A, Graham EM, Stroud MR, Bandisode V, Bhat AN, Crawford FA Jr, et al. Complete repair of conotruncal defects with an interatrial communication: oxygenation, hemodynamic status, and early outcome. Ann Thorac Surg. 2006;82(4):1286–91.

Lenox CC, Debich DE, Zuberbuhler JR. The role of coronary artery abnormalities in the prognosis of truncus arteriosus. J Thorac Cardiovasc Surg. 1992;104:1728–42.

Lev M, Saphir O. Truncus arteriosus communis persistens. J Pediatr. 1943;20:74.

Losay J, Planche C, Lacour-Gayet F, Touchot A, Bruniaux J. [Immediate and mid-term results of complete repair of truncus arteriosus during the first year of life]. Arch Mal Coeur Vaiss. 1991;84(5):691–5.

Marcelletti C, McGoon DC, Mair DD. The natural history of truncus arteriosus. Circulation. 1976;54(1):108–11.

Marcelletti C, McGoon DC, Danielson GK, Wallace RB, Mair DD. Early and late results of surgical repair of truncus arteriosus. Circulation. 1977;55(4):636–41.

Mavroudis C. Truncus arteriosus. In: Mavroudis C, Backer CL, editors. Atlas of pediatric cardiac surgery. London: Springer; 2015.

Mavroudis C, Backer CL. Surgical management of severe truncal insufficiency: experience with truncal valve remodeling techniques. Ann Thorac Surg. 2001;72:396–400.

Mavroudis C, Backer CL. Truncus arteriosus. In: Mavroudis C, Backer CL, editors. Pediatric cardiac surgery. 3rd ed. Philadelphia: Mosby; 2003. p. 339–52.

Mavroudis C, Backer CL. Truncus arteriosus. In: Mavroudis C, Backer CL, editors. Pediatric cardiac surgery. 4th ed. Wiley-Blackwell: Oxford; 2013.

Mavroudis C, Jonas RA, Bove EL, Aldo R. Castañeda lecture: personal glimpses into the evolution of Truncus Arteriosus repair. World J Pediatr Cong Heart Surg. 2015;6:226–38.

McElhinney DB, Reddy VM, Brook MM, Hanley FL. Repair of truncus arteriosus with intact ventricular septum (Van Praagh type B2) in a neonate. J Thorac Cardiovasc Surg. 1997;114(1):134–8.

McElhinney DB, Reddy VM, Rajasinghe HA, Mora BN, Silverman NH, Hanley FL. Trends in the management of truncal valve insufficiency. Ann Thorac Surg. 1998;65(2):517–24.

McGoon DC, Rastelli GC, Ongley PA. An operation for the correction of truncus arteriosus. JAMA. 1968;205:69–73.

McGoon DC, Danielson GK, Puga FJ, Ritter DG, Mair DD, Ilstrup DM. Late results after extracardiac conduit repair for congenital cardiac defects. Am J Cardiol. 1982;49(7):1741–9.

McKay R, Miyamoto S, Peart I, Battistessa SA, Wren C, Cunliffe M, et al. Truncus arteriosus with interrupted aortic arch: successful correction in a neonate. Ann Thorac Surg. 1989;48(4):587–9.

Mery CM, Guzman-Pruneda FA, DeLeon LE, Zhang W, Terwelp MD, Bocchini CE, Adachi I, Heinle JS, McKenzie ED, Fraser CD Jr. Risk factors for development of endocarditis and reintervention in patients undergoing right ventricle to pulmonary artery valved conduit placement. J Thorac Cardiovasc Surg. 2016;151:432–9.

Meyns B, Van Garsse L, Boshoff D, Eyskens B, Mertens L, Gewillig M, et al. The Contegra conduit in the right ventricular outflow tract induces supravalvular stenosis. J Thorac Cardiovasc Surg. 2004;128(6):834–40.

Mohamed G, Ott DA. Anterior translocation of the pulmonary confluence in the surgical treatment of truncus arteriosus. Tex Heart Inst J. 1993;20(4):285–7.

Mosca RS, Bove EL. Truncus arteriosus. In: Baue AE, Geha AS, Hammond GL, et al., editors. Glenn's thoracic and cardiovascular surgery. Appleton and Lange: Stamford; 1996.

Myers PO, Bautista-Hernandez V, del Nido PJ, Marx GR, Mayer JE, Pigula FA, Baird CW. Surgical repair of truncal valve regurgitation. Eur J Cardiothorac Surg. 2013;44(5):813–20.

Naimo PS, Fricke TA, Yong MS, d'Udekem Y, Kelly A, Radford DJ, Bullock A, Weintraub RG, Brizard CP, Konstantinov IE. Outcomes of truncus arteriosus repair in children: 35 years of experience from a single institution. Semin Thorac Cardiovasc Surg. 2016;28(2):500–11.

Naito Y, Fujita T, Manabe H, Kawashima Y. The criteria for reconstruction of right ventricular outflow tract in total correction of tetralogy of Fallot. J Thorac Cardiovasc Surg. 1980;80(4):574–81.

Nakae S, Kawada M, Kasahara S, Lin ZB, Hiraishi S, Yoshimura H. Truncus arteriosus with interrupted aortic arch: successful correction using autologous flap. Ann Thorac Surg. 1995;60(3):697–8.

Nemoto S, Ozawa H, Sasaki T, Katsumata T, Kishi K, Okumura K, Mori Y. Repair of persistent truncus arteriosus without a conduit: sleeve resection of the pulmonary trunk from the aorta and direct right ventricle-pulmonary artery anastomosis. Eur J Cardiothorac Surg. 2011;40(3):563–8.

Oddens JR, Boger AJ, Witsenburg M, et al. Anatomy of the proximal coronary arteries as a risk factor in primary repair of common arterial trunk. J Cardiovasc Surg. 1994;35:295–9.

Parenzan L, Crupi G, Alfieri O, Bianchi T, Vanini V, Locatelli G, et al. Surgical repair of persistent truncus arteriosus in infancy. Thorac Cardiovasc Surg. 1980;28(1):18–20.

Patrick WL, Mainwaring RD, Carrillo SA, Ma M, Reinhartz O, Petrossian E, Selamet Tierney ES, Reddy VM, Hanley FL. Anatomic factors associated with truncal valve insufficiency and the need for trun-

cal valve repair. World J Pediatr Congenit Heart Surg. 2016;7(1):9–15.
Pearl JM, Laks H, Drinkwater DC Jr, Milgalter E, Orrin Ailloni C, Giacobetti F, et al. Repair of truncus arteriosus in infancy. Ann Thorac Surg. 1991;52(4):780–6.
Pearl JM, Laks H, Drinkwater DC Jr, Loo DK, George BL, Williams RG. Repair of conotruncal abnormalities with the use of the valved conduit: improved early and midterm results with the cryopreserved homograft. J Am Coll Cardiol. 1992;20(1):191–6.
Perri G, Filippelli S, Polito A, Di Carlo D, Albanese SB, Carotti A. Repair of incompetent truncal valves: early and mid-term results. Interact Cardiovasc Thorac Surg. 2013;16(6):808–13.
Pretre R, Friedli B, Rouge JC, Kalangos A, Faidutti B. Anterior translocation of the right pulmonary artery to prevent bronchovascular compression in a case of truncus arteriosus and type A interrupted aortic arch. J Thorac Cardiovasc Surg. 1996;111(3):672–4.
Radford DJ, Perkins L, Lachman R, et al. Spectrum of Di George syndrome in patients with truncus arteriosus: expanded Di George syndrome. Pediatr Cardiol. 1988;9:95–101.
Raisky O, Ali WB, Bajolle F, Marini D, Metton O, Bonnet D, et al. Common arterial trunk repair: with conduit or without? Eur J Cardiothorac Surg. 2009;36:675–82.
Rajasinghe HA, McElhinney DB, Reddy VM, Mora BN, Hanley FL. Long-term follow-up of truncus arteriosus repaired in infancy: a twenty-year experience. J Thorac Cardiovasc Surg. 1997;113:869–79.
Ramirez-Marroquin S, Curi-Curi PJ, Calderon-Colmenero J, Garcia-Montes JA, Cervahtes-Salazar JL. Common arterial trunk repair by means of a handmade bovine pericardial-valved woven Dacron conduit. World J Pediatr Cong Heart Surg. 2017;8:69–76.
Rao IM, Swanson JS, Hovaguimian H, McIrvin DM, King DH, Starr A. Anterior pulmonary translocation for repair of truncus arteriosus with interrupted arch. Ann Thorac Surg. 1995;59(1):216–8.
Rastelli GC, Titus JL, McGoon DC. Homograft of ascending aorta and aortic valve as a right ventricular outflow: an experimental approach to the repair of truncus arteriosus. Arch Surg. 1967;95:698–708.
Reddy VM, Rajasinghe HA, McElhinney DB, Hanley FL. Performance of right ventricle to pulmonary artery conduits after repair of truncus arteriosus: a comparison of Dacron-housed porcine valves and cryopreserved allografts. Semin Thorac Cardiovasc Surg. 1995;7(3):133–8.
Ross DN, Somerville J. Correction of pulmonary atresia with a homograft aortic valve. Lancet. 1966;2(7479):1446–7.
Rowe RD, Freedom RM, Mehrizi A, Bloom KR. The neonate with congenital heart disease. Philadelphia: WB Saunders; 1981.
Russell HM, Jacobs ML, Anderson RH, et al. A simplified categorization for common arterial trunk. J Thorac Cardiovasc Surg. 2011;141:645–53.
Russell HM, Mavroudis CD, Backer CL, Mavroudis C. Long-term follow up after truncal valve repair. Cardiol Young. 2012a;22:718–23.
Russell HM, Pasquali SK, Jacobs JP, Jacobs ML, O'Brien S, Mavroudis C, Backer CL. Outcomes of common arterial trunk with truncal insufficiency: a review of the STS Congenital Heart Surgery Database. Ann Thorac Surg. 2012b;93:164–9.
Schaff HV, DiDonato RM, Danielson GK, Puga FJ, Ritter DG, Edwards WD, et al. Reoperation for obstructed pulmonary ventricle-pulmonary artery conduits. Early and late results. J Thorac Cardiovasc Surg. 1984;88(3):334–43.
Schaff HV, Danielson GK, Puga FJ. Truncus arteriosus. In: Arciniegas E, editor. Pediatric cardiac surgery. Chicago: Year Book Medical; 1985.
Shapiro PF. Truncus solitarius pulmonalis. A rare type of congenital cardiac anomaly. Arch Pathol. 1930;10:671.
Slavik Z, Keeton BR, Salmon AP, Sutherland GR, Fong LV, Monro JL. Persistent truncus arteriosus operated during infancy: long-term follow-up. Pediatr Cardiol. 1994;15(3):112–5.
Smith GW, Thompson WM Jr, Dammann JF Jr, Muller WH Jr. Use of the pulmonary artery banding procedure in treating type II truncus arteriosus. Circulation. 1964;29:108–13.
Sodian R, Hoerstrup SP, Sperling JS, Martin DP, Daebritz S, Mayer JE Jr, et al. Evaluation of biodegradable, three-dimensional matrices for tissue engineering of heart valves. ASAIO J. 2000;46(1):107–10.
Squarcia U, Squarcia A. Giancarlo Rastelli: the scientist, the man. Clin Cardiol. 2007;30:485–7.
Stark J, Gandhi D, de Leval M, Macartney F, Taylor JF. Surgical treatment of persistent truncus arteriosus in the first year of life. Br Heart J. 1978;40(11):1280–7.
Stock UA, Nagashima M, Khalil PN, Nollert GD, Herden T, Sperling JS, et al. Tissue-engineered valved conduits in the pulmonary circulation. J Thorac Cardiovasc Surg. 2000;119(4 Pt 1):732–40.
Thompson LD, McElhinney DB, Reddy M, Petrossian E, Silverman NH, Hanley FL. Neonatal repair of truncus arteriosus: continuing improvement in outcomes. Ann Thorac Surg. 2001;72(2):391–5.
Tiete AR, Sachweh JS, Roemer U, Kozlik-Feldmann R, Reichart B, Daebritz SH. Right ventricular outflow tract reconstruction with the Contegra bovine jugular vein conduit: a word of caution. Ann Thorac Surg. 2004;77(6):2151–6.
Tlaskal T, Hucin B, Kucera V, Vojtovic P, Gebauer R, Chaloupecky V, et al. Repair of persistent truncus arteriosus with interrupted aortic arch. Eur J Cardiothorac Surg. 2005;28(5):736–41.
Tlaskal T, Chaloupecky V, Hucin B, Gebauer R, Krupickova S, Reich O, Skovranek J, Tax P. Long-term results after correction of persistent truncus arteriosus in 83 patients. Eur J Cardiothorac Surg. 2010;37:1278–84.

Ullmann MV, Gorenflo M, Sebening C, Ulmer HE, Hagl S. Long-term results after repair of truncus arteriosus communis in neonates and infants. Thorac Cardiovasc Surg. 2003;51(4):175–9.
Urban AE, Sinzobahamvya N, Brecher AM, Wetter J, Malorny S. Truncus arteriosus: ten-year experience with homograft repair in neonates and infants. Ann Thorac Surg. 1998;66:S183–8.
Van Mierop LH, Patterson DF, Schnarr WR. Pathogenesis of persistent truncus arteriosus in light of observations made in a dog embryo with the anomaly. Am J Cardiol. 1978;41:755–62.
Van Praagh R, Van Praagh S. The anatomy of common aorticopulmonary trunk (truncus arteriosus communis) and its embryologic implications. A study of 57 necropsy cases. Am J Cardiol. 1965;16:406–25.
Victoria BE, Krovetz LJ, Elliott LP, et al. Persistent truncus arteriosus in infancy. Am Heart J. 1969;77:13–25.
Vohra HA, Whistance RN,,Chia AX, ,Janusauskas V,, Nikolaidis N,,Roubelakis A, Veldtman G, Haw MP. (2010) Long-term follow-up after primary complete repair of common arterial trunk with homograft: a 40-year experience. J Thorac Cardiovasc Surg, 140: 325–329.
Wallace RB, Rastelli GC, Ongley PA, Titus JL, McGoon DC. Complete repair of truncus arteriosus defects. J Thorac Cardiovasc Surg. 1969;57:95–107.
Weipert J, Meisner H, Mendler N, Haehnel JC, Homann M, Paek SU, et al. Allograft implantation in pediatric cardiac surgery: surgical experience from 1982 to 1994. Ann Thorac Surg. 1995;60(2 Suppl):S101–4.
Wesolowski SA. The healing of vascular prostheses. Surgery. 1965;57:319–24.
Wilson J. A description of a very unusual malformation of the human heart. Philos Trans R Soc Lond [Biol]. 1798;18:346–56.
Yokoyama S, Nagasaka S, Yoshida Y, Heima D, Soga Y, Kaneda K, Nishiwaki N. Truncus arteriosus communis with interrupted aortic arch: Successful repair using a novel technique. Ann Thorac Surg. 2013;95:714–6.

Complications Associated with Repair of Aortopulmonary Window

Constantine Mavroudis, Carl L. Backer, and Amy Heincker

Abstract

Aortopulmonary (AP) window is a communication between the main pulmonary artery and the ascending aorta in the presence of two separate semilunar valves. AP window is classified into three types: Proximal defect (type I), Distal defect (type II), and Total defect (type III). Although surgical complications of isolated AP window are uncommon, they may involve residual shunt or branch pulmonary artery stenosis. The presence of associated congenital heart defects with AP window increases the risk of surgical complications that may result in recurrent arch obstruction. This chapter will examine the surgical complications in the repair of AP window and offer solutions to avoid missteps.

Keywords

Congenital heart surgery · Aortopulmonary window · Complications · Outcomes

1 Anatomy and Classification

Aortopulmonary window is a rare congenital cardiac defect, representing approximately 0.2% of all congenital heart lesions (Richardson et al. 1979). It is the result of incomplete separation of the arterial trunk, creating an anatomic communication between the aorta and the pulmonary artery above the level of two separate semilunar valves (Richardson et al. 1979; Abbott 1936; Anderson et al. 2012; Cotton 1899; Elliotson 1830; Putnam and Gross 1966).

Although multiple classification systems exist (Richardson et al. 1979; Ho et al. 1994; Mori et al. 1978), the Mori classification (Fig. 1, types I, II, III), also adopted by the Congenital Heart Surgery Nomenclature and Database Project (Jacobs et al. 2000), is most often utilized to classify the anatomical variants into three main types. Figures 2, 3, 4, and 5 show more detailed color

C. Mavroudis (✉)
Chief of Pediatric Cardiothoracic Surgery (Retired), Peyton Manning Children's Hospital, Indianapolis, IN, USA

Professor Emeritus of Surgery, Johns Hopkins University School of Medicine, Baltimore, MD, USA

C. L. Backer
Chief, Section of Pediatric Cardiothoracic Surgery, UK Healthcare Kentucky Children's Hospital, Lexington, KY, USA

Cardiothoracic Surgery, Cincinnati Children's Hospital Medical Center, Cincinnati, OH, USA

A. Heincker
Pediatric and Congenital Heart Surgery, Peyton Manning Children's Hospital, Indianapolis, IN, USA

C. L. Backer, C. Mavroudis (eds.), *Complications in Pediatric and Congenital Heart Surgery*,
https://doi.org/10.1007/978-3-032-02661-3_11

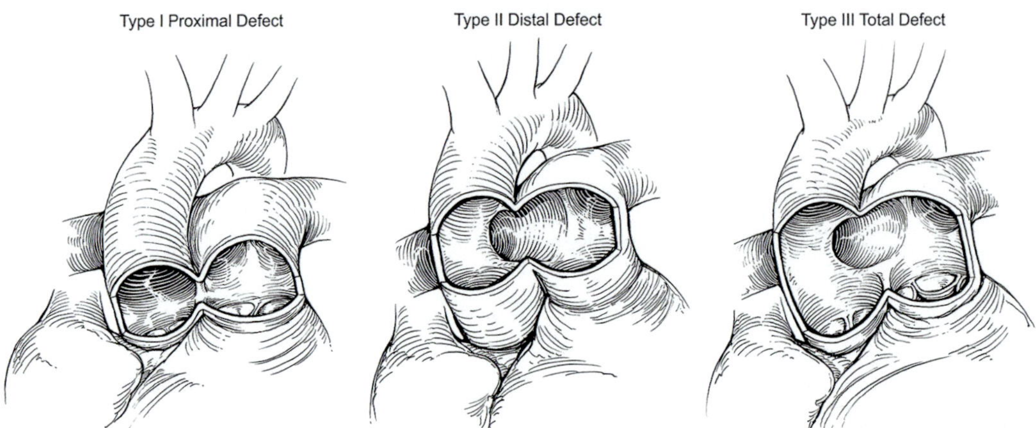

Fig. 1 Shows the Mori Classification which is based on the location and level of the aortopulmonary window. The Type I or Proximal Defect is noted in the left panel. The level of aortopulmonary connection is in the proximal ascending aorta and the pulmonary artery trunk. The type II Distal Defect is noted in the center panel which shows the aortopulmonary connection more superiorly than the Type I with an extension into the right proximal pulmonary artery. The Type III Total Defect involves an enlarged aortopulmonary window involving a combination of the proximal and distal defects ensemble. (With permission: Gaynor 2003)

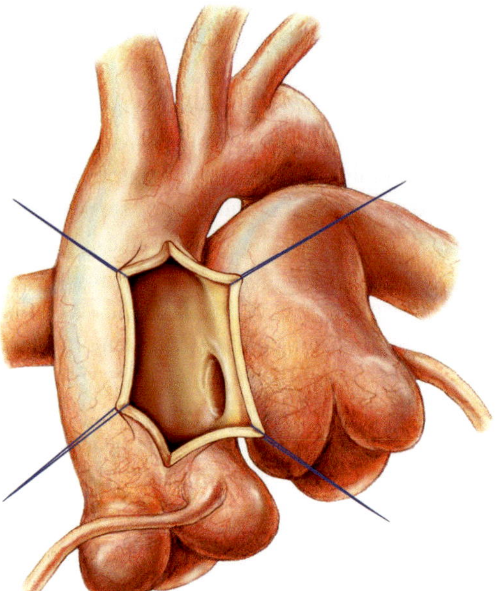

Fig. 2 Transaortic depiction of the Type I Proximal Defect which demonstrates the communicating defect above the semilunar valves. The defect is usually upstream to the orifice of the left main coronary artery which should be noted and respected in the event that there is an anomalous origin. (With permission: Backer and Mavroudis 2002)

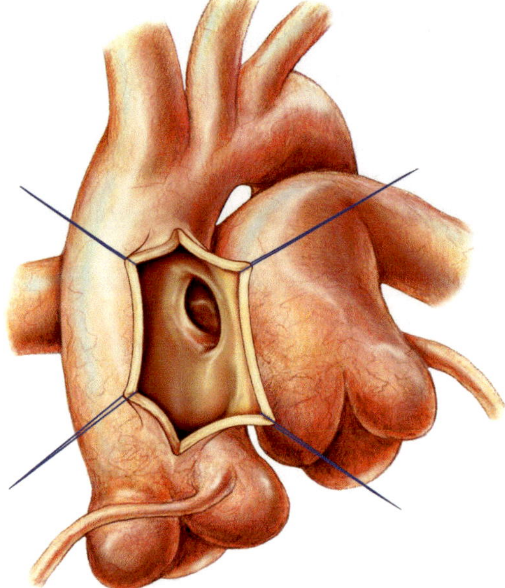

Fig. 3 Shows a longitudinal transaortic depiction of the Type II Distal Defect. The characteristics of the Type II Distal Defect are variable and may extend into the right pulmonary artery as shown in Fig. 4. The defect is well away from the semilunar valves and the origin of the coronary arteries. (With permission: Backer and Mavroudis 2002)

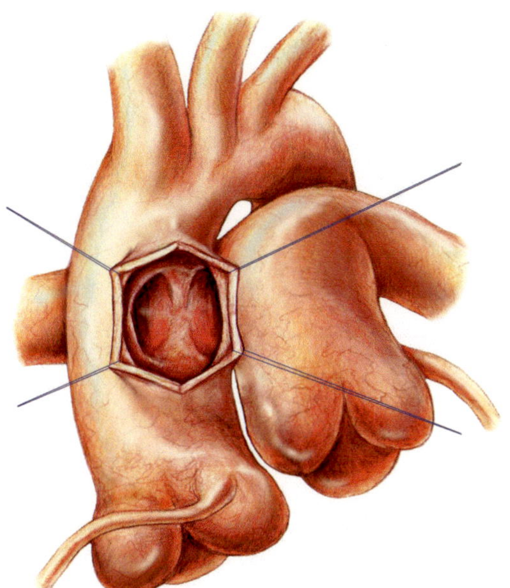

Fig. 4 Shows a longitudinal transaortic depiction of the Type II Distal Defect with extension into the origin of the right pulmonary artery. This type of defect is a variation of the Type II Distal Defect which is noted in Fig. 3. This defect is shown here to illustrate the large variation of the Type II Distal Defect which could be located at the distal aortopulmonary window or could extend into the right pulmonary artery. This distinction is important to perform the septation operation carefully to avoid right pulmonary artery stenosis. (With permission: Mavroudis 2015)

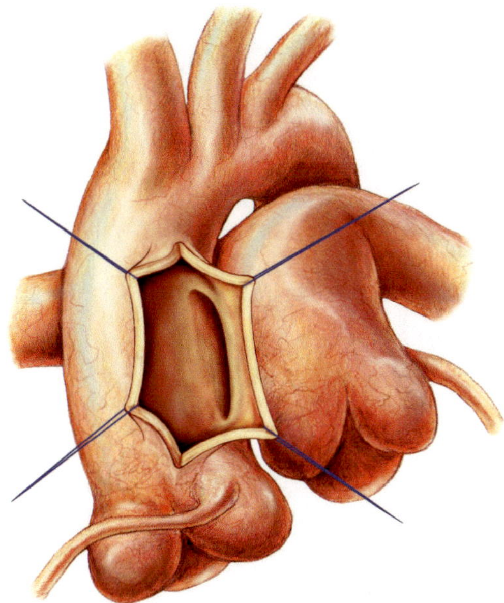

Fig. 5 Longitudinal transaortic depiction of the Type III Total Defect which anatomically is an extended combination of the Type I and Type II defects. (With permission: Backer and Mavroudis 2002)

depictions of the various types of aortopulmonary window based on the Mori Classification.

The Type I Proximal Defect (Fig. 2) is localized just above both semilunar valves. Type II Distal Defect is more variable. It is located upstream to involve the upper portion of the ascending aorta and the main pulmonary artery before the bifurcation (Fig. 3) or may involve the orifice of the right pulmonary artery as well (Fig. 4). The Type III Total Defect (Fig. 5) is a combination of the prior types and is usually much larger in cross sectional areas.

The physiologic effects are comparable to a large patent ductus arteriosus and truncus arteriosus in which the left-to-right shunt results in a wide pulse pressure and diastolic runoff into the pulmonary artery, often leading to congestive heart failure and pulmonary hypertension, depending on the size of the defect. Aortopulmonary window may occur in isolation or, commonly, in conjunction with other lesions, such as patent ductus arteriosus, ventricular septal defect, subaortic stenosis, interrupted aortic arch, tetralogy of Fallot, and single ventricle (Gangana et al. 2007).

2 Repair of Aortopulmonary Window and Associated Complications

Surgical repair is typically accomplished via patch closure of the defect; however, smaller lesions may be doubly ligated and divided (Talwar et al. 2017a). Repair is approached with standard transmediastinal cardiopulmonary bypass (Fig. 6) for a Type I Proximal Defect with control of the distal pulmonary arteries to prevent pulmonary artery runoff, similar to the approach for repair of Common Arterial Trunk (see Chapter "Complications Associated with Repair of Common Arterial Trunk"). Aortic cross-clamp is placed, and antegrade cardioplegia is adminis-

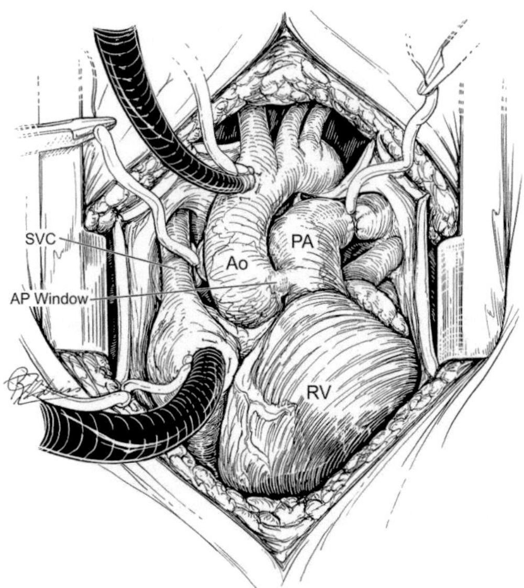

Fig. 6 Shows the cardiopulmonary bypass characteristics for repair of aortopulmonary window. In general, one arterial catheter and one atrial catheter with a left ventricular vent via the right superior pulmonary vein will be sufficient for repair unless there are other associated lesions such as a ventricular septal defect in which case bi-atrial cannulation will be required. As noted, immediately after the commencement of cardiopulmonary bypass, the right and left pulmonary arteries are controlled with snuggers to prevent pulmonary artery runoff, pulmonary overcirculation, and poor systemic perfusion. (With permission: Gaynor 2003). *Ao* aorta, *AP* aortopulmonary, *SVC* superior vena cava, *PA* pulmonary artery, *RV* right ventricle

tered with snuggers in place around the left and right pulmonary arteries to prevent runoff, ineffective cardioplegia, or poor visceral perfusion. The transaortic approach is best for visualization of the defect, which can extend into the right pulmonary artery, making the transpulmonary artery exposure difficult. Additionally, this view is best for visualizing and preserving the left coronary orifice. Many centers prefer to use a sandwiching technique via a trans-window approach (Figs. 7 and 8). Alternatively, an incision can be made through the aortopulmonary connection with individual patches being placed on the aorta and the pulmonary artery respectively (Naimo and Konstantinov 2015) We have preferred to use a polytetrafluoroethylene (PTFE) patch with running suture technique via a transaortic approach, incorporating the aortic and pulmonary artery

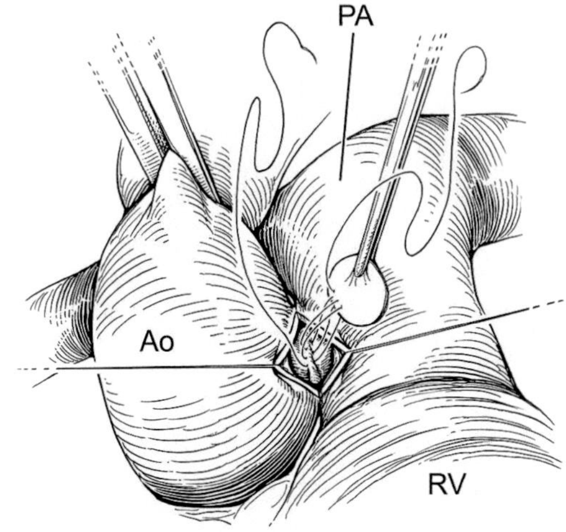

Fig. 7 Shows aortic cross-clamp and a trans-window approach using a sandwiching technique that can avoid a large transaortic incision. The suturing technique commences from the opposite side of the defect and carried to the anterior portion. Careful attention to the left coronary artery orifice is required. (With permission: Gaynor 2003). *Ao* aorta, *PA* pulmonary artery, *RV* right ventricle

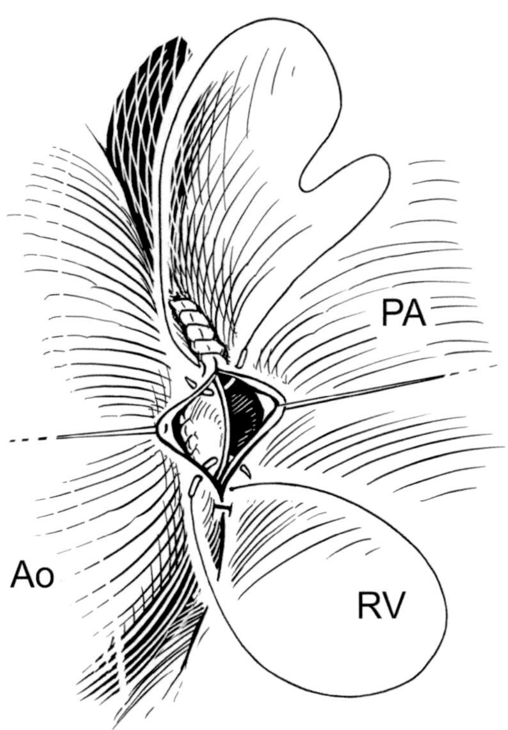

Fig. 8 Shows the continuation of the trans-window technique towards the anterior incision. (With permission: Gaynor 2003). *Ao* aorta, *PA* pulmonary artery, *RV* right ventricle

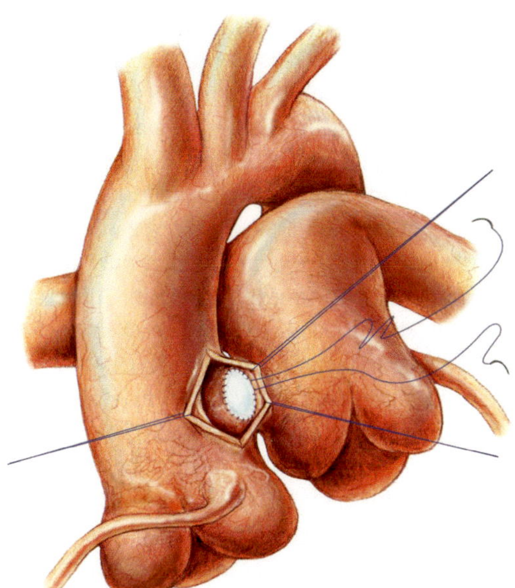

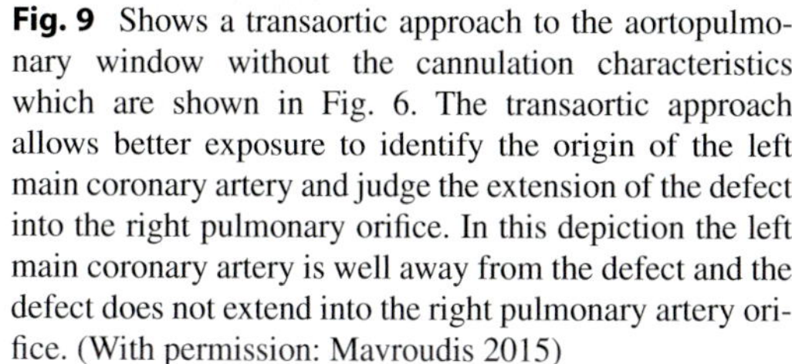

Fig. 9 Shows a transaortic approach to the aortopulmonary window without the cannulation characteristics which are shown in Fig. 6. The transaortic approach allows better exposure to identify the origin of the left main coronary artery and judge the extension of the defect into the right pulmonary orifice. In this depiction the left main coronary artery is well away from the defect and the defect does not extend into the right pulmonary artery orifice. (With permission: Mavroudis 2015)

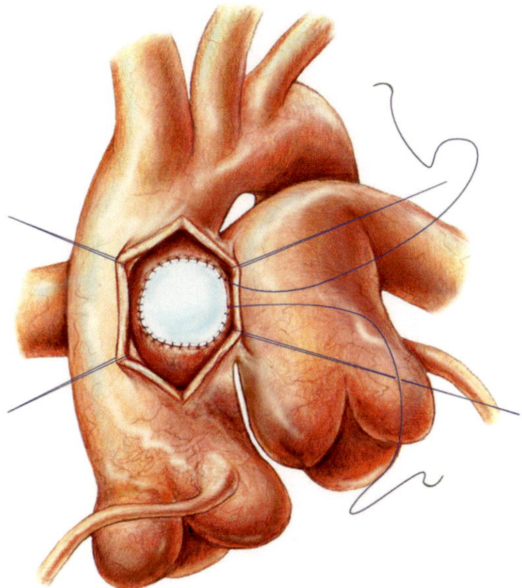

Fig. 10 Shows a transaortic approach to a Type II aortopulmonary window without the cannulation characteristics which are shown in Fig. 6. The transaortic approach allows better exposure to identify the origin of the left main coronary artery and judge the extension of the defect into the right pulmonary orifice. In this depiction the left main coronary artery is well away from the defect however, the defect extends into the orifice of the right pulmonary artery. As shown in the illustration, the transaortic approach allows repair with a large enough patch to prevent right pulmonary artery stenosis. (With permission: Mavroudis 2015)

walls into the repair for reinforcement (Johansson et al. 1978) (Fig. 9). Figure 10 shows the PTFE patch being seated to close a Type II Distal Defect when the hole involves the origin of the right pulmonary artery. Figure 11 depicts a similar technique for the larger Type III Total Defect. When dealing with a smaller, more restrictive defect, percutaneous device closure has been accomplished utilizing double disk closure devices (Demir et al. 2013; Giordano and Butera 2020).

Complications of late presentation of aortopulmonary window diagnosis are analogous to that of other large left-to-right shunts and include significant pulmonary hypertension or Eisenmenger's syndrome (Chen et al. 2020; Fotaki et al. 2017). Patients with late presentation of a significant lesion should undergo cardiac catheterization to accurately assess pulmonary artery hypertension and reversibility prior to repair (Naimo and Konstantinov 2015; Melby and Gandhi 2009).

Surgical complications of isolated aortopulmonary window repair are uncommon (Jansen et al. 2006; Naimo et al. 2014) but most frequently involve residual shunt or branch pulmonary artery stenosis (Barnes et al. 2011). Depending on the size of the residual aortopulmonary shunt, reintervention may be necessary. When the residual left-to-right shunt is identified by intraoperative transesophageal echocardiogra-

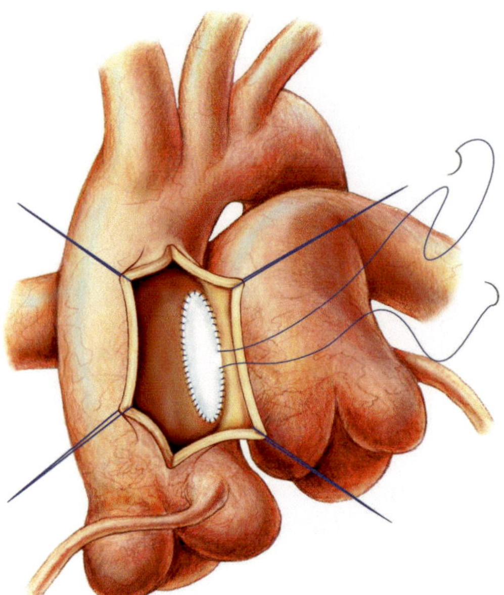

Fig. 11 Longitudinal transaortic depiction of the Type III Defect which is a combination of the proximal and distal defects. The characteristic of the drawing is similar to the surgical exposure for this anatomic variant without the cannulas and depictions of cardiopulmonary bypass, aortic cross-clamping, cardioplegic arrest, and transaortic patch repair. This approach allows excellent exposure of this large defect to respect the orifice of the left main coronary artery and allow the creation of a large enough patch to avoid right pulmonary artery stenosis. (With permission: Backer and Mavroudis 2002)

phy, reoperation should be undertaken. The reasons for the residual shunt can be caused by suture disruption due to ineffective suture placement during the running suture technique or by using a patch which proves to be too small resulting in a tear due to pressure load (Fig. 12). The repair should involve removal of the original patch with placement of a larger patch with effective suture placement. When the left-to-right shunt is not identified or when the leak is discovered late after hospital discharge, a cardiac catheterization will be required which may lead to reoperation. At the time of reoperation, the recurrent leak should be closed with another patch to avoid a second recurrence (Fig. 13). Distortion of the right pulmonary artery origin may also warrant reoperation (Talwar et al. 2017b). Branch pulmonary artery stenosis most often occurs in the right pulmonary artery, and, while amenable to balloon angioplasty (Fig. 14), a cautious approach is required so as not to recreate an aortopulmonary connection (Varan et al. 2019). Under these circumstances a repeat operation for pulmonary artery reconstruction may be needed. Additionally, coronary anatomy should be well-defined prior to intervention, and care should be taken while suturing near the coronary ostia to ensure coronary arteries are not excluded from the systemic circulation (Naimo and Konstantinov 2015). Finally, injury to the recurrent laryngeal nerve should be considered if the child demonstrates vocal hoarseness or choking with feeds following repair. Ultimately, early repair of an isolated aortopulmonary window typically results in an excellent long-term prognosis (Naimo and Konstantinov 2015).

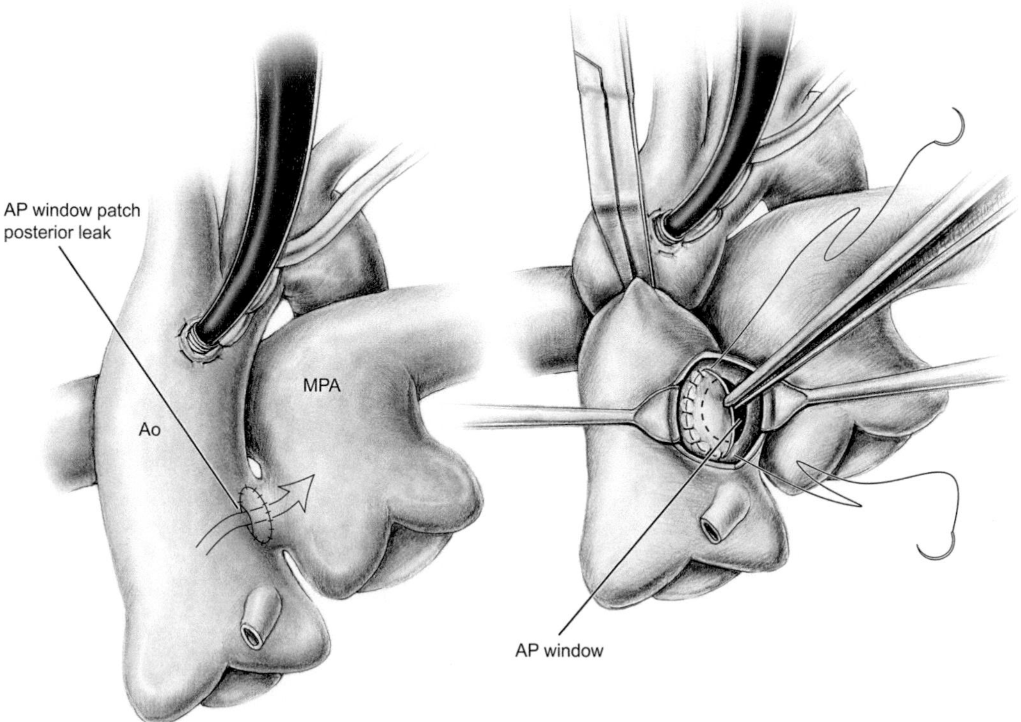

Fig. 12 Shows an intraoperative patch leak and residual left-to-right shunt after the initial operation (left panel). This situation can be identified immediately postoperatively in the operating room by transesophageal echocardiogram or much later in the postoperative period. The residual shunt can be caused by suture disruption caused by superficial purchase of the suture line or disruption caused by too small of a patch which was used for the repair. The repair (right panel) involves removal of the original patch and placement of a large patch to avoid the problem of patch disruption and recurrent left-to-right shunt. *Ao* aorta, *AP* aortopulmonary window, *MPA* main pulmonary artery

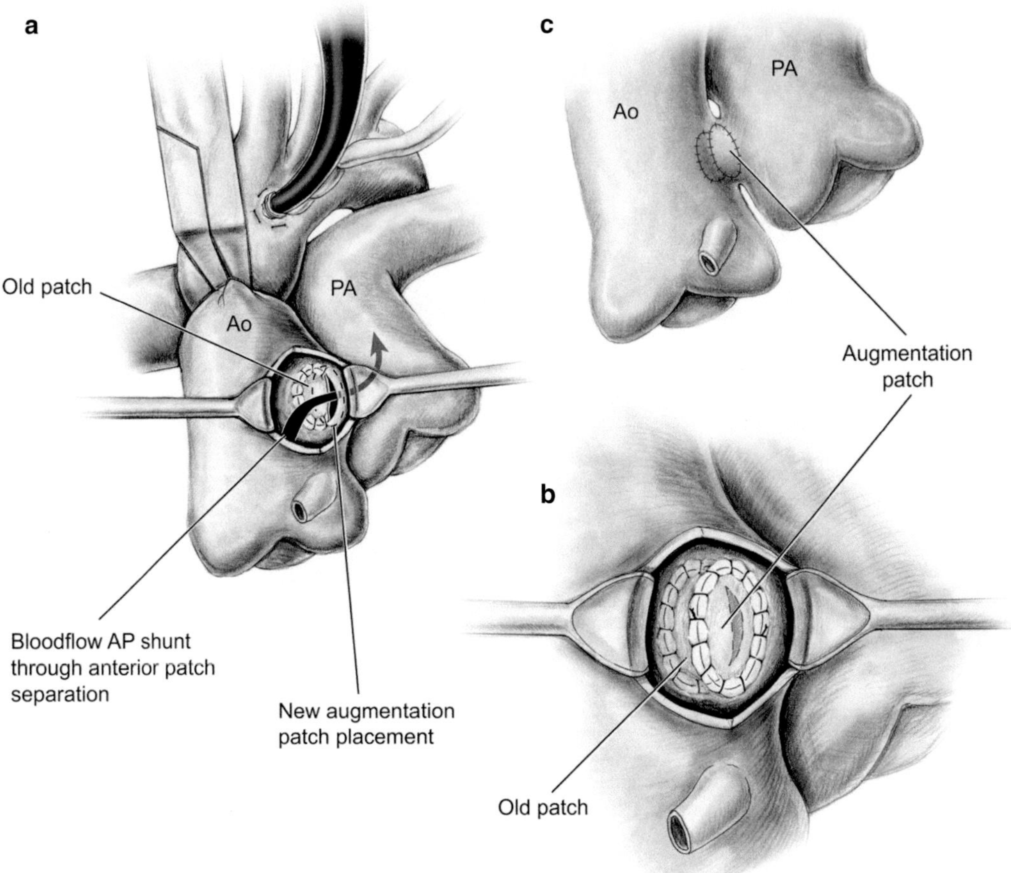

Fig. 13 Shows additional patch reinforcement of a residual left to right shunt which was caused by patch disruption during the original operation. Panel (**a**) depicts the patient with a chronic left to right shunt as a consequence of a disrupted patch at the original operation that was not discovered until a later time. Likely the cause of disruption was a small patch placed at the original operation which tore away from the arterial wall after systemic pressure was established. Panel (**b**) shows the placement of an augmentation patch at reoperation. Removal of the original patch could cause unwanted incision to the epicardium. Consequently, an additional patch is better to complete the separation of circulations. Panel (**c**) shows the completed re-repair in a ghosted manner after separation from cardiopulmonary bypass. Ao aorta, AP aortopulmonary, PA pulmonary artery

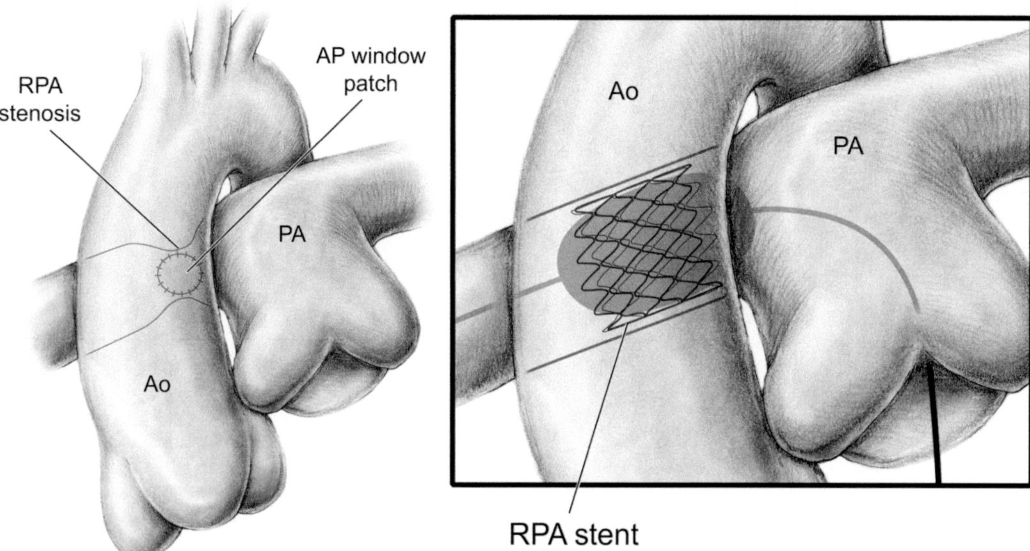

Fig. 14 Left panel shows the resultant right pulmonary artery stenosis likely caused by a small patch at the time of the original operation. The right panel shows the placement of a metal stent in the right pulmonary artery to treat right pulmonary stenosis which could have been caused by a small patch. The danger of using a stent in this location is patch disruption which can cause a recurrent aortopulmonary window. A covered stent in this location could be considered; however, when such a complication occurs, a reoperation for right pulmonary artery reconstruction and aortic reconstruction is recommended. *Ao* aorta, *AP* aortopulmonary, *PA* pulmonary artery, *RPA* right pulmonary artery

3 Repair of Aortopulmonary Window with Interrupted Aortic Arch and Associated Complications

The surgical approach to aortopulmonary window with interrupted aortic arch is largely the same as for common arterial trunk and interrupted aortic arch (See Chapter "Complications Associated with Repair of Common Arterial Trunk", Figs. 30, 31). Double arterial cannulation (ascending aorta and pulmonary artery) is not necessary since the aortopulmonary window allows for arterial flow to the ascending aorta and to the descending aorta through the patent arterial duct. Adequate perfusion and cooling are assured using this method. Figure 15 shows the cannulation technique for cardiopulmonary bypass progressing to deep hypothermia and circulatory arrest to repair the interrupted aortic arch. Alternatively, aortic cannulation via a PTFE graft to the innominate artery to achieve selective cerebral perfusion (Chapter "Complications Associated with Repair of Interrupted Aortic Arch", Figures A–E) can be utilized. Figure 16 shows the establishment of deep hypothermia and circulatory arrest with takedown of the aortopulmonary window, ligation of patent ductus arteriosus, mobilization of the descending aorta, and the planned (dotted line) incision into the

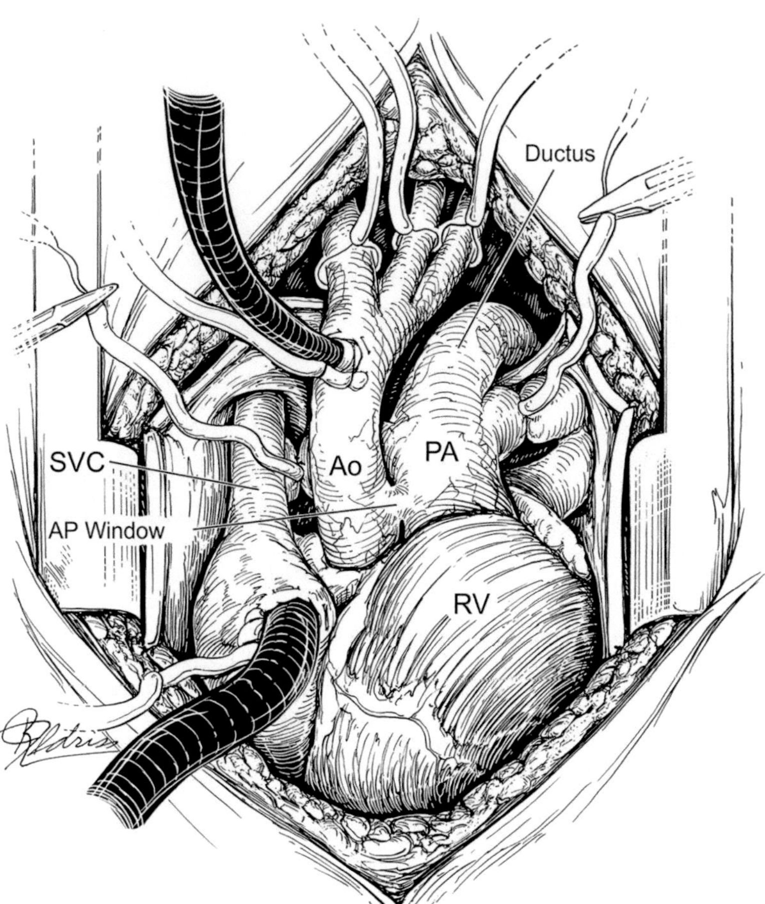

Fig. 15 Double arterial cannulation to assure systemic perfusion and cooling is not necessary for aortopulmonary window and interrupted aortic arch because the aortopulmonary window facilitates arterial flow to the ascending aorta and to the descending aorta through the patent arterial duct. Adequate perfusion and cooling are assured using this method. This drawing shows the cannulation which can assure total systemic perfusion and cooling en route to circulatory arrest and repair of interrupted aortic arch. Alternatively, aortic cannulation via a PTFE graft to the innominate artery to achieve selective cerebral perfusion can be used instead of the circulatory arrest technique. (With permission: Gaynor 2003). *Ao* aorta, *PA* pulmonary artery, *RV* right ventricle, *SVC* superior vena cava

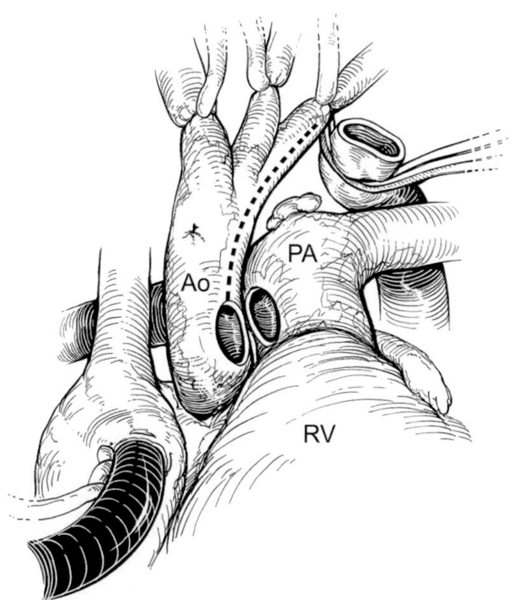

Fig. 16 Illustrates the result of deep hypothermia and circulatory arrest with takedown of the aortopulmonary window, ligation of patent ductus arteriosus, mobilization of the descending aorta, and the planned (dotted line) incision into the ascending aorta for the proposed neoaortic reconstruction. The aortic cannula has been removed to clearly show the anatomy and the proposed operation. (With permission: Gaynor 2003). *Ao* aorta, *PA* pulmonary artery, *RV* right ventricle

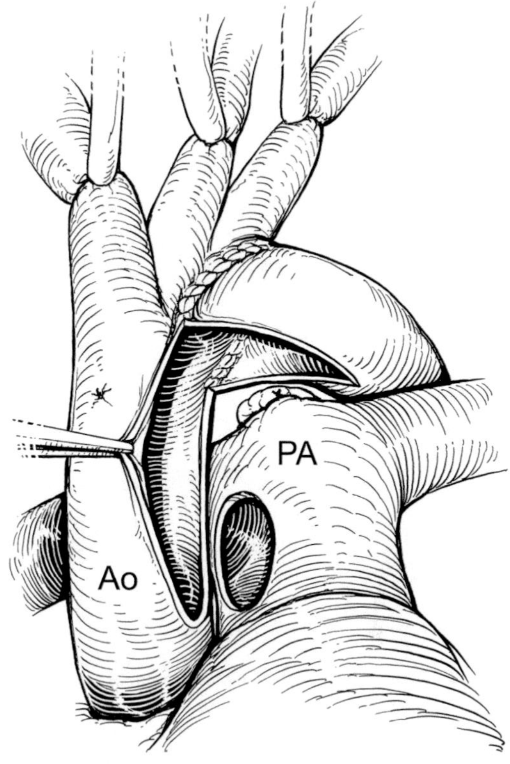

Fig. 17 Shows how the neoaortic transverse arch and ascending aorta are to be aligned and repaired by primary anastomosis and augmented with a patch. The partial primary aortic anastomosis between the descending aorta and the transverse arch is shown with a superior incision into the proximal left subclavian artery. (With permission: Gaynor 2003). *Ao* aorta, *PA* pulmonary artery, *RV* right ventricle

ascending aorta for the proposed neoaortic reconstruction. Figure 17 illustrates the initial partial aortic anastomosis between the descending aorta and the transverse arch and incised subclavian artery. The neoaortic reconstruction is augmented with a pulmonary or aortic homograft. The pulmonary artery defect which was initially part of the aortopulmonary defect is closed using a patch, thereby completing the repair (Fig. 18). The patient can then be placed on cardiopulmonary bypass or revert to total body circulation if selective cerebral perfusion was chosen for the arch reconstruction.

Understandably, the presence of associated complex congenital heart disease increases the risk of complications associated with repair

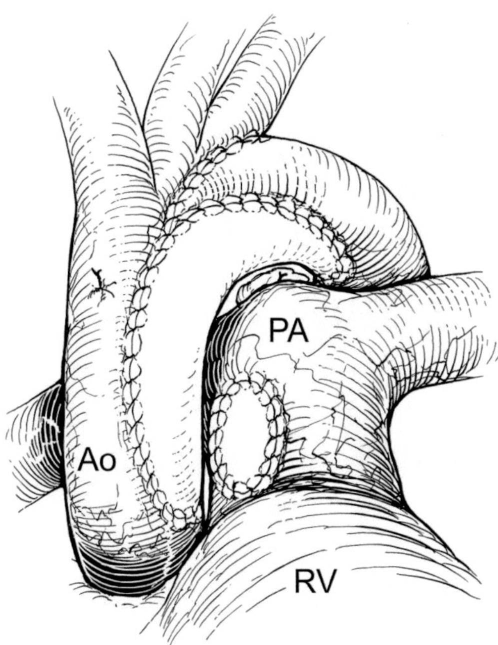

Fig. 18 Shows the result of neoaortic patch augmentation of the ascending and transverse aorta using a pulmonary or aortic homograft. The pulmonary artery defect which was initially part of the aortopulmonary defect is closed using a patch, thereby completing the reconstruction. (With permission: Gaynor 2003). *Ao* aorta, *PA* pulmonary artery, *RV* right ventricle

(Naimo et al. 2014; Konstantinov et al. 2006). Recurrent aortic arch obstruction is a known complication in this population and can require cardiac reoperation or balloon angioplasty. Figure 19 shows successful balloon dilatation of the stenotic segment (Demir et al. 2013; Konstantinov et al. 2006; Backer and Mavroudis 2002). Mild left ventricular dysfunction requiring postoperative diuretics and afterload reduction has been reported, as has residual pulmonary hypertension requiring sildenafil (Gowda et al. 2017). Additionally, one must be mindful of complications associated with the repair of concomitant lesions, such as injury to the conduction system, thoracic duct, or recurrent laryngeal nerve. Patients with more complex physiology tend to have lengthier hospital courses and increased morbidity and mortality but largely similar late survival rates (Talwar et al. 2017b). Overall, the outcomes following early and complete surgical repair of aortopulmonary window, even when associated with complex congenital cardiac defects, are quite favorable (Alsoufi et al. 2016; Bin-Moallim et al. 2020; Ghaderian 2012).

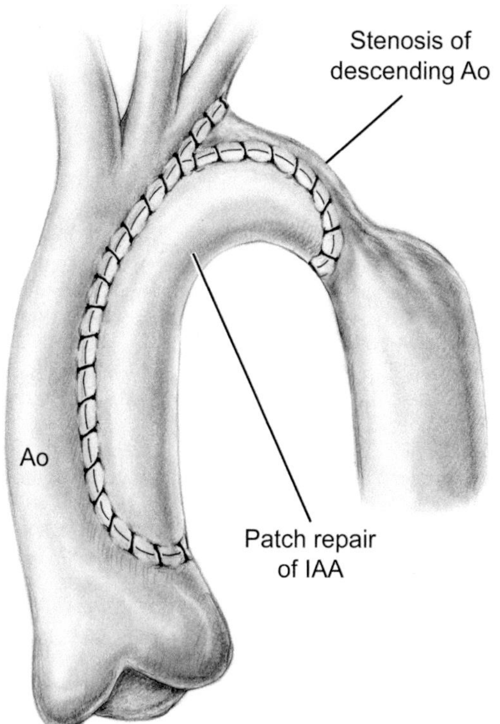

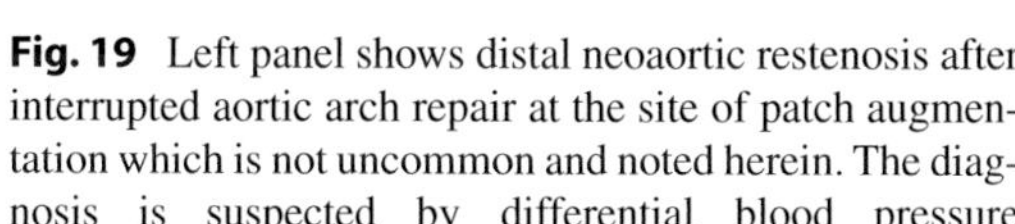

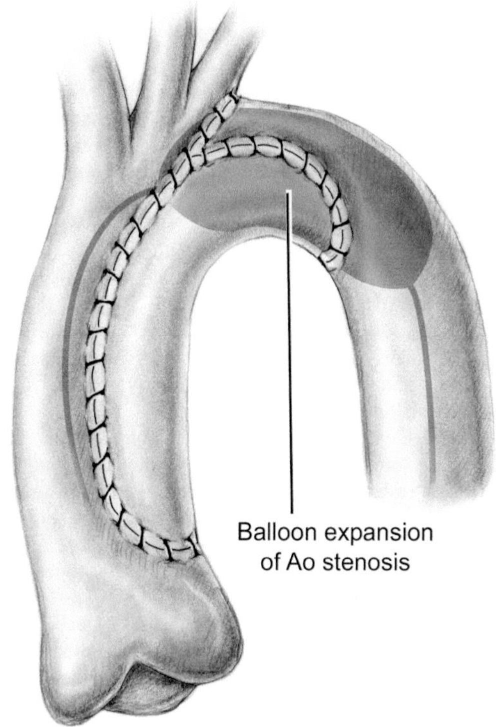

Fig. 19 Left panel shows distal neoaortic restenosis after interrupted aortic arch repair at the site of patch augmentation which is not uncommon and noted herein. The diagnosis is suspected by differential blood pressure measurements comparing the upper and lower extremities. The right panel shows a focused balloon dilatation of the stenotic segment which is generally sufficient in treating this problem. *Ao* aorta, *IAA* interrupted aortic arch

References

Abbott ME. Atlas of congenital cardiac disease. New York: American Heart Association; 1936.

Alsoufi B, Schlosser B, McCracken C, Kogon B, Kanter K, Border W, Sachdeva R. Current outcomes of surgical management of aortopulmonary window and associated cardiac lesions. Ann Thorac Surg. 2016;102:608–14.

Anderson RH, Chaudhry B, Mohun TJ, et al. Normal and abnormal development of the intrapericardial arterial trunks in humans and mice. Cardiovasc Res. 2012;95:108–15.

Backer CL, Mavroudis C. Surgical management of aortopulmonary window: a 40-year experience. Eur J Cardiothorac Surg. 2002;21:773–9.

Barnes ME, Mitchell ME, Tweddell JS. Aortopulmonary window. Semin Thorac Cardiovasc Surg Pediat Card Surg Ann. 2011;14:67–74.

Bin-Moallim M, Hamadah HK, Alhabshan F, Alghamdi AA, Kabbani MS. Aortopulmonary window: types, associated cardiovascular anomalies, and surgical outcome. Retrospective analysis of a single center experience. J Saudi Heart Assoc. 2020;32:127.

Chen J, Guo J, Cao S. Unexplained pulmonary hypertension: an overlooked aortopulmonary window. Eur Heart J. 2020;41:1217.

Cotton A. Report of a case of anuria. Trans Am Pediatr Soc. 1899;11:858–63.

Demir İH, Erdem A, Saritaş T, Demir F, Nurdan ER, Yücel İK, Aydemir NA, Çelebi A. Diagnosis, treatment and outcomes of patients with aortopulmonary window. Balkan Med. 2013:191–6.

Elliotson J. Case of malformation of the pulmonary artery and aorta. Lancet. 1830;1:247–51.

Fotaki A, Novaes J, Jicinska H, Carvalho JS. Fetal aortopulmonary window: case series and review of the literature. Ultrasound Obstet Gynecol. 2017;49:533–9.

Gangana CS, Malheiros AF, Alves EV, Azevedo MA, Bernardes RM, Simões LC. Aortopulmonary window: impact of associated lesions on surgical results. Arq Bras Cardiol. 2007;88:402–7.

Gaynor W. Aortopulmonary window and aortic origin of a pulmonary artery. In: Mavroudis C, Backer CL, editors. Pediatric cardiac surgery. 3rd ed. Philadelphia: Mosby; 2003.

Ghaderian M. Aortopulmonary window in infants. Heart Views. 2012;13:103.

Giordano M, Butera G. Percutaneous closure of an aortopulmonary window in a young adult patient: a case report of transcatheter closure with an occluder device. Eur Heart J-Case Rep Jun. 2020;4(3):1–4.

Gowda D, Gajjar T, Rao JN, Chavali P, Sirohi A, Pandarinathan N, Desai N. Surgical management of aortopulmonary window: 24 years of experience and lessons learned. Inter CardioVasc Thorac Surg. 2017;25:302–9.

Ho SY, Gerlis LM, Anderson C, Devine WA, Smith A. The morphology of aortopulmonary windows with regard to their classification and morphogenesis. Cardiol Young. 1994;4:146–55.

Jacobs JP, Quintessenza JA, Gaynor JW, Burke RP, Mavroudis C. Congenital heart surgery nomenclature and database project: aortopulmonary window. Ann Thorac Surg. 2000;1(69):44–9.

Jansen C, Hruda J, Rammeloo L, Ottenkamp J, Hazekamp MG. Surgical repair of aortopulmonary window: thirty-seven years of experience. Pediatr Cardiol. 2006;27:552–6.

Johansson L, Michaelsson M, Westerholm CJ, Åberg T. Aortopulmonary window: a new operative approach. Ann Thorac Surg. 1978;25:564–7.

Konstantinov IE, Karamlou T, Williams WG, Quaegebeur JM, del Nido PJ, Spray TL, Caldarone CA, Blackstone EH, McCrindle BW, Society CH. Surgical management of aortopulmonary window associated with interrupted aortic arch: a Congenital Heart Surgeons Society study. J Thorac Cardiovasc Surg. 2006;131:1136–341.

Mavroudis C. Aortopulmonary window. In: Mavroudis C, Backer CL, editors. Atlas of pediatric cardiac surgery. London: Springer; 2015.

Melby SJ, Gandhi SK. Current treatment of aortopulmonary window. Curr Treat Opt Cardiovasc Med. 2009;11:392–5.

Mori K, Ando M, Takao A, Ishikawa S, Imai Y. Distal type of aortopulmonary window. Report of 4 cases. Heart. 1978;40:681–9.

Naimo PS, Konstantinov IE. Aortopulmonary window repair in children. Oper Tech Thorac Cardiovasc Surg. 2015;1:370–83.

Naimo PS, Yong MS, d'Udekem Y, Brizard CP, Kelly A, Weintraub R, Konstantinov IE. Outcomes of aortopulmonary window repair in children: 33 years of experience. Ann Thorac Surg. 2014;98:1674–9.

Putnam TC, Gross RE. Surgical management of aortopulmonary fenestration. Surgery. 1966;59:727–35.

Richardson JV, Doty DB, Rossi NP, Ehrenhaft JL. The spectrum of anomalies of aortopulmonary septation. J Thorac Cardiovasc Surg. 1979;78:21–7.

Talwar S, Siddharth B, Gupta SK, Choudhary SK, Kothari SS, Juneja R, Saxena A, Airan B. Aortopulmonary window: results of repair beyond infancy. Inter CardioVasc Thorac Surg. 2017a;25:740–4.

Talwar S, Agarwal P, Choudhary SK, Kothari SS, Juneja R, Saxena A, Airan B. Aortopulmonary window: morphology, diagnosis, and long-term results. J Card Surg. 2017b;32:138–44.

Varan B, Yakut K, Tokel K, Özkan S, Aşlamacı S. A rare complication of balloon pulmonary angioplasty: aortopulmonary window and its treatment. Anat J Cardiol. 2019;21:46.

Complications Associated with Repair of Tetralogy of Fallot

Constantine Mavroudis

Abstract

The four anatomic features that characterize Tetralogy of Fallot (TOF) are: (1) stenosis of the pulmonary artery, (2) ventricular septal defect (VSD), (3) rightward deviation of the aortic root, and (4) right ventricular hypertrophy. Surgical measures to treat TOF have not been settled and questions still remain regarding timing of the intervention, pre-repair palliation, and valve preservation options. In this chapter complications associated with palliative procedures, right ventricular outflow tract obstruction, direct closure of the VSD, tricuspid disruption, aortic valve injury, chordal transection, and injury to the leaflets will be discussed and methods to resolve these complications will be addressed.

Keywords

Congenital heart surgery · Tetralogy of Fallot

C. Mavroudis (✉)
Chief of Pediatric Cardiothoracic Surgery (Retired), Peyton Manning Children's Hospital, Indianapolis, IN, USA

Professor Emeritus of Surgery, Johns Hopkins University School of Medicine, Baltimore, MD, USA

1 Introduction

While this book is written to describe and resolve complications that are associated with repair of congenital heart disease, it is useful to review historical, morphologic, and management aspects of disease patterns which will help to understand the basis of repair options and complications that can occur relevant to unusual anatomic structures.

2 Definition, Morphology, and Nomenclature

The history of tetralogy of Fallot is rich and extends back to 1671 in a report by the Danish monk Niels Stetson who noted the anatomy which would become tetralogy of Fallot in an ectopic fetal heart (Steno 1671). This discovery was followed by the French physician Etienne-Louis Fallot in 1888, who published his clinic-pathologic findings in his treatise, "Contribution à l'anatomie pathologique de la maladie bleue (Fallot 1888)". His description was the first to note the four elements of the "blue baby syndrome" and included pulmonary artery stenosis, ventricular septal defect, rightward deviation of the aortic root, and right ventricular hypertrophy (Fig. 1). In 1892, Ambrose Birmingham, Professor of Anatomy at the University of Dublin, Ireland, offered the description of the constellation of findings as the

C. L. Backer, C. Mavroudis (eds.), *Complications in Pediatric and Congenital Heart Surgery*,
https://doi.org/10.1007/978-3-032-02661-3_12

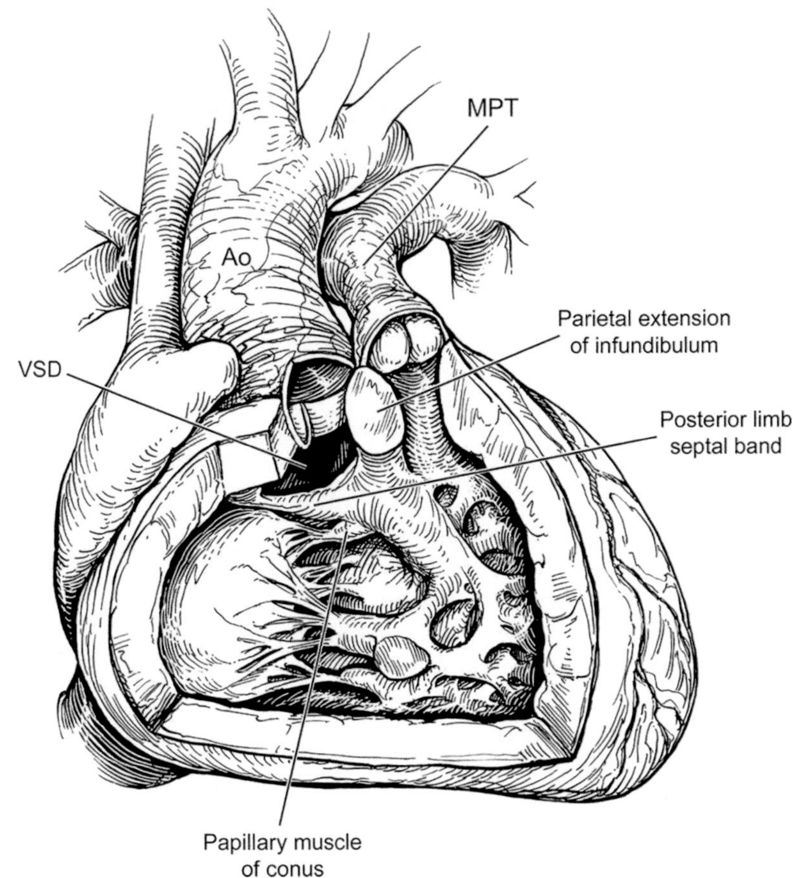

Fig. 1 Pathologic anatomy of tetralogy of Fallot demonstrating a nonrestrictive malalignment ventricular septal defect with aortic override. Right ventricular outflow tract obstruction caused by hypertrophied parietal and septal bands and the hypoplastic main pulmonary trunk and valve. (With permission: Hirsch and Bove 2003). *Ao* aorta, *MPT* main pulmonary trunk, *TV* tricuspid valve, *VSD* ventricular septal defect

"Pentalogy of Fallot" to account for the common presence of atrial septal defect (ASD) (Birmingham 1892). The accepted prevalent term, tetralogy of Fallot (TOF), was to be introduced by Maude Abbott, in the clinical classification of congenital heart defects which was published by Dawson and Abbott in 1924 (Abbott 1924).

Important embryological findings have led to fetal developmental theories that have lent more scientific considerations to the aforementioned anatomic findings of tetralogy of Fallot. These theories have centered on a single alteration in fetal cardiac development rather than the four-lesion set of the disease. Van Praagh and his associates described a theory that proposed underdevelopment of the subpulmonary infundibulum to be the primary lesion, noting this portion of the heart as "too narrow, too shallow, and too short" (Van Praagh 1989; Van Praagh et al. 1970). Further to this analysis, Anderson and colleagues noted that the infundibulum to be narrow and hypoplastic during embryologic development and variable in length to account for tetralogy hearts which have a longer than normal infundibulum (Becker et al. 1975; Howell et al. 1990). Their theory is consistent with their assertion that there is anterocephalad deviation of the insertion of the infundibular septum, relative to the septomarginal trabeculation. This accounts for the abnormal relation of the outlet septum to the septoparietal trabeculations, producing subpulmonary obstruction (Anderson and Weinberg 2005). One can imagine anteroseptal migration of the infundibulum septum that accounts for an overriding aorta and subpulmonary stenosis.

Common to the single embryologic development thesis is that the ventricular septal defect (VSD) in TOF, occurs due to the anterocephalad malalignment and deviation of the insertion of the infundibular septum, relative to the limbs of the septomarginal trabeculation. This results in an overriding aorta which straddles the ventricular septum. This type of VSD is described by Anderson as an outlet defect (Anderson and Weinberg 2005). Others describe this defect as a malaligned, conoventricular defect. Physiologically, the tetralogy associated VSD is large and nonrestrictive. The anatomic details for VSD closure, especially through a transatrial approach, are important to avoid heart block, VSD recurrence, tricuspid valve disruption, and aortic valve leaflet injury.

In keeping with the complexity of TOF, pulmonary stenosis is variable, is often associated with a bicuspid valve, and in extreme cases, pulmonary atresia can be present. These anatomic findings are very important when one is considering pulmonary valve sparing operations with repair of TOF and clearly enter in the overall discussion of potential complications in the management of right ventricular outflow tract obstruction.

Anatomic variability regarding right ventricular outflow associated with the spectrum of TOF with pulmonary stenosis is characterized by anatomic variants of anterior and cephalad deviation of the outlet septum (Dodge-Khatami et al. 2023). The localized narrowing of the os infundibulum can be identified at the inferior border of the right ventricular infundibulum. The pulmonary valve morphology is also variable and is usually characterized by thickened immobile leaflets, commissural fusion, leaflet tethering to the pulmonary artery wall, and has been reported to be bicuspid in over 50% of cases (Altrichter et al. 1989). Stenotic portions of the right ventricular outflow tract extend to the pulmonary trunk and the distal pulmonary arteries as well. Frequently, there is discrete narrowing caused by a fibrous shelf within the proximal left branch pulmonary artery at the level of the patent arterial duct/ligamentum insertion site. This reality has caused surgeons to extend the patch repair of the pulmonary outflow tract to an area well beyond the proximal right pulmonary artery or perform a resection and end-to-end anastomosis of the proximal left pulmonary artery. As noted by Dodge-Khatami and associates (Dodge-Khatami et al. 2023),

"The International Working Group for Mapping and Coding of Nomenclatures for Pediatric and Congenital Cardiac Disease adopted the following consensus definition in 2008:

> *Tetralogy of Fallot is defined as a group of malformations with biventricular atrioventricular alignments or connections characterized by antero-superior deviation of the conal or outlet septum or its fibrous remnant, narrowing or atresia of the pulmonary outflow, a ventricular septal defect of the malalignment type, and biventricular origin of the aorta. Hearts with tetralogy of Fallot will always have a ventricular septal defect, narrowing or atresia of the pulmonary outflow, and aortic override; hearts with tetralogy of Fallot will most often have right ventricular hypertrophy.* (Beland et al. 2004)

The diagnostic choices used for coding in the contemporary version of the Society of Thoracic Surgeons Congenital Heart Surgery Database are listed in Table 1 (Jacobs 2000)." Database nomenclature issues however do not distinguish in a hierarchical mode between VSD and pulmonary atresia and tetralogy. In other words, not all cases of pulmonary atresia with VSD can conclusively be characterized as a form of TOF. This is the reason why tetralogy in the database is noted as tetralogy with pulmonary stenosis to distinguish it from the other forms. Furthermore, other anatomical variants include the presence of additional VSDs, which occur in approximately 5% of cases (Dickinson et al. 1982). The most common variant of coronary artery anatomy with tetralogy is anterior descending coronary artery origin from the right coronary artery (Dabizzi

Table 1 The diagnostic short list of the version of The International Pediatric and Congenital Cardiac Code

TOF (tetralogy of Fallot)
TOF, Pulmonary stenosis
TOF, Absent pulmonary valve
TOF, AVC (AVSD)
DORV, TOF type
Pulmonary atresia, VSD (Including TOF, PA)
Pulmonary atresia, VSD-MAPCA (pseudo-truncus)

Derived from the International Congenital Heart Surgery Nomenclature and Database Project of The European Association for Cardio-Thoracic Surgery and The Society of Thoracic Surgeons et al. 1980; van Son 1995) which oftentimes dictates the type of repair. In these cases, the anterior descending coronary artery traverses the anterior surface of the right ventricular outflow tract in close proximity to the pulmonary annulus. The risk of injury is complicated by two circumstances. The first is that the artery has not been preoperatively diagnosed and not appreciated at the reparative operation. An intramyocardial course of the artery further complicates these circumstances. The second potential complication can occur from a camouflaged artery due to epicardial adhesions from a previous operation such as a systemic-to-pulmonary artery shunt. Specifically, arterial injury can occur from a ventriculotomy or from intracavitary tangential injury resulting in an arterial to right ventricular fistula during intraventricular muscle resection. In either case, significant interruption of myocardial perfusion can occur. Other less common coronary anomalies can occur as well. Dual supply to the anterior interventricular septum can occur from branches originating from both the right and left main coronary arteries. In addition, a single coronary artery can arise from the right sinus of Valsalva with anomalous arterial distribution. TOF is associated with other important congenital heart defects such as complete atrioventricular septal defect, patent foramen ovale (PFO), ostium secundum type ASD, patent arterial duct (PAD), persistent left superior vena cava, ductal origin of one branch pulmonary artery, and right-sided aortic arch (15%–25% of TOF patients) (Suzuki et al. 1990).

About 7% of patients with TOF have associated pulmonary atresia (PA), which can be further defined by those with PAD and those without PAD (Dodge-Khatami et al. 2023; Chiariello et al. 1975). The presence of a PAD in patients with TOF-PA is an important factor since it is generally the only source of pulmonary blood flow. Consequently, there may be pulmonary artery size variability to all right and left lung segments depending upon the extent of forward flow. In patients with TOF-PA and absence of the PAD, pulmonary artery arborization is much less predictable. Patient survival is therefore dependent on the degree and amount of multiple major aortopulmonary collateral arteries (MAPCAs). The clinical presentation and natural history of this type of TOF-PA is discussed in Chapter "Complications Associated with Pulmonary Atresia with Major Aortopulmonary Collateral Arteries" since many of the treatment options relate to pulmonary segment unifocalization with significant variability and challenging outcomes.

The incidence of TOF and associated variants has been determined to constitute about 10% of all types of congenital heart disease and a major cause of cyanotic heart disease along with transposition of the great arteries (Beland et al. 2004). Associated genetic syndromes are common (20%) with DiGeorge Syndrome comprising the majority (Michielon et al. 2006).

3 History of Surgical Management: How Associated Complications Influenced the Development Towards Intracardiac Repair

On November 29th, 1944, Drs. Alfred Blalock and Helen Taussig cooperated to introduce the celebrated Blalock-Taussig Shunt, which was named, "the blue baby operation" for cyanotic patients with significant pulmonary stenosis (Blalock and Taussig 1945). The collaboration was the stuff of a storied history. Blalock, with the help of Vivien Thomas, the director of the surgical laboratory at Hopkins, was experimenting with systemic arterial to pulmonary artery anastomosis to create pulmonary hypertension in an animal model. Taussig reasoned that this shunt could increase pulmonary blood flow which led to the operation which was performed by Blalock who was assisted by William P. Longmire (first assistant) and Denton Cooley (intern). Vivien Thomas stood behind Blalock in the operating room for consultation since he developed the anatomic approach in the laboratory. When the clamps were released, there was no demonstrable thrill, however, the patient became acyanotic and improved. Months later, because of increasing cyanosis, a repeat shunt was performed on the opposite side which was unsuccessful. As a result of this complication, it was determined that the operation is best performed in older patients which led to a high rate of success and by 1950, 1000 such operations had been performed by Blalock and his team (Taussig 1979).

Intrepid advances by other surgical pioneers applied the idea of increasing pulmonary artery flow using a number of methods. In London, in 1948, Thomas Holmes Sellors and Russell Claude Brock separately reported the use of genitourinary sounds to probe and dilate the right ventricular outflow tract (Brock 1948; Sellors 1948). These advances were duplicated by Charles Bailey who reported (1951) treating 8 patients with TOF in Philadelphia with the Brock procedure (Downing et al. 1951). In Chicago, Willis J. Potts performed an anastomosis between the descending thoracic aorta and the left pulmonary artery (Potts et al. 1946). Using a variation on a theme by Potts, David Waterston described and performed a posterior anastomosis of the ascending aorta to the right pulmonary artery (Waterston 1962). Both side-to-side anastomoses were relatively easy to perform, especially in younger patients which made them all the more attractive than the Blalock-Taussig shunt. Thousands of patients were improved by the Potts and Waterston shunts which at the time were thought to be long term palliation and preparation for the yet unreported safe and effective cardiopulmonary bypass. Nevertheless, complications were embedded in the process and would become significant problems relating to pulmonary hypertension due to long-standing pulmonary overcirculation and difficulty in subsequent takedown operations in association with complete repair.

It remained for C. Walton Lillehei, Richard Varco, and Herbert E Warden at the University of Minnesota on August 31, 1954 (Gott 1990), to perform the first complete repair of TOF using cross-circulation. Complications associated with direct closure of the VSD led to the development of a patch to close the VSD (Warden et al. 1954; Lillehei et al. 1955). One year later, John Kirklin who perfected the heart lung machine which was introduced by Gibbon, performed the first successful repair of TOF using cardiopulmonary bypass at the Mayo Clinic in 1955 (Kirklin et al. 1955).

4 Presentation, Diagnosis, and Medical Management

Patients with TOF present with cyanosis mostly in the neonatal period following PAD closure. If the resultant cyanosis is profound, the right ventricular outflow tract is very stenotic, and they are referred to as "blue TETs." Those with less stenosis and mild or no cyanosis are referred to as "pink TETs." When prostaglandin infusion is necessary to maintain adequate oxygen saturation after PAD closure, intervention by catheter stent placement, surgical systemic-to-pulmonary artery shunt, right ventricular outflow tract placement, or complete repair will become necessary.

The introduction and general use of prenatal echocardiography had been effective with in utero diagnosis of TOF, albeit with a less predictive account of pulmonary stenosis (Tongsong et al. 2005). Postnatal echocardiography with pulse oximetry has been effective in determining TOF diagnosis and the degree of pulmonary stenosis (Koppel et al. 2003; Sendelbach et al. 2008).

Electrocardiography is non-specific for diagnosis. The findings are marked by RV hypertrophy and right axis deviation. Chest x-ray may show the classic "boot shaped" heart resulting from RV hypertrophy and small main pulmonary artery (Fig. 2). In 15%–25% of cases, a right aortic arch is present and can be inferred on chest x-ray by the absence of an aortic knob. The lung fields are generally dark indicating under perfused parenchyma.

The diagnostic method of choice is echocardiography in most cases (Fig. 3). M-mode and Doppler echocardiography combine to evaluate the TOF anatomy (Dadlani et al. 2008; Gatzoulis et al. 2000a) which includes pressure gradient estimates of the right ventricular outflow tract and abnormal coronary artery patterns such as a left anterior descending artery arising from the right coronary artery, which is present in 3%–5% of patients (Need et al. 2000; Humes et al. 1987). Because echocardiography has been so accurate, cardiac catheterization (Fig. 4) has been reserved for those situations where there is unclear anatomy of the branch pulmonary arteries, discontinuous pulmonary arteries, and ductal-induced branch PA stenosis. In addition, if the observed oxygen saturation is out of proportion to the right ventricular outflow tract gradient, cardiac catheterization is indicated to evaluate the presence of aortopulmonary collateral arteries which will impact on the type of reparative operation.

Cardiac catheterization may also be indicated in those patients who have had a prior systemic-to-pulmonary artery shunt to screen for branch pulmonary artery stenosis or distortion at the site of anastomosis which will require patch repair. Other diagnostic techniques have been used as well. Axial imaging with three-dimensional reconstruction, which includes CT scan and magnetic resonance imaging (MRI), have an important role in preoperative evaluation of TOF and can be used as an alternative to cardiac catheterization to assess branch pulmonary artery anatomy, aortic arch configurations, and coronary artery anomalies. Furthermore, Cardiac MRI has been very useful in determining when pulmonary valve insertion is indicated (Fig. 5) (van den Berg et al. 2007; Geva et al. 1998; Roest et al. 2002; Therrien et al. 2005; Knauth and Landzberg 2005; Dave et al. 2005; Buechel et al. 2005; Hallbergson et al. 2015) based on volumetric

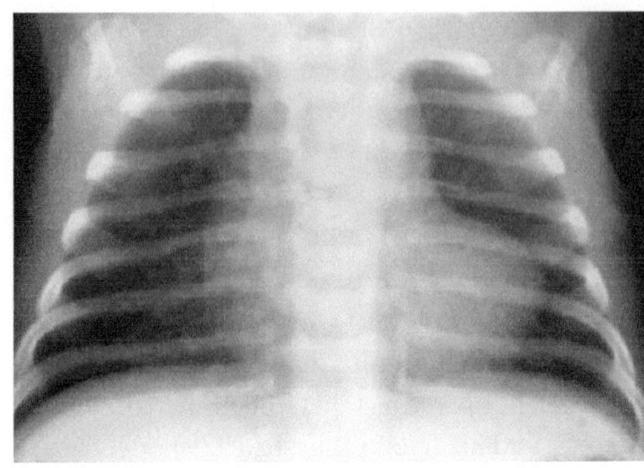

Fig. 2 Typical chest radiograph of the boot-shaped heart in a patient with tetralogy of Fallot. This appearance results from right ventricular hypertrophy and hypoplasia of the main pulmonary artery. (With permission: Hirsch and Bove 2003)

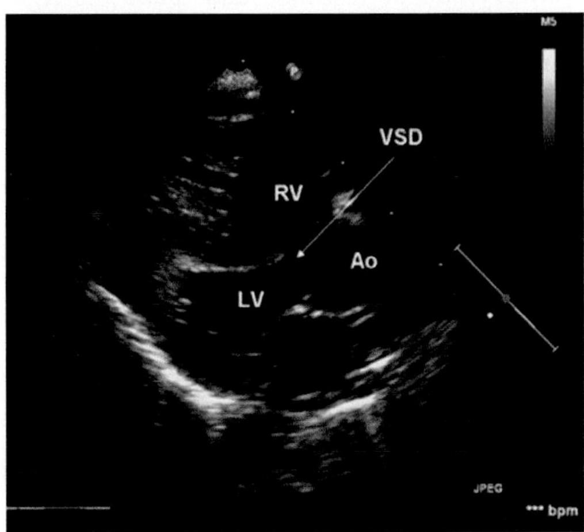

Fig. 3 Two-dimensional echocardiogram with a parasternal long access view of a patient with tetralogy of Fallot. The large unrestrictive malalignment ventricular septal defect is clearly evident with significant aortic override. (With permission: Dodge-Khatami et al. 2023). *Ao* aorta, *LV* left ventricle, *RV* right ventricle, *VSD* ventricular septal defect

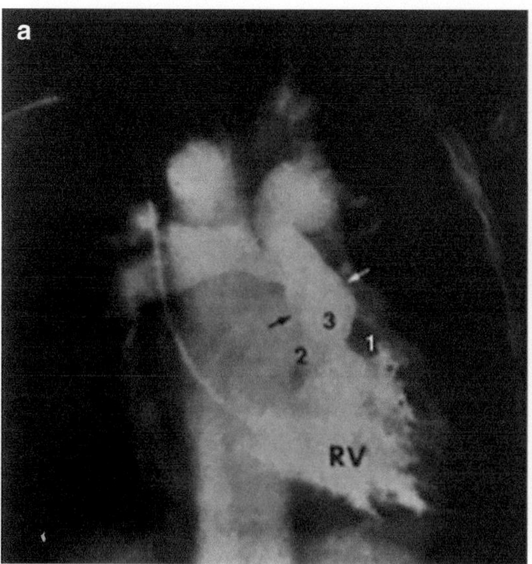

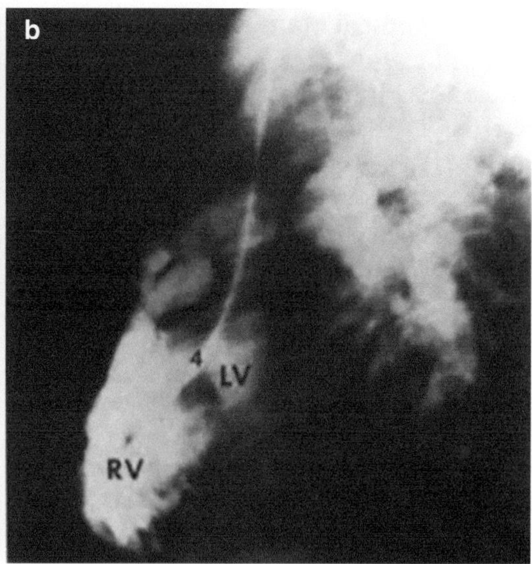

Fig. 4 Right ventricular angiograms in a patient with tetralogy of Fallot. (**a**) Frontal view demonstrating right ventricular obstruction caused by hypertrophied septal and parietal bands. There is mild stenosis of the right pulmonary artery origin and filling of the ascending aorta with contrast. The aortic arch is on the right and the left Blalock-Taussig-Thomas shunt is visible. (**b**) The lateral view demonstrates the right ventricular obstruction with anterior displacement of the infundibular (conal) septum. The stenotic pulmonary valve is seen. Contrast material outlines the ventricular septal defect and the left ventricle. (With permission: Hirsch and Bove 2003). *LV* left ventricle, *RV* right ventricle

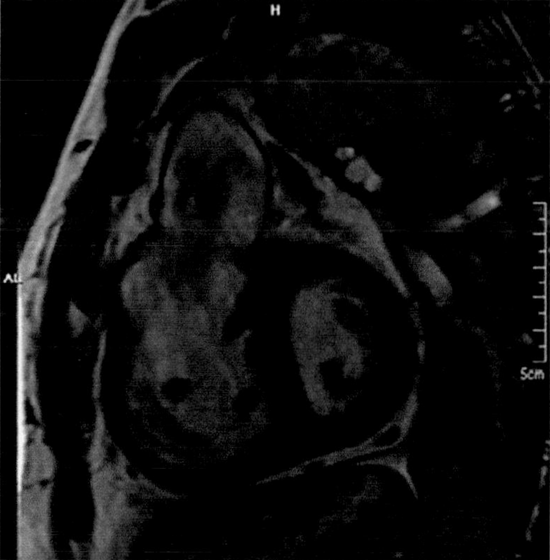

Fig. 5 Cardiac magnetic resonance image with a sagittal view of a patient with long-standing repaired tetralogy of Fallot. The right ventricle is significantly dilated, and there is severe pulmonary regurgitation. (With permission: Dodge-Khatami et al. 2023)

assessment of right ventricular end-diastolic volume index. Timely intervention for pulmonary valve insertion is an important issue since there is a metric that indicates a point after which pulmonary valve insertion is not effective. Most programs have settled on a range of 120–170 ml/m^2 as a favorable preoperative measurement that will allow remodeling and recovery of RV function after insertion of a competent pulmonary valve.

Failure to make an accurate diagnosis in the setting of TOF by echocardiography or by other techniques represents a complication of diagnosis and management which may lead to unwanted TET spells, extreme cyanosis, and acidosis in the short term and right ventricular functional preservation in the long term.

5 Medical Management

Medical management of TOF is palliative and reserved for those preoperative patients who require prostaglandin E1 (PGE1) for ductal patency in the neonatal period (Elliott et al. 1975) or right ventricular muscle relaxation (beta blockade) (Cumming 1966; Garson et al. 1981). While prostaglandin therapy has been very effective to ensure ductal patency and allow patient stabilization before surgical therapy, beta-blockade has been less so. The idea is that beta-blockade will reduce infundibular muscle spasm of the right ventricular outflow tract and allow better pulmonary blood flow. There are conflicting accounts of this therapeutic modality (Cumming 1966; Garson Jr et al. 1981). This therapy doesn't always work and more importantly, continued preoperative use can cause an increase in inotrope requirement and temporary pacing following surgical repair (Graham et al. 2008). If beta-blockade is to be used, the recommendation is to limit the therapeutic time period en route to surgical palliation or complete repair. Clearly, other important medical therapeutic interventions include supplemental oxygen, sedation, volume resuscitation, and the alpha-receptor antagonist phenylephrine, all of which have the combined hemodynamic effects of increasing oxygen saturation (Nudel et al. 1976; Tanaka et al. 2003). These aforementioned medical interventions and supportive care notwithstanding, TOF patients with repetitive hypercyanotic spells should undergo urgent surgical palliation or repair.

6 Complications Associated with Surgical Repair Options

Surgical measures to treat TOF have not been settled and questions still remain regarding timing of the intervention, pre-repair palliation, and valve preservation options, among others. In general, there are two options to consider. The first controversy involves the application of palliation or complete repair options in the surgical management of symptomatic (cyanotic) patients below a certain age or size. Complications are associated with both management schemes, especially in neonatal patients. The second controversy relates to asymptomatic (acyanotic) neonates and young infants who could be repaired at the time of diagnosis or whether they should wait until later in life when age and weight considerations are more favorable that might improve outcomes.

Early primary repair has many theoretical benefits that include (1) intervention to limit the longer cyanotic period with the associated negative impact of neurologic development, (2) lessening the degree of acquired right ventricular hypertrophy during a waiting period, (3) stimulating pulmonary artery and pulmonary alveolar development, and (4) limiting the therapeutic intervention to one reparative operation thereby avoiding the palliation and interstage problems that can occur relating to shunt malfunction and pulmonary artery distortion (Jonas 2009). Early complete repair has been proposed to avoid these potential problems with low mortality and excellent outcomes (Derby and Pizarro 2005; Di Donato et al. 1991; Hennein et al. 1995; Kolcz and Pizarro 2005; Parry et al. 2000; Pigula et al. 1999; Reddy et al. 1995; Tamesberger et al. 2008). Reports however are not uniform since others have noted increased morbidity, higher inotrope requirements, and prolonged mechanical ventilation after very early repair (Kanter et al. 2010; van Dongen et al. 2003) and higher rates of reinterventions and reoperations in infants who have undergone primary repair under 1 month of age (Hirsch et al. 2000). More granular data has been supplied by pediatric databases which have affirmed comparable outcomes and hospital charges for non-elective early primary repair compared with systemic-to-pulmonary artery shunting in symptomatic patients <90 days of age (Bacha 2018; Ramakrishnan et al. 2018).

The other side of this debate is the protagonist view that selective staged surgical management in neonates and infants with TOF is more favorable based on the unfavorable need for a transventricular approach for VSD closure and higher requirement for a transannular patch or pulmonary homograft, when performing an early primary repair. The data to support this position are gleaned from the extant literature comprised of retrospective studies with all the associated biases thereto pertaining. Nevertheless, these reports cannot be ignored. Authors have found that TOF patients less than 3 months of age receive a transannular patch in at least 50% of cases (van Dongen et al. 2003; Gustafson et al. 1988). This is in contrast to reports that document the use of a transannular patch or homograft in neonates (less than 1 month of age) in 84%–100% of cases (Hennein et al. 1995; Kolcz and Pizarro 2005; Tamesberger et al. 2008; Hirsch et al. 2000). While pulmonary regurgitation after TOF repair can be well tolerated for many years (Bacha et al. 2001; Kirklin et al. 1989), long-term observations have been well known and include an increased incidence of arrhythmia, decreased right ventricular function, and risk of sudden death (Horneffer et al. 1990; Ilbawi et al. 1987; Marie et al. 1992).

Despite the aforementioned studies that have espoused either early complete repair or staged repair, a settled clinical position has not been reached despite the advances of neonatal surgery, improved myocardial preservation techniques, and valve preservation techniques. There is however a hybrid trend towards the transatrial-transpulmonary approach for elective complete repair, with only selective systemic-to-pulmonary artery shunting of symptomatic neonates which has resulted in an increase in pulmonary valve sparing techniques with excellent outcomes (Fraser Jr et al. 2001; Karl et al. 1992; Stewart et al. 2005). There are still advantages and disadvantages of this hybrid approach. Namely, while studies have shown decreased ventricular arrhythmias and improved right ventricular function with the transatrial-transpulmonary approach, when compared with the transventricular approach (Stellin et al. 1995), it has been accompanied by higher rates of residual or recurrent right ventricular outflow tract obstruction with valve-sparing repairs. This has resulted in increased reintervention rates and progressive right ventricular hypertrophy (Bacha 2019; Kim et al. 2019). Some authors experimented with intraoperative balloon dilatation of the pulmonary valve annulus while trying to preserve pulmonary valve function. Early optimism, however, was short lived with results showing progressive pulmonary regurgitation and RV dilatation similar to the results of TOF patients with a transannular patch (Hofferberth et al. 2018; Lozano-Balseiro et al. 2019; Vida et al. 2014).

7 Complications Associated with Palliative Procedures

While complications involving palliative operations for cyanotic patients have been reviewed in Chapter "Complications Associated with Palliative Operations", this chapter will evaluate the specific options for additional pulmonary artery flow in TOF individuals. The modified Blalock-Taussig Shunt (MBTS) which was introduced by de Leval and associates in 1981 has been the mainstay of shunt procedures in this setting (de Leval et al. 1981). Other less used systemic-to-pulmonary artery shunts include the central aortopulmonary shunt with or without (Watterson et al. 1991) a Gore-Tex interposition graft. The original rationale for performing the MBTS through a thoracotomy was to leave the subsequent sternotomy free from the potential hazards of resternotomy. Median sternotomy for MBTS however allows the surgeon latitude to commence cardiopulmonary bypass in cases of hemodynamic collapse or profound hypoxia. In addition, sternotomy and cardiopulmonary bypass facilitates reconstruction of a stenotic left pulmonary artery due to ductal tissue or a pulmonary artery coarcted segment; repair of discontinuous pulmonary arteries; and inspection of the epicardial coronary artery anatomy. Repeat sternotomy, especially when Gore-Tex substernal membranes are used, has become more facile and commonplace owing to increased experience with staged neonatal repair for complex congenital heart disease. In most cases, the systemic-to-pulmonary artery shunts are performed without the use of cardiopulmonary bypass. The target vessels are the innominate artery and the right pulmonary artery. The PTFE graft is measured to size with a proximal bevel and straight edge distal cut; too short can result in tethering and pulmonary artery distortion; too long can result in compression localized pulmonary stenosis. In short, the graft should be constructed to the extant anatomy and not worry about future somatic growth since most of the time, the reparative operation will be performed within 6–8 months. For the most part, a 3.5 mm (preterm babies less than 3 kg) or 4-mm (term babies between 3 and 4 kg) Gore-Tex shunt is anastomosed end-to-side to the innominate artery and to the ipsilateral branch pulmonary artery. The systemic-to-pulmonary artery shunt is generally constructed opposite (contralateral) to the aortic arch. Consequently, an individual with a left aortic arch receives a right-sided MBTS. Associated maneuvers include ligation and division of the PAD, mobilization of the pulmonary artery and treatment of a pulmonary artery coarctation if present. The advantages of median sternotomy and cardiopulmonary bypass allow for probing both branch PAs through the opening made for distal shunt anastomosis. This maneuver can be used to assess PA size and absence of scarring by ductal tissue. There should be a low threshold to patch branch PAs at the same time of the shunt procedure.

Continuing with the primary repair vs. staged repair debate for neonates and young infants, there is evidence to show that systemic-to-pulmonary artery shunting may mitigate against transannular patching and improve the chances of pulmonary valve preservation at the initial repair. In one retrospective series (Stewart et al. 2005), only 40% of patients who were previously shunted required a transannular patch at the subsequent reparative operation. These results compare favorably with other reports which register nearly 100% use of transannular patch in association with complete repair. In a more granular analysis, Sousa and associates reported on 56 TOF patients who underwent repair younger than 6 months of age. Eight of these patients had prior palliative shunts. Interestingly and intuitively, the z-score of the pulmonary annulus in these 8 patients increased by a mean of 2.2 and only 1 of 8 infants repaired after shunt required a transannular patch (Sousa Uva et al. 1994). No shunt-related mortality was reported reflecting the experience of other reports (Fraser et al. 2001; Stewart et al. 2005).

So, how do these discordant policies and reports measure up when large database analyses are used in an attempt to resolve the equipoise, namely shunt or no shunt? The short answer is that no settled position has been reached despite 80 years of surgical experience. Perioperative mortality, interstage morbidity, and complications relating to shunt takedown and branch PA stenosis still persist (Dave 2016). The STS Congenital Heart Surgery database report has registered a 12.6% for all shunt procedures with a higher mortality rate associated with early shunt failure (31.9%) as opposed to those without (11.1%) (Do et al. 2018). Because of these findings, many centers are moving away from systemic-to-pulmonary artery shunts when there are other options. One consideration is a measured transannular patch which is not dependent on proximal and distal vascular anastomoses (Batlivala et al. 2018; Gerelli et al. 2014; Lenoir et al. 2017; Rabinowitz et al. 2017). Rather, the operation is performed on cardiopulmonary bypass with the creation of a limited right outflow muscle bundle resection resulting in a 6 mm opening, without VSD closure (Korbmacher et al. 2005; Seipelt et al. 2002). This has been shown to be better tolerated resulting in a reduced interstage mortality as long as the transannular patch is measured appropriately (Zhao et al. 2019).

In an attempt to offer less invasive procedures, authors have introduced percutaneous ballooning or stent placement of the right ventricular outflow tract (RVOT) and pulmonary valve. These procedures have been shown to be effective resulting in branch pulmonary artery growth, especially in very small infants or poor surgical candidates (Laudito et al. 2006; Wu et al. 2006). Complications however have been reported regarding irreversible damage to the pulmonary valve which obviates the possibility of a valve preservation procedure in the future (Dohlen et al. 2009). Moreover, the potential exists for more difficult stent removal, potential tricuspid valve injury, and branch pulmonary artery distortion at the time of complete repair.

At the present time, clinical equipoise has given way to a more settled position albeit with the potential for variation depending on the surgeon and surgical program. As noted in a previous report, "In our current practice, in the absence of contraindications to cardiopulmonary bypass, poor surgical candidacy from extracardiac malformations or syndromes, or diminutive pulmonary arteries, the primary goal is complete neonatal repair. In the presence of diminutive PAs, the modified right outflow tract procedure is the preferred palliation, and systemic-to-pulmonary artery shunts are avoided whenever possible" (Dodge-Khatami et al. 2023).

8 Complications Associated with Complete Repair

It is not too simplistic to affirm that any operation begins with the safe induction of anesthesia, proper monitoring, adherence to standard protocols, and alert operative staff. Anesthetic induction in patients with TOF can cause unwanted systemic vasodilation resulting in increased right to left shunting, profound hypoxemia, and potential hemodynamic collapse. These serious consequences can be averted by the maintenance of optimal volume states, a hemoglobin level of at least 10 mg/dL, use of a high inspired oxygen level, and avoidance of inhalational agents as they have a significant vasodilatory affect. Modern day intravenous anesthetic induction includes narcotics (Barankay et al. 1992) and ketamine (Tugrul et al. 2000) which do not have extreme vasodilation properties at appropriate doses. Complications can also occur from human mistakes. Introducing air bubbles through the venous lines during fluid and medication administration can result in myocardial ischemia or stroke (Horrow and Laucks 1982).

Transesophageal echocardiography (TEE) is generally employed for pre- and postoperative assessment in size appropriate patients. Esophageal perforation during TEE placement is a rare but dreaded complication which will require open surgical management or conservative measures depending on the extent of perforation (Miller et al. 2015). In the majority of patients who have suffered esophageal perforation the lesions occur in the hypopharynx or proximal esophagus (Elsayed et al. 2010). Gastrografin contrast swallow can demonstrate the leak in some cases; however, endoscopy is the procedure of choice which will identify the tear and lead to therapeutic options. While it is intuitive that early treatment of esophageal perforation is optimal, some studies have demonstrated little difference in overall mortality between early and late surgical interventions (Kotoulas 2010). In general, practitioners should have a high level of suspicion for esophageal perforation when conducting TEE, especially when the probe placement is attended with technical difficulty. In addition, any patient with postoperative swallowing difficulties should undergo timely evaluation.

Assuming that the anesthetic and TEE evaluation are uncomplicated, the patient is approached through a median sternotomy. Absence of the thymus is an important factor because of the potential association between TOF and DiGeorge syndrome, which will require careful long-term follow-up. In the event that a prior systemic-to-pulmonary artery shunt was performed, a careful dissection will be necessary to isolate the shunt after systemic heparinization and aortobicaval cannulation. At the initiation of cardiopulmonary bypass en route to moderate hypothermia (28–32 °C), the shunt is ligated proximally, distally and divided to avoid tethering or distortion of the branch pulmonary arteries. If preoperative evaluation showed localized pulmonary artery stenosis at the side of the shunt, the shunt is excised and pulmonary artery patch arterioplasty is performed with autologous pericardium or PTFE material. Figure 6 shows the cannulation technique which includes a left ventricular vent inserted via the right superior pulmonary vein. Figure 7 shows the progression of the operation which is illustrated by aortic cross-clamp and antegrade cold-blood cardioplegia. Depending upon the type of cardioplegia and systemic temperature, the cardioplegia should be readministered every 30–60 min or at any sign of cardiac activity. It should be the goal

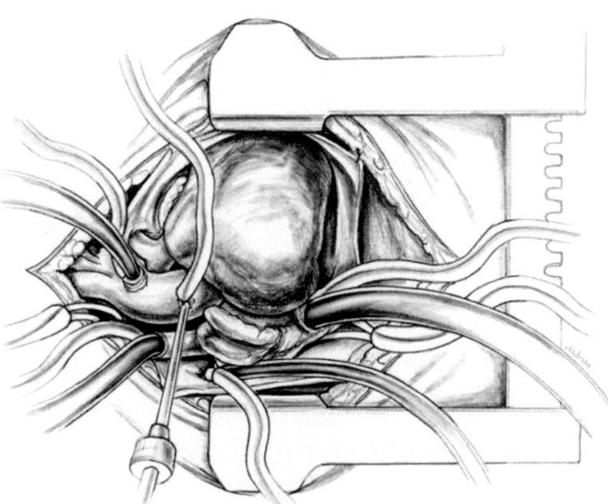

Fig. 6 Shows the cannulation technique that is established for aortobicaval cardiopulmonary bypass with left ventricular venting (right superior pulmonary vein) and antegrade cold blood cardioplegia. (With permission: Mavroudis 2015)

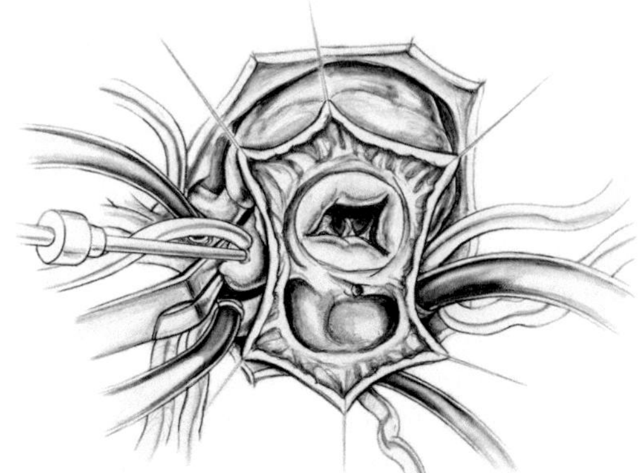

Fig. 7 This is the result of a right atrial incision that is performed from the base of the right atrial appendage, parallel to the atrioventricular groove and extending towards the coronary sinus medial to the inferior caval vein catheter. This incision will allow excellent tricuspid valve exposure by counterclockwise cardiac rotation and medial retraction. Through this exposure the surgeon can have a clear view of the right ventricular outflow tract. (With permission: Mavroudis 2015)

to perform this reparative operation through the right atrium with only a minimal ventricular outflow tract incision if a transannular patch is needed. After caval vein snares are applied, a medial right atriotomy is performed parallel to the atrioventricular groove with extension to the coronary sinus. This maneuver will enhance right ventricular exposure as noted in Figs. 7 and 8. Clearly, manual or suture exposure techniques will require retraction of the atrial wall and tricuspid valve for precise muscle resection and suture placement. However, unnecessary traction and roughness can be associated with malignant peri- and postoperative arrhythmias, such as junctional ectopic tachycardia (Dodge-Khatami et al. 2002a, b). The other point to remember is that retractors are moved for enhanced exposure multiple times during the operation. In fact, retraction is an important part of the operation with its own advantages and disadvantages as noted herein. Complications such as tricuspid disruption, aortic valve injury, and chordal transection can be avoided with close attention to the operation which includes optimal exposure. As shown in Fig. 8, the right ventricular outflow tract is exposed with landmarks and proposed areas for resection. Muscle resection requires careful excision of any endocardial fibroelastic tissue (generally off-white in color), which represents areas of turbulent flow. The hypertrophic muscle bundles projecting from the septomarginal, and septoparietal bands can be divided or partially excised. Smaller trabecular muscles that are causing obstruction can be completely excised. Excessive resection in the septal portion of the RVOT can result in injury to large perforating coronary arteries which can cause coronary cameral fistulas. When recognized, intracameral ligation of these vessels will prevent fistulas which if not managed can enlarge over time. Free wall disruption can also occur

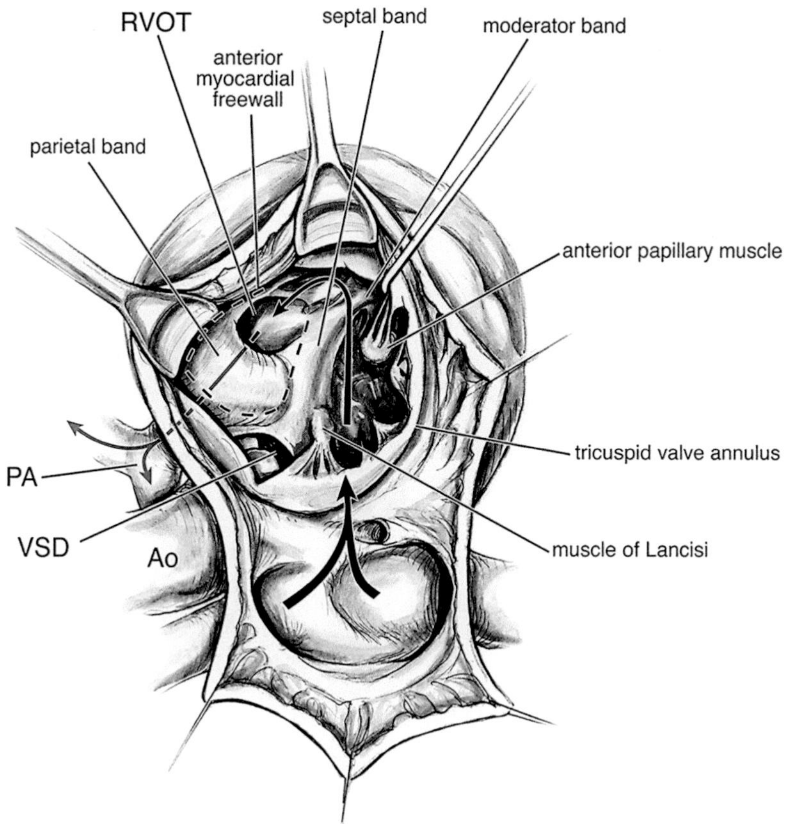

Fig. 8 Shows the exposure that will facilitate the obstructive right ventricular muscle resection. This exposure is accomplished by septal and anterior tricuspid leaflet manual retraction. A suction catheter (not shown) can be placed through the narrow ventricular outlet to provide a bloodless field and optimize the exposure by providing gentle downward traction. These maneuvers will expose the right ventricular outflow tract, minimize the blood in the field, and allow the surgeon to perform an accurate muscle resection. (With permission: Mavroudis 2015). *Ao* aota, *PA* pulmonary artery, *RVOT* right ventricular outflow tract, *VSD* ventricular septal defect

which will require patch repair of the RVOT as shown in Fig. 9. These complications can be avoided, for the most part, by keeping the dissection within the trabeculations of the RVOT which will facilitate identification of the pulmonary valve. Bimanual finger palpation can also help with the evaluation as long as the palpation maneuver does not disrupt the fine chordal attachments of the tricuspid valve. To this end, the subvalvar apparatus of the tricuspid valve must also be carefully noted and preserved during resection. Using proper retraction and exposure techniques most of the RVOT resection can be performed and accomplished through the right atrium and tricuspid valve as noted in Figs. 10 and 11. When necessary, additional

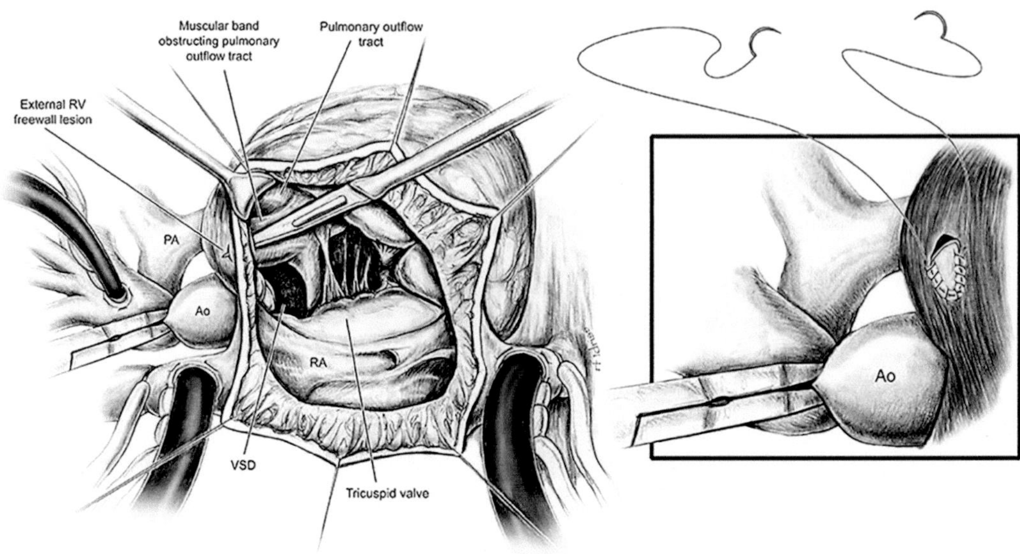

Fig. 9 Shows right atrial exposure and deep resection of the right ventricular outflow tract through the tricuspid valve with resultant unwanted perforation. The inset shows the transventricular hole that was made by deep dissection being repaired with a PTFE patch. *Ao* aorta, *PTFE* polytetrafluoroethylene, *RV* right ventricle, *VSD* ventricular septal defect

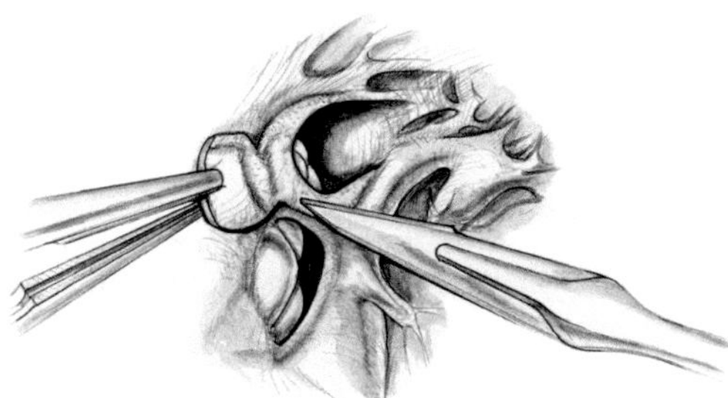

Fig. 10 Shows the technique of resection of the medial portion of the parietal band making sure to leave enough tissue for VSD closure while avoiding injury to the aortic valve. The resection is started at the base of the septal band as shown in the figure and extended toward the ventricular septal defect and superiorly towards the pulmonary outflow tract. The surgeon should be able to see the pulmonary valve once this resection is adequately accomplished. The resection should be extended as close to the pulmonary annulus as possible. (With permission: Mavroudis 2015)

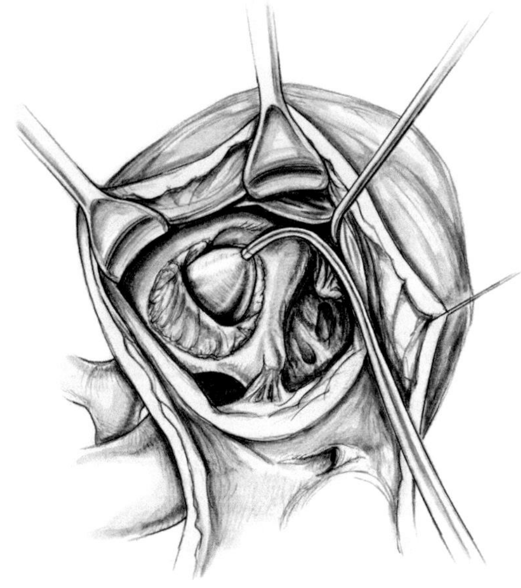

Fig. 11 Demonstrates a sized dilator being placed in the right ventricular outflow tract by direct vision. (With permission: Mavroudis 2015)

resection can be performed through the pulmonary valve which can be assessed by careful incision as noted in Figs. 12 and 13, or through a limited subvalvar ventriculotomy when tunnel stenosis of the RVOT is present. This infundibular incision is best managed and closed with a thin walled (0.4 mm) Gore-Tex patch.

A careful pulmonary arteriotomy will allow the possibility of pulmonary valve preservation assuming that the annulus is of good size. The dashed lines for this approach are noted in Fig. 12. A longitudinal pulmonary arteriotomy is made and continued into the two anterior sinuses in the case of a trileaflet valve or into the lateral sinuses of a vertically oriented bicuspid valve (Fig. 13). In those cases where there is a horizontally oriented bicuspid valve, the incision is not bifurcated but rather extended to the annulus (RV-PA junction). The pulmonary valvotomy is performed using a number 11 blade, dividing the partially fused commissures towards the arterial wall, insuring maximal opening through the preserved annulus. A measured probe is inserted and if the size is larger than −3 Z score, the annulus is left intact. Attention can then be directed to VSD closure which is noted in Figs. 14, 15, 16, and 17.

While there are many techniques for VSD closure, the editors prefer interrupted pledgetted suture technique. The anatomic borders of the VSD include the aortic valve annulus, the tricuspid valve annulus, the ventricular septum, and the area of the conduction system. Each location requires careful attention to the details of the operation. Suture placement at the septal muscle border of the VSD has been reviewed with focused drawings in Fig. 20 (VSD Chapter "Complications Associated with Ventricular Septal Defect Closure"). The drawing highlights the suturing technique to ensure firm septal mus-

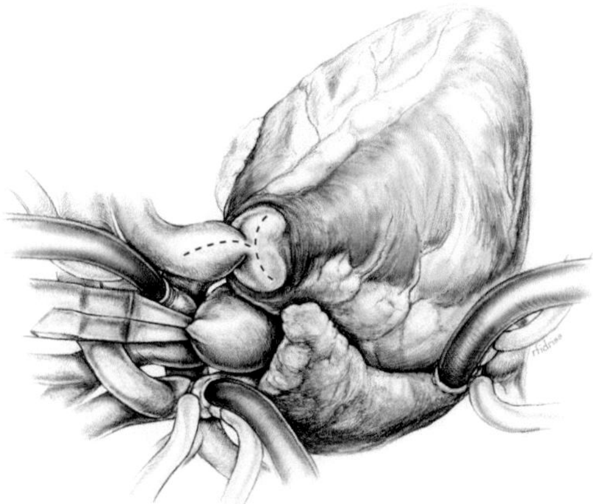

Fig. 12 Shows how the exposure can now be addressed to the surface of the main pulmonary artery where an inverted Y incision is planned (dotted lines) into the pulmonary valve sinuses of Valsalva. In the majority of cases, there is a supravalvar narrowing which when properly enlarged can help with the right ventricular muscle resection and form the basis for a valve preserving operation. The incision is commenced well into the main pulmonary artery and is carefully advanced towards the valve leaflets where an assessment can be made concerning the orientation and number of valve leaflets. If a three-leaflet pulmonary valve is encountered, the two anterior sinuses of Valsalva are incised to the annulus; if there is a bicuspid valve oriented anterior-posterior then the incisions are made in the existing sinuses of Valsalva; if the bicuspid valve is oriented in the horizontal position, the incision is made into the anterior sinus of Valsalva. (With permission: Mavroudis 2015)

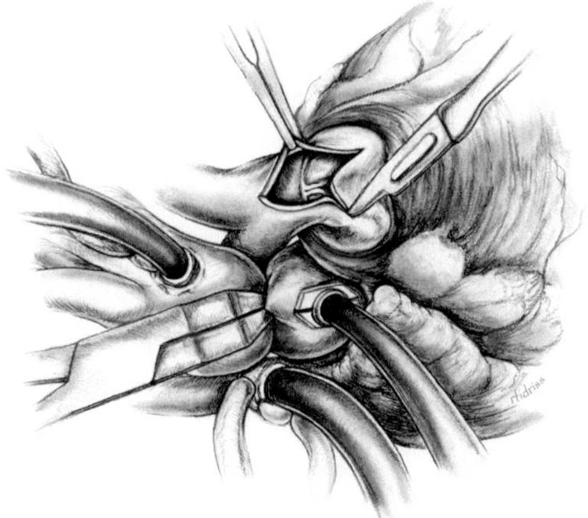

Fig. 13 Shows the inverted Y incision being made into the two existing sinuses of Valsalva in a bicuspid valve oriented in an anterior-posterior position. Careful commissurotomies can be performed to enlarge the valve orifice without sacrificing the integrity of the pulmonary valve apparatus. The leaflets should not be detached, only incised. The purpose is to maintain competency of the pulmonary valve. Through the valve, the right ventricular outflow tract muscle resection can be assessed and more resection through this exposure can be accomplished if needed. Measurements can be taken by sized dilators which should be introduced carefully in order to avoid valvar injury by excessive dilatation. (With permission: Mavroudis 2015)

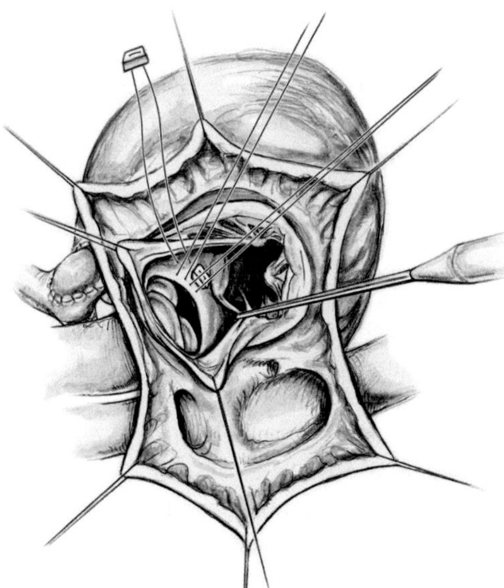

Fig. 14 Shows how attention can now be directed to the transatrial ventricular septal defect (VSD) closure. The figure demonstrates the exposure for a VSD closure. Interrupted pledgetted sutures are placed commencing at the crest of the right interventricular septum with special care to avoid injury to the tricuspid valve apparatus, the aortic valve, and the conduction system. (With permission: Mavroudis 2015)

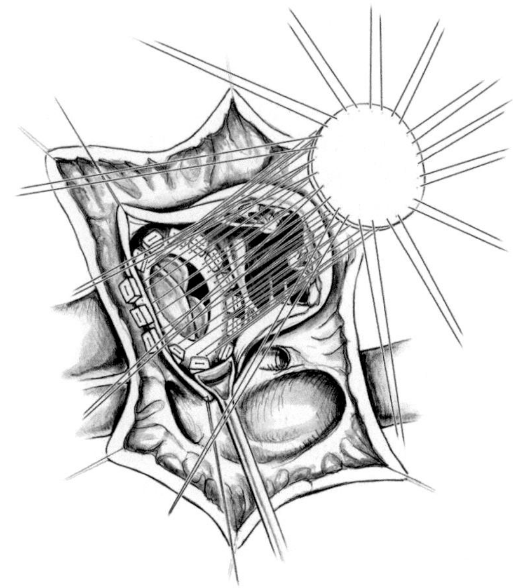

Fig. 16 Shows the hovering medical illustration technique that demonstrates the suture placement technique through the PTFE patch in anticipation of patch engagement with the ventricular septum. (With permission: Mavroudis 2015). *PTFE* polytetrafluoroethylene

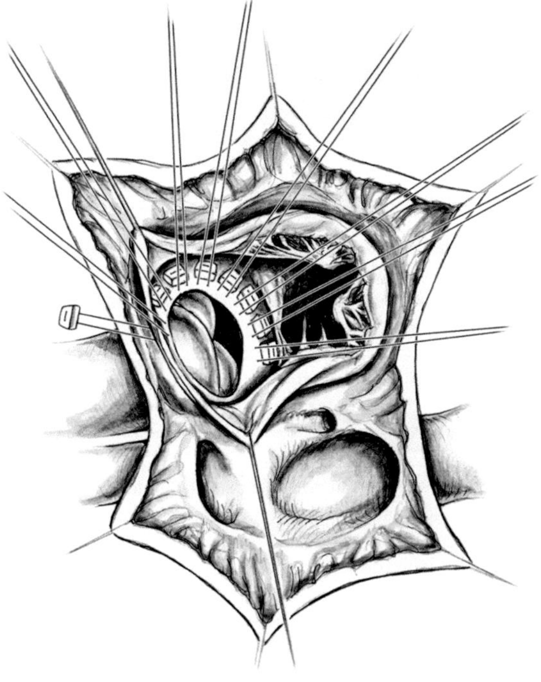

Fig. 15 Illustrates how the suture placement technique is continued as noted in the figure. Some sutures may need to be anchored in the right atrium at the tricuspid-aortic annular area. Careful suture placement will avoid septal leaflet and conduction system injury. (With permission: Mavroudis 2015)

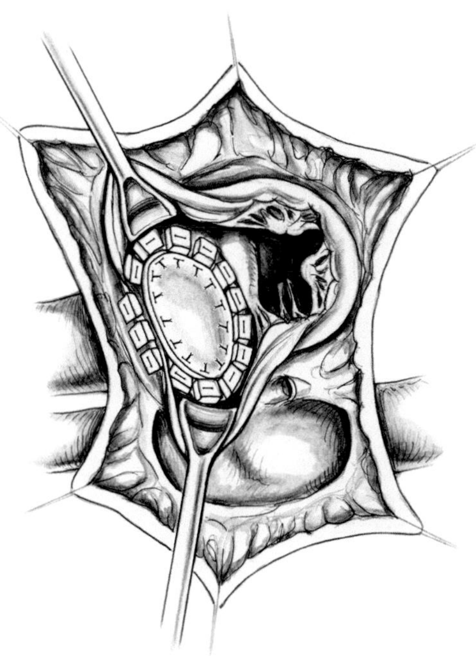

Fig. 17 After the sutures are placed through a PTFE patch, it is lowered into the area of the ventricular septal defect (VSD) and tied in place all the time assessing the tension of the tied knot with regard to dimpling of the pledgetted suture which is always kept in view. Sutures too loosely tied will result in a residual VSD; sutures too tightly applied will cause endocardial disruption and a residual VSD. The patent foramen ovale (PFO) can either be closed or left open depending on the patient's age (younger the age, the more likely that the PFO will be left open) to unload the right ventricle in the event of associated right ventricular postoperative dysfunction. The right atrium can be closed, the aortic cross-clamp can be removed taking care to perform all the air maneuvers, and attention can now be directed to the right ventricular outflow tract reconstruction. (With permission: Mavroudis 2015). *PTFE* polytetrafluoroethylene

cle engagement for snug patch apposition and proper closure. The conduction system is noted by a dashed line. The sutures are placed on the right ventricular side of the septum no deeper than 50% of its thickness. The surrounding structures are noted for visual perspective. In contrast, Fig. 21 (VSD Chapter "Complications Associated with Ventricular Septal Defect Closure" shows how ill-advised deep suture technique can endanger the conduction system in this location and cause heart block. The difference between suture placement in Fig. 20 (recommended) and Fig. 21 (ill-advised) is subtle, but extremely important to avoid heart block. The important landmarks for continued suture technique involve the area between the Muscle of Lancisi and the tricuspid valve annulus inferiorly. As noted, avoiding deep suture placement is critical to avoid damage to the AV node and Bundle of His. Several of the sutures are typically placed from the right atrial side of the tricuspid annulus which helps with retraction in this area. The VSD patch is cut in a slightly oversized configuration which avoids potential subaortic narrowing due to the malaligned VSD. Another potential problem with suture placement at the muscular septum is the entrapment of the tricuspid chords within the closure technique. Figure 22 shows how pledgetted sutures can entrap the tricuspid chords which will result in tricuspid regurgitation. Oftentimes, these entrapping sutures go unnoticed until the VSD has been closed and at the time of tricuspid valve evaluation by cold saline filled bulb syringe infusion. When severe tricuspid regurgitation is seen, resolution of this problem can be VSD patch revision to free the entrapped chords. If the regurgitation is minor, one can consider tricuspid repair by side-to-side repair in the area of leaking as noted in Figure 23. This maneuver can avoid an extension of the cross-clamp time. At the superior aspect of the VSD, sutures should be placed close to or into the aortic annulus (sparing the leaflets) to avoid residual defects through the trabeculations. Most of the time, the tricuspid valve can be retracted enough for suture placement. It is rare to incise the tricuspid valve in TOF patients to implement adequate exposure for these circumstances unless there is extensive aortic override as in cases of Double Outlet Right Ventricle-Tetralogy Type, which is often difficult to visualize from the right atrium. This anatomic configuration may require takedown of the anterior and parts of the septal leaflets of the tricuspid valve. Specifically, a radial incision from 2 o'clock counterclockwise back to the hinging point of the tricuspid valve and the inferior VSD border, which corresponds to approximately 8 o'clock, greatly increases access to the borders of the VSD, and allows for complete closure without undue traction (Mavroudis and Backer 2002). Complications that can occur in this location involve injuries to the aortic leaflets. Sometimes, secure suture purchase in this area can be performed by placing the pledgetted sutures from the right atrium and through the tricuspid-aortic shared annulus as noted in the left panel of Fig. 24. Including an unwanted amount of the tricuspid leaflet can result in leaflet shortening and tricuspid regurgitation as noted in the right panel of Fig. 24. The resolution of this problem, where severe, is suture revision to avoid the tricuspid leaflet entrapment. Another method to resolve mild regurgitation is tricuspid side-to-side suture technique in the area of leaking as illustrated in Fig. 25, Chapter "Complications Associated with Ventricular Septal Defect Closure").

In cases where tricuspid valve leaflet takedown has been performed, the leaflet is repaired and resuspended to the annulus in a radial fashion with a running suture technique and tested for competence with a saline infusion. A patent foramen ovale, which is often present, is closed primarily, unless the patient is a neonate in which case, it is advisable to leave it open. The right atrial incision is closed using two layers of running suture. The heart is carefully de-aired and the cross-clamp removed.

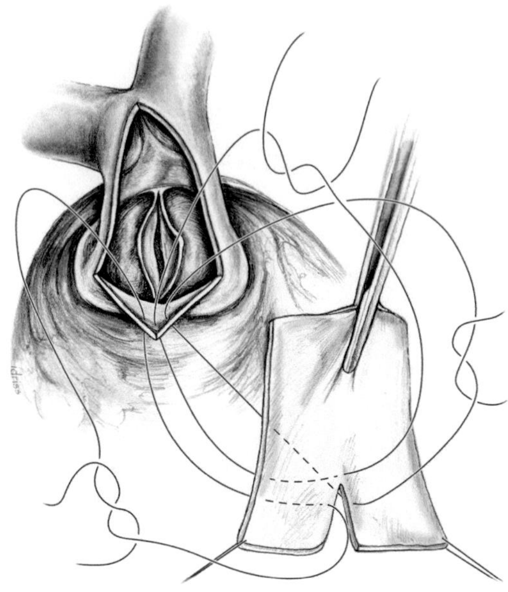

Fig. 18 Shows an autologous pericardial patch which was cut to size and in a pantaloon configuration to eventually fill out and augment the incised sinuses of Valsalva. Three interrupted sutures are placed at the incised apex of the pantaloon patch to align with the anterior pulmonary valve commissure and tied. The intent of these interrupted sutures is to avoid suture disruption in the event that the resultant right ventricular pressure proves to be too high which will require a transannular incision in the area of the interrupted sutures. The transannular incision will not disturb the integrity of the rest of the pericardial patch repair. (With permission: Mavroudis 2015)

The pulmonary arteriotomy is then closed with a pantaloon pericardial patch, which maximizes the size of the pulmonary root, completely relieving supravalvar obstruction (Figs. 18, 19, 20, and 21) (Dodge-Khatami et al. 2023; Bacha 2017). Inspection and evaluation of the branch pulmonary artery orifices is important, especially the left pulmonary artery (LPA), since it is frequently stenotic in TOF patients and can be corrected with an extension of the pericardial patch

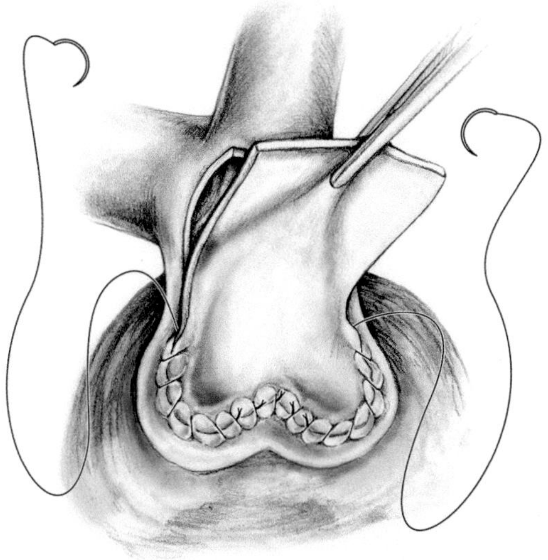

Fig. 19 Shows the pantaloon pericardial patch being sewn into place augmenting the supravalvar area. If performed correctly, the pericardial patch will be too large and redundant in the superior area of the reconstruction. Tapering the superior portion of the pericardial patch to the estimated exact size will risk supravalvar stenosis. (With permission: Mavroudis 2015)

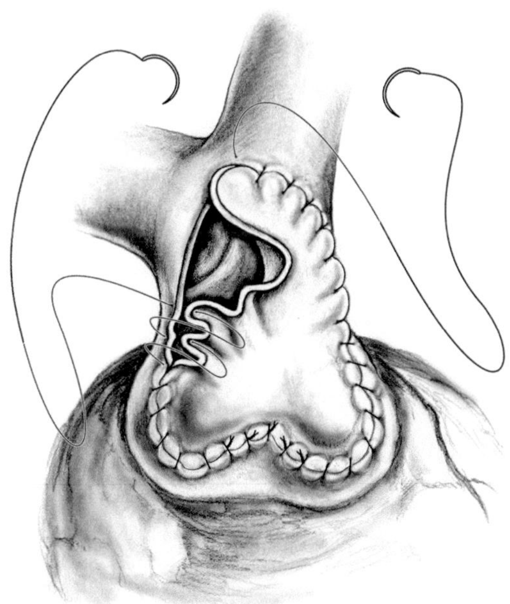

Fig. 20 Demonstrates the gathering technique that helps to match up the pericardium with the extant pulmonary artery wall. (With permission: Mavroudis 2015)

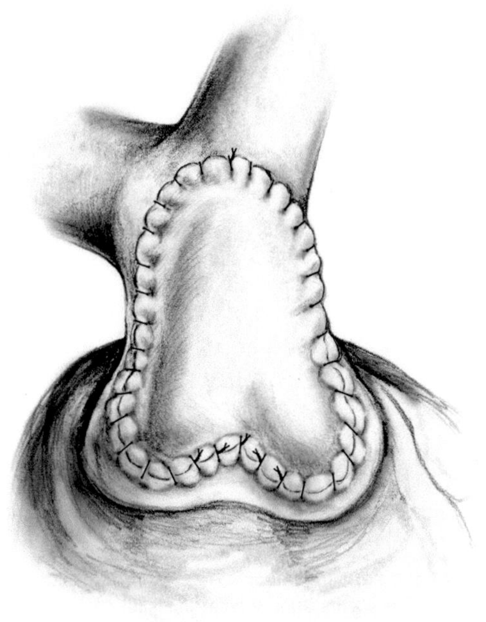

Fig. 21 Shows the completed supravalvar repair using the suture gathering technique. (With permission: Mavroudis 2015)

onto the branch PA, or a separate patch, as needed.

Even after a well-executed operation, further assessment is necessary. In particular, TEE can evaluate the presence of a residual VSD, ventricular function, and the presence of pulmonary regurgitation. RVOT pressure gradients are best determined by direct measurements after separation from cardiopulmonary bypass. Direct measurements of the RV and LV pressures are determined using a 21-gauge spinal needle attached to a pressure transducing line. If the RV/LV pressure ratio is greater than 0.7 (Hirsch et al. 2000; Stewart et al. 2005), the TEE is assessed for level of residual obstruction which can help to determine the reparative procedure if necessary. Some authors intervene to revise the RVOT if the RV/LV threshold is 50% (Bacha 2017). If the stenosis is predominately at the annulus, then cardiopulmonary bypass is recommenced and a transannular patch is created. The method for

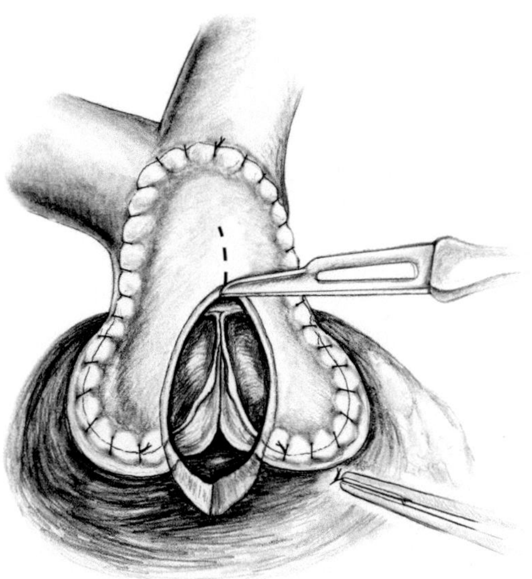

Fig. 22 In the case that post repair right ventricular hypertension occurs after separation from cardiopulmonary bypass, a transannular patch must be performed. Resumption of cardiopulmonary bypass is performed, and one or two interrupted sutures can be removed without disrupting supravalvar reconstruction as shown in the figure. The transannular incision is made with the intent of preserving the commissural attachments of the pulmonary valve anteriorly. The goal is to preserve the competency of the two now separated leaflets. Recent reports have emphasized this maneuver in the anticipation that these leaflets will grow over time and be available for possible valve restoration in the future by reapproximation thereby avoiding the placement of homografts, heterografts or PTFE pulmonary valves at subsequent operations. (With permission: Mavroudis 2015). *PTFE* polytetrafluoroethylene

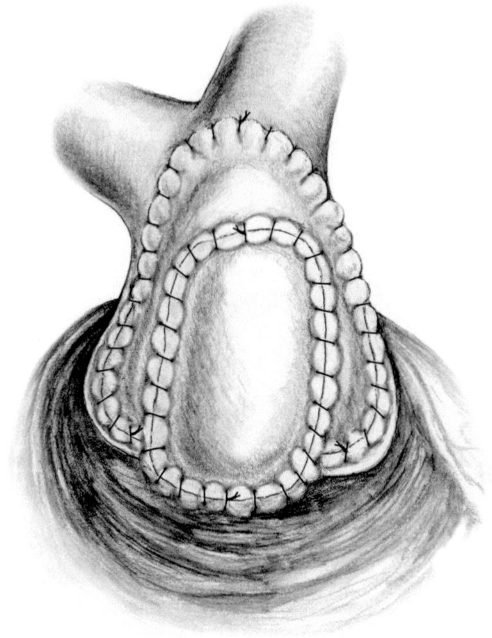

Fig. 23 Once the valve is preserved and the appropriately sized transannular incision into the ventricle is accomplished, then another pericardial patch can be placed to augment the original patch as noted in the figure. (With permission: Mavroudis 2015)

patch augmentation after a transannular patch is shown in Figs. 22 and 23. If the stenosis is subvalvar, then only an infundibular patch is inserted taking origin just below the annulus. In those patients who are known to have a pulmonary valve that is likely too small for even the most aggressive attempts at valve preservation, a planned transannular incision can be made across the anterior pulmonary valve commissure thereby preserving the leaflet attachments in the event that the valve grows in the future. Figures 24, 25, and 26 show the progression of the transannular operation that will preserve leaflets for future evaluation and possible pulmonary valve restoration.

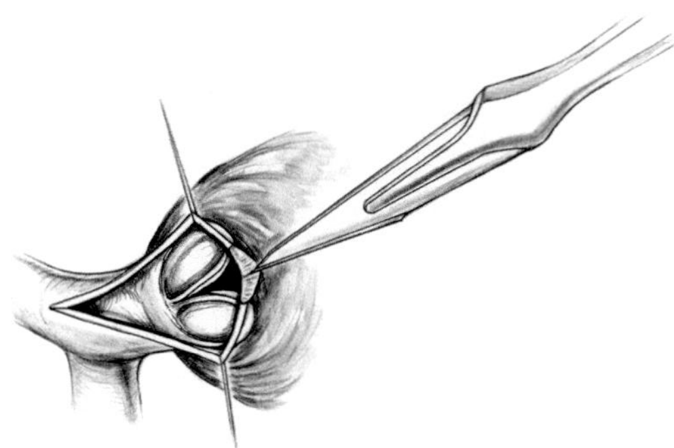

Fig. 24 When the pulmonary valve is deemed to be too small for any attempted valve sparing strategy, a primary transannular incision can be performed as noted in the figure. The tenets of valve preservation as noted previously in Fig. 18 are still operative and special care should be made to preserve the valve leaflets and commissures in the event that subsequent operations for pulmonary valve regurgitation may find these leaflets favorable for valve restoration. (With permission: Mavroudis 2015)

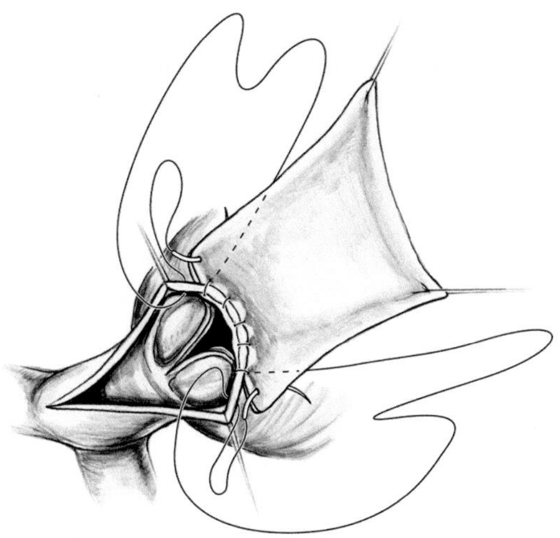

Fig. 25 Shows the limited transannular incision with placement of a pericardial transannular patch. (With permission: Mavroudis 2015)

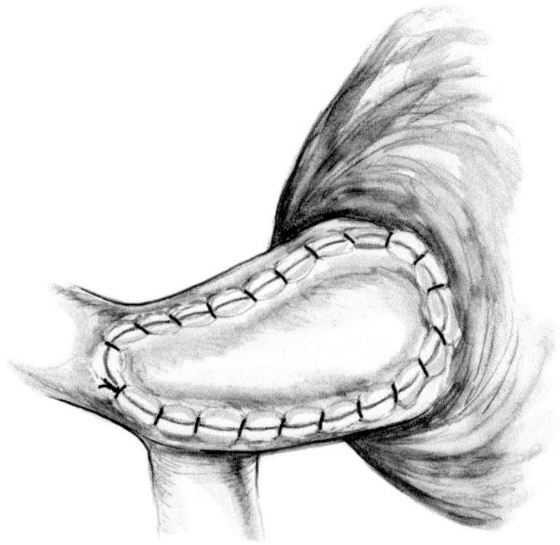

Fig. 26 Demonstrates the completed transannular repair. (With permission: Mavroudis 2015)

Complications associated with a transannular right ventricular outflow tract patch can also be due to an undiagnosed intramyocardial course of an anomalous origin of the left anterior descending coronary artery (Meyer et al. 1975; Mavroudis 2017). In most cases, this diagnosis is discovered by preoperative cardiac catheterization. Nevertheless, even if the anomalous coronary artery is not suspected, it is wise to perform the ventriculotomy from the mid ventricle and slowly progress towards the stenotic pulmonary valve. If an intramyocardial coronary artery is discovered, and if it is not injured, preparations should be made to perform a right ventricular to pulmonary artery conduit with great care to avoid injury to the coronary artery by careful suture placement at the proximal conduit anastomosis. If the artery is transected, a significant problem becomes manifest, especially if the artery is large enough to compromise perfusion to the myocardium. Ligating the artery will likely result in significant left ventricular dysfunction leading to ECMO and the problems relating thereto. A left internal thoracic artery bypass graft to the left anterior descending coronary artery should be considered (Mavroudis 2017; Mavroudis et al. 1996). Assuming that the cross-clamp has been removed, the internal thoracic artery can be dissected and prepared for bypass grafting. Cardioplegic arrest is then established and the arteriotomy in the LAD coronary artery can be performed. Fine monofilament (Prolene) 8-0 suture can then be used to perform the anastomosis (Fig. 7) from Chapter “Complications Associated with Repair of Double Outlet Ventricles with Two Adequate Ventricles” DORV]. Alternatively, interrupted suture technique can also be used (Mavroudis et al. 1996).

In cases not associated with an anomalous coronary artery, some surgeons prefer to use a valved conduit in the setting where a transannular patch would be necessary. Conduits that are too short or too long can result in coronary artery compression and distal pulmonary stenosis, respectively as noted in Chapter “Complications Associated with Repair of Common Arterial Trunk” (Common Arterial Trunk Chapter Figs. 16, 17, and 18). The editors’ first preference is to use a transannular patch under these circumstances unless there are complicating factors that indicate an extracardiac valved conduit placement such as right ventricular dysfunction, right ventricular outflow tract obstruction due to the VSD patch or anomalous coronary artery as noted herein.

When the time comes for mediastinal closure, it is important to be mindful of the potential for junctional ectopic tachycardia (JET) following

TOF repair. Temporary atrial and ventricular pacing wires are placed regardless of the rhythm after separation from bypass.

9 Results

9.1 Mortality

Mortality rates for complete repair of TOF have decreased steadily over the years owing to advances in surgical techniques, intensive care, and myocardial preservation (Murphy et al. 1993; Zhao et al. 1985; Nollert et al. 2003; Ebert and Turley 1983; Turley et al. 1982; Barratt-Boyes and Neutze 1973; Castaneda et al. 1977). A selective more recent historical review, shows that Roger Mee and colleagues reported a 0.5% hospital mortality among 366 patients with TOF between 1980 and 1991 using a transatrial, transpulmonary approach (Karl et al. 1992). There were no mortalities in the Editors' series of 102 cases (average age: 5.9 months) at Lurie Children's Hospital in Chicago between 1997 and 2004 (Stewart et al. 2005). More recent reports accounting for infant and neonatal TOF repair have similarly low rates of mortality ranging from 0% to 3% (Derby and Pizarro 2005; Kolcz and Pizarro 2005; Parry et al. 2000; van Dongen et al. 2003).

The long-term survival rate of patients with TOF is excellent and noteworthy which is highlighted by the 86% 32-year actuarial survival among 163 patients who had survived 30 days after complete repair of TOF at the Mayo Clinic before 1960. These results were compared to an expected rate of 96% in a control population matched for age and sex (Murphy et al. 1993). A similar report (1997) documented the results in a group of 490 survivors with repaired TOF and found an 89% 30-year actuarial survival (Nollert et al. 1997).

9.2 Morbidity

Noteworthy complications following TOF repair include arrhythmias, early reoperation, catheter reintervention, residual VSD, and heart block. Other complications include phrenic nerve injury, chylothorax, and delayed sternal closure.

Heart block requiring a pacemaker occurs between 0% and 2%, and occasionally develops late after the operation (Friedli 1999). Transient heart block, namely heart block after operation that resolves, is a risk factor for the development of late heart block (Hokanson and Moller 2001).

10 Early Reoperation and Reinterventions

Pulmonary regurgitation after transannular repair of TOF is well tolerated in the short and mid-term and generally does not lead to morbidity unless accompanied by residual VSD, residual RVOT obstruction and heart block. The most common indication for early reoperation after TOF repair is residual right ventricular outflow tract obstruction, which can occur at the infundibular level, valvar level, or in the branch pulmonary arteries. Branch pulmonary artery stenosis can be treated by catheter-based balloon dilatation and stent placement. RVOT obstruction, however, is highly dependent on the patient population at risk. The reported incidence of RVOT obstruction in electively repaired patients is relatively low. Mee and colleagues in 1991 reported a 5- and 10-year freedom from reoperation of 95% (Karl et al. 1992). Colleagues from Texas Children's Hospital reported a 3% early reoperative rate (Fraser Jr et al. 2001). When primary repair of TOF less than 4 months of age is considered, Tamesberger and associates reported a reoperation rate was 8%, and a 14% catheter reintervention rate at a mean follow-up of 4.7 years (Tamesberger et al. 2008).

Repaired symptomatic patients however had a reoperative rate that has been reported to be as high as 30% (Hirsch et al. 2000). Further long-term analysis revealed that a comparison of reoperative rates on the right ventricular outflow tract at 20 years for primary repairs versus staged repairs was not statistically different (Knott-Craig et al. 1998).

Residual RVOT obstruction at the conclusion of initial repair, as assessed by the RV/LV pressure ratio, is directly related to the incidence of reoperation. A comprehensive study from the University of Alabama, Birmingham (1982) determined that an RV/LV pressure ratio greater than 0.85 was associated with a 2.5 times increased risk of death, and a 7.3 times increased risk of reoperation (Katz et al. 1982). The Editors' report (2005) 4 of 7 reoperations occurred in patients who had an RV/LV pressure ratio between 0.7 and 0.8 (Stewart et al. 2005).

Other uncommon indications for early reoperation include a residual VSD, residual ASD, RVOT aneurysm, severe tricuspid regurgitation, heart block, phrenic nerve injury, and chylothorax. Residual VSD in TOF patients, especially when there is associated pulmonary regurgitation, is a significant source of right ventricular dysfunction and elevated central venous pressure. Tirilomis and associates have highlighted the problems that residual VSD can cause in TOF patients (Tirilomis et al. 2010). They reported on 914 patients who underwent TOF repair and documented 102 reoperations at 12.8 years after repair with half of the reoperations due to residual VSD.

11 Arrhythmias and Sudden Death

The most common cause of late mortality after TOF repair is sudden death, which is generally attributable to ventricular arrhythmias (Gatzoulis et al. 2000b). However, when considering arrhythmias in the early postoperative period, the most common electrocardiographic abnormality is right bundle branch block. This is caused by right ventricular outflow tract resection and deep sutures from the VSD repair. In addition, right bundle branch block is found in 90% of patients who had a ventriculotomy (Friedli 1996). As noted, complete heart block is an uncommon complication of TOF repair, with a reported incidence ranging from 1% to 3% (Kolcz and Pizarro 2005; Pigula et al. 1999; Tamesberger et al. 2008; Kanter et al. 2010).

The most common early arrhythmia following TOF repair is junctional ectopic tachycardia (JET). The incidence and severity of this arrhythmia varies considerably and depends on the age at surgery and surgical approach (Dodge-Khatami et al. 2002a). Selected literature reports seem to point to ventriculotomy as a significant risk factor for postoperative JET. In one report of patients under 3 months of age who had a transventricular repair, 29% had postoperative arrhythmias, of which 48% were JET and 17% had some form of supraventricular tachycardia (SVT) (Pigula et al. 1999). In contrast, the Editors' series of 102 patients who were repaired at a mean age of 6 months using a transatrial/transpulmonary approach, reported a 12% incidence of JET (Stewart et al. 2005). In a similar group of patients repaired at a mean age of 1 year by the same approach, the incidence of JET was only 6% (Fraser Jr et al. 2001).

JET can cause significant hemodynamic instability in the postoperative period which, although rare, can require ECMO for patient survival (Azzam and Fiore 1998). Therapeutic measures include, correction of electrolytes, mild hypothermia (34–36 °C), reduction or elimination of catecholaminergic infusions, sedation, and treatment with amiodarone (Dodge-Khatami et al. 2002b). Complications with amiodarone treatment are related to hypotension and decreased ventricular function. The recommended infusion for amiodarone is 5 mg/kg as a single bolus. In contrast, the Editors prefer multiple boluses of only 1 mg/kg over 20–30 min to avoid the negative inotropic effects of the drug. As noted, postoperative JET has been associated with maneuvers and causes which may be prevented by careful attention to technique and operative exposure. For instance, potential mechanisms which can induce JET include aggressive resection of the RVOT, and traumatic tissue handling to optimize VSD exposure (Elsayed et al. 2010). In contrast, gentle stay suture technique with focused tricuspid valve leaflet retraction to provide VSD exposure, and sharp muscle bundle division in the RVOT instead of blunt resection, have significantly reduced the Editors' incidence of postoperative JET in tetralogy patients.

Late arrhythmias after TOF repair are not uncommon and are characterized by supraventricular tachycardia (SVT) and ventricular tachycardias (VT). The Alliance for Adult Research in Congenital Cardiology conducted a multi-institutional retrospective study of 556 previously repaired TOF patients. They recorded 43% of patients to have a history of arrhythmias (Khairy et al. 2010) of which atrial tachyarrhythmias were present in 20% and ventricular tachyarrhythmias in 15%. Harrison and associates showed that sustained SVT was noted in 12% of 242 adult patients late after repair (Harrison et al. 2001). In another multi-institutional study of 793 patients who were reviewed at a mean of 21 years after repair, Gatzoulis and colleagues described an incidence of atrial and ventricular tachyarrhythmias in approximately 4% of patients with a disturbing incidence of sudden death in 2% of the cohort (Gatzoulis et al. 2000b).

Unfortunately, the surgical repair of TOF is attended by a persistent and long-term incidence of paroxysmal atrial tachyarrhythmias in as many as one-third of patients (Roos-Hesselink et al. 1995). Supraventricular tachycardia (SVT) is an inclusive term to describe the majority of the atrial tachyarrhythmias until the specific diagnosis is made. In the case of postoperative tetralogy patients, atrial reentry tachycardia is the most common type. Atrial reentry tachycardia requires two different substrates to create the intra-atrial circus movement, namely, an area of slow conduction and an area of unidirectional block. The area of slow conduction is mostly found at the isthmus between the tricuspid valve and the inferior vena cava (Le Gloan et al. 2010). The area of unidirectional block means that an atrial electrical impulse can proceed in only one direction which together with the area of slow conduction sets up the circus movement and atrial reentry tachycardia. Reentrant circuits can also develop in the areas of scar tissue around atrial incisions. Several risk factors are responsible for a higher incidence of SVT after TOF repair which include, older age at surgery, the presence of moderate or severe tricuspid regurgitation, right atrial enlargement, pulmonary regurgitation, poor right ventricular function, and hypertension (Khairy et al. 2010; Harrison et al. 2001; Roos-Hesselink et al. 1995; Le Gloan et al. 2010; Wessel et al. 1980).

Supraventricular arrhythmias are associated with less life-threatening events than ventricular tachyarrhythmias, however supraventricular arrhythmias are nevertheless responsible for significant morbidity, including decreased exercise capacity, heart failure, and stroke. Fortunately, there are a number of treatment options for patients with atrial arrhythmias after TOF repair which include pharmacologic agents, transcatheter ablation, and surgical ablation. The development and success of the various forms of the maze procedure in controlling atrial reentry arrhythmias has allowed more options in management (Deal et al. 2003; Stulak et al. 2006). In particular, TOF patients who require reoperation for pulmonary valve insertion and/or tricuspid repair/replacement should be evaluated for the presence of arrhythmias with a 24-h Holter monitor. Further, patients with any history of palpitations should be evaluated by an electrophysiologic study to elicit and characterize reentry pathways in the right or left atrium which can be obliterated with incision, cryotherapy, or radiofrequency ablation at the time of surgery.

Risk factors that have been associated with ventricular arrhythmias include older age at repair, ventriculotomy, transannular patch, severe PR, poor RV function, poor LV function, RV enlargement, and elongated QRS duration (Gatzoulis et al. 2000b; Khairy et al. 2004, 2010; Dietl et al. 1994). The risk of sudden death includes QRS duration greater than 180 msec, older age at repair, severe PR, history of sustained VT, and LV systolic dysfunction (Wessel et al. 1980; Ghai et al. 2002).

12 Long-Term Complications Following Repair of Tetralogy of Fallot

Long-term complications following repair of TOF are highly dependent on postoperative residual defects, which places significant responsibility on diagnosticians and surgeons to plan the optimal time of palliation/repair, complete closure of the VSD, transatrial repair, when possible, minimal ventriculotomy when needed, prudent transannular patch size, and resolution of branch pulmonary artery stenoses.

Residual lesions, for the most part, can be tolerated in the short-term, however the deranged physiology thereto pertaining can have major effects on the right ventricle that if not addressed in a timely manner can be irreversible. In particular, the long-term effects of volume overload due to pulmonary regurgitation, tricuspid regurgitation, and residual shunts become all the more problematic when associated with pressure load resulting from residual pulmonary stenosis. The clinical aftereffects of these combined conditions include right ventricular dysfunction, atrial and ventricular arrhythmias, sudden death, late left ventricular dysfunction, and aneurysmal dilation of the aorta.

Of these late residual lesions, pulmonary regurgitation is the most common and is related to the liberal use of transannular patch for TOF repair in the 1970s and 1980s. To illustrate the efficacy of chronic pulmonary regurgitation after TOF repair, several reports have demonstrated good long-term functional outcomes with a TAP (Bacha et al. 2001; Kirklin et al. 1989).

In a study of 44 TOF patients who had complete repair, Bacha and associates reported that the functional class was similar for TAP and valve-sparing procedures (Bacha et al. 2001). Another study by Kirklin and colleagues reported on 814 patients and noted that the risk of reoperation for pulmonary regurgitation at 20 years postoperatively was 7%. Interpretation of their favorable outcomes has been attributed to right ventricular adaptation qualities both with transannular patch and valve-sparing repairs (Kirklin et al. 1989). As more sensitive measurements of right ventricular function became available, the deleterious effects of pulmonary regurgitation become more manifest (Roest et al. 2002; Horneffer et al. 1990). Exercise testing (Horneffer et al. 1990; Carvalho et al. 1992; Singh et al. 1998) and Cardiac MRI (Roest et al. 2002; Singh et al. 1998) examination has been very effective in determining functional status in TOF patients who had transannular patch repair, even in asymptomatic patients. Frigiola and associates (Frigiola et al. 2004) (London), applied tissue Doppler assessments of isovolumetric myocardial acceleration to assess right ventricular function under varying volume loading conditions in patients with pulmonary regurgitation after TOF repair and found highly significant correlation with both right ventricular and left ventricular dysfunction. These data have led clinicians to offer timely pulmonary valve insertion to mitigate the negative effects of pulmonary regurgitation by ventricular remodeling resulting in symptomatic relief (Buechel et al. 2005; Discigil et al. 2001; Eyskens et al. 2000; Warner et al. 2003; Gengsakul et al. 2007; Therrien et al. 2001; Harrild et al. 2009; van Huysduynen et al. 2005; Oosterhof et al. 2007; van Straten et al. 2005; Geva 2006; Champsaur et al. 1998; Chan et al. 1994; Homann et al. 2000; Dave et al. 2006; Hawkins et al. 2009; Deorsola et al. 2010; Pragt et al. 2017).

13 Pulmonary Valve Restoration and Replacement Strategies

Early reports of improved right ventricular function notwithstanding, timing and effect of pulmonary valve insertion remains controversial. Warner and associates reported on matched cohorts of 82 patients with and without PVR. Interestingly, there were no sudden deaths in the PVR group, however the expected improvement in survival was not realized (Warner et al. 2003). The idea that improved right ventricular improvement in TOF patients could also decrease the incidence of ventricular tachycardia and sudden death, was also tested. To wit, Gengsakul and colleagues demonstrated a decrease in the incidence of ventricular tachycardia from 23% to 9% after PVR (Therrien et al. 2001). However, in a matched cohort of 98 patients, Harrild and associates showed that pulmonary valve insertion had no effect on the incidence of ventricular tachycardia or death (Harrild et al. 2009). These findings have emphasized the notion that correction of hemodynamic problems does not always impact the negative consequences of arrhythmias. Increased electrocardiographic QRS duration has been associated with ventricular dysfunction. Pulmonary valve insertion has had a positive effect on increased QRS duration. In particular, Therrien and associates noted that pulmonary valve insertion stabilized the duration of QRS interval (Therrien et al. 2001). but had no effect on decreasing the interval. Other authors have observed a QRS decrease in the early postoperative course after pulmonary valve insertion which correlates with an increase in right ventricular end diastolic volume (RVEDV) by MRI (Therrien et al. 2001). In addition to these reports, Oosterhof and associates demonstrated a temporary decrease in QRS duration after pulmonary valve insertion with an eventual increase in duration to >180 msec. This late increase in QRS duration was more likely to occur in those individuals who had a QRS > 180 msec duration before pulmonary valve insertion (Oosterhof et al. 2007).

A review on the effect of PVR on right ventricular function with regard to size and timing of the operation has been described by Dodge-Khatami (Dodge-Khatami et al. 2023), he notes:

"PVR has been shown to improve RV function and to decrease the size of the RV (Dave et al. 2005; Buechel et al. 2005; Therrien et al. 2001; van Straten et al. 2005), but this improvement appears to be limited when the RV has reached a critical size. In an analysis of patients after PVR, there was an improvement in RVEDV and RVESV; however, no patient with a RVEDDV > 170 mL/m^2 or a RVESD > 85 mL/m^2 achieved a normal RVEDV or RVESV, while 90% of those with RVEDV < 170 mL/m^2 before PRV had normal post-PRV in RV volumes (Roest et al. 2002). Most agree that symptoms of any kind are an indication for pulmonary valve replacement, regardless of RV dimensions or the degree of PR. In asymptomatic patients, the exact timing and indication remain controversial: most consider that PVR is an important intervention late after TOF repair, but if executed too late, may fail to achieve true benefit. Geva and colleagues have recommended general criteria for PVR in patients with moderate to severe PR (Warner et al. 2003): the presence of any two of the following represents an indication: RVEDD index > 160 mL/m^2; RVESD index > 70 mL/m^2; LVEDV index > 65 mL/m^2; RVEF < 45%; RVOT aneurysm; clinical symptoms or signs including syncope and ventricular tachycardia. In asymptomatic patients, our program currently proceeds with PVR at an RVEDV index of 150 ml/m^2. These indications will certainly evolve as more data are analyzed."

The technical aspects of pulmonary valve preservation, homograft replacement, valved conduit replacement, and bioprosthetic valve insertion in the orthotopic location with the creation of RVOT hood using Gore-Tex or heterograft pericardium are the options for valved right ventricular outflow tract reconstruction (Champsaur et al. 1998; Chan et al. 1994; Homann et al. 2000; Dave et al. 2006).

14 Pulmonary Valve Restoration

Pulmonary valve restoration is highly dependent on the previous TOF operation, the pulmonary valve anatomy, the method of right ventricular outflow tract reconstruction, and the growth of the pulmonary valve. It is not always clear therefore whether a valve preservation technique can be used. More often than not, patients are referred for transcatheter or operative placement of a pulmonary valve. When operative therapy is selected, resternotomy, cardiopulmonary bypass, careful management of a potential patent foramen ovale, and pulmonary valve insertion can usually be accomplished with homografts, heterographs, or constructed PTFE valve grafts.

The operation for pulmonary valve insertion, while complicated by resternotomy, can be performed safely by a number of techniques. Some surgeons use cardiopulmonary bypass with a single venous catheter in a beating non-working heart as long as a PFO is not detected. However, while transesophageal echocardiography can detect a PFO, it is not always accurate. If a small PFO is not detected, air embolism can occur with the beating heart technique due to the common use of suction assisted venous return which is used to enhance venous drainage and a decompressed right atrium. The PFO, under these circumstances, can come into direct contact with intracavitary air which can cause systemic air embolism, myocardial ischemia, and strokes. These potential complications have led many surgeons to use cardioplegic arrest to perform a pulmonary valve implant, even though it is a right ventricular operation. Previous operative reports, comprehensive echocardiography, and prudence are important factors to guide the operative team as to which technique to use.

Figure 27 shows the resternotomy, dissection, and exposure techniques in a patient who underwent transannular patch repair of tetralogy of Fallot with right ventricular dilatation. Hopefully, the TEE results can give the operative team some idea of valve leaflet preservation. Some surgeons left residual competent leaflets in place by resecting only the anterior leaflet while leaving the remaining leaflets in the event that some amount of resistance to backflow through partial valve competency would occur. This is the reason why leaflet evaluation should be part of the operation in the event that pulmonary valve preservation can be accomplished. To this end, the projected incision that will expose the right ventricular outflow tract is performed carefully and away from the valve leaflets. In this case, two competent leaflets are detected as noted in Fig. 28. These preserved leaflets are the remnants of a trileaflet pulmonary valve in which the anterior leaflet was resected in association with the original transannular patch. Figure 29 shows how the entire transannular patch can be carefully removed while preserving the valve commissures and allowing evaluation of the remaining leaflets for a competent bicuspid valve reconstruction without the need for a bioprosthetic valve replacement. So how does one preserve this valve without regurgitation and with only the minimal amount of stenosis? Good question. Figure 30 demonstrates how the anterior commissures can be approximated with pledgetted sutures to form a bicuspid pulmonary valve. After this maneuver, the reconstructed valve can be measured by sized dilators and compared with standard charts relating pulmonary valve size to body mass. Standard

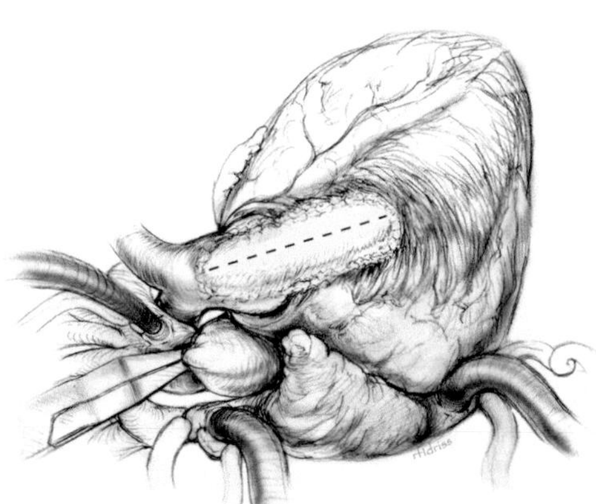

Fig. 27 Demonstrates mediastinal exposure after resternotomy, cardiopulmonary bypass, and cardioplegic arrest in a patient who underwent remote transannular repair of tetralogy of Fallot with right ventricular dilatation. The dotted line signifies the projected incision that will expose the right ventricular outflow tract and prepare for the projected pulmonary valve insertion. (With permission: Mavroudis 2015)

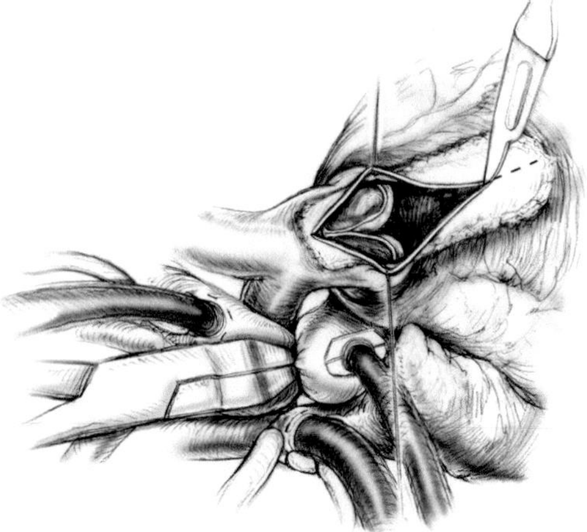

Fig. 28 During the incision to explore the nature and potential competency of the remaining pulmonary valve leaflets, two competent leaflets are discovered as noted in the figure. The leaflets are the remnants of a tricuspid pulmonary valve in which the anterior leaflet was resected in association with the original transannular patch. (With permission: Mavroudis 2015)

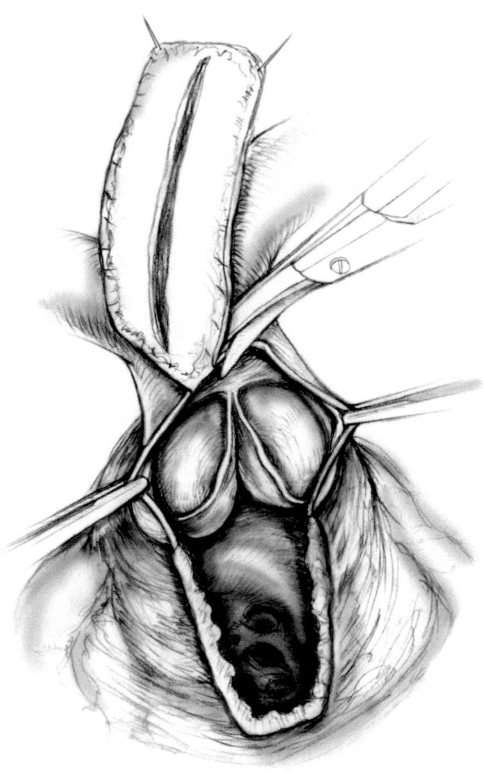

Fig. 29 The entire patch can be removed as noted in the figure, thereby exposing the extent that the remaining leaflets can be recruited to form a bicuspid valve without the need for bioprosthetic/prosthetic valve insertion. (With permission: Mavroudis 2015)

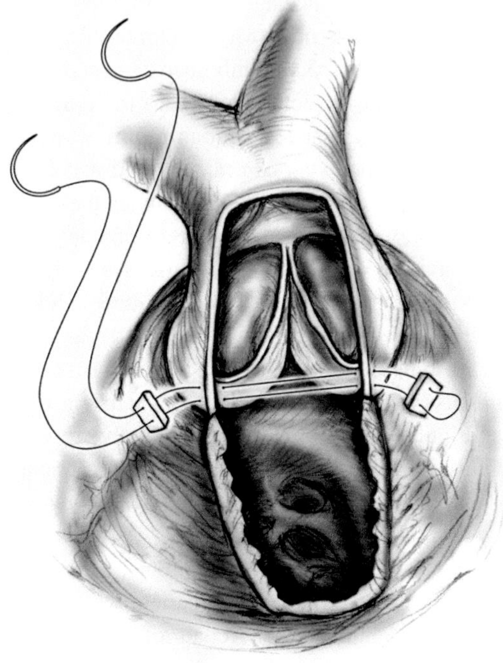

Fig. 30 Demonstrates placement of a pledgetted suture to approximate the anterior portions of the preserved pulmonary leaflets so as to recreate the anterior commissure. After this maneuver is performed, the reconstructed valve orifice is measured by sized dilators to determine the potential favorability of the newly constructed pulmonary valve in relationship to body mass. (With permission: Mavroudis 2015)

deviations away from the mean can be consulted to make an informed decision whether to carry on with valve preservation. The remaining parts of the operation are deliberately performed in sequence that will allow evaluation of the preserved pulmonary valve. Figures 31 and 32 show the placement of a supravalvar pulmonary artery patch for augmentation and to test for reconstructed valve competency using a saline filled bulb syringe or simply observing that the pulmonary back flow is contained. Figure 33 demonstrates the completed direct ventricular closure, which can also be accomplished with an augmentation patch. After separation from cardiopulmonary bypass, TEE evaluation and direct gradient measurements can be performed. In general, a gradient less than 30 mmHg should be within the acceptable range depending on the clinical circumstances.

In general, it is rare to have an opportunity to preserve the pulmonary valve after transannular patch. If this pathway is to be followed, surgeons should make efforts to preserve leaflets and the associated commissures at the original reparative operation, even if a transannular patch is necessary. Leaflet growth has been documented and competent neo-valve reconstruction is possible (Mavroudis et al. 2014). It is clearly worth the effort.

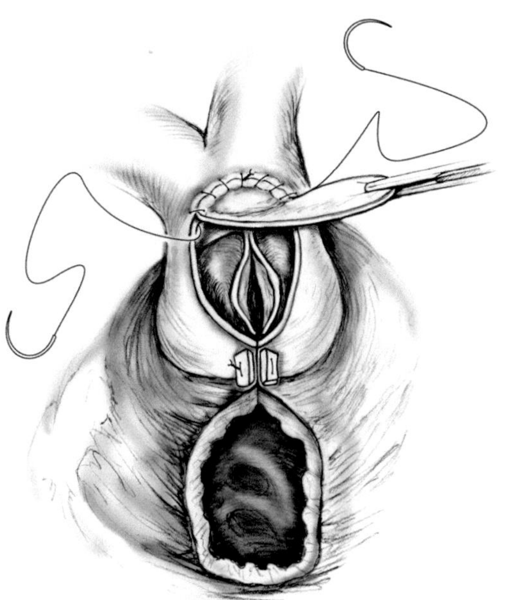

Fig. 31 Shows a supravalvar bioprosthetic patch being placed to augment the area and allow for testing of the reconstructed valve for competency. (With permission: Mavroudis 2015)

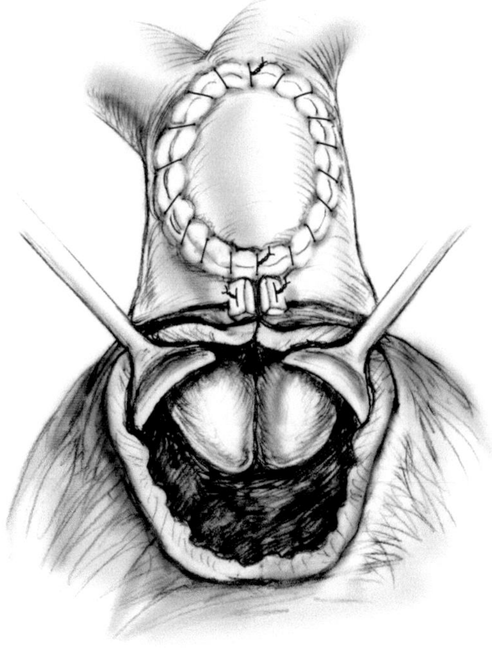

Fig. 32 With the right ventricular outflow tract open, the now reconstructed pulmonary valve as shown in the figure, can be tested for competency using a saline filled bulb syringe or simply noting that the pulmonary back flow is contained. (With permission: Mavroudis 2015)

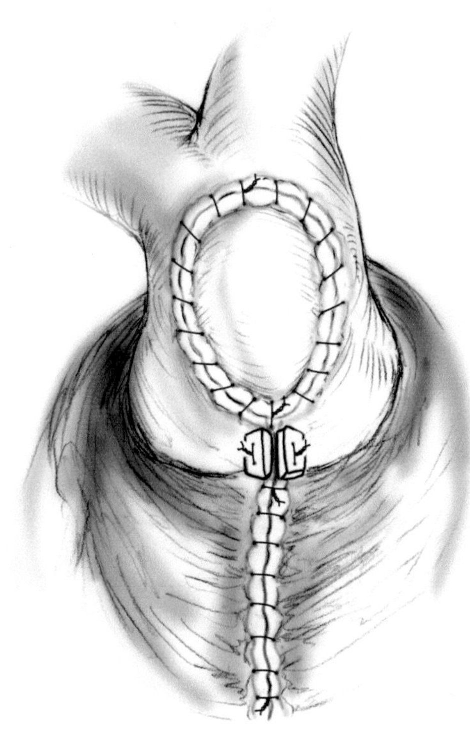

Fig. 33 Shows the completed ventricular closure, which in this case was performed primarily. Alternatively, the ventricle can be closed with a patch. (With permission: Mavroudis 2015)

15 Bioprosthetic Pulmonary Valve Insertion for Severe Pulmonary Regurgitation With and Without Pulmonary Stenosis

The previous sections have established the beneficial effects of pulmonary valve insertion in patients who had repaired tetralogy of Fallot by transannular patch. When planning pulmonary valve insertion, it is important to recognize the characteristics of the RVOT regarding size, as well as absence or presence of stenosis. The absence of stenosis with a wide-open outflow tract tends to be more common from the early eras of repair which emphasized large outflow tract reconstructions to avoid residual stenosis and not be concerned with free pulmonary regurgitation. Figures 34, 35, 36, and 37 demonstrate

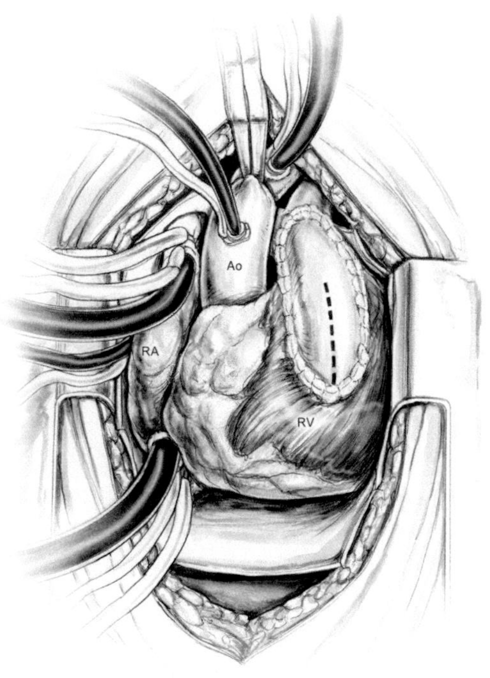

Fig. 34 Shows reoperative exposure in an adult patient with tetralogy of Fallot treated with a transannular patch. The operative principles are evident with aortobicaval cardiopulmonary bypass, left ventricular venting (right superior pulmonary vein), as well as aortic cross-clamping and cardioplegic arrest. The dotted line demonstrates the incision in the right ventricular outflow tract (RVOT) patch which extends upstream to the area of the previously incised pulmonary annulus. While this operation can be performed using aorto-uniatrial cardiopulmonary bypass in a beating heart, the recommended technique herein noted allows for a quiet, non-moving field which enhances suture placement accuracy, the elimination of unwanted systemic air embolism, and the ability to perform concomitant operations such as tricuspid valve repair, arrhythmia surgery, and right atrial wall reduction. Once the operative principles are established, the proximal RVOT patch is resected, and preparations are made for the bioprosthetic valve insertion. (With permission: Mavroudis and Dearani 2020). *Ao* aorta, *RA* right atrium, *RV* right ventricle

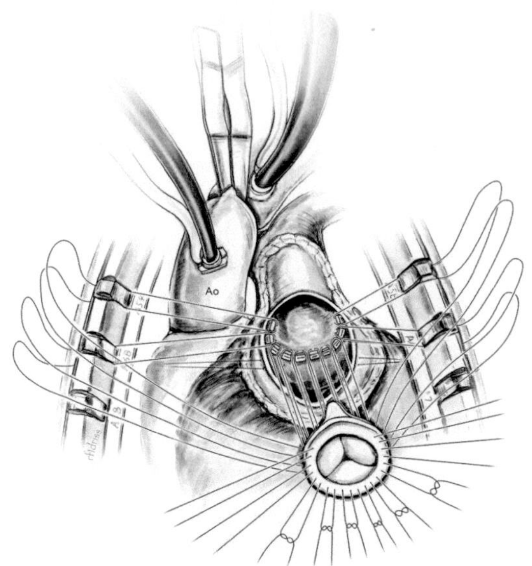

Fig. 35 This technique is interesting in so far that the pledgetted sutures are placed in such a manner that they are situated into the sewing ring and tied on the ventricular side and not the pulmonary artery side. The figure demonstrates the placement of interrupted pledgetted sutures in the posterior right ventricular outflow tract (RVOT) and simultaneously through the bioprosthetic valve sewing ring as noted. The outflow portion of the valve is oriented into the RVOT which will allow uncomplicated tying and careful implantation. (With permission: Mavroudis and Dearani 2020). *Ao* aorta

bioprosthetic valve insertion in a patient with wide open RVOT reconstruction after transannular TOF repair. In the majority of cases, proximal branch pulmonary stenosis was spared which allows a simplified pulmonary valve insertion owing to the large outflow tract patch. Consequently, the surgical team can plan to place a relatively large valve in the right ventricular outflow tract without worrying about proximal pulmonary artery stenosis.

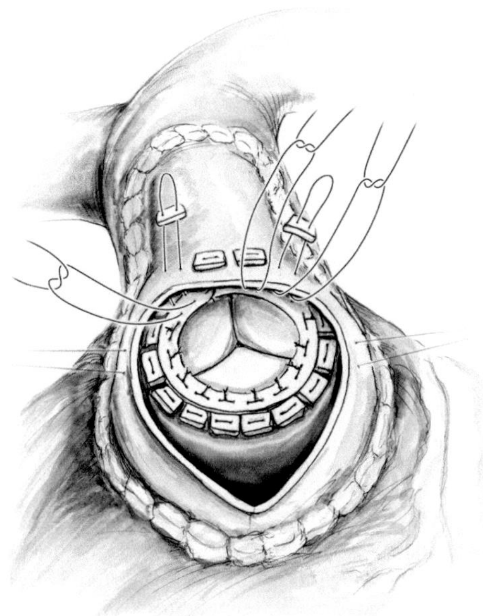

Fig. 36 Since the previously placed right ventricular outflow tract patch is generally large enough, the anterior sewing ring fixation can be performed by placing pledgetted sutures into the extant patch and through the sewing ring in the same manner as was used for the posterior sutures as shown in the figure. (With permission: Mavroudis and Dearani 2020)

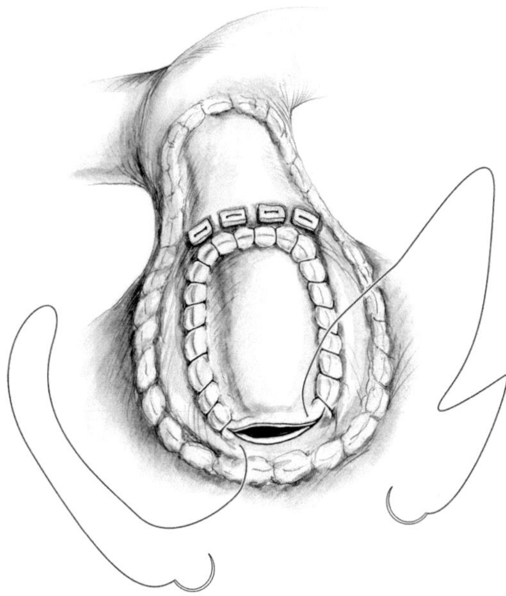

Fig. 37 The completion of the right ventricular outflow tract reconstruction and augmentation is performed by a separate patch as shown in the figure. Occasionally, a localized subvalvar muscle resection will be necessary to ensure an unobstructed pathway. (With permission: Mavroudis and Dearani 2020)

When considering pulmonary valve insertion late after repair of TOF with combined pulmonary stenosis and regurgitation, the surgical team must be mindful of the location of the pulmonary stenosis, the need for subvalvar muscular resection and appropriate patch augmentation. The particulars of pulmonary valve insertion in the presence of combined stenosis and regurgitation are noted in Figs. 38, 39, 40, 41, and 42.

Nevertheless, there are complications associated with pulmonary valve insertion and relate to resternotomy, associated bleeding, coronary artery injury, and unwanted bioprosthetic valve placement far into the RVOT which can cause

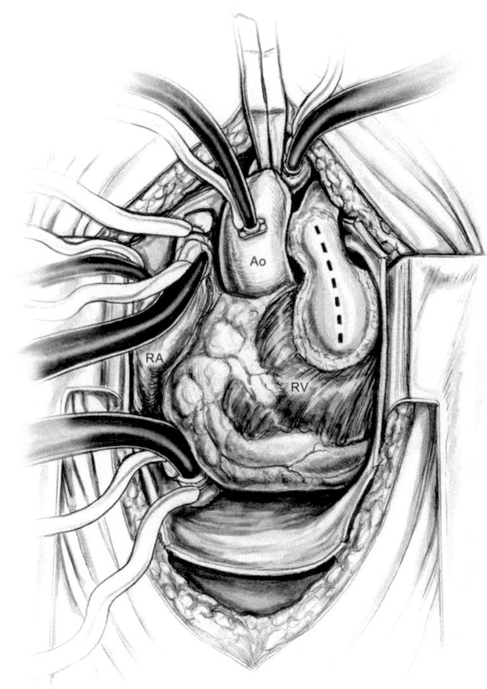

Fig. 38 In the majority of cases, the right ventricular outflow tract (RVOT) in a patient with tetralogy of Fallot treated with a transannular patch is both stenotic and regurgitant. When these patients develop symptoms and findings that require bioprosthetic pulmonary valve insertion, the same reoperative approach is used as noted above, namely, aortobicaval cardiopulmonary bypass, left ventricular venting, aortic cross-clamping, and cardioplegic arrest as shown in the figure. The anticipated incision in the RVOT, by necessity will be across the regurgitant area and the multiple levels of stenosis as noted in the drawing. The RVOT patch is removed and preparations are made for bioprosthetic valve implantation. (With permission: Mavroudis and Dearani 2020). *Ao* aorta, *RA* right atrium, *RV* right ventricle

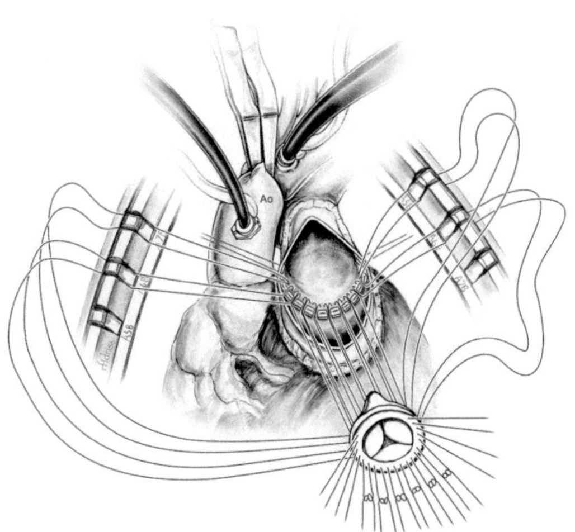

Fig. 39 Shows posterior right ventricular outflow tract placement of pledgetted sutures with simultaneous placement through the device sewing ring. The valve can then be anchored in place by tying the sutures. This leaves a significant moiety above and below the valve which can be repaired by a large PTFE patch. (With permission: Mavroudis and Dearani 2020)

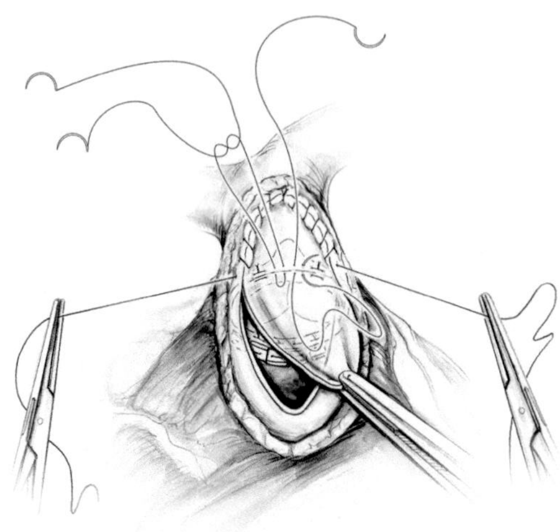

Fig. 41 Once the PTFE patch is aligned with the valve, the anterior sewing ring can be attached to the PTFE patch with interrupted pledgetted sutures thereby implanting the valve effectively as shown in the figure. (With permission: Mavroudis and Dearani 2020)

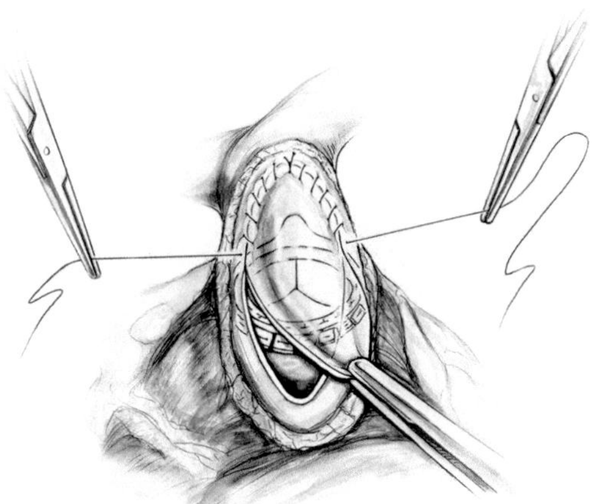

Fig. 40 Demonstrates the PTFE patch augmentation of the distal main pulmonary artery upstream to the bioprosthetic valve. (With permission: Mavroudis and Dearani 2020)

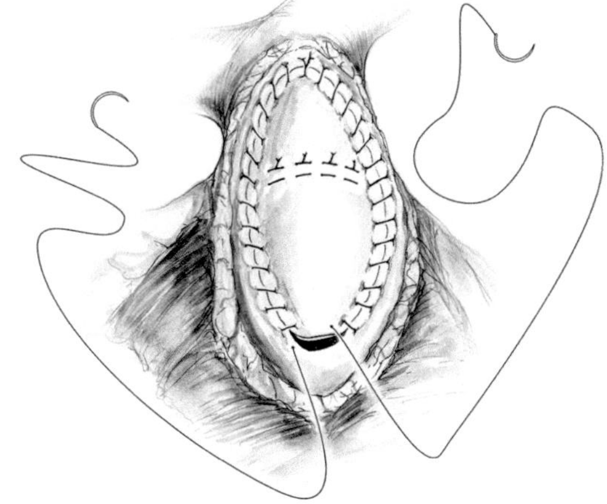

Fig. 42 The rest of the right ventricular outflow tract reconstruction is completed by attachment of the remaining lip of the patch to the edges of the right ventricular wall as shown in the figure. A conscientious evaluation of the ventricular outflow tract will determine whether a localized muscle resection will be necessary. (With permission: Mavroudis and Dearani 2020)

branch pulmonary artery stenosis. As compelling is the rare complication of bioprosthetic valve thrombosis and outflow tract stenosis (Reed et al. 2022). Regardless of intraoperative or postoperative risks, the clinical team must be mindful of the possible complications and be ready to intervene.

The aforementioned technical considerations have been successful, however there are no clear advantages regarding any particular technique. For example, other authors have successfully used stentless porcine valves for RVOT reconstruction (Hawkins et al. 2009). Mechanical valves have also been used for PVR; however, most surgeons avoid this strategy owing to the risks of valve thrombosis and anticoagulation requirement (Deorsola et al. 2010; Pragt et al. 2017).

Percutaneous transcatheter pulmonary valve replacement has gained efficacy over the recent era. Holzer and Hijazi have reviewed the extant literature as of 2016 and showed great promise in this modality. At the present time, there are two commercially available transcatheter pulmonary valve replacement valves which include the Edwards Sapien valve and the Medtronic Melody valve. More data has accrued for the Melody valve. Important findings that are relevant to complications included a 5% incidence of coronary artery anatomy that prohibited valve implantation, a 6% incidence of existing conduit disruption, and a freedom from stent fraction of the Melody valve stent of 60% at 30 months. In general, they found that short- and medium-term outcomes are comparable to surgical valve replacement (Holzer and Hijazi 2016) There has been, however, recent evidence suggesting that the incidence of infective endocarditis (IE) is higher in patients with congenital heart disease who have undergone implantation of Bovine Jugular Vein (BJV) grafts in the pulmonary position compared with other graft types. Specifically, the median cumulative incidence of IE was higher for BJV compared with other valves (5.4% vs. 1.2%, $p < 0.0001$). Interestingly, for patients with BJV valves, the incidence of IE was not different between surgical and catheter-based valve implantation. The authors concluded that, "There was no difference in the incidence of endocarditis between catheter-based bovine valves and surgically implanted bovine valves, suggesting that the substrate for future infection is related to the tissue rather than the method of implantation." (Sharma et al. 2017) The use of percutaneous PVR will certainly become more prevalent as engineering of newer devices improves. The indications for percutaneous PVR should be the same as for surgical PVR.

16 Neurological Outcomes

Assessments of children with repaired TOF have shown "inferior full-scale IQ than the general age-matched population (Miatton et al. 2007)." However, more granular data have clarified these conclusions. Namely, when repaired TOF children were considered and stratified by the presence or absence of a genetic lesion or syndrome, those without had scores within the normal limits for age (Zeltser et al. 2008). A report by Chow and associates noted that the incidence of stroke in adults with repaired TOF is higher than the general population. However, no clear etiology for these results have been demonstrated, leaving the scientific community to speculate regarding the prevalence of arrhythmias, clot embolization, and residual defects (Chow et al. 2005).

17 Aortic Valve and Root Issues

It has been well known that histopathologic changes in the ascending aorta can lead to aortic dilatation in patients with TOF (Chowdhury et al. 2008). Moreover, Seki and associates have documented aortic stiffness and aortic dilation in infants and children with TOF, even before corrective surgery (Seki et al. 2012). These findings often result in disease progression after TOF repair manifested by aortic root dilatation and aortic valve regurgitation (Niwa 2005; Niwa et al. 2002).

Consequently, these patients are being followed for complications that are generally more associated with adult acquired disease such as bicuspid aortic valve, connective tissue disorders, and atherosclerotic vascular disease. In order to lend some clarification on this issue several clinical and pathological studies have been performed. Zahka and colleagues evaluated 59 patients for pulmonary regurgitation 18 years after repair, and noted that 21% of patients had important aortic regurgitation (Zahka et al. 1988). Other authors have confirmed these findings and have shown that these aortic abnormalities in patients with TOF can occur even in childhood and documented by a high level of elastic fiber fragmentation seen in the aorta (Niwa et al. 2002; Chong et al. 2006). Tan and associates studied autopsy specimens from patients with TOF and found that the aorta had elastic fragmentation in 59%, medionecrosis in 29%, cystic medial necrosis in 35%, and fibrosis in 82% (Tan et al. 2005). These aortic histologic abnormalities can lead to the development of aortic aneurysms (Dimitrakakis et al. 2009) and aortic dissection (Kim et al. 2005) late after TOF repair. Notwithstanding these data, it is not clear what is the natural history and progression of aortic dilation in patients with TOF, especially when it pertains to prophylactic surgery. To investigate this clinical dilemma, Egbe and associates from the Mayo Clinic studied 453 adult repaired TOF patients at a mean age of 37 years at the time of imaging. Their results and conclusions are profound and worth quoting. They wrote,

"Results: Of the 453 consecutive patients (37 ± 13 years, men 216 (49%)) in the study, aortic aneurysm was present in 312 (69%) based on normative data; progressive aortic dilation occurred in 40 (9%), and there was no case of aortic dissection. Significant Aortic Valve Disease and Aortic Aneurysm, (AVD-AA) occurred in 52 (12%) patients; and 15 of them (29%) underwent aortic surgery without any surgical mortality. **Conclusions:** Although aortic aneurysm was common, progressive aortic dilation was uncommon and aortic dissection did not occur in our patients with TOF with significant aortic aneurysms who did not undergo aortic surgery. This has important clinical implication in deciding the frequency of imaging follow-up and timing of surgical intervention in this population. (Egbe et al. 2019)."

Clearly, aneurysmal progression in TOF patients requires evaluation depending on peculiar characteristics of their congenital heart disease. However, once indications for surgery are met, surgical intervention on aortic aneurysm and aortic valve disease in patients with repaired TOF are the same as in non-tetralogy patients (Crestanello et al. 2010; Nishimura et al. 2014).

18 Complications Associated with Repair of Tetralogy of Fallot with Absent Pulmonary Valve

Repair of tetralogy of Fallot with Absent Pulmonary Valve (TOF-APV), is a very challenging undertaking owing to the pathophysiology of TOF and the tracheobronchial obstructive consequences of the giant pulmonary arteries that have developed in utero owing to the prenatal pulmonary regurgitation. As a matter of incidence, about 2.5% of cases of TOF have near absence of the pulmonary valve leaflets (Zucker et al. 2004). It is important to review the anatomical characteristics of this anomaly since so many of the peculiarities will require surgical attention which increases the chances of significant complications. To begin with, the nomenclature is not entirely correct since these valves do have very rudimentary leaflets, which completely lack a three-dimensional cusp-like anatomy.

Furthermore, the leaflets have limited mobility and the cusps are centrally deficient with a large coaptation gap. The amalgamation of annular hypoplasia, leaflet immobility, and valvar tissue central deficiency combine to create the anatomic and physiologic conditions for combined pulmonary stenosis and insufficiency. Of surgical importance, the infundibulum is elongated and tubular. However, muscular right ventricular outflow obstruction is not generally a major part of this anomaly, which will limit the amount of muscular resection at the repair. In most cases of TOF-APV the main pulmonary trunk and central right and left branch pulmonary arteries are markedly dilated (Fig. 43) (Horrow and Laucks 1982). The aneurysmal characteristics of the central pulmonary arteries oftentimes extend into the pulmonary hilum, which makes the segmental branches emanating from the bulbous central aneurysm difficult to identify. The central aneurysmal pulmonary trunk and branch pulmonary arteries can cause severe compression of the tracheal-bronchial tree. As a consequence, in the most extreme instances, severe respiratory distress is present from birth. In addition to the anatomic aberrations, there is absence of a patent

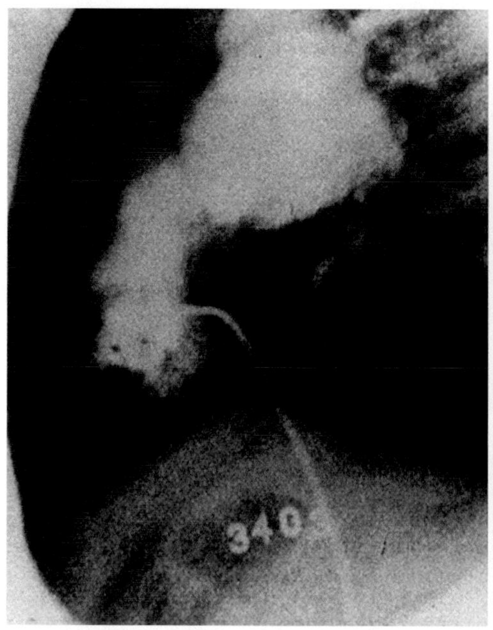

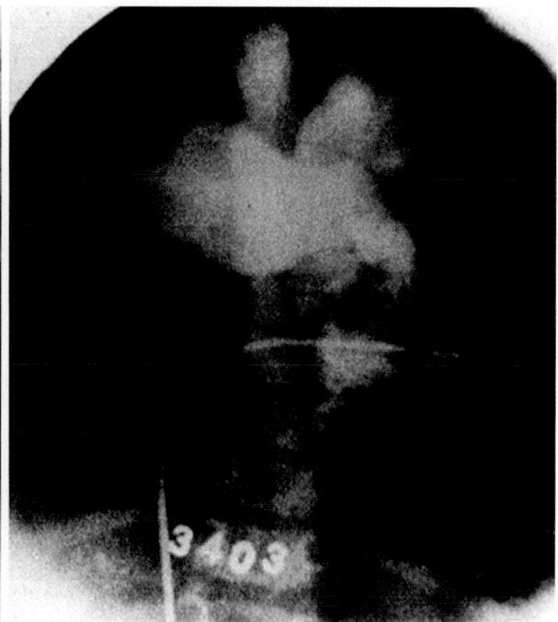

Fig. 43 Angiogram in a patient with tetralogy of Fallot and absent pulmonary valve. There is marked aneurysmal dilatation of the main, right, and left pulmonary arteries and absent pulmonary valve. (With permission: Hirsch and Bove 2003)

ductus or ductal ligament in the vast majority of cases, which is thought to be the consequential stimulus for in utero development of pulmonary artery aneurysmal dilatation. These unfortunate neonates are frequently ventilator-dependent and require early intervention. Those individuals with more favorable symptoms can have elective repair before 6 months of age, assuming that symptoms do not progress.

Because the early experience with transannular patch repair for TOF-APV was not optimal, surgeons initiated repair with VSD closure, right ventricular to pulmonary artery valved conduit, and pulmonary arterioplasty to reduce their size and relieve bronchial compression (Dodge-Khatami et al. 1999). While this approach became the classic approach used by the majority of surgeons, alternatives reemerged for complete repair with a transannular repair without a right ventricular to pulmonary artery valved conduit. The reasoning for this seemingly retrospective approach relates to a significantly longer interval before a required reoperation, since most infants will outgrow a valved conduit within the first few years of life (Chen et al. 2006). In circumstances when tracheobronchial compression is not relieved by pulmonary reduction arterioplasty, a Lecompte maneuver may help to alleviate the problem. The idea is to translocate the pulmonary arteries anteriorly to the aorta to provide significant relief from bronchial compression (Hraska et al. 2009). Other authors have approached this problem by resecting the pulmonary artery trunk and the dilated branch pulmonary arteries up to the respective hili and replacing it with a pulmonary homograft with the attached branch pulmonary arteries. (Hew et al. 2002).

Complications associated with this repair relate mostly to the management of the extant pulmonary artery compression of the tracheobronchial tree. The results of tracheobronchial relief by pulmonary artery reduction or translocation techniques can be assessed by intraoperative bronchoscopy and should be available during repair of TOF-APV. Figure 44 shows anterior and central pulmonary artery exposure after pulmonary artery trunk transection with the dashed lines indicating the area of the quadrangular

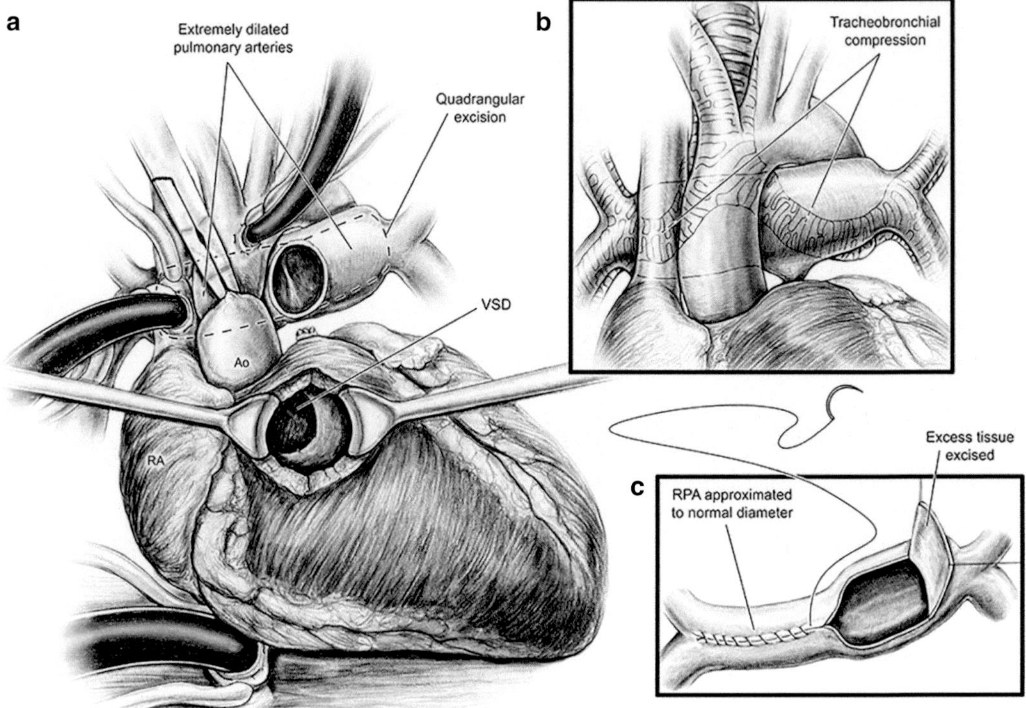

Fig. 44 (**a**) shows anterior and central pulmonary artery exposure after main pulmonary artery transection after cardiopulmonary bypass, aortic cross-clamping and cardioplegic arrest. The dashed lines show the proposed quadrangular excision. Also, the pulmonary artery stump is oversewn and a ventriculotomy is performed showing the open ventricular septal defect. Inset **b** shows the enlarged pulmonary artery and the tracheobronchial tree in hidden anatomy. Inset **c** shows right pulmonary artery excision and reanastomosis by anterior suture line. Also shown is the excised anterior pulmonary artery segment in anticipation of downstream reanastomosis and enough room for the recipient of the right ventricular to pulmonary artery valved conduit. *Ao* aorta, *RA* right atrium, *RPA* right pulmonary artery

resection to achieve pulmonary artery reduction arterioplasty to relieve the mass compression of the tracheobronchial tree. Figure 45 illustrates the result of pulmonary artery reduction arterioplasty and conduit placement with proximal anastomosis to the right ventricle in progress. The VSD has been closed and can be noted in the drawing. The expectation is that the pulmonary artery resection and conduit will result in a favorable outcome. However, this maneuver may not be helpful if the right ventricular to pulmonary artery conduit is too long as noted in Fig. 46 (left panel) The Fig. 46 right panel illustrates how the shortened conduit can relieve the pressure on the tracheobronchial tree. Deliberately making the conduit a little shorter than what would be considered normal, can effectively take the pressure off the tracheobronchial tree and relieve the compression. A more extensive and "bailout" procedure such as anterior tracheal suspension to the underside of the sternum can be helpful when all other measures prove to be ineffective. This technique is described conscientiously by Mitchell (Mitchell 2011) and should be consulted as needed. Mortality from repair of TOF-APV is approximately 5% (Alsoufi et al. 2007; Brown et al. 2006) with most of the deaths occurring in critically ill infants with significant airway compromise, related to tracheobronchial compression and persistent bronchial malacia.

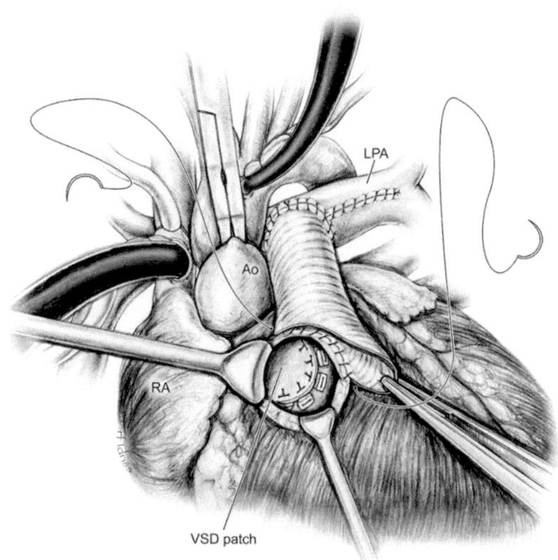

Fig. 45 Conduit is placed distally with completed reduction pulmonary artery arterioplasty. The closed ventricular septal defect is shown with the proximal conduit to the ventriculotomy being constructed. *Ao* aorta, *LPA* left pulmonary artery, *RA* right atrium, *VSD* ventricular septal defect

19 Tetralogy of Fallot and Atrioventricular Septal Defect

The association of TOF and AVSD (TOF-AVSD) occurs in about 3% of all tetralogy cases, the majority of whom have Trisomy 21 (Gatzoulis et al. 1994). Repair is usually performed between 4 and 6 months of age. Some anatomic and physiological characteristics are interesting and relate to surgical management. Physiologically, in contrast to the incidence of pulmonary hypertension which occurs in isolated AVSD, patients with TOF-AVSD are protected from pulmonary hypertension by RVOT obstruction. Anatomic considerations are important since retraction of the common anterior leaflet can be performed readily during VSD closure in patients with Rastelli type C TOF-AVSD. Absence of chordal attachments from the anterior bridging leaflet allows extensive exposure to the superior border of the VSD

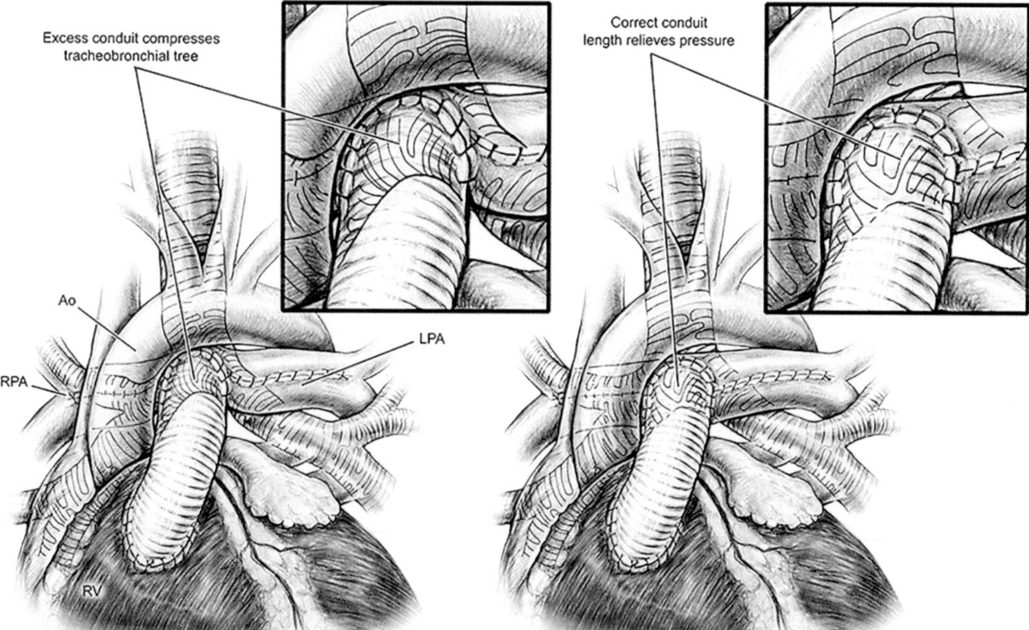

Fig. 46 Left panel shows how an elongated right ventricular to pulmonary artery conduit might result in continued pressure on the reconstructed pulmonary artery with resultant continued tracheobronchial obstruction. The right panel shows the shortened conduit which acts to pull the main pulmonary artery reconstruction away from the tracheobronchial tree thereby more effectively treating the tracheobronchial obstruction. *Ao* aorta, *LPA* left pulmonary artery, *RPA* right pulmonary artery, *RV* right ventricle

for accurate, safe, and secure suture placement for VSD closure. Like the approach for repair of AVSD, transatrial exposure is established through a right ventricular outflow tract resection can be done as well as VSD closure, and repair of the AVSD component. There are some interesting modifications that will be required to insure closure of the VSD without LVOT obstruction. In particular, a two-patch technique is most commonly used. The VSD patch is modified in the shape of a comma (Delius et al. 1997) with the larger and wider aspect to be placed in the superior portion of the malalignment tetralogy type of VSD at the area of the LVOT under the anterior common leaflet to allow accurate closure. The remaining geometric patch configuration is narrower and extends under the posterior bridging leaflet. As with all repairs of AVSD, competency of the atrioventricular valves is carefully considered and executed. While the left atrioventricular valve is the main focus of attention in patients with AVSD, conscientious repair of the right atrioventricular valve in patients with tetralogy of Fallot and complete atrioventricular canal is important to avoid right ventricular unwanted hemodynamic consequences, especially if a transannular patch is required for significant RVOT obstruction.

Early reports concerning TOF-AVSD repair were attended by a mortality up to 10%, however more recent outcomes have reported much better results with no mortality in 20 patients (Hoohenkerk et al. 2008).

20 Conclusion

Surgical repair of TOF is attended by favorable outcomes, durable long-term survival, and excellent functional status. Many centers are proponents of complete repair in infancy rather than staged repair after initial palliation. Those favoring early infant repair without prior palliation have extolled the virtues of a single operation for cure. However, there are drawbacks such as almost universal ventriculotomy for VSD closure, the length of which has not been measured or evaluated regarding right ventricular function. On the other hand, those proponents of staged palliation and later repair point to the greater possibility of pulmonary valve preservation, atrial repair, and fewer ventriculotomies. However, there continues to be morbidity, mortality, and interstage attrition associated with this approach. Palliation methods have been evolving in many centers away from the systemic-to-pulmonary artery shunt in favor of a more hemodynamically stable modified right ventricular outflow tract procedure, which is open enough for better perfusion and restrictive enough to replicate banded VSD physiology.

Early complications have been addressed and can be ameliorated and resolved by many of the methods that have been discussed such as residual VSD, coronary bypass for anomalous coronary artery injury, resolution of intraoperative sustained RVOT obstruction, and avoidance of arrhythmias.

Late complications include right ventricular dysfunction, atrial and ventricular arrhythmias, and sudden death. Pulmonary valve insertion by surgical and transcatheter methods has shown great efficacy with improved hemodynamic and functional outcomes.

As with all repairs of an atrioventricular canal, the competency of the atrioventricular valves is carefully considered. Although the left atrioventricular valve is the main focus of attention in patients with a simple atrioventricular canal, conscientious repair of the right atrioventricular valve in patients with tetralogy of Fallot and complete atrioventricular canal will be important to avoid right ventricular failure, especially if a transannular patch is required for significant RVOT obstruction.

References

Abbott MD. The clinical classification of congenital cardiac disease. Int Clin. 1924;4:156–88.

Alsoufi B, et al. Surgical outcomes in the treatment of patients with tetralogy of Fallot and absent pulmonary valve. Eur J Cardiothorac Surg. 2007;31(3):354–9.

Altrichter PM, et al. Surgical pathology of the valve: a study of 116 cases spanning 15 years. Mayo Clin Proc. 1989;64(11):1352–60.

Anderson RH, Weinberg PM. The clinical anatomy of tetralogy of Fallot. Cardiol Young. 2005;15(Suppl 1):38–47.

Azzam FJ, Fiore AC. Postoperative junctional ectopic tachycardia. Can J Anaesth. 1998;45(9):898–902.

Bacha E. Valve-sparing or valve reconstruction options in tetralogy of Fallot surgery. Semin Thorac Cardiovasc Surg Pediatr Card Surg Annu. 2017;20:79–83.

Bacha EA. Management of symptomatic infants with tetralogy of Fallot. World J Pediatr Congenit Heart Surg. 2018;9(5):546–7.

Bacha EA. Increased reinterventions after valve-sparing tetralogy of Fallot repair: is it the price to pay? Semin Thorac Cardiovasc Surg. 2019;31(2):264–5.

Bacha EA, et al. Long-term results after early primary repair of tetralogy of Fallot. J Thorac Cardiovasc Surg. 2001;122(1):154–61.

Barankay A, et al. Total intravenous anesthesia for infants and children undergoing correction of tetralogy of Fallot: sufentanil versus sufentanil-flunitrazepam technique. J Cardiothorac Vasc Anesth. 1992;6(2):185–9.

Barratt-Boyes BG, Neutze JM. Primary repair of tetralogy of Fallot in infancy using profound hypothermia with circulatory arrest and limited cardiopulmonary bypass: a comparison with conventional two stage management. Ann Surg. 1973;178(4):406–11.

Batlivala SP, et al. Staged palliation of cyanotic obstructive lesions with a modified right ventricular outflow procedure. World J Pediatr Congenit Heart Surg. 2018;9(1):68–73.

Becker AE, Connor M, Anderson RH. Tetralogy of Fallot: a morphometric and geometric study. Am J Cardiol. 1975;35(3):402–12.

Beland MJ, et al. Update from the International Working Group for Mapping and Coding of Nomenclatures for Paediatric and Congenital Heart Disease. Cardiol Young. 2004;14(2):225–9.

Birmingham A. Extreme anomaly of the heart and great vessels. J Anat Physiol. 1892;27(Pt 1):139–50.

Blalock AT, Taussig H. The surgical treatment of malformations of the heart in which there is pulmonary stenosis or pulmonary atresia. JAMA. 1945;128:189–202.

Brock RC. Pulmonary valvulotomy for the relief of congenital pulmonary stenosis; report of three cases. Br Med J. 1948;4562:1121–6.

Brown JW, et al. Surgical treatment of absent pulmonary valve syndrome associated with bronchial obstruction. Ann Thorac Surg. 2006;82(6):2221–6.

Buechel ER, et al. Remodelling of the right ventricle after early pulmonary valve replacement in children with repaired tetralogy of Fallot: assessment by cardiovascular magnetic resonance. Eur Heart J. 2005;26(24):2721–7.

Carvalho JS, et al. Exercise capacity after complete repair of tetralogy of Fallot: deleterious effects of residual pulmonary regurgitation. Br Heart J. 1992;67(6):470–3.

Castaneda AR, et al. Repair of tetralogy of Fallot in infancy. Early and late results. J Thorac Cardiovasc Surg. 1977;74(3):372–81.

Champsaur G, et al. Long-term clinical and hemodynamic evaluation of porcine valved conduits implanted from the right ventricle to the pulmonary artery. J Thorac Cardiovasc Surg. 1998;116(5):793–804.

Chan KC, et al. Right ventricular outflow reconstruction with cryopreserved homografts in pediatric patients: intermediate-term follow-up with serial echocardiographic assessment. J Am Coll Cardiol. 1994;24(2):483–9.

Chen JM, et al. Superior outcomes for repair in infants and neonates with tetralogy of Fallot with absent pulmonary valve syndrome. J Thorac Cardiovasc Surg. 2006;132(5):1099–104.

Chiariello L, et al. Intracardiac repair of tetralogy of Fallot. Five-year review of 403 patients. J Thorac Cardiovasc Surg. 1975;70:529–35.

Chong WY, et al. Aortic root dilation and aortic elastic properties in children after repair of tetralogy of Fallot. Am J Cardiol. 2006;97(6):905–9.

Chow CK, Amos D, Celermajer DS. Cerebrovascular events in young adults after surgical repair of tetralogy of Fallot. Cardiol Young. 2005;15(2):130–2.

Chowdhury UK, et al. Histopathologic changes in ascending aorta and risk factors related to histopathologic conditions and aortic dilatation in patients with tetralogy of Fallot. J Thorac Cardiovasc Surg. 2008;135(1):69–77.

Crestanello JA, et al. Medial necrosis in aortic root aneurysm after repair of tetralogy of Fallot. J Card Surg. 2010;25(2):230–2.

Cumming GR. Relief of dyspnoeic attacks in Fallot's tetralogy with propranolol. Lancet. 1966;1:519–22.

Dabizzi RP, et al. Distribution and anomalies of coronary arteries in tetralogy of Fallot. Circulation. 1980;61:95–102.

Dadlani GH, John JB, Cohen MS. Echocardiography in tetralogy of Fallot. Cardiol Young. 2008;18(Suppl 3):22–8.

Dave HH. Modified Blalock-Taussig shunt: simple but unpredictable. Eur J Cardiothorac Surg. 2016;50(1):178–9.

Dave HH, et al. Early insertion of a pulmonary valve for chronic regurgitation helps restoration of ventricular dimensions. Ann Thorac Surg. 2005;80(5):1615–21.

Dave H, et al. Modified technique for heterotopic implantation of a right ventricular outflow tract conduit. Ann Thorac Surg. 2006;81(6):2321–3.

de Leval MR, et al. Modified Blalock-Taussig shunt. Use of subclavian artery orifice as flow regulator in prosthetic systemic-pulmonary artery shunts. J Thorac Cardiovasc Surg. 1981;81(1):112–9.

Deal BJ, Mavroudis C, Backer CL. Beyond Fontan conversion: surgical therapy of arrhythmias including patients with associated complex congenital heart disease. Ann Thorac Surg. 2003;76(2):542–54.

Delius RE, et al. Atrioventricular septal defect and tetralogy of Fallot: a 15-year experience. Eur J Cardiothorac Surg. 1997;12(2):171–6.

Deorsola L, et al. Pulmonary valve replacement with mechanical prosthesis: long-term results in 4 patients. Ann Thorac Surg. 2010;89(6):2036–8.

Derby CD, Pizarro C. Routine primary repair of tetralogy of Fallot in the neonate. Expert Rev Cardiovasc Ther. 2005;3(5):857–63.

Di Donato RM, et al. Neonatal repair of tetralogy of Fallot with and without pulmonary atresia. J Thorac Cardiovasc Surg. 1991;101(1):126–37.

Dickinson DF, et al. Variations in the morphology of the ventricular septal defect and disposition of the atrioventricular conduction tissues in tetralogy of Fallot. Thorac Cardiovasc Surg. 1982;30:243–9.

Dietl CA, et al. Life-threatening arrhythmias and RV dysfunction after surgical repair of tetralogy of Fallot. Comparison between transventricular and transatrial approaches. Circulation. 1994;90(5 Pt 2):II7–II12.

Dimitrakakis G, et al. Aortic aneurysm formation five decades after tetralogy of Fallot repair. Ann Thorac Surg. 2009;88(3):1000–1.

Discigil B, et al. Late pulmonary valve replacement after repair of tetralogy of Fallot. J Thorac Cardiovasc Surg. 2001;121(2):344–51.

Do N, et al. Shunt failure-risk factors and outcomes: an analysis of The Society of Thoracic Surgeons Congenital Heart Surgery Database. Ann Thorac Surg. 2018;105(3):857–64.

Dodge-Khatami A, et al. Complete repair of Tetralogy of Fallot with absent pulmonary valve including the role of airway stenting. J Card Surg. 1999;14(2):82–91.

Dodge-Khatami A, et al. Impact of junctional ectopic tachycardia on postoperative morbidity following repair of congenital heart defects. Eur J Cardiothorac Surg. 2002a;21(2):255–9.

Dodge-Khatami A, et al. Surgical substrates of postoperative junctional ectopic tachycardia in congenital heart defects. J Thorac Cardiovasc Surg. 2002b;123(4):624–30.

Dodge-Khatami A, Chen P, Mavroudis C. Tetralogy of Fallot. In: Mavroudis C, Backer CL, editors. Pediatric cardiac surgery. 5th ed. London: Wiley Blackwell; 2023.

Dohlen G, et al. Stenting of the right ventricular outflow tract in the symptomatic infant with tetralogy of Fallot. Heart. 2009;95(2):142–7.

Downing DF, Bailey CP, Glover RP. Brock procedure for the relief of pulmonary stenosis in the tetralogy of Fallot. Pediatrics. 1951;7:230–9.

Ebert PA, Turley K. Surgery for cyanotic heart disease in the first year of life. J Am Coll Cardiol. 1983;1(1):274–9.

Egbe AC, et al. Aortic disease and interventions in adults with tetralogy of Fallot. Heart. 2019;105(12):926–31.

Elliott RB, Starling MB, Neutze JM. Medical manipulation of the ductus arteriosus. Lancet. 1975;1(7899):140–2.

Elsayed H, Page R, Agarwal S, Chalmers J. Oesophageal perforation complicating intraoperative transoesophageal echocardiography: suspicion can save lives. Interact Cardiovasc Thorac Surg. 2010;11:380–2.

Eyskens B, et al. Homograft insertion for pulmonary regurgitation after repair of tetralogy of fallot improves cardiorespiratory exercise performance. Am J Cardiol. 2000;85(2):221–5.

Fallot E. Contribution a l'anatomie pathologique de la maladie bleue. Marseille Med. 1888;25:77–138.

Fraser CD Jr, McKenzie ED, Cooley DA. Tetralogy of Fallot: surgical management individualized to the patient. Ann Thorac Surg. 2001;71(5):1556–63.

Friedli B. [Arrhythmia after surgery for congenital cardiopathies. What studies? What treatment?]. Arch Mal Coeur Vaiss. 1996;89(3):351–7.

Friedli B. Electrophysiological follow-up of tetralogy of Fallot. Pediatr Cardiol. 1999;20(5):326–30.

Frigiola A, et al. Pulmonary regurgitation is an important determinant of right ventricular contractile dysfunction in patients with surgically repaired tetralogy of Fallot. Circulation. 2004;110(11 Suppl 1):II153–7.

Garson A Jr, Gillette PC, McNamara DG. Propranolol: the preferred palliation for tetralogy of Fallot. Am J Cardiol. 1981;47(5):1098–104.

Gatzoulis MA, et al. Complete atrioventricular septal defect with tetralogy of Fallot: diagnosis and management. Br Heart J. 1994;71(6):579–83.

Gatzoulis MA, et al. Right and left ventricular systolic function late after repair of tetralogy of Fallot. Am J Cardiol. 2000a;86(12):1352–7.

Gatzoulis MA, et al. Risk factors for arrhythmia and sudden cardiac death late after repair of tetralogy of Fallot: a multicentre study. Lancet. 2000b;356(9234):975–81.

Gengsakul A, et al. The impact of pulmonary valve replacement after tetralogy of Fallot repair: a matched comparison. Eur J Cardiothorac Surg. 2007;32(3):462–8.

Gerelli S, et al. Neonatal right ventricle to pulmonary connection as a palliative procedure for pulmonary atresia with ventricular septal defect or severe tetralogy of Fallot. Eur J Cardiothorac Surg. 2014;45(2):278–88.

Geva T. Indications and timing of pulmonary valve replacement after tetralogy of Fallot repair. Semin Thorac Cardiovasc Surg Pediatr Card Surg Annu. 2006:11–22.

Geva T, et al. Evaluation of regional differences in right ventricular systolic function by acoustic quantification echocardiography and cine magnetic resonance imaging. Circulation. 1998;98(4):339–45.

Ghai A, et al. Left ventricular dysfunction is a risk factor for sudden cardiac death in adults late after repair of tetralogy of Fallot. J Am Coll Cardiol. 2002;40(9):1675–80.

Gott VL. C. Walton Lillehei and total correction of tetralogy of Fallot. Ann Thorac Surg. 1990;49:328–32.

Graham EM, et al. Effect of preoperative use of propranolol on postoperative outcome in patients with tetralogy of Fallot. Am J Cardiol. 2008;101(5):693–5.

Gustafson RA, et al. Early primary repair of tetralogy of Fallot. Ann Thorac Surg. 1988;45(3):235–41.

Hallbergson A, et al. Right ventricular remodeling after pulmonary valve replacement: early gains, late losses. Ann Thorac Surg. 2015;99(2):660–6.

Harrild DM, et al. Pulmonary valve replacement in tetralogy of Fallot: impact on survival and ventricular tachycardia. Circulation. 2009;119(3):445–51.

Harrison DA, et al. Sustained atrial arrhythmias in adults late after repair of tetralogy of Fallot. Am J Cardiol. 2001;87(5):584–8.

Hawkins JA, et al. Stentless porcine valves in the right ventricular outflow tract: improved durability? Eur J Cardiothorac Surg. 2009;35(4):600–5.

Hennein HA, et al. Intermediate results after complete repair of tetralogy of Fallot in neonates. J Thorac Cardiovasc Surg. 1995;109(2):332–43.

Hew CC, et al. Valved homograft replacement of aneurysmal pulmonary arteries for severely symptomatic absent pulmonary valve syndrome. Ann Thorac Surg. 2002;73(6):1778–85.

Hirsch JC, Bove EL. Tetralogy of Fallot. In: Mavroudis C, Backer CL, editors. Pediatric cardiac surgery. 3rd ed. Philadelphia: Mosby Inc.; 2003. p. 383–97.

Hirsch JC, Mosca RS, Bove EL. Complete repair of tetralogy of Fallot in the neonate: results in the modern era. Ann Surg. 2000;232(4):508–14.

Hofferberth SC, et al. Valve-sparing repair with intraoperative balloon dilation in tetralogy of Fallot: midterm results and therapeutic implications. J Thorac Cardiovasc Surg. 2018;155(3):1163–73.

Hokanson JS, Moller JH. Significance of early transient complete heart block as a predictor of sudden death late after operative correction of tetralogy of Fallot. Am J Cardiol. 2001;87(11):1271–7.

Holzer RJ, Hijazi ZM. Transcatheter pulmonary valve replacement: state of the art. Catheter Cardiovasc Interv. 2016;87(1):117–28.

Homann M, et al. Reconstruction of the RVOT with valved biological conduits: 25 years experience with allografts and xenografts. Eur J Cardiothorac Surg. 2000;17(6):624–30.

Hoohenkerk GJ, et al. 28 years' experience with transatrial-transpulmonary repair of atrioventricular septal defect with tetralogy of Fallot. Ann Thorac Surg. 2008;85(5):1686–9.

Horneffer PJ, et al. Long-term results of total repair of tetralogy of Fallot in childhood. Ann Thorac Surg. 1990;50(2):179–85.

Horrow JC, Laucks SO. Coronary air embolism during venous cannulation. Anesthesiology. 1982;56(3):212–4.

Howell CE, et al. Variations within the fibrous skeleton and ventricular outflow tracts in tetralogy of Fallot. Ann Thorac Surg. 1990;50(3):450–7.

Hraska V, et al. A novel approach to the repair of tetralogy of Fallot with absent pulmonary valve and the reduction of airway compression by the pulmonary artery. Semin Thorac Cardiovasc Surg Pediatr Card Surg Annu. 2009:9–62.

Humes RA, et al. Tetralogy of Fallot with anomalous origin of left anterior descending coronary artery. Surgical options. J Thorac Cardiovasc Surg. 1987;94(5):784–7.

Ilbawi MN, et al. Factors that exaggerate the deleterious effects of pulmonary insufficiency on the right ventricle after tetralogy repair. Surgical implications. J Thorac Cardiovasc Surg. 1987;93(1):36–44.

Jacobs ML. Congenital Heart Surgery Nomenclature and Database Project: tetralogy of Fallot. Ann Thorac Surg. 2000;69(4 Suppl):S77–82.

Jonas RA. Early primary repair of tetralogy of Fallot. Semin Thorac Cardiovasc Surg Pediatr Card Surg Annu. 2009:39–47.

Kanter KR, et al. Symptomatic neonatal tetralogy of Fallot: repair or shunt? Ann Thorac Surg. 2010;89(3):858–63.

Karl TR, Sano S, Pornviliwan S, Mee RB. Tetralogy of Fallot: favorable outcome of nonneonatal transatrial, transpulmonary repair. Ann Thorac Surg. 1992;54(5):903–7.

Katz NM, et al. Late survival and symptoms after repair of tetralogy of Fallot. Circulation. 1982;65(2):403–10.

Khairy P, et al. Value of programmed ventricular stimulation after tetralogy of fallot repair: a multicenter study. Circulation. 2004;109(16):1994–2000.

Khairy P, et al. Arrhythmia burden in adults with surgically repaired tetralogy of Fallot: a multi-institutional study. Circulation. 2010;122(9):868–75.

Kim WH, et al. Aortic dissection late after repair of tetralogy of Fallot. Int J Cardiol. 2005;101(3):515–6.

Kim DH, et al. Optimal pulmonary valve annulus diameter for annulus preservation in tetralogy of fallot may be far smaller than normal annulus size. Semin Thorac Cardiovasc Surg. 2019;31(2):253–63.

Kirklin JW, et al. Intracardiac surgery with the aid of a mechanical pump-oxygenator system (gibbon type): report of eight cases. Proc Staff Meet Mayo Clin. 1955;30:201–6.

Kirklin JK, et al. Effect of transannular patching on outcome after repair of tetralogy of Fallot. Ann Thorac Surg. 1989;48(6):783–91.

Knauth AG, Landzberg K. Right ventricular size and function and age at repair predict major adverse outcomes late after tetralogy of Fallot repair (abstr). Circulation. 2005;112:681.

Knott-Craig CJ, et al. A 26-year experience with surgical management of tetralogy of Fallot: risk analysis for mortality or late reintervention. Ann Thorac Surg. 1998;66(2):506–11.

Kolcz J, Pizarro C. Neonatal repair of tetralogy of Fallot results in improved pulmonary artery development without increased need for reintervention. Eur J Cardiothorac Surg. 2005;28(3):394–9.

Koppel RI, et al. Effectiveness of pulse oximetry screening for congenital heart disease in asymptomatic newborns. Pediatrics. 2003;111:451–5.

Korbmacher B, et al. Evidence for palliative enlargement of the right ventricular outflow tract in severe tetralogy of Fallot. Eur J Cardiothorac Surg. 2005;27(6):945–8.

Kotoulas C. Transoesophageal echocardiography and oesophageal perforation. Inter CardioVasc Thorac Surg. 2010;11(3):382.

Laudito A, et al. Right ventricular outflow tract stent as a bridge to surgery in a premature infant with tetralogy of Fallot. Ann Thorac Surg. 2006;81(2):744–6.

Le Gloan L, et al. Clinical assessment of arrhythmias in tetralogy of Fallot. Expert Rev Cardiovasc Ther. 2010;8(2):189–97.

Lenoir M, et al. Outcomes of palliative right ventricle to pulmonary artery connection for pulmonary atresia with ventricular septal defect. Eur J Cardiothorac Surg. 2017;52(3):590–8.

Lillehei CW, et al. Direct vision intracardiac surgical correction of the tetralogy of Fallot, pentalogy of Fallot, and pulmonary atresia defects; report of first ten cases. Ann Surg. 1955;142:418–42.

Lozano-Balseiro M, Garcia-Vieites M, Martínez-Bendayán I, et al. Valve-sparing tetralogy of Fallot repair with intraoperative dilation of the pulmonary valve. Mid-term results. Semin Thorac Cardiovasc Surg. 2019;31(4):828–34.

Marie PY, et al. Right ventricular overload and induced sustained ventricular tachycardia in operatively "repaired" tetralogy of Fallot. Am J Cardiol. 1992;69(8):785–9.

Mavroudis C. Tetralogy of Fallot. In: Mavroudis C, Backer CL, editors. Atlas of pediatric cardiac surgery. London: Springer; 2015.

Mavroudis C. Coronary artery bypass grafting in infants, children, and young adults for acquired and congenital lesions. Congenit Heart Dis. 2017;12(5):644–6.

Mavroudis C, Backer CL. Closure of ventricular septal defect. Op Tech Thorac Cardiovasc Surg. 2002;7:11–21.

Mavroudis C, Dearani JA. Tetralogy of Fallot. In: Mavroudis C, Dearani JA, editors. Atlas of adult congenital heart surgery. Cham: Springer Nature; 2020.

Mavroudis C, Backer CL, Muster AJ, Pahl E, Sanders JH, Zales VR, Gevitz M. Expanding indications for pediatric coronary artery bypass. J Thorac Cardiovasc Surg. 1996;111(1):181–9.

Mavroudis CD, Jacobs JP, Frost J, Mavroudis C. Pulmonary valve preservation and restoration strategies for tetralogy of fallot repair. Cardiol Young. 2014;24:1088–94.

Meyer J, Peul GJ Jr, Chiarello L, Hallman GL, Cooley DA. Anomalous origin and distribution of coronary arteries. Review of 38 patients who underwent operation. J Cardiovasc Surg. 1975;16(5):500–5.

Miatton M, et al. Intellectual, neuropsychological, and behavioral functioning in children with tetralogy of Fallot. J Thorac Cardiovasc Surg. 2007;133(2):449–55.

Michielon G, et al. Genetic syndromes and outcome after surgical correction of tetralogy of Fallot. Ann Thorac Surg. 2006;81:968–75.

Miller JW, Hart CK, Statile CJ. Oesophageal perforation in a neonate during transoesophageal echocardiography for cardiac surgery. Cardiol Young. 2015;25(5):1015–8.

Mitchell ME. Anterior tracheal ssupension. Oper Tech Thorac Cardiovasc Surg. 2011;16:331–9.

Murphy JG, et al. Long-term outcome in patients undergoing surgical repair of tetralogy of Fallot. N Engl J Med. 1993;329(9):593–9.

Need LR, et al. Coronary echocardiography in tetralogy of fallot: diagnostic accuracy, resource utilization and surgical implications over 13 years. J Am Coll Cardiol. 2000;36(4):1371–7.

Nishimura RA, et al. AHA/ACC guideline for the management of patients with valvular heart disease: executive summary: a report of the American College of Cardiology/American Heart Association Task Force on Practice Guidelines. J Am Coll Cardiol. 2014;63(22):2438–88.

Niwa K. Aortic root dilatation in tetralogy of Fallot long-term after repair—histology of the aorta in tetralogy of Fallot: evidence of intrinsic aortopathy. Int J Cardiol. 2005;103(2):117–9.

Niwa K, et al. Progressive aortic root dilatation in adults late after repair of tetralogy of Fallot. Circulation. 2002;106(11):1374–8.

Nollert G, et al. Long-term survival in patients with repair of tetralogy of Fallot: 36-year follow-up of 490 survivors of the first year after surgical repair. J Am Coll Cardiol. 1997;30(5):1374–83.

Nollert GD, et al. Risk factors for sudden death after repair of tetralogy of Fallot. Ann Thorac Surg. 2003;76(6):1901–5.

Nudel DB, Berman MA, Talner NS. Effects of acutely increasing systemic vascular resistance on oxygen tension in tetralogy of Fallot. Pediatrics. 1976;58(2):248–51.

Oosterhof T, et al. Long-term effect of pulmonary valve replacement on QRS duration in patients with corrected tetralogy of Fallot. Heart. 2007;93(4):506–9.

Parry AJ, et al. Elective primary repair of acyanotic tetralogy of Fallot in early infancy: overall outcome and impact on the pulmonary valve. J Am Coll Cardiol. 2000;36(7):2279–83.

Pigula FA, et al. Repair of tetralogy of Fallot in neonates and young infants. Circulation. 1999;100(19 Suppl):II157–II161.

Potts WJ, Smith S, Gibson S. Anastomosis of the aorta to a pulmonary artery in certain types of congenital heart disease. Case Rep Child Meml Hosp Chic. 1946;5:704–18.

Pragt H, et al. Mechanical valves in the pulmonary position: an international retrospective analysis. J Thorac Cardiovasc Surg. 2017;154(4):1371–8.

Rabinowitz EJ, et al. Promoting pulmonary arterial growth via right ventricle-to-pulmonary artery connection in children with pulmonary atresia, ventricular septal defect, and hypoplastic pulmonary arteries. World J Pediatr Congenit Heart Surg. 2017;8(5):564–9.

Ramakrishnan KV, et al. Symptomatic tetralogy of Fallot in young infants: primary repair or shunt-pediatric health information system database analysis. World J Pediatr Congenit Heart Surg. 2018;9(5):539–45.

Reddy VM, et al. Routine primary repair of tetralogy of Fallot in neonates and infants less than three months of age. Ann Thorac Surg. 1995;60(6 Suppl):S592–6.

Reed AK, Villaba JA, Cameron DE, Bloom JP. Early failure of a bioprosthetic valve in the pulmonary position causing panic. Ann Thorac Surg. 2022;114(1):e13–5.

Roest AA, et al. Exercise MR imaging in the assessment of pulmonary regurgitation and biventricular function in patients after tetralogy of fallot repair. Radiology. 2002;223(1):204–11.

Roos-Hesselink J, et al. Atrial arrhythmias in adults after repair of tetralogy of Fallot. Correlations with clinical, exercise, and echocardiographic findings. Circulation. 1995;91(8):2214–9.

Seipelt RG, et al. Antegrade palliation for diminutive pulmonary arteries in Tetralogy of Fallot. Eur J Cardiothorac Surg. 2002;21(4):721–4.

Seki M, et al. Aortic stiffness and aortic dilation in infants and children with tetralogy of Fallot before corrective surgery: evidence for intrinsically abnormal aortic mechanical property. Eur J Cardiothorac Surg. 2012;41(2):277–82.

Sellors TH. Surgery of pulmonary stenosis; a case in which the pulmonary valve was successfully divided. Lancet. 1948;1(6513):988.

Sendelbach DM, et al. Pulse oximetry screening at 4 hours of age to detect critical congenital heart defects. Pediatrics. 2008;122:e815–20.

Sharma A, Cote AT, Hosking MCK, Harris KC. A systematic review of infective endocarditis in patients with bovine jugular vein valves compared with other valve types. JACC Cardiovasc Interv. 2017;10(14):1449–58.

Singh GK, et al. Right ventricular function and exercise performance late after primary repair of tetralogy of Fallot with the transannular patch in infancy. Am J Cardiol. 1998;81(11):1378–82.

Sousa Uva M, et al. Surgery for tetralogy of Fallot at less than six months of age. J Thorac Cardiovasc Surg. 1994;107(5):1291–300.

Stellin G, et al. Repair of tetralogy of Fallot in the first six months of life: transatrial versus transventricular approach. Ann Thorac Surg. 1995;60(6 Suppl):S588–91.

Steno N. Anatomicus regij Halniensis, Embryo monstro affinis Parisiis dissectus. In: Bartholin T, editor. Acta Medica et Philosophia Hafniencia; 1671. p. 200–3.

Stewart RD, et al. Tetralogy of Fallot: results of a pulmonary valve-sparing strategy. Ann Thorac Surg. 2005;80(4):1431–9.

Stulak JM, et al. Right-sided Maze procedure for atrial tachyarrhythmias in congenital heart disease. Ann Thorac Surg. 2006;81(5):1780–5.

Suzuki A, et al. Further morphologic studies on tetralogy of Fallot, with particular emphasis on the prevalence and structure of the membranous flap. J Thorac Cardiovasc Surg. 1990;99(3):528–35.

Tamesberger MI, et al. Early primary repair of tetralogy of fallot in neonates and infants less than four months of age. Ann Thorac Surg. 2008;86(6):1928–35.

Tan JL, et al. Intrinsic histological abnormalities of aortic root and ascending aorta in tetralogy of Fallot: evidence of causative mechanism for aortic dilatation and aortopathy. Circulation. 2005;112(7):961–8.

Tanaka K, et al. Phenylephrine increases pulmonary blood flow in children with tetralogy of Fallot. Can J Anaesth. 2003;50(9):926–9.

Taussig HB. Neuhauser Lecture: Tetralogy of Fallot: early history and late results. AJR Am J Roentgenol. 1979;133:422–31.

Therrien J, et al. Impact of pulmonary valve replacement on arrhythmia propensity late after repair of tetralogy of Fallot. Circulation. 2001;103(20):2489–94.

Therrien J, et al. Optimal timing for pulmonary valve replacement in adults after tetralogy of Fallot repair. Am J Cardiol. 2005;95(6):779–82.

Tirilomis T, et al. Indications for reoperation late after correction of tetralogy of Fallot. Cardiol Young. 2010;20(4):396–401.

Tongsong T, et al. Prenatal sonographic diagnosis of tetralogy of fallot. J Clin Ultrasound. 2005;33:427–31.

Tugrul M, et al. Ketamine infusion versus isoflurane for the maintenance of anesthesia in the prebypass period in children with tetralogy of Fallot. J Cardiothorac Vasc Anesth. 2000;14(5):557–61.

Turley K, Mavroudis C, Ebert PA. Repair of congenital cardiac lesions during the first week of life. Circulation. 1982;66(2 Pt 2):I214–1219.

van den Berg J, et al. Diastolic function in repaired tetralogy of Fallot at rest and during stress: assessment with MR imaging. Radiology. 2007;243(1):212–9.

van Dongen EI, et al. The influence of perioperative factors on outcomes in children aged less than 18 months after repair of tetralogy of Fallot. J Thorac Cardiovasc Surg. 2003;126(3):703–10.

van Huysduynen BH, et al. Reduction of QRS duration after pulmonary valve replacement in adult Fallot patients is related to reduction of right ventricular volume. Eur Heart J. 2005;26(9):928–32.

Van Praagh R. Etienne-Louis Arthur Fallot and his tetralogy: a new translation of Fallot's summary and a modern reassessment of this anomaly. Eur J Cardiothorac Surg. 1989;3(5):381–6.

Van Praagh R, et al. Tetralogy of Fallot: underdevelopment of the pulmonary infundibulum and its sequelae. Am J Cardiol. 1970;26(1):25–33.

van Son JA. Repair of tetralogy of Fallot with anomalous origin of left anterior descending coronary artery. J Thorac Cardiovasc Surg. 1995;110:561–2.

van Straten A, et al. Time course of diastolic and systolic function improvement after pulmonary valve replacement in adult patients with tetralogy of Fallot. J Am Coll Cardiol. 2005;46(8):1559–64.

Vida VL, et al. Evolving strategies for preserving the pulmonary valve during early repair of tetralogy of Fallot: mid-term results. J Thorac Cardiovasc Surg. 2014;147(2):687–96.

Warden HE, et al. Controlled cross circulation for open intracardiac surgery: physiologic studies and results of creation and closure of ventricular septal defects. J Thorac Surg. 1954;28:331–43.

Warner KG, et al. Expanding the indications for pulmonary valve replacement after repair of tetralogy of fallot. Ann Thorac Surg. 2003;76(4):1066–72.

Waterston D. [Treatment of Fallot's tetralogy in children under 1 year of age]. Rozhl Chir. 1962;41:181–3.

Watterson KG, et al. Very small pulmonary arteries: central end-to-side shunt. Ann Thorac Surg. 1991;52(5):1132–7.

Wessel HU, et al. Prognostic significance of arrhythmia in tetralogy of Fallot after intracardiac repair. Am J Cardiol. 1980;46(5):843–8.

Wu ET, et al. Balloon valvuloplasty as an initial palliation in the treatment of newborns and young infants with severely symptomatic tetralogy of Fallot. Cardiology. 2006;105(1):52–6.

Zahka KG, et al. Long-term valvular function after total repair of tetralogy of Fallot. Relation to ventricular arrhythmias. Circulation. 1988;78(5 Pt 2):III14–9.

Zeltser I, et al. Genetic factors are important determinants of neurodevelopmental outcome after repair of tetralogy of Fallot. J Thorac Cardiovasc Surg. 2008;135(1):91–7.

Zhao HX, et al. Surgical repair of tetralogy of Fallot. Long-term follow-up with particular emphasis on late death and reoperation. J Thorac Cardiovasc Surg. 1985;89(2):204–20.

Zhao D, et al. Outcomes of different rehabilitative procedures in patients with pulmonary atresia, ventricular septal defect and major aortopulmonary collateral arteries. Eur J Cardiothorac Surg. 2019;55(5):837–44.

Zucker N, et al. Clinical presentation, natural history, and outcome of patients with the absent pulmonary valve syndrome. Cardiol Young. 2004;14(4):402–8.

Complications Associated with Pulmonary Atresia with Major Aortopulmonary Collateral Arteries

Arvind Bishnoi and Michael Ma

Abstract

Pulmonary atresia (PA), ventricular septal defect (VSD), with major aortopulmonary collateral arteries (MAPCAs) is an extreme variant of tetralogy of Fallot characterized by a lack of luminal continuity between the right ventricle and pulmonary artery tree, with pulmonary blood flow sourced through isolated MAPCAs, or a combination of MAPCAs and a unilateral ductus arteriosus, including absent development of central hilar pulmonary arteries. Anomalies in pulmonary artery architecture and arborization are common. This heterogeneity underlies the nuances in peri- and intraoperative decision-making.

Keywords

Congenital heart surgery · Pulmonary atresia · Major aortopulmonary collateral arteries · Tetralogy of Fallot

1 Anatomic Variation: Sources of Pulmonary Blood Flow

1. Patent ductus arteriosus. When the ductus provides flow to a single laterality, it can be associated with confluent or nonconfluent pulmonary arteries. Interestingly, the ductal-supplied lung is invariably of normal distal arborization.
2. Major aortopulmonary collateral arteries (MAPCAs). These are embryologic blood vessels from the aorta or other systemic arterial branches that supply the lung. Most of these arise from the upper thoracic aorta from the aortic arch to the T8 level. However, abdominal aortic origin is not uncommon. Other sources may include coronary arteries and tributaries of the head vessels. MAPCAs travel the mediastinum, enter the lung hilum, and continue as pulmonary arteries. When a MAPCA supplies a territory with no competi-

A. Bishnoi · M. Ma (✉)
Pediatric Cardiac Surgery, Stanford University School of Medicine, Stanford, CA, USA
e-mail: mma@stanford.edu

C. L. Backer, C. Mavroudis (eds.), *Complications in Pediatric and Congenital Heart Surgery*,
https://doi.org/10.1007/978-3-032-02661-3_13

tive flow from a secondary source, these are deemed single or sole supply. Conversely, MAPCAs that derive a secondary flow source are deemed a dual or redundant supply. MAPCAs are known to have intimal cushions leading to stenosis over time. Conversely, unguarded vessels that do not stenose can result in overcirculation to the distal lung bed and, ultimately, irreversible pulmonary vascular obstructive disease.

Acquired collaterals form at the site of adhesions between the lung and parietal pleura or in the mediastinum in long-term cyanosis. Although individual collaterals may be small, their number can be enormous, leading to significant volume overload. These thin-walled vessels are not amenable for use in complex pulmonary artery (PA) reconstruction and are typically left in situ to regress or controlled and eliminated during surgery.

2 Natural History

The natural history of each patient is variable because of the great variation in pulmonary blood flow. Although long-term survivors are known, mortality without treatment is high (Leonard et al. 2000). The diagnosis of tetralogy of Fallot (TOF), pulmonary atresia (PA), or MAPCA itself is considered an indication for treatment.

3 Comprehensive Management Algorithm

Various groups have described the different approaches to this pathology (Duncan et al. 2003; Ishibashi et al. 2007). Multiple vs. single stage are two different strategies to achieve a common goal of recruiting MAPCAs to allow complete septation of the heart with unobstructed blood supply to all 20 segments of the lung at the lowest possible pulmonary afterload. Stanford has pioneered the single-stage unifocalization applicable in most patients and developed protocols and techniques in a three-decade experience (Reddy et al. 1995; Ma et al. 2018), which will be elaborated upon in this chapter.

Treatment Protocol (Bauser-Heaton et al. 2017)

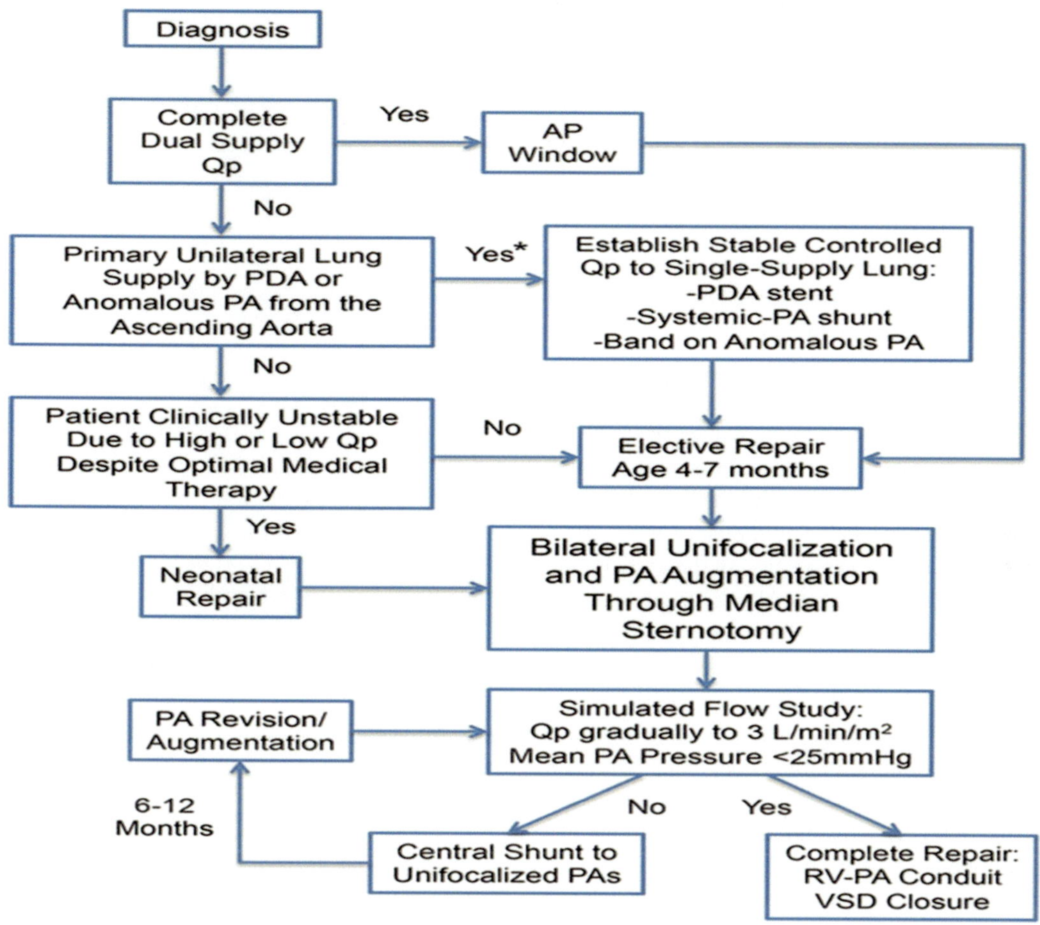

4 Preoperative Evaluation

All patients undergo echocardiography and computed tomographic (CT) angiography within a few days of birth, irrespective of the adequacy of pulmonary blood flow. These modalities can delineate two anatomic indications for neonatal intervention: (1) confluence of central PAs with all or primarily dual-supply MAPCAs, and (2) ductal supply to a single lung with contralateral MAPCAs. If neither finding is present, a patient is deferred to 3–6 months of age for single-stage repair unless physiologic indications prompt sooner intervention (i.e., pulmonary overcirculation and heart failure or pulmonary undercirculation and cyanosis). A cardiac catheterization is necessary prior to complex PA reconstruction. CT scans and cardiac catheterization complement each other and provide valuable information for surgical planning.

4.1 Cardiac Catheterization

Cardiac catheterization and angiography aim to delineate all the sources of blood supply in detail. All collaterals must be defined from origin to insertion. An attempt must be made to selectively catheterize every collateral and define its attachment to the pulmonary vasculature. Single and dual supply must be understood. Every bronchopulmonary segment of the lung should be defined for its blood supply in anteroposterior and lateral views. All stenoses in collaterals and central pulmonary arteries should be demonstrated. In cases where lung territories are not delineated by antegrade injection, retrograde venography is performed. Abdominal aorta imaging should be included to avoid missing collaterals.

4.2 Computed Tomography Angiography and Three-Dimensional (3D) Reconstruction

CT is an adjunct to cardiac catheterization. CT helps in surgical planning and mapping the collateral course, especially in the interdigitating airway, esophageal, and pulmonary venous structures. If an axial cross-section of the aorta is considered a clock face, MAPCA origins can be labeled by their takeoff from the aorta to enable localization. Intraoperatively, dissection must be completed around the trachea, esophagus, and behind the left atrium, which is not a common area of exploration in most congenital heart surgical operations. A thorough preoperative sense of the anatomy is essential for expeditious and safe conduct.

A useful preoperative exercise involves being able to describe the existing pulmonary artery tree as follows:

> MAPCA 1 arises from the first part of the right subclavian artery and travels parallel to the carotid artery before making a hairpin turn and coming close to the right paratracheal space. This MAPCA has stenoses at the hairpin turn. It travels further in the right paratracheal space to the cephalad border of the right bronchus and divides into two branches. The upper branch enters the lung hilum and supplies the right upper lobe as the sole supply. The lower branch continues anterior to the right bronchus and joins the central pulmonary artery. Both branches have ostial stenosis. Distal pressure in both branches is low (Fig. 1).

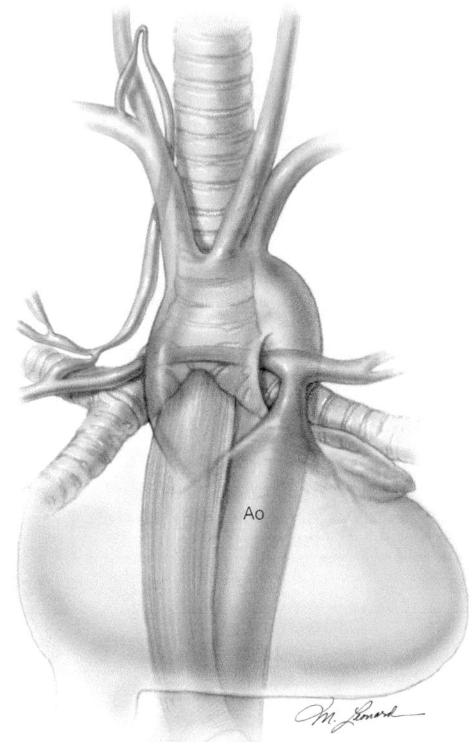

Fig. 1 Preoperative angiography and axial imaging provide a mental anatomic roadmap for each MAPCA and PA for a given patient. The focus should be on the vessel origin, turns, mediastinal course, branching patterns, points of stenosis, and relation to anatomic landmarks. *Ao* aorta, *MAPCA* major aortopulmonary collateral arteries, *PA* pulmonary artery

> MAPCA 2 arises from the descending thoracic aorta around the T5 thoracic vertebra at the 9 o'clock position and emanates about 2 cm below the caudal aspect of the carina of the trachea. It travels in cephalad fashion behind the esophagus and makes a caudal turn to reach the inferior border of the right bronchus. It gives two branches at this level to supply the right middle and lower lobes. Both branches appear as single supply. There is stenosis at the aortic origin, and the pressure is low distal to this stenosis (Fig. 2).

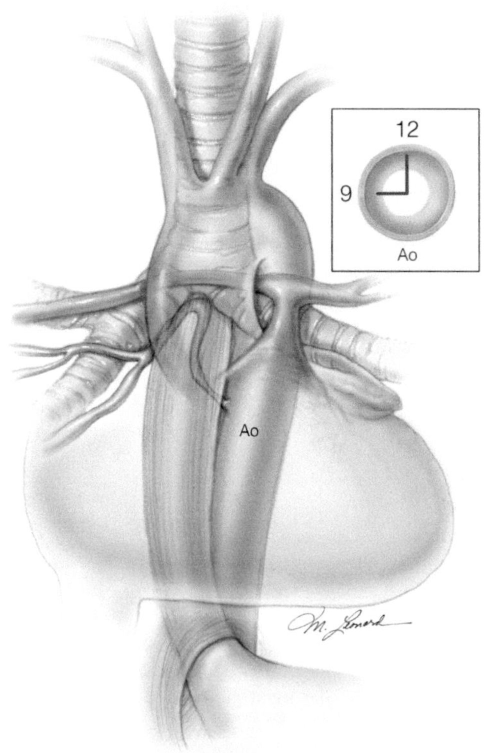

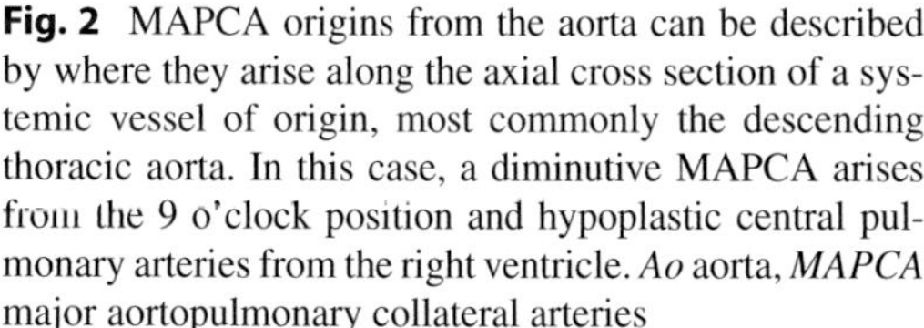
Fig. 2 MAPCA origins from the aorta can be described by where they arise along the axial cross section of a systemic vessel of origin, most commonly the descending thoracic aorta. In this case, a diminutive MAPCA arises from the 9 o'clock position and hypoplastic central pulmonary arteries from the right ventricle. *Ao* aorta, *MAPCA* major aortopulmonary collateral arteries

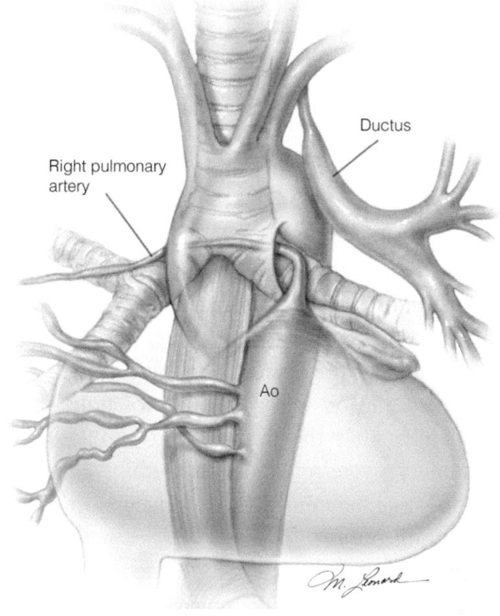

Fig. 3 In certain anatomic variants, MAPCAs may supply one lung and a ductus the other. In this example, the ductus supplies the entirety of the left lung, with MAPCAs to the right. Inadequate stabilization of the ductus, by stenting or shunt, can result in complete loss of one lung. *Ao* aorta, *MAPCA* major aortopulmonary collateral arteries

A ductus from the undersurface of the left subclavian artery supplies the entire left lung through a normal-appearing left pulmonary artery. All segments of the left lung are accounted for via this source of flow, and several MAPCAs are seen exiting the aorta to supply portions of the right lung (Fig. 3).

5 Operative Techniques, Complications, and Pitfalls

5.1 Palliation for Staged Repair

AP window: Neonates with hypoplastic central pulmonary arteries and all dual supply MAPCAs are candidates for aortopulmonary window creation (Mainwaring et al. 2012), with the aim of the procedure to promote antegrade PA flow for growth of the entire native PA tree. MAPCAs are ligated in the same operation or coiled in the cath lab depending on the assessment of pulmonary blood flow after the procedure to regulate any pulmonary overcirculation and reduce competitive flow that may reduce the efficacy of the antegrade connections.

The operation begins with a median sternotomy. The thymus is dissected and excised in totality. The pericardium is opened, and breaching the pleura is avoided. Hypoplastic main pulmonary artery (MPA) and branch pulmonary arteries are dissected (Fig. 4). Dissection is carried to the intrapericardial pleural reflections bilaterally to enhance branch PA mobility. However, extensive lobar multifurcations are not mobilized to reduce adhesions for the reoperative complete PA reconstruction. There can be small collaterals from the right or left coronary arteries supplying the main pulmonary artery, which needs to be addressed. The surgeon should be careful of thermal injury to the main trunk of the coronary while coagulating these collaterals.

One should use the main pulmonary artery to avoid branch pulmonary artery stenosis after window creation. The left main coronary artery is intimately related to the proximal main pulmonary artery, and cautious ligation/division of this is necessary to avoid coronary artery distortion. The patient is heparinized, and branch pulmonary arteries are test occluded. Unrecognized trivial antegrade flow from a rudimentary right ventricle connection will lead to pressurization of the pulmonary artery root, and this should be controlled prior to main pulmonary artery division to reduce blood loss. Once the main pulmonary artery is divided, it is positioned near the lesser curvature of the aorta to mark the anastomosis site on the aorta (Fig. 5a–c). Poorly selected sites can lead to branch pulmonary stenosis, rendering the procedure futile. An overly anterior or midline posterior anastomosis can lead to branch pulmonary artery stenosis, especially to the right pulmonary artery (Fig. 5d). A side-biting clamp is placed on the lesser curvature of the aorta, which may require full mobilization of the ascending aorta and arch to allow adequate torsion of the aorta. Care must be taken to avoid excess side clamping resulting in significant system afterload, coronary insufficiency, and/or aortic valve insufficiency (Mainwaring et al. 2012) (Fig. 5e). The main pulmonary artery is spatulated, without traversing too closely to the right pulmonary artery ostium.

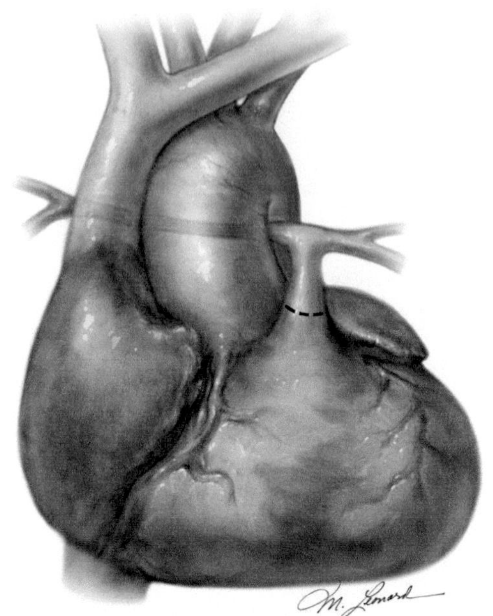

Fig. 4 Hypoplastic pulmonary arteries and main pulmonary stump. This illustration demonstrates the intended site of division of the main pulmonary artery, which is near the pulmonary annulus to provide maximal length for aortopulmonary window creation

An aortic incision is made along the line of the aorta at the previously marked site, and a small strip of tissue is excised. This aortotomy is created to be slightly larger than the main pulmonary artery size. A running 8–0 is used to create an end-to-side anastomosis. Occluding neuroclips are removed from the branch pulmonary

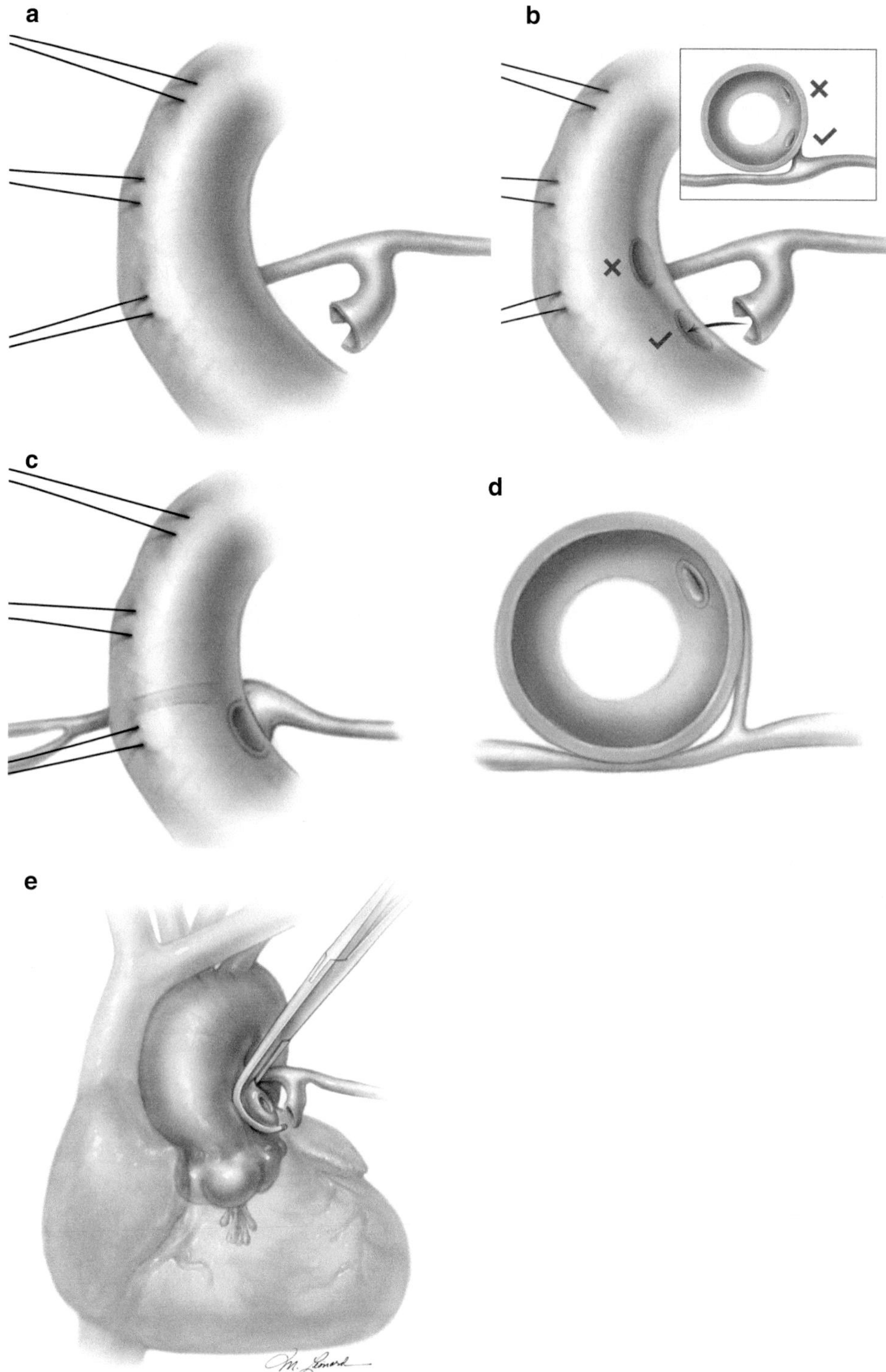

Fig. 5 (**a**–**e**) Aortopulmonary window creation requires careful selection on the aorta for the site of anastomosis. (**a**) Longitudinal dissection of the ascending aorta with stay suture placement allows aggressive rotation of the aorta to expose the left lateral posterior surface without hemodynamic compromise. (**b**) The appropriate aortotomy should be positioned left lateral posteriorly to avoid tension to the branch pulmonary arteries, with the (**c**) anastomosis resting posteriorly at conclusion. (**d**) An anteriorly displaced aortopulmonary window results typically in attenuation of the right pulmonary artery, resulting in inadequate growth to this lung and possible overcirculation to the left. (**e**) Aortic insufficiency due to side biting clamp

arteries, and the aortic clamp is removed. The lie and orientation of branch pulmonary arteries are assessed. Diastolic pressure falls with increasing pulmonary blood flow. If diastolic pressure is less than 30 with more than 90% saturation at 21% FiO2, we proceed with dual-supply MAPCA ligation.

Alternative, Unrecommended, Procedures to Promote Antegrade Flow

Right Ventricular Outflow Tract Augmentation

In our experience, improved PA growth occurs with a similar flow rate that occurs continuously in systole and diastole, as opposed to the same flow rate with a more pulsatile, primarily systolic pattern. Additionally, the significant regurgitant volume load and flow, combined with the systemic right ventricular systolic pressure, drives pseudoaneurysm formation (Rosenthal et al. 1972; Tomasulo et al. 2021) (Fig. 6a–d), which is very challenging for reoperation, especially since we avoid heparinization during the dissection phase of complex PA reconstruction. The geometry of the right ventricle (RV) outflow tract augmentation is generally unfavorable to promote ongoing branch PA flow and growth.

Non-native Shunt

Blalock Taussig-Thomas or central shunt also performs the same function as aortopulmonary window physiologically (d'Udekem 2019). However, the stiff, noncompliant graft leads to stenosis and thrombosis of hypoplastic pulmonary arteries (Gladman et al. 1997) (Figs. 7a, b) and the obligate mismatch in vessel size between the shunt and the ongoing diminutive branch PA does not lend well to flow and growth. An AP window is also a naturally growing systemic-pulmonary connection auto-regulated at the hypoplastic branch PA level. At the same time, an artificial shunt ultimately becomes the primary restrictor to flow with somatic growth.

MAPCA and/or Pulmonary Artery Stenting

Stenting should be completely avoided unless it is necessary as a temporary salvage for a patient presenting with extreme cyanosis and unstable for operative intervention. Our programmatic approach is to recruit as much "raw material" as possible, whether native PA or MAPCA in

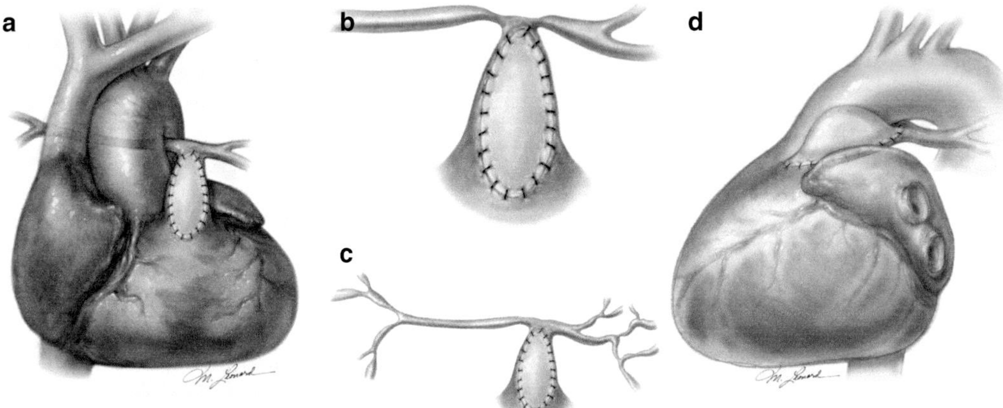

Fig. 6 (**a–d**) (**a**) RVOT augmentation is an alternative, but unrecommended, method for encouraging native confluent branch pulmonary artery growth. (**b**, **c**) The significantly increased degree of hypoplasia that is noted in transition from the diminutive main pulmonary artery into the extremely diminutive branch pulmonary arteries results in an exaggerated mismatched caliber change that creates distortion of the branch PAs that do not lend well to promoting confluent PA growth. (**d**) Pseudoaneurysm formation is an additional complication with this approach, with the high pressure proximal MPA creating a challenging environment at time of future resternotomy and pulmonary artery dissection. *MPA* main pulmonary artery, *PA* pulmonary artery, *RVOT* right ventricular outflow tract

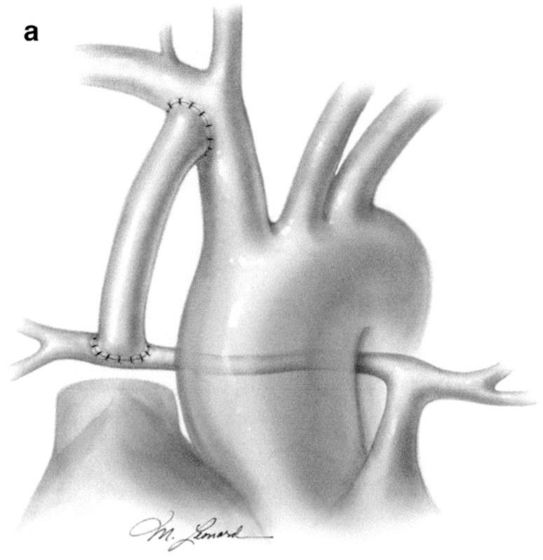

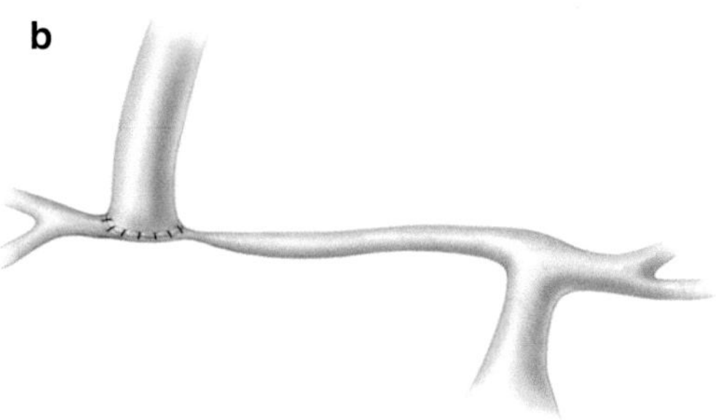

Fig. 7 (**a**, **b**). (**a**) Aortopulmonary shunting is yet another common, albeit unrecommended, strategy for encouraging confluent branch PA growth. Although physiologically like a native aortopulmonary window, this remains a fixed resistor without the potential for interval growth and requires use of an artificial graft with mismatch in compliance and size to the ongoing branch PA. (**b**) Hypoplasia along the confluent PA system is commonly seen. *PA* pulmonary artery

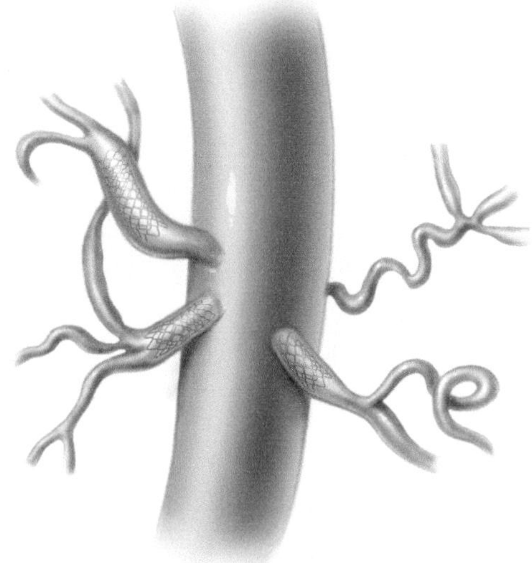

Fig. 8 MAPCA stenting is strongly discouraged in the management of this lesion. The proximal MAPCAs, although not entirely healthy, serve as important native tissue connections that do have ongoing growth potential after unifocalization. Distal MAPCAs have multiple branch points that can be compromised or "jailed" by an overly aggressively positioned stent. Surrounding airways and mediastinal structures can succumb to extensive stent-related adhesion, fibrosis, and surgical injury at the time of operation. *MAPCA* major aortopulmonary collateral arteries

embryologic origin, ultimately for use in complex PA reconstruction. Stented portions of these vessels lose their growth potential and attract intimal fibrosis, which are unattractive characteristics that reduce their usability (Fig. 8).

5.2 Complete Midline Unifocalization

Phase 1—Dissection

Median sternotomy and subtotal thymectomy are performed. The pericardium is opened in the midline, and a patch of pericardium is harvested for ventricular septal defect (VSD) closure. Next, the bilateral pleurae are opened widely to identify the phrenic nerves. We place three 5–0 Prolene sutures just above and parallel to the phrenic nerve (Fig. 9) on the pericardium, passing from the pleural side to the cardiac side. These stay sutures serve the dual purpose of pericardial stay and phrenic nerve markers.

Next, attention is paid to the confluent pulmonary arteries, if present. The aorta is retracted to the right side, and the main pulmonary artery and central pulmonary arteries are dissected. Great care is needed for all handling and dissection of PA and MAPCA vessels, given their fragility and sensitivity to diathermy injury. The superior vena cava (SVC) is mobilized through the innominate vein junction. Two to three 5–0 stay sutures are placed on the medial side of the SVC to assist in retraction and exposure. To access the posterior mediastinum and descending thoracic aorta, the subcarinal space is entered, with the aid of sev-

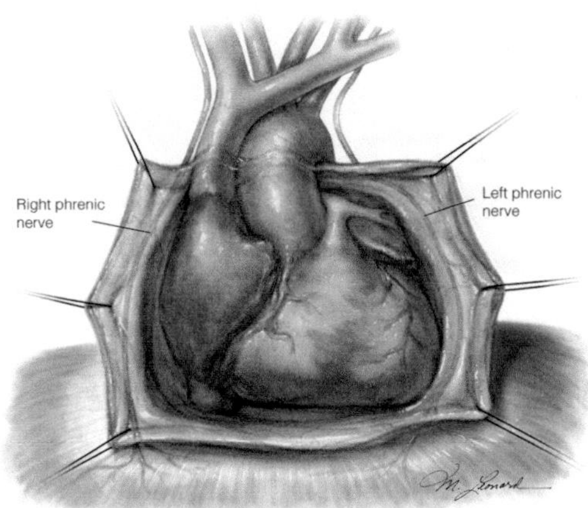

Fig. 9 Anterior view of the heart and pericardium after sternotomy, with attention to the bilateral phrenic nerve courses, just anterior to the pulmonary hila and near the head and neck vessels. Note the position of holding sutures just anterior to the phrenic nerve, which provides retraction and marks the nerves to reduce iatrogenic injury

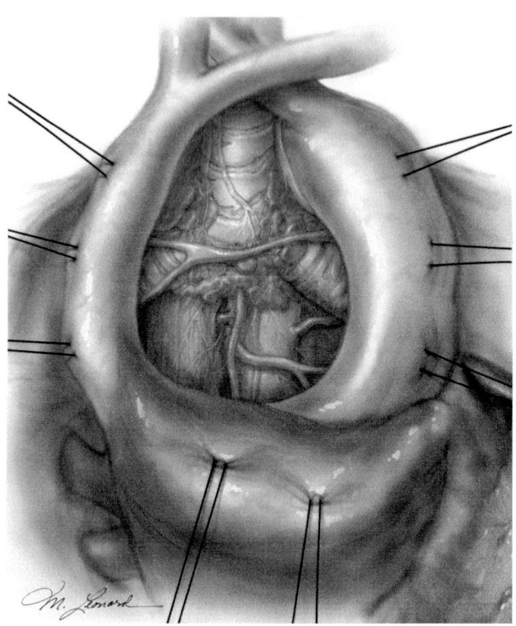

Fig. 10 The dissection phase of the unifocalization operation requires extensive retraction to expose the posterior mediastinum. Three holding sutures on the medial surface of the superior vena cava and three holding sutures on the right surface of the ascending aorta are used to pull these two in opposite directions. Additional holding sutures on the roof of the atrium pull the right atrium in a caudal direction to create more space. Central pulmonary arteries are meticulously dissected, and paratracheal, pretracheal, and subcarinal lymph nodes are removed. MAPCAs are tortuous and can run intimately with lymph nodes, and lymphadenectomy must be done cautiously to avoid MAPCA injury. *MAPCA* major aortopulmonary collateral arteries

eral retracting sutures (Fig. 10). A separate set of retracting sutures on the leftward ascending aorta can be utilized to access the leftward hilum (Fig. 11).

With appropriate exposure, dissection to delineate MAPCAs is commenced. A posterior mediastinal lymphadenectomy is helpful in the paratracheal and subcarinal spaces. Total excision of lymph nodes avoids partial transection and lymphatic leak or persistent oozing, which can be irritating during operation and insidiously life-threatening if chyle leaks persist postoperatively. MAPCAs are often closely intimated with lymph nodes, and great care must be taken to avoid injury to these vessels for ultimate reconstruction. Once these lymph nodes are removed, collaterals from the head, neck, aortic arch, and descending thoracic aorta can be easily located. Each MAPCA is dissected individually from its origin to its intrapulmonary course. Airways and pulmonary veins may be closely interdigitated with MAPCAs, and injury to these structures must be avoided. The esophagus is in close proximity during this, and an indwelling transesophageal echocardiography (TEE) probe or nasogastric tube or temperature probe should be withdrawn to provide greater ease of mobilizing the esophagus as the MAPCAs are identified and dissected. Hasty blunt dissection should be avoided, as it can lead to persistent oozing and thoracic duct injury and hamper further dissection of collaterals. We do not hesitate to encircle the esophagus with a silastic tape to help in dissection.

Complications

Nerve Injury

Phrenic Nerve Phrenic nerves run just above the hilum of both lungs. Extensive dissection is required around the lung hilum for MAPCA delineation and later dissection. Phrenic nerve

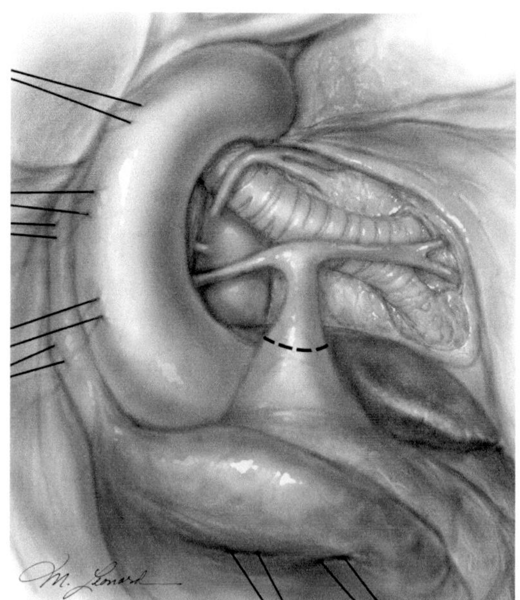

Fig. 11 Additional exposure to the leftward coursing PA and MAPCAs may be facilitated by retracting the aorta to the patient's right. Three holding sutures on the left side of the aorta are utilized to pull the ascending aorta rightward. Collaterals arising from the aortic arch often travel along the trachea and bronchus, can be very adherent, and more so in reoperative cases. Airway or MAPCA injury requires very precise dissection. *MAPCA* major aortopulmonary collateral arteries, *PA* pulmonary artery

injury, especially bilateral, can lead to significant morbidity even if the rest of the operation is perfect (Greene et al. 2018). Marking stay sutures is an essential step to prevent this complication.

Recurrent Laryngeal Nerve The recurrent laryngeal nerve runs around the ductus arteriosus. Patients with pulmonary atresia may or may not have a ductus, and it may be challenging to locate recurrent nerves. Some patients have collaterals arising from the right subclavian artery, and dissection of these collaterals can also jeopardize the right recurrent nerve. Dissection around the right subclavian origin must be avoided in patients without a ductus. Bilateral injury can lead to the need for tracheostomy.

Vagus Nerve Vagus nerve trunks run on both sides of the esophagus, and at least one nerve trunk must be protected. Division of bilateral trunks leads to gastrointestinal complications like delayed gastric emptying, gastroesophageal reflux, aspiration, and dumping syndrome. These complications can lead to significant morbidity in the postoperative period, necessitating expert care (Koth et al. 2018).

Autonomic Nervous Plexus Unifocalization requires extensive dissection in the posterior mediastinum, and the autonomic nerve plexus around the trachea and esophagus is often disturbed. Extensive dissection can lead to bronchospasm in the postoperative period, leading to respiratory complications (Schulze-Neick et al. 2000). Blunt dissection should be avoided; a very focused dissection should be considered as much as possible.

Airway Injury

Tracheobronchial Injuries MAPCAs are intimately related to the trachea and bronchus. They travel along the segmental bronchus in the lung parenchyma. Diathermy injury, especially to the membranous trachea, can be initially unrecognized but severely problematic in the postoperative period. This is much more common in reoperative cases due to loss of natural planes and scarring. Diathermy in cutting mode is recommended when working around the airway to limit heat-related injury to the wider area beyond the actual defect. If recognized, this is immediately repaired and confirmed to be improved using intraoperative bronchoscopy.

Occult Tracheobronchial Malacia This can become apparent after extensive dissection around the airways, clinically silent before surgery (Sganga et al. 2022; Yamagishi et al. 2002). Extensive dissection circumferentially leads to an unsupported membranous trachea, leading to the collapse of the airways.

Air Leaks Lung parenchyma injury is very common after extensive dissection of MAPCAs and pulmonary arteries. If there is no tracheobronchial injury, these will subside quickly in the immediate postoperative period.

Esophageal Injury

MAPCAs may rarely traverse through the muscular wall of the esophagus, which requires very careful dissection to reduce the risk of iatrogenic esophageal perforation (Mainwaring et al. 2016). This may be unrecognized intraoperatively, and transesophageal echo probe manipulation can exacerbate or reveal the issue. Gentle tissue handling around the esophagus is paramount to reduce this complication. Once injury is noted to have occurred, the mucosa is repaired with absorbable sutures and muscle with Prolene.

MAPCA Injury

Collaterals cross different parts of the mediastinum in their course. While changing from deep to superficial, they may be hidden just behind lymph nodes. Lymph node excision can lead to injury to these fragile MAPCAs and may cause a loss of supply to those distributions of the lung. MAPCAs may also provide minute tributaries to airways and can bleed if avulsed. Careful dissection is again warranted.

Lymphatic Injury

The thoracic duct runs in relation to the descending aorta and esophagus. Blunt dissection can lead to injury and a major lymph leak. We must look for a lymph leak at the end of the dissection before proceeding further. If identified, this must be controlled.

Phase 2: Cardiopulmonary Bypass

Cardiopulmonary bypass is initiated after full heparinization, which is avoided if at all possible during the dissection phase (Margetson et al. 2022). This includes a distal aortic, bicaval, and superior pulmonary vein cannula. The SVC cannula is placed cephalad, to enable working on the right lung hilum without resulting in obstruction to SVC return. With initiation of bypass, we immediately ligate MAPCAs at their systemic origins to reduce systemic runoff (Fig. 12). All patients are cooled to 25 °C for maximal end-organ protection. At this stage, the heart is on cardiopulmonary bypass and beating. Sometimes, the heart fibrillates with cooling, and is actively defibrillated. If unsuccessful after repeated attempts, perfusion pressure is ensured and the heart is allowed to stay in a fibrillated and empty state.

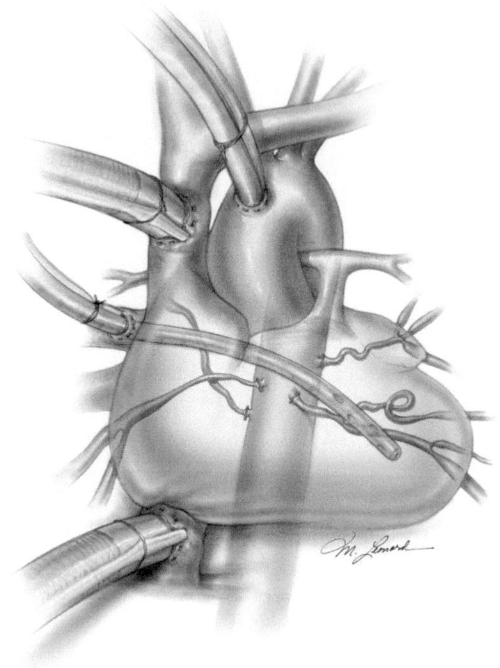

Fig. 12 All MAPCAs are clipped as soon as cardiopulmonary bypass is commenced to prevent runoff and systemic hypoperfusion. *MAPCA* major aortopulmonary collateral arteries

Complications

1. MAPCA reconstruction requires extensive time. Care must be taken to avoid cardiac compromise during aggressive retraction of intramediastinal contents, especially exposing the left hilum.
2. Long bypass times with excessive intrapericardial cardiotomy suction leads to hemolysis. Hemostasis should be ensured at each step.

Phase 3: Reconstruction

Reconstruction can be started from either the left or right side and often alternates side-side, but usually from the most posterior and inferior vessels working toward the most anterior superior vessels, with the final portion of the reconstruction being an extended hilum-hilum pulmonary artery homograft patch augmentation. All the previously dissected collaterals to both lungs are divided at the origin from the aorta, and stay sutures are placed on each MAPCA to prevent torsion of the vessels. Saline infusion can help pressurize the collateral temporarily to visualize its natural lay and reduce torsion. All the previously dissected branches of MAPCA and native pulmonary arteries are controlled with neuro clips to prevent back bleeding. Attention is turned to each collateral individually to evaluate branch ostial stenosis using probes. If stenoses are present, the vessel is opened longitudinally to one large branch, allowing visualization of any ostial stenoses in others. Stenotic ostia are enlarged by Heineke-Mikulicz V-plasty (Mainwaring et al. 2019). Once all stenotic ostia are dealt with, the entire length of MAPCA is augmented with a homograft pulmonary artery patch (Fig. 13). If a MAPCA and its branches are not stenotic, no augmentation is performed at this time (Fig. 14). Once all the MAPCAs are evaluated and adequately dealt with, as discussed, an anastomosis to create a neopulmonary artery begins. A common mistake is to perform end (of MAPCA) to side anastomosis (of the native pulmonary artery) or very short distance side-to-side anastomosis of MAPCA with each other. Longitudinal native-native anastomoses should be prioritized (Figs. 13, 14 and 15). There are two reasons for this. (1) Even if a MAPCA has no stenosis in an extrapulmonary course at the time of unifocalization, suture-line tissue is prone to delayed stenosis. (2) Limited anastomosis will create very short segments of central pulmonary artery and capacitance vessels. There is always the dilemma of dealing with a MAPCA crossing behind the bronchus. Rerouting such a vessel anteriorly makes a future reoperation simpler at the expense of potentially kinking such a vessel (Fig. 13). This is an intraoperative decision based on a surgeon's assessment of overall geometry. Once full reconstruction is complete, the neopulmonary artery bed is inflated with saline to ensure no significant leak or kink. All distal neuroclips are removed. In sizing the neocentral pulmonary

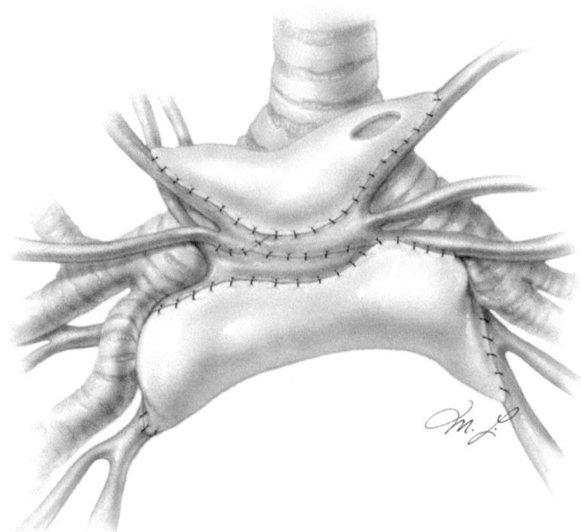

Fig. 13 All MAPCAs that are stenotic distally are augmented using native-native or homograft patch augmentation. In this example, the lower lobar MAPCAs are augmented inferiorly with PA homograft prior to amalgamation of the many interdigitating MAPCAs. Once the reconstruction is complete and deemed adequate, an appropriate size hole is created in the anterior patch on the left side of the aorta for implantation of a right ventricle-to-pulmonary artery conduit. Note that several branches are still posterior to the airways; intraoperative judgment is necessary to determine which vessels to reroute and which to leave in situ. *MAPCA* major aortopulmonary collateral arteries, *PA* pulmonary artery

arteries, we aim to create a central pulmonary artery system near z + 2 to ensure adequate capacitance with an anterior homograft onlay patch. An extraordinarily oversized central reconstruction can reduce laminar outflow and cause compression to branch airways.

Complications

Heineke-Mikulicz V plasty

This is an excellent technique for handling ostial stenosis at the branch point (Mainwaring et al. 2019). As the angle between branches increases however, the chances of iatrogenic narrowing of both branches increase. If the angle is less than 45 degrees long, V plasty can be safely performed; however, if the angle is wider, we must restrict it to near the ostium only. Angles more than 80 degrees are not suitable for V plasty, and patch augmentation is recommended.

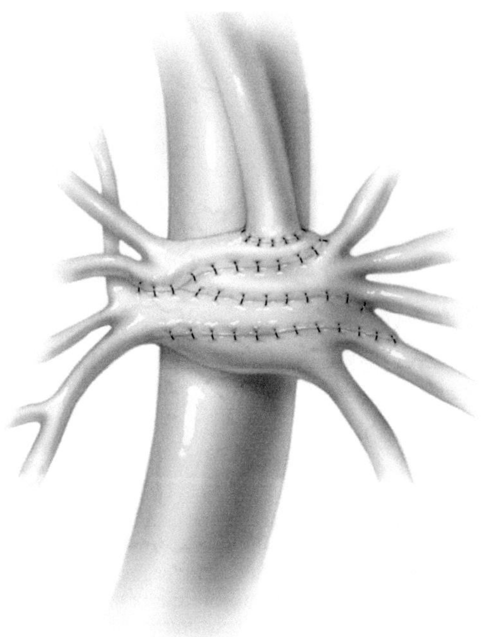

Fig. 14 A completed unifocalization, with the pulmonary artery end of a central shunt in situ. Note the extended side-side native-native anastomoses that are utilized in completing the reconstruction. Full lengths of collaterals are utilized to provide a neocentral pulmonary artery confluence with maximal capacitance and growth potential

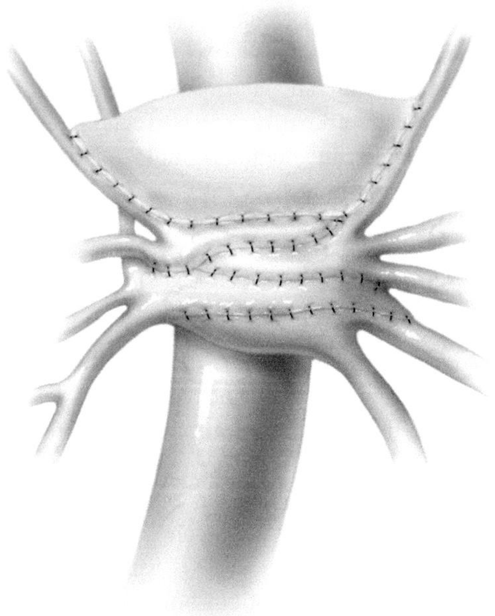

Fig. 15 A hilum-hilum anterior pulmonary artery homograft patch is utilized to complete the reconstruction. We ensure that the final reconstruction provides at minimum branch PA diameter z + 2 for a given patient. *PA* pulmonary artery

Phase 4: Assessment of Reconstructed Pulmonary Artery Bed (Flow Study)

An intraoperative flow study in selected patients can be performed (Reddy et al. 1997). The pulmonary artery confluence is cannulated with an appropriately sized cannula and connected to a primed circuit from the cardiopulmonary bypass machine. A pressure monitoring line is placed in the right pulmonary artery and calibrated. The lungs are ventilated gently, and the left atrial vent is maximized. Gradually, the aortic flow is reduced to 50 ml/kg, and the pulmonary artery flow increased in 20% increments. At each steady state of flow, pulmonary artery pressure is measured. A total target pulmonary artery flow of 3.0 L/m/m2 cardiac index with a mean pulmonary artery pressure of <25–30 mmHg is an excellent predictor of low pulmonary vascular resistance (Margetson et al. 2022), and adequacy of the pulmonary artery reconstruction for septation. If the pulmonary artery pressure is more than 30 mm Hg at any stage, the flow study is aborted, and a central aortopulmonary shunt is recommended.

Complications

False flow study readings may arise if residual bleeding at the reconstruction is not well-controlled. Uncontrolled acquired aortopulmonary collaterals may also falsely pressurize the reconstruction and impact the flow study.

Phase 5: Intracardiac Repair or Central Shunt

An appropriately-sized aortic valve homograft is thawed. The aorta is cross-clamped, and cardioplegia is delivered in the aortic root. Right ventriculotomy is performed, and muscular resection is completed to ensure an adequate right ventricular outflow opening. The VSD is closed with a glutaraldehyde-treated pericardial patch. An atrial level shunt can be closed retrograde from the RV through the tricuspid valve or through a separate right atriotomy. The left heart is de-aired and the cross-clamp removed for prompt cardiac reanimation. The thawed conduit is then anastomosed to the reconstructed pulmonary arteries distally and the RV infundibulotomy proximally, usually with an anterior hood augmentation. Once rewarming is complete, cardiopulmonary bypass is terminated, and postoperative echo and hemodynamics are assessed.

In patients with inadequate reconstructions for intracardiac repair, the heart is never arrested, and a central shunt placed from the ascending aorta to the reconstructed pulmonary artery system (Fig. 13). This shunt is typically larger than those used for other indications since the distal pulmonary vascular resistance is higher.

Phase 6: Hemostasis

Extensive suture lines, delicate tissues, and inaccessible locations can make hemostasis challenging. At every step of reconstruction, a meticulous technique must not be compromised. The pulmonary artery system is at low pressure after appropriate reconstruction. Surgical packing and topical hemostatic agents (typically Gelfoam with recombinant thrombin) are used until heparin is neutralized with protamine, and medical procoagulants (platelets, fresh frozen plasma, and cryoprecipitate) are administered. All topical agents are removed prior to case completion, as even absorbable retained materials can swell and compress the delicate distal aspects of the reconstruction and lead to vessel thrombosis. When bleeding remains challenging, packing may be retained for 24 h to allow an interval washout without ongoing high transfusion requirement.

Postoperative Complications

Reperfusion Pulmonary Edema and Other Airway Complications

Correction of stenosis in pulmonary blood supply with reestablishing the total cardiac output can lead to pulmonary edema in the early postoperative period (Asija et al. 2014), especially in segments with more severe stenosis. This can lead to prolonged ventilation and respiratory complications in the postoperative period. In severe cases, veno-venous extracorporeal oxygenation may be needed transiently.

Bronchial Compression

Large patches on reconstructed pulmonary arteries and large right ventricle-to-pulmonary artery conduits can lead to bronchial compression. In severe cases, this may require aortopexy, the LeCompte maneuver (Greene et al. 2019), or bronchial stenting.

Biomaterials

For pulmonary artery and MAPCA reconstruction, pulmonary artery homograft appears to be optimal. This is guided by ease of handling, compliance, and hemostasis. Theoretically, autologous or homograft pericardium, bovine pericardium, homograft femoral vein grafts, and/or PTFE patches can be used at the expense of one or the other of our choice criteria.

For right ventricle-to-pulmonary artery conduit, aortic valved homograft is recommended. The aortic homograft is less prone to dilation in the long run if there is elevated pulmonary artery pressure.

Summary

Pulmonary atresia, VSD, with MAPCAs is a complex defect, driven by heterogeneity in anatomy and physiology, derived from the behavior of the various individual sources of pulmonary blood flow. A comprehensive management algorithm is provided to account for this variance, with the ultimate goal for salvaging and unifying as many of these sources of blood flow to yield (1) low resistance to the right ventricle and (2) balanced and physiologic flow to as much lung territory as possible. The palliative and corrective operations herein prioritize this philosophy, and so that complications can be avoided, as with most lesions, via a thorough anatomic and physiologic understanding coupled with technical experience.

References

Asija R, Roth SJ, Hanley FL, Peng L, Liu K, Abbott J, et al. Reperfusion pulmonary edema in children with tetralogy of Fallot, pulmonary atresia, and major aortopulmonary collateral arteries undergoing unifocalization procedures: a pilot study examining potential pathophysiologic mechanisms and clinical significance. J Thorac Cardiovasc Surg. 2014;148(4):1560–5.

Bauser-Heaton H, Borquez A, Han B, Ladd M, Asija R, Downey L, et al. Programmatic approach to management of tetralogy of Fallot with major aortopulmonary collateral arteries: a 15-year experience with 458 patients. Circ Cardiovasc Interv. 2017;10(4):e004952. https://doi.org/10.1161/CIRCINTERVENTIONS.116.004952.

d'Udekem Y. Rehabilitation of pulmonary arteries in pulmonary atresia, VSD and Mapcas. Oper Tech Thorac Cardiovasc Surg. 2019;24(2):121–32.

Duncan BW, Mee RB, Prieto LR, Rosenthal GL, Mesia CI, Qureshi A, et al. Staged repair of tetralogy of Fallot with pulmonary atresia and major aortopulmonary collateral arteries. J Thorac Cardiovasc Surg. 2003;126(3):694–702.

Gladman G, McCrindle BW, Williams WG, Freedom RM, Benson LN. The modified Blalock-Taussig shunt: clinical impact and morbidity in Fallot's tetralogy in the current era. J Thorac Cardiovasc Surg. 1997;114(1):25–30.

Greene CL, Mainwaring RD, Sidell D, Yarlagadda VV, Patrick WL, Hanley FL. Impact of phrenic nerve palsy and need for diaphragm plication following surgery for pulmonary atresia with ventricular septal defect and major aortopulmonary collaterals. Semin Thorac Cardiovasc Surg. 2018;30(3):318–24.

Greene CL, Mainwaring RD, Sidell D, Palmon M, Hanley FL. Lecompte procedure for relief of severe airway compression in children with congenital heart disease. World J Pediatr Congenit Heart Surg. 2019;10(5):558–64.

Ishibashi N, Shin'oka T, Ishiyama M, Sakamoto T, Kurosawa H. Clinical results of staged repair with complete unifocalization for pulmonary atresia with ventricular septal defect and major aortopulmonary collateral arteries. Eur J Cardiothorac Surg. 2007;32(2):202–8.

Koth AM, Sakarovitch C, Sidell DR, Schultz LM, Freccero A, Rizzuto S, et al. Postoperative feeding problems in patients with tetralogy of Fallot, pulmonary atresia, and major aortopulmonary collaterals undergoing unifocalisation surgery. Cardiol Young. 2018;28(11):1329–32.

Leonard H, Derrick G, O'Sullivan J, Wren C. Natural and unnatural history of pulmonary atresia. Heart. 2000;84(5):499–503.

Ma M, Mainwaring RD, Hanley FL. Comprehensive management of major aortopulmonary collaterals in the repair of tetralogy of Fallot. Semin Thorac Cardiovasc Surg. 2018;21:75–82.

Mainwaring RD, Reddy VM, Perry SB, Peng L, Hanley FL. Late outcomes in patients undergoing aortopulmonary window for pulmonary atresia/stenosis and major aortopulmonary collaterals. Ann Thorac Surg. 2012;94(3):842–8.

Mainwaring RD, Patrick WL, Carrillo SA, Ibrahimye AN, Muralidaran A, Hanley FL. Prevalence and anatomy of retroesophageal major aortopulmonary collateral arteries. Ann Thorac Surg. 2016;102(3):877–82.

Mainwaring RD, Patrick WL, Hanley FL. Surgical management of pulmonary atresia with ventricular septal defect and major aortopulmonary collateral arteries: part II—midline unifocalization and unifocalization revision. Oper Tech Thorac Cardiovasc Surg. 2019;24(1):56–79.

Margetson T, Mainwaring RD, Hanley FL. Overview of cardiopulmonary bypass techniques and the incidence of postoperative complications in pediatric patients undergoing complex pulmonary artery reconstruction. J Extra Corpor Technol. 2022;54(4):330–7.

Reddy VM, Liddicoat JR, Hanley FL. Midline one-stage complete unifocalization and repair of pulmonary atresia with ventricular septal defect and major aortopulmonary collaterals. J Thorac Cardiovasc Surg. 1995;109(5):832–45.

Reddy VM, Petrossian E, McElhinney DB, Moore P, Teitel DF, Hanley FL. One-stage complete unifocalization in infants: when should the ventricular septal defect be closed? J Thorac Cardiovasc Surg. 1997;113(5):858–68.

Rosenthal A, Gross RE, Pasternac A. Aneurysms of right ventricular outflow patches. J Thorac Cardiovasc Surg. 1972;63(5):735–40.

Schulze-Neick I, Ho SY, Bush A, Rosenthal M, Franklin RC, Redington AN, et al. Severe airflow limitation after the unifocalization procedure: clinical and morphological correlates. Circulation. 2000;102(19):III142–7.

Sganga D, Meister K, Sidell DR, Wise-Faberowski L, Shek J, Ma M, et al. Airway characteristics of patients with 22q11 deletion undergoing pulmonary artery reconstruction surgery: retrospective cohort study. Pediatr Crit Care Med. 2022;23(5):371–7.

Tomasulo CE, Ravishankar C, Natarajan S, Mascio CE, Glatz AC. Large aneurysms and pseudoaneurysms of surgically reconstructed right ventricular outflow tracts. Cardiol Young. 2021;31(9):1522–4.

Yamagishi H, Maeda J, Higuchi M, Katada Y, Yamagishi C, Matsuo N, et al. Bronchomalacia associated with pulmonary atresia, ventricular septal defect and major aortopulmonary collateral arteries, and chromosome 22q11.2 deletion. Clin Genet. 2002;62(3):214–9.

Complications Associated with Repair of Transposition of the Great Arteries and Associated Lesions

Constantine Mavroudis

Abstract

Transposition of the great arteries (TGA) is a congenital heart defect in which there is malalignment of the aorta and pulmonary artery where the right ventricle (RV) gives rise to the aorta and the left ventricle (LV) gives rise to the pulmonary artery. There are three main groups of TGA: (1) TGA with intact interventricular septum (TGA-IVS), (2) TGA with ventricular septal defect (TGA-VSD), and (3) TGA with VSD and pulmonary stenosis (TGA-VSD-PS). This chapter will review the operative steps of the arterial switch operation. These steps include (1) great vessel dissection/mobilization, (2) coronary artery button transfer to the neoaorta, (3) neoaortic reconstruction, and (4) neopulmonary artery reconstruction. Each of these steps is attended by potential complications. This chapter will depict the anatomic complications and the solutions thereto pertaining.

Keywords

Congenital heart surgery · Transposition of the great arteries · Arterial switch operation · Complications · Outcomes

1 Introduction

Analysis of potential complications associated with repair options for transposition of the great arteries (TGA) and associated lesions requires a review of the unusual anatomy and physiology of TGA (Peacock 1866; Shaner 1962; Grant 1962; Bremer 1942; de Vries and Saunders 1962; Van Mierop et al. 1963; Van Mierop and Wiglesworth 1963; Van Praagh and Van Praagh 1966; Idriss et al. 1977; Jex et al. 1990; Sohn et al. 1998; Moene et al. 1983, 1985; Mavroudis and Backer 2023). Indeed, recognizing the complex anatomy and the surgical interventions will allow the reader to understand the important steps of each operation and appreciate the complications that can occur during the execution of the challenging maneuvers leading to complete repair. As discussed in other chapters, these complications don't occur until they do occur. Under these circumstances the surgeon is wise to consider the reparative measures that will help to resolve the complication and result in a competent repair.

C. Mavroudis (✉)
Chief of Pediatric Cardiothoracic Surgery (Retired), Peyton Manning Children's Hospital, Indianapolis, IN, USA

Professor Emeritus of Surgery, Johns Hopkins University School of Medicine, Baltimore, MD, USA

C. L. Backer, C. Mavroudis (eds.), *Complications in Pediatric and Congenital Heart Surgery*, https://doi.org/10.1007/978-3-032-02661-3_14

2 Anatomy and Physiology

Transposition of the great arteries (TGA) is a congenital heart defect in which there is anatomic malalignment of the aorta and pulmonary artery (Peacock 1866; Shaner 1962; Grant 1962; Bremer 1942; de Vries and Saunders 1962; Van Mierop et al. 1963; Van Mierop and Wiglesworth 1963; Van Praagh and Van Praagh 1966; Idriss et al. 1977; Jex et al. 1990; Sohn et al. 1998; Moene et al. 1983, 1985; Mavroudis and Backer 2023). Consequently, the right ventricle gives rise to the aorta and the left ventricle gives rise to the pulmonary artery (Peacock 1866; Shaner 1962; Grant 1962; Bremer 1942; de Vries and Saunders 1962; Van Mierop et al. 1963; Van Mierop and Wiglesworth 1963; Van Praagh and Van Praagh 1966). Described in further anatomic terms, there is atrioventricular concordance and ventricular to great vessel discordance; the result of which is cyanosis (Peacock 1866; Shaner 1962; Grant 1962; Bremer 1942; de Vries and Saunders 1962; Van Mierop et al. 1963; Van Mierop and Wiglesworth 1963; Van Praagh and Van Praagh 1966; Idriss et al. 1977; Jex et al. 1990; Sohn et al. 1998; Moene et al. 1983, 1985; Mavroudis and Backer 2023). There are three main groups of TGA (Bremer 1942; de Vries and Saunders 1962; Van Mierop et al. 1963; Van Mierop and Wiglesworth 1963; Van Praagh and Van Praagh 1966). The most common category (50%) is TGA with intact interventricular septum (TGA-IVS). These types of cases present at birth with cyanosis due to inadequate circulatory mixing at the atrial level. Those with profound cyanosis often leading to metabolic lactic acidosis will require a transcatheter balloon atrial septostomy to stabilize the hemodynamic conditions (Rashkind and Miller 1966). In general, patients can be stabilized and treated by an arterial switch operation (ASO) in the neonatal period as depicted in Figs. 1, 2 and 34.

The second type in this nomenclature system is transposition of the great arteries with ventricular septal defect (TGA-VSD) which occurs in 25% of cases (Moene et al. 1985; Huhta et al. 1982). These cases can be approached in the same manner as those with TGA-IVS with the notable exception that the VSD must be closed (see chapter "Complications Associated with Ventricular Septal Defect Closure"). In general, the VSD closure is performed first and followed by the arterial switch operation to avoid disruption of the arterial switch reconstruction when the VSD is performed first owing to the retraction maneuvers that are required for the closure. A transcatheter balloon septostomy may or may not be indicated since there is mixing due to the presence of a VSD. This condition is usually treated by ASO and concomitant VSD closure in the neonatal period.

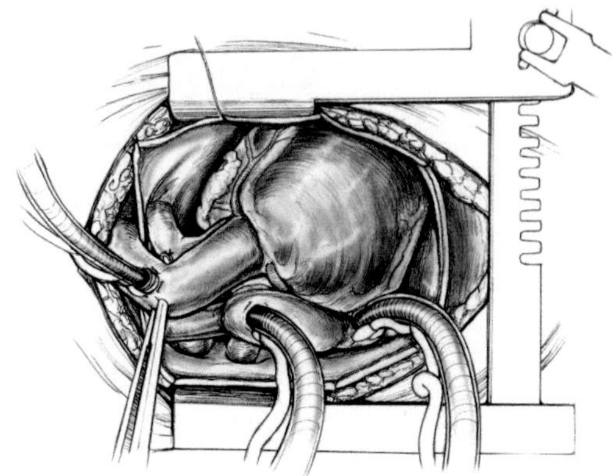

Fig. 1 shows aortobicaval cannulation and the commencement of cardiopulmonary bypass in a patient with transposition of the great arteries. Aortic cannulation is performed high on the ascending aorta just downstream of the innominate artery to faciliate the arterial switch operation. (With permission: Mavroudis 2015)

The third type is TGA with VSD and pulmonary stenosis (left ventricular outflow tract stenosis) (TGA-VSD-PS) which is present in 25% of cases of TGA (Peacock 1866; Shaner 1962; Grant 1962; Bremer 1942; de Vries and Saunders 1962; Van Mierop et al. 1963; Van Mierop and Wiglesworth 1963; Van Praagh and Van Praagh 1966; Rastelli et al. 1969). Management of this condition is based on the severity of the left ventricular outflow tract obstruction, the degree of cyanosis, and the cause of the left ventricular outflow tract obstruction. Usually, a systemic-to-pulmonary artery shunt is placed and followed by a Rastelli operation (Rastelli et al. 1969) later on in life. This lesion has been approached by many reconstruction solutions which largely require

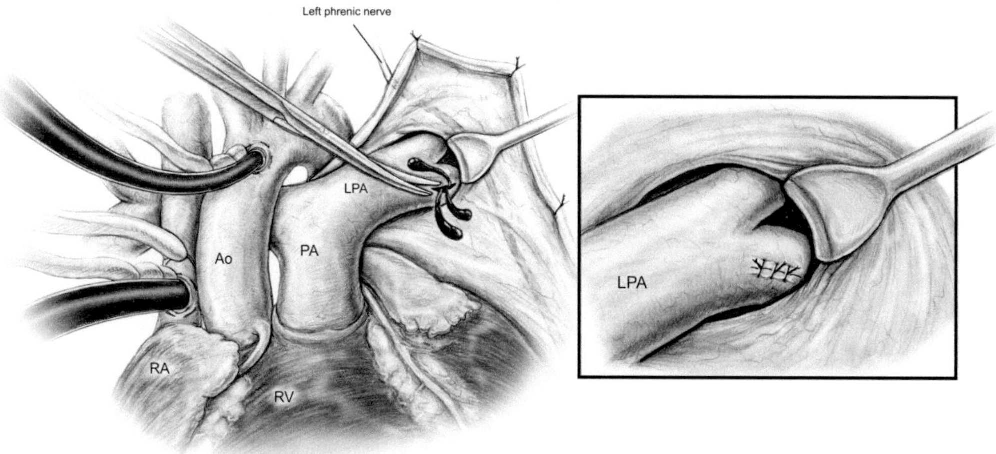

Fig. 2 shows localized distal pulmonary artery disruption caused by rough scissor dissection. The figure shows longitudinal disruption but horrizontal disruption can occur as well. In the event that this complication happens, it is wise to commence cardiopulmonary bypass to avoid hemodynamic compromise. Interrupted suture technique as shown in the inset should be performed to avoid the pursestring effect of running suture technique. *Ao* aorta, *LPA* left pulmonary artery, *PA* pulmonary artery, *RA* right atrium, *RV* right ventricle

left intraventricular tunneling to the aorta with right ventricular-to-pulmonary artery continuity by various types of conduits, both valved and nonvalved (Fiore et al. 1983; Lecompte et al. 1982). These reconstructive solutions are discussed in the latter half of this chapter. In some rare cases, pulmonary stenosis is subvalvar with a normal pulmonary valve. This situation is amenable to subpulmonic resection, VSD closure and arterial switch (Idriss et al. 1988a).

The arterial switch operation has had a dramatic effect on the treatment of all the types of transposition resulting in anatomic and physiologic correction (Idriss et al. 1988b; O'Byrne et al. 2018; Cain et al. 2014; Anderson et al. 2014; Ahlström et al. 2019; Skinner et al. 2008; Lim et al. 2019; Backer et al. 1989a; Bove 1989; Castaneda et al. 1984, 1988; Kreutzer et al. 1977; Mavroudis et al. 1991; Backer et al. 1991; Lecompte et al. 1981; Mavroudis 1987, 1989; Muster et al. 1987; Kirklin et al. 1992; Lupinetti et al. 1992; Norwood et al. 1988; Pacifico et al. 1983; Planché et al. 1988, 1998; Quaegebeur et al. 1986; Serraf et al. 1993; Sidi et al. 1983; Wernovsky et al. 1995; Yacoub et al. 1976, 1980; van der Palen et al. 2021).

3 Complications Associated with the Arterial Switch Operation with and Without Ventricular Septal Defect

The arterial switch operation for TGA-IVS is performed in the first 2 weeks of life to take advantage of the physiologic pulmonary artery hypertension of the newborn since the left ventricle will be expected to take over the work of systemic circulation. As noted, the operative steps of the operation and potential complications are shown in Figs. 1, 2, 3, 4, 5, 6, 7, 8, 9, 10, 11, 12, 13, 14, 15, 16, 17, 18, 19, 20, 21, 22, 23, 24, 25, 26, 27, 28, 29, 30, 31, 32, 33, and 34. Most of these figures and legends are quoted from our *Atlas of Pediatric Cardiac Surgery* (Mavroudis and Backer 2015) in order to establish the normal execution of the operation in contrast to the complications that can occur and resolution thereof, which are illustrated by new drawings.

The arterial switch operation is a complex array of multiple steps each of which is attended by potential complications that can impact unfa-

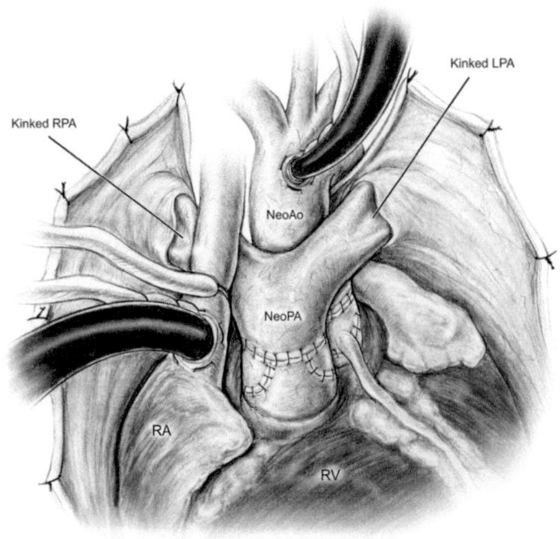

Fig. 3 shows the result of incomplete dissection of the distal right and left main pulmonary arteries whch can result in distal stenosis and right ventricular hypertension. In general, the dissection should be taken to the first branches of the distal pulmonary arteries with circumferential mobilization to ensure a proper anatomic and physiologic result after the maneuver of Lecompte. *Ao* aorta, *LPA* left pulmonary artery, *PA* pulmonary artery, *RA* right atrium, *RPA* right pulmonary artery, *RV* right ventricle

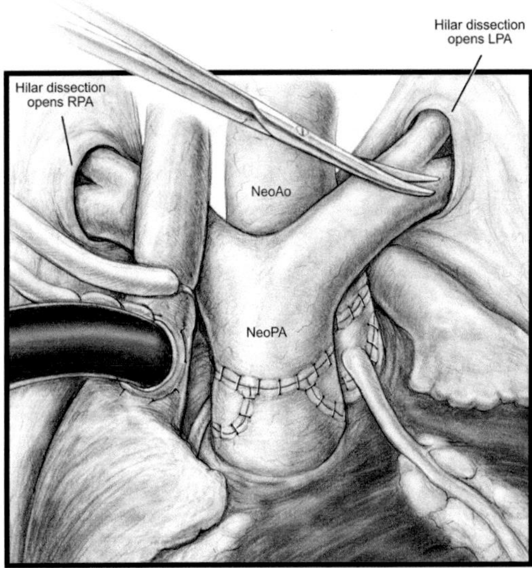

Fig. 4 shows the result of complete circumferenital dissection of the distal right and left main pulmonary arteries whch extend into the respective bifurcations. This extended dissection ensures a favorable anatomic configuration to prevent distal stenosis and right ventricular hypertension. *Ao* aorta, *LPA* left pulmonary artery, *PA* pulmonary artery, *RPA* right pulmonary artery

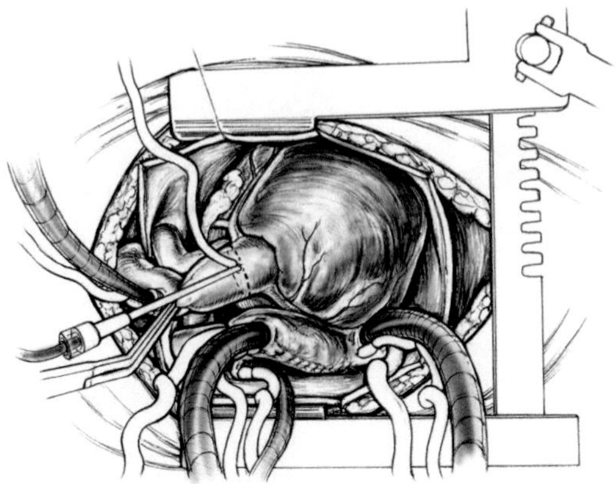

Fig. 5 demonstrates cardiopulmonary bypass, left ventricular vent in the right superior pulmonary vein, application of the aortic cross-clamp, and administration of antegrade cardioplegia in the aortic root. The right atrial suture line represents the atrial entry for patent foramen ovale or atrial septal defect closure. (With permission: Mavroudis 2015)

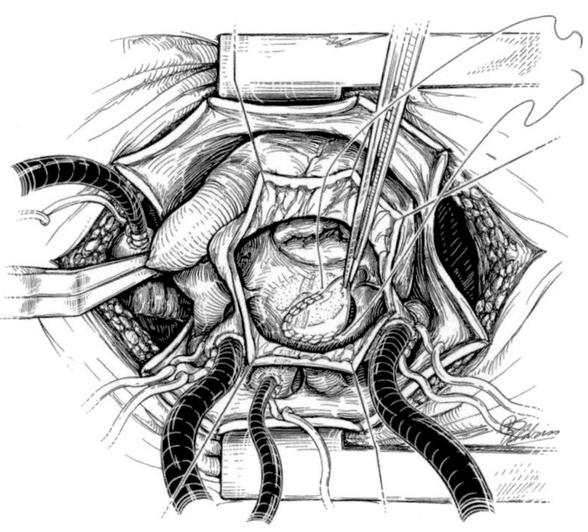

Fig. 6 shows right atrial exposure and closure of the atrial septal defect caused by the atrial septostomy using a pericardial patch. Most often, the septum primum can be repaired primarily without a patch. Some surgeons prefer to leave the septum open for the neoaortic reconstruction since it can allow improved left ventricular drainage (via the vent) and facilitate exposure through a bloodless field. Other surgeons close the right atrium at this point and rely on the left ventricular vent to maximize ventricular drainage. When there is an associated ventricular septal defect (VSD), the VSD is approached and closed through the right atrium before the arterial switch operation is performed for fear of disrupting the reconstruction due to exposure techniques. (With permission: Mavroudis 2015)

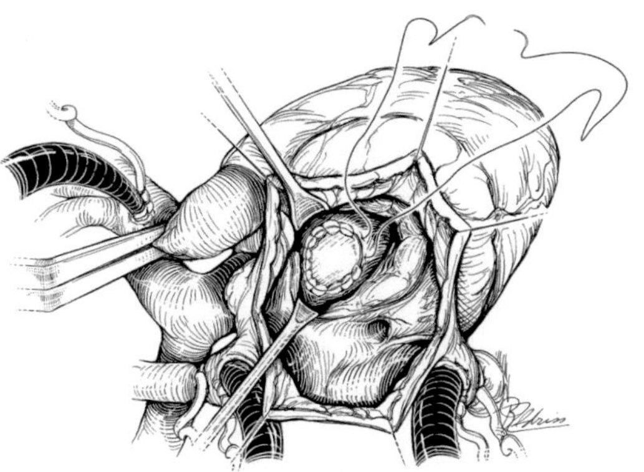

Fig. 7 When there is an associated ventricular septal defect (VSD), the VSD is approached and closed through the right atrium before the arterial switch operation is performed for fear of disrupting the reconstruction due to exposure techniques. Oftentimes, running suture technique is elected due to the projected prolonged cross-clamp time. Optimal cardioplegia strategies will ensure myocardial protection during this time period. (With permission: Mavroudis 2015)

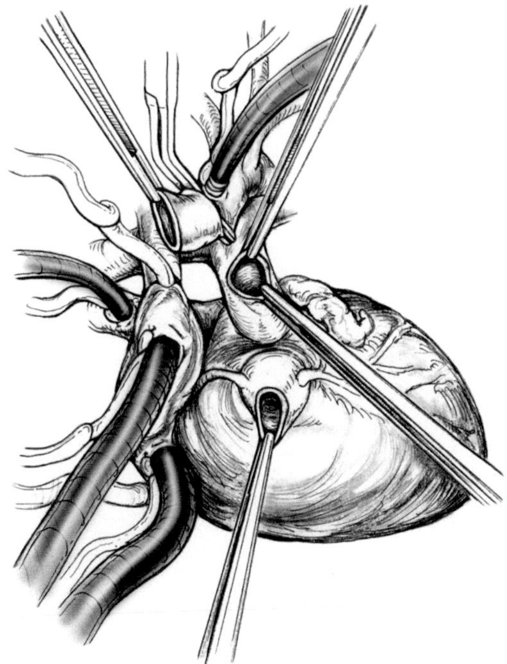

Fig. 8 shows the transected and retracted aorta with scissor transection of the main pulmonary artery. (With permission: Mavroudis 2015)

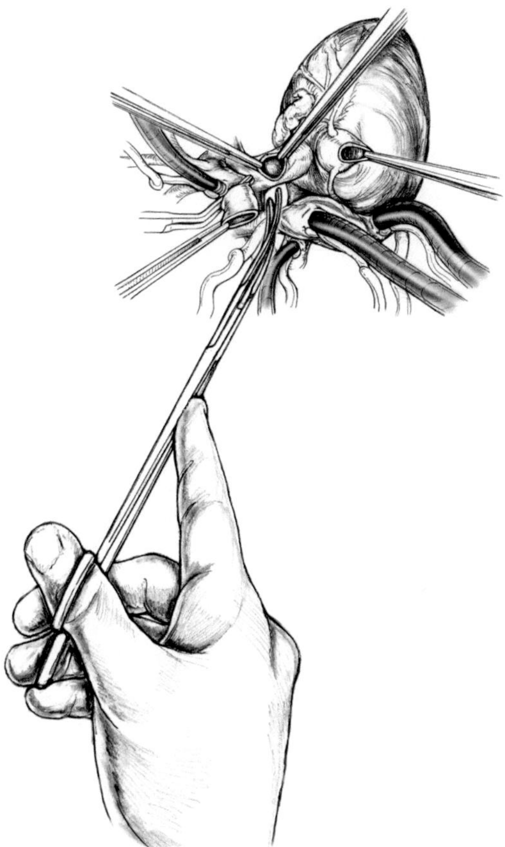

Fig. 9 depicts the same exposure which highlights a more distant view with the surgeon's hand in focus. Care is taken to adjust the left ventricular vent to maximize drainage and maintain a bloodless field for the neoaortic reconstruction. (With permission: Mavroudis 2015)

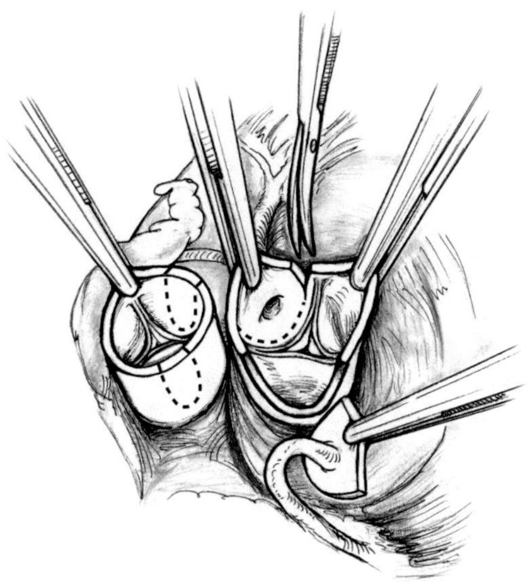

Fig. 10 shows the already dissected right coronary artery (forceps) and scissor dissection of the left main coronary artery. The dotted lines on the pulmonary artery, soon to become the neoaorta, represent the excisions (approximately 2/3 of the estimated area of the coronary buttons) that are performed to transfer the coronary artery buttons to the respected sinus of Valsalva to complete the proximal neoaortic reconstruction. (With permission: Mavroudis 2015)

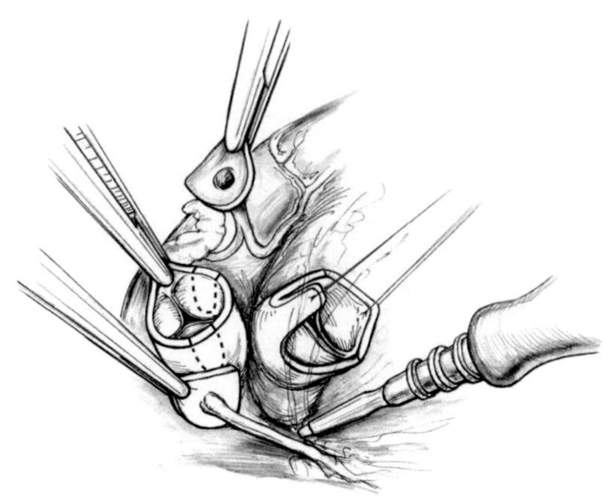

Fig. 12 demonstrates the electrocautery (very low setting) mobilization technique that will avoid tension or kinking at the coronary anastomosis. (With permission: Mavroudis 2015)

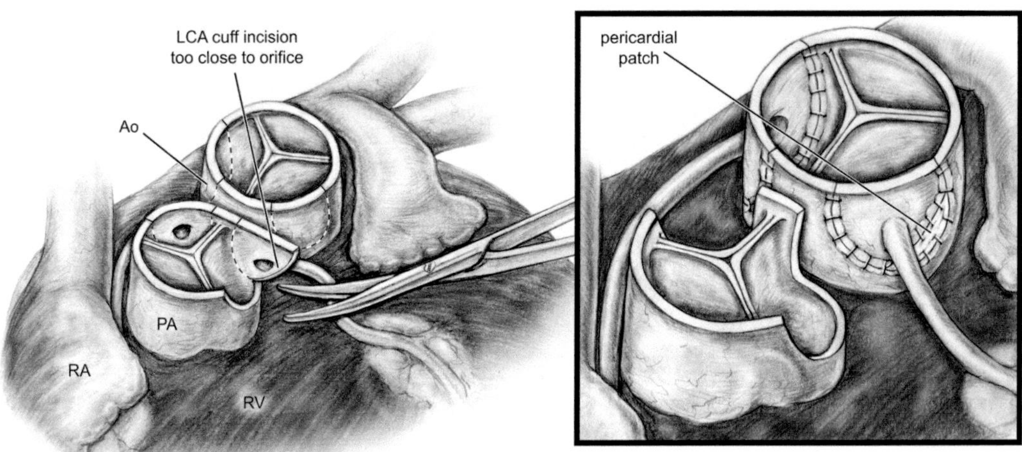

Fig. 11 shows a cut too close to the cornary artery origin which can complicate the coronary button translocation. The inset shows how this problem can be repaired by pericardial patch neoaortoplasty to ensure proper coronary button alignment and optimal flow. *Ao* aorta, *RA* right atrium, *LCA* left coronary artery, *PA* pulmonary artery, *RV* right ventricle

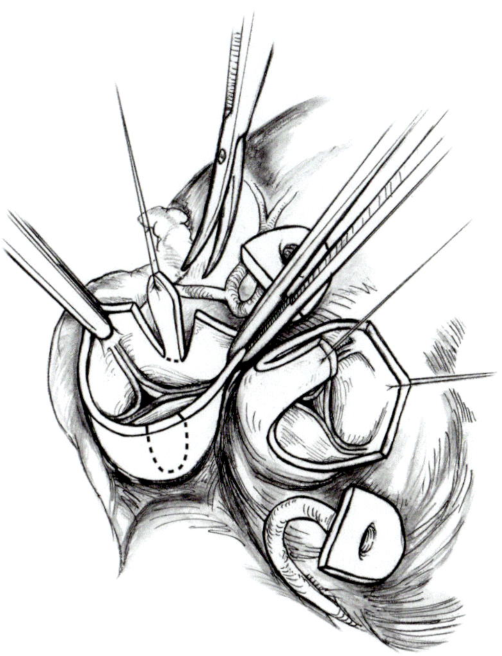

Fig. 13 shows the localized pulmonary artery at the respective sinus of Valsalva being resected to make ready the coronary transfer. (With permission: Mavroudis 2015)

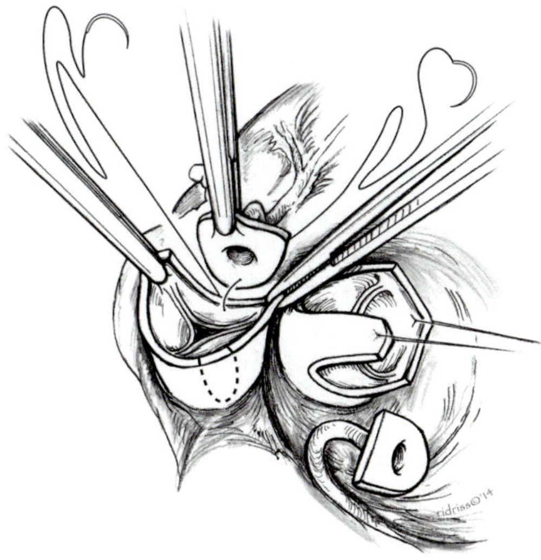

Fig. 14 shows the left main coronary button anastomosis being commenced at the center point of the coronary button and the sinus of Valsalva. Some surgeons prefer to rotate the coronary button to achieve a "best lie" configuration. These preferences are left to the operating surgeon to decide on the best anatomic arrangement that will optimize flow after reconstruction. (With permission: Mavroudis 2015)

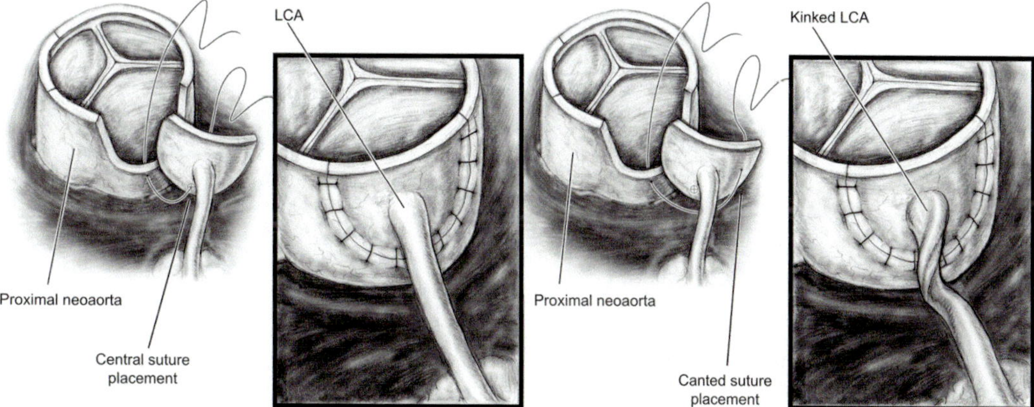

Fig. 15 Left panel shows how the coronary artery button is accurately aligned for the implantation which will result in an unobstructed reconstruction as noted in the left panel inset. When the planned anastomosis is not properly aligned and malrotated, coronary kinking can occur. The right panel shows the initial inaccurate placement of the suture for the anastomotic reconstruction. If this situation is not recognized the completion anastomosis will result in twisting, kinking, and an obstructive pattern which can result in poor perfusion, myocardial ischemia, and ventricular dysfunction. *LCA* left coronary artery

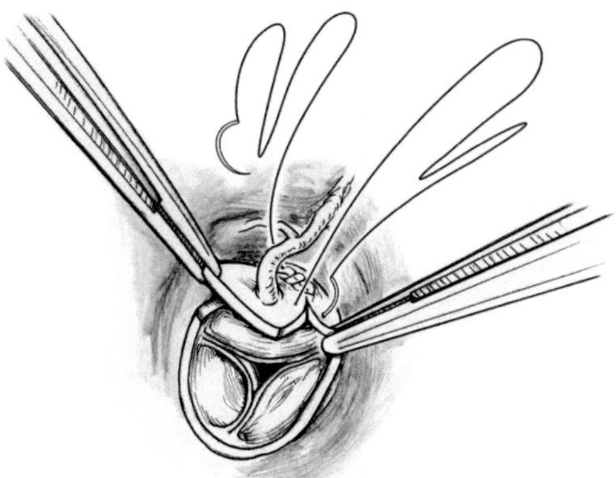

Fig. 16 shows the suture line being continued on one side with 8–0 running monofilament suture (With permission: Mavroudis 2015)

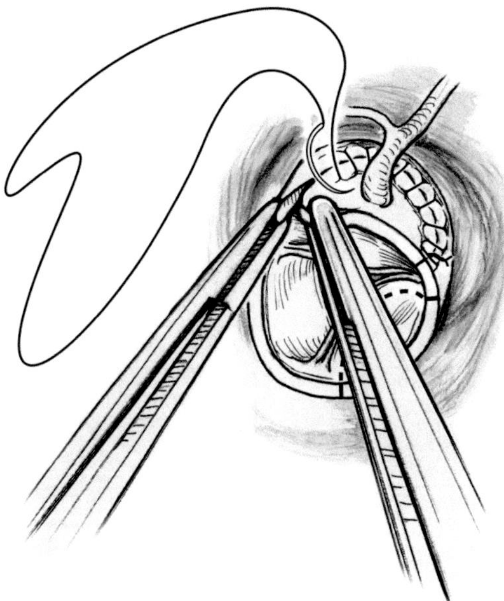

Fig. 17 shows the completion of the anastomosis in progress on the opposite side of the original suture line. Individual sutures at the top of the anastomosis are used to anchor the running suture. The surgeon should know which suture represents the running suture that was used for the anastomosis, and which one represents the anchoring suture which was placed at the top of the anastomosis. In this way, the surgeon will know whether to redo the entire anastomosis if one of the sutures snaps during the tie. If the anchoring suture snaps, then the other one can be used to anchor the suture line. If the running suture snaps, then the entire anastomosis may need to be redone to avoid unwanted unraveling. (With permission: Mavroudis 2015)

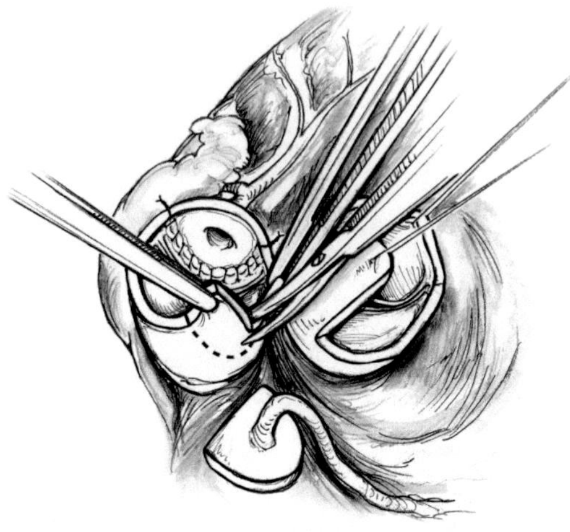

Fig. 18 shows the right coronary sinus being prepared for coronary transfer by local wall resection as was performed for the left neocoronary artery sinus. (With permission: Mavroudis 2015)

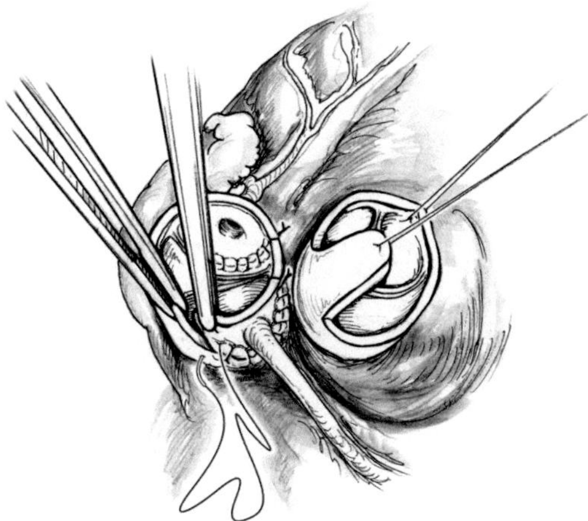

Fig. 19 highlights the same surturing technique as was applied for the left coronary artery anastomosis. (With permission: Mavroudis 2015)

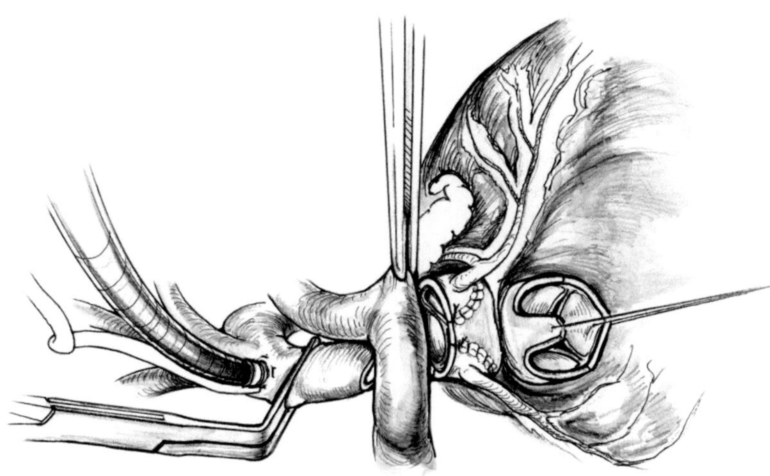

Fig. 20 shows the first stage of the Lecompte maneuver which is performed by the assistant to retract anteriorly the distal confluence of pulmonary arteries. The aortic cross-clamp is shown in preparation for the replacement of the clamp to the other side of the transposed pulmonary artery confluence. (With permission: Mavroudis 2015)

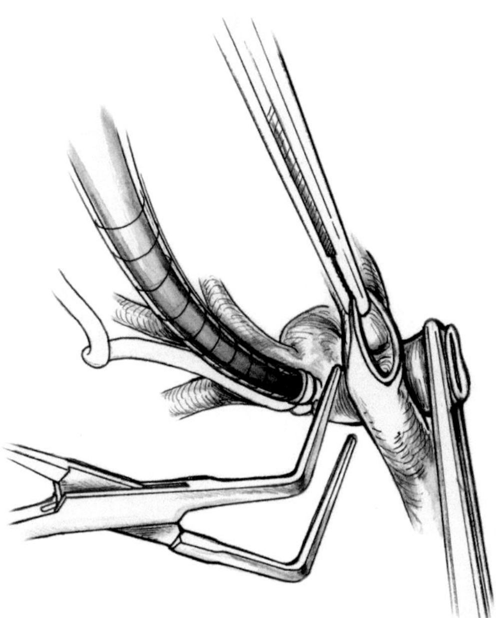

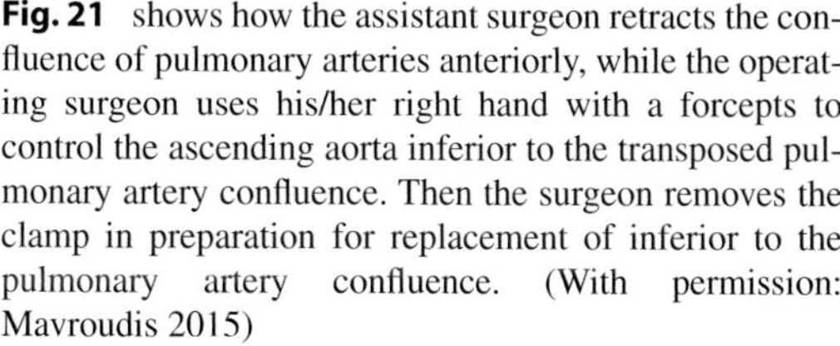

Fig. 21 shows how the assistant surgeon retracts the confluence of pulmonary arteries anteriorly, while the operating surgeon uses his/her right hand with a forcepts to control the ascending aorta inferior to the transposed pulmonary artery confluence. Then the surgeon removes the clamp in preparation for replacement of inferior to the pulmonary artery confluence. (With permission: Mavroudis 2015)

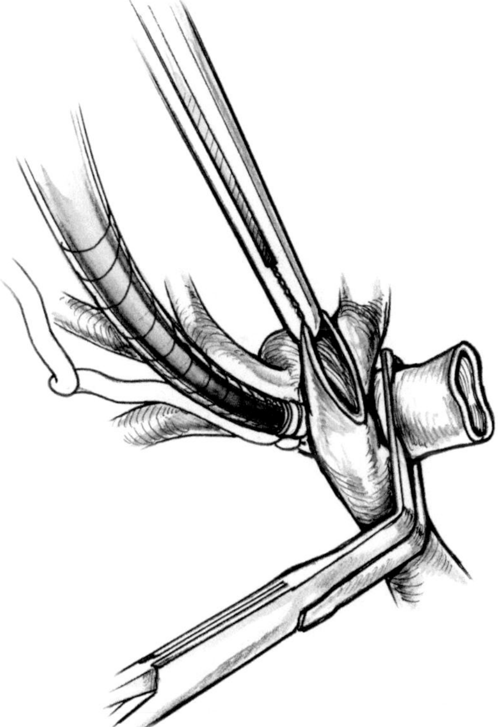

Fig. 22 shows the released aortic cross-clamp being moved and reclamped in front of the transposed confluence of pulmonary arteries thereby completing the maneuver of Lecompte. This maneuver assures the position of the pulmonary artery in front of the neoaorta during the completion of the neoaortic anastomosis. (With permission: Mavroudis 2015)

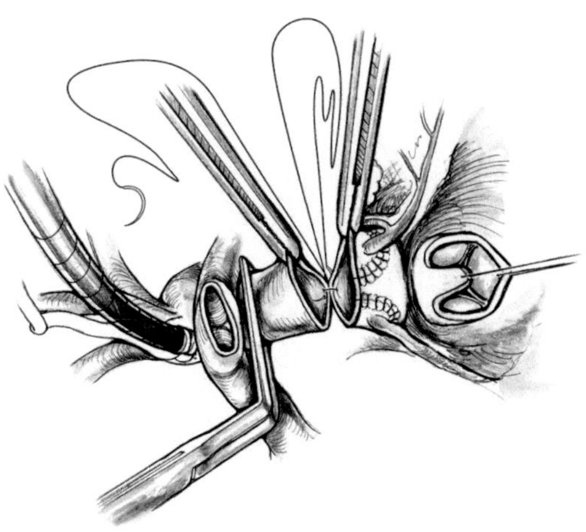

Fig. 23 depicts the neoaortic anastomosis being commenced at the posterior position making sure that the two structures align accurately. Failure to perform this will result in a poor reconstruction which can cause coronary artery kinking and neoaortic regurgitation due to anastomotic malrotation and mismatch. The neoaortic anastomosis is usually performed with running suture technique. (With permission: Mavroudis 2015)

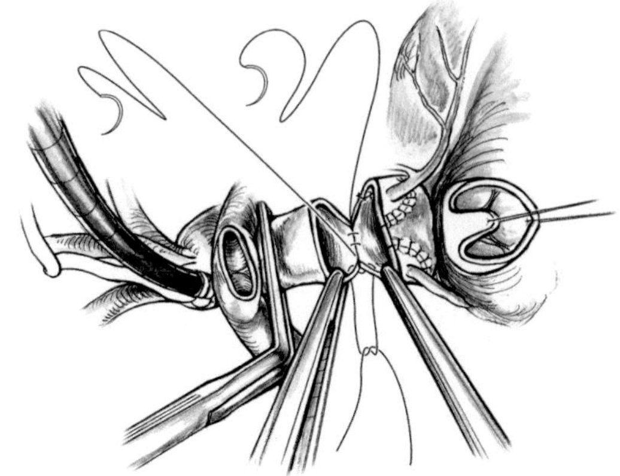

Fig. 25 shows an interrupted suture being placed along the extant suture line. This is used when the surgeon recognizes poor apposition of the suture line especially in the area of the coronary artery button anchoring stitch. An interrupted suture in this location will ensure hemostasis and is well worth the effort. (With permission: Mavroudis 2015)

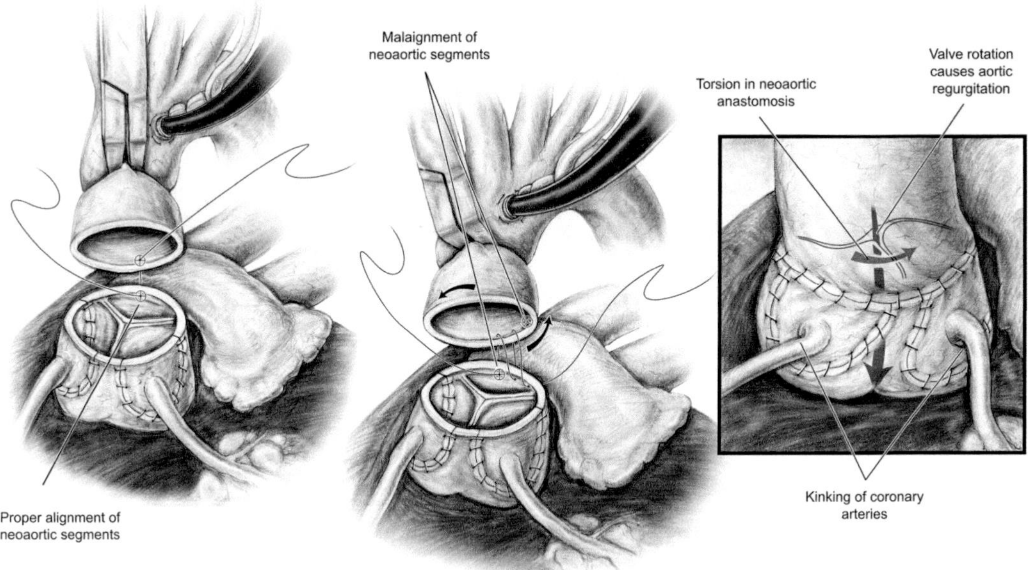

Fig. 24 Left panel shows the beginning of the malrotation of the neoaortic anastomosis. This can be caused by inaccurate suture placement owing to the placement of the aortic cross- clamp in association with the Lecompte maneuver. The right panel shows how the progression of the aortic anastomosis can result in malrotation which can cause coronary kinking and neoarotic leaflet distortion. This situation can occur if the proximal neoaorta and the distal aorta are not aligned properly. As noted, this can happen due to improper clamp placement after the maneuver of Lecompte or inaccurate estimation of posterior suture placement that should align both structures. If this problem is identified before the completion of the anastomosis, the anastomotic suture line should be taken down and replaced with a more suitable suture line that will result in proper alignment. As shown in the right panel, if the malrotation of the neoaortic reconstruction is completed (horizontal arrow), coronary perfusion problems (straight lines) and/or neoaortic regugitation (ghosted arrow into the left ventricle) can be identified by electrocardiographic findings and ventricular distention as the case may be. Prompt recognition of the problem(s) and reanastomosis will generally resolve these signficant potential hemodynamic catastophes

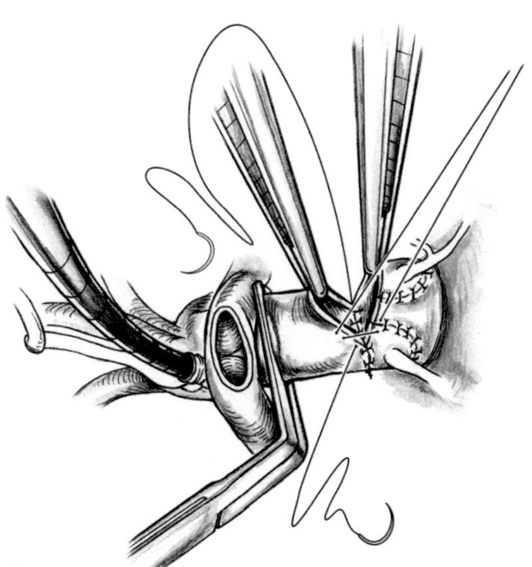

Fig. 26 demonstrates how the completion neoarotic reconstruction is performed while maintaining the suturing principles as noted in Fig. 19. (With permission: Mavroudis 2015)

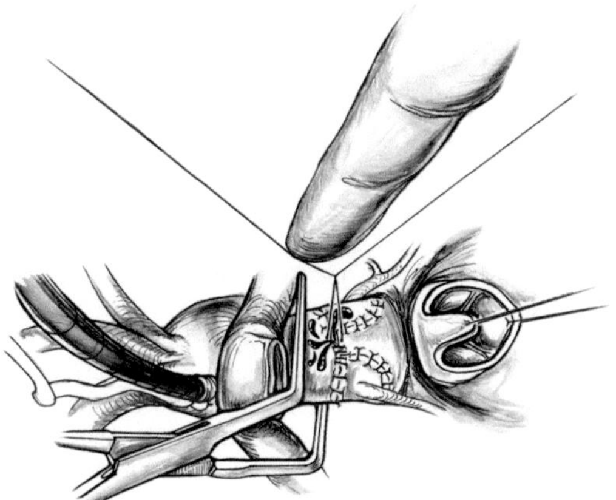

Fig. 27 shows the de-airing maneuvers being performed in tandem with release of the cross-clamp before the final suture line is tied. The patient can then be rewarmed while the neopulmonary artery is performed. (With permission: Mavroudis 2015)

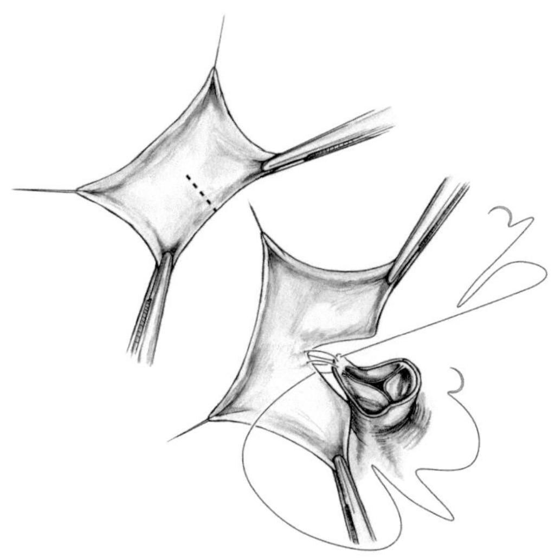

Fig. 28 shows the proximal aorta, soon to become the neopulmonary artery, with the dissected sinuses of Valsalva. A rectangular piece of pericardium is incised centrally to construct a pantaloon patch which when sutured appropriately, will fill out the dissected sinuses of Valsalva. The suture is being placed at the apex of the incised pericardium and approximated to the apex of the posterior commissure. Running suture technique (7–0 monofilament suture) is used for this reconstruction. (With permission: Mavroudis 2015)

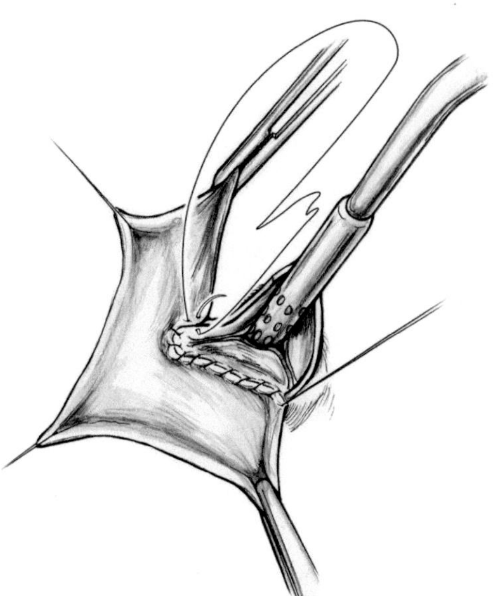

Fig. 29 shows the anastomosis in progress with a sucker in the orifice of the neopulmonary artery to facilitate exposure. Once this is finished, the very important tapering of the pericardial patch is performed as is shown in Fig. 24. (With permission: Mavroudis 2015)

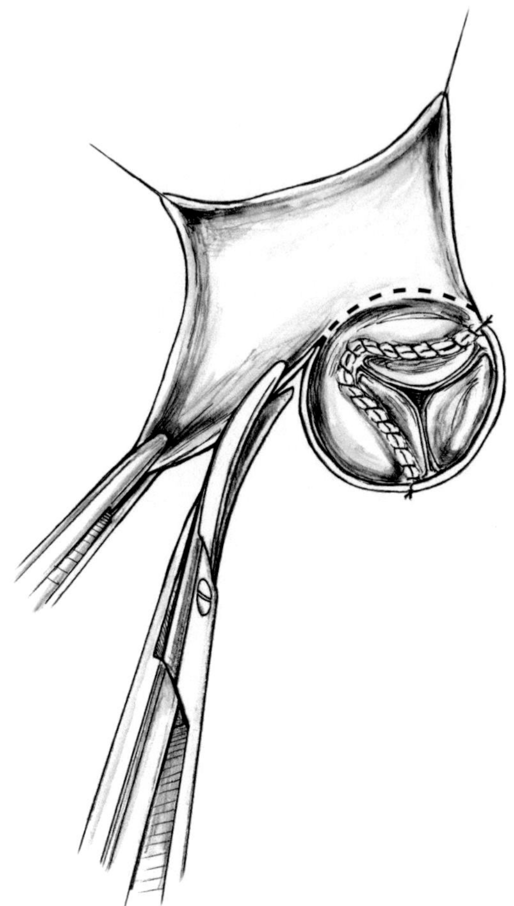

Fig. 30 There are two principles to this technique that are shown in the figure. First, the posterior portion of the pericardial patch is intentionally left approximately 3–4 mm longer in order to decrease any chances of coronary artery compression from the neopulmonary artery. This extra distance allows a favorable match between the neopulmonary artery and the distal pulmonary artery without posterior compression of the coronary arteries. Secondly, the patch is cut in a semicircular crescent shaped configuration; not in a straight line from commissure to commissure. This maneuver ensures redundant neosinuses of Valsalva (Fig. 25) that mitigates against the development of supravalvar pulmonary stenosis which was the most common complication of arterial switch prior to the institution of this redundant pantaloon pericardial patch. (With permission: Mavroudis 2015)

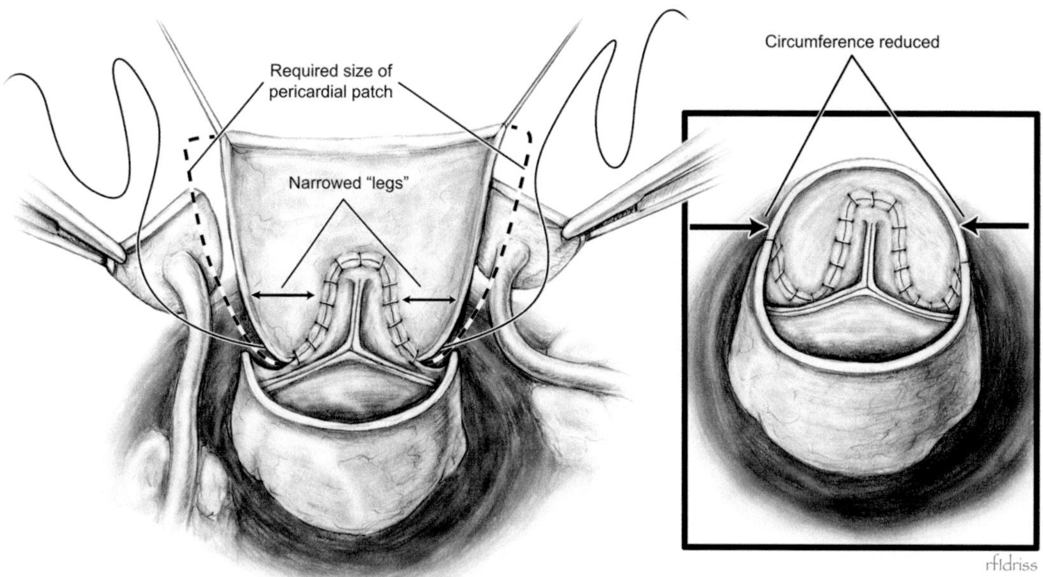

Fig. 31 shows how an undersized and narrow pericardial patch used to augment the sinuses of Valsalva for the neopulmonary artery reconstruction can result in surpravalvar neopulmonary artery stenosis. The pantaloon pericardial patch is shown with narrow dimensions for each of the legs of the pericardial patch. The dotted lines show the acceptable size of the legs of the pantaloon patch that will avoid supravalvar neopulmonary stenosis. The coronary artery buttons are shown for anatomic relevance. In general, the coronary artery buttons would have been attached to the neoaorta before the neopulmonary artery reconstruction. The inset demonstrates how supravalvar neopulmonary artery stenosis can occur if the undersized and narrow pantaloon patch is sewn into place. If recognized intraoperatively, it is better to take the patch down and replace it with an appropriately sized pantaloon patch that will prevent supravalvar neopulmonary artery stenosis

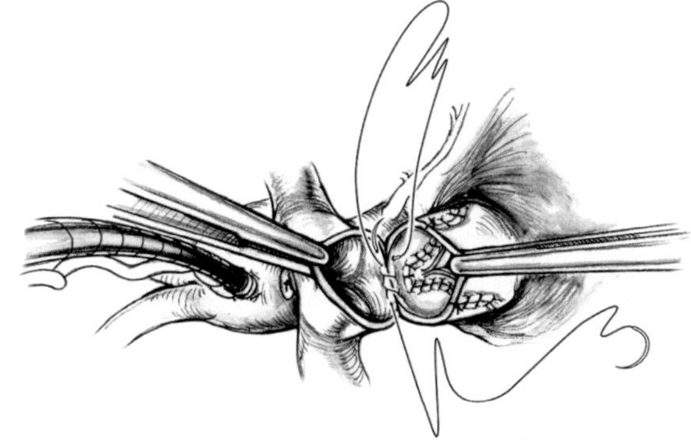

Fig. 32 shows the neopulmonary artery being reconstructed using the priniciples that have been noted in Figs. 28, 29 and 30. The anastomosis is commenced posteriorly to accurately align the two structures and to prevent unwanted malrotation and neopulmonary artery regurgitation. (With permission: Mavroudis 2015)

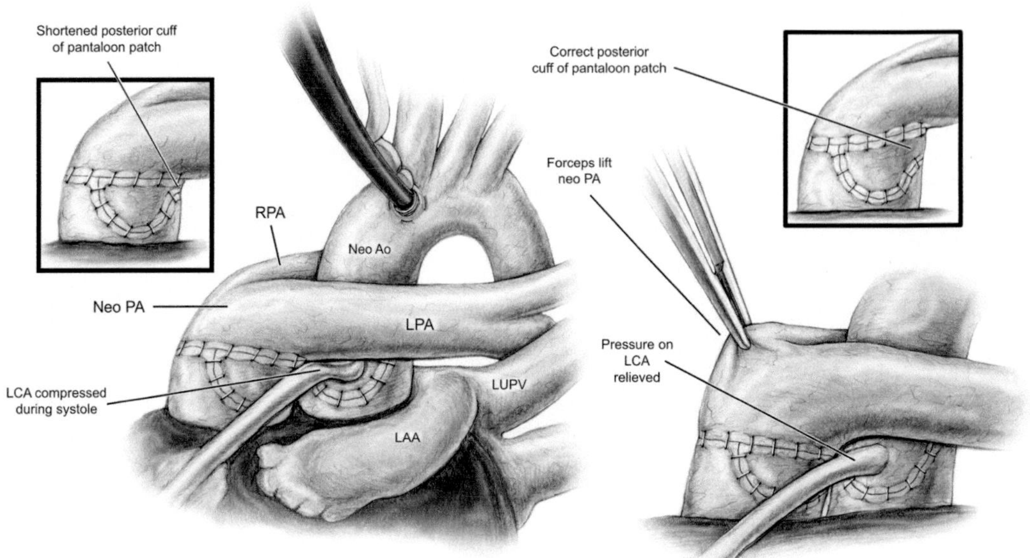

Fig. 33 Left Panel and inset show how the shortened neopulmonary artery reconstruction can cause anastomotic tension and complicating coronary artery compression. ST-T wave electrocardiographic changes can be noted during separation from cardiopulmonary bypass thereby alerting the surgeon of myocardial ischemia. Epicardial inspection can determine the problem. The right panel shows how anterior forceps retraction of the neopulmonary artery will result in improved hemodynamic circumstances which should lead to recommencement of cardiopulmonary bypass and neopulmonary artery anastomotic revision as shown in the right inset. *Ao* aorta, *LAA* left atrial appendage, *LCA* left coronary artery, *LPA* left pulmonary artery, *LUPV* left upper pulmonary vein, *PA* pulmonary artery, *RPA* right pulmonary artery

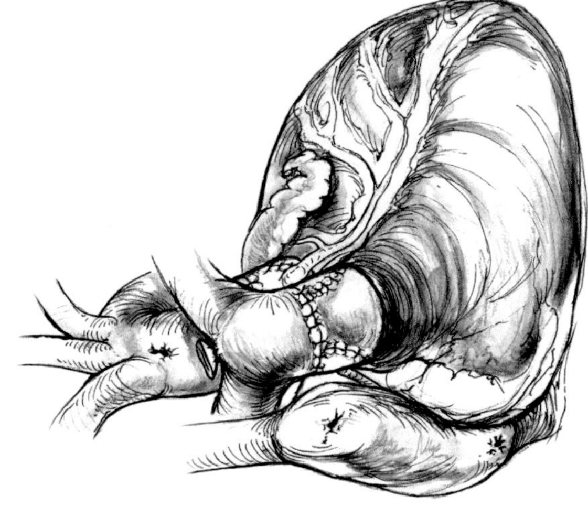

Fig. 34 shows the complete repair after separation from cardiopulmonary bypass and decannulation. Note the absence of coronary artery conpression and the fullness of the neopulmonary artery reconstruction which will prevent supravalvar pulmonary artery stenosis in the long-term. (With permission: Mavroudis 2015)

vorably on the end result. These steps include (1) great vessel dissection/mobilization, (2) coronary artery button transfer to the neoaorta, (3) neoaortic reconstruction, and (4) neopulmonary artery reconstruction. This discussion will build upon the extant procedural figures and add new drawings which will depict the anatomic complications and the solutions thereto pertaining.

The initial part of the operation, namely the dissection and mobilization of the great vessels can be complicated by patent ductal disruption, coronary artery injury, and pulmonary artery mobilization.

Oftentimes, the surgeon will want to mobilize the patent arterial duct to facilitate dissection of the aorta and pulmonary artery and avoid an increased cardiopulmonary bypass time. There are several issues that need to be addressed concerning the management of the patent arterial duct. First of all, even if no complications with ductal dissection are encountered, ligation and division of the duct can lead to acute and unfavorable cyanosis especially if a preoperative atrial balloon septostomy was not performed. This will require immediate heparinization and commencement of cardiopulmonary bypass to avoid the consequences of lactic acidosis. Secondly, during dissection the ductal tissue may rupture resulting in troublesome bleeding. Efforts to control the bleeding with suture technique can lead to recurrent laryngeal nerve injury, neocoarctation at the aortic ductal origin, and pulmonary artery distortion (see chapters "Complications Associated with Ligation of Patent Arterial Duct (Patent Ductus Arteriosus)", "Complications Associated with Repair of Coarctation of the Aorta", and "Complications Associated with Repair of Interrupted Aortic Arch"). Complications can also occur during the pulmonary artery dissection and mobilization at each respective hilum where the pulmonary artery bifurcates into the distal branches. Rough digital or scissor dissection and high setting of the electrocautery probe can result in localized distal pulmonary artery disruption and potential uncontrolled bleeding. Figure 2 shows how rough dissection of the distal pulmonary arteries can cause localized disruption. The inset shows how the problem can be repaired. Prudence will determine what is the best manner to repair such an injury either with direct suture repair or pericardial patch augmentation arterioplasty. On the other hand, limited dissection of the distal pulmonary arteries could cause distal distortion and obstruction resulting in right ventricular hypertension as shown in Fig. 3. The solution to this problem is to dissect the distal main pulmonary arteries into their respective hilli which generally involve identification and mobilization of the first branch pulmonary arteries as shown in Fig. 4.

Some surgeons prefer to dissect the proximal coronary arteries before aortic cross- clamping and coronary button mobilization. These maneuvers could cause unwanted coronary injury and bleeding. The best way to repair this problem is to institute cardiopulmonary bypass, aortic cross-clamping, and cardioplegic arrest. This will allow a proper view of the injury allowing the surgeon to perform the best non-obstructive repair solution which will ensure coronary perfusion after the coronary button transfer to the neoaorta.

Complications associated with coronary artery button harvesting can be fatal if the problems are not recognized early and repaired effectively. Figure 10 shows how the coronary artery button can be harvested by careful sharp dissection making sure to respect the boundaries of the aortic valve leaflets (neopulmonary artery leaflets), the aortic annulus, and the coronary artery orifice. If, however, the incision drifts too closely to the coronary artery orifice, a potential coronary artery malperfusion situation presents itself (Fig. 11). Trying to perform the coronary transfer to the neoaorta with intraluminal sutures might work but may be hazardous in the construction especially if there is bleeding after the cross-clamp is removed. Better to use a well-placed pericardial patch to augment the area where the unwanted close incision occurred. Figure 11 inset shows how the pericardial patch can augment the neoaortic reconstruction which will improve the anatomic reconstruction and thus improve coronary perfusion.

Another coronary artery problem that may arise is unwanted rotation of the coronary button during neoaortic reconstruction which could cause twisting of the proximal coronary artery resulting in malperfusion. Figure 14 shows the proper orientation of the coronary artery button for neoaortic reconstruction. If the visual calculation of the first suture is not applied accurately an unwanted rotation of the coronary button could result in twisting of the proximal coronary artery causing stenosis and hypoperfusion. If this problem is not identified and rectified, postoperative myocardial ischemia and ventricular dysfunction may occur. Avoidance of this problem was considered in the early days of introduction of the arterial switch operation by Farouk Idriss (Idriss et al. 1988a, b). He advanced the idea that once the coronary artery button is harvested, the optimal orientation could be determined by simply placing the coronary button, without sutures, near the intended anastomotic location while determining a "best lie" configuration. This obviously is a simple way to best determine proper button orientation. It has the benefit of being inherently clear and intuitively obvious. Figure 15 left panel shows how the coronary artery button is oriented in a "best lie" configuration with the first stitch being placed to commit to the proper orientation. The left panel insert shows the completed anastomosis without rotation. However, unwanted button rotation resulting in myocardial ischemia can happen. Figure 15 right panel shows how an inappropriate first suture can commit the anastomosis to an unwanted rotation which, when completed, will result in coronary artery twisting, kinking, and an obstructive orientation as noted in the right panel insert. When recognized the anastomotic suture must be taken down and reperformed with an accurate orientation.

Acquired postoperative coronary stenosis after neoaortic reconstruction can also occur due to anastomotic malrotation which occurs by the initial suture placement that is mistakenly placed resulting in malalignment of the completed neoaortic anastomosis. Figure 24 shows how malrotation of the neoaortic reconstruction can result in coronary stenosis due to kinking and neoaortic regurgitation caused by leaflet distortion. This situation can result in myocardial malperfusion and important neoaortic regurgitation that can be identified by an increase in left ventricular distention and/or increased flow from the left ventricular vent. Prompt recognition of the problems with anastomotic takedown, neoaortic realignment, and proper reanastomosis will resolve the issue.

4 Neopulmonary Artery Problems

Neopulmonary artery distortion can occur during the reconstruction that deserves mention since the most common long-term complication of the arterial switch operation is supravalvar pulmonary artery stenosis (Spector et al. 2018; Khairy et al. 2013; Raju et al. 2013; Loke et al. 2019; Belhadjer et al. 2020). Other less common complications involve neopulmonary artery compression of the transferred coronary artery buttons and distal pulmonary artery stenosis owing to suboptimal distal pulmonary artery dissection and mobilization. The pantaloon pericardial patch as shown in Fig. 28 was introduced by Farouk Idriss (Idriss et al. 1988a, b) to accomplish three objectives.

The first objective is to construct a singular oversized pericardial patch that will fill in the sinuses of Valsalva of the neopulmonary reconstruction. The pericardial "pantaloons" are generally made to be larger than the estimated size of the pulmonary artery moieties. The pericardial edges are sutured in such a way as to gather the pericardium in a 2:1 ratio (pericardium-to-pulmonary artery edge) which will ensure hemostasis while resulting in a large balloon-like outpouching that will help to avoid supravalvar stenosis. Failure to ensure a large pericardial patch for the sinuses of Valsalva can result in immediate supravalvar pulmonary artery stenosis as noted in Fig. 31. When this is recognized, taking down the patch with a larger replacement is indicated.

The second objective is to leave a pericardial extension to increase the length of the neopulmonary artery reconstruction as noted in Fig. 32. This extra length will avoid coronary artery compression by ensuring enough length so that the proximal neopulmonary artery anastomosis to the distal pulmonary artery will not cause undue tension and resultant compression of the transferred coronary artery buttons which, by design, arise anteriorly from the neoaorta. Figure 33 shows how the shortened neopulmonary artery reconstruction can result in anastomotic tension and eventual coronary artery compression. This situation should be suspected if ST-T electrocardiographic changes are noted during separation from cardiopulmonary bypass. The condition can be identified readily since the problem is anterior and can be evaluated by epicardial inspection. Usually, anterior forceps retraction of the neopulmonary artery will result in improved hemodynamic conditions which will lead the surgeon to recommencement of cardiopulmonary bypass and neopulmonary artery anastomotic revision.

The third objective is to properly dissect and mobilize the distal pulmonary arteries as noted earlier in the chapter. The potential difficulties with this dissection are injury to the pulmonary arteries and the phrenic nerve. It is for these reasons that the surgeon may choose not to extend the hilar mobilization to avoid complications. Avoiding complications is what this book is about; however, failure to complete the distal pulmonary artery mobilization may cause distal pulmonary artery kinking and right ventricular hypertension as noted in Fig. 3 Once this problem is identified, a more robust hilar dissection and mobilization can resolve the problem (Fig. 4). Of course, careful attention to vessel integrity to avoid bleeding and careful attention to the course of the phrenic nerve are necessary. The completed arterial switch operation should compare to that noted in Fig. 34 to ensure the best outcome.

5 Coronary Artery Anomalies

Coronary artery anomalies are frequent in patients with TGA and can consist of every conceivable configuration (Gittenberger-de Groot et al. 1986, 2018; Jatene et al. 1982; Kurosawa et al. 1991; Smith et al. 1986; Pasquini et al. 1987, 1994; Tamisier et al. 1997; Mavroudis et al. 1999; Tanel et al. 1995; Arensman et al. 1985; Goor et al. 1982; Rowlatt 1962; Yacoub and Radley-Smith 1978; Ebels et al. 1989; Mariani et al. 1998; Mayer Jr et al. 1990; Chiu et al. 1995; Shukla et al. 2000; Sim et al. 1994; van Son 1996; Day et al. 1992; Rossi et al. 1986; Chang et al. 2005; Zheng et al. 2008; Moll et al. 2017; Asou et al. 1994; Li et al. 2000; Cleuziou et al. 2008; Mavroudis et al. 2011; Parry et al. 1999; Ou et al. 2013; Michalak et al. 2019; van Wijk et al. 2017). While there are a number of classifications, the Leiden Classification (Gittenberger-de Groot et al. 2018) has simplified the nomenclature by naming the sinuses 1 and 2 and is characterized by imagining a surgeon standing in the noncoronary cusp of the aorta looking posteriorly. The surgeon's right hand will signify sinus 1 and the left hand will signify sinus 2. This description allows for all types of configurations to be classified by simply noting which coronaries arise from each of the sinuses. The Leiden classification can account for the majority of coronary artery anomalies which include, inverted coronary arteries, single coronary arteries and intramural coronary arteries by simple description using the sinus 1, sinus 2 method.

Each of the anomalous coronary artery configurations featured herein Figs. 35, 36, 37, 38, 39, 40, 41, 42, 43, 44, 45, 46, 47, 48, 49, 50, and 51 have a unique reconstructive solution for effective resolution and optimal myocardial perfusion. In general terms, the principles of management require careful intraoperative diagnosis, appropriate cardioplegic techniques consistent with the anticipated longer cross-clamp time which may involve retrograde cardioplegia or intracoronary administration, and extensive mobilization of the coronary artery buttons for eventual transfer to the neoaorta. Depending on the favorable or unfavorable anatomic lie, small pericardial patches may be necessary to create a satisfactory reconstruction, especially for those patients with single coronary artery buttons which cannot be transferred easily.

Combination of coronary artery lesions are not rare and will require special attention when they are discovered. For instance, Figs. 35 and 36 show how both coronary arteries arise from sinus 2 in patients with TGA. In addition, however, the

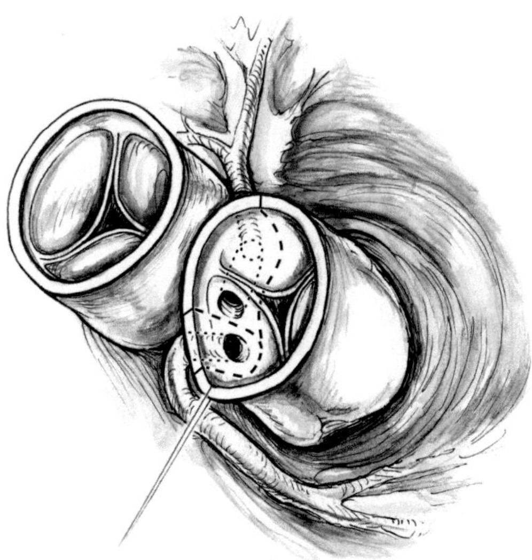

Fig. 35 shows a Sinus 1–0 and Sinus 2 left anterior descending (LAD), Circumflex, right coronary artery origins. In addition, the left main coronary artery has an intramural route that courses across the commissure into Sinus 1 where it emerges as the left main coronary artery. This is a very challenging artery to reconstruct. (With permission: Mavroudis 2015)

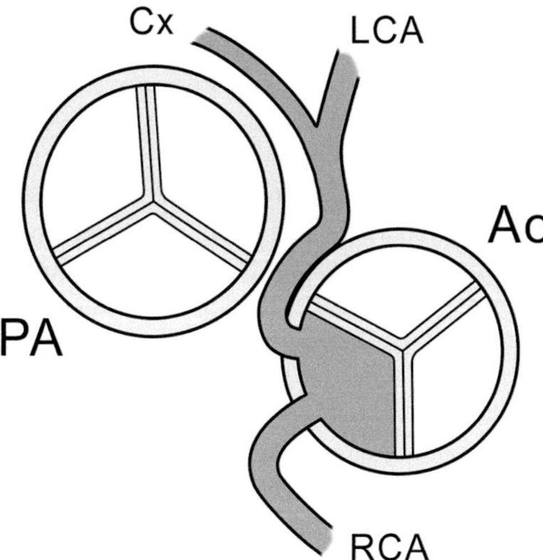

Fig. 36 shows the surgeon's diagrammatic view of the coronary artery anatomy which is reverse of the anatomist's convention which views the anatomy from the feet up. The surgeon views the anatomy from the head down. From the outset and before any incisions are made, the surgeon has to decide whether there is enough room between the orifices of the two coronary arteries to form two distinct buttons. Most of the time, two buttons can be formed. (With permission: Mavroudis 2015)

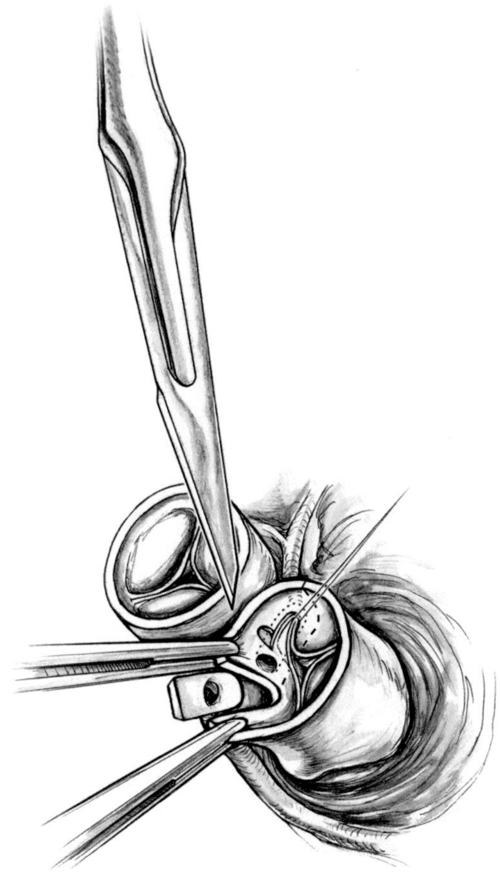

Fig. 37 shows the right coronary artery button being mobilized after it has been detached from the common aortic wall and the other coronary artery. The mobilization of this coronary button is less complex than the left main coronary button. (With permission: Mavroudis 2015)

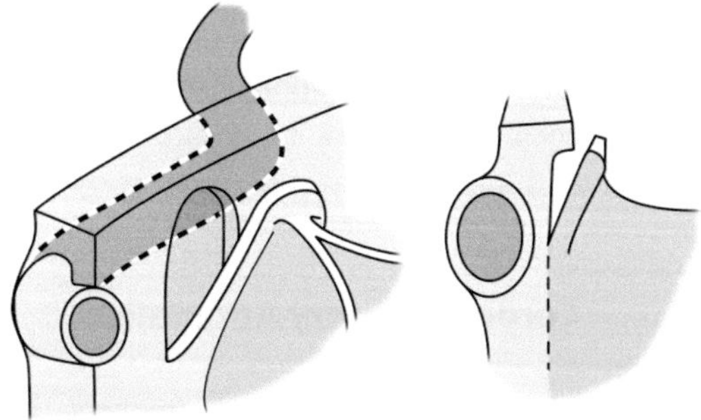

Fig. 38 The remaining coronary button must be separated from the aortic wall and the posterior commissure where the leaflets are attached. This is performed by sharp dissection and mobilizing the commissural attachment with a portion of the aortic wall to allow for eventual reconstruction. (With permission: Mavroudis 2015)

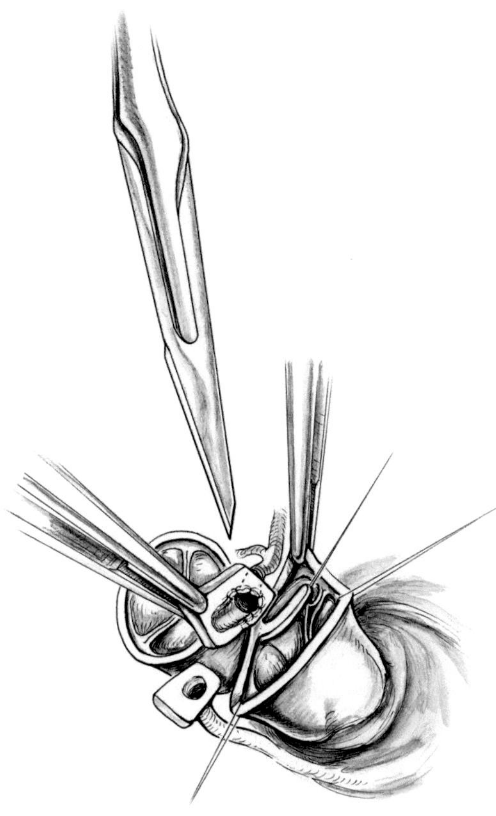

Fig. 39 The intramural segment is then unroofed and tacking sutures are placed at the neo-orifice to insure the integrity of the orifice and to avoid dissection and occlusion. (With permission: Mavroudis 2015)

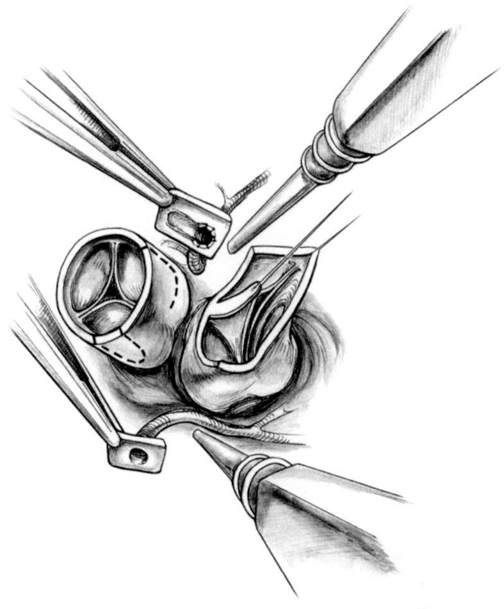

Fig. 40 The coronary artery is then mobilized with careful low setting electrocautery techniques. The surgeon must decide whether to unroof the intramural course. In this set of drawings, the intramural course of the coronary artery is unroofed and sutured to avoid dissection. In times past, the unroofing was not always performed owing to fear of disruption and dissection. Nowadays, the wisdom is to always unroof the course of the intramural artery to avoid any problems in the future. (With permission: Mavroudis 2015)

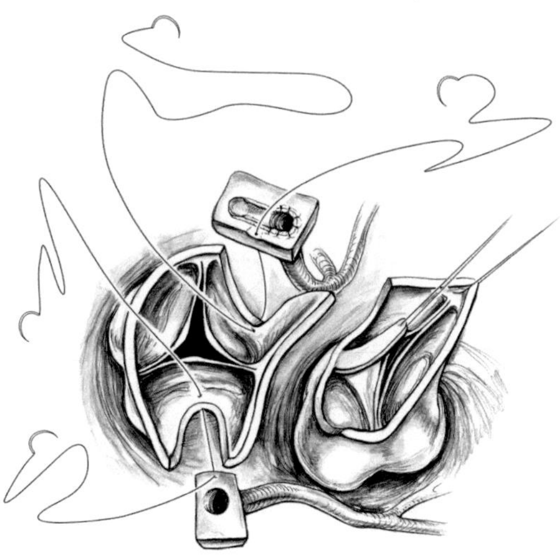

Fig. 41 depicts the coronary artery buttons being implanted to the ascending neoaorta using techniques previously noted in this chapter. (With permission: Mavroudis 2015)

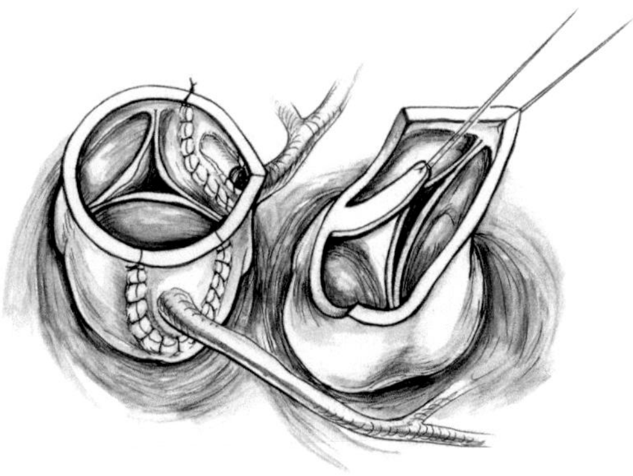

Fig. 42 shows the reconstructed proximal neoaorta with unobstructed coronary artery anatomy and respective courses. The original aortic root, now to become the neopulmonary artery after reconstruction is being retracted to show the neoaorta. (With permission: Mavroudis 2015)

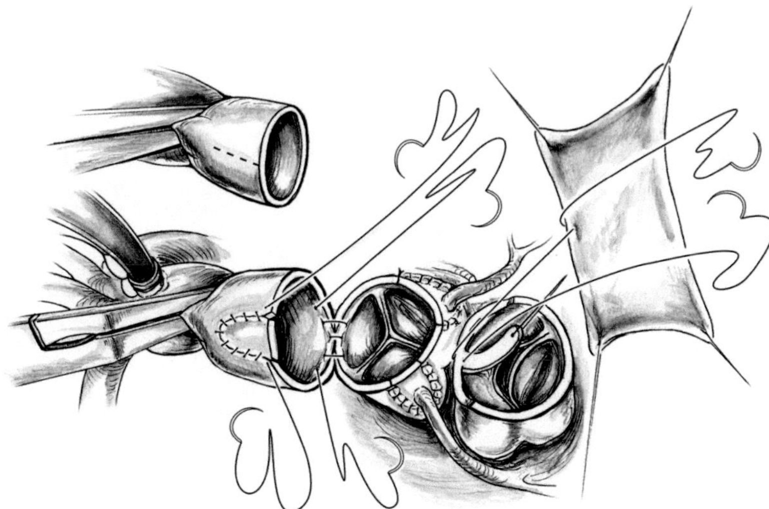

Fig. 43 Oftentimes, the proximal neoaortic reconstruction is much larger than the distal aorta especially when the coronary buttons are anomalous and require more space for reimplantation. Under these circumstances, the ascending aorta can be enlarged by linear incision and pericardial patch augmentation. This will allow a more appropriate anastomotic alignment that will avoid coronary artery restriction and neoaortic valve infringement. The neopulmonary artery reconstruction is commenced with the pericardial patch which, in this case, is not cut into a pantaloon configuration since the coronary artery detachment involved much of the posterior pulmonary artery wall. The pericardium is therefore sewn to the edges of the remaining neopulmonary artery wall in anticipation of commissural reattachment to the implanted pericardium. (With permission: Mavroudis 2015)

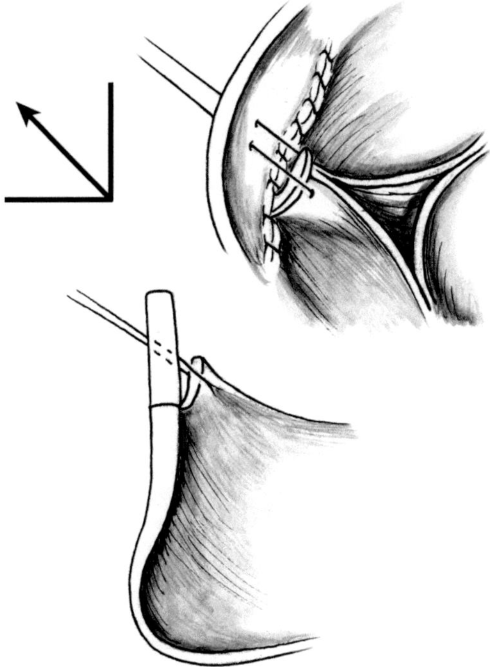

Fig. 44 Once the pericardium is sewn in place, the posterior commissure of the neopulmonary valve can be reattached to the pericardial wall with interrupted suture technique. The surgeon can determine the height and number of sutures that will be required to effect a competent valve. (With permission: Mavroudis 2015)

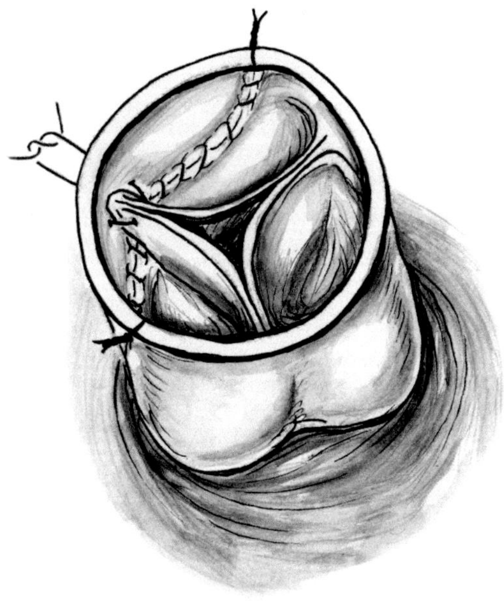

Fig. 45 illustrates the completed reconstruction of the proximal neopulmonary artery with pericardial patch sinus of Valsalva augmentations and leaflet attachment. This can be followed by the end-to-end anastomosis between the reconstructed proximal neopulmonary artery and the distal pulmonary artery. (With permission: Mavroudis 2015)

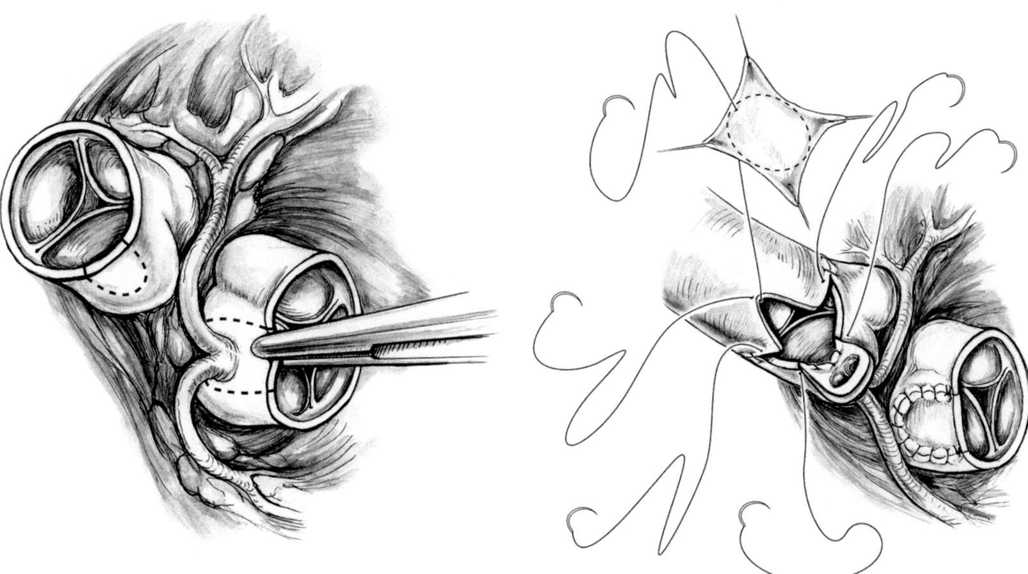

Fig. 46 Some single coronary artery anomalies are not amenable to division and individual reimplantation to the neoaorta due to the close proximity of the coronary artery origins. Such is the case with a single coronary artery origin from Sinus 2 as noted in the figure. The dashed lines depict the area of dissection and separation of the coronary artery button from the aorta. The area of reimplantation into the pulmonary artery soon to become the neoaorta is shown by dashed lines. In order to reimplant the coronary artery button directly into the neoaorta without any patches, the coronary button would have to be rotated 180° which would cause a complete obstruction due to kinking. (With permission: Mavroudis 2015)

Fig. 48 Since a 180° rortation of the coronary artery button is fraught with obstructive complications an acceptable alternative to this situation is to mobilize the branches of both coronary arteries and rotate the coronary artery button 90° by suturing the superior edge of the coronary artery button to the inferior portion of the incised sinus of Valsalva. The figure shows how the pericardial patch is engaged to form a funnel and establish unobstructed flow when the reconstruction is finished. (With permission: Mavroudis 2015)

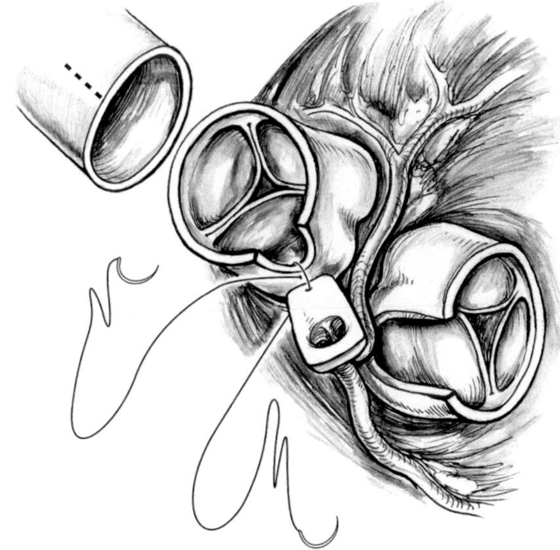

Fig. 47 shows aortobicaval cannulation and the commencement of cardiopulmonary bypass in a patient with transposition of the great arteries. Aortic cannulation is performed high on the ascending aorta just downstream of the innominate artery to faciliate the arterial switch operation. (With permission: Mavroudis 2015)

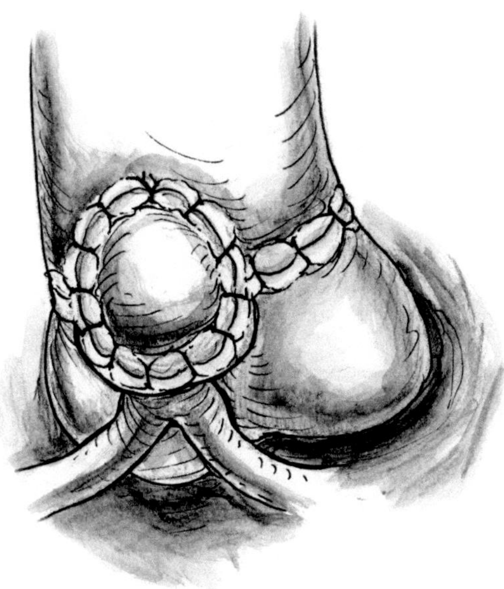

Fig. 49 shows the completed reconstruction of the single coronary artery to the ascending neoaorta using the rotated artery and pericardial patch technique. The pericardium is used to create a hood thereby ensuring a patent and non-obstructive pathway to the coronary arteries. Other coronary artery configurations may require more creative solutions. The principles are the same however and require close attention to myocardial preservation, coronary mobilization, and tension free anastomoses which will enhance flow. (With permission: Mavroudis 2015)

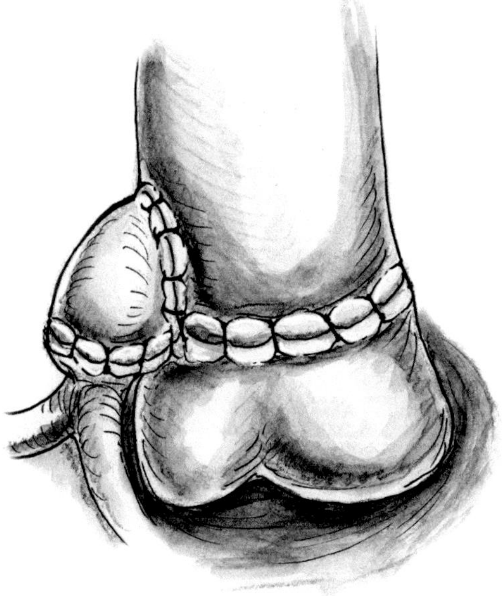

Fig. 50 demonstrates the lateral view of the single coronary artery transfer and reconstruction. The rotated coronary artery button, when dissected conscientiously will allow unobstructed flow using this technique. (With permission: Mavroudis 2015)

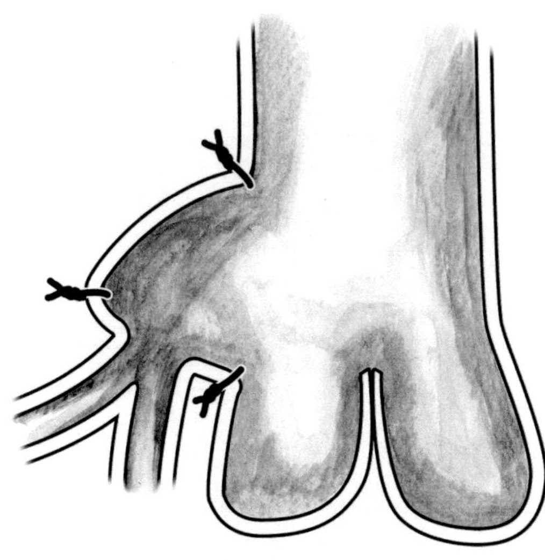

Fig. 51 shows the coronal view of that which is depicted in Fig. 41. Emphasis is placed on the suture attachments. (With permission: Mavroudis 2015)

left main coronary artery proceeds intramurally towards sinus 1 before branching to the left anterior descending and circumflex coronary arteries. The initial approach towards reconstructive resolution is to create separate coronary artery buttons by separating the right coronary artery button from the left main coronary artery button as shown in Figs. 37 and 38. The potential complications associated with this maneuver center around unwanted excision lines that are too close to the coronary orifice or direct injury to the course of the coronary artery. Careful and direct scalpel incision and scissor dissection should help the surgeon to avoid these complications. Electrocautery dissection, if needed to control collateral bleeding, should be used sparingly and at low settings since an inadvertent application can easily result in coronary artery injury. In this particular case, the surgeon, either preoperatively or intraoperatively, is confronted with an intramural left coronary artery which traverses across the aortic (neopulmonary root) commissure. When this is discovered, the surgeon must make plans for an extended cross-clamp time which may consist of lowering the systemic temperature (perhaps to 28 ° C) and ensuring that the retrograde coronary sinus catheter is well situated for cardioplegia delivery. The management of the coronary artery button starts with the commissural takedown of the involved aortic commissure (to become the neopulmonary root) as shown in Fig. 38. This part of the operation should be performed with a Beaver blade to find the correct plane between the course of the coronary artery and the aortic wall to preserve the commissure. Obviously, technical complications can occur to both the course of the coronary artery and the commissure if the division is not performed carefully and deliberately. Injury to the coronary artery is not the worst situation since the artery will require unroofing as noted in Fig. 39. Injury to the commissure and neopulmonary valve root is not catastrophic since the neopulmonary valve will eventually be subject to lower pressures and mild to moderate pulmonary regurgitation is better tolerated than in the aortic position. Figure 39 also shows how the course of the intramural coronary artery was unroofed and reinforced with tacking sutures in order to avoid coronary dissection and disruption. The process of unroofing an intramural coronary artery, especially in a newborn, can be problematic especially if the unroofing procedure is carried too far into and through the intimal layer of the coronary artery. While it can be identified and seemingly repaired with interrupted sutures, it will not be identified until the coronary button is transferred, and the cross-clamp is removed. Bleeding at the area of the previous intimal repair is rarely resolved by further interrupted sutures. More often than not, the attempted repair will result in a larger hole and further, more robust bleeding. This situation can lead to disastrous coronary complications and must be taken seriously. Repeat cross-clamp and cardioplegic arrest will allow the surgeon to assess the problem, take down the repair sutures, freshen the edges of the leak, and apply a pericardial patch to augment the disrupted area with a hemostatic repair that will ensure coronary flow. This problem has been discussed and shown in chapter "Complications Associated with Repair of Congenital and Acquired Coronary Artery Anomalies" in the section of Anomalous Aortic Origin of the Coronary Arteries. The proposed transfer of the coronary arteries to the neoaorta is shown in Fig. 40. Each coronary artery button transfer will require its own method of reimplantation. For instance, shown in the figure is the "J" incision for the unroofed left main coronary artery button. The "J" flap will allow more neoaortic tissue for the anastomosis and a better anatomic lie for optimal coronary flow. The right coronary button is transferred in the usual fashion. The potential complications regarding coronary button transfer are reviewed in Figs. 10, 11, 12, 13, 14, 15, 16, 17, 18, 19, 20, 21, 22, 23, 24, and 25. The optimal coronary artery button transfer in this case is shown in Figs. 41 and 42.

In circumstances where the proximal neoaortic reconstruction proves to be too large to align with the ascending aorta as is often the case with complex coronary artery button transfer, the surgeon may want to augment the ascending aorta with a patch prior to the neoaortic reconstruction as is noted in Fig. 43. The potential malalignment problems which can cause coronary kinking and neoaortic regurgitation as described in Figs. 23, 24, 25, 26 and 27 are appropriate in this situation as well. The ascending aortic patch may cause the surgeon to miscalculate the correct alignment for accurate anastomosis. The best way to avoid this problem is to align the posterior aspects of the proximal neoaorta and the distal aorta as the starting point for the anastomosis, thereby not paying attention as much to the ascending aortic augmentation patch. Figure 43 also shows the proximal neopulmonary artery root reconstruction. Notice that the pericardial patch is not configured in a pantaloon manner like that used for the standard arterial switch operation without coronary artery anomalies. As noted in Figs. 38 and 39, the posterior commissure was taken down within the aortic wall to harvest without injury to the left main coronary artery. As a result, the classic pantaloon patch to fill out the sinuses of Valsalva will not have enough satisfactory suture purchase to complete this style of reconstruction. Alternatively, Fig. 44 shows the reattachment of the posterior commissure to the pericardial patch at the appropriate height and suture strength to ensure pulmonary valve function with the absence of pulmonary regurgitation. Figure 45 shows the completed proximal completed neopulmonary artery reconstruction en route to anastomosis to the distal pulmonary artery.

Complications associated with this maneuver is the tearing of the pulmonary valve leaflets, resultant pulmonary regurgitation, and right ventricular outflow tract obstruction owing to the prolapsed posterior commissure.

Management of the single coronary artery in association with the arterial switch operation is a challenging undertaking requiring careful dissection and operator stereovision to achieve an unusual anastomotic resolution. Figure 46 shows the standard coronary artery harvest from the aorta with the standard and optimal location on the neoaorta for the coronary artery button. All is not standard by any means, however. Once the coronary artery button is mobilized to the surface of the epicardium with special care to avoid injury to the branches, the button is turned 180 degrees so that the superior portion of the button now becomes the inferior part for the anastomosis. This maneuver is nicely shown in Fig. 47. Clearly, the most important step of this maneuver is to avoid coronary artery kinking by extensive mobilization without injuring the branch coronary arteries. The idea is to reconstruct the inverted coronary button by posterior neoaortic anastomosis and pericardial patch aortoplasty as shown in Fig. 48. As a result, the resultant reconstruction shows the coronary artery button rotated only 45 degrees which together with coronary artery mobilization will ensure coronary artery flow and myocardial perfusion as shown in Figs. 49, 50, and 51. The potential complications associated with this maneuver and neoaortic reconstruction are bleeding and coronary kinking owing to inadequate mobilization. Fortunately, the reconstruction is anterior and easily visible for resolution of bleeding and coronary kinking.

6 Left Ventricular Training and Delayed Arterial Switch

The arterial switch operation is based on the capacity of the left ventricular muscle and contractile power to undertake the pressure requirements of the systemic circulation. The ASO when applied to neonates takes advantage of the physiologic pulmonary hypertension that normally occurs in the first 2 weeks of life. Under these circumstances the left ventricle is prepared for the eventual arterial switch which will allow the left ventricle to take over the systemic circulation. Consequently, it is for these reasons that the arterial switch operation for patients with intact ventricular septum (TGA-IVS) is performed within the first 2 weeks of life. For patients with TGA-VSD the arterial switch operation with VSD closure can be delayed as long as the VSD is large enough to maintain systemic left ventricular pressure (Mavroudis and Backer 2023).

Some patients with TGA-IVS or TGA with a small VSD present late in life. Over time, left ventricular pressure recedes due to the fall in pulmonary artery resistance (Mavroudis and Backer 2023). Predictably, the anatomic left ventricle performs just like the right ventricle in patients with normal hearts; namely, the left ventricular pressure in TGA patients falls over time. This situation, however, does not preclude performing an atrial baffle operation (Senning or Mustard). Under these circumstances, the cyanosis is corrected but leaves the right ventricle as the systemic pumping chamber that eventually will fail (Ohtake et al. 1989, 1990). There are other options however that involve “training” the left ventricle by way of pulmonary artery banding strategies that will induce left ventricular hypertrophy. This careful preparation will allow the ventricle to hypertrophy for favorable pressure requirements that will support systemic flow (Mee 1986; de Jong et al. 1995; Reisman et al. 1999; Shinebourne et al. 1994; Mavroudis and Backer 2000; Maeda et al. 2016).

7 Pulmonary Artery Band and Systemic-to-Pulmonary Artery Shunt

For patients who present late in life for TGA-IVS or TGA with small VSD, pulmonary artery banding can serve to increase left ventricular afterload and induce left ventricular hypertrophy. Since pulmonary artery banding can cause cyanosis due to decreased pulmonary artery flow, a systemic-to-pulmonary artery shunt is performed prior to the pulmonary artery band to ensure appropriate systemic oxygen saturations.

There are, however, potential complications associated with this procedure that are worth discussing. In most cases, inotropic support will be required during and after the pulmonary artery band procedure as noted in Fig. 52. Increasing need for inotropic support in the operating room or in the early postoperative period should signal the possibility of significant

left ventricular afterload which may be poorly tolerated. Echocardiography will show decreased left ventricular function with decreased systemic pressure. This situation will require immediate return to the operating room for pulmonary artery

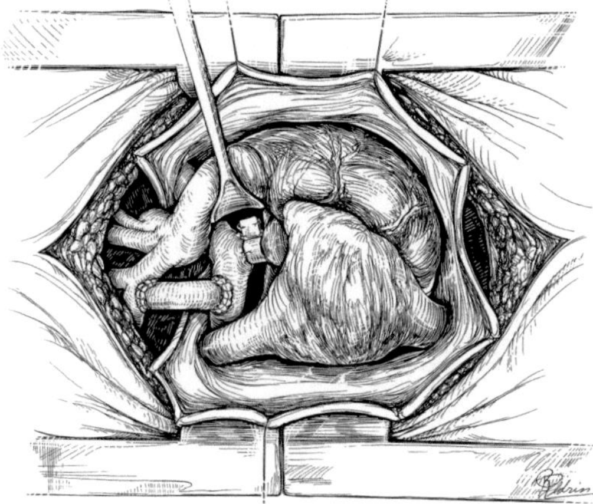

Fig. 52 shows the completed pulmonary artery band and systemic-to-pulmonary artery shunt in a patient with transposition of the great arteries-intact ventricular septum who presented late for the arterial switch operation. In general, the systemic-to-pulmonary artery shunt is performed first (see chapter "Complications Associated with Palliative Operations") and is followed by the pulmonary artery band procedure (see chapter "Complications Associated with Palliative Operations"). The band is constricted to raise the proximal pulmonary artery pressure to approximately 75% of the systemic pressure. Oftentimes, pressor agents are required in the short term. The left ventricle quickly accommodates, especially in the infant who is 2 months or older allowing the process to be "fast-tracked" which can result in an arterial switch operation within 2–4 weeks. When performed in older children, the interval between pulmonary artery band and the arterial switch operation can be longer. Echocardiography, left ventricular wall thickness, and left ventricular function guide the physician as to the optimal time for intervention to perform the arterial switch operation. (With permission: Mavroudis 2015)

band adjustment. It is not unusual for multiple attempts for pulmonary artery banding to cause gradual left ventricular hypertrophy. The operative team should be cognizant of these situations and use the pulmonary artery band technique judiciously and patiently (Mee 1986; de Jong et al. 1995; Reisman et al. 1999; Shinebourne et al. 1994; Mavroudis and Backer 2000; Maeda et al. 2016).

8 Mustard/Senning Takedown; Arterial Switch Operation

Left ventricular training using pulmonary artery banding in patients with existing Mustard or Senning operations en route to the arterial switch operation is not often used nowadays since these atrial switch operations have given way to the more physiologic anatomic repair by arterial switch (Stark 1984; Yacoub 1979). Left ventricular training however is used for congenitally corrected transposition of the great arteries in anticipation of the double switch operation (Ibrahimiye et al. 2017). This topic will be discussed in the appropriate chapter on the subject (Chapter "Complications Associated with Repair of Congenitally Corrected Transposition of the Great Arteries").

In any case, it is useful to discuss the complications associated with left ventricular training, atrial baffle takedown and arterial switch for those rare patients who present late with hemodynamic problems.

In general, when patients who had atrial baffle operations for transposition of the great arteries present late after atrial switch with right ventricular failure, tricuspid regurgitation, and arrhythmias, consideration can be given to conversion to arterial switch after staged left ventricular training by pulmonary artery banding (Mee 1986; de Jong et al. 1995; Reisman et al. 1999; Shinebourne et al. 1994; Mavroudis and Backer 2000; Maeda et al. 2016). Unlike transposition patients who present late without prior operations, patients with existing atrial baffles operations are physiologically corrected. As a result, there is little or no cyanosis. Consequently, left ventricular training can be performed by pulmonary artery banding without addition of a systemic-to-pulmonary artery shunt. The principles of staged constriction of the pulmonary artery are well described and should be adhered to during the operation to prevent acute ventricular decompensation. These principles are shown in Fig. 53 In particular, placement of the pulmonary artery band can cause immediate shifting of the interventricular septum towards the right ventricle which will favorably affect the tricuspid valve apparatus and decrease the amount of tricuspid regurgitation. Care must be taken not to overly tighten the pulmonary artery band which could cause immediate or remote biventricular failure (Mee 1986; de Jong et al. 1995; Reisman et al. 1999; Shinebourne et al. 1994; Mavroudis and Backer 2000; Maeda et al. 2016). In many cases, the pulmonary artery band will require staged constriction over time to avoid unsustainable increased left ventricular afterload. These issues can be avoided (Ibrahimiye et al. 2017; Cochrane et al. 1993; Benzaquen et al. 2004) by careful intraoperative gradient measurements and transesophageal function determinations.

Atrial switch takedown and conversion to arterial switch can be performed when left ventricular free wall dimensions and cardiac catheterization show satisfactory left ventricular function and favorable adaptability to the new circulation. However, there are notable exceptions to this management scheme. As noted, these patients often present with right ventricular dysfunction, tricuspid regurgitation, and severe congestive symptoms. Patient selection is very important since pulmonary artery banding in the

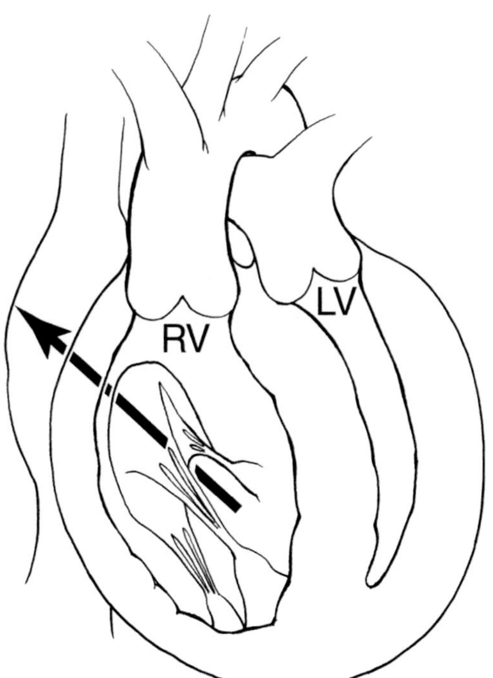

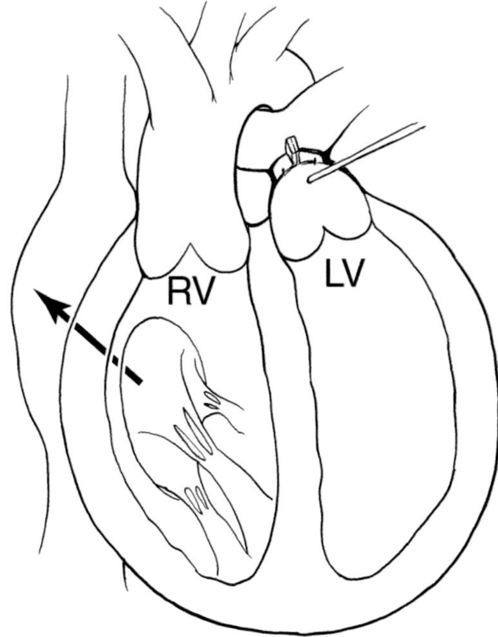

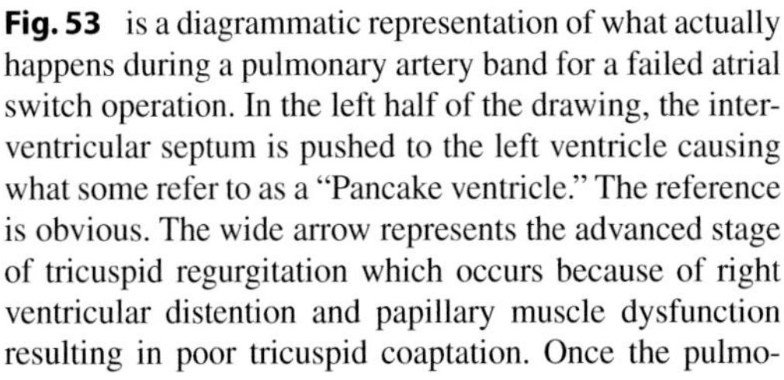

Fig. 53 is a diagrammatic representation of what actually happens during a pulmonary artery band for a failed atrial switch operation. In the left half of the drawing, the interventricular septum is pushed to the left ventricle causing what some refer to as a "Pancake ventricle." The reference is obvious. The wide arrow represents the advanced stage of tricuspid regurgitation which occurs because of right ventricular distention and papillary muscle dysfunction resulting in poor tricuspid coaptation. Once the pulmonary artery band is placed a dramatic shift of the interventricular septum occurs towards the right ventricle resulting in better papillary function, improved tricuspid valve coaptation, and decreased tricuspid insufficiency. This change can be appreciated by transesophageal echocardiography in the operating room. The patients usually require pressor agents for a few days and controlled ventilation. (With permission: Mavroudis 2015). *LV* left ventricle, *RV* right ventricle

presence of biventricular failure can result in cardiac decompensation, ventricular assist, and possible death. Authors have shown that in adult patients selected to undergo a 2-stage arterial switch procedure after a failed atrial baffle operation, acute pulmonary artery banding to achieve near-systemic subpulmonary left ventricular pressure leads rapidly to ventricular failure and failure of this treatment strategy. They recommended that a more gradual and staged approach to pulmonary artery banding may be required to achieve a successful outcome (Benzaquen et al. 2004) Fortunately, as discussed earlier, the transition to arterial switch has resulted in the rare application of this operative scheme. Nevertheless, it is useful to review the operative techniques and complications associated with this operative technique.

Figures 54, 55, 56 and 57 show the methods of Senning and Mustard operation takedown as well as application of a right-sided maze procedure for those frequent patients who have troubling atrial arrhythmias (Mavroudis et al. 2015). Complications associated with these maneuvers include unwanted transatrial epicardial excursion which if not recognized can cause pesky postoperative bleeding which will usually lead to a return to cardiopulmonary bypass, cardioplegic arrest and intra-atrial control of bleeding. Careful attention to the baffle incision line and intra-atrial repair as necessary will avoid these complications. The lines of ablation that will likely be necessary for atrial reentry tachycardia will require careful placement to avoid complete heart block. These principles are carefully reviewed in chapter "Complications Associated with Mechanical Circulatory Support for Pediatric and Congenital Heart Surgery". The atria are generally separated by a polytetrafluoroethylene (PTFE) or tissue patch since the autologous pericardium is generally not available for use. The complications of atrial septation are reviewed in chapter "Complications Associated with Atrial Septal

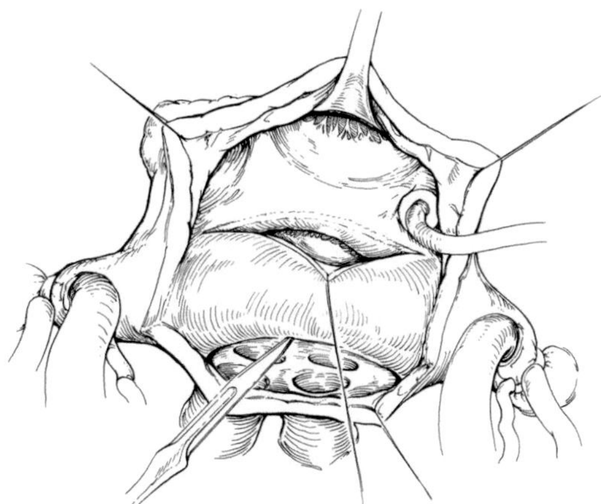

Fig. 54 Once left ventricular training is adequate as noted by echocardiographic evidence of left ventricular free wall dimensions and cardiac catheterization, the patient can undergo atrial baffle takedown and arterial switch. The figure shows the result of aortobicaval cardiopulmonary bypass, aortic cross-clamping, and cardioplegic arrest. Note the retrograde catheter for cardioplegic administration. This particular exposure shows the takedown of a Senning operation by careful entry into the previously constructed baffle. (With permission: Mavroudis 2015)

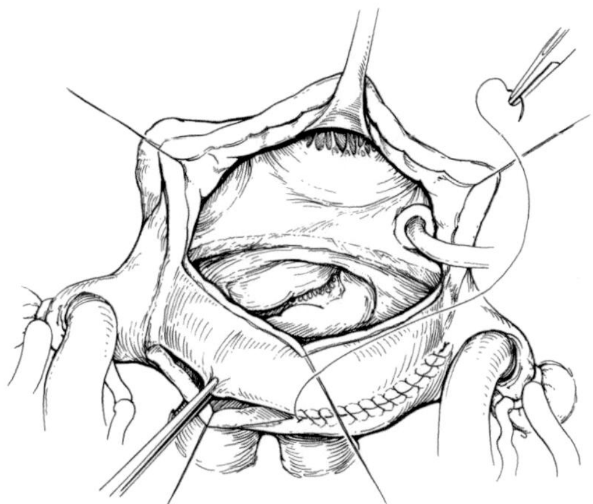

Fig. 55 shows mobilization of the previously constructed baffle and the posterior portion being reattached to the atrial wall. Dissection and mobilization of the baffle requires careful attention to depth of incisions to avoid unwanted incisions to the epicardial surface. (With permission: Mavroudis 2015)

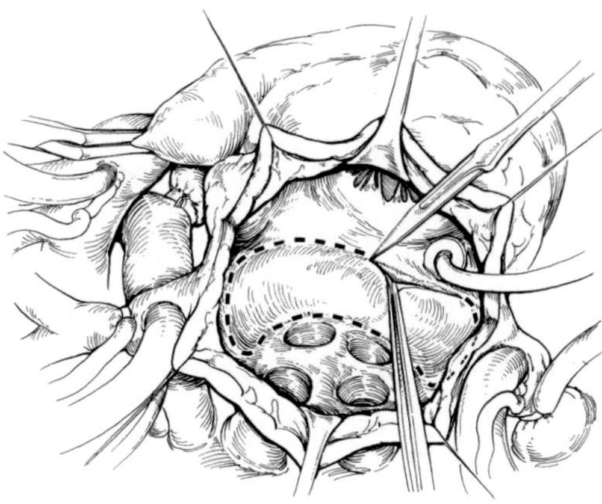

Fig. 56 In the case of a previously constructed Mustard operation, the approach is very similar to mobilization of the previously performed Senning operation except that the baffle need not be preserved. The figure shows the pericardial baffle in place with the dotted lines indicating the area where the baffle can be resected. (With permission: Mavroudis 2015)

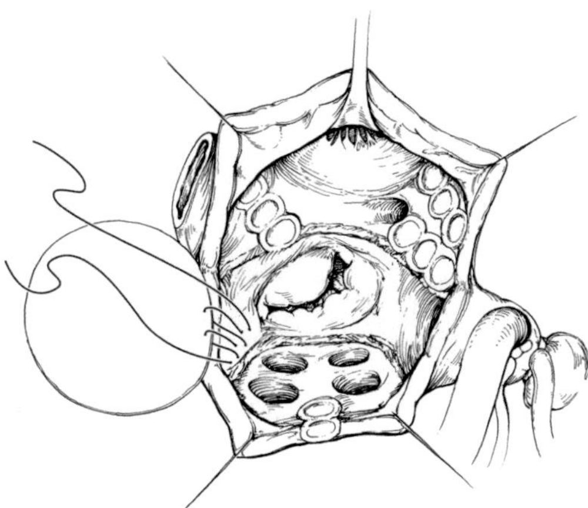

Fig. 57 Once the baffle is either reattached to the atrial wall or resected, cryoablation lesions can be placed if the patient has atrial reentry tachycardia which is prevalent in this patient population. The figure shows the completed cryoablation lesions in the right atrium which constitute a right atrial maze procedure as a therapeutic procedure for atrial reentry tachycardia. Prophylactic lesions can also be placed, but the lesion set that is recommended is the cavotricuspid isthmus instead of the comprehensive right sided maze that is noted in the fig. A large piece of PTFE or biologic material can be used to reconstruct the atrial septum with special care to avoid injury to the atrioventricular node. (With permission: Mavroudis 2015)

Defect, Partial Anomalous Pulmonary Venous Return, and Scimitar Syndrome Repairs". Careful attention to suture placement and inflow separation of systemic and pulmonary veins will ensure proper anatomic and physiologic alignment. No one wants to inadvertently tunnel the inferior vena cava flow to the left atrium. The neo-atrial septation is performed before the ASO to avoid suture line disruption which may occur during the atrial procedure due to retraction. The arterial switch operation can be performed taking care to avoid the associated complications as noted in Figs. 1, 2, 3, 4, 5, 6, 7, 8, 9, 10, 11, 12, 13, 14, 15, 16, 17, 18, 19, 20, 21, 22, 23, 24, 25, 26, 27, 28, 29, 30, 31, 32, 33 and 34. The reader will take note that the proximal neoaortic reconstruction in Fig. 58 shows Dacron patch supravalvar valve sparing neoaortic reconstruction with the coronary artery buttons anastomosed to the Dacron patch. In some cases, the pulmonary artery band, that was used for left ventricular training, can

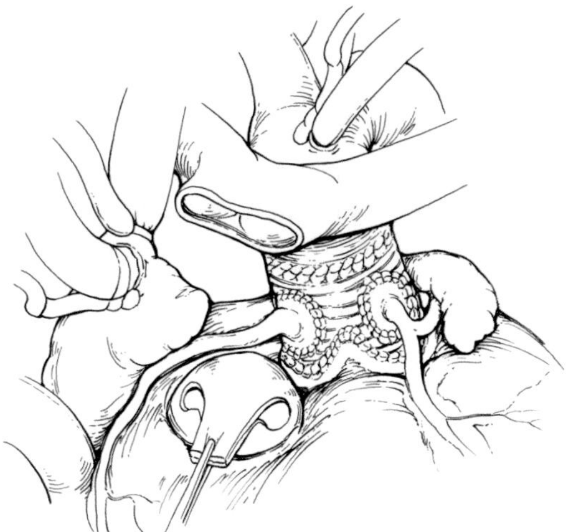

Fig. 58 demonstrates how a straightforward arterial switch can be performed after the atrial baffle reconstruction is performed. The figure shows the neoaortic reconstruction completed using a Dacron tube reconstruction to ensure neoaortic valve competence which can occur after long term pulmonary artery banding. The neopulmonary artery reconstruction is being prepared for completion. (With permission: Mavroudis 2015)

cause proximal wall distention and distal fibrosis. Using this distended and fibrous tissue for the neoaortic reconstruction may prove to be problematic for anastomotic hemostasis and neoaortic valve regurgitation. Better to take the time to perform a valve sparing patch augmentation to ensure proper coronary artery alignment and neoaortic function.

9 Complications of the Arterial Switch Operation

9.1 Supravalvar Neopulmonary Artery Stenosis

Like the introduction of many avante garde operations, the arterial switch operation experience resulted in complications that became evident and required reparative operations. The intraoperative coronary and neopulmonary artery complications are considered earlier in this chapter. However, the most common long-term complication of the arterial switch operation turned out to be supravalvar neopulmonary artery stenosis (Nellis et al. 2016). This complication is less frequent nowadays due to the extended pantaloon pericardial patch. Nevertheless, supravalvar neopulmonary artery stenosis can occur and is worth discussing. Figure 59 shows the supravalvar pulmonary artery stenosis likely caused by small pericardial patches that were placed at the original operation. The dotted lines depict the lines of incision that will be necessary to augment the sinuses of Valsalva. Figures 60 and 61 show the progression of supravalvar repair by fibrous resection and comprehensive pulmonary artery sinuses of Valsalva patch augmentation. Complications associated with these maneuvers involve unwanted neopulmonary valve injury during incision into the sinuses of Valsalva and unwanted suture entrapment during patch augmentation. In the event of pulmonary leaflet injury, the alert surgeon will recognize the injury and use interrupted fine sutures with or without a tissue patch to repair the damage. Unfortunately, suture entrapment of the neopulmonary valve leaflet may not be discovered until separation from cardiopulmonary bypass and intraoperative transesophageal echocardiogram (TEE) interrogation. If there is any question of valve dysfunction due to this mishap, reinstitution of cardiopulmonary bypass, anastomotic takedown, and valve assessment should be made.

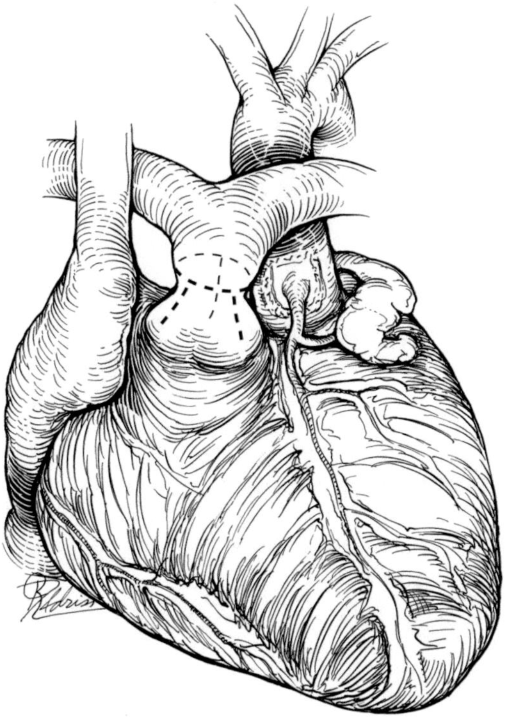

Fig. 59 Early on in the experience of the arterial switch operation, the most common long-term complication was supravalvar neopulmonary artery stenosis. While this complication has been less frequent owing to the extended pantaloon pericardial patch, supravalvar neopulmonary artery stenosis can occur. The figure shows the artist's preoperative depiction of supravalvar neopulmonary artery stenosis with the proposed incisions (dotted lines) into the three sinuses of Valsalva and the projected resection of the localized stenotic segment above the valve leaflets. (With permission: Mavroudis 2015)

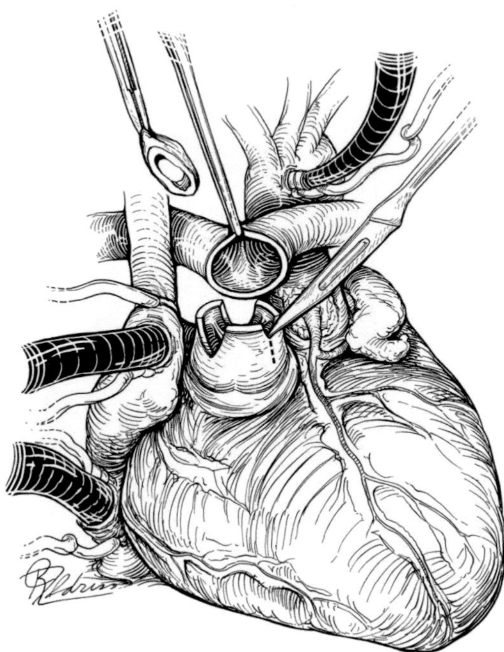

Fig. 60 illustrates the establishment of aortobicaval cardiopulmonary bypass with transection/excision of the supravalvar stenotic segment and linear incisions into the three sinuses of Valsalva for the purpose of sinus augmentation. (With permission: Mavroudis 2015)

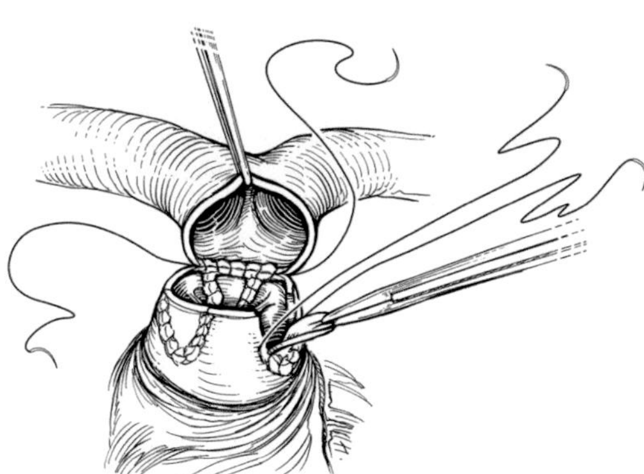

Fig. 61 shows the completed biological patch augmentation of the three sinuses of Valsalva of the neopulmonary artery and the initiation of the end-to-end anastomosis between the neopulmonary artery and the distal pulmonary artery. These maneuvers have been durable and long lasting, with the hope that no further intervention would be necessary. (With permission: Mavroudis 2015)

10 Valve Sparing Procedure for Neoaortic Regurgitation

TGA patients most likely to develop neoaortic regurgitation after the ASO are those with (1) associated VSD and proximal neoaorta and distal aorta anatomic mismatch, (2) complex coronary artery transfer techniques which resulted in extensive reconstructive augmentation patch material and asymmetric commissural dilatation, and (3) prior pulmonary artery banding (Mavroudis et al. 2011; Co-Vu et al. 2013; Ma et al. 2016). Frequently, the regurgitant neoaortic valve can be repaired by a valve sparing operation as described by Tirone David (2012) and noted in Figs. 62, 63, 64, 65, 66, 67, 68 and 69. This operation will avoid prosthetic valve replacement and the associated problems of systemic anticoagulation. There are however complications associated with this complex operation that should be noted.

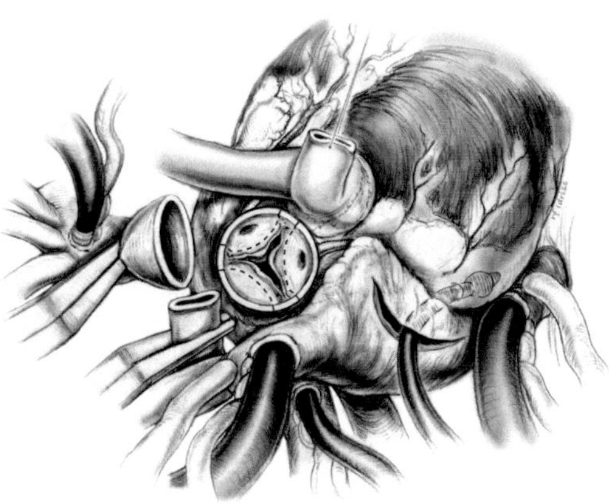

Fig. 62 shows optimized neoaortic root exposure after aortobicaval cardiopulmonary bypass, aortic cross-clamp, antegrade and retrograde blood cardioplegia, and right pulmonary artery transection. The right pulmonary artery transection is performed to visualize more clearly the origin of the transferred coronary artery buttons. The dotted lines represent incisions in the sinus of Valsalva neoaortic wall that facilitate coronary artery button dissection and mobilization. (With permission: Mavroudis 2015)

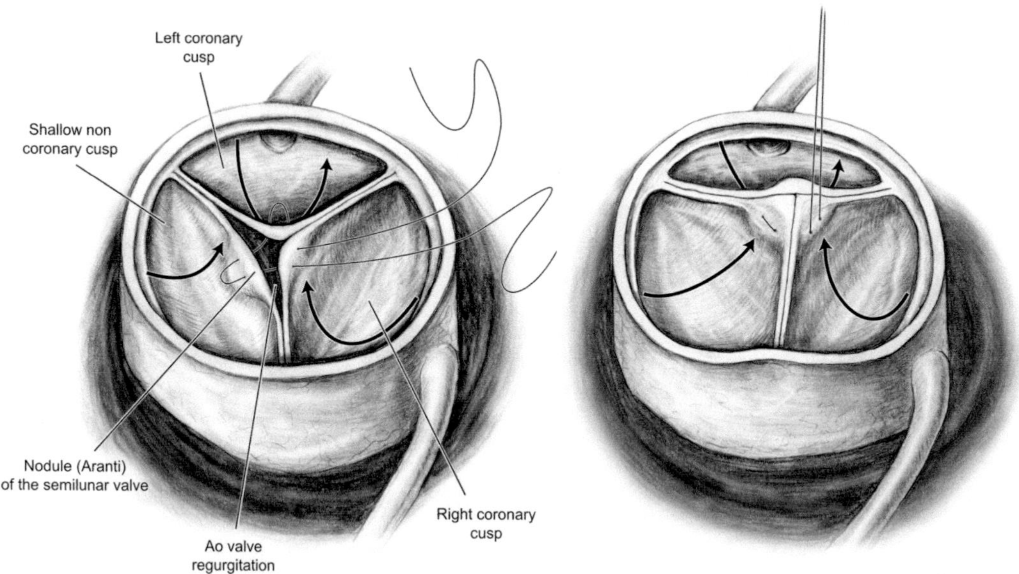

Fig. 63 Figure shows assessment of the neoaortic valve for preoperative evaluation to achieve postoperative competency. The method of evaluating cusp depth and therefore potential competence is to apply temporary sutures at the nodules of Arantius and offer a slight tug superiorly to guage the depth of the coronary cusps. The idea is to identify a superficial cusp that could be amenable to commissure valvuloplasty and or patch augmentation. The left panel shows the temporary placement of a fine suture to approximate the nodules of Arantius. The curved arrows are more acute and circular to indicate deeper cusps in the left and right coronary sinuses of Valsalva. The right panel shows that the right and left coronary cusps are deeper than the noncoronary cusp as shown by the acute curvilinear lines as apposed to the flatter curve as shown in the noncoronary cusp. The corrective maneuvers for this type of valve are explained in the narrative. *Ao* aorta

Fig. 64 depicts pledgetted sutures being placed at the neoaortic annulus midway between the commissures and anchored in the Dacron graft which allows fixation over the neoaorta. The coronary buttons are preserved and evaluated for transfer to the Dacron graft. Further mobilization may be necessary for the eventual implantation. (With permission: Mavroudis 2015)

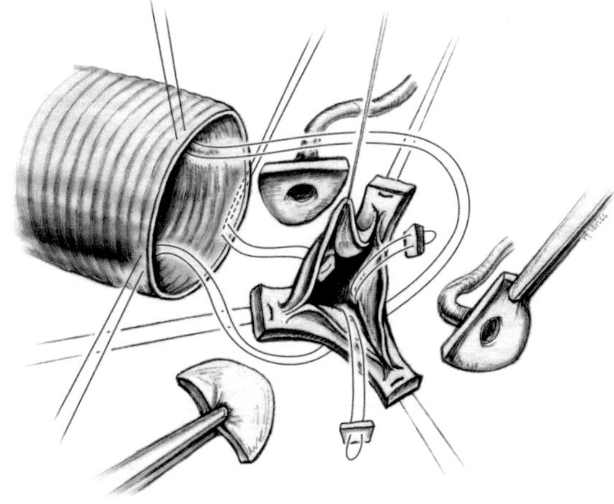

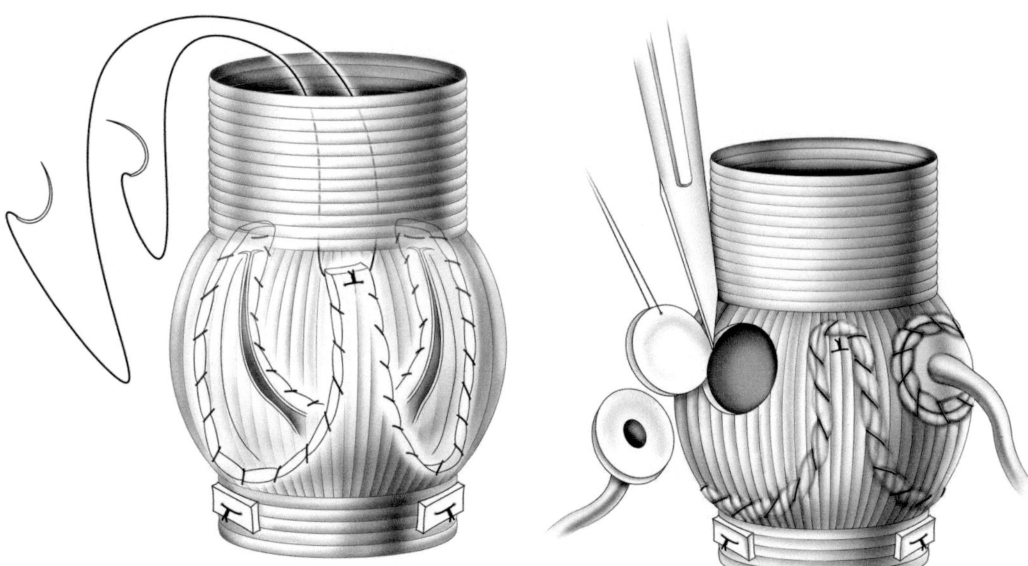

Fig. 65 The affixed Dacron graft is shown with the act of suturing the dissected and tapered neoaortic wall to the inner portion of the graft. These suture lines attach the walls of the neoaorta to the graft and solidify the reconstruction. This part of the operation depends on estimating the appropriate height of the commissures for attachment to the graft. Failure to perform this maneuver correctly will result in unwanted neoaortic regurgitation. (With permission: Mavroudis 2015)

Fig. 66 shows the creation of an orifice to accept the coronary button on one side and the completed coronary-to-graft anastomosis on the other side. It remains then for the proximal neoaorta-to-ascending aorta anastomosis to be completed. Deairing procedures and cross-clamp removal complete the process. (With permission: Mavroudis 2015)

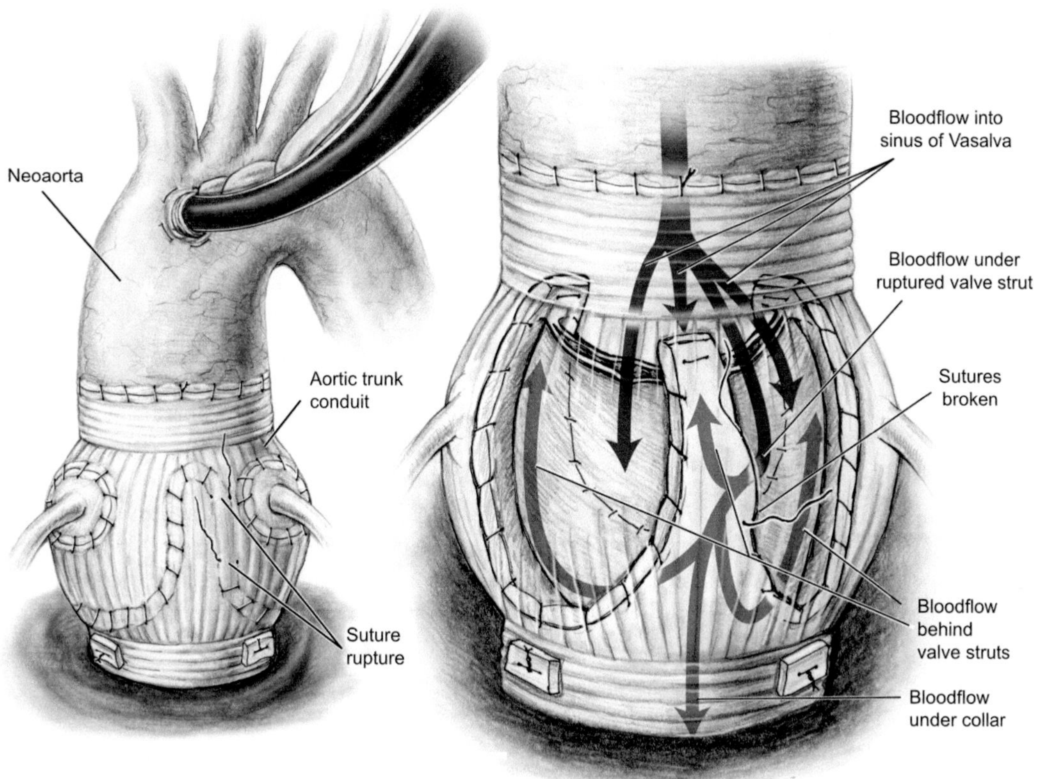

Fig. 67 Left panel shows internal suture disruption of the attached scalloped neoarotic valve to the surrounding aortic graft. This situation allows diastolic flow to enter the area between the attached valve and the graft which can enlarge and cause significant neoaortic regurgitation. The right panel demonsgtrates by arrows the flow patterns that can result from suture disruption. After separation from cardiopulmonary bypass, intraoperative transesophageal echocardiography will be able to identify this ptentially devestating complication and signal a return to cardiopulmonary bypass, cardioplegic arrest and re-repair

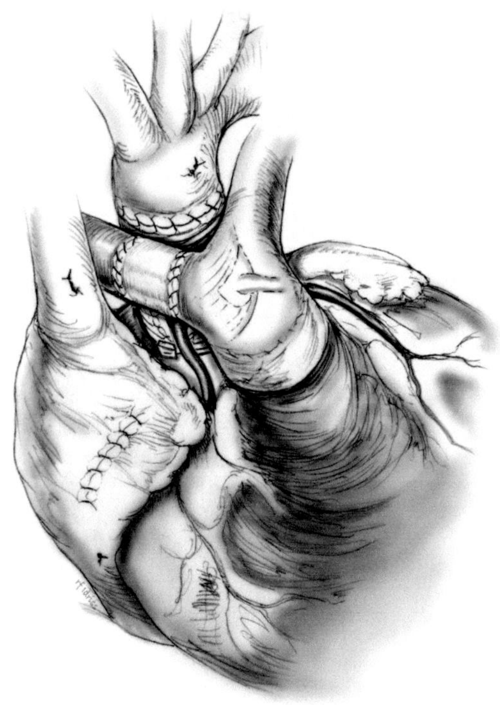

Fig. 68 shows the completed repair with a PTFE interposition graft for the right pulmonary artery reconstruction. A direct anastomosis may cause unwanted tension on the coronary anastomoses. The right pulmonary artery extension allows for appropriate reinstitution of unobstructed right pulmonary artery flow without the possibility of coronary artery compression. (With permission: Mavroudis 2015)

The first dilemma regarding the execution of this valve sparing operation is the preoperative and intraoperative assessment of the neoaortic valve regurgitation and the probability that a valve sparing operation can be performed with an acceptable outcome. TEE can determine the amount of individual leaflet prolapse, leaflet retraction, and leaflet perforation (Meyerowitz et al. 1993). Suture approximation of the noduli of Arantii as noted in Fig. 63 will help to evaluate the valve by annular assessment, sinus cupping depth, and leaflet apposition (Svensson 2021). A recent publication by Lars Svensson has provided guidelines for assessment and repair of regurgitant aortic valves (Tables 1 and 2 (Svensson 2021). Clearly, neoaortic valve assessment and possible repair is the mainstay for a valve sparing operation. Performing this complex valve sparing operation with an intraoperative failure will only result in operative conversion to a Bentall opera-

Table 1 CLASS schema

C	Commissures
L	Leaflets
A	Annulus
S	Sinuses
S	Sinotubular junction

With permission: Svensson (2021)

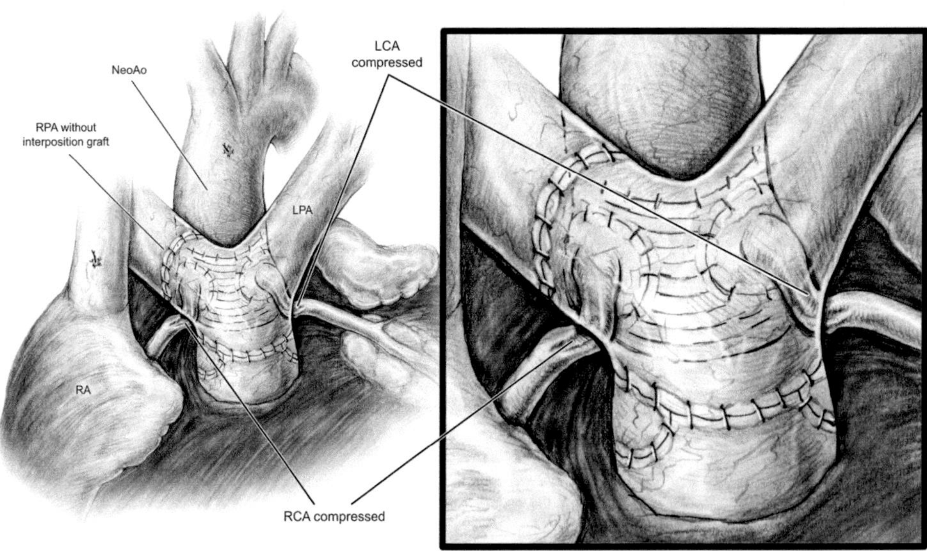

Fig. 69 shows the coronary artery compression when the right pulmonary artery inerposition graft is not used. By necessity, transection and reanastomosis will cause a shortened reconstruction which can have an unwanted compression of the translocated coronary arteries in association with arterial switch. *Ao* aorta, *LCA* left coronary artery, *LPA* left pulmonary artery, *RA* right atrium, *RCA* right coronary artery, *RPA* right pulmonary artery

Table 2 Assessment of the valve unit

	Assessment	Possible solutions
Commissures	Height, orientation, apposition, tears, fusion	Figure-of-8[a], Cabrol stitch[b], tissue excision[c]
Leaflets	Tears, perforations, prolapse, incomplete fusion, thickness, edge, noduli of Arantii, cupping depth	Repairs, Trussler stitch, running edge[d], suture plication, shaving
Annulus	Size (eg, CT area, diameter, radius, concentricity); subannular stenosis/LVOT obstruction	Annular reduction with a Hegar dilator, bracing, myectomy, rarely annular enlargement for repair
Sinuses	Both native and artificial with reimplantation or remodeling	Division of raphe[e], rarely patch, create new sinuses with reimplantation
Sinotubular junction	Splayed or narrow? Will figure-of-8 stitch be accommodated?	Narrow with reimplantation, splay with bicuspid remodeling, tailor or smaller for tricuspid valve repairs

With permission: Svensson (2021)

CT Computed tomography, *LVOT* left ventricular outflow tract

[a]Used most commonly for repairs

[b]For a large annulus, either bicuspid- or trileaflet-associated valve, and no reimplantation

[c]For an ideal unicuspid valve that can be turned into a bicuspid valve

[d]This can be used to try to reduce late prolapse in the thicker bicuspid valve leaflets, in combination with tying the suture around a Hegar dilator

[e]This should be a deep cut to free up the body of the conjoint leaflet

tion (prosthetic valve root replacement) with significant extension of the cross-clamp time and possible ischemic ventricular dysfunction.

The second dilemma regarding this valve sparing operation involves proper seating of the tube graft over the scalloped neoaortic valve as noted in Fig. 64 (Aalaei-Andabili et al. 2019) The pledgetted anchoring sutures need to be placed in the annulus at the nadir of each sinus. Failure to perform this part of the operation will result in poor seating and annular disruption leading to neoaortic regurgitation and coronary kinking. Once the graft is seated appropriately, reattachment of the commissures to the graft and suture attachment of the scalloped valve edges are performed as noted in Fig. 65. It remains for the coronary artery buttons to be attached to the proximal valve sparing reconstruction as shown in Fig. 66. Complications associated with this part of the operation involve bleeding at the anastomotic sites such as the coronary button attachments, which is generally amenable to suture repair, and internal dissection between the attached scallops of the neoaorta and the enveloping graft as shown in Fig. 67. In general, this situation can be identified by TEE. This should signal a return to cardiopulmonary bypass, aortic cross-clamping, and cardioplegic arrest to take down the neoaortic anastomosis and repair the problem.

The third dilemma regarding this valve sparing operation involves the neopulmonary reconstruction. Figure 68 correctly shows the right pulmonary artery interposition graft in place to avoid pulmonary artery stenosis and compression of the involved coronary arteries which are originating from the neoaorta. Figure 69 demonstrates what could happen if the right pulmonary artery interposition graft is not used. Notice the distortion of the right pulmonary artery and the compression of the neopulmonary artery on the right and left coronary arteries. Such a situation can be rectified by placement of the right pulmonary artery interposition graft as nicely shown in Fig. 68.

11 Bentall Procedure for Neoaortic Regurgitation

In those cases where the neoaortic valve cannot be repaired owing to leaflet foreshortening, prolapse, and annular dilatation, a Bentall procedure requires consideration. Most surgeons prefer to implant a prosthetic valve conduit for this reconstruction which requires lifelong coagulation (Mookhoek et al. 2016). Some patients, however, would prefer a lifestyle without systemic anticoagulation. Under these circumstances, a biologic prosthetic valve can be placed within a prosthetic graft to construct a bioprosthetic valve conduit. Both prosthetic and biologic graft implantation techniques are similar and are subject to the same complications of residual bleeding and coronary artery button distortion. Figures 70, 71 and 72 show a prosthetic valve conduit being placed with coronary artery reimplantation and right pulmonary artery interposition graft which prevents pulmonary artery distortion and coronary artery compression as noted in Figs. 68 and 69. Intraoperative TEE will help to determine any prosthetic or biologic valve dysfunction and possible return to cardiopulmonary bypass for repair.

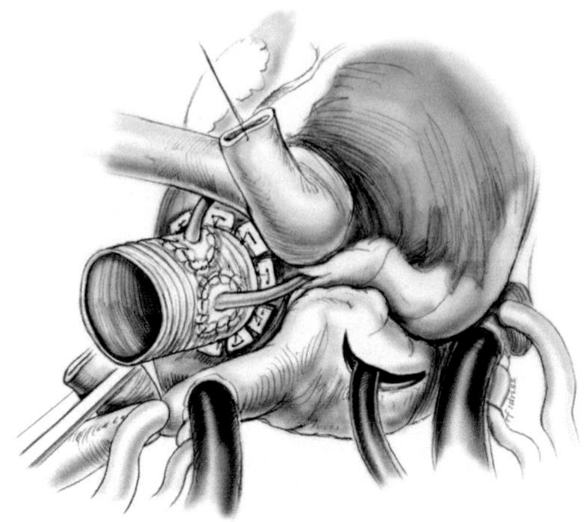

Fig. 71 shows prosthetic valve conduit implanted with reanastomosis of the coronary buttons to the graft. (With permission: Mavroudis 2015)

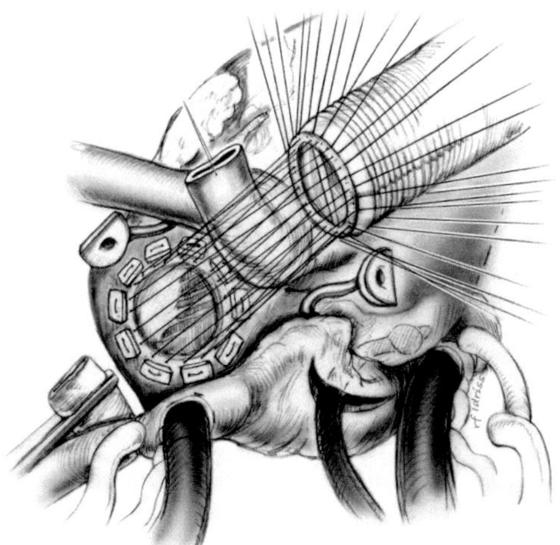

Fig. 70 shows neoaortic root exposure after aortobicaval cardiopulmonary bypass with antegrade/retrograde cardioplegia, and neoaortic as well as right pulmonary artery transection. Pledgetted sutures are anchored at the neoaortic annulus and sutured to the sewing ring of the prosthetic valve conduit. (With permission: Mavroudis 2015)

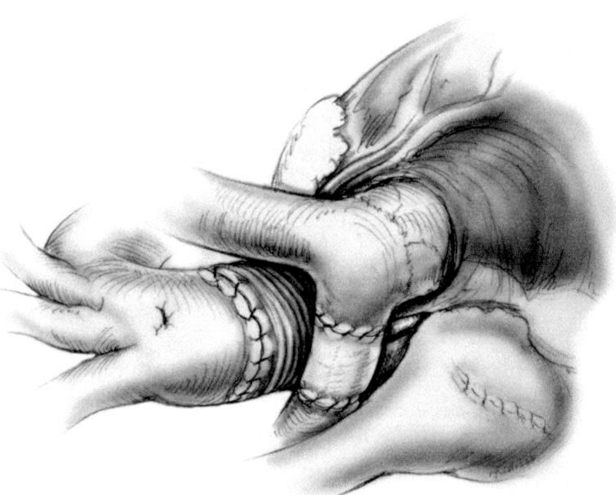

Fig. 72 depicts the completed reconstruction with a PTFE interposition graft to augment the course of the right pulmonary artery and prevent coronary artery compression. (With permission: Mavroudis 2015)

12 Coronary Artery Revascularization Late After the Arterial Switch Operation

12.1 Internal Thoracic Artery to Coronary Artery Bypass

Late coronary artery stenosis after the arterial switch operation has been reported (Mavroudis et al. 1999) which is generally caused by technical complications occurring at the original operation. Oftentimes, the technical mishaps are well tolerated for many months and years, and become manifest owing to somatic growth, increased myocardial oxygen demand, and chronic fibrous orifice encroachment. Anatomic reasons for these physiologic developments include: malrotation of the coronary button, coronary stretching, aneurysmal formation, and transfer of an intramural coronary artery that was not unroofed (Mavroudis and Backer 2023; Mavroudis et al. 2011). The therapeutic options for resolution of the problems are proximal coronary button patch arterioplasty, coronary bypass, or both as well as unroofing of an untreated intramural artery. The anatomic details and chances of success will dictate which procedures to apply (Mavroudis and Backer 2023; Mavroudis et al. 2011).

In particular, there has been some controversy about whether to address proximal coronary stenosis by patch arterioplasty or coronary bypass or both. Authors have extolled the notion that malrotation of the coronary button without anatomic coronary artery distortion can be repaired with takedown of the coronary button and repair with appropriate rotational repair coupled with patch aortoplasty (Mavroudis and Backer 2023; Mavroudis et al. 2011). Some have advocated simultaneous coronary bypass to ensure myocardial perfusion if the proximal coronary button repair fails over time (Mavroudis and Backer 2023; Mavroudis et al. 2011). When the coronary obstruction pattern extends into the anatomic coronary artery distal to the button implantation, proximal exploration is not recommended, the preference being coronary bypass using the internal thoracic artery (Mavroudis 2017) as noted in Fig. 73.

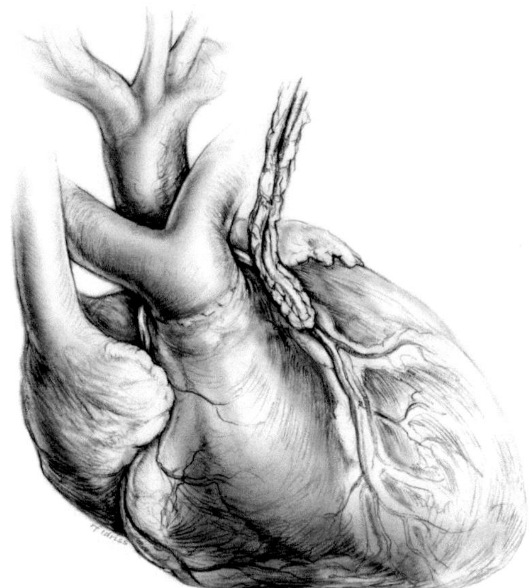

Fig. 73 shows an internal thoracic artery to left anterior coronary artery bypass graft in a patient who had a remote arterial switch operation complicated by proximal left main coronary artery occlusion that was tolerated after the initial operation owing to abundant collaterals from the right coronary artery. No effort was made to perform a left main coronary artery arterioplasty due to the fibrous tissue at the original anastomosis. In other cases, proximal left main coronary artery arterioplasty can be coupled with coronary bypass to ensure patency of coronary flow, the idea being that if one of the reconstructions does not work, the other will. This is a pants and suspenders solution to a difficult problem. Not all surgeons agree with this approach concentrating their efforts on one or the other reconstructive solutions. (With permission: Mavroudis 2015)

12.2 Coronary Unroofing for Unrecognized Intramural Coronary

In some cases, a coronary artery button with an intramural coronary artery can be transferred to the neoaorta without associated unroofing. It is understandable that a surgeon may not want to unroof this segment because of intraoperative assessment that the course of the coronary artery will not cause future problems. In addition, the arterial switch operation is complicated enough. Any further surgical maneuvers, especially with coronary artery manipulations, might be deemed unnecessary and possibly cause irreparable damage to the coronary artery. Nevertheless, coronary problems due to unroofing a coronary artery in association with the arterial switch can be problematic and life threatening (Mavroudis and Backer 2023). Such a case has been described years after the arterial switch operation in which the intramural coronary artery was not unroofed resulting in myocardial ischemia, hypotension, institution of ECMO, lower extremity amputation, and eventual coronary unroofing with an excellent result (Mavroudis and Backer 2023; Mavroudis 2017). Figures 74, 75, 76 and 77 show the course of coronary unroofing in a patient who had transposition repair without unroofing the left coronary artery. The principles of the operation are appropriate cardiopulmonary bypass, antegrade and retrograde cardioplegic arrest, and proper neoaortic exposure for the coronary artery unroofing technique that is used for patients with anomalous aortic origin of the coronary arteries (Chapter "Complications Associated with Repair of Congenital and Acquired Coronary Artery Anomalies"). The figure legends describe with some accuracy the steps of the operation and basically how to avoid complications. And as described in earlier redo operations for neoaortic exposure, the right pulmonary artery is reconstructed using an interposition graft to avoid pulmonary artery stenosis and coronary artery compression.

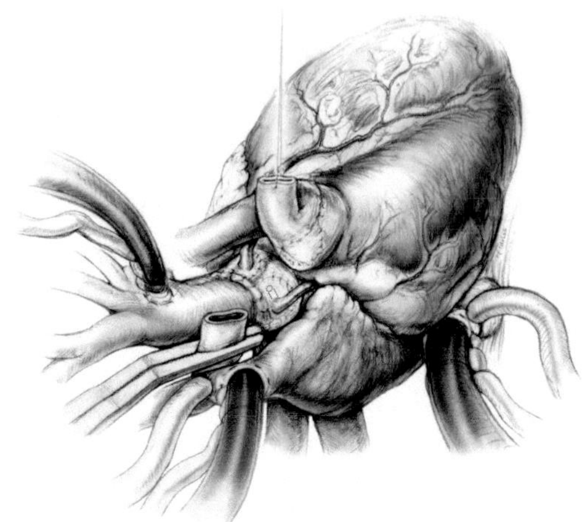

Fig. 74 Rarely, intramural coronary artery buttons can be transferred to the neoaorta without coronary artery unroofing. While flow can be established in this manner, the patient is at risk for a coronary artery event owing to the slit-like orifice associated with intramural coronary arteries. One such patient had an intramural right coronary transferred to the neoaorta without unroofing. Nineteen years later he suffered a myocardial infarction, cardiac arrest, and was placed on extracorporeal membrane oxygenation. After the anatomy was confirmed, he underwent an unroofing procedure. The figure shows aortobicaval cardiopulmonary bypass, aortic cross-clamping, and antegrade/retrograde cardioplegic arrest with right pulmonary artery transection for neoaortic root exposure. (With permission: Mavroudis 2015)

12.3 Bronchial Compression After the Arterial Switch Operation

Obstruction and compression of the tracheobronchial tree is well described mostly by innominate artery compression and vascular rings (Backer et al. 1989b; Berlinger et al. 1983). Tracheobronchial compression after the arterial switch operation is rare (Worsey et al. 1994; Toker et al. 2000). Worsey, del Nido and associates described a case of left main bronchial obstruction after the arterial switch (Worsey et al. 1994). The stridor in their patient was noted at 3 months of age and was followed until the patient reached 16 months of age which resulted in diagnostic bronchoscopy as noted in Fig. 78 (Worsey et al. 1994) and MRI (Fig. 79) (Worsey et al. 1994). Their reparative operative procedure involved aortic suspension as noted herein.

> The aorta was approached by excision of the cartilaginous section of the second rib up to the costochondral joint on the left. The ascending aorta was

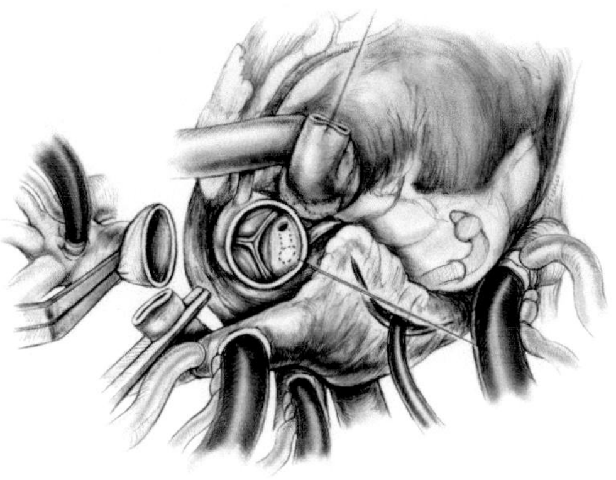

Fig. 75 shows neoaortic transection and exposure of the transferred intramural coronary artery by the dotted lines. It is important to achieve a bloodless field by a left ventricular vent and transection of the neoaorta which enhances the exposure by allowing the proximal neoaorta to be raised into the field of vision for a more accurate unroofing procedure. (With permission: Mavroudis 2015)

suspended up to the undersurface of the sternum, using two mattress sutures placed through the adventitia of the aorta just distal to the left pulmonary artery. The sutures were passed through the sternum and tightened under bronchoscopic guidance until relief of the anterior compression of the left bronchus was observed. After this maneuver, however, bronchoscopy revealed persistent posterior compression (Fig lB), which was attributed to the descending aorta. This was relieved by posterior suspension of the descending aorta to the prevertebral fascia, as confirmed by repeat bronchoscopy (Fig 1C). Postoperatively, all clinical signs of airway obstruction resolved, and repeat magnetic resonance imaging (Fig 3) showed that the aorta no longer compressed the left bronchus, but there was a discrete 50% residual narrowing, probably secondary to chondromalacia. Two years of follow-up has been uneventful. (Worsey et al. 1994).

Fig. 76 shows the unroofing procedure using sharp dissection which is followed by intimal tacking sutures to avoid postoperative dissection. (With permission: Mavroudis 2015)

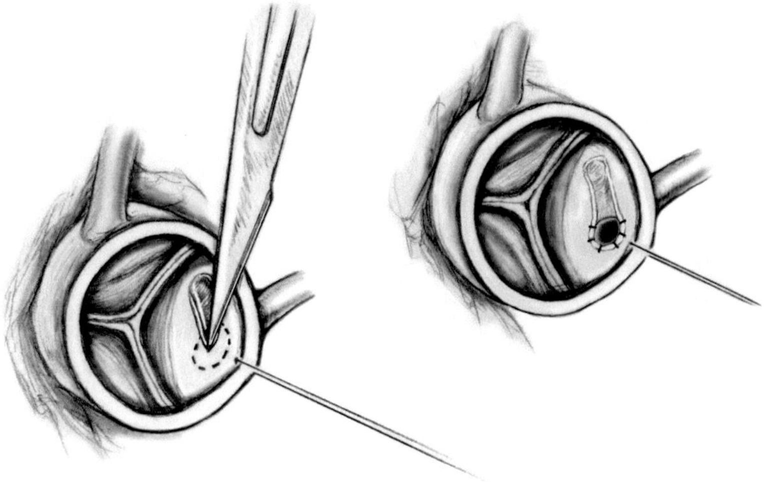

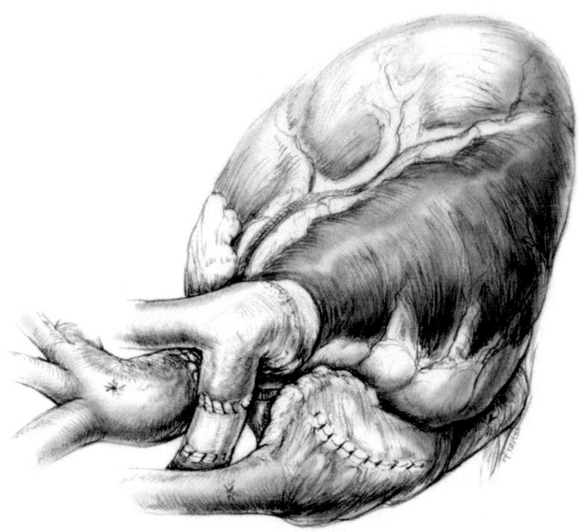

Fig. 77 As in the previous reconstructive techniques this figure shows the right pulmonary artery augmented with an interposition PTFE graft to prevent pulmonary artery stretching and coronary artery compression. (With permission: Mavroudis 2015)

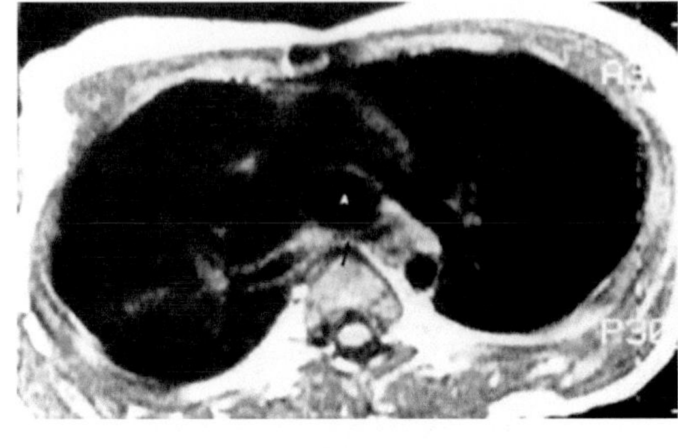

Fig. 79 Preoperative magnetic resonance image showing near-total occlusion of left main bronchus (arrow) by aortic arch. (With permission: Worsey et al. 1994)

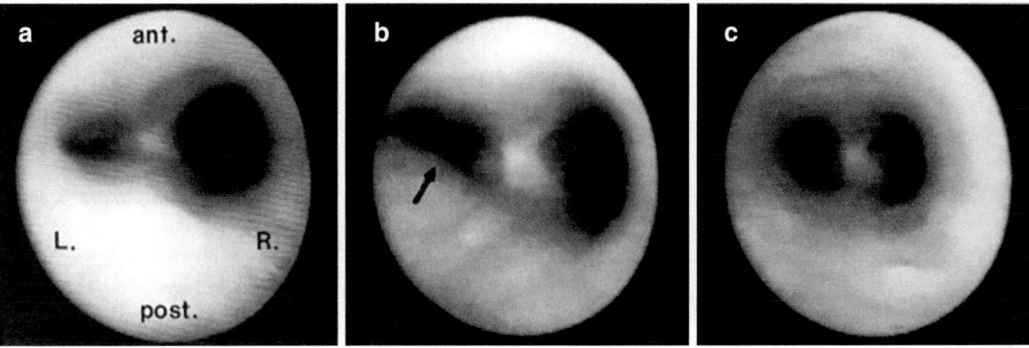

Fig. 78 (a) Bronchoscopy of left main bronchus at 3 months. (b) Intraoperative bronchoscopy after anterior aortic suspension (arrow illustrates posterior compression). (c) Intraoperative bronchoscopy after posterior suspension. (ant. = anterior; L. = left; post. = posterior; R = right.) (With permission: Worsey et al. 1994)

As noted by the authors, repair of tracheobronchial compression after the arterial switch operation requires careful follow-up, comprehensive preoperative evaluation, and creative intraoperative decision making that will arrive at the desired result. There is no 'one size fits all" approach. However, when necessary, surgeons should be aware of tracheobronchial compression and should not hesitate to operate and repair when indicated.

13 Transposition with VSD and Left Ventricular Outflow Tract Obstruction (Pulmonary Stenosis)

13.1 Rastelli Operation

The Rastelli operation was developed on the principle that intraventricular tunneling and extracardiac connections can be used to address biventricular and physiologic repair of complex congenital heart disease (Mavroudis et al. 1992; Marcelletti et al. 1976; Moulton et al. 1981; Toyoda et al. 2017; Barron et al. 2019; Huang et al. 2019). Historically, this operation was first used to repair patients with TGA-VSD-PS because the traditional transannular patch connecting the right ventricle to the pulmonary artery was impossible to perform due to the aortopulmonary anterior-posterior anti-anatomic configuration (Peacock 1866; Shaner 1962; Grant 1962; Bremer 1942; de Vries and Saunders 1962; Van Mierop et al. 1963; Van Mierop and Wiglesworth 1963; Van Praagh and Van Praagh 1966). The concept was therefore that the left ventricle could be tunneled to the anterior aorta and the posterior pulmonary artery with a large interventricular patch. The main pulmonary artery is then transected, the proximal portion oversewn, and right ventricular-to-pulmonary artery continuity could be established by an extracardiac valved conduit. This concept and application were subsequently applied to patients with truncus arteriosus as well as other congenital defects which required right ventricular-to-pulmonary artery extracardiac continuity (see chapter "Complications Associated with Repair of Common Arterial Trunk"). Examples include VSD and pulmonary atresia and tetralogy patients with anomalous course of the left anterior coronary artery among others. The Rastelli operation accordingly became the moniker that was given to any operative solution for complex congenital heart disease that required a right ventricular-to-pulmonary artery conduit.

The Rastelli operation for TGA-VSD-PS is noted in Figs. 80, 81, 82 and 83 with legend descriptions that guide the surgeon towards a successful operation. Probably the most difficult

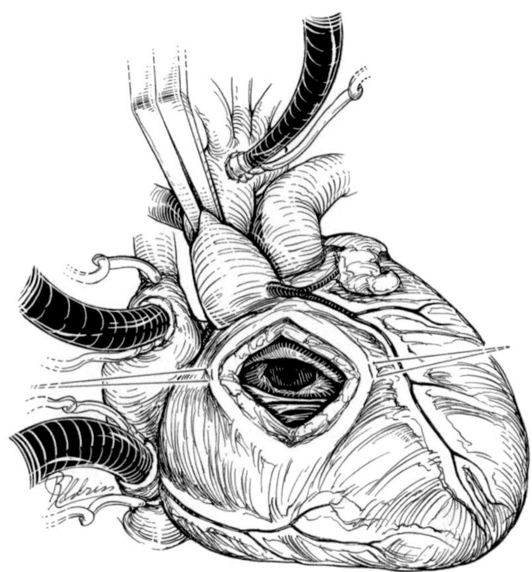

Fig. 80 When the Rastelli operation is applied to transposition of the great arteries-ventricular septal defect-pulmonary stenosis (TGA-VSD-PS), cannulation is performed in the usual manner using aortobicaval cardiopulmonary bypass and left ventricular venting after systemic-to-pulmonary artery shunts are controlled as necessary. The aorta is then clamped, antegrade cardioplegia is administered and a right ventriculotomy is performed away from the course of the left anterior descending coronary artery and the right ventricular branches. Care is taken to avoid injury to the aortic valve which lies anterior and is subject to injury. The best way to avoid this complication is to make the ventriculotomy at the mid-portion of the anterior right ventricular wall for cavitary entry. Scissors dissection and muscular incision with the aortic valve in constant view can help to avoid valvar injury. Some surgeons prefer to place a large dilator through the aorta to better define the pulmonary annulus and guide the infundibular resection. The infundibular muscle is then assessed as noted in the figure which shows the obstructing muscle mass below the aortic valve. (With permission: Mavroudis 2015)

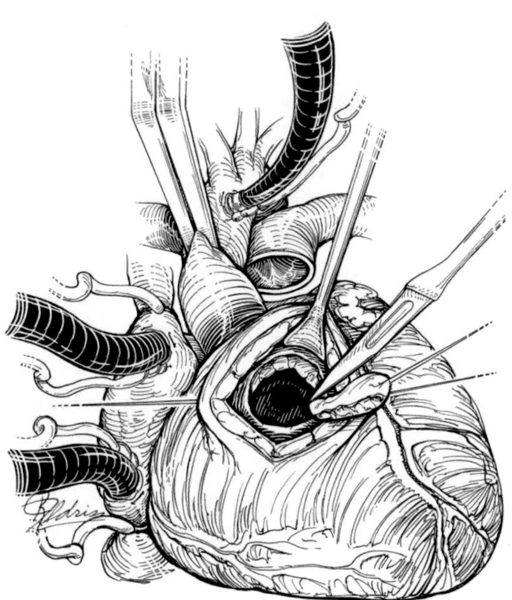

Fig. 81 demonstrates the infindibulum being carefully resected to avoid injury to the aortic valve and to avoid extraventricular excursions (making an unwanted hole) as shown in the figure. Preparations can now be made for ventricular septal defect closure. (With permission: Mavroudis 2015)

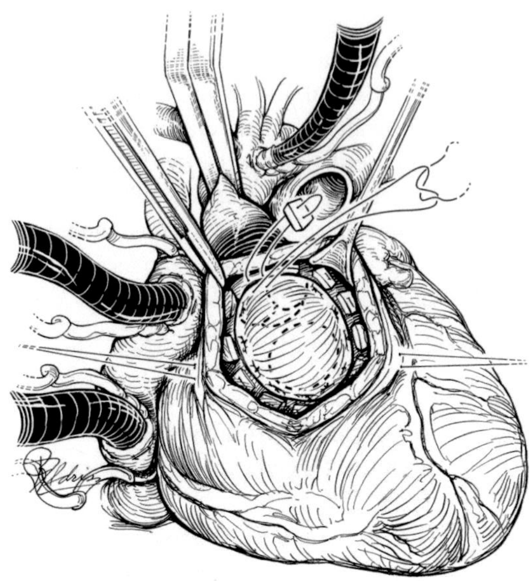

Fig. 82 A large ventricular septal defect patch can then be configured to close the VSD using interrupted pledgetted sutures thereby establishing the tunnel from the left ventricle to the aorta as shown in the figure. While not shown in the drawing, some surgeons, including this author, prefer to selectively transect the aorta and insert a Hagar dilator through the aortic valve into the left ventricle to assure that no stenosis is created by the VSD patch. This maneuver makes some sense since common long-term complications of the Rastelli operation include left ventricular outflow track obstruction and left ventricular hypertrophy. In addion to this maneuver, the surgeon should be mindful that a large patch will be necessary for the left ventricular outflow tract to avoid short-term and long-term stenosis. Sizing and configuring the patch is discussed in chapter "Complications Associated with Repair of Double Outlet Ventricles with Two Adequate Ventricles". (With permission: Mavroudis 2015)

and injury prone part of the operation is the resection of the infundibular septum that is needed to enlarge the left ventricular outflow to the aorta as shown in Fig. 81. The aortic valve is very close to the resection plane and should be respected by slow, accurate, and deliberate incisions. This maneuver is very nicely shown in Fig. 15.1 Chapter "Complications Associated with Repair of Double Outlet Ventricles with Two Adequate Ventricles" which highlights the infundibular resection associated with repair of double outlet right ventricle. Unwanted injury to the aortic valve leaflet will require immediate suture repair or a pericardial patch if the injury is large. The VSD patch placement and configuration is noted in Fig. 82 and highlighted in chapter "Complications Associated with Repair of Double Outlet Ventricles with Two Adequate Ventricles". The idea is to place a large, curved patch to avoid left ventricular outflow tract obstruction. The operation is completed by a right ventricular-to-pulmonary artery conduit as noted in Fig. 83. The particulars of conduit type, size, and potential complications are discussed in chapters "Complications Associated with Repair of Double Outlet Ventricles with Two Adequate Ventricles" and "Complications Associated with Right Ventricular Outflow Tract Reconstruction for Congenital Heart Disease in Children and Adults".

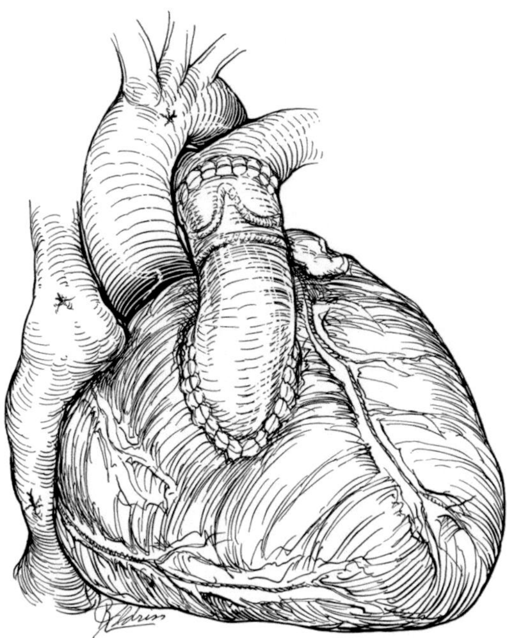

Fig. 83 Once the left ventricular outflow tract is constructed, the cross-clamp can be removed, the patient rewarmed, and right ventricular to pulmonary artery continuity can be established by an extracardiac valved conduit as shown in the figure. (With permission: Mavroudis 2015)

14 Reparation a L'etage Ventriculaire

Yves Lecompte and Pascal Vouhe introduced the operation that is called Reparation a l'Etage Ventriculaire (REV procedure) in 1980 to address the problems of left ventricular outflow tract development and a valveless right ventricular-to-pulmonary artery connection. Their assertion was that this was not a Rastelli procedure without a conduit (Vouhé et al. 1992; Lecompte 1991; Di Carlo et al. 2011). The REV procedure was designed to improve on some of the problems of the Rastelli operation, namely, (1) the development of left ventricular outflow tract obstruction and left ventricular hypertrophy and (2) the quest to extend right ventricular-to-pulmonary artery durability by a valveless reconstruction. In their words,

> The REV procedure allows some of the anatomic contraindications to biventricular repair to be overcome and, much more importantly, to decrease the incidence of the late complications associated with classical repair (i.e., deterioration of LV function) and the development of subaortic stenosis (Lecompte et al. 1993; Prêtre et al. 2001). The final advantage of avoiding the use of a circular conduit for reconstructing the POT is, in our experience, of secondary importance. For this reason, the intracardiac step of the REV procedure will be described in great detail in this article. Although the REV procedure can be indicated in many types of anomalies of ventriculo-arterial connection, the description will be limited to the most frequent anatomy: "classical" transposition of the great arteries, with fibrous continuity between the atrioventricular valves and the pulmonary artery, and a well-developed subaortic infundibulum. (Lecompte and Vouhe 2003)

The conduct of the REV procedure is noted in Figs. 84, 85, 86, 87, 88 and 89 and the respective legend descriptions. Complications associated with the REV operation regarding infundibular resection have been reviewed in the figures in chapter "Complications Associated with Repair of Double Outlet Ventricles with Two Adequate Ventricles" which involve aortic valve injury and repair. The Lecompte maneuver may also be associated with complications owing to ineffective distal pulmonary artery dissection and pulmonary artery draping over the existing aorta as noted in Fig. 3 of this chapter. The problems of residual VSD, heart block, and ventricular dysfunction may be avoided by interrupted and carefully applied pledgetted sutures for the VSD closure, knowledge of the conductions system regarding wayward suture placement, and appropriate cardioplegia administration.

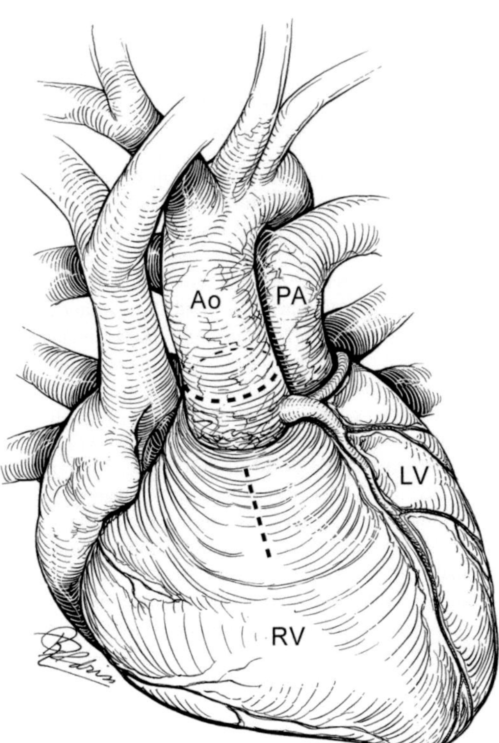

Fig. 84 The reparation a l'etage ventriculaire (REV) is a variation of the Rastelli operation with important modifications. The French moniker was introduced in the initial publication describing this technique and has been universally accepted. Figure 71 shows the anatomic details of TGA-VSD-PS with proposed dotted lines that will eventually result in aortic transection, pulmonary artery transection, right ventriculotomy, extensive infundibular resection, ventricular septal defect closure, Lecompte maneuver. and valveless right ventricular-to-pulmonary artery connection. (With permission: Mavroudis 2015)

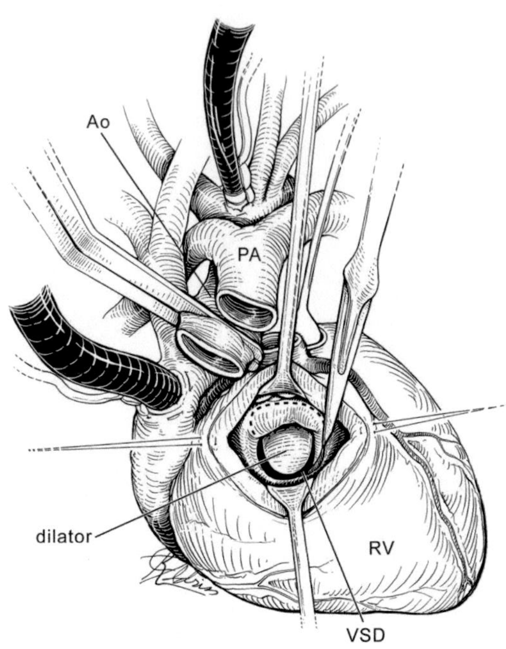

Fig. 85 shows the result of aorto-uniatrial cardiopulmonary bypass with left ventricular venting, antegrade and retrograde administration of cardioplegia (not shown), completed aortic/pulmonary artery transection, Lecompte maneuver, and right ventriculotomy. The line of infundibular resection is noted through the right ventriculotomy. (With permission: Mavroudis 2015). *Ao* aorta, *PA* pulmonary artery, *RV* right ventricle, *VSD* ventricular septal defect

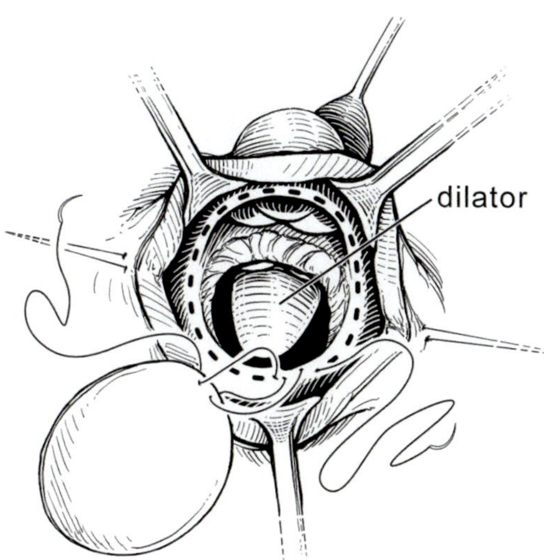

Fig. 86 Once the infundibulectomy is performed as shown in the figure, a Hagar dilator is placed through the pulmonary artery into the left ventricle to assess for the possibility of left ventricular outflow tract obstruction during the ventricular septal defect patch placement. The patch is being placed using running suture technique which some surgeons prefer. The Editors, however, use interrupted pledgetted sutures for such a complex patch to prevent dehiscence. (With permission: Mavroudis 2015)

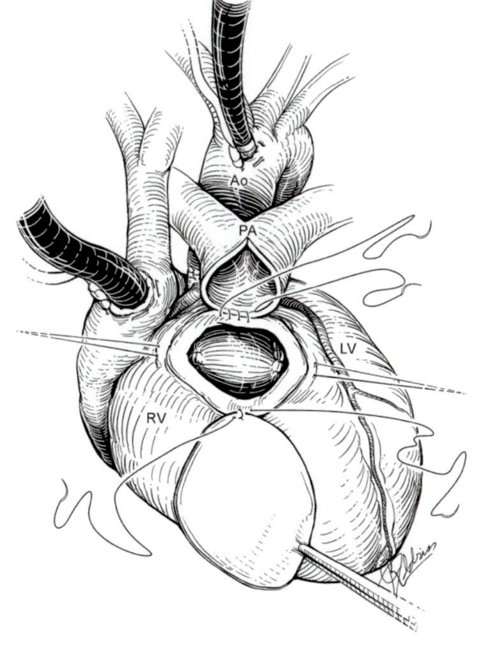

Fig. 88 demonstrates the aortic reanastomosis with the aortic suture line posterior to the neopulmonary artery reconstruction and the untethered main pulmonary artery trunk being connected to the right ventriculotomy. (With permission: Mavroudis 2015)

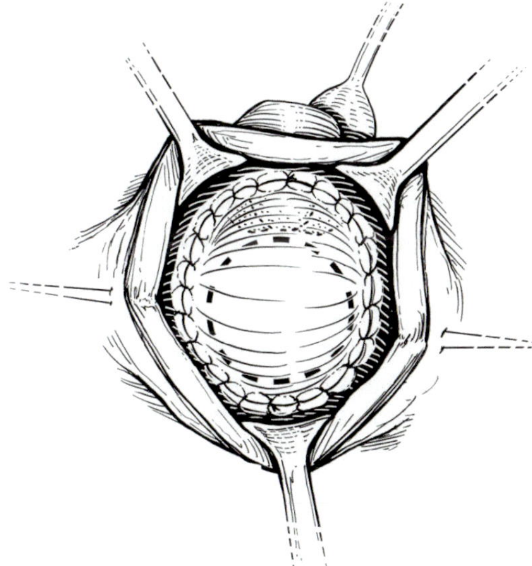

Fig. 87 shows the completed ventricular septal defect patch in place. The aorta can then be reconstructed (not shown). The reparation a l'etage ventriculaire operation includes ascending aorta shortening before reanastomosis by a small circumferential aortic resection. This will allow the pulmonary artery to have a more favorable anatomic configuration after the Lecompte maneuver, which will allow easier connection to the right ventricle. (With permission: Mavroudis 2015)

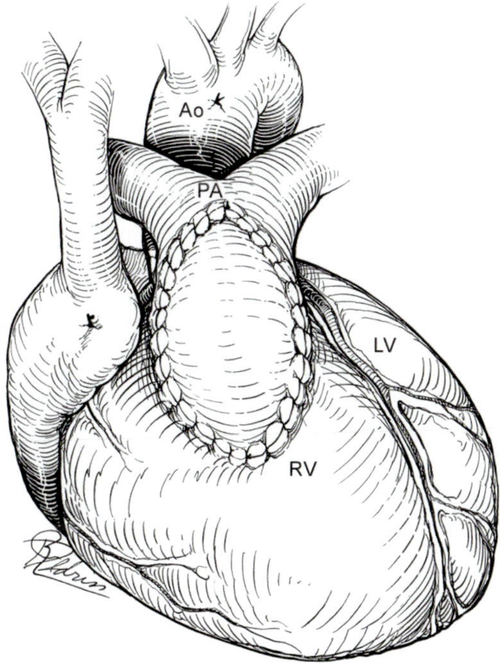

Fig. 89 shows how a patch can be used to complete the anterior valveless reconstruction. (With permission: Mavroudis 2015). *Ao* aorta, *LV* left ventricle, *RV* right ventricle

15 The Nikaidoh Procedure

Like the REV procedure, the Nikaidoh procedure was introduced to create a more direct left ventricle-to-aorta connection thereby limiting the problems of left ventricular outflow tract obstruction and the development of left ventricular hypertrophy (Bautista-Hernandez et al. 2007; Hazekamp et al. 2007; Morell 2013; Morell and Wearden 2007; Nikaidoh 1984; Sayin et al. 2006; Kramer et al. 2014; Raju et al. 2015; Ventosa-Fernández et al. 2017). In addition to repair of TGA-VSD-PS, this technique can be used to repair other congenital heart lesions with similar features of malposed great vessels and pulmonary outflow tract obstruction. The theoretical principles are attractive (Bautista-Hernandez et al. 2007; Hazekamp et al. 2007; Morell 2013; Morell and Wearden 2007; Nikaidoh 1984; Sayin et al. 2006; Kramer et al. 2014; Raju et al. 2015; Ventosa-Fernández et al. 2017), and the clinical results in experienced centers are favorable (Bautista-Hernandez et al. 2007; Hazekamp et al. 2007; Morell 2013; Morell and Wearden 2007; Nikaidoh 1984; Sayin et al. 2006; Kramer et al. 2014; Raju et al. 2015; Ventosa-Fernández et al. 2017). However, the operation is very challenging owing to the process of aortic root translocation, coronary artery relocation, ventricular septation, and pulmonary artery reconstruction. Nevertheless, when performed properly and without complications, the resultant anatomic configuration is favorable and in some surgeons' minds more favorable than the other operations applied to this set of patients (Agarwal and Vaidyanathan 2021). Figures 90, 91, 92, 93, 94, 95 and 96 show the progression of the Nikaidoh procedure. The principles of aortobicaval cardiopulmonary bypass, antegrade/retrograde cardioplegia, coronary artery dissection/mobilization, and management of the enlarged VSD are respected. In general, the Nikaidoh procedure is performed in several steps which include (1) aortic root mobilization by removing the valve and aortic root from the right ventricle as noted in Figs. 90 and 91, (2) pulmonary root incision/excision to create an enlarged area for anterior aorta translocation to the more posterior pulmonary annulus anatomically situated over the left ventricle, and (3) coronary artery mobilization from the epicardial surfaces to allow posterior translocation of the aorta. Some authors have

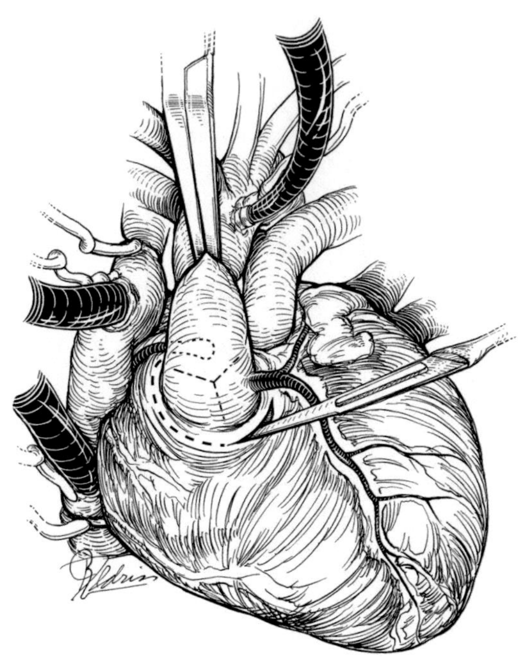

Fig. 90 shows a patient with transposition of the great arteries, ventricular septal defect, and pulmonary stenosis (TGA-VSD-PS) undergoing aortobicaval cardiopulmonary bypass, a left ventricular vent, aortic cross-clamping and the commencement of disconnection of the aortic root from the right ventricular outflow tract with its intact circumferential conus. Some surgeons can perform this part of the operation without an aortic cross-clamp in which the aortic conus is disconnected leaving the coronary arteries and the perfusion system intact. (With permission: Mavroudis 2015)

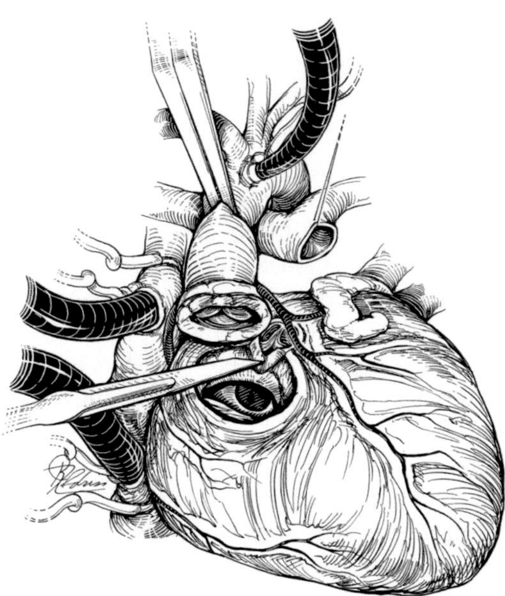

Fig. 91 The coronary arteries can then be mobilized without interruption of flow for the eventual translocation to the left ventricular outflow tract as shown in the figure. Alternatively, the coronary artery buttons can be removed from their respective sinuses of Valsalva under cardioplegic arrest and reimplanted after the aortic root has been translocated posteriorly in the left ventricular outflow tract. (With permission: Mavroudis 2015)

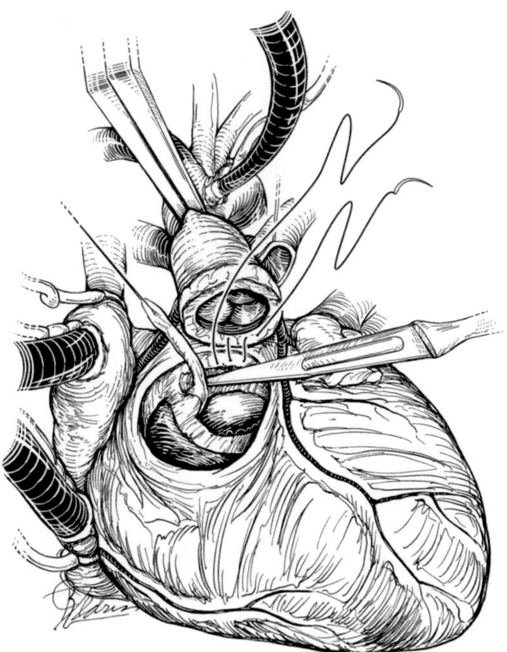

Fig. 92 shows the progression of the operation after aortic root mobilization with a longitudinal incision across the septum that connects the pulmonary artery annulus with the right ventricular outflow tract. This allows further resection of the infundibulum and repositioning of the aortic root posteriorly to better align with the left ventricular outflow tract. (With permission: Mavroudis 2015)

identified variants of this operation that consider reimplantation of one or both coronary artery buttons (Bautista-Hernandez et al. 2007; Hazekamp et al. 2007; Morell 2013; Morell and Wearden 2007; Nikaidoh 1984; Sayin et al. 2006; Kramer et al. 2014; Raju et al. 2015; Ventosa-Fernández et al. 2017). Further, the area between the VSD and the posterior pulmonary annulus is connected by incision as noted in Fig. 91 This creates an enlarged translocation site for the aorta which will lie anatomically over the left ventricular outflow tract as noted in Fig. 92. The completion of left ventricular outflow tract is shown in progress (Fig. 93) which includes the translocated aorta and the extended VSD patch. The figures show the best case scenario of this operation. Complications, however, can occur and can be life threatening like any procedure that requires coronary manipulation and aortic root translocation. During the translocation, malrotation of the aortic root can result in aortic valve regurgitation or coronary artery kinking or both. Figure 94 (three panels) shows a dramatic representation of aortic regurgitation of the translocated aorta and coronary artery kinking after the cross-clamp has been removed. This situation will result in significant left ventricular distention owing to the aortic valve leak and ventricular dysfunction due

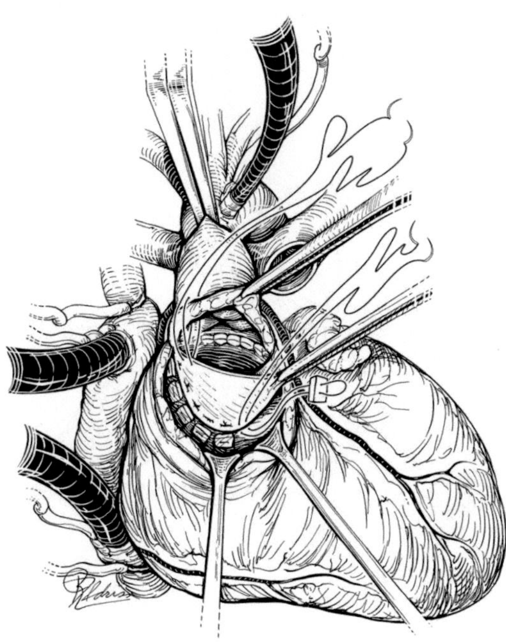

Fig. 93 also shows the repositioned aortic root being sewn to the posterior pulmonary annulus. The left ventricular outflow tract is then completed by fashioning a patch to close the ventricular septal defect and to serve as the anterior anchoring neo-annulus for the remaining aortic root. This maneuver requires careful attention to detail to avoid aortic regurgitation due to rotational problems and coronary artery stretching. Once completed, the cross-clamp is removed, the patient rewarmed, and the right ventricular outflow tract is reconstructed. Right ventricular outflow tract reconstruction under these circumstances is variable. Some surgeons prefer to use a valved conduit, while others prefer a valveless reconstruction as originally reported by Nikaidoh. (With permission: Mavroudis 2015)

to the kinked coronary arteries. Such a situation should immediately signal the operating team to reapply the cross-clamp, administer retrograde cardioplegia, and inspect the nature of the aortic root malrotation and address the problems. What does "address the problems" mean? The first problem is to correct the malrotation and adjust the translocation in such a way that will eliminate the aortic regurgitation. This maneuver will require takedown of the aortic implantation and visually realign the "best lie" formation to avoid aortic regurgitation. If this adjustment still causes coronary kinking, then the surgeon should consider removal of the coronary button in question and reimplant the coronary button in a more favorable position in another sinus of Valsalva. Some surgeons (Bautista-Hernandez et al. 2007; Hazekamp et al. 2007; Morell 2013; Morell and Wearden 2007; Nikaidoh 1984; Sayin et al. 2006; Kramer et al. 2014; Raju et al. 2015; Ventosa-Fernández et al. 2017; Agarwal and Vaidyanathan 2021) selectively remove the coronary buttons and reimplant them after the aorta has been translocated to avoid coronary kinking. The surgeon should research the pros and cons of this operation regarding coronary artery translocation before attempting this operation. In addition to the aortic root translocation problem is the possibility of residual VSD. This book has espoused the benefits of interrupted pledgetted suture technique for VSD closure (see chapter

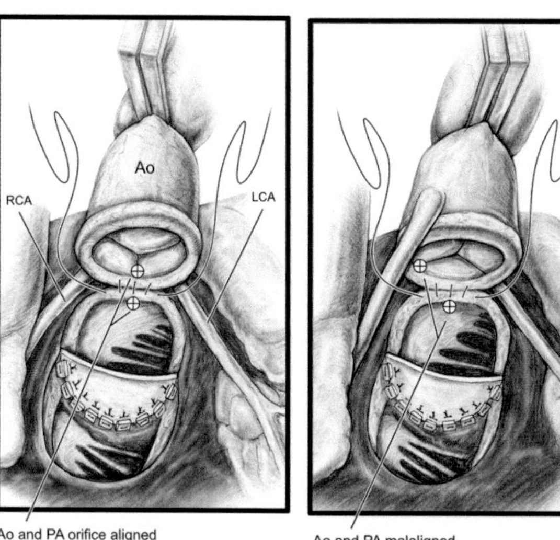

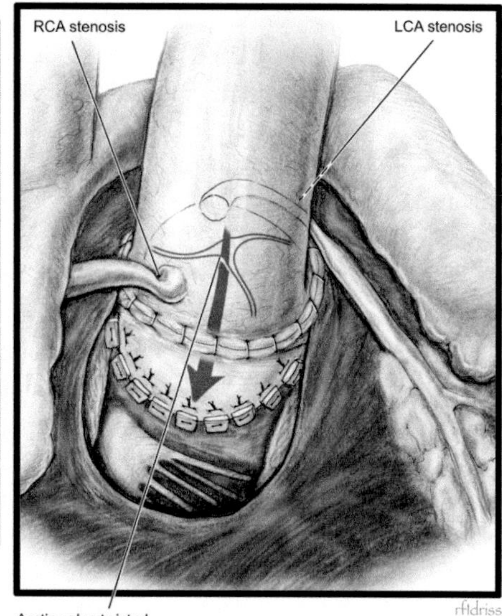

Fig. 94 shows malrotation of the completed posterior aortic translocation and coronary kinking. The left panel demonstrates correct alignmnet of the aorta and attached left and right coronary arteries. The middle panel shows the initial malalignment of the translocated aorta in a counterclockwise manner which when finished will result in the configuration that is shown in the right panel. The resultant reconstruction after initial malalignment demonstrates how coronary kinking and aortic regurgitation can occur simply by mismanaging the initial suture line as shown in the middle panel

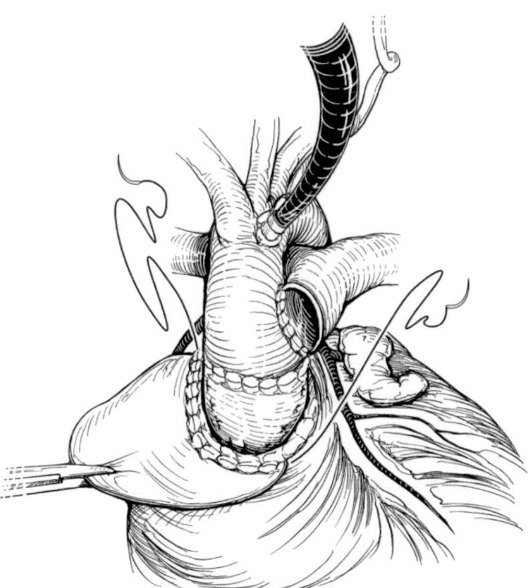

Fig. 95 demonstrates the right wall of the pulmonary artery sutured to the ascending aorta with a large patch being configured to complete the right ventricular-to-pulmonary artery continuity. (With permission: Mavroudis 2015)

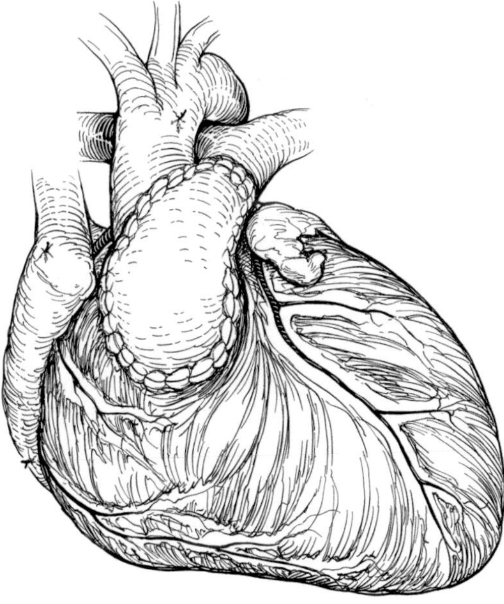

Fig. 96 shows the completed reconstruction after separation from cardiopulmonary bypass. (With permission: Mavroudis 2015)

"Complications Associated with Ventricular Septal Defect Closure"). This VSD has been enlarged and the resultant edges do not conform to a circular pattern. Interrupted pledgetted sutures will allow careful placement and assessment which should avoid to a great extent a residual defect as shown in Fig. 93.

In the majority of patients who had a successful and uncomplicated aortic translocation and those who had a successful aortic translocation revision, the right ventricular-to-pulmonary artery connection can be performed. Depending on the specific needs of the patient and the programmatic preferences a right ventricular-to-pulmonary valved conduit can be performed or other non-valve solutions such as are shown in Figs. 83.

In general, the reader should recognize that the specific operation that is applied for repair of TGA-VSD-PS depends on the patient's anatomic characteristics and the experience of the surgical program. There are many extant anatomic variations that suggest a case-by-case analysis be considered with application of the optimal operation.

15.1 Arterial Switch for Transposition, Ventricular Septal Defect, and Pulmonary Stenosis in Selected Patients

In some patients with TGA-VSD-PS, the LVOTO is caused by tricuspid valve accessory tissue which prolapses through the VSD causing subpulmonic stenosis in an otherwise normal left ventricular outflow tract and a normal pulmonary valve (Kumar et al. 2018). The tenets for a successful arterial switch operation are based on the demonstration that the left ventricle is well prepared, that the accessory tricuspid valve can be reduced, and that the pulmonary valve is normal. An arterial switch procedure can be performed in association with reduction of the accessory tricuspid valve and VSD closure. No specific drawings to illustrate this procedure are offered since the principles in the VSD and Transposition chapters show these techniques adequately. However, the potential complications are noteworthy in so far that the (1) left ventricle may not actually take over the systemic circulation due to ineffective preparation, (2) the pulmonary valve to become the neoaorta was too small and resulted in severe neoaortic stenosis, and (3) the prolapsed tricuspid valve may result in tricuspid regurgitation that will require tricuspid valvuloplasty. These potential complications can be avoided by careful and operative preparation which include cardiac catheterization, magnetic resonance imaging, and modeling techniques if available.

These cases are very rare but comprehensive assessment and careful attention to the operative principles will yield excellent results.

References

Aalaei-Andabili SH, Martin TD, Hess PJ, Karimi A, Bavry AA, Arnaoutakis GJ, Beaver TM. The Florida sleeve procedure is durable and improves aortic valve function. Aorta (Stamford). 2019;7(2):49–55.

Agarwal V, Vaidyanathan S. Aortic root translocation: the Bex-Nikaidoh procedure. Indian J Thorac Cardiovasc Surg. 2021;37(Suppl 1):36–41.

Ahlström L, Odermarsky M, Malm T, Johansoon Ramgren J, Hanseus K, Liuba P. Surgical age and morbidity after arterial switch for transposition of the great arteries. Ann Thorac Surg. 2019;108:1242–7.

Anderson BR, Ciarleglio AJ, Hayes DA, Quaegebeur JM, Vincent JA, Bacha EA. Earlier arterial switch operation improves outcomes and reduces costs for neonates with transposition of the great arteries. J Am Coll Cardiol. 2014;63:481–7.

Arensman FW, Sievers HH, Lange P, et al. Assessment of coronary and aortic anastomoses after anatomic correction of transposition of the great arteries. J Thorac Cardiovasc Surg. 1985;90:597–604.

Asou T, Karl TR, Pawade A, Mee RB. Arterial switch: translocation of the intramural coronary artery. Ann Thorac Surg. 1994;57:461–5.

Backer CL, Ilbawi MN, Ohtake S, et al. Transposition of the great arteries: a comparison of results of the mustard procedure versus the arterial switch. Ann Thorac Surg. 1989a;48:10–4.

Backer CL, Ilbawi MN, Idriss FS, DeLeon SY. Vascular anomalies causing tracheoesophageal compression. Review of experience in children. J Thorac Cardiovasc Surg. 1989b;97(5):725–31.

Backer CL, Idriss FS, Mavroudis C. Surgical techniques and intraoperative judgments to facilitate the arterial switch operation in transposition with intact ventricular septum. In: Mavroudis C, Backer CL, editors. Arterial switch. Cardiac surgery: state of the art review, vol. 5. Philadelphia, PA: Hanley & Belfus; 1991.

Barron DJ, Mehsood DK, Kutty RS, et al. Fate of the left ventricular outflow tract after Rastelli with selective infundibular muscle resection. Ann Thorac Surg. 2019;107:1226–31.

Bautista-Hernandez V, Marx GR, Bacha EA, del Nido PJ. Aortic root translocation plus arterial switch for transposition of the great arteries with left ventricular outflow tract obstruction: intermediate-term results. J Am Coll Cardiol. 2007;49:485–90.

Belhadjer Z, Soulat G, Ladouceur M, et al. Neopulmonary outflow tract obstruction assessment by 4D flow MRI in adults with transposition of the great arteries after arterial switch operation. J Magn Reson Imaging. 2020;51:1699–705.

Benzaquen BS, Webb GD, Colman JM, Therrien J. Arterial switch operation after Mustard procedures in adult patients with transposition of the great arteries: is it time to revise our strategy? Am Heart J. 2004;147(3):E8. https://doi.org/10.1016/j.ahj.2003.09.015.

Berlinger NT, Long C, Foker J, Lucas RV Jr. Tracheobronchial compression in acyanotic congenital heart disease. Ann Otol Rhinol Laryngol. 1983;92(4 Pt 1):387–90.

Bove EL. Current technique of the arterial switch procedure for transposition of the great arteries. J Card Surg. 1989;4:193–9.

Bremer JL. Transposition of the aorta and the pulmonary artery: an embryologic study of its cause. Arch Pathol. 1942;34:1016–30.

Cain MT, Cao Y, Ghanayem NS, et al. Transposition of the great arteries—outcomes and time interval of early neonatal repair. World J Pediatr Congenit Heart Surg. 2014;5:241–7.

Castaneda AR, Norwood WI, Jonas RA, Colon SD, Sanders SP, Lang P. Transposition of the great arteries and intact ventricular septum: anatomical repair in the neonate. Ann Thorac Surg. 1984;38:438–43.

Castaneda AR, Trusler GA, Paul MH, Blackstone EH, Kirklin JW. The early results of treatment of simple transposition in the current era. J Thorac Cardiovasc Surg. 1988;95:14–28.

Chang YH, Sung SC, Lee HD, Kim S, Woo JS, Lee YS. Coronary reimplantation after neoaortic reconstruction can yield better result in arterial switch operation: comparison with open trap door technique. Ann Thorac Surg. 2005;80:1634–40.

Chiu IS, Chu SH, Wang JK, et al. Evolution of coronary artery pattern according to short-axis aortopulmonary rotation: a new categorization for complete transposition of the great arteries. J Am Coll Cardiol. 1995;26:250–8.

Cleuziou J, Hörer J, Henze R, Schreiber C, Lange R. Surgical management of single intramural coronary artery in Taussig-Bing anomaly detected at arterial switch operation. Thorac Cardiovasc Surg. 2008;56:170–2.

Cochrane AD, Karl TR, Mee RB. Staged conversion to arterial switch for late failure of the systemic right ventricle. Ann Thorac Surg. 1993;56(4):854–62.

Co-Vu JG, Ginde S, Bartz PJ, Frommelt PC, Tweddell JS, Earing MG. Long-term outcomes of the neoaorta after arterial switch operation for transposition of the great arteries. Ann Thorac Surg. 2013;95:1654–9.

David TE. Aortic valve sparing operations: a review. Korean J Thorac Cardiovasc Surg. 2012;45(4):205–12.

Day RW, Laks H, Drinkwater HC. The influence of coronary anatomy on the arterial switch operation in neonates. J Thorac Cardiovasc Surg. 1992;104:706–12.

de Jong PL, Bogers AJ, Witsenburg M, Bos E. Arterial switch for pulmonary venous obstruction complicating Mustard procedure. Ann Thorac Surg. 1995;59:1005–7.

de Vries PA, Saunders JB. Development of the ventricles and spiral outflow tract in the human heart. Contrib Embryol. 1962;37:89–114.

Di Carlo D, Tomasco B, Cohen L, Vouhé P, Lecompte Y. Long-term results of the REV (reparation a l'etage ventriculaire) operation. J Thorac Cardiovasc Surg. 2011;142:336–43.

Ebels T, Meuzelaar K, Gallandat Huet RC, et al. Neonatal arterial switch operation complicated by intramural left coronary artery and treated by left internal mammary artery bypass graft. J Thorac Cardiovasc Surg. 1989;97:473–5.

Fiore AC, Peigh PS, Robison RJ, Glant MD, King H, Brown JW. Valved and nonvalved right ventricular--pulmonary arterial extracardiac conduits. An experimental comparison. J Thorac Cardiovasc Surg. 1983;86(4):490–7.

Gittenberger-de Groot AC, Sauer U, Quaegebeur J. Aortic intramural coronary artery in three hearts with transposition of the great arteries. J Thorac Cardiovasc Surg. 1986;91:566–71.

Gittenberger-de Groot AC, Koenraadt WMS, Bartelings MM, et al. Coding of coronary arterial origin and branching in congenital heart disease: the modified Leiden convention. J Thorac Cardiovasc Surg. 2018;156:2260–9.

Goor DA, Shem-Tov A, Neufeld HN. Impeded coronary flow in anatomic correction of transposition of the great arteries: prevention, detection, and management. J Thorac Cardiovasc Surg. 1982;83:747–54.

Grant RP. The morphogenesis of transposition of the great vessels. Circulation. 1962;26:819–40.

Hazekamp M, Portela F, Bartelings M. The optimal procedure for the great arteries and left ventricular outflow tract obstruction. An anatomical study. Eur J Cardiothorac Surg. 2007;31:879–87.

Huang ES, Herrmann JL, Rodefeld MD, Turrentine MW, Brown JW. Rastelli operation for D-transposition of the great arteries, ventricular septal defect, and pulmonary stenosis. World J Pediatr Congenit Heart Surg. 2019;10:157–63.

Huhta JC, Edwards WD, Danielson GK, Feldt RH. Abnormalities of the tricuspid valve in complete transposition of the great arteries with ventricular septal defect. J Thorac Cardiovasc Surg. 1982;83:569–76.

Ibrahimiye AN, Mainwaring RD, Patrick WL, Downey L, Yarlagadda V, Hanley FL. Left ventricular retraining and double switch in patients with congenitally corrected transposition of the great arteries. World J Pediatr Congenit Heart Surg. 2017;8(2):203–9.

Idriss FS, DeLeon SY, Nikaidoh H, et al. Resection of left ventricular outflow obstruction in d-transposition of the great arteries. J Thorac Cardiovasc Surg. 1977;74:343–51.

Idriss FS, Ilbawi MN, DeLeon SY, et al. Arterial switch in simple and complex transposition of the great arteries. J Thorac Cardiovasc Surg. 1988a;95:29–36.

Idriss FS, Ilbawi MN, DeLeon SY, et al. Transposition of the great arteries with intact ventricular septum. Arterial switch in the first month of life. J Thorac Cardiovasc Surg. 1988b;95:255–62.

Jatene AD, Fontes VF, Souza LC, Paulista PP, Neto CA, Sousa JE. Anatomic correction of transposition of the great arteries. J Thorac Cardiovasc Surg. 1982;83:20–6.

Jex RK, Puga FJ, Julsrud PR, Weidman WH. Repair of transposition of the great arteries with intact ventricular septum and left ventricular outflow tract obstruction. J Thorac Cardiovasc Surg. 1990;100:682–6.

Khairy P, Clair M, Fernandes SM, et al. Cardiovascular outcomes after the arterial switch operation for D-transposition of the great arteries. Circulation. 2013;127:331–9.

Kirklin JW, Blackstone EH, Tchervenkov CI, Castaneda AR. Clinical outcomes after the arterial switch operation for transposition. Patient, support, procedural, and institutional risk factors. Congenital Heart Surgeons Society. Circulation. 1992;86:1501–15.

Kramer P, Ovroutski S, Hetzer R, Hübler M, Berger F. Modified Nikaidoh procedure for the correction of complex forms of transposition of the great arteries with ventricular septal defect and left ventricular outflow-tract obstruction: mid-term results. Eur J Cardiothorac Surg. 2014;45:928–34.

Kreutzer G, Neirotti R, Galindez E, Coronel AR, Kreutzer E. Anatomic correction of transposition of the great arteries. J Thorac Cardiovasc Surg. 1977;73:538–42.

Kumar B, Jayant A, Munirathinam GK, Mahajan S. Tricuspid valve straddling: an uncommon cause of left ventricular outflow tract obstruction in transposition of great artery with ventricular septal defect. Ann Card Anaesth. 2018;21(1):61–4.

Kurosawa H, Imai Y, Kawada M. Coronary arterial anatomy in regard to the arterial switch procedure. Cardiol Young. 1991;1:54–62.

Lecompte Y. Reparation a l'Etage Ventriculaire—the REV procedure: technique and clinical results. Cardiol Young. 1991;1:63–70.

Lecompte Y, Vouhe P. Reparation a l'Etage Ventriculaire (REV procedure): not a Rastelli procedure without a conduit. Oper Tech. 2003;8:150–9.

Lecompte Y, Zannini L, Hazan E, et al. Anatomic correction of transposition of the great arteries. J Thorac Cardiovasc Surg. 1981;82:629–31.

Lecompte Y, Neveux JY, Leca F, et al. Reconstruction of the pulmonary outflow tract without prosthetic conduit. J Thorac Cardiovasc Surg. 1982;84:727–33.

Lecompte Y, Batisse A, Di Carlo D. Double-outlet right ventricle: a surgical synthesis. In: Advances in cardiac surgery, vol. 4. Mosby Year Book; 1993. p. 109–36.

Li J, Tulloh RM, Cook A, Schneider M, Ho SY, Anderson RH. Coronary arterial origins in transposition of the great arteries: factors that affect outcome. A morphological and clinical study. Heart. 2000;83:320–5.

Lim JM, Porayette P, Marini D, et al. Associations between age at arterial switch operation, brain growth, and development in infants with transposition of the great arteries. Circulation. 2019;139:2728–38.

Loke YH, Capuano F, Mandell J, et al. Abnormal pulmonary artery bending correlates with increased right ventricular afterload following the arterial switch operation. World J Pediatr Congenit Heart Surg. 2019;10:572–81.

Lupinetti FM, Bove EL, Minich LL, et al. Intermediate–term survival and functional results after arterial repair for transposition of the great arteries. J Thorac Cardiovasc Surg. 1992;103:421–7.

Ma K, Li S, Hu S, et al. Neoaortic valve regurgitation after arterial switch: ten years outcomes from a single center. Ann Thorac Surg. 2016;02:636–42.

Maeda T, Sakamoto T, Nagashima M, Hiramatsu T, Yamazaki K. Long-term outcome of arterial switch operation conversion after failed Senning/Mustard procedure. Ann Thorac Surg. 2016;102:1573–9.

Marcelletti C, Mair DD, McGoon DC, Wallace RB, Danielson GK. The Rastelli operation for transposition of the great arteries. Early and late results. J Thorac Cardiovasc Surg. 1976;72:427–34.

Mariani MA, Waterbolk TW, Ebels T. Transposition of the great arteries and isolated origin of the sinus node artery. Ann Thorac Surg. 1998;66:2087–9.

Mavroudis C. Anatomical repair of transposition of the great arteries with intact ventricular septum in the neonate: guidelines to avoid complications. Ann Thorac Surg. 1987;43:495–501.

Mavroudis C. Transposition of the Great Arteries. In: Mavroudis C, Backer CL, editors. Atlas of pediatric cardiac surgery. London: Springer; 2015.

Mavroudis C. Coronary artery bypass grafting in infants, children, and young adults for acquired and congenital lesions. Congenit Heart Dis. 2017;12(5):644–6.

Mavroudis C, Backer CL. Arterial switch after failed atrial baffle procedures for transposition of the great arteries. Ann Thorac Surg. 2000;69:851–7.

Mavroudis C, Backer CL, editors. Pediatric cardiac surgery. 5th ed. London: Wiley-Blackwell Inc.; 2023.

Mavroudis C, Arensman FW, Rees AH. Anatomical repair of transposition of the great arteries with intact ventricular septum in the neonate. In: Kron IL, Mavroudis C, editors. Innovations in congenital heart surgery. Cardiac surgery: state of the art review, vol. 3. Philadelphia, PA: Hanley & Belfus; 1989.

Mavroudis C, Backer CL, Idriss FS. Special considerations for and reoperations after the arterial switch operation. In: Mavroudis C, Backer CL, editors. Arterial switch. Cardiac surgery: state of the art review, vol. 5. Philadelphia, PA: Hanley & Belfus; 1991.

Mavroudis C, Backer CL, Idriss FS. Arterial switch for transposition of the great arteries and associated malposition anomalies. In: Karp RB, Laks H, Wechsler AS, editors. Advances in cardiac surgery. St Louis: Mosby; 1992.

Mavroudis C, Backer CL, Duffy CE, Pahl E, Wax DF. Pediatric coronary artery bypass for Kawasaki congenital, post arterial switch, and iatrogenic lesions. Ann Thorac Surg. 1999;68:506–12.

Mavroudis C, Stewart RD, Backer CL, Rudra H, Vargo P, Jacobs ML. Reoperative techniques for complications after arterial switch. Ann Thorac Surg. 2011;92:1747–55.

Mavroudis C, Stulak JM, Ad N, Siegel A, Giamberti A, Harris L, Backer CL, Tsao S, Dearani J, Weerasena N, Deal BJ. Prophylactic arrhythmia surgery in association with congenital heart operations: a critical review and recommendations. Ann Thorac Surg. 2015;99:352–9.

Mayer JE Jr, Sanders SP, Jonas RA, Castaneda AR, Wernovsky G. Coronary artery pattern and outcome of arterial switch operation for transposition of the great arteries. Circulation. 1990;82(Suppl 5):IV139–45.

Mee RB. Severe right ventricular failure after Mustard or Senning operation. Two-stage repair: pulmonary artery banding and switch. J Thorac Cardiovasc Surg. 1986;92(3 Pt 1):385–90.

Meyerowitz CB, Jacobs LE, Kotler MN, Wertheimer JH, Ioli A, Janzer S, Chandrasekaran K. Assessment of aortic regurgitation by transesophageal echocardiography: correlation with angiographic determination. Echocardiography. 1993;10(3):269–78.

Michalak KW, Sobczak-Budlewska K, Moll JJ, et al. Can we predict potentially dangerous coronary patterns in patients with transposition of the great arteries after an arterial switch operation? Cardiol Young. 2019;29:1350–5.

Moene RJ, Oppenheimer-Dekker A, Bartelings MM. Anatomic obstruction of the right ventricular outflow tract in transposition of the great arteries. Am J Cardiol. 1983;51:1701–4.

Moene RJ, Oppenheimer-Dekker A, Wenink AC, Bartelings MM, Gittenberger-de Groot AC. Morphology of ventricular septal defect in complete transposition of the great arteries. Am J Cardiol. 1985;55(13 Pt 1):1566–70.

Moll M, Michalak KW, Sobczak-Budlewska K, et al. Coronary artery anomalies in patients with transposition of the great arteries and their impact on postoperative outcomes. Ann Thorac Surg. 2017;104:1620–8.

Mookhoek A, Korteland NM, Arabkhani B, Di Centa I, Lansac E, Bekkers JA, Bogers AJ, Takkenberg JJ. Bentall procedure: a systematic review and meta-analysis. Ann Thorac Surg. 2016;101(5):1684–9.

Morell VO. Aortic translocation for TGA with VSD and PS. CTSNet Congenital Cardiac Expert Techniques, March 21, 2013. Available at: https://www.ctsnet.org/article/aortic-translocation-tga-vsd-and-ps. Accessed 10 June 2020.

Morell VO, Wearden PD. Aortic translocation for the management of transposition of the great arteries with a ventricular septal defect, pulmonary stenosis, and hypoplasia of the right ventricle. Eur J Cardiothorac Surg. 2007;31(3):552–4.

Moulton AL, de Leval MR, Macartney FJ, Taylor JF, Stark J. Rastelli procedure for transposition of the great arteries, ventricular septal defect, and left ventricular outflow tract obstruction. Early and late results in 41 patients (1971 to 1978). Br Heart J. 1981;45:20–8.

Muster AJ, Berry TE, Ilbawi MN, DeLeon SY, Idriss FS. Development of neo-coarctation in patients with transposed great arteries and hypoplastic aortic arch after Lecompte modification of anatomical correction. J Thorac Cardiovasc Surg. 1987;93:276–80.

Nellis JR, Turek JW, Aldoss OT, Atkins DL, Ng BY. Intervention for supravalvar pulmonary stenosis after the arterial switch operation. Ann Thorac Surg. 2016;102:154–62.

Nikaidoh H. Aortic translocation and biventricular outflow tract reconstruction. A new surgical repair for transposition of the great arteries associated with ventricular septal defect and pulmonary stenosis. J Thorac Cardiovasc Surg. 1984;88:365–72.

Norwood WI, Dobell AR, Freed MD, Kirklin JW, Blackstone EH. Intermediate results of the arterial switch repair. A 20-institution study. J Thorac Cardiovasc Surg. 1988;96:854–63.

O'Byrne ML, Glatz AC, Song L, et al. Association between variation in preoperative care before arterial switch operation and outcomes in patients with transposition of the great arteries. Circulation. 2018;138:2119–29.

Ohtake S, Idriss FS, Ilbawi MN, et al. Severe systemic right ventricular dysfunction after mustard operation for transposition. Circulation. 1989;80(Suppl II):70.

Ohtake S, Idriss FS, Backer CL, et al. Fate of tricuspid valve as a systemic atrioventricular valve: a 20-year follow-up of TGA with Mustard repair. J Am Coll Cardiol. 1990;15:79A.

Ou P, Khraiche D, Celermajer DS, et al. Mechanisms of coronary complications after the arterial switch for transposition of the great arteries. J Thorac Cardiovasc Surg. 2013;145:1263–9.

Pacifico AD, Stewart RW, Bargeron LM Jr. Repair of transposition of the great arteries with ventricular septal defect by an arterial switch operation. Circulation. 1983;68(3 Pt 2):II49–55.

Parry AJ, Thurm M, Hanley FL. The use of 'pericardial hoods' for maintaining exact coronary artery geometry in the arterial switch operation with complex re anatomy. Eur J Cardiothorac Surg. 1999;15:159–65.

Pasquini L, Sanders SP, Parness IA, Colan SD. Diagnosis of coronary artery anatomy by two-dimensional echocardiography in patients with transposition of the great arteries. Circulation. 1987;75:557–64.

Pasquini L, Sanders SP, Parness IA, et al. Coronary echocardiography in 406 patients with d-loop transposition of the great arteries. J Am Coll Cardiol. 1994;24:763–8.

Peacock TB. On malformations of the human heart, with original cases and illustrations. 2nd ed. London: John Churchill and Sons; 1866.

Planché C, Bruniaux J, Lacour-Gayet F, et al. Switch operation for transposition of the great arteries in neonates. A study of 120 patients. J Thorac Cardiovasc Surg. 1988;96:354–63.

Planché C, Lacour-Gayet F, Serraf A, et al. Anatomical repair in transposition of great vessels. Bull Acad Natl Med. 1998;182(8):1739–55.

Prêtre R, Gendron G, Tamisier D, et al. Results of the Lecompte procedure in malposition of the great arteries and pulmonary obstruction. Eur J Cardiothorac Surg. 2001;19:283–9.

Quaegebeur JM, Rohmer J, Ottenkamp J, et al. The arterial switch operation. An eight-year experience. J Thorac Cardiovasc Surg. 1986;92(3 Pt 1):361–84.

Raju V, Burkhart HM, Durham LA 3rd, et al. Reoperation after arterial switch: a 27-year experience. Ann Thorac Surg. 2013;95:2105–13.

Raju V, Myers PO, Quinonez LG, et al. Aortic root translocation (Nikaidoh procedure): intermediate follow-up and impact of conduit type. J Thorac Cardiovasc Surg. 2015;149:1349–55.

Rashkind WJ, Miller WW. Creation of an atrial septal defect without thoracotomy. A palliative approach to complete transposition of the great arteries. JAMA. 1966;196:991–2.

Rastelli GC, Wallace RB, Ongley PA. Complete repair of transposition of the great arteries with pulmonary stenosis. A review and report of a case corrected by using a new surgical technique. Circulation. 1969;39:83–95.

Reisman M, Rosengart RM, Degner TL, Sintek C, Khonsari S. Post-Mustard procedure pulmonary venous obstruction: an opportunity for anatomic correction with a one-stage arterial switch. Pediatr Cardiol. 1999;20:301–3.

Rossi MB, Ho SY, Anderson RH, Rossi Filho RI, Lincoln C. Coronary arteries in complete transposition: the significance of the sinus node artery. Ann Thorac Surg. 1986;42:573–7.

Rowlatt UF. Coronary artery distribution in complete transposition. JAMA. 1962;179:269–78.

Sayin OA, Ugurlucan M, Saltik L, Sungur Z, Tireli E. Modified Nikaidoh procedure for transposition of great arteries, ventricular septal defect and left ventricular outflow tract obstruction. Thorac Cardiovasc Surg. 2006;54:558–60.

Serraf A, Lacour-Gayet F, Bruniaux J, et al. Anatomic correction of transposition of the great arteries in neonates. J Am Coll Cardiol. 1993;22:193–200.

Shaner RF. Comparative development of the bulbus and ventricles of the vertebrate heart with special reference to Spitzer's theory of heart malformations. Anat Rec. 1962;142:519–29.

Shinebourne EA, Jahangiri M, Carvalho JS, Lincoln C. Anatomic correction for post-Mustard pulmonary venous obstruction. Ann Thorac Surg. 1994;57:1655–6.

Shukla V, Freedom RM, Black MD. Single coronary artery and complete transposition of the great arteries: a technical challenge resolved? Ann Thorac Surg. 2000;69:568–71.

Sidi D, Heurtematte Y, Kachaner J, et al. Problems posed by preparation of the left ventricle for anatomical correction in simple transposition of the great vessels. Arch Mal Coeur Vaiss. 1983;76:575–83.

Sim EK, van Son JA, Edwards WD, Julsrud PR, Puga FJ. Coronary artery anatomy in complete transposition of the great arteries. Ann Thorac Surg. 1994;57:890–4.

Skinner J, Hornung T, Rumball E. Transposition of the great arteries: from fetus to adult. Heart. 2008;94:1227–35.

Smith A, Arnold R, Wilkinson JL, Hamilton DI, McKay R, Anderson RH. An anatomical study of the patterns of the coronary arteries and sinus nodal artery in complete transposition. Int J Cardiol. 1986;12(3):295–307.

Sohn YS, Brizard CP, Cochrane AD, Wilkinson JL, Mas C, Karl TR. Arterial switch in hearts with left ventricular outflow and pulmonary valve abnormalities. Ann Thorac Surg. 1998;66:842–8.

Spector LG, Menk JS, Knight JH, et al. Trends in long-term mortality after congenital heart surgery. J Am Coll Cardiol. 2018;71:2434–46.

Stark J. Transposition of the great arteries: which operation? Ann Thorac Surg. 1984;38:429–31.

Svensson LG. The art of aortic valve repair. JTCVS Tech. 2021;7:121–5.

Tamisier D, Ouaknine R, Pouard P, et al. Neonatal arterial switch operation: coronary artery patterns and coronary events. Eur J Cardiothorac Surg. 1997;11:810–7.

Tanel RE, Wernovsky G, Landzberg MJ, Perry SB, Burke RP. Coronary artery abnormalities detected at cardiac catheterization following the arterial switch operation for transposition of the great arteries. Am J Cardiol. 1995;76:153–7.

Toker A, Tireli E, Bostanci K, Ozcan V, Dayioğlu E. Uncommon complication of arterial switch operation: tracheobronchial compression. Ann Thorac Surg. 2000;69(3):927–9.

Toyoda Y, Hiramatsu T, Nagashima M, Matsumura G, Yamazaki K. Long-term effect of enlargement of a ventricular septal defect in the Rastelli procedure. Semin Thorac Cardiovasc Surg. 2017;29:215–20.

van der Palen RLF, Blom NA, Kuipers IM, Rammeloo LAJ, Jongbloed MRM, Konings TC, Bouma BJ, Koolbergen DR, Hazekamp MG. Long-term outcome after the arterial switch operation: 43 years of experience. Eur J Cardiothorac Surg. 2021;59(5):968–77.

Van Mierop LH, Wiglesworth FW. Pathogenesis of transposition complexes. II. Anomalies due to faulty transfer of the posterior great artery. Am J Cardiol. 1963;12:226–32.

Van Mierop LH, Alley RD, Kausel HW, Stranahan A. Pathogenesis of transposition complexes. I. Embryology of the ventricles and great arteries. Am J Cardiol. 1963;12:216–25.

Van Praagh R, Van Praagh S. Isolated ventricular inversion. A consideration of the morphogenesis, definition and diagnosis of nontransposed and transposed great arteries. Am J Cardiol. 1966;17:395–406.

van Son JA. Classification of origin and proximal epicardial course of coronary arteries in transposition of the great arteries. J Cardiovasc Surg. 1996;37:251–4.

van Wijk SWH, van der Stelt F, Ter Heide H, et al. Sudden death due to coronary artery lesions long-term after the arterial switch operation: a systematic review. Can J Cardiol. 2017;33:1180–7.

Ventosa-Fernández G, Pérez-Negueruela C, Mayol J, Paradela M, Caffarena-Calvar JM. The Nikaidoh procedure for complex transposition of the great arteries: short-term follow-up. Cardiol Young. 2017;27(5):945–50.

Vouhé PR, Tamisier D, Leca F, Ouaknine R, Vernant F, Neveux JY. Transposition of the great arteries, ventricular septal defect, and pulmonary outflow tract obstruction. Rastelli or Lecompte procedure? J Thorac Cardiovasc Surg. 1992;103:428–36.

Wernovsky G, Mayer JE Jr, Jonas RA, et al. Factors influencing early and late outcome of the arterial switch operation for transposition of the great arteries. J Thorac Cardiovasc Surg. 1995;109:289–302.

Worsey J, Pham SM, Newman B, Park SC, del Nido PJ. Left main bronchus compression after arterial switch for transposition. Ann Thorac Surg. 1994;57(5):1320–2.

Yacoub MH. The case for anatomic correction of transposition of the great arteries. J Thorac Cardiovasc Surg. 1979;78:3–6.

Yacoub MH, Radley-Smith R. Anatomy of the coronary arteries in transposition of the great arteries and methods for their transfer in anatomical correction. Thorax. 1978;33:418–24.

Yacoub MH, Radley-Smith R, Hilton CJ. Anatomical correction of complete transposition of the great arteries and ventricular septal defect in infancy. Br Med J. 1976;1:1112–4.

Yacoub M, Bernhard A, Lange P, et al. Clinical and hemodynamic results of the two-stage anatomic correction of simple transposition of the great arteries. Circulation. 1980;62(2 Pt 2):I190–6.

Zheng JH, Xu ZW, Liu JF, Su ZK, Ding WX. Arterial switch operation with coronary arteries from a single sinus in infants. J Card Surg. 2008;23:606–10.

Complications Associated with Repair of Double Outlet Ventricles with Two Adequate Ventricles

Constantine Mavroudis

Abstract

Double-outlet right ventricle (DORV) is a type of ventriculoarterial connection in which both great vessels arise entirely or predominantly from the right ventricle. Many controversies associated with DORV relate to its anatomic definition, and surgical management. The complications associated with repair of these variable effects relate to the management of the ventricular septal defect (residual defects), acquired heart block, atrial and ventricular arrhythmias, aortic and pulmonary valve injury during subarterial resection, coronary artery rotational problems and myocardial ischemia associated with arterial switch, inappropriate intraventricular tunneling, and acquired subarterial stenosis. These complications will be identified, discussed, and be the focus of resolution.

Keywords

Congenital heart surgery · Double outlet right ventricle · Double outlet right ventricle tetralogy of Fallot type · Double outlet right ventricle transposition type · Complications · Outcomes

1 Introduction

Double outlet right ventricle (DORV) is an anatomic term to describe a cardiac malformation that is characterized by ventriculoarterial connections resulting in both great vessels arising entirely or principally from the right ventricle. The anatomic variations have been defined, categorized, and debated by informed anatomists, embryologists, and surgeons. Nomenclature schemes have been developed each with their own advantages and disadvantages. The controversies associated with the nomenclature of DORV relate to its anatomic definition, surgical management, and characterization of its multiple phenotypes (Lev et al. 1972; Tynan et al. 1979; Piccoli et al. 1983; Kirklin et al. 1986; Tabry et al. 1978; Taussig and Bing 1949; Van Praagh 1968; Van Praagh et al. 1980; Ebadi et al. 2017; Howell et al. 1991; Peacock 1866; Rokitansky 1875; Braun et al. 1952; Kirklin et al. 1964; Witham 1957; Engle and Steinberg 1961). In general terms, presuming that there are two functional left and right ventricles, DORV can be a tetralogy type or a transposition type with many associated subtypes in each category (Neufeld et al. 1961a, b, 1962). The in utero development of DORV anatomy relates to the embryologic

C. Mavroudis (✉)
Chief of Pediatric Cardiothoracic Surgery (Retired), Peyton Manning Children's Hospital, Indianapolis, IN, USA

Professor Emeritus of Surgery, Johns Hopkins University School of Medicine, Baltimore, MD, USA

C. L. Backer, C. Mavroudis (eds.), *Complications in Pediatric and Congenital Heart Surgery*,
https://doi.org/10.1007/978-3-032-02661-3_15

rotation of the aorta and pulmonary artery above the right ventricular outflow tract and the relationship to the ventricular septal defect (VSD) (Angelini and Leachman 1976; Anderson 1978; Anderson et al. 1974a; Goor and Lillehei 1975; Okamoto 1980; Van Praagh 1973; van Mierop and Wiglesworth 1963; van Mierop and Gessner 1972; Bartelings and Gittenberger-de Groot 1989). The most commonly associated cardiac malformations that are found with DORV add to the complexity of the defect and include: concordant atrioventricular connections (Wilcox et al. 1981; Anderson et al. 1983), atrioventricular and arterial valve atresia, and atrial isomerism. DORV is frequently associated with functionally single ventricle; however, this chapter will focus on DORV with two functioning ventricles. The complications associated with repair of these variable effects relate to the management of the VSD (residual defects), acquired heart block, atrial and ventricular arrhythmias, aortic and pulmonary valve injury during subarterial resection, coronary artery rotational problems and myocardial ischemia associated with arterial switch, inappropriate intraventricular tunneling, acquired subarterial stenosis, and many more. These complications will be identified, discussed, and be the focus of resolution.

The types of DORV will dictate the surgical management schemes and will be approached by the indicated operation and the associated complications that might be encountered (De Azevedo et al. 1956; Beuren 1960; Daicoff and Kirklin 1967; Hightower et al. 1969; Patrick and McGoon 1968; Kawashima et al. 1971; Sakata et al. 1988; Lecompte et al. 1993; Sondheimer et al. 1977; Danielson et al. 1978; Ruttenberg et al. 1964; Alfieri et al. 1978; Lauer et al. 1960; Cheng 1962; Serratto et al. 1967; Mason et al. 1969; Lavoie et al. 1971; Marin-Garcia et al. 1978; Matsuoka et al. 1987; Zamora et al. 1975; Sridaromont et al. 1978; Walters III and Pacifico 2003; Edwards 1981; Stewart et al. 1979; Danielson et al. 1972; Shafer et al. 1967; Anderson et al. 1975; Mehrizi 1965).

2 Complications Associated with Repair of Double Outlet Right Ventricle, Ventricular Septal Defect Type

Patients with DORV, VSD type without pulmonary stenosis are characterized by an overriding aorta (>90% or >50%, depending on the nomenclature scheme) and aortic to mitral annular discontinuity (not always recognized as required for the diagnosis of DORV) (Mahle et al. 2008; Artrip et al. 2006; Freedom and Yoo 2000; Belli et al. 1998; Walters III et al. 2000; Franklin et al. 2002; Sridaromont et al. 1976; Yoo and van Arsdell 2018; Yoo et al. 2015; Oladunjoye et al. 2020; Backer 2016, 2020; Bradley et al. 2007; Tchervenkov et al. 1995; Luber et al. 1983; Li et al. 2014; Brown et al. 2001; Tchervenkov et al. 2000). Whatever nomenclature is used to describe this entity, this repair can be accomplished using the techniques of tetralogy of Fallot repair with certain exceptions that are noted in the following drawings.

Figure 1 depicts the anatomy associated with DORV-VSD. The repair in this drawing is approached through a right ventriculotomy. However, the operation can be accomplished through a right atriotomy that exposes the entire tricuspid valve which will allow adequate valve leaflet retraction to identify and accomplish the repair (see chapter "Complications Associated with Ventricular Septal Defect Closure"). Unlike most perimembranous VSDs, the VSD in patients with DORV, VSD type without pulmonary stenosis is often restrictive due to a hypertrophied infundibulum. As noted in the figure, the hypertrophied infundibulum is being resected to avoid injury to the aortic valve and the conduction system. During the subaortic infundibular resection, the aortic valve is prone to injury if the resection is misjudged. The difficulty with this resection plane is that the aortic valve is not always apparent owing to its location behind the muscular infundibular ridge. A staged approach with intermittent inspection will prove to be the best

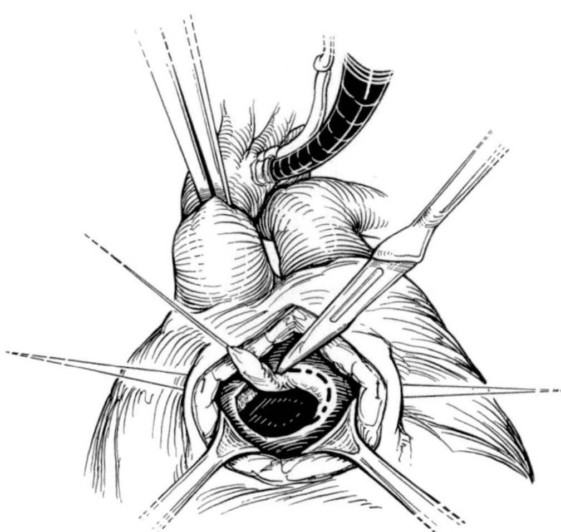

Fig. 1 Shows a patient with DORV undergoing aortobicaval cardiopulmonary bypass (not shown), left ventricular venting (not shown), and aortic cross-clamping. The relevant anatomy is approached through a right ventriculotomy, although exposure through a right atriotomy is also possible. The VSD in patients with DORV, VSD type without pulmonary stenosis is often restrictive owing to a hypertrophied infundibulum. The drawing shows the resection starting in the subaortic area and being extended to the medial portion thereby enlarging the VSD. Care must be taken to ensure that the aortic leaflets are preserved at the beginning of the resection and that the resection extension is not carried out too far into the inferior rim of the VSD where the conduction system can be injured. This is a delicate balance; not enough infundibular resection will result in subaortic stenosis and too much infundibular resection will result in left ventricular dysfunction. In general, the resultant VSD after the resection should approximate the size of the aorta. DORV, double outlet right ventricle; VSD, ventricular septal defect. (With permission: Walters III and Pacifico 2003)

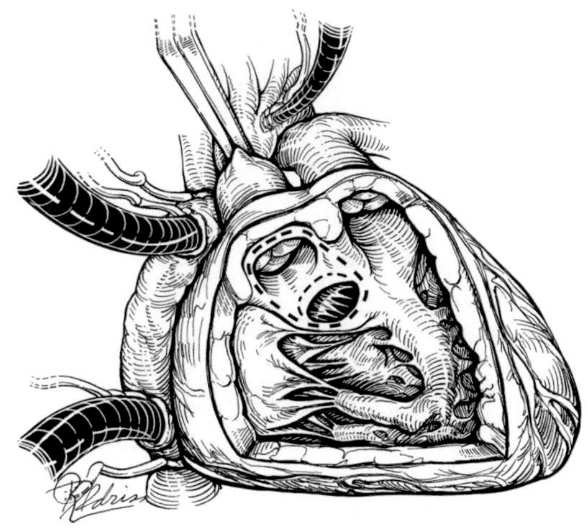

Fig. 2 This is a coronal view of the right ventricle with exclusion of the right ventricular free wall to highlight the anatomy. The infundibulum has been resected and the proposed suture line for the VSD patch is shown by the dashed lines. Once the patch is placed the intraventricular tunnel will direct left ventricular flow to the aorta. Abbreviation: VSD, ventricular septal defect. (With permission: Walters III and Pacifico 2003)

method to avoid aortic valve injury. In addition, intermittent cardioplegic administration will identify the valve, note the degree of competence, and guide the subsequent resection pathway to avoid valve injury. If the valve is injured by an unwanted incision, immediate measures should be taken to repair the valve by interrupted suture technique or patch repair depending on the extent of the injury (see chapter "Complications Associated with Ventricular Septal Defect Closure"). The rest of the resection will require care to avoid injury to the conduction system which is located at the inferior rim of the VSD. The infundibular resection should approximate the size of the aorta to prevent postoperative subaortic stenosis (Mavroudis et al. 1996a). Figure 2 shows the relevant coronal anatomy of the right ventricle after the infundibular resection indicating the suture placement (dashed lines) for tunneling of the left ventricular flow to the aorta. Aortobicaval cardiopulmonary bypass is established with aortic cross-clamping and left ventricular venting (not shown). Figure 3 shows the completed intraventricular tunnel using an incised corrugated vascular graft. Interrupted pledgetted sutures are best for anchoring an oversized or corrugated patch to insure unobstructed aortic flow. However, the patch should not be so large as to obstruct pulmonary artery flow. Figure 4 depicts the resultant outcome of placing a small tunnelling patch that can result in a flattened structure without a curved configuration. Such a patch might be well suited for a VSD closure; however, it will not be optimal for this repair since it will cause left ventricular outflow tract obstruction. The best solution to mitigate this type of complication is to oversize the patch so that it maintains a curved pattern as noted in Figs. 3 and 4 (right panel). A longitudinally incised corrugated vascular graft is tailor-made

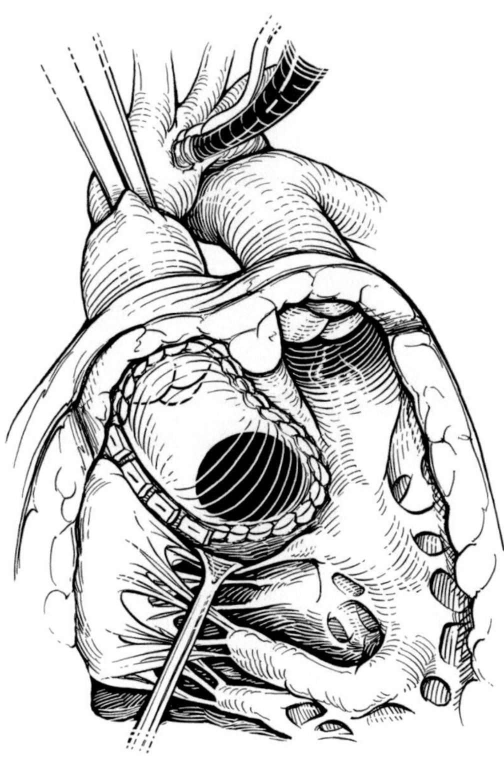

Fig. 3 This illustration demonstrates how interrupted pledgetted sutures are best used for anchoring an oversized patch to insure unobstructed aortic flow. The patch however should not be so large as to obstruct pulmonary artery flow. (With permission: Walters III and Pacifico 2003)

for this reconstruction since it maintains its configuration so that an internal intraventricular baffle can be formed without left ventricular outflow tract stenosis.

After the repair is completed, the right ventricle or right atrium is closed, the air maneuvers can be accomplished, the aortic cross-clamp can be removed, and the patient can be rewarmed. The obvious potential complication that can occur with these maneuvers is the management of retained intracardiac air (Quintero et al. 2019). Most surgeons have mastered a particular technique that was learned during residency or fellowship. In this particular case air can be easily trapped within the oversized baffle. Care should be taken to perform the air maneuvers with great care and attention to remove all the air by venous line constriction. This will facilitate blood flow through the heart with negative pressure at the cardioplegia line connecting to the ascending aorta combined with pulmonary Valsalva maneuvers. After separation from cardiopulmonary bypass, the repair can be assessed. Transesophageal echocardiography (TEE) can evaluate the right and left ventricular outflow tracts as well as the presence or absence of a ventricular residual shunt. The team can then determine whether return to bypass for repair revision will be necessary. The important intraoperative complications relate to a residual left-to-right shunt, pulmonary stenosis, and heart block. A residual left- to-right shunt can be evaluated by TEE and differential oxygen saturation measurements from the right atrium and pulmonary artery. The determination of the residual left-to-right shunt is reviewed and discussed in chapter "Complications Associated with Ventricular Septal Defect Closure". In general, calculated shunts of 1.5:1 or less together with a residual anatomic shunt of 1.25 mm or less will likely close within a 6-month period and will not require immediate reoperation. Residual pulmonary stenosis is an important factor to consider. The clinical team will have to distinguish between flow acceleration at the pulmonary valve and pulmonary stenosis caused by an oversized VSD patch that is encroaching anteriorly on the right ventricular outflow tract (Fig. 5 left panel). If the calculated pressure determination exceeds 40 mmHg and if the TEE findings corroborate these findings of right ventricular outflow tract obstruction, then consideration should be given to a subpulmonary artery ventricular patch augmentation which will require return to cardiopulmonary bypass for re-repair as noted in Fig. 5 right panel.

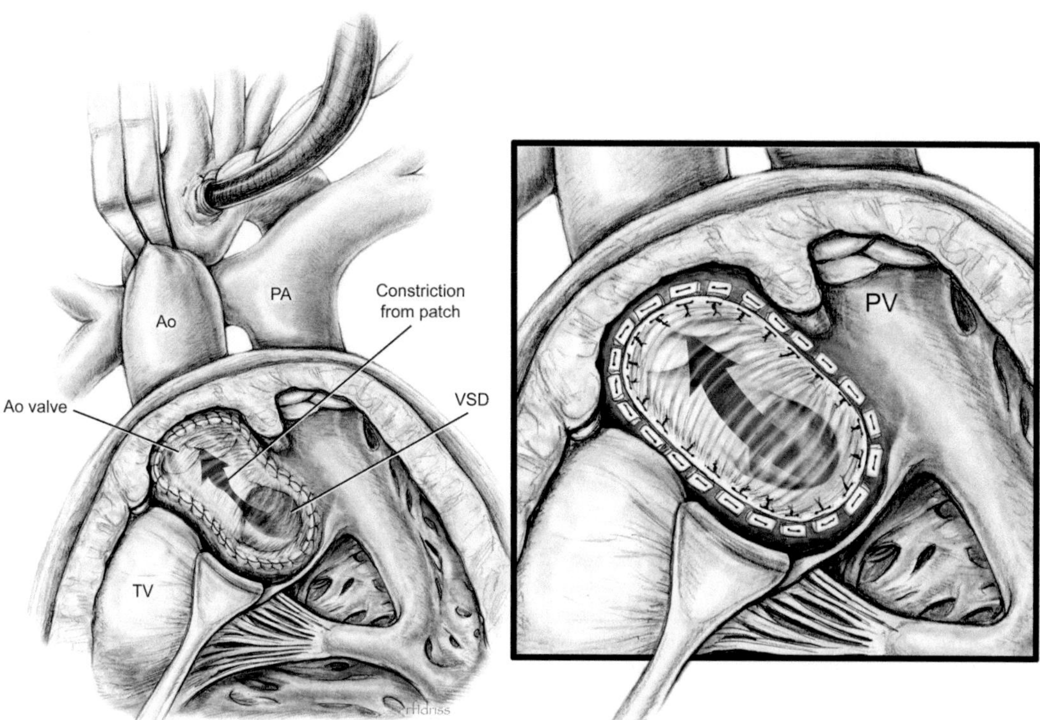

Fig. 4 (Left panel) shows how a small tunnelling patch can result in a flattened structure without a curved configuration. While this patch can be well suited for a VSD closure, it will not suffice for this repair since it will cause left ventricular outflow tract obstruction. The best way to avoid this type of complication is to oversize the patch so that it maintains a curved pattern as noted in the right panel. A longitudinally incised corrugated vascular graft is tailor-made for this reconstruction since it holds its configuration to form an internal intraventricular baffle. *Ao* aorta, *PA* pulmonary artery, *TV* tricuspid valve, *VSD* ventricular septal defect

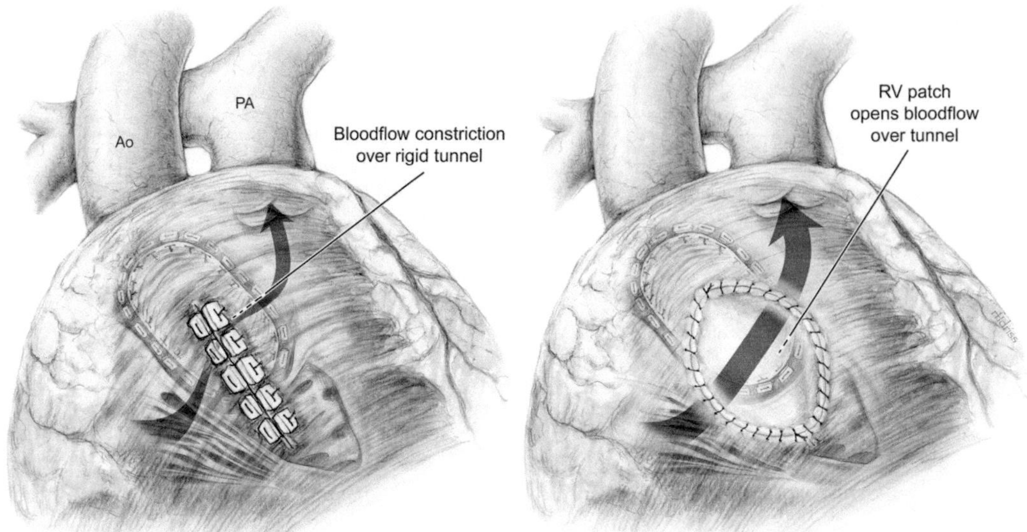

Fig. 5 After repair of DORV with subaortic VSD, residual pulmonary stenosis can occur as is shown in the left panel and the arrow which is full sized for normal flow and undersized for stenotic flow. It is important to distinguish between flow acceleration at the pulmonary valve and pulmonary stenosis caused by an oversized VSD patch that is encroaching anteriorly on the right ventricular outflow tract. If the pressure gradient exceeds 40 mmHg with collaborative TEE findings, then ventricular patch augmentation should be considered by resuming cardiopulmonary bypass for re-repair. The right panel in this illustration shows the completed re-repair of right ventricular outflow tract obstruction using a subpulmonic right ventricular patch. *Ao* aorta, *DORV* double outlet right ventricle, *PA* pulmonary artery, *RV* right ventricle, *TEE* transesophageal echocardiography, *TV* tricuspid valve, *VSD* ventricular septal defect

3 Complications Associated with Repair of Double Outlet Right Ventricle, Tetralogy Type

In the case of DORV associated with pulmonary stenosis, also known as DORV, tetralogy type, the repair is largely the same as for DORV, VSD type without pulmonary stenosis (Kleinert et al. 1997). The major difference for this repair is the management of the stenotic right ventricular outflow tract in much the same way that tetralogy of Fallot is repaired. When appropriate, a pulmonary valve sparring operation using techniques noted in chapter "Complications Associated with Repair of Tetralogy of Fallot" (tetralogy Chapter) can be applied as long as the pulmonary valve annulus is large enough (z-score larger than −3). In most cases however a right ventricular outflow tract patch will be necessary. Figure 6 shows the completed repair of DORV, tetralogy type with a right ventricular transannular outflow tract patch. The complications associated with a transannular right ventricular outflow tract patch stem from the undiagnosed intramyocardial course of an anomalous origin of the left anterior descending coronary artery (Meyer et al. 1975; Mavroudis 2017). Ordinarily, this situation would be discovered by a preoperative cardiac catheterization. However, it is wise to perform the ventriculotomy from the mid-ventricle and slowly progress towards the stenotic pulmonary valve. If an intramyocardial coronary artery is discovered, and if it is not injured, preparations should be made to perform a right ventricular-to-pulmonary artery conduit with great care to avoid injury to the coronary artery by careful suture placement at the proximal conduit anastomosis. If the artery is

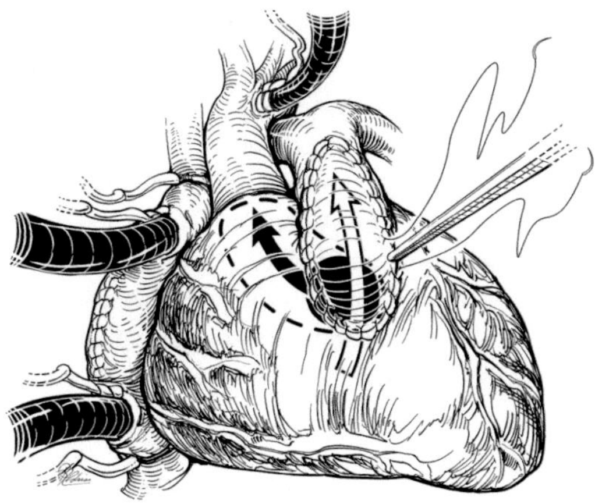

Fig. 6 Demonstrates a transannular right ventricular outflow tract patch. Alternatively, a pulmonary valve sparring operation can be applied as long as the pulmonary valve annulus is large enough (z-score larger than −3). (With permission: Walters III and Pacifico 2003)

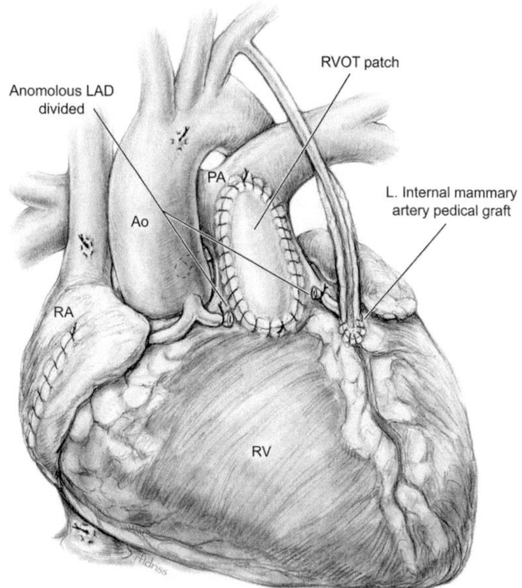

Fig. 7 This drawing demonstrates left internal thoracic artery to left anterior descending coronary artery bypass for a patient with unwanted left anterior coronary artery transection that was ligated with resultant internal thoracic artery bypass graft in place. This drawing represents how coronary bypass can be performed in infants and children when needed in emergency situations to preserve ventricular function and preserve life. When an anomalous left anterior descending coronary artery is severed because of inaccurate preoperative diagnosis or unwanted operative mishaps, coronary bypass should be considered. *Ao* aorta, *LAD* left anterior descending, *PA* pulmonary artery, *RA* right atrium, *RV* right ventricle, *RVOT* right ventricular outflow tract

transected, a significant problem becomes manifest, especially if the artery is large enough to compromise perfusion to the myocardium. Ligating the artery will likely result in significant left ventricular dysfunction leading to extracorporeal membrane oxygenation (ECMO) and the problems relating thereto. A left internal thoracic artery bypass graft to the left anterior descending coronary artery should be considered (Mavroudis 2017; Mavroudis et al. 1996b). Assuming the cross-clamp has been removed, the internal thoracic artery can be dissected and prepared for the bypass graft. Cardioplegic arrest is then established and the arteriotomy in the left anterior descending coronary artery can be performed. Fine monofilament (Prolene) 8–0 suture can then be used to perform the anastomosis (Fig. 7). Alternatively, interrupted suture technique can also be used (Mavroudis et al. 1996b).

Some surgeons prefer to use a valved conduit in the setting where a transannular patch would be necessary as noted in Fig. 6. Conduits that are too short or too long can result in coronary artery compression and distal pulmonary stenosis, respectively as noted in chapter "Complications Associated with Repair of Common Arterial Trunk". Our first preference is to use a transannular patch under these circumstances unless there are complicating factors that indicate an extracardiac valved conduit placement (Fig. 8) such as right ventricular dysfunction, right ventricular outflow tract obstruction due to the VSD patch, or anomalous coronary artery as noted herein.

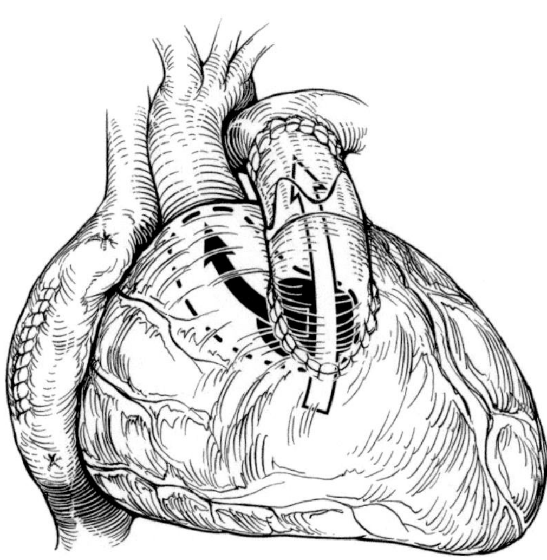

Fig. 8 Shows the completed repair of DORV, tetralogy type using a valved right ventricular to pulmonary artery conduit. The choice to use a conduit centers around right ventricular dysfunction, severe right ventricular outflow tract obstruction not amenable to transannular patch, and anomalous coronary artery. The black arrow shows the left ventricular to aortic flow pattern while the white arrow shows the right ventricular to pulmonary artery flow pattern through the right ventricular to pulmonary artery conduit. (With permission: Walters III and Pacifico 2003)

4 Complications Associated with Repair of Double Outlet Right Ventricle, Transposition Type, Without Pulmonary Stenosis and Subaortic VSD by VSD Closure and Arterial Switch

Further categorization of DORV, Transposition Type without pulmonary stenosis depends on the type of VSD and its location (Brown et al. 2001; Tchervenkov et al. 2000; Kleinert et al. 1997). In other words, is the VSD subaortic or subpulmonic? The modern-day approach to DORV, Transposition Type, and subaortic VSD without pulmonary stenosis is arterial switch and VSD closure to tunnel the left ventricle to the neoaorta. The complications associated with this operation have been described based on the VSD closure (Fig. 3) and arterial switch (Chapter "Complications Associated with Repair of Transposition of the Great Arteries and Associated Lesions"). In general, the complications have been discussed and relate to residual VSD, pulmonary stenosis, acquired heart block, coronary artery distortion and hypoperfusion, neoaortic regurgitation, and supravalvar neopulmonary artery stenosis. The difference with this operation is the extended cross-clamp time and induced cardioplegic arrest which must be managed efficiently and carefully to limit ischemia time while performing an accurate operation free of complications.

5 Repair of Double Outlet Right Ventricle, Transposition Type with Subpulmonic VSD (Taussig-Bing Malformation) with Side-by-Side Vessels by Intraventricular Tunnel Kawashima Repair

The previous discussion regarding DORV repairs centered on those patients with DORV, VSD type with subaortic or subarterial VSD and no pulmonary stenosis as well as those patients with DORV, tetralogy type (pulmonary stenosis) with subaortic or subarterial VSD. These anatomic subtypes or variants have been, more or less, normally related to great vessel anatomy that allows intraventricular tunneling of the left ventricle to the aorta and a right ventricular outflow tract that can be managed conservatively by valvar preservation, valve repair, or a transannular patch in much the same way that classic tetralogy patients are treated. The complications relating to these repairs have been discussed herein and in the tetralogy chapter (Chapter "Complications Associated with Repair of Tetralogy of Fallot").

The range of DORV anatomy however is a continuum from normally related great vessel anatomy as noted in the previous paragraph to transposed great arteries which starts with side-by-side great arteries and extends to transposed great arteries with various types of VSD (Lopez et al. 1966). Those patients with TGA, subpulmonic VSD, and side-by-side vessels can be treated by arterial switch and VSD closure (Lopez et al. 1966; van Buchem et al. 1950; Goor and Ebert 1975;

Gittenberger-de Groot et al. 1983; Ottino et al. 1980; Wedemeyer et al. 1970; Smith et al. 1982; Binet et al. 1983; Pacifico et al. 1986; Harvey et al. 1977; Agarwala et al. 1973; Stewart 1977; Metras et al. 1984; Doty 1986; Abe et al. 1984; Danielson 1984; Kanter et al. 1986; Soszyn et al. 2011; Alsoufi et al. 2008; Griselli et al. 2007; Wetter et al. 2004; Hayes et al. 2013; Sinzobahamvya et al. 2007) or by the intraventricular tunneling Kawashima technique (Mavroudis et al. 1996a; Kawashima et al. 1993; Kawahira et al. 1999).

The Kawashima procedure is characterized by extensive infundibular resection and left ventricular to aortic tunneling (Mavroudis et al. 1996a; Kawashima et al. 1993; Kawahira et al. 1999). Since the left ventricle is tunneled to the aorta, an arterial switch operation is not necessary because it avoids the attendant problems of coronary artery translocation and supravalvar neopulmonary artery reconstruction. Figure 9 shows a coronal view of the right ventricle with right ventricular wall exclusion. The anatomic characteristics show a heart with side-by-side great vessels and subpulmonic VSD.

The small, dashed line depicts the area and extent of resection of the infundibulum which will help to avoid an obstructed pathway from the left ventricle to the aorta. The larger dashed lines demonstrate the location where the pledgetted sutures are placed to accomplish a firm attachment of the patch for the tunnel reconstruction. Figure 10 shows how the extensive resection of the malaligned infundibular septum is performed. The semilunar valves are retracted superiorly to avoid injury. Figure 11 shows the completed intraventricular patch reconstruction with a detailed description of the possible complications that can occur with this repair which include heart block, tricuspid valve regurgitation, patch dehiscence, and semilunar valve injury.

Preoperative assessment pertaining to the distance between the pulmonary annulus and the tricuspid annulus to ensure proper distance for left ventricular outflow is crucial for the success of this operation. In general, the distance should

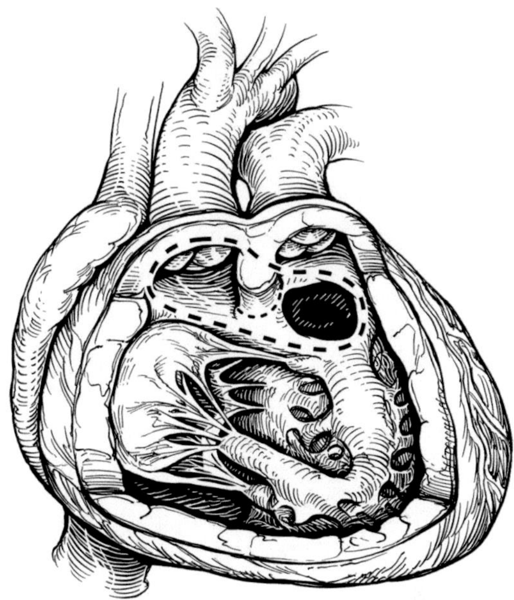

Fig. 9 This is a coronal view of the anatomic details in a patient with transposition of the great arteries, subpulmonic ventricular septal defect, and side-by-side great arteries. The small, dashed line demonstrates the extensive resection of the infundibulum which is required for an unobstructed tunnel from the left ventricle to the aorta. The larger dashed lines show where the pledgetted sutures are to be placed for the tunnel reconstruction. (With permission: Walters III and Pacifico 2003)

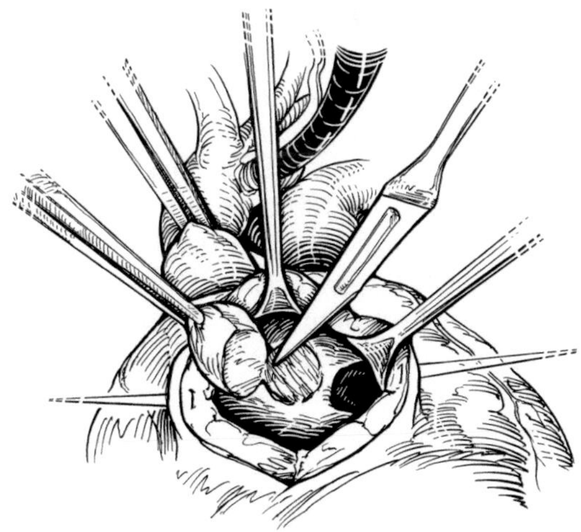

Fig. 10 Shows the extensive resection of the malaligned infundibular septum. This maneuver requires careful attention to both semilunar valves to avoid injury. (With permission: Walters III and Pacifico 2003)

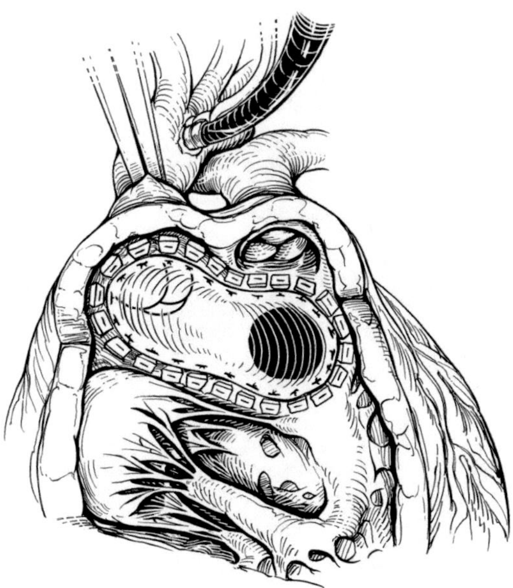

Fig. 11 Illustrates pledgetted sutures which are shown together with the completed intraventricular tunnel. These sutures require careful placement around the edges of the subpulmonic ventricular septal defect to avoid heart block, near the tricuspid valve to avoid valvar regurgitation, directly into the anterior aortic valve annulus to strengthen the purchase thereby avoiding dehiscence, and directly into the inferior course of the pulmonary annulus for the same reasons. (With permission: Walters III and Pacifico 2003)

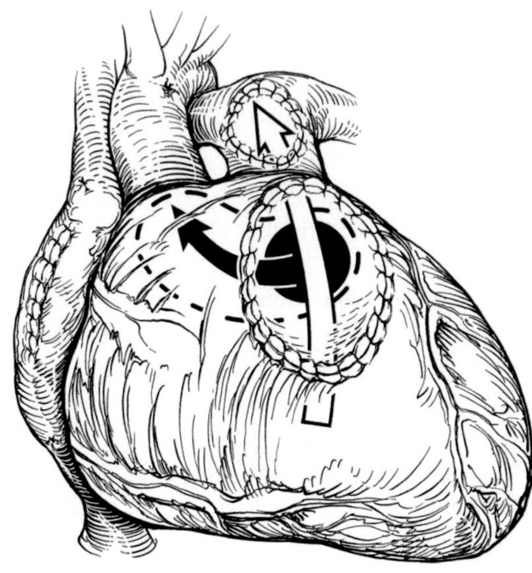

Fig. 12 This illustration depicts the completed repair of the Kawashima operation noting left ventricular to aortic flow by the black arrow and right ventricular to pulmonary flow by the white arrow. Preoperative measurements are important to insure unobstructed left ventricular to aortic flow patterns. The preoperative distance between the pulmonary annulus and tricuspid annulus should be at least the size of the aorta with a proper patch size to maintain unobstructed flow. Right ventricular patch augmentation will avoid turbulent flow to the pulmonary artery. (With permission: Walters III and Pacifico 2003)

be determined to be at least the size of the aortic annulus (Raisky and Vouhé 2013). Oftentimes, right ventricular patch augmentation is needed to maintain unobstructed right ventricular outflow as noted in Fig. 12. This operation, while complex, avoids coronary transfer that is associated with the arterial switch operation but has a short and long-term risk of subaortic and tunnel stenosis. In the present era, this operation is rarely used since most surgeons prefer to perform VSD closure and arterial switch which is discussed in the next section.

6 Repair of Double Outlet Right Ventricle, Transposition Type with Subpulmonic VSD (Taussig-Bing Malformation) by VSD Closure and Arterial Switch

The repair of DORV, transposition type with subpulmonic VSD (Taussig-Bing Malformation) is conceptually similar to the other types of conotruncal malformations which require arterial switch for anatomic repair (Lopez et al. 1966; van Buchem et al. 1950; Goor and Ebert 1975; Gittenberger-de Groot et al. 1983; Ottino et al. 1980; Wedemeyer et al. 1970; Smith et al. 1982; Binet et al. 1983; Pacifico et al. 1986; Harvey et al. 1977; Agarwala et al. 1973; Stewart 1977; Metras et al. 1984; Doty 1986; Abe et al. 1984; Danielson 1984; Kanter et al. 1986; Soszyn et al. 2011; Alsoufi et al. 2008; Griselli et al. 2007; Wetter et al. 2004; Hayes et al. 2013; Sinzobahamvya et al. 2007). Figures 13, 14, 15, 16, 17 and 18 show a comprehensive display of the arterial switch operation with VSD closure associated with DORV, transposition type with subpulmonic VSD (Taussig-Bing Malformation). This series of drawings focuses on the arterial switch operation and the possible complications thereto related. The drawings and legends recount the comprehensive and important steps of the operation including coronary mobilization, great vessel reorientation (note that the Lecompte maneuver is not usually performed for this type of DORV), and VSD closure. The management of cardiopulmonary bypass is straightforward assuming that no cannulation or perfusion problems arise. Most surgeons take the time of systemic cooling to perform ligation and division of the patent arterial duct, perform comprehensive dissection of the great vessels, and assess the coronary artery origins. While these maneuvers seem easy enough, patent arterial duct disruption, great vessel perforation, and coronary laceration could occur and cause significant problems even before the main part of the operation. And as noted in previous chapters, these complications generally do not occur until they do. The principles of careful and deliberate dissection, attention to detail, and management of complications will serve the surgeon and his/her patient well.

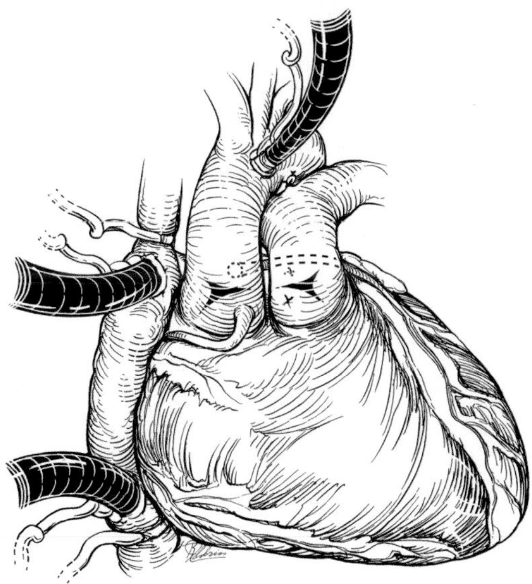

Fig. 13 Shows a patient undergoing aortobicaval cardiopulmonary bypass, left ventricular venting (not shown) in preparation for the reparative operation. The left coronary artery is shown ghostlike with the dotted lines and the x inclusions mark the spots where the coronary artery buttons will be transferred. No matter the great vessel orientation, the coronary artery configuration is almost always suitable for favorable coronary transfer and arterial switch. (With permission: Walters III and Pacifico 2003)

Patent arterial duct disruption should be managed by careful ligation of the pulmonary artery component and great attention given to the aortic side to avoid recurrent laryngeal nerve injury and neocoarctation in the event of aggressive suture repair causing aortic obstruction. Comprehensive great vessel mobilization in anticipation of the arterial switch including the distal right and left pulmonary arteries requires attention to detail to avoid unwanted pulmonary and aortic entry and bleeding. Each situation is different and can be managed by judicious clamp placement and suture repair or institution of cardiopulmonary bypass to repair the bleeding areas. In the event that the bleeding is emanating from the aortic disruption at the patent arterial duct, cardiopulmonary bypass, hypothermia, and low flow techniques may be required for an accurate and complication free repair. Some surgeons prefer to use epicardial coronary artery dissection to facilitate mobilization after aortic cross-clamping and aortic transection. These maneuvers should be carried out with blunt instruments and low setting electrocautery in the event of superficial bleeding in preparation for more mobilization during the arterial switch. Any unwanted injury to the coronary artery should be attended by expeditious cardiopulmonary bypass, aortic cross-clamping, and careful repair by fine interrupted suture technique. Efforts to attempt coronary artery laceration

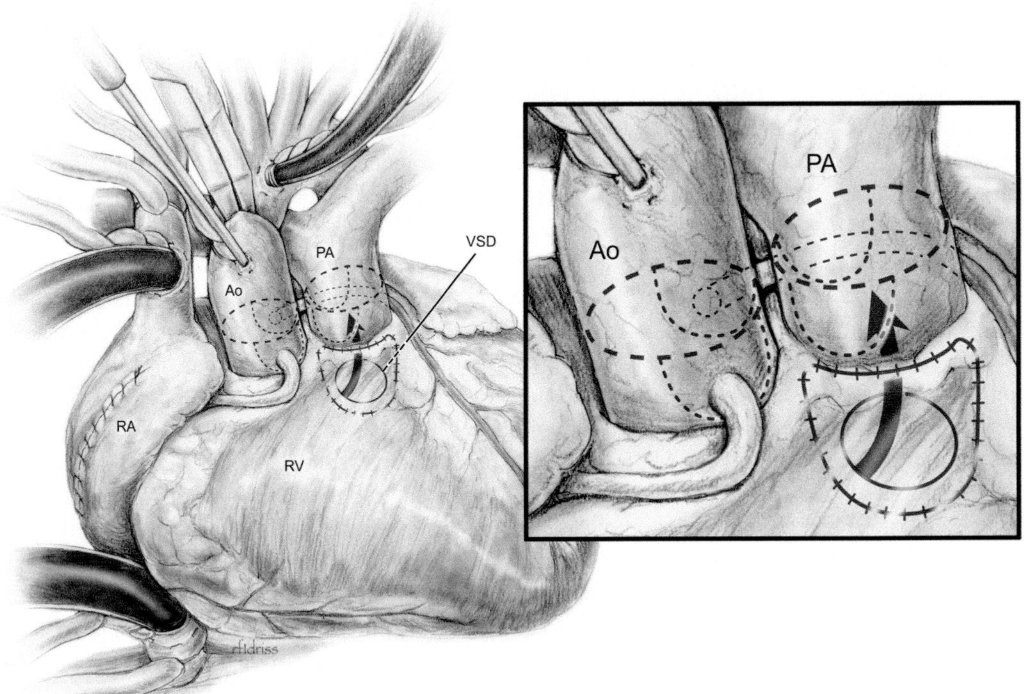

Fig. 14 Depicts aortic cross-clamping, antegrade cardioplegia and the numerous dotted lines that indicate incisions, transections, coronary artery excision and mobilization, and location of ventricular septal defect (VSD) suture placement en route to compete repair. This drawing shows more or less side-by-side vessels; however, the pulmonary artery can lie more posteriorly as well. The arrow shows the eventual left ventricular flow pattern to the pulmonary artery which is to become the neoaorta after arterial switch. The VSD closure can be accomplished through a right atriotomy or right ventriculotomy. The infundibular resection, if necessary, can be accomplished by either approach. The VSD is closed before the arterial switch is performed owing to the possibility of neoaortic disruption during the course of VSD closure which may involve tricuspid retraction for exposure. The surgeon may choose to use a combination of antegrade and retrograde cardioplegia in this kind of operation because of the extended cross-clamp time that is necessary for an accurate repair. The inset shows a magnified view. *Ao* aorta, *PA* pulmonary artery, *RA* right atrium, *RV* right ventricle, *VSD* ventricular septal defect

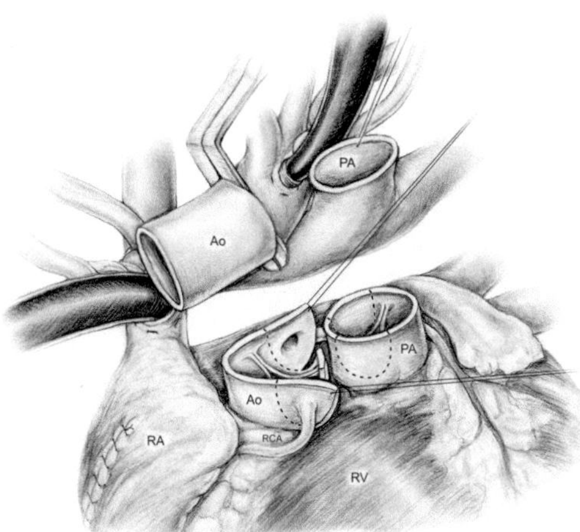

Fig. 15 Shows the transected great arteries, and the dotted lines depict the coronary button harvesting and the proposed sinuses of Valsalva attachment sites to form the neoaorta. Because the vessels are more or less side-by-side in orientation, the surgeon may elect not to perform the Lecompte maneuver as is being noted in this set of drawings. *Ao* aorta, *PA* pulmonary artery, *RA* right atrium, *RCA* right carotid artery, *RV* right ventricle

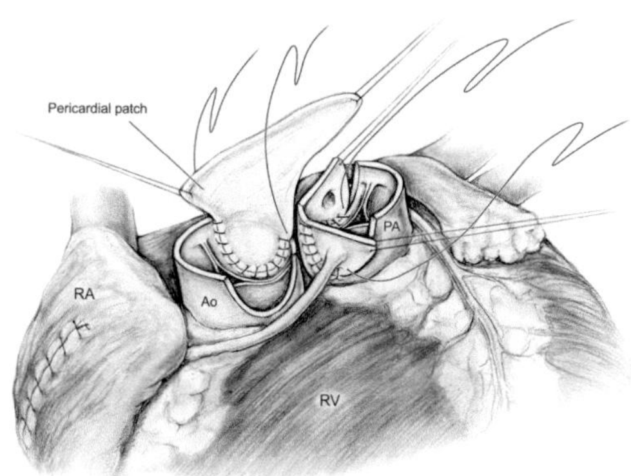

Fig. 16 This illustration depicts the transected aorta and pulmonary artery with coronary artery mobilization en route to coronary button reimplantation to the neoaorta. The coronary artery buttons are shown being transferred using an excision technique. Some surgeons use a circular button technique for reimplantation into the proposed site of the coronary transfer (not shown). This circular button technique is popular with many surgeons who use this for all their arterial switch operations. Clearly, coronary button transfer can be performed by a number of techniques that ensure coronary patency after cross-clamp removal. In like manner the neopulmonary artery can be repaired with separate pericardial patches instead of the large pantaloon patch technique (shown herein) that was introduced by Idriss and his colleagues and is shown in chapter "Complications Associated with Repair of Transposition of the Great Arteries and Associated Lesions". *Ao* aorta, *PA* pulmonary artery, *RA* right atrium, *RV* right ventricle

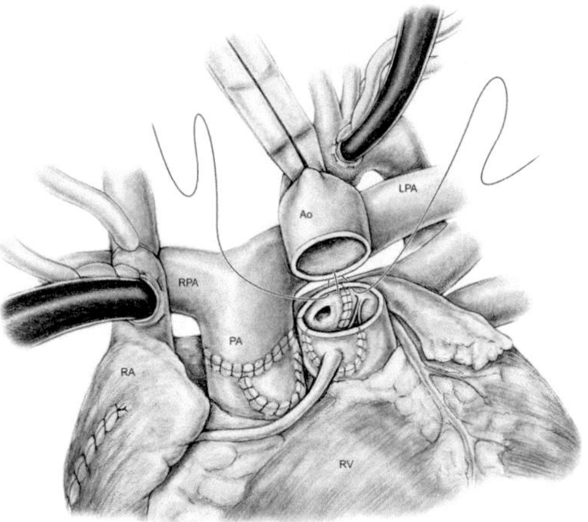

Fig. 17 Shows the neopulmonary artery reconstruction already performed and then neoaortic reconstruction in progress. Ordinarily, one would perform the neoaortic reconstruction before the neopulmonary artery reconstruction, thereby saving cross-clamp time. However, nowadays, the myocardial preservation strategies have allowed longer cross-clamp times and the depicted approach can be used especially if the surgeon anticipates more problems with the neopulmonary artery reconstruction than the neoaortic reconstruction. *Ao* aorta, *LPA* left pulmonary artery, *PA* pulmonary artery, *RA* right atrium, *RPA* right pulmonary artery, *RV* right ventricle

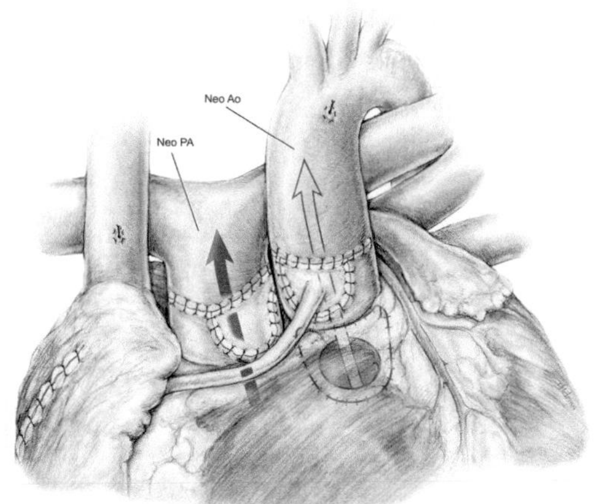

Fig. 18 This drawing illustrates the completed repair after separation from cardiopulmonary bypass. The white arrow depicts the left ventricle to neoaorta flow, and the black arrow shows the right ventricle to neopulmonary artery flow

repair without aortic cross-clamping and optimal exposure can lead to further disruption, inaccurate repair, and myocardial infarction

7 Repair of Double Outlet Right Ventricle, Transposition Type with Subpulmonic VSD (Taussig Bing Malformation) and Aortic Arch Obstruction by VSD Closure, Arterial Switch, and Arch Repair

Taussig-Bing malformation is often associated with a small ascending aorta and coarctation of the aorta. The repair for these patients is very challenging due to great vessel size discrepancy and the need for aortic arch repair, which often requires a period of deep hypothermia and circulatory arrest or regional perfusion techniques which have been described in chapters "Complications Associated with Repair of Interrupted Aortic Arch", "Complications Associated with Repair of Common Arterial Trunk", and "Complications Associated with Repair of Transposition of the Great Arteries and Associated Lesions". Figure 19 demonstrates the anatomic characteristics of the Taussig-Bing abnormality with coarctation of the aorta. The dashed lines show the areas of incision, transection, and coronary artery harvesting for the eventual complete repair.

In general, aortobicaval cardiopulmonary bypass, left ventricular venting, and a combination of antegrade/retrograde cardioplegia strategies with systemic cooling to 18–20 C° is employed. If the ascending aorta is very small, we prefer to use a PTFE graft sewn to the innominate artery which will facilitate regional perfusion techniques. The cardioplegia can be then given by an antegrade technique after aortic cross-clamping, and the arterial duct can be ligated and removed from the transverse arch.

Figure 20 shows the important supracardiac diagrammatic visualization of the incisions, excisions, and coronary mobilization that is required for the continuation and completion of the operation. The intent is to depict what needs to be done

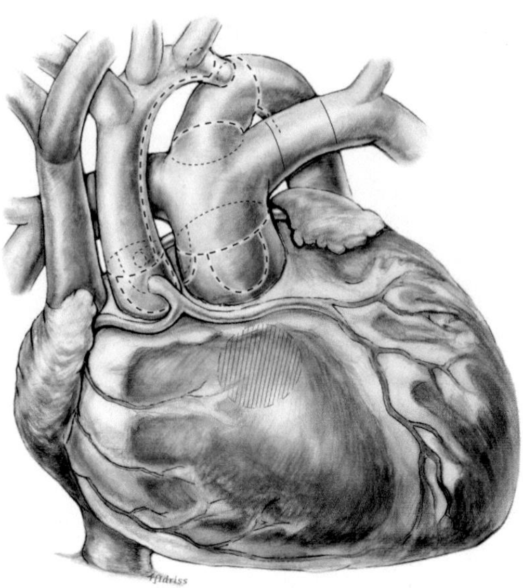

Fig. 19 Depicts the anatomic details and the prospective incisions, transections, and coronary button harvests that attend this operation. (With permission: Mavroudis 2015)

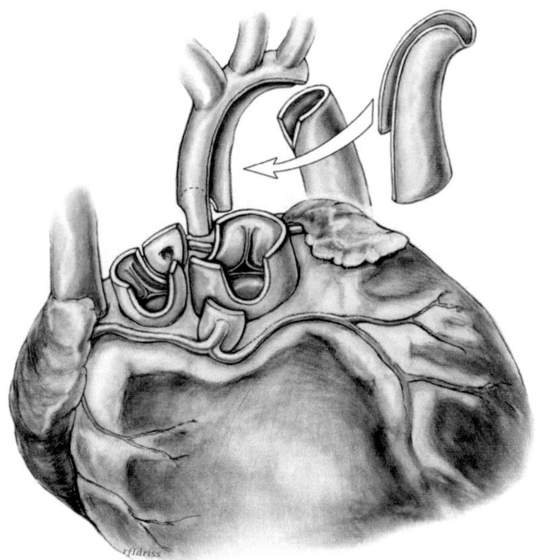

Fig. 20 Shows the relevant extracardiac diagrammatic repair segments for the Taussig-Bing Anomaly. These segmental maneuvers are to be performed in an organized fashion to accomplish the repair. When the transverse arch at the coarctation site is too narrow, all the ductal tissue is removed, and the posterior portion is re-approximated after adequate distal aorta mobilization. The transverse and ascending aortic arch is then augmented using a homograft patch configured to compliment the curve of the arch. This maneuver will also enlarge the proximal ascending aortic orifice for the neoaortic reconstruction (old pulmonary artery) which is always large owing to the great artery discrepancy that has been described in the text. (With permission: Mavroudis 2015)

but not in the proper order. A synopsis of the steps of the operation is noted in the figure. The potential complications associated with all of these maneuvers have been noted and include semilunar valve injury during the coronary artery button removal (Chapter "Complications Associated with Repair of Transposition of the Great Arteries and Associated Lesions"), coronary artery injury, ductal disruption (Chapters "Complications Associated with Repair of Coarctation of the Aorta" and "Complications Associated with Repair of Interrupted Aortic Arch"), great vessel injury during the dissection (Chapter "Complications Associated with Repair of Coarctation of the Aorta"), recurrent laryngeal nerve injury (Chapters "Complications Associated with Ligation of Patent Arterial Duct" and Complications Associated with Repair of Coarctation of the Aorta), and thoracic duct injury (Chapter "Complications Associated with Repair of Coarctation of the Aorta"). These complications have been discussed in these previous chapters. Precautions and resolution of these problems apply in this case as well.

Figure 21 shows the completed operation comprised of VSD closure, arterial switch with the Lecompte maneuver, and aortic arch reconstruction.

Besides the aforementioned procedural mishaps, other potential intraoperative complications for this complex and challenging procedure are neopulmonary artery stenosis due to the small caliber of the neopulmonary valve (old aortic valve) and left pulmonary artery stenosis due to the draping effect of the left pulmonary artery over the course of the augmented ascending aorta as both are shown in Fig. 22.

Selected studies have recommended that surgeons accept a reasonable amount of stenosis after this operation reasoning that the stenosis will abate with time (Yoo and Park 2013). Practical wisdom reflects that after a long and complex operation, immediate reinstitution of cardiopulmonary bypass to repair the right ventricular outflow tract and achieve a perfect result may be imprudent and could result in compromising postoperative ventricular dysfunction.

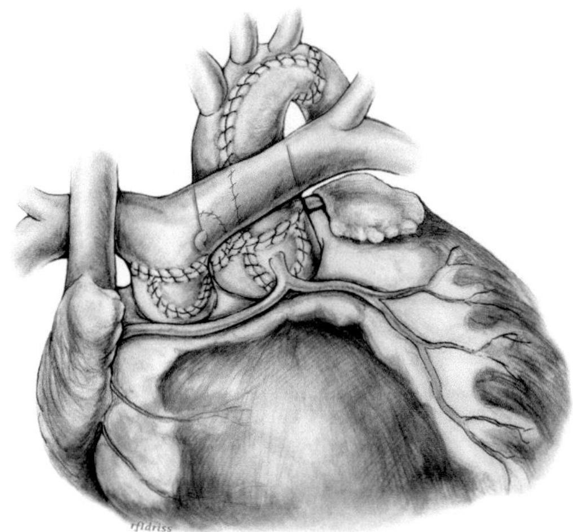

Fig. 21 The coronary transfer and Lecompte maneuver are accomplished before the neoaortic reconstruction, and the cross-clamp is removed. The patient can then be rewarmed while the neopulmonary artery reconstruction is being performed. (With permission: Mavroudis 2015)

If the decision to forego further reparative measures proves to be incorrect, the right pulmonary artery obstruction can be approached and repaired at a subsequent operation as noted in Fig. 23. The right ventricular outflow tract stenosis (annular stenosis) should be tolerated as much as possible (right ventricular pressure less than 70% of the left ventricular pressure) since repair will oftentimes require a right ventricular-to-pulmonary artery conduit to repair the stenosis and avoid injury to the crossing right coronary artery.

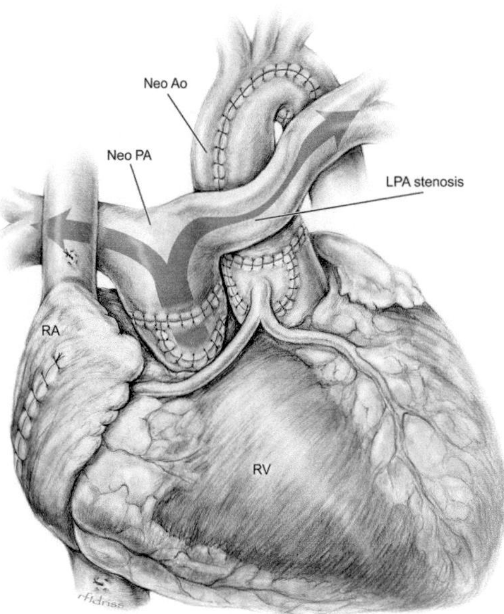

Fig. 22 This drawing demonstrates the potential problems with the repair resulting in left pulmonary artery stenosis due to left pulmonary artery draping over the ascending neoaorta. The arrow shows the decreased flow noted by narrower width over the neoaorta. This situation can cause right ventricular hypertension, hypertrophy, and differential pulmonary artery flow

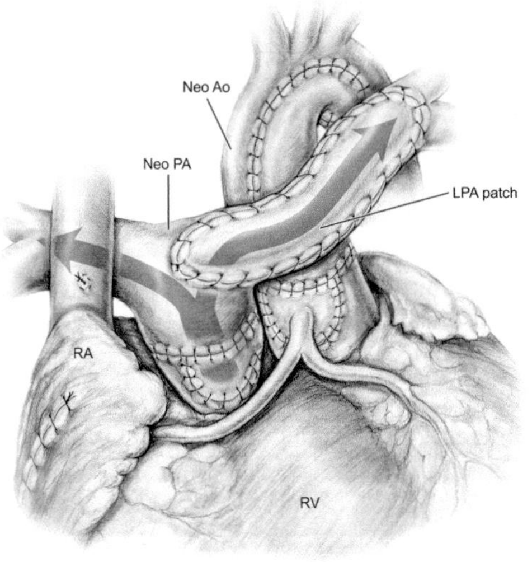

Fig. 23 Shows the repair of left pulmonary artery by patch augmentation over the course of the ascending neoaorta

8 Repair of Double Outlet Right Ventricle with Distant VSD by Complex Patch VSD Closure and Arterial Switch

When considering repair options for DORV with remote VSD, the opposing issues center on the controversial decision to apply a complex operation resulting in a two ventricular repair with pulsatile pulmonary artery flow versus single ventricle repair with nonpulsatile pulmonary artery flow (Fontan physiology). The alternatives involve a higher operative mortality achieving a biventricular repair compared with the lower operative mortality and reasonable lifestyle associated with Fontan physiology. Both options have their own sets of problems. The Fontan operation is relatively easy to visualize, and while some surgeons suggest that Fontan physiology might be better tolerated in patients with two competent ventricles, the results have proved otherwise (Marathe et al. 2019). Further to this, there is no getting around the reality that there are significant drawbacks of long-term Fontan physiology which include arrhythmias, protein-losing enteropathy, and pathway obstructions (Chungsomprasong et al. 2011; Frigiola and Lo Rito 2017; Kverneland et al. 2018). This can lead to atrioventricular valve regurgitation, unfavorable ventricular interaction, and eventual Fontan failure.

On the other hand, the benefits of an operation that result in a two-ventricular physiology is attractive. There is an adage that supports the idea that any two-ventricular repair is better than an excellent univentricular repair. There are several drawbacks to this theory, namely that the early mortality for the two-ventricular repair is higher, the chance for heart block is greater, and the possibility for future reoperations including VSD patch obstruction and left ventricular outflow tract obstruction are not insignificant (Delius et al. 1996). The controversy has not been settled. At the present time, prospective studies to resolve this controversy are nonexistent.

The determining anatomic factors that can help surgeons to decide the strategy for the two-ventricular repair in this entity are centered around the type of remote VSD, whether it be the atrioventricular septal defect type of VSD (inlet VSD) or large muscular VSD type without any anatomic association with either of the great arteries. In addition to this decision lies the importance of the intended pathway that will tunnel the left ventricular flow to the neoaorta after the arterial switch in anticipation of the arterial switch. These operations are not performed frequently. Consequently, surgeon experience and familiarity with the anatomy is required for a successful operation. Those who attempt this operation generally find that the inlet type of VSD is more amenable to a two-ventricular solution than the large muscular VSD (Lacour-Gayet et al. 2002; Belli et al. 1999; Lacour-Gayet 2008; Luisi et al. 1980; Kirklin and Castaneda 1977; Barbero-Marcial et al. 1999; Sridaromont et al. 1975; Bharati et al. 1980; Pacifico et al. 1980; Villemain et al. 2016); however, there are surgeons who do not hesitate to perform the two-ventricular repair to both types of VSD (Lacour-Gayet et al. 2002; Belli et al. 1999; Lacour-Gayet 2008; Luisi et al. 1980; Kirklin and Castaneda 1977; Barbero-Marcial et al. 1999; Sridaromont et al. 1975; Bharati et al. 1980; Pacifico et al. 1980; Villemain et al. 2016).

Figure 24 is an important depiction showing the interrelational anatomy of a patient with DORV with a remote atrioventricular type of VSD. The crossed line inferior to the inlet VSD shows the conduction system which is located on the left ventricular side of the VSD. The dashed line shows the area of potential VSD enlargement should the surgeon find it necessary. Also noted in the drawing is the prominent muscular conus which will require resection to prepare for an unobstructed pathway from the left ventricle to the intended neoaorta which is shown as the pulmonary artery. A complex two-cavity approach is essential for this repair oftentimes requiring two individual patches which can be connected after the anticipated pathway is formed. The right atrial exposure is preferred to form and establish the intraventricular tunnel in the same manner that is used to repair a tetralogy and atrioventricular septal defect. The superior part of the patch requires a focused expansion (larger patch in the outflow area), extension, and rotational reconstruction which is best approached and completed through a limited right ventriculotomy. Figure 25 shows the completed reconstruction. Not shown is the infundibular resection which is performed by careful attention to preserve the semilunar valves and limit the amount of ventricular resection at the inlet which can cause left ventricular dysfunction if the ventricular resection proves to be too extensive.

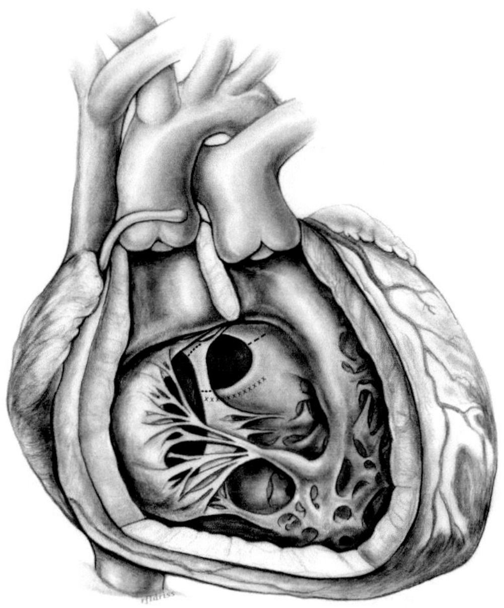

Fig. 24 Shows a coronal view of the relevant anatomy of a patient with DORV and remote VSD of the inlet (atrioventricular canal) type. The interrupted crossed line shows the course of the conduction system along the left ventricular side of the septum. The dashed line represents the area of intended VSD enlargement should it be needed. This location is away from the conduction system and if performed will have a lower chance of heart block than other locationsThis repair often requires a two-cavity approach (right atrium and right ventricle) and a complex patch which often requires two distinct patches which can be connected after the anticipated pathway is formed. The right atrial exposure is required to form the intraventricular tunnel in much the same way that it is used to repair a tetralogy and atrioventricular septal defect. The superior part of the patch requires a complex expansion (larger patch in the outflow area), extension, and rotational reconstruction which is best completed through a limited right ventriculotomy. (With permission: Mavroudis 2015)

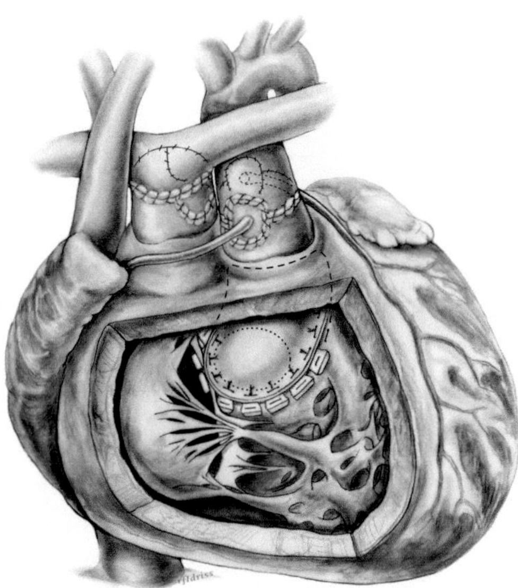

Fig. 25 Shows a coronal view of the repair by VSD closure using complex tunneling techniques involving two separate patches. One patch is performed through the right atrium in much the same way as is used for tetralogy with atrioventricular septal defect repair and the other patch is performed as an extension to the neoaorta through a limited right ventriculotomy. The patch edges are anchored by individual and interrupted pledgetted suture technique. (With permission: Mavroudis 2015)

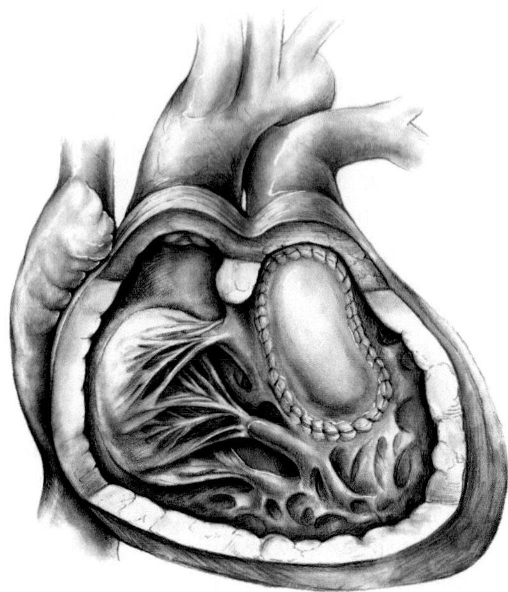

Fig. 26 Shows the completion of the complex intraventricular tunnel after the infundibular resection to allow an unobstructed pathway from the left ventricle to the pulmonary artery which is to become the neoaorta after arterial switch which is not shown. (With permission: Mavroudis 2015)

After the extensive patch is performed, antegrade and retrograde cardioplegia is readministered and the arterial switch operation can be performed using the Lecompte maneuver. Cavitary closure follows, cross-clamp and vent are removed, and separation from cardiopulmonary bypass is performed. For those patients who have a more favorably located large muscular VSD, a localized infundibular resection can prepare the outflow tract for a satisfactory intraventricular tunnel to connect the left ventricle with the pulmonary artery (neoaorta). Figure 26 shows the completion of the infundibular resection and tunnel reconstruction before the arterial switch operation is performed.

9 Repair of Double Outlet Left Ventricle by VSD Closure and Pulmonary Artery Translocation

Double outlet left ventricle (DOLV) is an infrequent congenital cardiac malformation with a ventriculoarterial connection that is defined by both great arteries arising entirely or mostly from the morphologic left ventricle (Bharati et al. 1978; Sakakibara et al. 1967; Paul et al. 1970; Kerr et al. 1971; Anderson et al. 1974b; Sharratt et al. 1976; Goor et al. 1972; Van Praagh et al. 1972; Van Praagh and Weinberg 1983; DeLeon et al. 1995; Chiavarelli et al. 1992; McElhinney et al. 1997; Brandt et al. 1976). To make things more complicated, associated lesions can occur and include pulmonary stenosis, situs inversus, atrioventricular discordance, and variations of the relationship of the pulmonary artery to the aorta. The classical approach to these patients, assuming two normal sized ventricles and atrioventricular concordance, has traditionally been based on the Rastelli principle which can be accomplished by VSD closure and right ventricular-to-pulmonary artery conduit. There are two methods to complete the right ventricular-to-pulmonary artery continuity based on the amount of pulmonary artery stenosis. For those patients with pulmonary artery stenosis, a ventricular-to-pulmonary valved conduit is necessary since the extant anatomy prohibits a right ventricular transannular patch. For those without pulmonary artery stenosis, a pulmonary artery root harvest can be moved from the left ventricular outflow to the right ventricular outflow with a well-placed VSD patch (pulmonary artery root translocation).

Figure 27 shows the cannulation technique for subpulmonic VSD closure en route to right ventricular-to-pulmonary artery conduit or pulmonary root translocation. Preliminary exposure is performed by aortobicaval cardiopulmonary bypass, left ventricular venting, aortic cross-clamping with cardioplegic arrest, and right ventriculotomy. The initial evaluation is to confirm the extant great vessel anatomy by placing a curved clamp through the VSD to make sure that both great vessels are originating from the left ventricle as noted in Fig. 27. The left panel shows the curved clamp through the VSD to identify the pulmonary artery. The right panel shows the curved clamp through the VSD to identify the aorta.

Patients with associated pulmonary stenosis can undergo transventricular VSD closure with secure suture placement that includes the subpul-

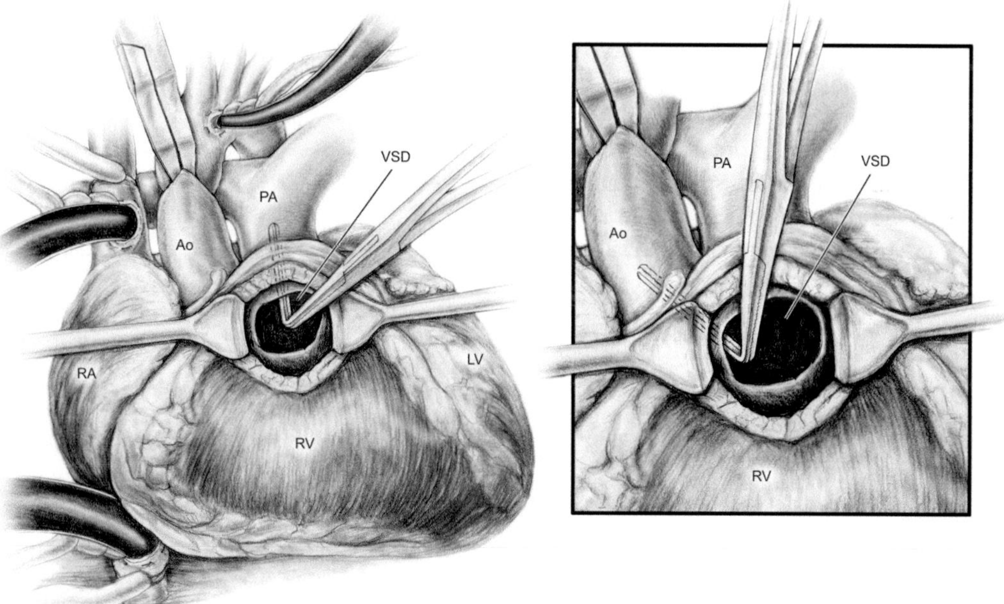

Fig. 27 Shows aortobicaval cardiopulmonary bypass, aortic cross-clamping with cardioplegic arrest, and left ventricular venting in a patient with DOLV. After a right ventriculotomy is performed a curved clamp is placed through the VSD to identify the pulmonary artery (left panel) and the aorta (right panel) to make sure that VSD closure will tunnel the left ventricle to the aorta and the pulmonary artery. This will allow the pulmonary artery to be transected with proximal oversewing and establishing a right ventricular to pulmonary conduit. *Ao* aorta, *LV* left ventricle, *PA* pulmonary artery, *RA* right atrium, *RV* right ventricle, *VSD* ventricular septal defect

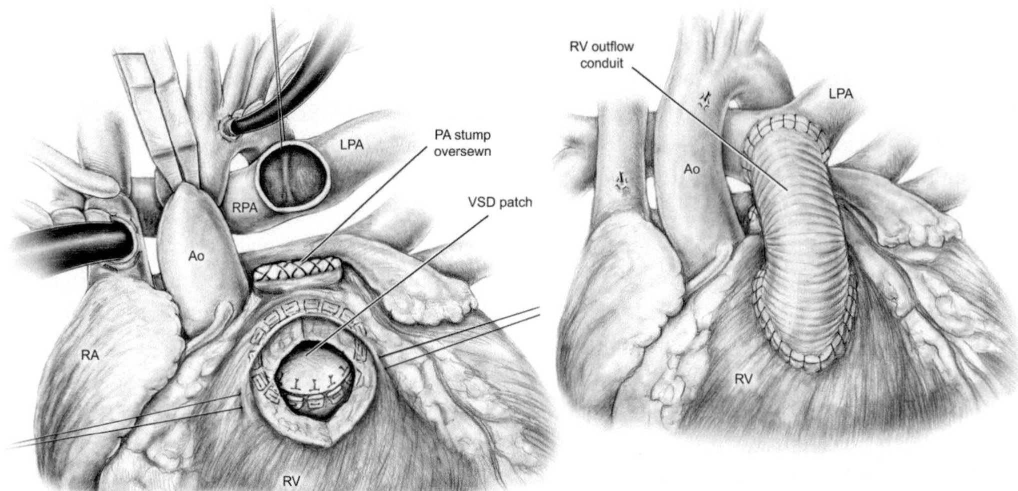

Fig. 28 Shows the DOLV repair completion by VSD closure using interrupted pledgetted suture technique (left panel) and right ventricle to pulmonary artery conduit after appropriate establishment of left ventricular to aortic continuity (Right Panel). *Ao* aorta, *LPA* left pulmonary artery, *PA* pulmonary artery, *RA* right atrium, *RPA* right pulmonary artery, *RV* right ventricle, *VSD* ventricular septal defect

monic conus as shown in Fig. 28 (left panel). The operation is completed by an extracardiac right ventricular-to-pulmonary artery conduit (Fig. 28 Right Panel). Those patients for whom pulmonary stenosis is not a contributing factor, pulmonary artery translocation from the left ventricular outflow to the right ventricle can be entertained as long as the course of the left main coronary artery can be avoided by the translocation. The VSD closure is very complicated in this situation since the patch involves the ventricular septum with extension to the area from where the pulmonary artery trunk arose. It is here where the coronary artery could be damaged. If the operation can be safely performed the pulmonary artery trunk can then be attached to the right ventricle with an augmentation patch.

References

Abe T, Sugiki K, Izumiyama O, et al. A successful procedure for correction of the Taussig-Bing malformation. J Thorac Cardiovasc Surg. 1984;87:403–9.

Agarwala B, Doyle EF, Danilowicz D, et al. Double outlet right ventricle with pulmonic stenosis and anteriorly positioned aorta (Taussig-Bing variant). Report of a case and surgical correction. Am J Cardiol. 1973;32:850–4.

Alfieri O, Crupi G, Vanini V, Parenzan L. Successful surgical repair of double outlet right ventricle with situs inversus, l-loop, l-malposition and subaortic VSD in a 16-month-old patient. Eur J Cardiol. 1978;7:41–7.

Alsoufi B, Cai S, Williams WG, et al. Improved results with single-stage total correction of Taussig-Bing anomaly. Eur J Cardiothorac Surg. 2008;33:244–50.

Anderson RH (1978) The morphogenesis of ventriculoarterial discordance. In: Van Mierop LHS, Oppenheimer-Dekker A, Bruins CLD, eds. Embryology and tetralogy of the heart and great arteries Leiden University Press, The Hague.

Anderson RH, Wilkinson JL, Arnold R, Becker AE, Lubkiewicz K. Morphogenesis of bulboventricular malformations. II. Observations on malformed hearts. Br Heart J. 1974a;36:948–70.

Anderson R, Galbraith R, Gibson R, et al. Double outlet left ventricle. Br Heart J. 1974b;36:554–8.

Anderson RH, Pickering D, Brown R. Double outlet right ventricle with L-malposition and uncommitted ventricular septal defect. Eur J Cardiol. 1975;3:133–42.

Anderson RH, Becker AE, Wilcox BR, Macartney FJ, Wilkinson JL. Surgical anatomy of double-outlet right ventricle–a reappraisal. Am J Cardiol. 1983;52:555–9.

Angelini P, Leachman RD. The spectrum of double outlet right ventricle: an embryologic interpretation. Cardiovasc Dis. 1976;3:127–49.

Artrip JH, Sauer H, Campbell DN, Mitchell MB, Haun C, Almodovar MC, Hraska V, Lacour-Gayet F. Biventricular repair in double outlet right ventricle: surgical results based on the STS-EACTS international nomenclature classification. Eur J Cardiothorac Surg. 2006;29:545–50.

Backer CL. Double outlet right ventricle: where are we now? Semin Thorac Cardiovasc Surg. 2016;28:79–80.

Backer CL. Commentary: double-outlet right ventricle revisited. J Thorac Cardiovasc Surg. 2020;159:265.

Barbero-Marcial M, Tanamati C, Atik E, Ebaid M. Intraventricular repair of double-outlet right ventricle with noncommitted ventricular septal defect: advantages of multiple patches. J Thorac Cardiovasc Surg. 1999;118:1056–67.

Bartelings MM, Gittenberger-de Groot AC. The outflow tract of the heart–embryologic and morphologic correlations. Int J Cardiol. 1989;22:289–300.

Belli E, Serraf A, Lacour-Gayet F, Prodan S, Piot D, Losay J, Petit J, Bruniaux J, Planché C. Biventricular repair for double-outlet right ventricle. Results and long-term follow-up. Circulation. 1998;98(Suppl 19):II360–7.

Belli E, Serraf A, Lacour-Gayet F, et al. Double-outlet right ventricle with non-committed ventricular septal defect. Eur J Cardiothorac Surg. 1999;15:747–52.

Beuren A. Differential diagnosis of the Taussig-Bing heart from complete transposition of the great vessels with a posteriorly overriding pulmonary artery. Circulation. 1960;21:1071–87.

Bharati S, Lev M, Stewart R, et al. The morphologic spectrum of double outlet left ventricle and its surgical significance. Circulation. 1978;58:558–65.

Bharati S, Kirklin JW, McAllister HA Jr, et al. The surgical anatomy of common atrioventricular orifice associated with tetralogy of Fallot, double outlet right ventricle and complete regular transposition. Circulation. 1980;61:1142–9.

Binet JP, Lacour-Gayet F, Conso JF, et al. Complete repair of the Taussig-Bing type of double-outlet right ventricle using the arterial switch operation without coronary translocation. Report of one successful case. J Thorac Cardiovasc Surg. 1983;85:272–5.

Bradley TJ, Karamlou T, Kulik A, et al. Determinants of repair type, reintervention, and mortality in 393 children with double-outlet right ventricle. J Thorac Cardiovasc Surg. 2007;134:967–73.

Brandt PW, Calder AL, Barratt-Boyes BG, Neutze JM. Double outlet left ventricle. Morphology, cineangiocardio-graphic diagnosis and surgical treatment. Am J Cardiol. 1976;38:897–909.

Braun K, De Vries A, Feingold DS, Ehrenfeld NE, Feldman J, Schorr S. Complete dextroposition of the aorta, pulmonary stenosis, interventricular septal defect, and patent foramen ovale. Am Heart J. 1952;43:773–80.

Brown JW, Ruzmetov M, Okada Y, Vijay P, Turrentine MW. Surgical results in patients with double outlet right ventricle: a 20-year experience. Ann Thorac Surg. 2001;72:1630–5.

Cheng TO. Double outlet right ventricle: diagnosis during life. Am J Med. 1962;32:637–44.

Chiavarelli M, Boucek MM, Bailey LL. Arterial correction of double-outlet left ventricule by pulmonary artery translocation. Ann Thorac Surg. 1992;53:1098–100.

Chungsomprasong P, Soongswang J, Nana A, Durongpisitkul K, Loahaprasitiporn D, Vijansorn C, Sriyodchartti S. Medium and long-term outcomes of Fontan operation. J Med Assoc Thail. 2011;94:323–30.

Daicoff GR, Kirklin JW. Surgical correction of Taussig-Bing malformation. Report of three cases. Am J Cardiol. 1967;19:125. (abst)

Danielson GK. A successful procedure for correction of the Taussig-Bing malformation. (invited commentary). J Thorac Cardiovasc Surg. 1984;87:403.

Danielson GK, Ritter DG, Coleman HN 3rd, DuShane JW. Successful repair of double-outlet right ventricle with transposition of the great arteries (aorta anterior and to the left), pulmonary stenosis, and subaortic ventricular septal defect. J Thorac Cardiovasc Surg. 1972;63:741–6.

Danielson GK, Tabry IF, Ritter DG, Maloney JD. Successful repair of double-outlet right ventricle, complete atrioventricular canal, and atrioventricular discordance associated with dextrocardia and pulmonary stenosis. J Thorac Cardiovasc Surg. 1978;76:710–7.

De Azevedo AC, Toledo AN, De Carvalho AA, Roubach R. Transposition of the aorta and levoposition of the pulmonary artery (Taussig-Bing syndrome). Am Heart J. 1956;52:249–56.

DeLeon SY, Ow EP, Chiemmongkoltip P, et al. Alternatives in biventricular repair of double-outlet left ventricle. Ann Thorac Surg. 1995;60:213–6.

Delius RE, Rademecker MA, de Leval MR, Elliott MJ, Stark J. Is a high-risk biventricular repair always preferable to conversion to a single ventricle repair? J Thorac Cardiovasc Surg. 1996;112:1561–8.

Doty DB. Correction of Taussig-Bing malformation by intraventricular conduit. J Thorac Cardiovasc Surg. 1986;91:133–8.

Ebadi A, Spicer DE, Backer CL, Fricker FJ, Anderson RH. Double-outlet right ventricle revisited. J Thorac Cardiovasc Surg. 2017;154:598–604.

Edwards WD. Double-outlet right ventricle and tetralogy of Fallot. Two distinct but not mutually exclusive entities. J Thorac Cardiovasc Surg. 1981;82:418–22.

Engle MA, Steinberg I. Angiocardiography in diagnosis of transposition of aorta with subaortic ventricular septal defect (origin of both great vessels from right ventricle). Circulation. 1961;24:927. (abst)

Franklin RC, Anderson RH, Daniels O, et al. Report of the coding Committee of the Association for European paediatric cardiology. Cardiol Young. 2002;12:611–8.

Freedom RM, Yoo SJ. Double-outlet right ventricle: pathology and angiocardiography. Semin Thorac Cardiovasc Surg Pediatr Card Surg Annu. 2000;3:3–19.

Frigiola A, Lo Rito M. Le complicanze tardive dell'intervento di Fontan [Late complications of Fontan operation]. G Ital Cardiol (Rome). 2017;18:625–30. Italian

Gittenberger-de Groot AC, Sauer U, Oppenheimer-Dekker A, et al. Coronary arterial anatomy in transposition of the great arteries: a morphologic study. Pediatr Cardiol. 1983;4(Suppl I):15–24.

Goor DA, Ebert PA. Left ventricular outflow obstruction in Taussig-Bing malformation. J Thorac Cardiovasc Surg. 1975;70:69–75.

Goor DA, Lillehei CW. Congenital malformations of the heart. New York: Grune & Stratton; 1975.

Goor DA, Dische R, Lillehei CW. The conotruncus. I. Its normal inversion and conus absorption. Circulation. 1972;46:375–84.

Griselli M, McGuirk SP, Ko C, et al. Arterial switch operation in patients with Taussig-Bing anomaly—influence of staged repair and coronary anatomy on outcome. Eur J Cardiothorac Surg. 2007;31:229–35.

Harvey JC, Sondheimer HM, Williams WG, et al. Repair of double-outlet right ventricle. J Thorac Cardiovasc Surg. 1977;73:611–5.

Hayes DA, Jones S, Quaegebeur JM, et al. Primary arterial switch operation as a strategy for total correction of Taussig-Bing anomaly: a 21-year experience. Circulation. 2013;128(11 Suppl 1):S194–8.

Hightower BM, Barcia A, Bargeron LM Jr, Kirklin JW. Double-outlet right ventricle with transposed great arteries and subpulmonary ventricular septal defect. The Taussig-Bing malformation (abstr). Circulation. 1969;39(5 Suppl 1):I207–13.

Howell CE, Ho SY, Anderson RH, Elliott MJ. Fibrous skeleton and ventricular outflow tracts in double-outlet right ventricle. Ann Thorac Surg. 1991;51:394–400.

Kanter K, Anderson R, Lincoln C, et al. Anatomic correction of double-outlet right ventricle with subpulmonary ventricular septal defect (the "Taussig-Bing" anomaly). Ann Thorac Surg. 1986;41:287–92.

Kawahira Y, Yagihara T, Uemura H, et al. Ventricular outflow tracts after Kawashima intraventricular rerouting for double outlet right ventricle with subpulmonary ventricular septal defect. Eur J Cardiothorac Surg. 1999;16:26–31.

Kawashima Y, Fujita T, Miyamoto T, Manabe H. Intraventricular rerouting of blood for the correction of Taussig-Bing malformation. J Thorac Cardiovasc Surg. 1971;62:825–9.

Kawashima Y, Matsuda H, Yagihara T, et al. Intraventricular repair for Taussig-Bing anomaly. J Thorac Cardiovasc Surg. 1993;105:591–7.

Kerr AR, Barcia A, Bargeron LM Jr, et al. Double-outlet left ventricle with ventricular septal defect and pulmonary stenosis: report of surgical repair. Am Heart J. 1971;81:688–93.

Kirklin JK, Castaneda AR. Surgical correction of double-outlet right ventricle with noncommitted ventricular septal defect. J Thorac Cardiovasc Surg. 1977;73:399–403.

Kirklin JW, Harp RA, McGoon DC. Surgical treatment of origin of both vessels from right ventricle, including cases of pulmonary stenosis. J Thorac Cardiovasc Surg. 1964;48:1026–36.

Kirklin JW, Pacifico AD, Blackstone EH, Kirklin JK, Bargerson LM Jr. Current risks and protocols for operations for double-outlet right ventricle. Derivation from an 18 year experience. J Thorac Cardiovasc Surg. 1986;92:913–30.

Kleinert S, Sano T, Weintraub RG, et al. Anatomic features and surgical strategies in double-outlet right ventricle. Circulation. 1997;96:1233–9.

Kverneland LS, Kramer P, Ovroutski S. Five decades of the Fontan operation: a systematic review of international reports on outcomes after univentricular palliation. Congenit Heart Dis. 2018;13:181–93.

Lacour-Gayet F. Intracardiac repair of double outlet right ventricle. Semin Thorac Cardiovasc Surg Pediatr Card Surg Annu. 2008;11:39–43.

Lacour-Gayet F, Haun C, Ntalakoura K, et al. Biventricular repair of double outlet right ventricle with non-committed ventricular septal defect (VSD) by VSD rerouting to the pulmonary artery and arterial switch. Eur J Cardiothorac Surg. 2002;21:1042–8.

Lauer RM, DuShane JW, Edwards JE. Obstruction of left ventricular outlet in association with ventricular septal defect. Circulation. 1960;22:110–24.

Lavoie R, Sestier F, Gilbert G, Chameides L, Van Praagh R, Grondin P. Double outlet right ventricle with left ventricular outflow tract obstruction due to small ventricular septal defect. Am Heart J. 1971;82:290–9.

Lecompte Y, Batisse A, DiCarlo D. Double-outlet right ventricle: a surgical synthesis. In: Advances in cardiac surgery, vol. 4. St Louis: Mosby-Yearbook, Inc; 1993. p. 109–36.

Lev M, Bharati S, Meng CC, Liberthson RR, Paul MH, Idriss F. A concept of double-outlet right ventricle. J Thorac Cardiovasc Surg. 1972;64:271–81.

Li S, Ma K, Hu S, et al. Surgical outcomes of 380 patients with double outlet right ventricle who underwent biventricular repair. J Thorac Cardiovasc Surg. 2014;148:817–24.

Lopez FN, Dobben GG, Rabinowitz M, et al. Taussig-Bing complex with pulmonary stenosis. Dis Chest. 1966;50:1–12.

Luber JM, Castaneda AR, Lang P, et al. Repair of double-outlet right ventricle: early and late results. Circulation. 1983;68:II144–7.

Luisi VS, Pasqué A, Verunelli F, Eufrate S. Double outlet right ventricle, non-committed ventricular septal defect and pulmonic stenosis. Anatomical and surgical considerations. Thorac Cardiovasc Surg. 1980;28:368–70.

Mahle WT, Martinez R, Silverman N, Cohen MS, Anderson RH. Anatomy, echocardiography, and surgical approach to double outlet right ventricle. Cardiol Young. 2008;18(Suppl 3):39–51.

Marathe SP, Zannino D, Shi WY, du Plessis K, Kehr J, Perumal G, Sun J, Gentles TL, Ayer J, Sholler GF, Verrall CE, Alphonso N, Andrews D, d'Udekem Y, Winlaw DS. Two ventricles are not better than one in the Fontan circulation: equivalent late outcomes. Ann Thorac Surg. 2019;107:852–9.

Marin-Garcia J, Neches WH, Park SC, Lenox CC, Zuberbuhler JR, Bahnson HT. Double-outlet right ventricle with restrictive ventricular septal defect. J Thorac Cardiovasc Surg. 1978;76:853–8.

Mason DT, Morrow AG, Elkins RC, Friedman WF. Origin of both great vessels from the right ventricle associated with severe obstruction to left ventricular outflow. Am J Cardiol. 1969;24:118–24.

Matsuoka Y, Akimoto K, Sennari E, Hayakawa K. Double outlet right ventricle with severe left ventricular outflow tract obstruction due to small ventricular septal defect and anomalous adherence of the mitral valve to the ventricular septum. Jpn Circ J. 1987;51:1335–40.

Mavroudis C. Double-outlet ventricles (with two adequate ventricles). In: Mavroudis C, Backer CL, editors. Atlas of pediatric cardiac surgery. London: Springer; 2015.

Mavroudis C. Coronary artery bypass grafting in infants, children, and young adults for acquired and congenital lesions. Congenit Heart Dis. 2017;12:644–6.

Mavroudis C, Backer CL, Muster AJ, et al. Taussig-Bing anomaly: arterial switch versus Kawashima intraventricular repair. Ann Thorac Surg. 1996a;61:1330–8.

Mavroudis C, Backer CL, Muster AJ, Pahl E, Sanders JH, Zales VR, Gevitz M. Expanding indications for pediatric coronary artery bypass. J Thorac Cardiovasc Surg. 1996b;111:181–9.

McElhinney DB, Reddy VM, Hanley FL. Pulmonary root translocation for biventricular repair of double-outlet left ventricle with absent subpulmonic conus. J Thorac Cardiovasc Surg. 1997;114:501–3.

Mehrizi A. The origin of both great vessels from the right ventricle. I with pulmonic stenosis. Clinicopathological correlation in 18 autopsied cases. Bull Johns Hopkins Hosp. 1965;117:75.

Metras D, Coulibaly AO, Ouattara K. Successful intraventricular repair of Taussig-Bing anomaly in infancy: report of a case. J Thorac Cardiovasc Surg. 1984;88:311–2.

Meyer J, Peul GJ Jr, Chiarello L, Hallman GL, Cooley DA. Anomalous origin and distribution of coronary arteries. Review of 38 patients who underwent operation. J Cardiovasc Surg. 1975;16:500–5.

Neufeld HN, DuShane JW, Edwards JE. Origin of both great vessels from the right ventricle. II With pulmonary stenosis. Circulation. 1961a;23:603–12.

Neufeld HN, DuShane JW, Wood EH, Kirklin JW, Edwards JE. Origin of both great vessels from the right ventricle. I. Without pulmonary stenosis. Circulation. 1961b;23:399–412.

Neufeld HN, Lucas RV Jr, Lester RG, Adams P Jr, Anderson RC, Edwards JE. Origin of both great vessels from the right ventricle without pulmonary stenosis. Br Heart J. 1962;24:393–408.

Okamoto N. Congenital anomalies of the heart. Embryologic, morphologic and experimental teratology. Tokyo: Igaku-Shoin; 1980.

Oladunjoye O, Piekarski B, Baird C, et al. Repair of double outlet right ventricle: midterm outcomes. J Thorac Cardiovasc Surg. 2020;159:254–64.

Ottino G, Kugler JD, McNamara DG, et al. Taussig-Bing anomaly: total repair with closure of ventricular septal defect through the pulmonary artery. Ann Thorac Surg. 1980;29:170–6.

Pacifico AD, Kirklin JW, Bargeron LM Jr. Repair of complete atrioventricular canal associated with tetralogy of Fallot or double-outlet right ventricle: report of 10 patients. Ann Thorac Surg. 1980;29:351–6.

Pacifico AD, Kirklin JK, Colvin EV, et al. Intraventricular tunnel repair for Taussig-Bing heart and related cardiac anomalies. Circulation. 1986;74:I53–60.

Patrick DL, McGoon DC. An operation for double-outlet right ventricle with transposition of the great arteries. J Cardiovasc Surg. 1968;9:537–42.

Paul MH, Muster AJ, Sinha SN, et al. Double-outlet left ventricle with an intact ventricular septum. Clinical and autopsy diagnosis and developmental implications. Circulation. 1970;41:129–39.

Peacock TB. Malformations of the human heart. 2nd ed. London: J. Churchill and Sons; 1866.

Piccoli G, Pacifico AD, Kirklin JW, Blackstone EH, Kirklin JK, Bargerson LM Jr. Changing results and concepts in the surgical treatment of double-outlet right ventricle: analysis of 137 operations in 126 patients. Am J Cardiol. 1983;52:549–54.

Quintero OL, Giraldo JC, Sandoval NF. Successful management of massive air embolism during cardiopulmonary bypass using multimodal neuroprotection strategies. Semin Cardiothorac Vasc Anesth. 2019;23:324–32.

Raisky O, Vouhé PR. Pitfalls in repair of conotruncal anomalies. Semin Thorac Cardiovasc Surg Pediatr Card Surg Annu. 2013;16:7–12.

Rokitansky K. Die Defecte der Scheidewande des Herzens: Pathologisch-anatomische Abhandlung. Wein: Wilhelm Braumuller; 1875.

Ruttenberg HD, Anderson RC, Elliott LP, Edwards JE. Origin of both great vessels from the arterial ventricle: a complex with ventricular inversion. Br Heart J. 1964;26:631–41.

Sakakibara S, Takao A, Arai T, et al. Both great vessels arising from the left ventricle. Bull Heart Inst Jpn. 1967;11:66–86.

Sakata R, Lecompte Y, Batisse A, Borromée L, Durandy Y. Anatomic repair of anomalies of ventriculoarterial connection associated with ventricular septal defect. I. Criteria of surgical decision. J Thorac Cardiovasc Surg. 1988;95:90–5.

Serratto M, Arevalo F, Goldman EJ, Hastreiter A, Miller RA. Obstructive ventricular septal defect in double outlet right ventricle. Am J Cardiol. 1967;19:457–63.

Shafer AB, Lopez JF, Kline IK, Lev M. Truncal inversion with biventricular pulmonary trunk and aorta from right ventricle (variant of Taussig-Bing complex). Circulation. 1967;36:783–8.

Sharratt GP, Sbokos CG, Johnson AM, et al. Surgical "correction" of solitus-concordant, double-outlet left ventricle with L-malposition and tricuspid stenosis with hypoplastic right ventricle. J Thorac Cardiovasc Surg. 1976;71:853–8.

Sinzobahamvya N, Blaschczok HC, Asfour B, et al. Right ventricular outflow tract obstruction after arterial switch operation for the Taussig-Bing heart. Eur J Cardiothorac Surg. 2007;31:873–8.

Smith EE, Pucci JJ, Walesby RK, et al. A new technique for correction of the Taussig-Bing anomaly. J Thorac Cardiovasc Surg. 1982;83:901–4.

Sondheimer HM, Freedom RM, Olley PM. Double outlet right ventricle: clinical spectrum and prognosis. Am J Cardiol. 1977;39:709–14.

Soszyn N, Fricke TA, Wheaton GR, et al. Outcomes of the arterial switch operation in patients with Taussig-Bing anomaly. Ann Thorac Surg. 2011;92:673–9.

Sridaromont S, Feldt RH, Ritter DG, et al. Double-outlet right ventricle associated with persistent common atrioventricular canal. Circulation. 1975;52:933–42.

Sridaromont S, Feldt RH, Ritter DG, et al. Double outlet right ventricle: hemodynamic and anatomic correlations. Am J Cardiol. 1976;38:85–94.

Sridaromont S, Ritter DG, Feldt RH, Davis GD, Edwards JE. Double-outlet right ventricle. Anatomic and angiocardiographic correlations. Mayo Clin Proc. 1978;53:555–77.

Stewart S. Double-outlet right ventricle (S,D,D), VSD related to pulmonary artery, and pulmonic stenosis absent. Correction with an intraventricular conduit in infancy. J Thorac Cardiovasc Surg. 1977;74:70–2.

Stewart RW, Kirklin JW, Pacifico AD, Blackstone EH, Bargerson LM Jr. Repair of double-outlet right ventricle. An analysis of 62 cases. J Thorac Cardiovasc Surg. 1979;78:502–14.

Tabry IF, McGoon DC, Danielson GK, Wallace RB, Davis Z, Maloney JD. Surgical management of double-outlet right ventricle associated with atrioventricular discordance. J Thorac Cardiovasc Surg. 1978;76:336–44.

Taussig HB, Bing RJ. Complete transposition of the aorta and a levoposition of the pulmonary artery; clinical, physiological, and pathological findings. Am Heart J. 1949;37:551–9.

Tchervenkov CI, Marelli D, Beland MJ, et al. Institutional experience with a protocol of early primary repair of double-outlet right ventricle. Ann Thorac Surg. 1995;60(Suppl 6):S610–3.

Tchervenkov CI, Walters HL 3rd, Chu VF. Congenital heart surgery nomenclature and database project: double outlet left ventricle. Ann Thorac Surg. 2000;69(Suppl 4):S264–9.

Tynan MJ, Becker AE, Macartney FJ, Jiménez MQ, Shinebourne EA, Anderson RH. Nomenclature and classification of congenital heart disease. Br Heart J. 1979;41:544–53.

van Buchem FSP, van Wermeskerken JL, Orie NGM. Transposition of the aorta (Taussig's syndrome). Acta Med Scand. 1950;137:66–77.

van Mierop LH, Gessner IH. Pathogenetic mechanisms in congenital cardiovascular malformations. Prog Cardiovasc Dis. 1972;15:67–85.

van Mierop LH, Wiglesworth FW. Pathogenesis of transposition complexes. II. Anomalies due to faulty transfer of the posterior great artery. Am J Cardiol. 1963;12:226–32.

Van Praagh R. What is the Taussig-Bing malformation? Circulation. 1968;38:445–9.

Van Praagh R. Conotruncal malformations. In: Barratt-Boyes BG, Neutze JM, Harris EA, editors. Heart disease in infancy. Edinburgh: Churchill Livingstone; 1973.

Van Praagh R, Weinberg PM. Double outlet left ventricle. In: Adams FH, Emmanouilides GC, editors. Heart disease in infants, children, and adolescents. 3rd ed. Baltimore: Williams & Wilkins; 1983.

Van Praagh R, Calder AL, Delisle G. Transposition of the great arteries with overriding aorta and pulmonary stenosis. New entity and its surgical management (abstr). Circulation. 1972;46(Suppl II):II96.

Van Praagh R, David I, Wright GB, Van Praagh S. Large RV plus small LV is not single RV. Circulation. 1980;61:1057–9.

Villemain O, Bonnet D, Houyel L, et al. Double-outlet right ventricle with noncommitted ventricular septal defect and 2 adequate ventricles: is anatomical repair advantageous? Semin Thorac Cardiovasc Surg. 2016;28:69–77.

Walters HL III, Pacifico AD. Double outlet ventricles. In: Mavroudis C, Backer CL, editors. Pediatric cardiac surgery. 3rd ed. Philadelphia: Mosby Inc; 2003. p. 408–41.

Walters HL III, Mavroudis C, Tchervenkov CI, et al. Congenital heart surgery nomenclature and database project: double outlet right ventricle. Ann Thorac Surg. 2000;69(Suppl 4):S249–63.

Wedemeyer AL, Lucas RV Jr, Castaneda AR. Taussig-Bing malformation, coarctation of the aorta, and reversed patent ductus arteriosus. Operative correction in an infant. Circulation. 1970;42:1021–7.

Wetter J, Sinzobahamvya N, Blaschczok HC, et al. Results of arterial switch operation for primary total correction of the Taussig-Bing anomaly. Ann Thorac Surg. 2004;77:41–7.

Wilcox BR, Ho SY, Macartney FJ, Becker AE, Gelis LM, Anderson RH. Surgical anatomy of double-outlet right ventricle with situs solitus and atrioventricular concordance. J Thorac Cardiovasc Surg. 1981;82:405–17.

Witham AC. Double outlet right ventricle; a partial transposition complex. Am Heart J. 1957;53:928–39.

Yoo BW, Park HK. Pulmonary stenosis and pulmonary regurgitation: both ends of the spectrum in residual hemodynamic impairment after tetralogy of Fallot repair. Korean J Pediatr. 2013;56:235–41. [Published correction appears in Korean J Pediatr. 2016 Sep;59(9):384-385]

Yoo SJ, van Arsdell GS. 3D printing in surgical management of double outlet right ventricle. Front Pediatr. 2018;5:289.

Yoo SJ, Thabit O, Kim EK, et al. 3D printing in medicine of congenital heart diseases. 3D Print Med. 2015;2(1):3.

Zamora R, Moller JH, Edwards JE. Double-outlet right ventricle. Anatomic types and associated anomalies. Chest. 1975;68:672–7.

Complications Associated with Repair of Congenitally Corrected Transposition of the Great Arteries

Constantine Mavroudis and Tom R. Karl

Abstract

Congenitally corrected transposition of the great arteries (ccTGA) is a complex congenital heart defect that is defined by reversed (discordant) atrioventricular (AV) and ventriculoarterial (VA) connections. Physiologic (leaving the right ventricle in the systemic circuit and the left ventricle in the pulmonary circuit) and anatomic (placing the right ventricle in the pulmonary circuit and the left ventricle in the systemic circuit) repairs have been used. This chapter will discuss the multiple operations for ccTGA including anatomic correction via the double switch operation, Senning or Mustard, and intra-atrial baffle plus translocation of the great vessels. In addition, we will examine the roles of the Fontan operation and cardiac transplantation for complex ccTGA. The attendant complications related to these procedures will be explored.

Keywords

Congenital heart surgery · Congenitally corrected transposition of the great arteries · Physiologic repair · Anatomic repair · Double switch operation · Atrial switch operation · Rastelli procedure · Outcomes

1 Introduction

Congenitally corrected transposition of the great arteries (ccTGA) is a complex cardiac malformation which is characterized by reversed (discordant) atrioventricular (AV) and ventriculo-arterial (VA) connections. There are many other descriptive terms to describe this anomaly including corrected transposition, discordant transposition, AV and VA discordance, physiologically corrected transposition, double discordance, AV discordance with transposition, L-transposition, and inverted transposition, among others. Figure 1 with the associated legend reviews the nomenclature characteristics related to the informative illustration (Mavroudis 2015). In addition to these classification schemes there is a standard segmental nomenclature which also has been used to describe the variants (Karl and Jacobs 2023). When considering the segmental approach, the most common configuration is atrial situs solitus with left ventricular loop and left TGA {S,L,L}. Less common is ccTGA with atrial situs

C. Mavroudis (✉)
Chief of Pediatric Cardiothoracic Surgery (Retired), Peyton Manning Children's Hospital, Indianapolis, IN, USA

Professor Emeritus of Surgery, Johns Hopkins University School of Medicine, Baltimore, MD, USA

T. R. Karl
Queensland Pediatric Cardiac Service, University of Queensland, Brisbane, Australia

C. L. Backer, C. Mavroudis (eds.), *Complications in Pediatric and Congenital Heart Surgery*, https://doi.org/10.1007/978-3-032-02661-3_16

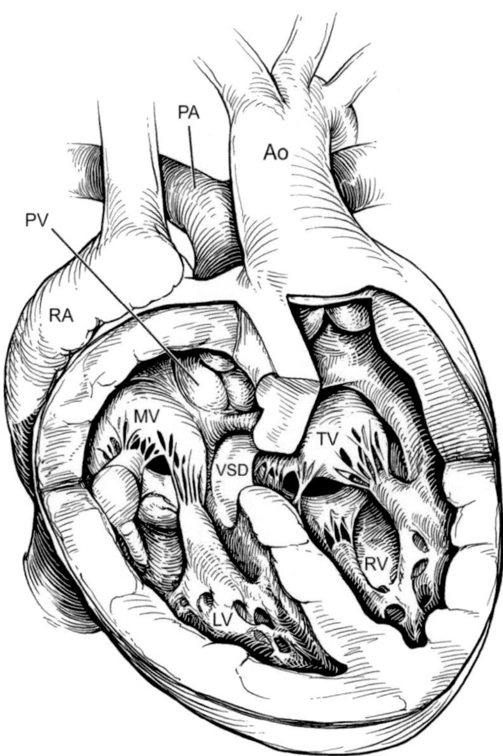

Fig. 1 Congenitally corrected transposition of the great arteries (ccTGA) is a complex congenital heart defect that is defined by atrioventricular and ventriculoarterial discordance. The figure shows a coronal view of a heart with ccTGA, and ventricular septal defect (VSD). The morphologic right atrium (systemic collecting chamber) is connected to the morphologic left ventricle through a mitral valve, which is connected to the pulmonary artery. The morphologic left atrium (pulmonary venous collecting chamber) is connected to the morphologic right ventricle through a tricuspid valve which is connected to the aorta. This arrangement results in physiologically corrected but not anatomically corrected circulation. Associated lesions are generally responsible for circulatory aberrations and include VSDs, pulmonary stenosis or atresia, and tricuspid valve abnormalities. Congenitally corrected transposition may occur in association with situs solitus (normal atrial situs) or situs inversus. In addition, the conduction system in patients with ccTGA is notably atypical. The incidence of spontaneous heart block is high even without surgical correction. (With permission: Karl and Cochrane 2003). *Ao* aorta, *LV* left ventricle, *MV* mitral valve, *PA* pulmonary artery, *PV* pulmonary valve, *RA* right atrium, *RV* right ventricle, *TV* tricuspid valve, *VSD* ventricular septal defect

inversus {I,D,D}. Discordance between the atrial situs and the position of the cardiac apex (i.e., ventricular apex pointing toward caval axis) is frequent in ccTGA (as compared with concordant TGA). This convoluted classification issue was addressed by the Congenital Heart Surgery Nomenclature and Database Project (Wilkinson et al. 2000). After a full review, the term congenitally corrected transposition of the great arteries (ccTGA) was adopted and has become a widely accepted term (Wilkinson et al. 2000).

For the purpose of discussing complications involving repair of ccTGA with two ventricles, single or unbalanced ventricular variants with L-loop embryology but without a discordant AV connection are excluded from this discussion. In their chapter on ccTGA (Karl and Jacobs 2023), Karl and Jacobs offered the following:

> The morphologic features common to hearts with ccTGA are as follows:
>
> 1. The systemic venous atrium (morphologic right atrium) is connected to the morphologic left ventricle (LV) through a mitral valve.
> 2. The LV is connected to the pulmonary artery (PA) through the pulmonary valve.
> 3. The pulmonary venous atrium (morphologic left atrium) is connected to the morphologic right ventricle (RV) through a tricuspid valve (TV) (which functions as the systemic AV valve).
> 4. The RV is connected to the aorta via the aortic valve (Fig. 1) (Karl and Jacobs 2023)

Associated cardiac anomalies are frequently present (99% of cases) in patients with ccTGA, as noted in Fig. 2. The most common of these anomalies are VSD, pulmonary valve and/or subpulmonary stenosis (resulting in LVOT obstruction), and tricuspid valve malformations (resulting in systemic AV valve insufficiency). The anomalies associated with ccTGA create important anatomic and physiologic considerations when planning the approach to management. Whichever therapeutic course is taken, the accompanying potential for short-term and long-term complications requires thoughtful analysis.

In Fig. 3 the course of the conduction system is highlighted which is susceptible to spontaneous or surgically induced heart block. Fig. 3 inset shows how individual pledgetted sutures can be placed to avoid heart block (Jonker et al. 2015; Waldo et al. 1975).

- Dextrocardia ± situs abnormalities
- Malalignment of atrial and ventricular septa
- Mitral-pulmonary continuity (usually) with subaortic conus, parallel outflow tracts
- LVOTO (valvar or multilevel)
- VSD perimembranous / malalignment multiple VSDs
- TV leaflet and tensor anomalies
- Straddling AV valves
- Overriding AV valves
- Ventricular hypoplasia
- Coronary anomalies
- Interruption of abnormally situated conduction pathway (→ spontaneous or surgically induced AV block)
- Systemic RV with circumferential contraction (as compared to longitudinal in systemic LV)

Fig. 2 Anomalies associated with ccTGA. The majority of cases (99%) of ccTGA have anatomic abnormalities that could complicate the discordant AV and VA connections. These additional anomalies can have an important influence on the natural history, the timing of surgery, and the choice of surgical options. *AV, atrioventricular; LV, left ventricle; LVOTO, left ventricular outflow tract obstruction; RV, right ventricle; TV, tricuspid valve; VSD, ventricular septal defect.* (With Permission: Karl and Jacobs 2023)

Further to the discussion of anatomic variants, the presence of left ventricular outflow tract (LVOT) obstruction is an important determinant of surgical strategy, since both physiologic and anatomic repair are adversely affected. Specifically, the LVOT in patients with ccTGA is located between the tricuspid valve and the mitral valve, which creates either dynamic or fixed LVOT obstruction in 30%–50% of cases (El-Zein et al. 2015). Coronary artery anomalies are frequently found in patients with ccTGA and can influence the conduct of any reparative procedure for ccTGA. The most common orientation of coronary anatomy according to the Leiden classification is 1R, 2LCx (Quaegebeur et al. 1986). Anatomic studies of coronary artery distribution for ccTGA have noted that 45% of ccTGA coronary patterns can add complexity to anatomic surgical repairs (Karl et al. 1997; Ismat et al. 2002; Unolt et al. 2013) (Fig. 4).

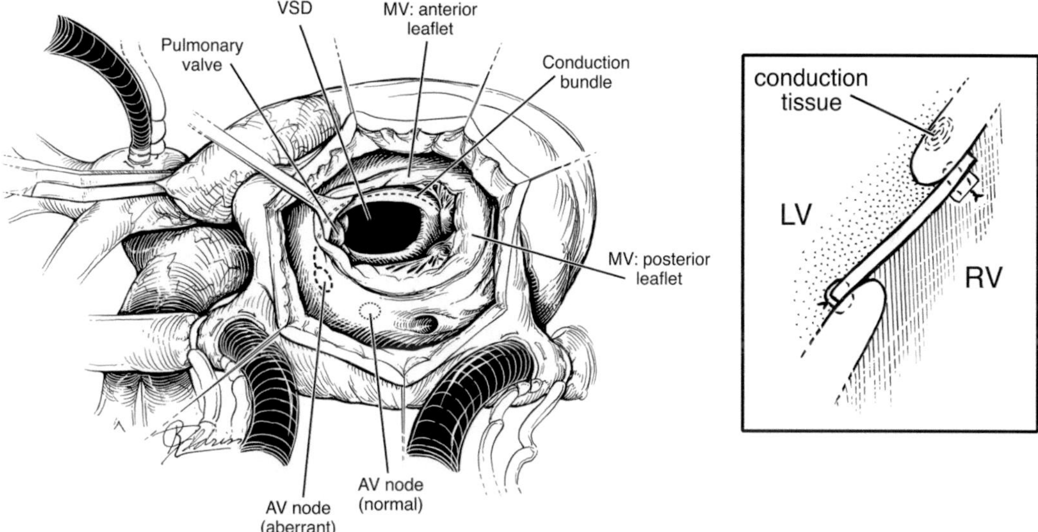

Fig. 3 Shows a patient with ccTGA, ventricular septal defect (VSD) and situs solitus undergoing aortobicaval cardiopulmonary bypass with aortic cross-clamping and cardioplegic arrest. The relevant right atrial and morphological left ventricular anatomy is depicted with retraction of the mitral valve for transatrial perimembranous VSD closure. The location of the normally positioned atrioventricular (AV) node is included to emphasize the abnormal location of the aberrant AV node (also shown) and the pathway of the bundle of His as it passes anterior to the pulmonary annulus along the morphologic left ventricular crest of the ventricular septum. The conduction system can be avoided during VSD closure by anchoring interrupted pledgetted sutures on the right ventricular side of the VSD over the course of the conduction system as noted in the inset which shows how sutures can be placed on the left ventricular side of the septum at the inferior margin of the VSD, which is safely away from the conduction system. The sutures can then be taken through a prosthetic patch and individually tied to effectively close the VSD. (With permission: Karl and Cochrane 2003). *AV, atrioventricular; LV, left ventricle; MV, mitral valve; RV, right ventricle; VSD, ventricular septal defect*

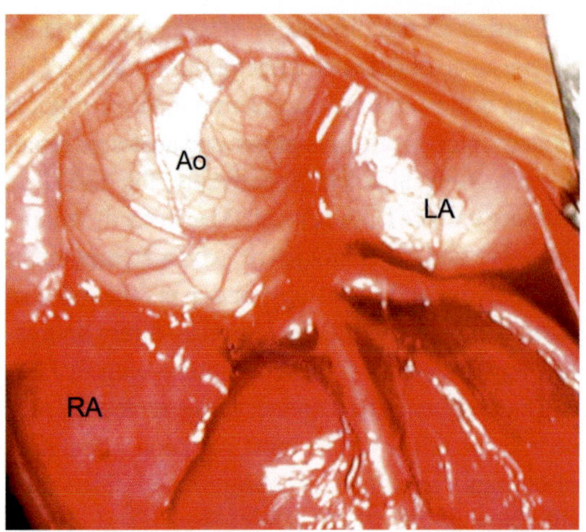

Fig. 4 Coronary anomaly in ccTGA. This example shows a single coronary arising from a nonfacing sinus, an extremely rare variant in both concordant and discordant TGA. (*Ao* aorta, *LA* left atrium, *RA* right atrium). (With Permission: Karl and Jacobs 2023). *Ao* aorta, *LA* left atrium, *RA* right atrium

2 Important Historical Aspects

The first anatomist to describe the characteristics of ccTGA was von Rokitansky (1875) (von Rokitansky 1875). Further to this, Monckeberg (1913) reported the important anterior AV node position, and Walmsley (1931) described the mirror image coronary arterial branching pattern and the position of the central fibrous body (Monckeberg 1913; Walmsley 1931). Schiebler and associates (1961) proposed the "ccTGA" terminology (Schiebler et al. 1961). Early surgical repairs were primarily physiologic; the first being performed by Anderson et al. (1957). It took some time for surgeons to attempt and report anatomic repairs. It was Imai and colleagues (1989), and Mee and co-workers (1989) who independently described various anatomic repair strategies, including what is now known as the double switch operation (Senning and Arterial Switch Operation) (Imai et al. 2001; Helvind et al. 1998). The association of pulmonary stenosis (PS) and LVOT obstruction made repair by double switch untenable. To address this issue, Ilbawi (1990) described the Rastelli + atrial baffle approach to ccTGA with ventricular septal defect (VSD) and LVOT obstruction (Ilbawi et al. 1990). Another approach to ccTGA with LVOT obstruction was offered by Mavroudis et al. (1999) who performed a 1.5 ventricular repair employing a bidirectional Glenn shunt which was subsequently incorporated into anatomic repairs as well. Aortic and pulmonary root translocation in ccTGA have been described independently by multiple groups over the past 2 decades, based in part on the principles of the Nikaidoh operation for concordant TGA patients with VSD and LVOTO (Karl and Jacobs 2023; Kwak et al. 2010; Davies et al. 2008a; Ikai et al. 2012).

3 Diagnosis

Two-dimensional echocardiography (Fig. 5) can generally form the basis of ccTGA diagnosis including VSD location, great vessel orientation, and LVOT obstruction. Cardiac catheterization is very informative and can further delineate anatomic relationships and pulmonary artery (PA) morphology. Angiography can establish the site and number of VSDs, the morphology of the ventricular chambers, the nature of the LVOTO, and most associated anomalies. Added to these diagnostic modalities are imaging strategies such as computed tomographic imaging (CTA), magnetic resonance imaging (MRI), and 3D modeling. It is important to define the outflow tracts to rule out double outlet ventricles which can complicate the operation. Knowing if there is double outlet ventricle will allow the surgeon to plan effectively, since the VSD baffling to a great artery will be more complicated. Also, closing a VSD in double outlet right ventricle (DORV) would leave both outlets on one side of the septum resulting in a lethal complication.

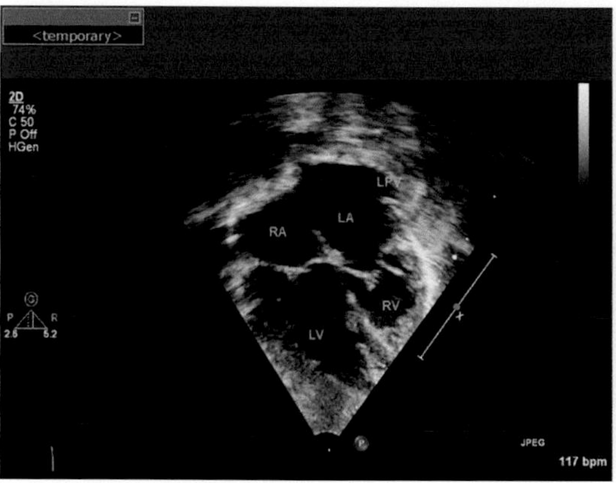

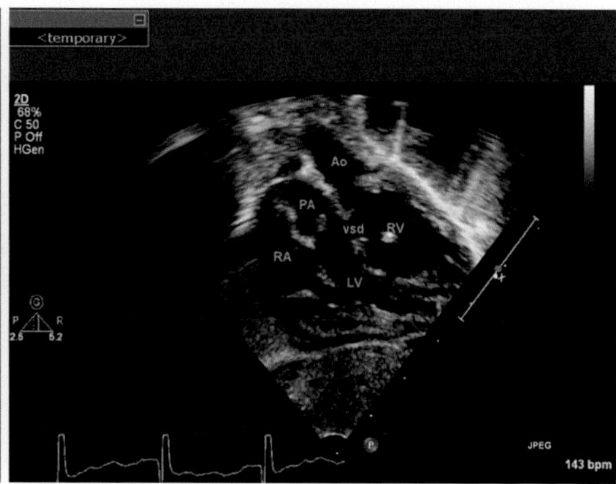

Fig. 5 2D echocardiography imaging in ccTGA. Four chamber (left) and subcostal images (right) from the same child are shown. The discordant AV connection is well seen. There is reverse offset of the AV valves (TV more apically displaced than MV). The great vessels have a parallel (rather than spiral) proximal course. A perimembranous VSD is also present. (*Ao* aorta, *LA* left atrium, *LPV* left pulmonary valve, *LV* left ventricle, *PA* pulmonary artery, *RA* right atrium, *RV* right ventricle, *VSD* ventricular septal defect). (Echo images kindly provided by Dr. Thieu Nguyen, JH-ACH.) (With Permission: Karl and Jacobs 2023)

4 Natural History and Clinical Presentation

The natural history of ccTGA is highly variable and is decidedly dependent on associated cardiac malformations. Those infants with severe pulmonary stenosis or pulmonary atresia and those with severe left-sided (tricuspid valve) regurgitation oftentimes present early in life. On the other hand, some individuals with ccTGA (approximately 1%–2% of patients with no associated defects) can remain asymptomatic for many years and may even experience successful pregnancies (Yamagishi et al. 2003; Wissocque et al. 2016; Karl 2016; Kowalik et al. 2014). Even so, survival for all patients with ccTGA, regardless of palliation, surgical repair, or close observation, is significantly poorer than that of the normal population, from early infancy onward. In particular, signs and symptoms in the short- and long-term are related to abnormal pulmonary blood flow, systemic AV valve insufficiency, bradycardia from heart block, or systemic (right) ventricular dysfunction.

The aforementioned ccTGA associated lesions can cause significant physiologic problems and can become manifest at any age. In particular, ccTGA can cause cyanosis in infancy owing to LVOT obstruction and intracardiac shunts. When LVOT obstruction is not present, patients suffering from severe tricuspid regurgitation (TR) with or without a large VSD may present at any time from infancy to early childhood with congestive heart failure. Further complicating these associated anomalies and physical findings is the development of spontaneous heart block and bradycardia, the incidence of which increases by 2% per year (Deal 2016).

Tricuspid regurgitation in patients with ccTGA is multifactorial,and challenges clinicians who seek medical and surgical options in both operated and unoperated individuals. The multifactorial aspects of tricuspid regurgitation involve congenital leaflet abnormalities (Ebstein-like anomaly), papillary muscle dysfunction, dilated tricuspid valve annulus, papillary muscle elongation owing to intraventricular septal shift, and asynchronous ventricular contraction caused by atrioventricular arrhythmias. Some important pathophysiologic interactions have been summarized by Karl and Jacobs (2023):

> The features of Ebstein anomaly as seen in concordant hearts (such as thinning of the atrialized portion of the RV and severe tethering of leaflets) are not generally present in ccTGA. Furthermore, the typical surgical treatments of Ebstein anomaly in

AV concordant hearts (e.g., cone repair) may not be applicable in ccTGA. Hence, the term "Ebsteinoid" is most often applied to the TV in ccTGA, acknowledging that the morphology is significantly different. In some cases of ccTGA, RV hypertrophy eventually gives way to dilation, so the TV papillary muscles are distracted. The short, tethered TV chords and displaced leaflets fail to coapt, and tricuspid insufficiency becomes progressive and self-perpetuating. Tricuspid insufficiency can also be exacerbated by surgical relief of LVOT obstruction, due to unfavorable septal shift that occurs when the LV pressure drops. Pulmonary artery band placement may have the opposite effect and move the septum to a more favorable midline location improving tricuspid valve function.

5 Surgical Indications and Options

The first attempts at repair of ccTGA were reported by Anderson et al. (1957). Figure 6. highlights the historic and currently used surgical approaches regarding palliation and interim solutions that may be applicable in selected situations. Physiologic (maintenance of the RV as systemic pumping chamber) and anatomic (complex solutions to establish the LV as the pumping chamber) have been applied for definitive treatment. However, owing to the unfavorable outcomes of children with ccTGA and a systemic RV resulting in RV failure, more complex operations have been developed toward anatomic repair which utilizes the LV as the systemic pumping chamber. While not the present-day norm, univentricular and 1.5 ventricular repairs have also been employed selectively (Karl 2011).

6 Interim (Palliative or Nondefinitive) Operations for ccTGA

Modern day palliation for patients with ccTGA is mostly aimed at control of pulmonary artery flow and consists of systemic-to-pulmonary artery modified Blalock-Taussig-Thomas (BTT) shunts and PA banding. The conduct of the procedures and associated complications are noted and explained in chapter "Complications Associated with Palliative Operations". Other procedures, such as isolated TV repair or replacement, as well as pacemaker implantation and cardiac resynchronization for heart block (Deal 2016), can improve hemodynamic conditions en route to further palliation, physiologic repair, or anatomic reconstruction.

As previously noted, the modified BTT shunt is a useful strategy for ccTGA patients with VSD

Fig. 6 Taxonomy of some operative strategies used for ccTGA. Bold type implies systemic LV, italic type implies systemic RV and LV) (With Permission: Karl and Jacobs 2023)

1. PA band:
   a. *control of CHF in ccTGA + VSD*
   b. LV conditioning
   c. for definitive treatment of TV insufficiency
   d. open ended palliation
2. Physiological repairs:
   a. VSD closure
   b. VSD closure + LV-PA conduit
   c. relief of LVOTO + BCPS (1.5 ventricle)
3. **Anatomic repairs:**
   a. **ASO + atrial repair (double switch) (± VSD closure)**
   b. **Rastelli + atrial repair + RV-PA connection (± conduit)**
   c. **Aortic root translocation + atrial repair + RV-PA connection (± conduit)**
   d. **Rastelli + hemi-Mustard + BCPS**
   e. **Rastelli + PA root translocation + atrial repair + RV-PA connection ((± conduit)**
   f. **En bloc Truncal rotation**
   g. **Patrick McGoon repair + atrial repair**
4. *Univentricular repairs:*
   a. *Fontan operation*
      i. *primary*
      ii. *surgical completion following BCPS*
      iii. *interventional completion following modified BDPS*
5. Tricuspid valve surgery:
   a. Repair
   b. Replacement

and LVOT obstruction in preparation for physiologic or anatomic repair with an extracardiac conduit when size and conditions dictate. In addition, the modified BTT shunt can be performed in patients with ccTGA, VSD, and LVOT obstruction who are not candidates for biventricular repair due to unbalanced ventricles, straddling AV valves, or multiple unfavorable VSDs. These patients are more likely to be candidates for a univentricular pathway (Fontan procedure) (Karl 2011; Karl et al. 2016).

Most patients with ccTGA have their cardiac apex located on the same side as the inferior vena cava (IVC), which results in some natural limitation of pulmonary blood flow and usually obviates, in most cases, the need for PA band (Karl et al. 2016). However, other complex considerations may require a preliminary PAB en route to further therapeutic solutions. For instance, PAB may be indicated in patients with a large VSD in whom a double switch (arterial switch and atrial baffle procedure) are planned. Recently, however, some authors have advocated double switch in infancy without preliminary PAB (Hoashi et al. 2013; Marathe et al. 2022). In unoperated patients with ccTGA-IVS (intact ventricular septum) who develop tricuspid regurgitation and RV failure, a PAB may be employed for LV training and eventual double switch operation or as a palliative operation to reduce tricuspid regurgitation.

As a matter of historical review, Yacoub and associates first employed LV conditioning for patients with TGA-IVS (Yacoub et al. 1977). Further advances with this strategy by Mee and others allowed surgeons to accumulate experience with LV conditioning in unoperated patients with ccTGA-IVS (Ohye et al. 2015). Subsequent clinical studies have determined that the likelihood of success with pulmonary artery banding is inversely related to age, specifically that early infancy is the most reliable time period to induce LV hypertrophy (Myers et al. 2013). More recent advances have added to this experience. Zartner and associates have proposed that a loose PA band in combination with creation of an ASD is a more efficient and reliable way to condition and induce subpulmonary LV hypertrophy, through a physiologic combination of augmented preload and afterload (Zartner et al. 2016). Induction of LV hypertrophy and subsequent double switch can also be performed in selected patients with ccTGA who had prior physiologic repair. Pulmonary artery banding can also be used as "destination therapy" or "open ended palliation" (Cools et al. 2012) in ccTGA patients with tricuspid regurgitation owing to an unfavorable shift in the interventricular septum. This maneuver has been shown to improve tricuspid regurgitation by a rightward repositioning of the septum with more favorable papillary muscle function. The clinical basis for this strategy was observed by Mee and associates, who noticed improved tricuspid function during their experience with LV conditioning en route to atrial baffle to arterial switch conversion (Mee 1986). Another early palliative intervention for infants with ccTGA-IVS involves placement of an adjustable pulmonary artery (PA) band (tightened to induce LV/RV = 50%) that could maintain LV mass and stabilize TV function (Metton et al. 2010; Malekzadeh-Milani et al. 2016; Talwar et al. 2016; Termignon et al. 1996; Hraska et al. 2005). This strategy can allow subsequent conversion to double switch depending on the clinical course and management circumstances. The benefits of such an approach are based on the adjustable or dilatable PA band that will allow the proper amount of LV hypertrophy to maintain RV function and TV competence. Helsen and associates suggest that such a surgical strategy is as effective as that of anatomic repairs (Helsen et al. 2015). Long-term outcomes will determine the efficacy of all the aforementioned applications of PA banding.

7 Complications Associated with Reparative Operations for ccTGA

Because of the anatomic and physiologic conditions associated with the variants of ccTGA, the best surgical strategy for complete repair is debatable. Numerous operations have been advanced at all age groups, by proponents who champion their management choices based on early survival, long-term survival, and freedom from significant complications. Comparative studies to evaluate all of the possible surgical applications have been few owing to the rarity of the lesion. Timing of treatment ranges from infancy to adulthood with reports describing repair as late as the fifth decade of life (Ma et al. 2014; Baruah et al. 2016). As has been noted and emphasized in this chapter, the choice between physiologic and anatomic repair is highly dependent on the anatomy, associated lesions, and experience of the surgical team. Conditions that have been cited to favor the physiologic approach include competence of both AV valves, balanced ventricular size, and excellent RV function. Conditions that favor the anatomic approach include ventricular size disparity, poor RV function, tricuspid regurgitation, and an appropriate systemic LV pressure conditioned by LVOT obstruction, secondary pulmonary hypertension, or following PA banding) (Karl and Jacobs 2023).

These issues notwithstanding, anatomic correction are more complex than physiologic repair, but may be associated with better long-term outcomes. So, what are the data supporting anatomic versus physiologic repair, even from database comparisons with limited granularity? Congenital heart operations have been assessed by complexity scores and anticipated mortality scores. Both the Aristotle Complexity Score and the Society of Thoracic Surgeons - European Association for Cardio-Thoracic Surgery Congenital Heart Surgery Mortality Score (STAT) are useful tools (Karl 2011; Baruah et al. 2016; Lacour-Gayet et al. 2005). The double switch operation (anatomic repair including repair of all associated lesions), for example, has a STAT mortality category of 5 (highest expected level of mortality), and an Aristotle Complexity Score of 13.8, rising to 18.8 in a patient with prior trans-sternal PA banding for LV conditioning. In comparison, STAT mortality categories for a physiologic correction involving isolated VSD closure in ccTGA or VSD closure with LV-PA conduit placement are 3 and 4 respectively, suggesting a significant difference in early mortality risk (Karl and Jacobs 2023; Lacour-Gayet et al. 2005; Jacobs et al. 2016).

The comparison continues, but it is hampered by the fact that follow-up time accrual for physiologic repair is greater than anatomic repair, making definitive comparisons unreliable and largely theoretical. Nevertheless, current reports which have shown decreased early mortality for anatomic repair suggest that this approach is better for patients in the long-term owing to the aforementioned benefits (El-Zein et al. 2015; Miller et al. 2022).

The other choice for division of the pulmonary and systemic circuits is the Fontan operation, which has been advanced for patients with ccTGA and complicated anatomic conditions in which the risk of ventricular septation outweighs the benefits. The indications for the Fontan pathway are mostly obvious and include those with important straddling of an AV valve, unbalanced ventricular size, and multiple unfavorable VSDs. The authors have also employed an interventional strategy for the Fontan operation after appropriate preparation at the bidirectional cavopulmonary shunt (BCPS) stage (Prabhu et al. 2017). There is much to consider when choosing the Fontan pathway. At first consideration is that the STAT score is 2 for all single ventricle patients. Although it has not been verified, it is likely that those patients who have biventricular Fontan operations will fare better than those patients with complex univentricular anatomy (El-Zein et al. 2015). Furthermore, the Fontan operation when applied to patients with the variants of ccTGA may result in an event-free survival advantage when compared with physiologic and anatomic biventricular repair options. These advantages include similar or better exercise capacity and improved quality of life, even for patients who, theoretically, could undergo biventricular repair (Malekzadeh-Milani et al. 2016; Hsu et al. 2016; Talwar et al. 2013). Studies documenting the long-term outcome of well-selected Fontan patients have been favorable, especially for those individuals with ccTGA, VSD, and LVOT obstruction. Unresolved is the long-term fate of the tricuspid valve and right ventricle with this strategy (Miller et al. 2022; d'Udekem et al. 2014) resulting in active controversy and equipoise (El-Zein et al. 2015; Malekzadeh-Milani et al. 2016; Talwar et al. 2016; Miller et al. 2022; Hsu et al. 2016) regarding risk factors which pertain to the morphologic RV or the surgical strategy (Malekzadeh-Milani et al. 2016; Talwar et al. 2016).

As noted, each management pathway, including surgical intervention or medical observation, for treatment of patients with ccTGA has the potential for significant complications. One notable example concerns the treatment or nontreatment options regarding the asymptomatic or mildly symptomatic older patient with ccTGA, intact ventricular septum, no outlet obstruction, moderate tricuspid regurgitation, and mild RV dilatation. A patient with these anatomic characteristics may survive well into adult life with no surgical treatment. Alternatively, surgical correction, when considered, involves a 2-stage operative approach, with PA banding and double switch procedures. Complicating this strategy is the possibility that PA banding may not prove to be effective resulting in further operations for sequential tightening to avoid the induction of LV fibrosis and myocardial edema (Talwar et al. 2013; d'Udekem et al. 2014; Ma et al. 2016; Hsu and Chang 2016). Advancing age is also a risk factor for the PA band-anatomic conversion option. Moreover, LV dysfunction and neoaortic regurgitation 1 year following anatomic repairs is more common in patients who had preliminary PA banding (Davies et al. 2008a; Hörer et al. 2008). Regarding these confounding risks of operation vs. observational management, it is almost universally accepted that these patients described above will do better without operative therapy.

8 Management of Systemic Right Ventricular Failure in ccTGA

Right ventricular failure in the mid- and long-term management of ccTGA is common, especially in unoperated patients and in those individuals with physiologic repairs (Termignon et al. 1996). There are, however, other options which include continued medical therapy, cardiac resynchronization, TV repair or replacement, palliative PA banding, ventricular assist devices, and cardiac transplantation (Karl and Jacobs 2023).

When considering tricuspid valve surgery as an isolated procedure, the results are most effective in patients with severe tricuspid regurgitation and preserved RV systolic function. Repair options tend to be difficult both in the preoperative assessment and in the technical procedure, owing to the variability of tricuspid valve anatomy in these patients. Tricuspid valve replacement tends to be a better option and may result in prompt improvement assuming that there is preexisting preserved right ventricular function (Talwar et al. 2016; Hsu and Chang 2016). Transcatheter TV edge-to-edge repair in patients with ccTGA has been reported in adults, but its role has yet to be determined (Picard et al. 2017).

9 Specific Surgical Techniques for ccTGA Physiologic Repair for ccTGA with VSD with or Without LVOT Obstruction

Physiologic repair by VSD closure in patients with ccTGA without LVOT obstruction can generally be performed by right atrial exposure

(Fig. 3) with few complications assuming that the conduction system is respected as noted in (Fig. 3, Inset). This technique has been shown to be very effective in avoiding heart block, but the inherent risk of heart block in these patients cannot eliminate the problem entirely. The principles of VSD closure using cardiopulmonary bypass with moderate hypothermia, cardioplegic arrest, right atrial exposure, AV valve retraction and closure by interrupted suture technique are described in chapter "Complications Associated with Ventricular Septal Defect Closure" (VSD Chapter). Care must be taken to avoid heart block, chordal entrapment leading to mitral valve regurgitation, pulmonary valve injury by the VSD sutures, and mitral leaflet disruption owing to excessive retraction. These complications and the drawings relating thereto are noted in chapter "Complications Associated with Ventricular Septal Defect Closure".

Before the advent of anatomic repair, patients with ccTGA with VSD without LVOT obstruction had traditionally undergone physiologic repair with an LV-to-pulmonary artery conduit, owing to the variation of LVOT obstruction and coronary artery anatomy. The extent and anatomic characteristics of the LVOT stenosis in ccTGA are highly variable, caused by a combination of annular, leaflet, and subvalvar components. Direct muscular resection relief of the LVOT is generally unsatisfactory, due to the posterior position of the pulmonary outflow tract, which is wedged between the AV valves. In addition, the right coronary artery proceeds in proximity to the pulmonary annulus making it vulnerable to injury. The third major impediment is the risk of heart block due to the presence of the penetrating bundle in the proposed area of resection. Figure 7 shows the transventricular closure of the VSD in preparation for the LV-to-PA conduit. The figure legend describes the anatomical reasons for this approach as noted herein.

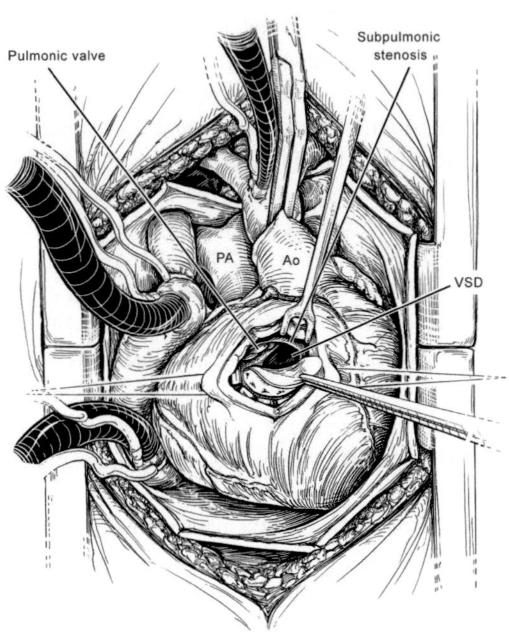

Fig. 7 Before the introduction of the double switch procedures (arterial switch and atrial switch; Rastelli and atrial switch), physiologic repair was popular. It entailed simple ventricular septal defect (VSD) closure as described in the previous section or by VSD closure and left ventricular-to-pulmonary artery conduit for left ventricular outflow tract obstruction (pulmonary stenosis). The figure shows a patient with ccTGA, VSD and pulmonary stenosis undergoing aortobicaval cardiopulmonary bypass with aortic cross-clamping and cardioplegic arrest. The location of the pulmonary annulus is not favorably located for a transannular patch due to the course of the right coronary artery and the conduction system which traverses this area en route to the interventricular septum and the bundle of His. (With permission: Karl and Cochrane 2003). *Ao* aorta, *PA* pulmonary artery, *VSD* ventricular septal defect

The left ventricular-to-pulmonary artery conduit in these circumstances is warranted, as shown in Fig. 8, but complications loom large. In the first place, coronary artery distribution to the anterior wall of the displaced LV is clearly different from the anatomic RV which can tolerate ventriculotomy in most cases. LV ventriculotomy is poorly tolerated owing to interruption of

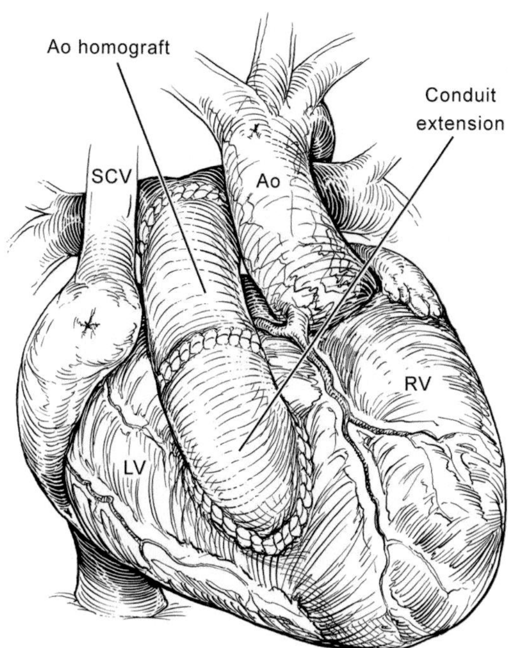

Fig. 8 Under these circumstances, surgeons have closed the ventricular septal defect and performed a left ventricular-to-pulmonary artery conduit reconstruction, allowing for a physiologic but not an anatomic correction as shown in the figure. The difficulty with this approach is that the right ventricle fails with time owing to right ventricular dilatation, resultant tricuspid regurgitation due to papillary muscle stretching, and arrhythmias. Interestingly, those patients with acquired conduit stenosis with resultant left ventricular hypertension tend to do better since the interventricular septum maintains its neutral position. Consequently, the cascade leading to right ventricular failure doesn't occur; namely, the interventricular septum does not bow into the left ventricle, the right ventricle does not correspondingly dilate, and the tricuspid valve doesn't become regurgitant. When the time comes for conduit replacement, two issues become important. The first is that the left ventricle becomes decompressed thereby allowing the interventricular septum to bow to the left and cause tricuspid regurgitation. The second is avoiding coronary artery injury due to left ventricular free wall incision for the larger conduit. This problem doesn't usually happen in the right ventricle because the right anterior ventricular wall is not rich with large coronary arteries. The left ventricular free wall however is a different issue with many ventricular branches arising from the course of the right coronary artery. Interruption of these vessels during conduit replacement can have an additive negative effect on ventricular interaction and overall ventricular function. Cardiac transplantation may be the only solution to these unfortunate series of events. (With permission: Karl and Cochrane 2003). *Ao* aorta, *LV* left ventricle, *RV* right ventricle, *SVC* superior vena cava

coronary artery distribution and interventricular septal discoordination (DiBernardo et al. 1998). In the mid- to long-term, left ventriculotomy in ccTGA patients can cause a shift in the interventricular septum away from the RV causing chordal stretching and papillary muscle dysfunction which results in systemic tricuspid valve regurgitation as noted in Fig. 9. This situation may lead to heart failure and cardiac transplantation. Alternatively, it may be possible to partially relieve the LVOT obstruction resulting in moderately elevated LV pressure. This situation would eliminate the need for a LV-to-PA conduit, and obviate the potential injury to the coronary artery distribution to the LV. Furthermore, the interventricular septum is maintained in a neutral position thereby preventing the deleterious effects of RV chordal stretching and papillary muscle dysfunction leading to important TR. Another surgical application as noted in Fig. 10 is partial LVOT obstruction relief by careful transpulmonary artery valvotomy and limited subvalvar resection, VSD closure if present, and bidirectional Glenn shunt which acts to reduce the LV volume load and limit the pressure gradient across the LVOT (Mavroudis et al. 1999) The end result of this surgical strategy is shown in (Fig. 11). The important issue, regardless of adjunct bidirectional Glenn application is that residual mild to moderate LVOT obstruction may be beneficial in the long term for maintenance of TV function (Karl and Jacobs 2023; Mavroudis et al. 1999).

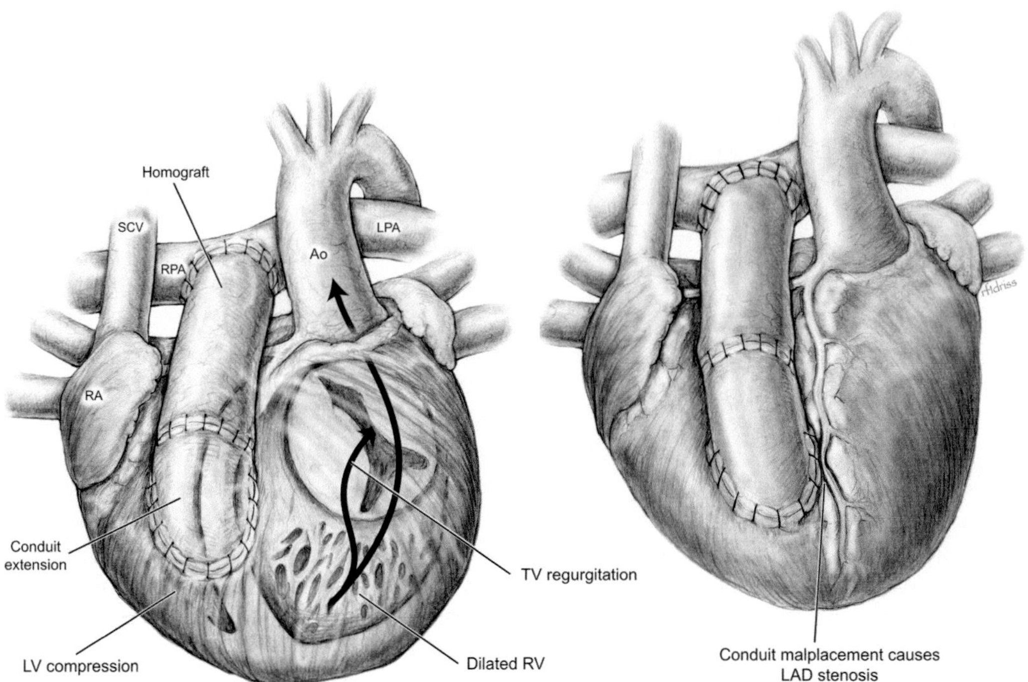

Fig. 9 The left panel shows ventricular septal deviation thereby causing tricuspid regurgitation and ventricular failure. The right panel shows the medial suture line of the left ventricular-to-pulmonary artery conduit encroaching upon the course of the left anterior coronary artery. Other coronary artery branches are also at risk of injury. Encroachment of the left anterior descending artery can lead to left and right ventricular dysfunction, heart failure, and eventual cardiac transplantation. *Ao* aorta, *LPA* left pulmonary artery, *LV* left ventricle, *RA* right atrium, *RPA* right pulmonary artery, *RV* right ventricle, *SCV* superior caval vein, *TV* tricuspid valve

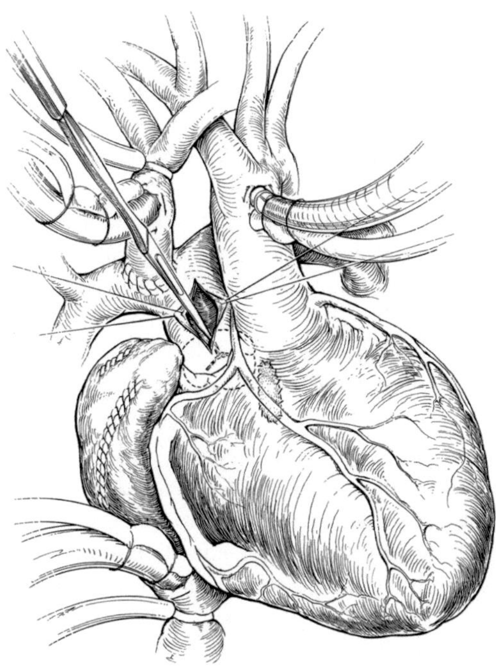

Fig. 10 Shows a patient with ccTGA, ventricular septal defect (VSD), and moderate pulmonary stenosis who has undergone aortobicaval cardiopulmonary bypass, transatrial VSD closure, infundibular resection (subpulmonic resection) away from the conduction system, and bidirectional Glenn shunt. The operative drawing shows the performance of a localized sharp pulmonary valvotomy. The bidirectional Glenn shunt functions to unload the left ventricle in order to lower the developed pressure to sub-systemic levels, but high enough to maintain favorable interventricular interactions. (With permission: Mavroudis 2015)

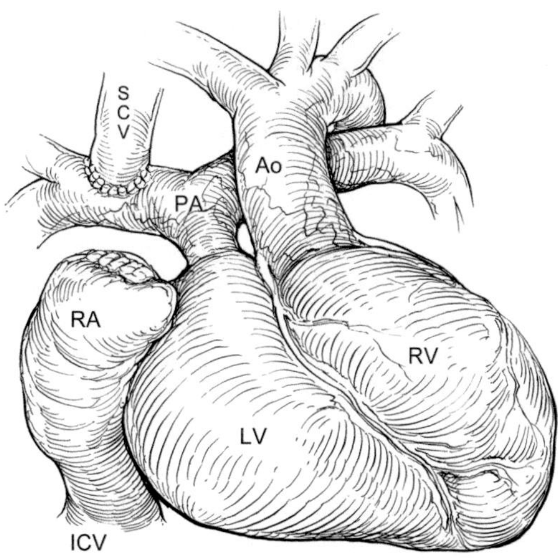

Fig. 11 Shows the completed repair, which has been successful in a handful of patients over a 10-year period. This operation can only be applied to a minority of patients who must have the right constellation of lesions with moderate pulmonary stenosis who might benefit from this type of physiology. (With permission: Mavroudis 2015). *Ao* aorta, *IVC* inferior vena cava, *LV* left ventricle, *PA* pulmonary artery, *RA* right atrium, *RV* right ventricle, *SVC* superior vena cava

10 Complications Associated with Anatomic Correction of ccTGA via the Double Switch Operation

The double switch operation combines an atrial baffle procedure (Senning or Mustard operation) with an arterial switch operation to achieve anatomic correction of ccTGA, assuming that certain anatomic and physiologic criteria are met. This strategy was introduced independently by Imai and co-workers in 1989 in Tokyo (Imai et al. 2001) and Mee and associates in Melbourne (Mee 2005). The indications and criteria for inclusion regarding this strategy has been noted by Karl and Jacobs (2023) and includes the following:

> Based on experience since that era, candidates for double switch generally should meet the following minimal criteria:
>
> 1. No obstruction between either ventricle or its respective semilunar valve
> 2. Balanced ventricular size
> 3. Heart that can be septated without major AVV straddling
> 4. Translocatable coronary arteries that can be safely transferred to the neoaorta
> 5. LV pressure > 75% of RV pressure, with good LV contractile function (this may be a consequence of a large VSD, PA band, or passive pulmonary hypertension related to RV failure). In such cases indexed LV free wall thickness will usually approach normal, but there are no universally accepted criteria (Karl and Jacobs 2023)

The double switch operation can be performed in neonates. To this end, Bove and associates have expressed the idea that the double switch operation can be performed even in asymptomatic neonates assuming that the modified Senning operation (in situ pericardial baffle for the pulmonary venous return) is used as the right atrial augmentation technique (Bove 2022). The more conventional option however is to perform this operation later in infancy or early childhood owing to technical issues. This strategy may require preliminary PA banding in neonates with a large VSD, congestive heart failure, and systemic PA pressure, to defer repair to 6–12 months of age. In keeping with the variability of patients with ccTGA, other individuals with a restrictive VSD or intact ventricular septum may require PA banding to induce systemic LV pressure prior to double switch.

The order of the operation is debatable. Some surgeons prefer to perform the atrial baffle operation first to be followed by the arterial switch operation. The idea is that performing the arterial switch operation first might be disrupted by the retraction required for the atrial baffle operations. There are no data for this approach and it is surgeon specific. This chapter will describe performance of the arterial switch operation first followed by the atrial baffle part of the operation, the idea being that gentle retraction required for the atrial baffle operation will be used in a way that will preserve the integrity of the arterial switch reconstruction.

Figure 12 shows the epicardial anatomy of ccTGA with VSD and no PS with coronary artery distribution characteristics. Figure 13 shows a coronal view of the left ventricle which highlights the VSD in the subpulmonic area. The right coronary artery is depicted traversing the anterior margin of the pulmonary artery and annulus.

The operation starts with aortobicaval cardiopulmonary bypass, moderate/deep hypothermia, and cardioplegic arrest in preparation for VSD closure and arterial switch (Fig. 14). Exposure for the VSD closure has been noted in Fig. 3, using appropriate suturing technique to avoid heart block. Alternatively, the VSD can be approached through the aortic valve after great vessel transection in preparation for the arterial switch operation as noted in Fig. 15. The advantage of this approach is that the sutures are placed on the right ventricular side of the interventricular septum, reducing the risk of heart block. Once the VSD is completed, the arterial switch operation can proceed using a technique similar to that used for concordant TGA as outlined in chapter "Complications Associated with Repair of Transposition of the Great Arteries and Associated

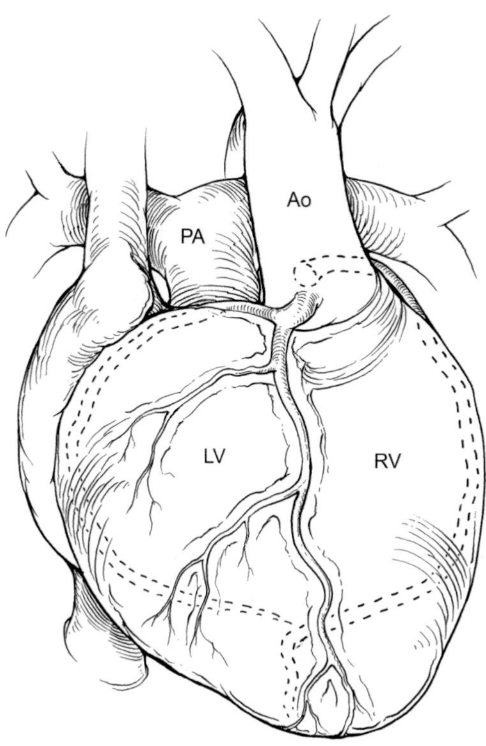

Fig. 12 Shows the epicardial anatomic details of ccTGA with ventricular septal defect and no pulmonary stenosis. The coronary arteries generally require extensive dissection, mobilization, and modified implantation techniques to accomplish a tension free anastomosis. When this operation was being conceived, anatomic dissections were performed in ccTGA cadaver specimens to determine whether coronary transfer could be accomplished safely. The initial assessment was not supportive perhaps because the specimens were fixed and not amenable to mobilization. It was subsequently performed successfully in the clinical setting making the operation feasible and applicable to this group of patients. (With permission: Mavroudis 2015). *Ao* aorta, *LV* left ventricle, *PA* pulmonary artery, *RV* right ventricle

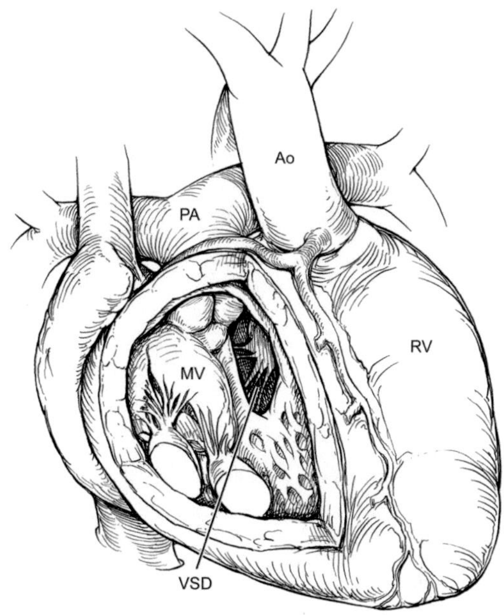

Fig. 13 Shows a coronal view of the left ventricle with the noted landmarks. The ventricular septal defect is highlighted in the subpulmonic area. The right coronary artery traverses across the anterior margin of the pulmonary artery. (With permission: Mavroudis 2015). *Ao* aorta, *MV* mitral valve, *PA* pulmonary artery, *RV* right ventricle, *VSD* ventricular septal defect

Lesions" (TGA chapter). The complications of the transaortic VSD repair are heart block, residual VSD, and aortic (neopulmonary) leaflet injury. Aortic leaflet injury during repair of VSD is reviewed in chapter "Complications Associated with Ventricular Septal Defect Closure" (VSD Chapter). The difference in this case is that the injury will be to the neopulmonary valve leaflets which does not hold the same severity as does injury to the neoaortic leaflets. Nevertheless, attention to detail will avoid such a complication. A residual VSD can be avoided by careful placement of interrupted pledgetted sutures with appropriate spacing, careful tying to avoid disruption, and post closure inspection (see chapter "Complications Associated with Ventricular Septal Defect Closure", VSD).

While arterial switch in patients with ccTGA is similar to arterial switch for concordant TGA, there are some notable differences. Coronary transfer can be challenging owing to the distance between the facing sinuses of the semilunar valves. In general, coronary translocation is possible for all coronary patterns using large medially based rectangular flaps, and in extreme cases

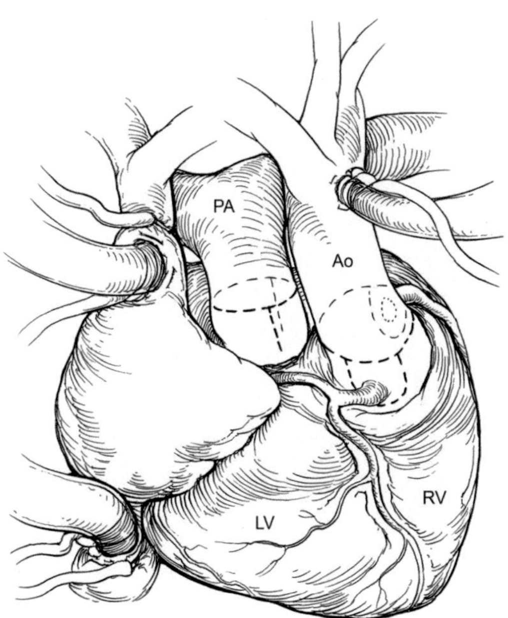

Fig. 14 The drawing illustrates cardiopulmonary bypass in anticipation for the arterial switch operation (ASO), which will be performed before the Senning operation in this case. Some surgeons elect to perform the atrial baffle procedure before the arterial switch to avoid ASO disruption that could occur with overzealous atrial wall retraction during the atrial baffle operation. The dashed lines represent the paths of great artery transection, coronary artery button formation, and reimplantation sites on the pulmonary artery (neoaorta). (With permission: Mavroudis 2015). *Ao* aorta, *LV* left ventricle, *PA* pulmonary artery, *RV* right ventricle

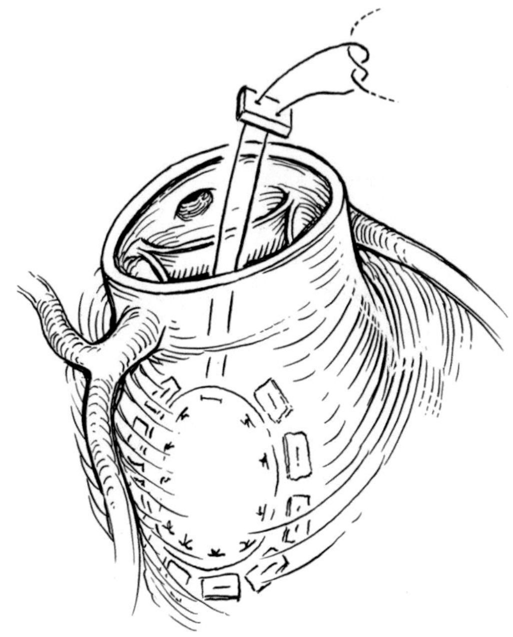

Fig. 15 Shows transaortic closure of the ventricular septal defect before the arterial switch operation and atrial baffle operation en route to complete anatomic and physiologic repair. (With permission: Mavroudis 2015)

with the addition of biologic material to the neoaortocoronary anastomoses (Fig. 16). Figure 16 inset shows the "trap door" technique for coronary transfer which is used to optimize the coronary flow pattern. In cases involving patients with ccTGA, the "trap door" technique is very helpful in avoiding complications. Complications associated with coronary transfer are noted in chapter "Complications Associated with Repair of Transposition of the Great Arteries and Associated Lesions", (Transposition) and involve coronary button harvest too close to the orifice, injury to the coronary artery, and malrotation of the implanted coronary button which can cause coronary artery stenosis. While the Lecompte maneuver is generally employed as noted in Fig. 17, rare cases involving a posterior aorta may dictate a different reconstruction without the Lecompte maneuver as noted in the legend for

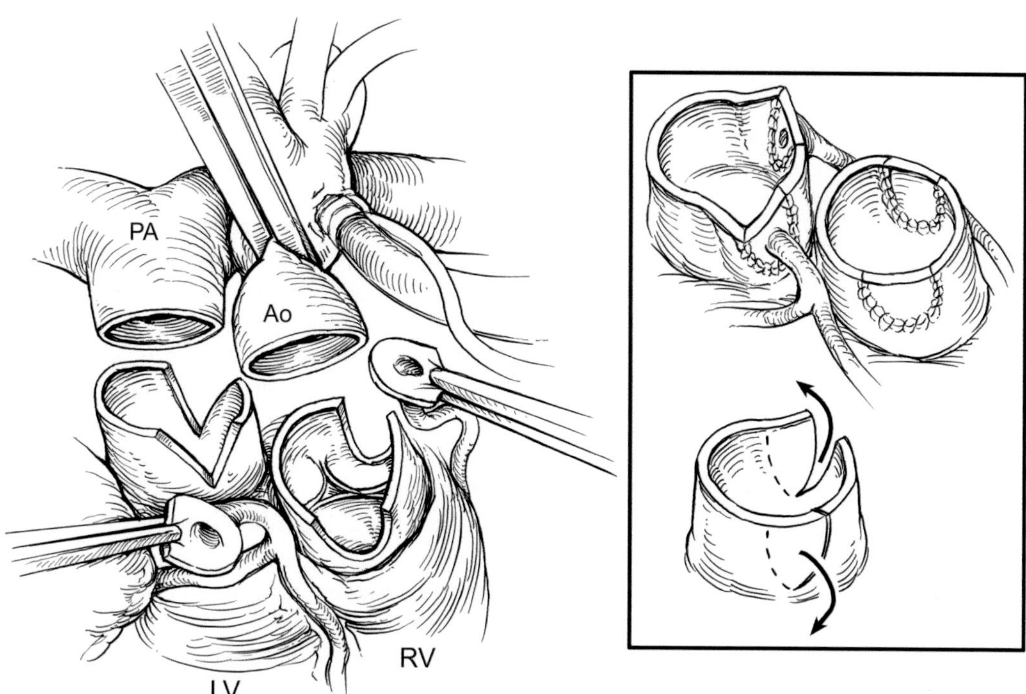

Fig. 16 Shows the proper placement of the aortic cross-clamp with great artery transection and coronary artery mobilization. The linear incisions in the pulmonary artery are made in preparation for direct coronary translocation technique. The "trap door" type of implantation technique is shown in the inset. The "trap door" technique is used to optimize the coronary flow pattern since the coronary arteries need to be mobilized for a considerable distance for this operation; more than for the usual pattern that is used for arterial switch for simple TGA. *Ao, aorta; LV, left ventricle; PA, pulmonary artery; RV, right ventricle.* (With permission: Mavroudis 2015)

Fig. 17. As previously noted, VSD closure is undertaken through the right atrium and mitral valve, or with a trans-left atrial trans-tricuspid valve approach in some cases with situs solitus and dextrocardia. In keeping with physiologic repairs, the de Leval technique can be used to avoid injury to the anterosuperior conduction system (de Leval et al. 1979) (Fig. 3). As previously noted, VSD closure via the transected aorta is also possible, and is likely the best technique to avoid heart block.

Most surgeons prefer the Senning technique in ccTGA with the addition of pulmonary venous chamber enlargement for atrial reconstruction, in combination with the arterial switch operation (Fig. 18a–e) (Malhotra et al. 2011). In some cases, however, an inadvertently placed small right atrial patch will cause pulmonary venous return obstruction as shown in the left panel of Fig. 19. Once systemic venous return problems such as baffle leak or stenosis, have been excluded, the "red tube" pathway (pulmonary

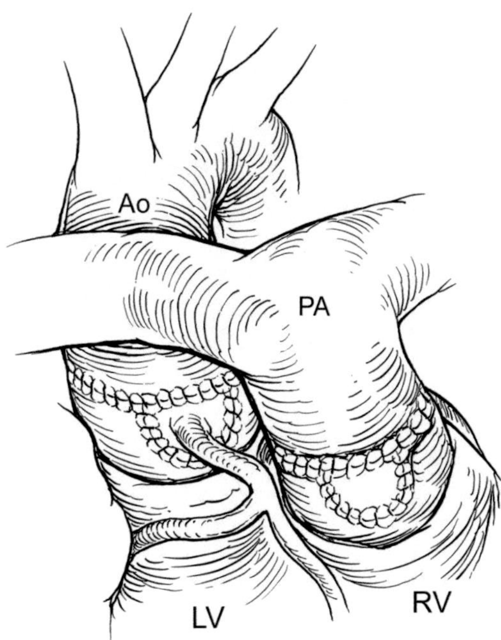

Fig. 17 The neopulmonary artery reconstruction can then be accomplished by separate pericardial patches as noted in the figure or by a pantaloon pericardial patch described previously in chapter "Complications Associated with Repair of Transposition of the Great Arteries and Associated Lesions". The figure also shows the completed arterial switch operation after the Lecompte maneuver was performed prior to great artery reconstruction. Some surgeons will prefer not to perform the maneuver of Lecompte in some circumstances where the expectant anatomic configuration is not favorable. This is a personal choice and best left up to the surgeon who is performing the operation. *Ao* aorta, *LV* left ventricle, *PA* pulmonary artery, *RV* right ventricle. (With permission: Mavroudis 2015)

venous return) can be repaired by a large pericardial or PTFE patch as noted in the right panel of Fig. 19. Figure 20 shows the modified Senning operation in progress which involves an improved technique of forming the pulmonary venous return "red tube" atrial augmentation and unobstructed flow by employing in situ pericardium in a side-to-side patch reconstruction. This in situ pericardial patch augmentation technique has been shown to have better results without pulmonary venous obstruction. The preference for the Senning procedure reflects general familiarity with the technique, applicability to all types of atrial arrangements, and demonstrated superiority to the Mustard procedure in many historical concordant TGA series. However, some surgical programs have registered success using the Mustard technique for these patients with ccTGA (Davies et al. 2008a) as shown in Figs. 21 and 22). The acute complications associated with double switch (arterial switch + Senning procedure or Mustard procedure) are mostly caused by problems due to coronary artery translocation causing ischemia and poor ventricular function, oftentimes leading to ECMO as highlighted in Figs. 15, 16, 17, 18, 19, 20, 21, 22, 23 and 24 (Chapter "Complications Associated with Repair of Transposition of the Great Arteries and Associated Lesions", Transposition). Mid-term complications following the arterial switch and Mustard operations are usually caused by baffle leaks and/or pulmonary venous baffle obstructions as noted

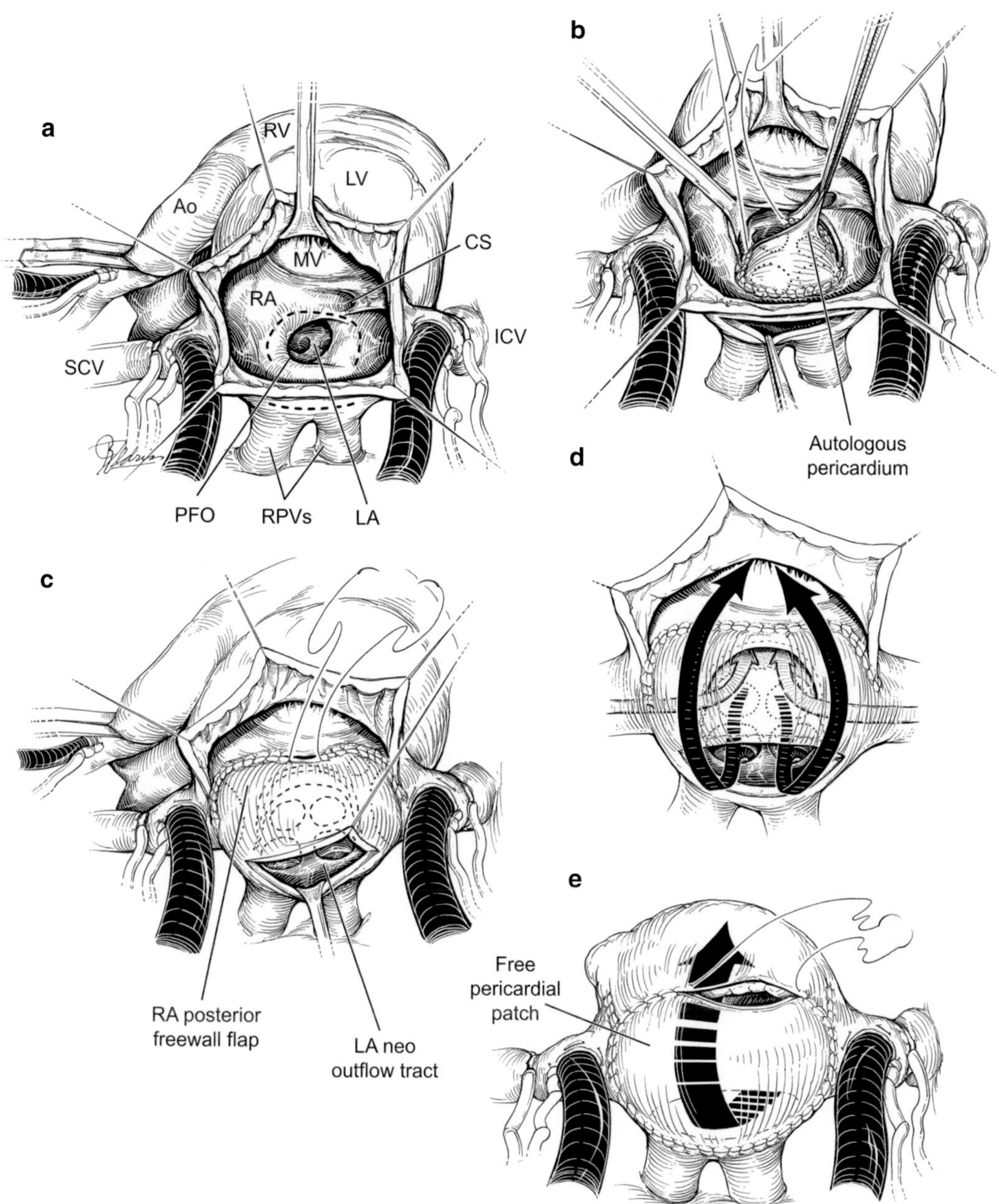

Fig. 18 Once the ventricular septal defect closure and arterial switch operations are accomplished, right atrial exposure for the Senning operation is commenced. Fig. a shows the incisions in the atrial septum which together with the pericardial extension (Fig. b) will form the posterior extension of the systemic venous return connecting the superior and inferior caval veins to the tricuspid orifice and thence to the right ventricle. Fig. c illustrates the formation of the systemic return baffle utilizing the right atrial wall. The confluence of pulmonary veins are shown in the posterior area of the atrium as noted in Fig. d with arrows to depict the flow characteristics of the pulmonary venous return around the right atrial tube into the mitral valve and thence to the left ventricle. Fig. e shows free pericardial augmentation of the right atrium to allow unobstructed flow from the confluence of the pulmonary veins into the left ventricle. *Ao* aorta, *CS* coronary sinus, *ICV* inferior caval vein, *LA* left atrium, *LV* left ventricle, *MV* mitral valve, *PFO* patent foramen ovale, *RA* right atrium, *RPVs* right pulmonary veins, *RV* right ventricle, *SCV* superior caval vein

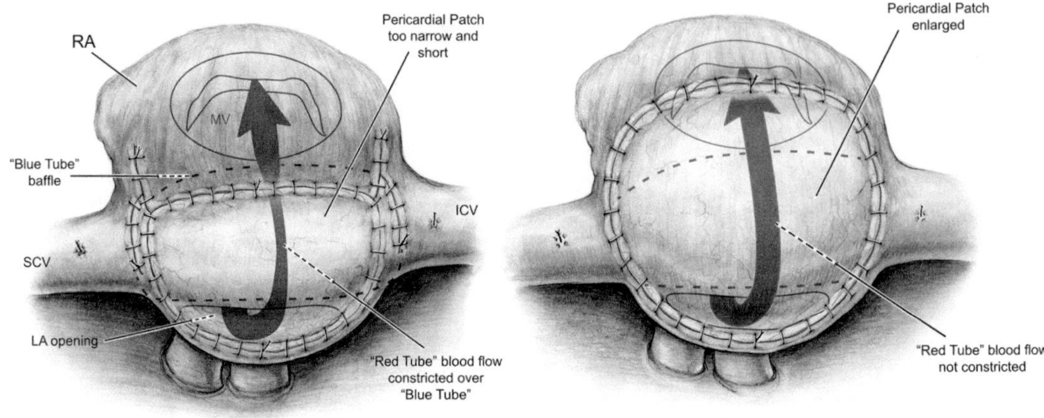

Fig. 19 Classic Senning operation with a small free pericardial patch can result in pulmonary vein stenosis (red tube stenosis) as noted in the left panel. Once systemic venous return "Blue Tube" problems such as baffle stenosis or disruption have been excluded, a right atrial augmentation patch using pericardium or polytetrafluoroethylene (PTFE) can be used to enlarge the "Red Tube" pathway as noted in the right panel. *ICV* inferior caval vein, *LA* left atrium, *MV* mitral valve, *RA* right atrium, *RPVs* right pulmonary veins, *SCV* superior caval vein

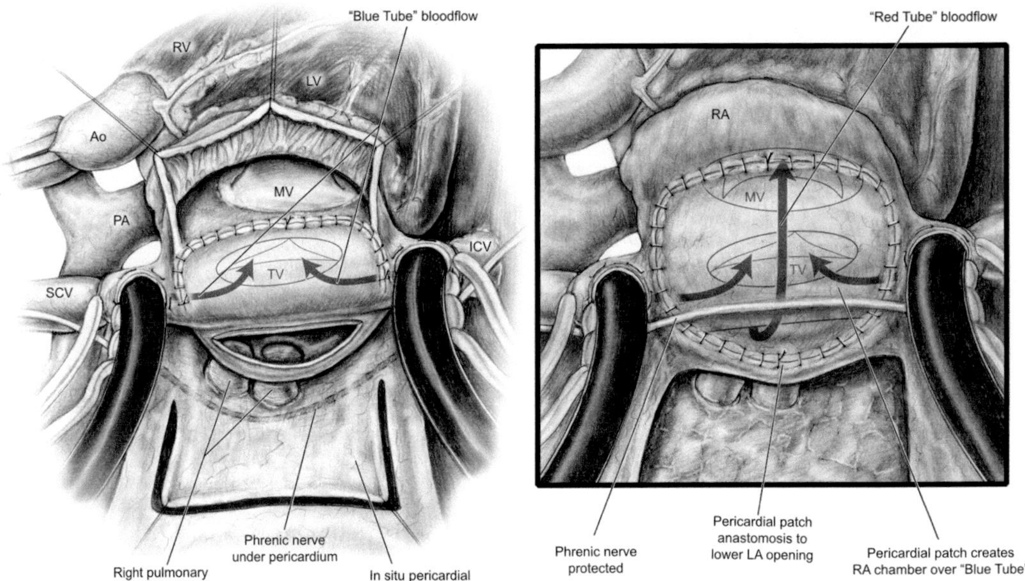

Fig. 20 Shows the right atrial wall baffle in the process of being sewn into place at the posterior portion of the atrial wall baffle. The atrial wall baffle size is important since it must form an appropriately sized pathway for the systemic venous return to the tricuspid valve/right ventricle and allow an appropriately sized pathway for the pulmonary venous return to flow unimpeded towards the mitral valve and into the left ventricle. Once the systemic venous baffle is completed, there is no access to the coronary sinus for retrograde cardioplegia administration. Therefore, aortic antegrade cardioplegic administration will be optimal. The left panel illustrates the appropriate size of the atrial wall baffle with arrows indicating the systemic venous return into the tricuspid valve. The systemic venous return pathway is noted as the "Blue Tube" to indicate the unoxygenated systemic venous return. The right panel shows the modified technique of forming the pulmonary venous return "Red Tube" which is a sobriquet for oxygenated blood return to the left ventricle. The right panel shows the modified technique of right atrial augmentation to ensure unobstructed flow is constructed using intact pericardium in a side-to-side patch augmentation. This arrangement has been shown to have better results thereby avoiding progressive pulmonary venous pathway obstruction. *Ao* aorta, *ICV* inferior caval vein, *LA* left atrium, *LV* left ventricle, *MV* mitral valve, *PA* pulmonary artery, *RA* right atrium, *RV* right ventricle, *SCV* superior caval vein, *TV* tricuspid valve

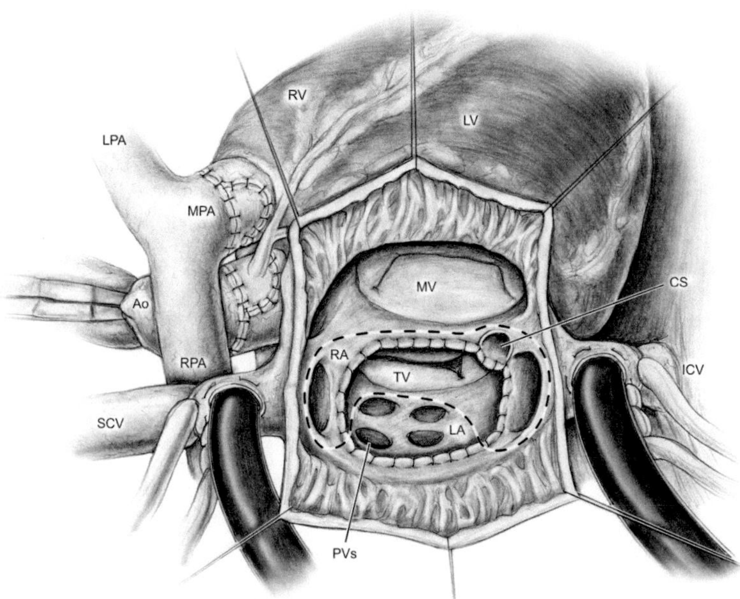

Fig. 21 Revision shows a patient who had had the arterial switch operation and ventricular septal defect (VSD) closure before the atrial baffle operation for ccTGA repair. Once the VSD is accomplished, right atrial exposure for the atrial switch operation is commenced. In this case, we elected to show the Mustard operation, although the majority of surgeons nowadays prefer the Senning operation for reasons that are expressed in previous drawings. The figure demonstrates a patient undergoing aortobicaval cardiopulmonary bypass, aortic cross-clamping and cardioplegic arrest after arterial switch. The anatomic details are shown with the dotted lines projecting the suture line that will be necessary to implant the pericardial baffle. Note that the coronary sinus is incised into the left atrium to ensure drainage. The baffle therefore serves to direct systemic venous blood flow towards the tricuspid valve and into the right ventricle. *Ao* aorta, *CS* coronary sinus, *ICV* inferior caval vein, *LA* left atrium, *LPA* left pulmonary artery, *LV* left ventricle, *MPA* main pulmonary artery, *MV* mitral valve, *PVs* pulmonary veins, *RA* right atrium, *RPA* right pulmonary artery, *RV* right ventricle, *SCV* superior caval vein, *TV* tricuspid valve

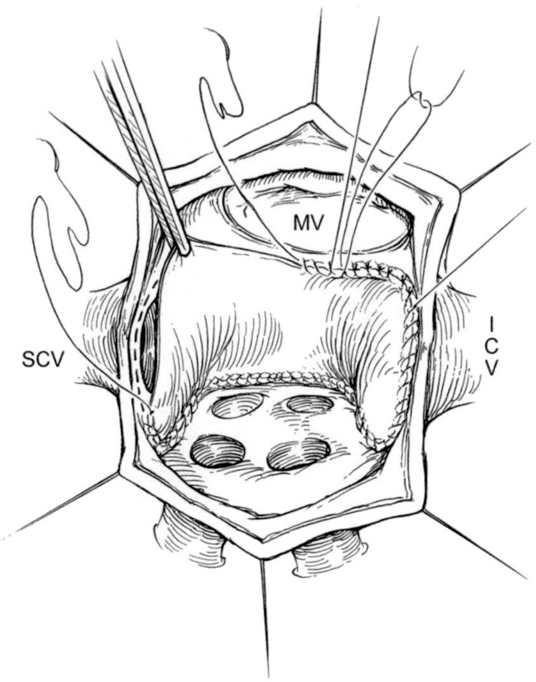

Fig. 22 The baffle is being sewn into place as noted in the figure leaving space for the pulmonary venous return to flow unimpeded towards the mitral valve and into the left ventricle. Cardioplegia administration can still be accomplished after the arterial switch operation. *IVC* inferior vena cava, *MV* mitral valve, *SVC* superior vena cava. (With permission: Mavroudis 2015)

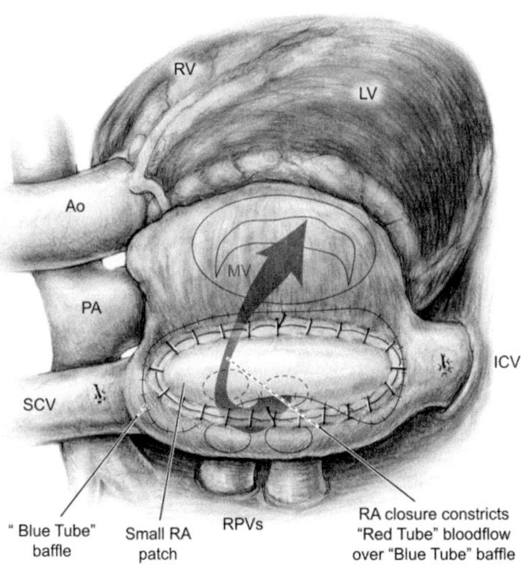

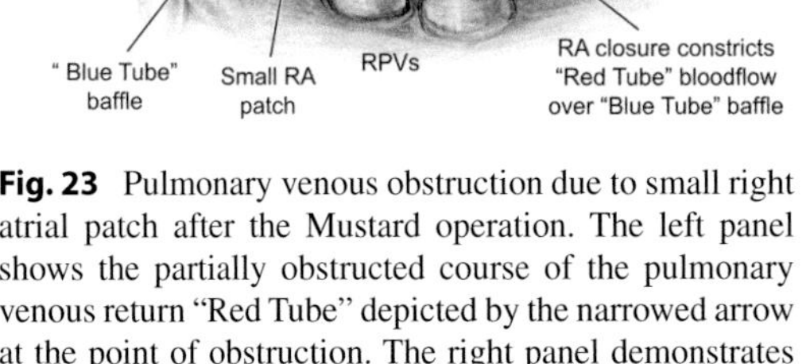

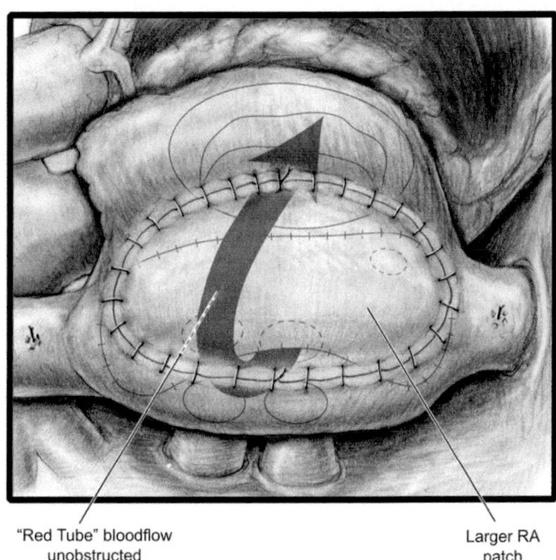

Fig. 23 Pulmonary venous obstruction due to small right atrial patch after the Mustard operation. The left panel shows the partially obstructed course of the pulmonary venous return "Red Tube" depicted by the narrowed arrow at the point of obstruction. The right panel demonstrates the resolution of the obstructed "Red Tube" pathway by an augmentation patch depicted by the unobstructed arrow. *Ao* aorta, *ICV* inferior caval vein, *LV* left ventricle, *MV* mitral valve, *PA* pulmonary artery, *RA* right atrium, *RV* right ventricle, *SCV* superior caval vein

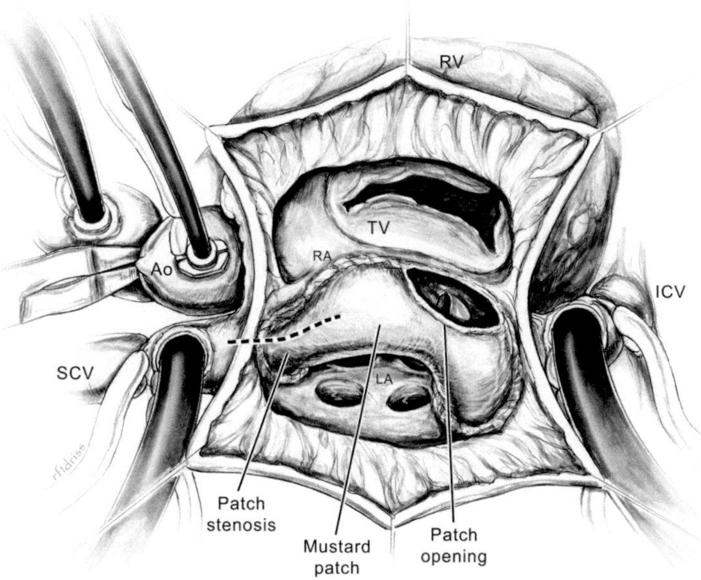

Fig. 24 In general, the operative approach for patients with baffle obstructions and/or leaks is similar. Aortobicaval cardiopulmonary bypass is established with direct cannulation of the superior and inferior caval veins. Once cardioplegic arrest is performed, an atrial incision is performed inferior to the superior caval vein, with entry into the neopulmonary venous atrium. This incision is extended parallel to the superior and inferior caval veins to expose the atrial baffle that was previously constructed using the Mustard or Senning technique. At this point, inspection determines the site of baffle stenosis or baffle leak. The figure illustrates both problems in one drawing: a stenotic superior caval vein baffle pathway and a baffle leak, which is shown closer to the inferior caval vein at the attachment near the tricuspid valve. Generally, only one of these problems is noted in any given patient, but these drawings show both problems and their operative solutions in the same drawing. In the case of a baffle leak, it is imperative to determine whether the baffle leak is also associated with a baffle stenosis. The best approach to this anatomic dilemma is to extend the baffle leak by incision to the os of the superior or inferior caval vein, whichever is closer to the baffle leak as shown by dashed line. *Ao* aorta, *ICV* inferior caval vein, *LA* left atrium, *RA* right atrium, *RV* right ventricle, *SCV* superior caval vein, *TV* tricuspid valve. (With permission: Mavroudis and Dearani 2020)

in Figs. 23, 24, 25, 26 and 27. These problems, if not corrected in a timely manner can result in sudden death.

Further to treatment options are patients with a low PA pressure (e.g., following PA banding) who can undergo adjunct bidirectional Glenn shunt in association with baffling the IVC to the TV as shown in Fig. 28. This anatomic reconstruction alternative may simplify atrial baffling and reduce the chance of superior vena cava (SVC) obstruction, which in historical terms, has been a significant disadvantage of the Mustard operation for TGA. In patients with a small RV, this technique is an important adjunct, but surgical programs advocate the approach as a more routine choice (Malhotra et al. 2011). This strategy, generally known as the hemi-Mustard + BCPS, revives in small measure the principles of the Baffes operation, an early palliative approach for concordant TGA (Mavroudis et al. 2014). The potential complications concerning this approach are baffle leaks, pathway stenosis, and atrial arrhythmias.

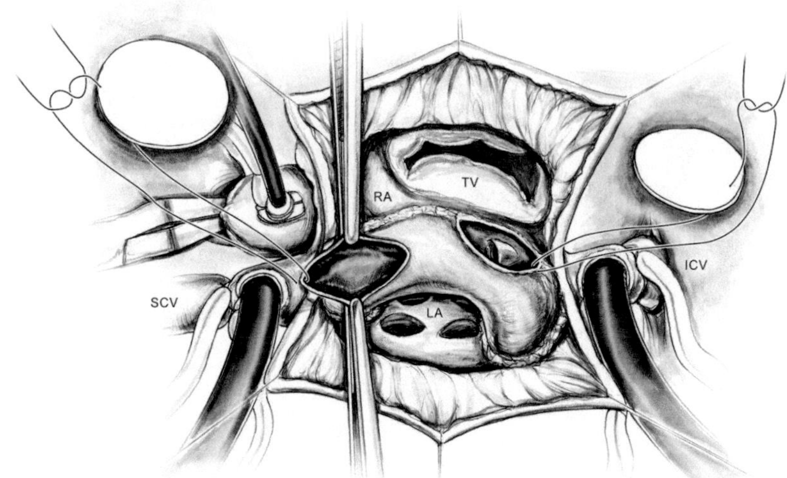

Fig. 25 Once the atrial incision is performed, biologic materials are used to simultaneously close the leak and augment the baffle pathway, using the running suture technique as shown in the figure. In the case of a baffle leak without stenosis, the leak can be repaired with a biologic patch, as noted in the baffle disruption near the inferior caval vein in the same drawing. *ICV* inferior caval vein, *LA* left atrium, *RA* right atrium, *SCV* superior caval vein, *TV* tricuspid valve. (With permission: Mavroudis and Dearani 2020)

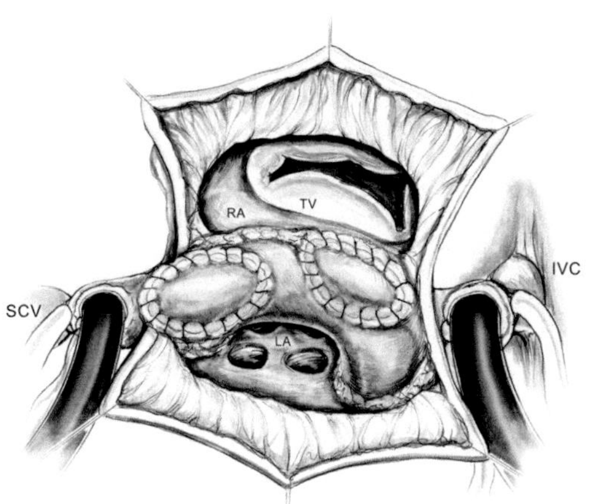

Fig. 26 Shows the completed repairs, with both patches in place. *IVC* inferior vena cava, *LA* left atrium, *RA* right atrium, *SCV* superior caval vein, *TV* tricuspid valve. (With permission: Mavroudis and Dearani 2020)

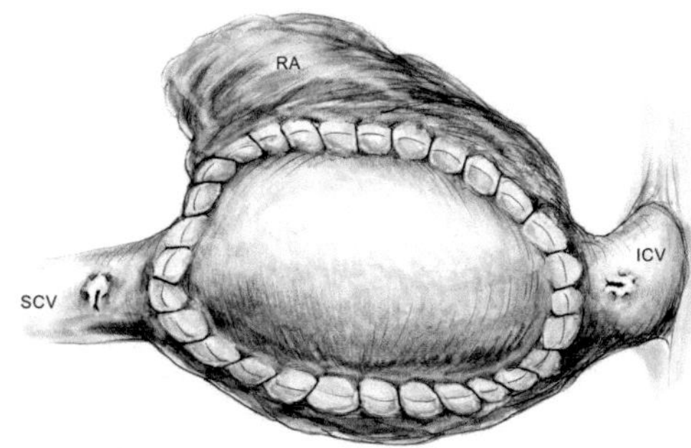

Fig. 27 Shows how the pulmonary venous chamber is augmented with a biologic or synthetic PTFE patch to ensure a proper and unobstructed pathway of the pulmonary venous atrium. A pulmonary venous vent in the right atrial appendage can aid in cavitary air removal before release of the cross-clamp; alternatively, opening the slings around the caval veins with manual propulsion of venous flow through the heart, the lungs, and out the aortic vent can also be effective for air removal. *ICV* inferior caval vein, *RA* right atrium, *SCV* superior caval vein. (With permission: Mavroudis and Dearani 2020)

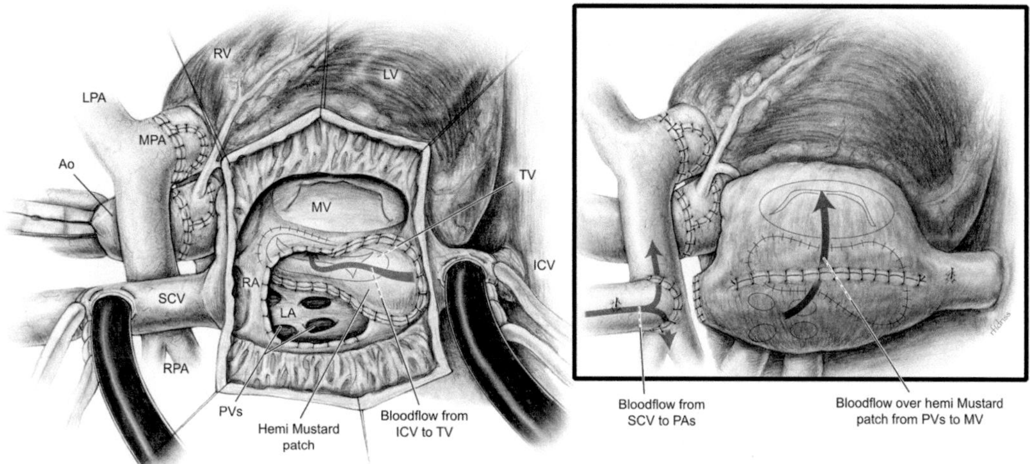

Fig. 28 Shows the hemi-Mustard operation that can be performed in association with the arterial switch operation for ccTGA. Note that the pericardial baffle directs inferior caval vein flow to the tricuspid valve leaving the superior caval vein to be connected to the systemic venous return via concurrent bidirectional Glenn anastomosis. Patients with low pulmonary artery pressure (e.g., following pulmonary artery banding) or significant subpulmonary stenosis are candidates for anatomic configuration. This anatomic reconstruction alternative may simplify the creation of the atrial baffling and reduce the chance of superior caval vein obstruction, which in historical terms, has been a significant disadvantage of the Mustard operation for transposition of the great arteries. In addition, patients with a small right ventricle can be treated in this manner. Potential complications concerning this approach are baffle leaks, pathway stenosis, and atrial arrhythmias. *Ao* aorta, *ICV* inferior caval vein, *LA* left atrium, *LPA* left pulmonary artery, *LV* left ventricle, *MPA* main pulmonary artery, *MV* mitral valve, *PVs* pulmonary veins, *RA* right atrium, *RPA* right pulmonary artery, *RV* right ventricle, *SCV* superior caval vein, *TV* tricuspid valve

11 Anatomic Correction of ccTGA via Senning or Mustard Plus Rastelli Operation

Patients with ccTGA and LVOT obstruction are not suitable subjects for the double switch operation as herein described; however, anatomic repair is still possible using a complex strategy which consists of an atrial baffle, intraventricular baffling of the VSD to the aorta, and RV-PA conduit placement (Ilbawi et al. 1990). This combined Mustard (Figs. 21 and 22) or Senning (Figs. 18) with the principles of the Rastelli operation (Figs. 29, 30, 31, 32, 33, 34, 35, 36, 37, 38, 39, 40, 41, 42 and 43) are reviewed. The Rastelli part of this combined operation is characterized by an intraventricular baffle to connect the LV with both the aorta and pulmonary artery, followed by proximal PA division and right ventricular-to-pulmonary artery conduit placement. The VSD may have to be enlarged to ensure an unobstructed pathway between the LV and aorta, respecting the location and course of the conduction system. Other options to manage the restrictive VSD include root translocation (ensuing paragraphs), and an adjunct Damus-Kaye-Stansel connection (El-Zein et al. 2015). Whatever the solution regarding LV-to-Ao pathway connection, the intraventricular baffle will require careful attention to detail to avoid subaortic stenosis. This potential complication and its resolution are noted in Figs. 1, 2, 3, 4 and 5 (DORV chapter). Essentially, the patch must be large enough to create a curved configuration to enhance the flow pattern. A corrugated Dacron graft cut longitudinally will create an excellent patch with the appropriate curved configuration to avoid subaortic stenosis as noted in Fig. 38. RV-to-PA continuity is established using an extracardiac valved conduit. Figure 43 shows the completed right ventricular-to-pulmonary artery

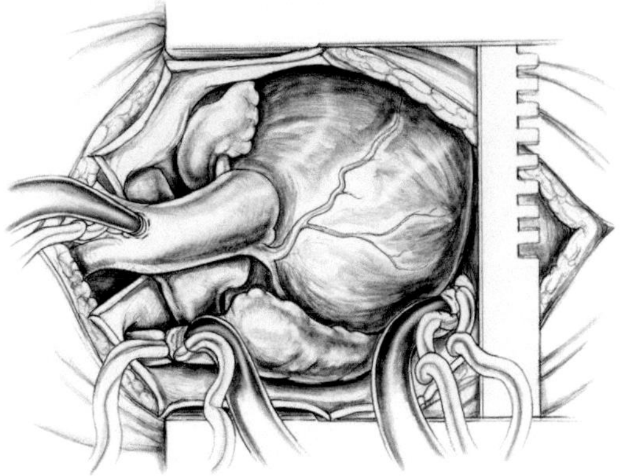

Fig. 29 The atrial switch-Rastelli operation was designed to create an anatomic and physiologic repair of ccTGA with ventricular septal defect and left ventricular outflow tract obstruction. The atrial switch can be accomplished by the Mustard operation or the Senning operation. There are advantages and disadvantages of both procedures. Historically, the Senning operation was first described in 1959. The complex flaps proved challenging to most surgeons and it was not until Mustard's 1964 innovation that the atrial switch operation gained popularity. In the ensuing decades, surgeons debated the efficacy of both operations. Nowadays, some surgeons favor the Senning operation because the atrial flaps can grow. Others feel that the Mustard operation is easier to visualize and execute, especially since this operation is not performed frequently in the present era. The operating surgeon should elect a procedure based on past experience and familiarity with the procedure. We have performed both operations and cannot offer one as being superior to the other. We demonstrate the Mustard operation herein. The principles of repair are very similar for both atrial switch operations. No matter which procedure is used, of primary importance is the creation of obstruction-free venous pathways. The figure shows aortobicaval cardiopulmonary bypass being instituted. (With permission: Mavroudis 2015)

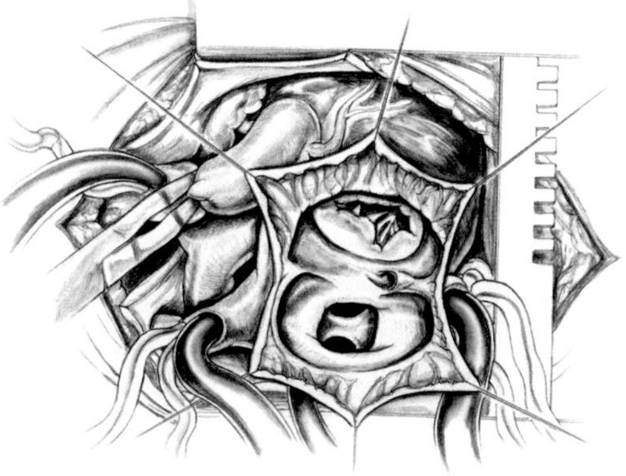

Fig. 30 Shows aortic cross-clamping, cardioplegic arrest, and right atrial exposure. A foramen ovale is noted in the fossa ovalis. (With permission: Mavroudis 2015)

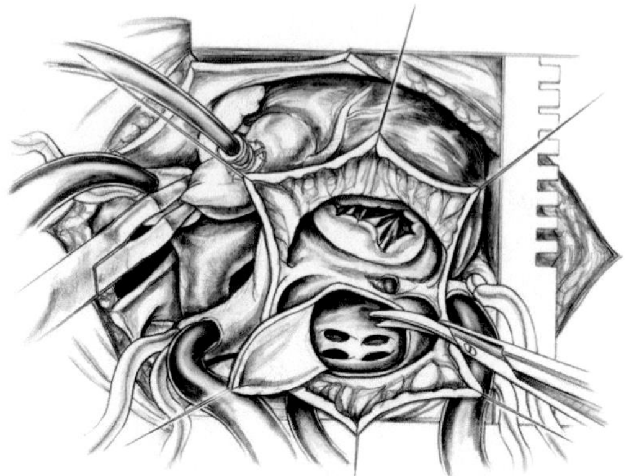

Fig. 31 Demonstrates the resection of the septum secundum (with special care to avoid injury to the conduction system) in order to facilitate creation of the superior portion of the pericardial baffle. (With permission: Mavroudis 2015)

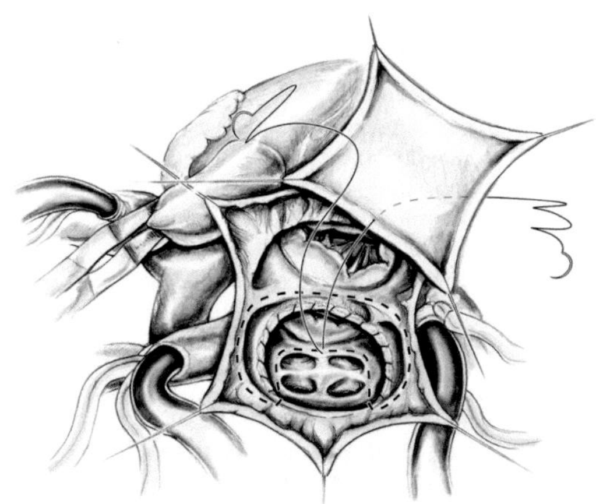

Fig. 32 Shows a number of important considerations. First, one can notice the suture line that reapproximates the endocardial surface from where the septum secundum was resected. This part of the operation is not always accomplished by surgeons. Some prefer to leave the resected area alone while others just reapproximate the edges of the resected septum secundum. This is a rather important consideration since during the resection, the atrial wall can be inadvertently excised thereby causing a large hole which may or may not be appreciated during the operation. Reapproximating the endocardial edges will emphasize this possibility and will correct the problem if present. Also depicted in this drawing are the dotted lines which visualize the course and extent of the pericardial baffle which is to be sutured in place. The pericardium is noted with a suture that starts the implantation technique midway between the posterior mitral valve annulus and left-sided confluence of pulmonary veins. Notice that the pericardial patch is not cut to size or shape at the outset of the implantation procedure. The patch can be cut and shaped as the suturing takes place accounting for optimal placement, large enough for the systemic venous pathway and small enough not to obstruct the pulmonary venous pathway. (With permission: Mavroudis 2015)

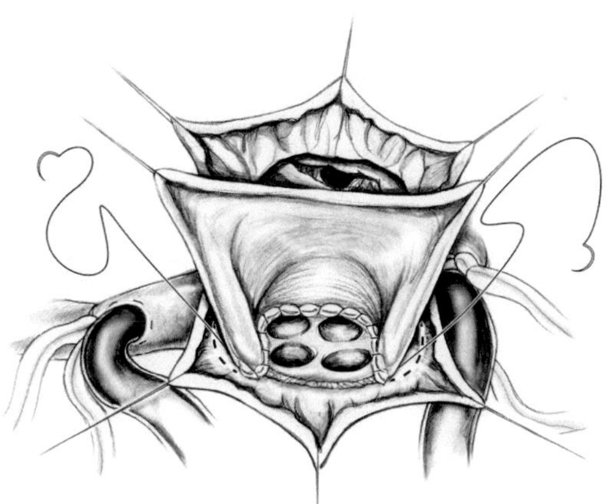

Fig. 33 Shows the posterior half of the baffle being placed. At this point, the pericardial patch can be cut to shape and size for the remainder of the baffle formation. (With permission: Mavroudis 2015)

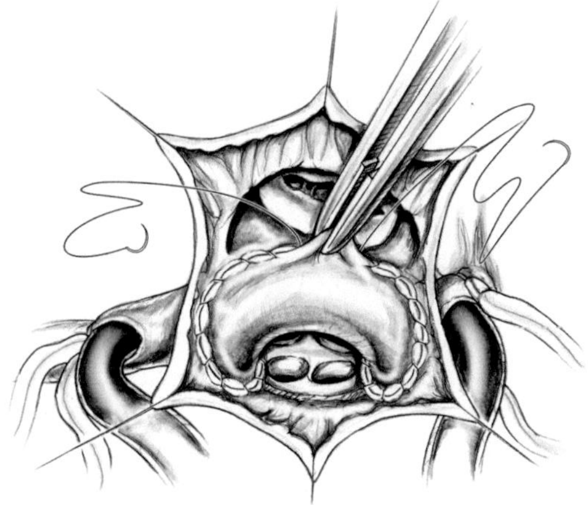

Fig. 34 Shows the near completion of the pericardial baffle with the last stitches being placed. At this point, one can either accept the result based on past experience or one could release the superior and inferior vena cava slings and allow the baffle to fill and assume the position that it would have during separation from cardiopulmonary bypass. Some surgeons prefer to perform this maneuver and assess the baffle, which could result in baffle revision if deemed necessary. The drawback for this maneuver is that the heart will fill with warmer systemic blood and compromise the extent of cardioplegic arrest if not recognized and countered by another administration of cardioplegic solution. These rather subtle maneuvers will allow for an optimally sized baffle and enhanced myocardial preservation. (With permission: Mavroudis 2015)

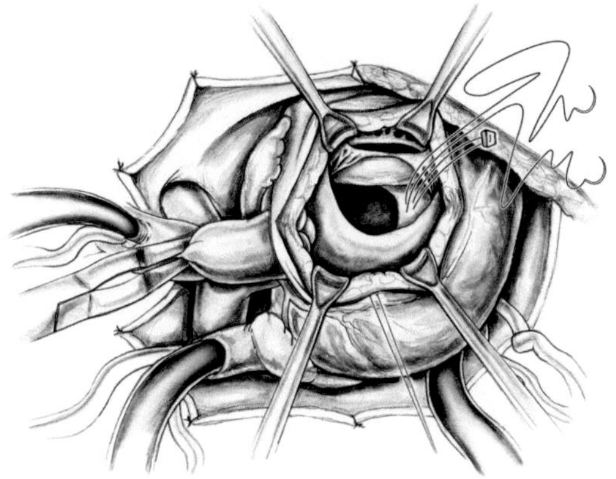

Fig. 35 The Rastelli part of the Mustard-Rastelli or Senning-Rastelli operation starts with the right ventriculotomy with special consideration to the course of the coronary arteries. In this situation, it must be remembered that the morphologic right ventricle is towards the left. The figure shows the placement of interrupted pledgetted sutures around the edges of the ventricular septal defect. Care is taken to avoid injury to the tricuspid valve and conduction system which is demonstrated in Fig. 24. (With permission: Mavroudis 2015)

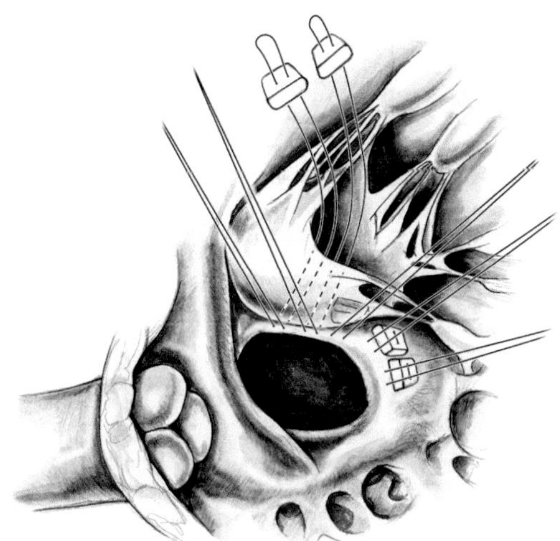

Fig. 36 Shows further placement of interrupted pledgetted ventricular septal defect (VSD) sutures with care being taken to recognize the path of the tricuspid valve and the conduction system which courses along the superior portion of the VSD on the morphologic surface of the left ventricle. (With permission: Mavroudis 2015)

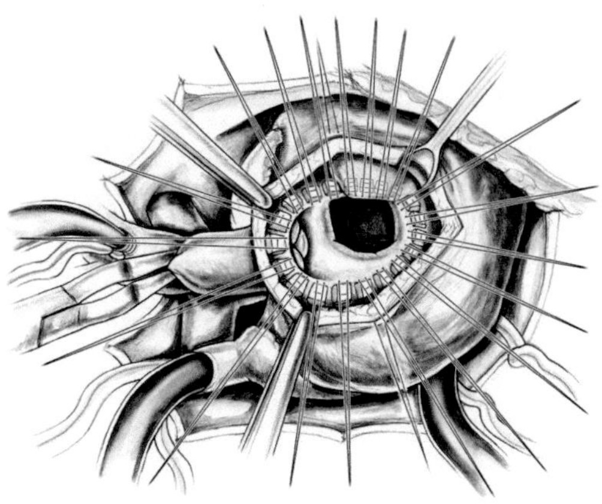

Fig. 37 Shows the completion of the pledgetted suture placement in preparation for the ventricular baffle. Some surgeons prefer fewer pledgetted sutures or a running suture technique. The choice of suture repair of a complicated ventricular septal defect (VSD) is left to the operating team. Because the course of the left ventricle to the aorta can be potentially obstructed with a flat patch, some surgeons use a divided corrugated Dacron graft that maintains its favorable shape for an unobstructed pathway from the left ventricle, through the VSD, and into the right ventricular outflow tract (subaortic area). (With permission: Mavroudis 2015)

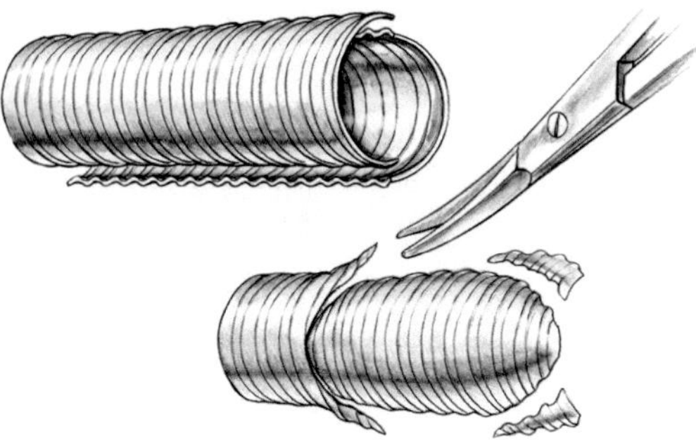

Fig. 38 Shows the preparation of the graft with the proper length and fashioning for the implantation. (With permission: Mavroudis 2015)

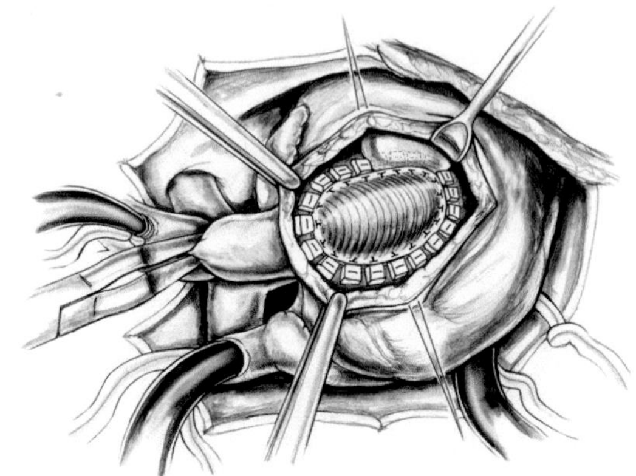

Fig. 39 Shows the completed ventricular baffle in place which assures left ventricular to aortic unobstructed continuity without impinging on right ventricular volume which will facilitate right ventricular-to-pulmonary artery continuity by a valved conduit. The pulmonary artery trunk should be transected with oversewing of the proximal trunk in preparation for the conduit placement. (With permission: Mavroudis 2015)

conduit which is shown to the left side of the aorta. This maneuver will allow conduit positioning to the left of the closed sternum thereby avoiding conduit compression and dangerous reentry in the event of conduit replacement in the future. Figure 44 shows the conduit being placed to the right side of the aorta with obligatory conduit course across the midline which carries both risks (Fig. 44, inset). Alternatively, direct RV-to-PA connection may be facilitated by the Lecompte maneuver which will more easily bring into apposition the two structures (PA and RV). Even with this reconstruction, however, sternal reentry is still a risk factor. The connection can be modified with a monocusp-bearing patch placed anteriorly. Atrial ventricular concor-

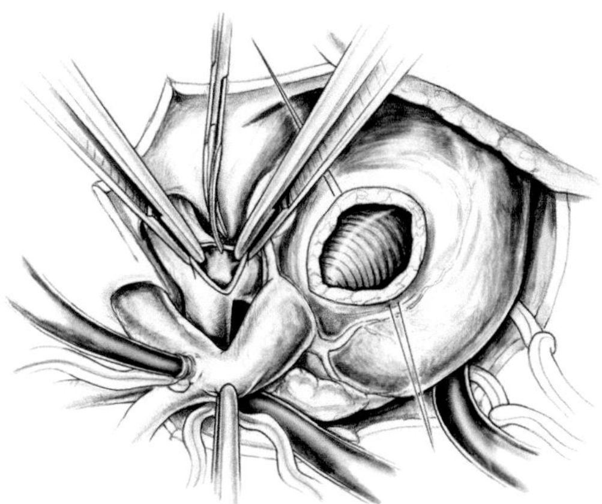

Fig. 40 Shows transection of the pulmonary artery trunk after the cross-clamp has been removed. Some surgeons would not release the cross clamp until the proximal pulmonary artery trunk is oversewn to ensure that no air is introduced into the left side. Others reason that the shortened cross-clamp time is worth the risk. They note that there is a left ventricular vent in place, and a working rhythm is not likely to return immediately after cross-clamp removal. In addition, some surgeons use insufflated CO_2 into the operative field that will minimize entry of ambient air into the left ventricle during this time. Obviously, there are no data to challenge either approach and it is left up to the surgeon and his/her practical wisdom to do what seems to be correct. (With permission: Mavroudis 2015)

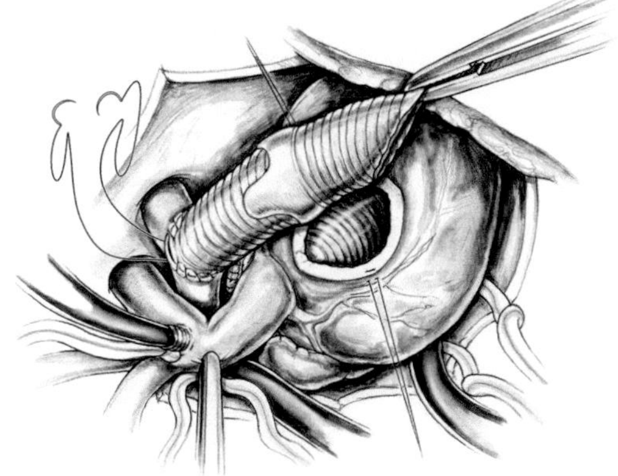

Fig. 42 Once the distal anastomosis is performed, the right ventricular-to-pulmonary artery conduit can be measured to size and cut on a bevel as noted in the figure. This is a rather important part of the operation. Too long a segment can result in distal pulmonary artery compression and right ventricular hypertension. Too short of a segment can result in undue anastomotic tension which can lead to disruption in the short term or false aneurysm in the long term. The corrugated graft allows for some leeway in this regard since the graft was manufactured with a certain amount of stretch potential. The surgeon can be comforted that while an accurate measurement is preferable, it is often not necessary because of the inherent graft specifications. (With permission: Mavroudis 2015)

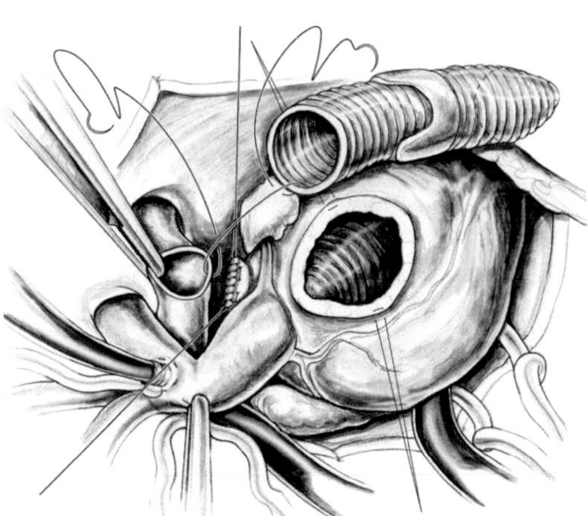

Fig. 41 The pulmonary artery does not often lie in such a favorable position as noted in the Figs. 29 and 30, however. Oftentimes, the main pulmonary orifice must be closed with a separate patch and the right ventricular-to-pulmonary artery conduit must be placed in the body of the left pulmonary artery to optimize the conduit pathway. In this projection, the artist depicts the distal pulmonary artery reconstruction in a favorably placed distal main pulmonary artery. (With permission: Mavroudis 2015)

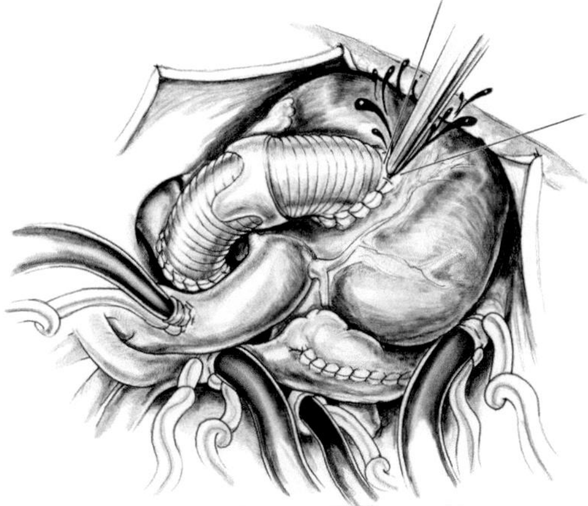

Fig. 43 Shows the completed right ventricular-to-pulmonary artery valved conduit with the deairing maneuvers. The deairing maneuver on the right side of the heart can be accomplished by release of the vena cava slings (not shown in the drawing) and intentional decrease of venous return to the bypass circuit. This will shift blood return to the heart that will facilitate the deairing maneuver. After separation from cardiopulmonary bypass the conduit should lie toward the left thoracic cavity. This anatomic configuration will help to avoid sternal compression and facilitate mediastinal reentry when conduit replacement becomes necessary. (With permission: Mavroudis 2015)

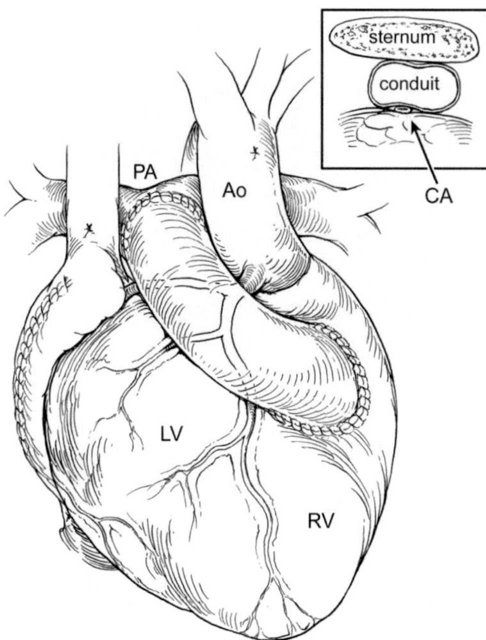

Fig. 44 Shows the result of a right ventricular-to-pulmonary conduit placement to the right of the ascending aorta which traverses across the midline. The inset illustrates the conduit being compressed by the closed sternum which has the disadvantages of conduit stenosis and unfavorable position during resternotomy for conduit replacement. *Ao, aorta; CA, coronary artery; LV, left ventricle; PA, pulmonary artery; RV, right ventricle.* (With permission: Mavroudis 2015)

dance is created by the Senning or Mustard baffle with simultaneous pulmonary venous pathway augmentation using in situ pericardium. Alternatively, the hemi-Mustard + bidirectional Glenn shunt approach, as noted herein, may be used in suitable cases to simplify this part of the procedure and improve SVC drainage.

12 Anatomic Correction using Intra-atrial Baffle Plus Translocation of the Great Vessels

Anatomic correction for ccTGA and LVOT obstruction can be performed by many methods depending on the specific anatomy and experience of the surgical team. In particular, anatomic correction under these circumstances with or without VSD can incorporate atrial baffling with various current techniques such as modified Rastelli or aortic translocation techniques which have been used in concordant TGA variants (Mavroudis et al. 2014). Aortic translocation, mostly known as the modified Nikaidoh operation can be combined with either Senning, Mustard, or hemi-Mustard + bidirectional Glenn Shunt (Ikai et al. 2012; Mavroudis et al. 2014; Hu et al. 2007; Nikaidoh 2016; Morell et al. 2005; Hraska 2008; Mair et al. 2016; Tateishi et al. 2013; Da Silva et al. 2015).

Aortic root translocation may obviate the need for a complex intraventricular baffle and outflow tract resection owing to difficult VSD anatomy remote from the aorta, confounding straddling tensor apparatus, hypertrophied RV, and volume limited RV which will not accommodate protrusion of the large interventricular baffle into the right ventricular outflow tract, causing RVOT obstruction. The beneficial anatomic construction of aortic translocation allows for a short and straight pathway from the LV to the aorta which has been highlighted in patients with concordant TGA. Aortic root translocation in patients with ccTGA is performed by coronary artery button

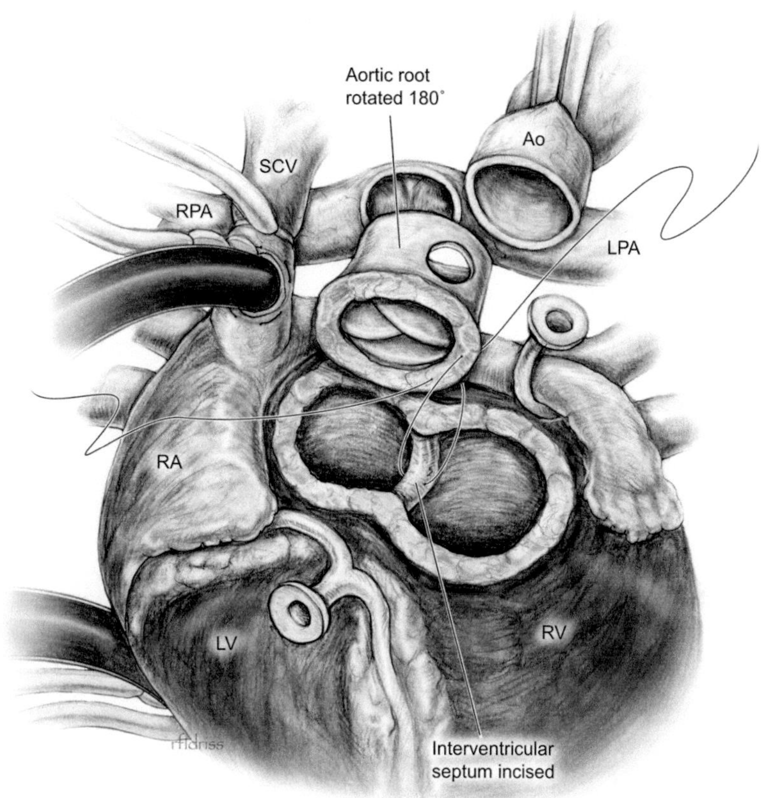

Fig. 45 Shows aortic root translocation in ccTGA. A modified Nikaidoh procedure is employed in conjunction with a Senning, Mustard, or hemi-Mustard/bidirectional cavopulmonary shunt atrial repair. The excised aortic root is moved to lie over the left ventricle, sutured to the pulmonary valve orifice and septal crest. Coronary mobilization and translocation is usually required to perform the neoaortic reconstruction as is noted in the drawing. *Ao* aorta, *LPA* left pulmonary artery, *LV* left ventricle, *RA* right atrium, *RPA* right pulmonary artery, *RV* right ventricle, *SCV* superior caval vein

excisions, aortic root mobilization (with an intact aortic annulus and leaflets) 180-degree rotation and posterior relocation after excision of the PA annulus and pulmonary valve leaflets. The aortic bloc is sutured to the PA annulus as noted in Fig. 45. The coronary buttons can then be reimplanted to avoid twisting or kinking as described in Figs. 90, 91, 92, 93, 94, 95 and 96, Chapter "Complications Associated with Repair of Transposition of the Great Arteries and Associated Lesions", TGA. In patients whose LVOT is obstructed by a small annulus, the LVOT can be enlarged by incising the infundibular septum in its midportion into the VSD if present (Ikai et al. 2012) as shown in Fig. 45. The anterior rim of the translocated aortic root is sutured to the ventricular septum, with or without interposing a VSD patch, depending on the size and complexity of the VSD. Conduction tissue is avoided since the suturing technique around the anterior root is limited in most cases to the anatomic RV myocardium. The repair is completed by a right ventricular-to-pulmonary artery conduit as noted in Fig. 46. Note that the conduit that is used is an

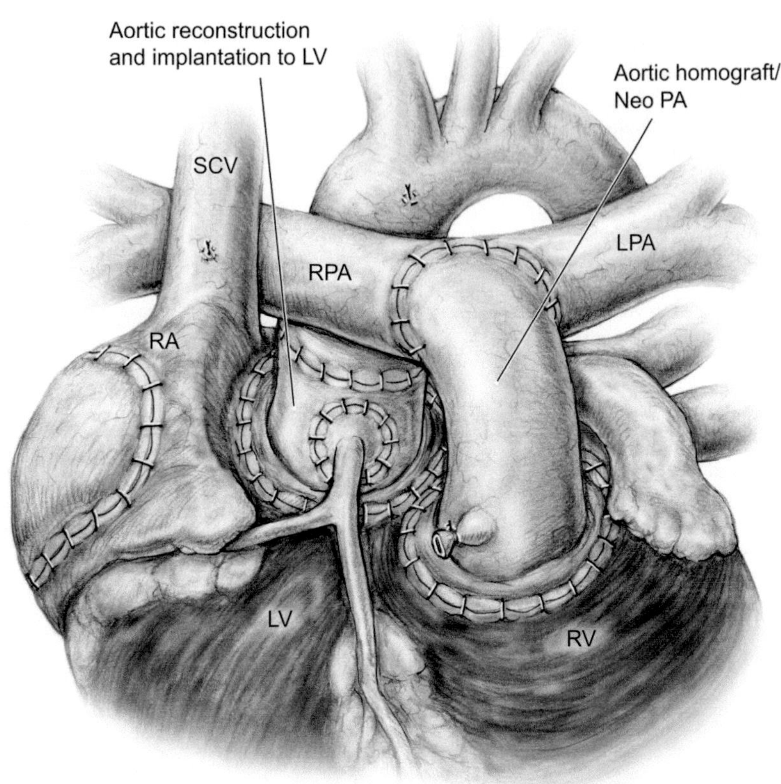

Fig. 46 Shows the completed repair of the modified Nikaidoh operation for congenitally corrected transposition of the great arteries. In this illustration, an aortic homograft has been depicted for right ventricular-to-pulmonary artery continuity after the Lecompte maneuver. A pulmonary homograft can also be used. Note that the modified intact pericardial patch is employed for right atrial patch augmentation. *LPA* left pulmonary artery, *LV* left ventricle, *PA* pulmonary artery, *RA* right atrium, *RPA* right pulmonary artery, *RV* right ventricle, *SCV* superior caval vein

aortic homograft in the fig. A pulmonary homograft or bioprosthesis also can be used for this purpose. Also note that the modified intact pericardial patch is used for right atrial patch augmentation to ensure unobstructed flow from the pulmonary venous inflow to the mitral valve and left ventricle.

Another technique for aortic translocation for septation and ventriculoarterial reconstruction in patients with ccTGA is the Yamagishi operation which involves en bloc rotation of the entire truncal root (Ikai et al. 2012; Tateishi et al. 2013) as depicted in Figs. 47, 48, 49, 49 and 50. This technique addresses the advantages of the Nikaidoh operation while simultaneously allowing the use of both native arterial roots, which eliminates the need for an extracardiac conduit. Figure 48 shows the rotated en bloc truncal root being implanted to the respective right and left outflow tracts. Proper mobilization of the right and left coronary arteries will promote accurate reimplantation to their respective aortic sinuses. The figure also shows how the pulmonary artery root can be enlarged using tetralogy techniques in the event that the pulmonary trunk proves to be too small. Complicating factors with this en bloc rotation

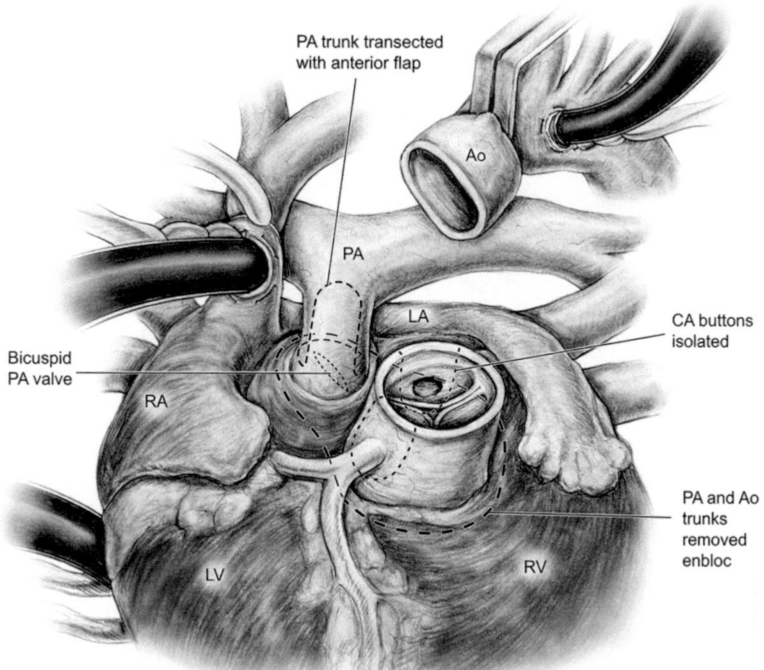

Fig. 47 Shows the anatomic details of the proposed Yamagishi operation which involves an en bloc rotation of the entire truncal root, coronary reimplantation, and use of the native pulmonary artery trunk, assuming that the pulmonary trunk is large enough to avoid pulmonary outflow tract obstruction. After aortobicaval cardiopulmonary bypass and cardioplegic arrest, the aorta is transected above the coronary arteries. The coronary buttons are then harvested from their positions in the aortic root. The supravalvar pulmonary artery trunk is resected as noted by the small, dashed lines. Once this is performed the entire truncal root can be excised as noted by the long, dashed lines with special care to avoid coronary artery injury. *Ao* aorta, *CA* coronary artery, *LA* left atrium, *LV* left ventricle, *PA* pulmonary artery, *RA* right atrium, *RV* right ventricle

involve coronary artery relocation which can result in ischemic episodes. Other important issues to avoid are aortic root distortion and regurgitation, as well as heart block. Attention to detail and planning will help to avoid these complications. Figure 49 shows the completed truncal root implantation with coronary artery reimplantation and cross-clamp release. At this point the operating team should look for any coronary artery distortion and kinking, which may necessitate reimplementation of cardioplegic arrest and re-exploration to correct the problem. The drawing in this case shows excellent anatomic characteristics resulting in favorable flow patterns. Also, the drawing shows the reparative procedure that might be needed if the pulmonary annulus proves to be too small to achieve favorable flow characteristics. The pulmonary annulus has been divided at the anterior commissure, assuming a bicuspid pulmonary valve. This allows a larger outflow tract much the same way that is performed for a tetralogy of Fallot repair. Figure 50 illustrates the completed operation with a transannular pulmonary outflow tract

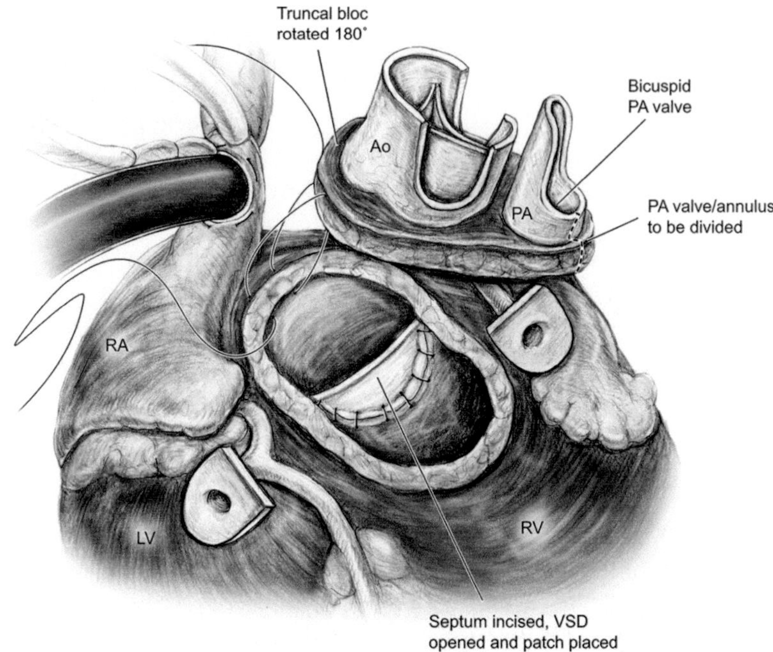

Fig. 48 Shows the en bloc rotation of the truncal root in ccTGA (Yamagishi operation) in the process of implantation. The two roots are excised as one autograft, and the coronaries are mobilized. After 180-degree rotation the roots are sutured to the outlet myocardium and crest of the ventricular septal defect patch. Coronaries are reimplanted, and standard tetralogy techniques can be used to augment the new right ventricular outflow tract obstruction as needed. Atrial repair can proceed or follow the Nikaidoh operation as determined by the operating team. *Ao* aorta, *LV* left ventricle, *PA* pulmonary artery, *RA* right atrium, *RV* right ventricle, *VSD* ventricular septal defect

Fig. 49 Shows the completed reversed truncal implantation, coronary artery reimplantation and cross-clamp removal. The small pulmonary artery root has been enlarged at the area between the anterior commissure to enlarge the right ventricular outflow tract. *Ao* aorta, *LPA* left pulmonary artery, *LV* left ventricle, *PA* pulmonary artery, *RA* right atrium, *RPA* right pulmonary artery, *RV* right ventricle

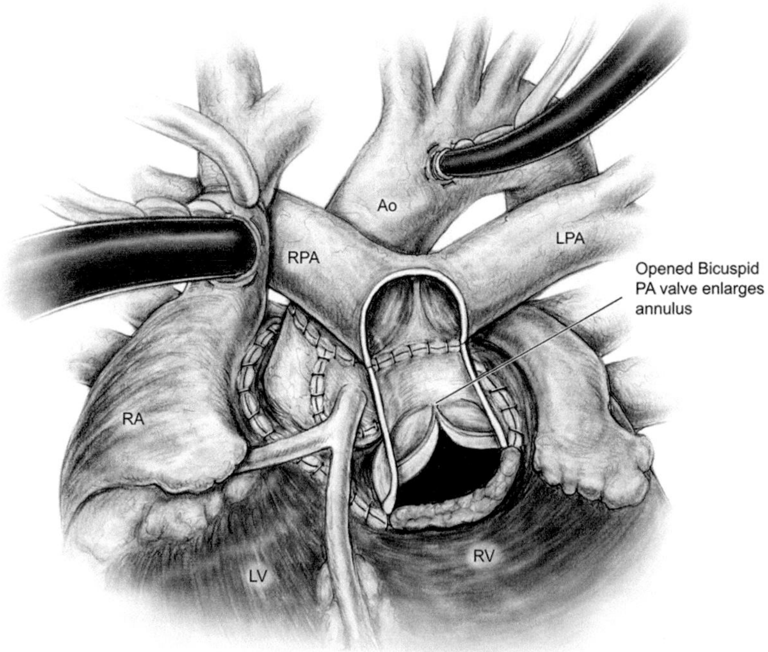

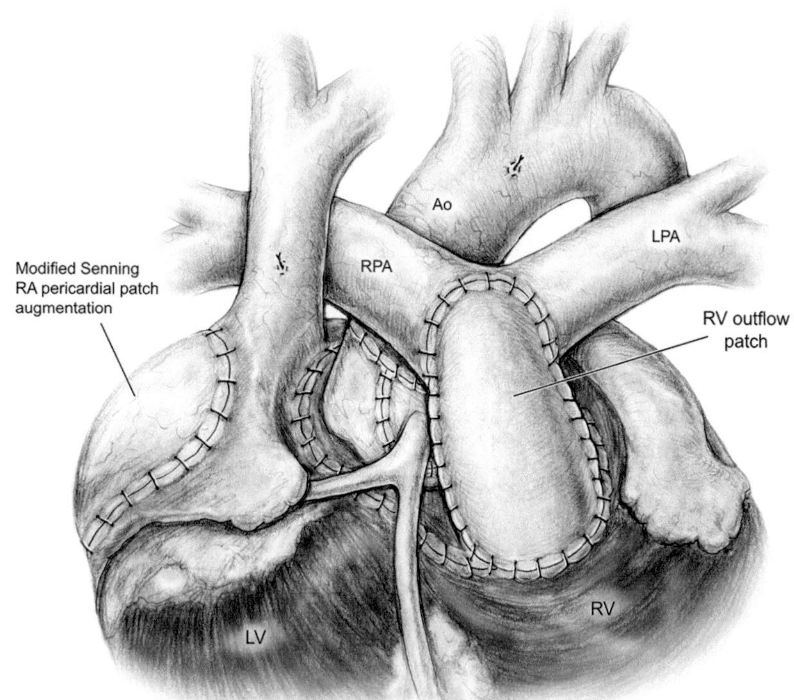

Fig. 50 Shows the completed operation with a transannular right ventricular outflow tract patch augmentation. The modified Senning right atrial intact pericardial patch augmentation is clearly seen. *Ao* aorta, *LPA* left pulmonary artery, *LV* left ventricle, *RA* right atrium, *RPA* right pulmonary artery, *RV* right ventricle

patch and the modified Senning right atrial intact pericardial patch augmentation.

Excision, mobilization, and reimplantation of the pulmonary root onto the RV has been utilized for both concordant and discordant TGA, in combination with Rastelli type septation (Tateishi et al. 2013; Da Silva et al. 2015). The process involves closure of the PA origin on the LV with a patch with the aorta remaining in the original position. The pulmonary artery trunk is then anastomosed to the right ventricle thereby avoiding the use of an extracardiac TV-to-PA conduit. Mobilization of the pulmonary valve is facilitated because the pulmonary valve is not in continuity with the mitral valve in ccTGA (Da Silva et al. 2015). Enlargement of the pulmonary valve and main PA may be required. Since the pulmonary valve now arises from the right ventricular free wall, standard tetralogy of Fallot techniques can be employed (Karl and Jacobs 2023).

While extensive experience has not accrued with translocation strategies for anatomic repair of ccTGA, preliminary reports have been favorable. Tam and associates (2021) have reported on 8 patients with a mean follow up of 52 months (Tam et al. 2021). Their abstracted analysis is as follows:

> Associated anomalies included situs inversus (n = 2), dextrocardia (n = 6), multiple muscular VSDs (n = 2), abnormal or straddling atrioventricular valve chords (n = 5), and branch pulmonary artery stenosis (n = 3). Four of 8 had previous systemic arterial shunts. Mean cardiopulmonary bypass was 487 min, and mean cardiac ischemic time was 307 min. Additional procedures included repair of branch pulmonary artery stenoses and closure of multiple muscular VSDs. There was no hospital death. One patient was supported with extracorporeal membrane oxygenation because of junctional tachycardia on postoperative day 5. One patient required pacemaker placement for first-degree heart block. Median hospital length of stay was 31 days. Mean length of follow-up was

52 months. All patients remain well with mild or no aortic regurgitation. The first patient underwent a repeat surgical operation for pulmonary venous baffle obstruction 2 years after Senning with aortic translocation (Tam et al. 2021).

Clearly, this operation is challenging due to technical complexity. However, patient outcomes have been satisfactory. Longer term follow-up will determine the need for late intervention. As surgeons master the technique of aortic translocation and repair of associated lesions, the role of the Nikaidoh and truncal rotation options will likely be used in routine cases which are also suitable for a Senning-Rastelli approach (Tateishi et al. 2013; Da Silva et al. 2015; Tam et al. 2021; Davies et al. 2008b).

As noted herein, the Nikaidoh operation for concordant hearts with TGA has been well illustrated in chapter "Complications Associated with Repair of Transposition of the Great Arteries and Associated Lesions", Figs. 90, 91, 92, 93, 94, 95 and 96. In particular Fig. 94 shows how complications leading to root malrotation, translocated aortic regurgitation, and coronary artery kinking can occur. Careful attention to accurate anatomic rotation, coronary artery reimplantation, and VSD closure will help surgeons to avoid these problems.

13 Cavopulmonary Connection Technique in ccTGA

The Fontan operation and associated potential complications is reviewed in chapter "Complications Associated with Bidirectional Glenn, Fontan Operations, and Arrhythmia Surgery". In particular complications associated with the Fontan procedure are noted in Figs. 11, 14, 19, 20, 22, 35, 36, and 72. The operation can be performed with or without fenestrations or previously established bidirectional Glenn shunt (Miller et al. 2022). The success of Fontan operations are highly dependent on the extant anatomic and hemodynamic characteristics of each patient. Oftentimes, especially in Fontan conversion operations, associated lesions will require attention and resolution such as arrhythmia surgery, aneurysm repair, atrioventricular valvar repair, and pathway stenoses resolution. There is however controversy as to how aggressive surgeons should be in treating mild AV valve regurgitation at the time of the Fontan operation. Karl and associates have noted that progression of native tricuspid insufficiency is unusual in this setting, as has been suggested by others (Karl 2011; Malekzadeh-Milani et al. 2016).

Other partial cavopulmonary surgical options for children with ccTGA and LVOT obstruction have been proposed and assessed by Mavroudis and co-workers who have employed a bidirectional Glenn shunt as an adjunct to pulmonary valvotomy in ccTGA with LVOT obstruction (Mavroudis et al. 1999) (Fig. 11). As previously noted, LV volume preload and pressure are reduced by diverting all superior caval venous blood to the confluent PAs.

This physiologic strategy in patients with ccTGA with LVOT obstruction is simple to perform and does not expose the patient to the complex operation of anatomic repair. The idea is to maintain the position of the interventricular septum by higher LV pressures which will allow proper TV and RV function without the risks of chordal stretching and papillary muscle dysfunction which attends patients with ccTGA when there is a disadvantageous shift of the interventricular septum. Consequently, this is an attractive approach for selected patients with good TV and RV function with a suitable LV outflow tract. The role of hemi-Mustard + bidirectional Glenn shunt has been discussed.

14 Pacemakers in ccTGA

The potential risk for spontaneous heart block or bradyarrhythmias for patients with ccTGA (L-looped hearts) is present with uni- and biventricular morphology. The need for pacemaker insertion in patients with ccTGA can therefore reach 38% by 40 years of age. The asynchronous cardiac rhythm can cause a decline in RV systolic function (Kwak et al. 2010; Kowalik et al. 2014; Graham Jr et al. 2000; Dobson et al. 2013). Cardiac synchronicity is extremely important in patients with ccTGA, not only for RV and TV function, but also for maintenance of LV function after anatomic repair. Dual chamber biventricular pacing has been shown to be beneficial, but there is controversy regarding resource allocation resulting in cost-benefit implications (Kowalik et al. 2014). In an attempt to create indications for dual chamber pacing, vector velocity echocardiographic imaging has emerged to analyze dyssynchrony in these patients as a guide to indications and lead positioning. In the majority of patients, the optimal ventricular pacing site in ccTGA with a systemic RV is on the LV side of the septum, at mid-ventricular level (El-Zein et al. 2015) similar to what is shown in Fig. 85 (Fontan Chapter). It is not altogether clear whether prophylactic atrial and ventricular epicardial leads should be placed at the reparative operation for ccTGA patients, even if the operation results in sinus rhythm. The propensity of future spontaneous heart block may cause some to place prophylactic leads to avoid resternotomy in the event that pacemaker therapy is indicated.

15 Cardiac Transplantation in ccTGA

Despite the aforementioned reparative methods for physiologic and anatomic treatment of patients with ccTGA, cardiac transplantation may become necessary, especially in those who develop ventricular failure. The indications and contraindications (mostly untreatable pulmonary hypertension) for transplantation in patients with ccTGA are no different than for others with advanced congenital heart disease. The techniques are similar to those used in concordant hearts. Most associated anatomic abnormalities do not preclude cardiac implantation as long as the great vessels are extensively mobilized. Individual aortic, PA, and caval anastomoses, with additional donor vascular tissue as required can be performed without too much difficulty. The main technical and therapeutic problems regarding cardiac transplantation in these patients, aside from effective donor harvest and ischemic time, are the challenges of resternotomy, safe dissection, and hemostasis, which are likely to increase the risk proportionally (Lewis et al. 2016; Sano et al. 1995). Complications associated with cardiac transplantation are discussed in chapter "Complications Associated with Pediatric Heart Transplantation". The general principles of cardiac transplantation which are presented therein apply in concept and practice to patients with ccTGA as well.

16 Outcome Analysis for ccTGA: Physiologic Repair

As Karl and Jacobs have written (Karl and Jacobs 2023),

> Historically, reported mortality for classical repairs has ranged from 4% to 33%. In the Melbourne series of operations designed to leave the RV in the systemic circuit (originally reported in 1995), 28 patients had VSD closure as an isolated procedure (n = 7), with direct relief of LVOT obstruction (n = 5), or with placement of an LV-PA conduit (n = 16. Hospital mortality was 4% and actuarial survival at 10 years was 83%. Twenty of the 24 long-term survivors were in New York Heart Association (NYHA) class I and 3 were in class II. Sixteen of 24 had important tricuspid insufficiency, and 12 of 22 had deterioration of RV function. These changes were noted within 3 years of operation in 75% of cases, and pre-repair $Q_p/Q_s > 1$ was a risk factor for both (related) problems ($p < .05$). This initial experience was what led Mee and his team to explore the possibility of anatomic correction for ccTGA, especially for patients with high pulmonary blood flow. Not all of the world's experience with classical repairs has been unfavorable, however, which further complicates the issue (Karl and Jacobs 2023).

The aforementioned paragraph by Karl and Jacobs not only summarizes the results of physiologic repair from one institution, but also provides the considered reasons for proceeding with the possibilities of anatomic repairs.

17 Anatomic Repair

In 1997, Karl and associates reported the initial Melbourne results for the arterial switch operation plus Senning repair in a group of 14 patients, age range 0.5–120 months who had ccTGA (Karl et al. 1997). Thirteen patients had an LV/RV pressure ratio of greater than 0.7 due to a large VSD (with or without prior PA band), severe congestive heart failure due to RV dysfunction and tricuspid insufficiency, or a PA band placed for ventricular conditioning following failed classic repair. Of the original 14 patients, 10 were not candidates for classic repair owing to RV hypoplasia, RV dysfunction, or tricuspid regurgitation. There was one hospital death and the amount of regurgitation improved from 3/4 preoperatively to 1/4 postoperatively. In addition, RV function normalized in 11 patients.

In 2013, Hoashi, Ichikawa and colleagues from Osaka reported 47 cases of anatomic correction with ccTGA, VSD, and LVOT obstruction or atresia, with either a Mustard or Senning atrial baffle. Of interest, the mean follow-up was 11 years. There was a 70.2% 20-year survival with no mortality since 1997. The 20-year freedom from reoperation was 49.7%. The only significant risk factor was era of operation (Hoashi et al. 2013).

The current world experience is summarized in Table 1 (Karl and Jacobs 2023). Significantly, TV function has improved significantly in the majority of patients who had dysfunction before operation. The long-term fate of LV function under these circumstances has been of some concern, especially in patients who had pre-repair PA banding. However, when compared with matched strategies in patients unsuitable for other types of repairs, the aforementioned results seem favorable. Nevertheless, cardiac transplantation will need to be considered for those patients who have LV failure.

A recent analysis by Drs. Karl and Jacobs (2023) have considered both EACTS Congenital Database and STS Congenital Heart Surgery Database results and offered a thoughtful approach to the potential long-term outcomes of physiologic and anatomic repair of ccTGA. They note,

> Results in the EACTS Congenital Database (to 2017) suggest that the contemporary hospital mortality for the double switch is 11.46% (n = 158) and for the atrial repair + Rastelli operation 16.67% (n = 90). Ischemic times and cardiopulmonary bypass durations were 160/256 and 145/232 minutes, respectively, for the two strategies. While individual teams have reported better results than those represented in multi-institutional pooled data, this information highlights again the complexity of anatomic repairs, and the relative infrequency with which they are performed worldwide. Complementary results from the STS Congenital Heart Surgery Database also suggest a significant operative risk, especially for Rastelli + atrial repair (n = 60, mortality = 10%). It is also notable that the primary diagnosis of ccTGA applies to only 0.1% of all operations listed in the database (Karl and Jacobs 2023).

Table 1 Results for anatomic repairs of ccTGA, as reported in the world literature

Authors, (year of publication)	City of origin	N	Early mortality (95% CL)
Karl et al. (1997)	Melbourne	14	7% (1.6–32)
Imai (1997)	Tokyo	44	9% (3–21)
Langley et al. (2003)	Birmingham	54	5.6% (2–15)
Duncan and Mee (2005)	Cleveland	73	1.5% (0.3–7)
Bautista-Hernandez et al. (2006)	Boston	44	4.5% (2–15)
Alghamdi et al. (2006)	Toronto (meta-analysis)	94	6.4% (3–13)
Gaies et al. (2009)	Ann Arbor	65	13.8% (8–24)
Ly et al. (2009), Gaies et al. (2009)	Paris	20	0 (0–16)
Sharma et al. (2009)	Bangalore	68	15% (8–25)
Hoashi et al. (2013)	Osaka	47	0 (0–14) for last 21 cases 70.2%, 20 year survival
All 2 stage (Cui et al. 2014)	Beijing	14	14% (4–40)
Bilal et al. (2016)	Istanbul	16	6.3% (1–28)
Hsu et al. (2016)	Taipei	18	22% (9–45), 53% 13-year survival
Tocharoenchok et al. (2016)	Bangkok	22	9% (2–28)

In general, enthusiasm for anatomic repairs is based on the known poor long-term outcome following classical repair in some patients, more than a well-documented favorable outcome for anatomic repairs over the same follow-up interval. Although anatomic repair can be performed with short-term outcomes similar to those achieved after physiologic repair, a full understanding of the long-term risks and benefits of anatomic repair is lacking. Moreover, in some series freedom from important LV dysfunction after anatomic repair is only about 50%–75% at 10 years, with the worst outcome observed in children requiring LV conditioning. Likewise, late freedom from reoperation has not improved significantly, owing partly (but not completely) to the use of extracardiac conduits."

18 Univentricular Repair and Extant Comparisons with Physiologic and Anatomic Repairs

Physiologic and anatomic repair options for ccTGA should be considered in light of the Fontan operation which has been proposed for some variants of ccTGA as noted in previous sections of this chapter. The Fontan operation in the recent era has been evaluated in the Australia New Zealand Fontan Registry with outcome for 220 lateral tunnel Fontan operations performed from 1987–1991. The results showed a 91% actuarial survival and 87% freedom of reoperation at 10 years (d'Udekem et al. 2014). In the current era, Fontan operative mortality for all anatomic subtypes remains very low and approaches zero in many experienced programs. Moreover, when considering relative complications between anatomic/physiologic repairs and the Fontan pathway, acquired heart block, LVOT obstruction, atrial baffle obstruction, and progressive TV and RV dysfunction are less germane to the Fontan operation for ccTGA.

Clearly, not all Fontan patients are the same and it appears that ccTGA patients may represent a favourable group owing to biventricular anatomy. Hsu and associates from Taipei (Hsu et al. 2016) have presented very important comparative data regarding follow-up in 56 ccTGA patients who had Fontan operations (n = 23), physiologic repair (n = 15) and anatomic repair (n = 18), in 2016. They presented 23 complex ccTGA patients who underwent univentricular palliations, largely for non-septatable hearts, with a survival of 100% at 16 years follow-up. In comparison, survival for 15 patients undergoing physiologic repair and 18 undergoing anatomic repair over a similar interval was 80% and 53%, respectively (92% and 64% when operative mortality was excluded) (Hsu et al. 2016). They concluded that single ventricle palliation showed good results in ccTGA patients with complex anatomy, assuming that long-term results are maintained. Furthermore, anatomic repair is the choice operation only for those with favorable anatomy. The more complicated intracardiac repairs have unfavorable outcomes due to LVOT obstruction, various degrees of atrioventricular block, systemic or pulmonary venous return obstruction and the lack of an ideal valved conduit for the Rastelli reconstruction. Consequently, they favored single ventricle palliation in ccTGA patients with complex and unfavorable anatomy.

In 2016, De Leon and associates from Texas Children's Hospital reported 97 patients with variants of ccTGA who were divided into 4 cohorts, namely, (1) those with systemic RV who had physiologic repair or no operation, (2) those with an anatomic repair, (3) those who had Fontan palliation, and (4) those who received a pulmonary artery band or systemic-to-pulmonary artery shunt only. The ten-year transplant free survival was 93%, 86%, 100%, and 79%, respectively, leading the authors to conclude that transplant free survival was essentially the same for patients with a systemic RV, anatomic repair, and Fontan procedure with systemic RV being a risk factor for death and transplantation (De León et al. 2017).

Anatomic repairs accomplished by aortic, pulmonary, and combined root translocation have not accrued outcome follow up times that have been attained by other anatomic repairs yet. However, the early operative mortality results are encouraging and comparable with other techniques. (Mair et al. 2016; Tateishi et al. 2013; Da Silva et al. 2015; Tam et al. 2021; Davies et al. 2008b).

The most effective short- and long-term operation for ccTGA patients with LVOT obstruction who could be suitable for several types of repairs is uncertain (Imai 1997; Langley et al. 2003; Bautista-Hernandez et al. 2006; Alghamdi et al. 2006; Gaies et al. 2009; Ly et al. 2009; Sharma et al. 2009; Cui et al. 2014; Bilal et al. 2016; Duncan and Mee 2005; Tocharoenchok et al. 2016). This therapeutic dilemma will be difficult to resolve without a formal prospective clinical study which is unlikely in our specialty. The eventual optimal treatment plan will be determined by thoughtful and unbiased comparison of modern-day Fontan outcomes with Senning-Rastelli or root translocation strategies.

19 Summary

The aforementioned anatomic variation, surgical analysis, and understanding of potential complications that can occur with repair of the diverse types of ccTGA have highlighted the challenging aspects of each of the multiple operations that offer physiologic, anatomic, and single ventricle palliation. The available literature reviews have supported anatomic repair over physiologic repair, which may improve the long-term outlook of patients with ccTGA. For complex ccTGA, the Fontan operation will play a major role in long term survival. An understanding of the many complexities of this lesion is critical for strategic planning and optimal outcome. And always in the future, cardiac transplantation will be required in those patients with complications of RV/LV failure, AV valve pathology, and the eventual complications of Fontan physiology. Lifelong surveillance, irrespective of operative approach, will be necessary.

References

Alghamdi AA, McCrindle BW, Van Arsdell GS. Physiologic versus anatomic repair of congenitally corrected transposition of the great arteries: meta-analysis of individual patient data. Ann Thorac Surg. 2006;81:1529–35.

Anderson RC, Lillehei CW, Lester RG. Corrected transposition of the great vessels of the heart: a review of 17 cases. Pediatrics. 1957;20:626–46.

Baruah SD, Marwah A, Dalvi B, Sharma R. Anatomical repair of congenitally corrected transposition in the fifth decade of life. Indian Heart J. 2016;68(Suppl 2):S57–9.

Bautista-Hernandez V, Marx GR, Gauvreau K, Mayer JE Jr, Cecchin F, del Nido PJ. Determinants of left ventricular dysfunction after anatomic repair of congenitally corrected transposition of the great arteries. Ann Thorac Surg. 2006;82:2059–66.

Bilal MS, Avşar MK, Yıldırım Ö, et al. Double switch procedure and surgical alternatives for the treatment of congenitally corrected transposition of the great arteries. J Card Surg. 2016;31:231–6.

Bove EL. Current strategies for AV discordance. Presented at the inaugural John W. and Carol Ann Brown Lectureship for Congenital Heart Surgery Visiting Professor, Indiana University. November 2, 2022. Personal Communication; 2022.

Cools B, Brown SC, Louw J, Heying R, Meyns B, Gewillig M. Pulmonary artery banding as 'open end' palliation of systemic right ventricles: an interim analysis. Eur J Cardiothorac Surg. 2012;41:913–8.

Cui B, Li S, Yan J, et al. The results of a two-stage double switch operation for congenital corrected transposition of the great arteries with a deconditioned morphologically left ventricle. Interact Cardiovasc Thorac Surg. 2014;19:921–5.

Da Silva JP, Da Silva LF, Baumgratz JF, Castro RM, Bezerra RF, Guilhen JC. Root translocation in congenitally corrected transposition of the great arteries with ventricular septal defect and pulmonary stenosis, and other lesions. Semin Thorac Cardiovasc Surg Pediatr Card Surg Annu. 2015;18:34–9.

Davies B, Oppido G, Wilkinson JL, Brizard CP. Aortic translocation, Senning procedure and right ventricular outflow tract augmentation for congenitally corrected transposition, ventricular septal defect and pulmonary stenosis. Eur J Cardiothorac Surg. 2008a;33:934–6.

De León LE, Mery CM, Verm RA, et al. Mid-term outcomes in patients with congenitally corrected transposition of the great arteries: a single center experience. J Am Coll Surg. 2017;224:707–15.

de Leval MR, Bastos P, Stark J, Taylor JF, Macartney FJ, Anderson RH. Surgical technique to reduce the risks of heart block following closure of ventricular septal defect in atrioventricular discordance. J Thorac Cardiovasc Surg. 1979;78:515–26.

Deal BJ. Can patients with congenitally corrected transposition of the great arteries live better electrically? J Thorac Cardiovasc Surg. 2016;151:140–2.

DiBernardo LR, Kirshbom PM, Skaryak LA, Quarterman RL, Johnson RL, Davies MJ, Gaynor JW, Ungerleider RM. Acute functional consequences of left ventriculotomy. Ann Thorac Surg. 1998;66(1):159–65.

Dobson R, Danton M, Nicola W, Hamish W. The natural and unnatural history of the systemic right ventricle in adult survivors. J Thorac Cardiovasc Surg. 2013;145(6):1493–503.

d'Udekem Y, Iyengar AJ, Galati JC, et al. Redefining expectations of long-term survival after the Fontan procedure: twenty-five years of follow-up from the entire population of Australia and New Zealand. Circulation. 2014;130(11 Suppl 1):S32–8.

Duncan BW, Mee RB. Management of the failing systemic right ventricle. Semin Thorac Cardiovasc Surg. 2005;17(2):160–9.

El-Zein C, Subramanian S, Ilbawi M. Evolution of the surgical approach to congenitally corrected transposition of the great arteries. Semin Thorac Cardiovasc Surg Pediatr Card Surg Annu. 2015;18:25–33.

Gaies MG, Goldberg CS, Ohye RG, Devaney EJ, Hirsch JC, Bove EL. Early and intermediate outcome after anatomic repair of congenitally corrected transposition of the great arteries. Ann Thorac Surg. 2009;88:1952–60.

Graham TP Jr, Bernard YD, Mellen BG, et al. Long-term outcome in congenitally corrected transposition of the great arteries: a multi-institutional study. J Am Coll Cardiol. 2000;36:255–61.

Helsen F, De Meester P, Van Keer J, et al. Pulmonary outflow obstruction protects against heart failure in adults with congenitally corrected transposition of the great arteries. Int J Cardiol. 2015;196:1–6.

Helvind MH, McCarthy JF, Imamura M, et al. Ventriculo-arterial discordance: switching the morphologically left ventricle into the systemic circulation after 3 months of age. Eur J Cardiothorac Surg. 1998;14:173–8.

Hoashi T, Kagisaki K, Miyazaki A, et al. Anatomic repair for corrected transposition with left ventricular outflow tract obstruction. Ann Thorac Surg. 2013;96:611–20.

Hörer J, Schreiber C, Krane S, et al. Outcome after surgical repair/palliation of congenitally corrected transposition of the great arteries. Thorac Cardiovasc Surg. 2008;56:391–7.

Hraska V. Anatomic correction of corrected transposition {I,D,D} using an atrial switch and aortic translocation. Ann Thorac Surg. 2008;85:352–3.

Hraska V, Duncan BW, Mayer JE Jr, Freed M, del Nido PJ, Jonas RA. Long-term outcome of surgically treated patients with corrected transposition of the great arteries. J Thorac Cardiovasc Surg. 2005;129:182–91.

Hsu KH, Chang CI. Reply to Ma et al. Eur J Cardiothorac Surg. 2016;49:1294–5.

Hsu KH, Chang CI, Huang SC, Chen YS, Chiu IS. 17-year experience in surgical management of congenitally corrected transposition of the great arteries: a single-centre's experience. Eur J Cardiothorac Surg. 2016;49:522–7.

Hu SS, Li SJ, Wang X, et al. Pulmonary and aortic root translocation in the management of transposition of the great arteries with ventricular septal defect and left ventricular outflow tract obstruction. J Thorac Cardiovasc Surg. 2007;133:1090–2.

Ikai A, Koizumi J, Kin H, et al. Aortic translocation using the hemi-mustard procedure for corrected transposition. Ann Thorac Surg. 2012;94:996–8.

Ilbawi MN, DeLeon SY, Backer CL, et al. An alternative approach to the surgical management of physiologically corrected transposition with ventricular septal defect and pulmonary stenosis or atresia. J Thorac Cardiovasc Surg. 1990;100:410–5.

Imai Y. Double-switch operation for congenitally corrected transposition. Adv Card Surg. 1997;9:65–86.

Imai Y, Seo K, Aoki M, Shin'oka T, Hiramatsu K, Ohta A. Double-switch operation for congenitally corrected transposition. Semin Thorac Cardiovasc Surg Pediatr Card Surg Annu. 2001;4:16–33.

Ismat FA, Baldwin HS, Karl TR, Weinberg PM. Coronary anatomy in congenitally corrected transposition of the great arteries. Int J Cardiol. 2002;86:207–16.

Jacobs JP, He X, Mayer JE Jr, et al. Mortality trends in pediatric and congenital heart surgery: an analysis of the Society of Thoracic Surgeons Congenital Heart Surgery Database. Ann Thorac Surg. 2016;102:1345–52.

Jonker V, Atallah J, Horne D, Rebeyka IM. A novel surgical technique for repair of congenitally corrected transposition of the great arteries with atrioventricular septal defect: avoiding damage to the conduction system. Ann Thorac Surg. 2015;100:1121–3.

Karl TR. The role of the Fontan operation in the treatment of congenitally corrected transposition of the great arteries. Ann Pediatr Cardiol. 2011;4:103–10.

Karl TR. Re: Late diagnosis of isolated congenitally corrected transposition of the great arteries in a 92-year old woman. Eur J Cardiothorac Surg. 2016;49:1526.

Karl TR, Cochrane AD. Congenitally corrected transposition of the great arteries. In: Mavroudis C, Backer CL, editors. Pediatric cardiac surgery. 3rd ed. Philadelphia: Mosby; 2003. p. 476–95.

Karl T, Jacobs JP. Congenitally corrected transposition of the great arteries. In: Mavroudis C, Backer CL, editors. Pediatric cardiac surgery. 5th ed. West Sussex: Wiley-Blackwell; 2023. p. 581–600.

Karl TR, Weintraub RG, Brizard CP, Cochrane AD, Mee RB. Senning plus arterial switch operation for discordant (congenitally corrected) transposition. Ann Thorac Surg. 1997;64:495–502.

Karl TR, Quintessenza J, Jacobs J. Anatomic repair for congenitally corrected transposition: the promise and the reality. Eur J Cardiothorac Surg. 2016;49:528–9.

Kowalik E, Klisiewicz A, Biernacka EK, Hoffman P. Pregnancy and long-term cardiovascular outcomes in women with congenitally corrected transposition of the great arteries. Int J Gynaecol Obstet. 2014;125:154–7.

Kwak JG, Lee CH, Lee C, Park CS. Aortic root translocation with atrial switch: another surgical option for congenitally corrected transposition of the great arteries with isolated pulmonary stenosis. J Thorac Cardiovasc Surg. 2010;139:1652–3.

Lacour-Gayet F, Clarke DR, Aristotle Committee. The Aristotle method: a new concept to evaluate quality of care based on complexity. Curr Opin Pediatr. 2005;17:412–7.

Langley SM, Winlaw DS, Stumper O, et al. Midterm results after restoration of the morphologically left ventricle to the systemic circulation in patients with congenitally corrected transposition of the great arteries. J Thorac Cardiovasc Surg. 2003;125:1229–41.

Lewis M, Ginns J, Schulze C, et al. Outcomes of adult patients with congenital heart disease after heart transplantation: impact of disease type, previous thoracic surgeries, and bystander organ dysfunction. J Card Fail. 2016;22:578–82.

Ly M, Belli E, Leobon B, et al. Results of the double switch operation for congenitally corrected transposition of the great arteries. Eur J Cardiothorac Surg. 2009;35:879–84.

Ma K, Gao H, Hua Z, et al. Palliative pulmonary artery banding versus anatomic correction for congenitally corrected transposition of the great arteries with regressed morphologic left ventricle: long-term results from a single center. J Thorac Cardiovasc Surg. 2014;148:1566–71.

Ma K, Qi L, Li S. Tricuspid regurgitation in single ventricular palliation for corrected transposition. Eur J Cardiothorac Surg. 2016;49:1294.

Mair R, Sames-Dolzer E, Innerhuber M, Tulzer A, Grohmann E, Tulzer G. Anatomic repair of complex transposition with *en bloc* rotation of the truncus arteriosus: 10-year experience. Eur J Cardiothorac Surg. 2016;49:176–82.

Malekzadeh-Milani S, Jalal Z, Tamisier D, Boudjemline Y. Dilatable pulmonary artery band: Safety and efficacy of balloon dilatation. Catheter Cardiovasc Interv. 2016;88:446–51.

Malhotra SP, Reddy VM, Qiu M, et al. The hemi-Mustard/bidirectional Glenn atrial switch procedure in the double-switch operation for congenitally corrected transposition of the great arteries: rationale and midterm results. J Thorac Cardiovasc Surg. 2011;141:162–70.

Marathe SP, Chávez M, Schulz A, Sleeper LA, Marx GR, Emani SM, Del Nido PJ, Baird CW. Contemporary outcomes of the double switch operation for congenitally corrected transposition of the great arteries. J Thorac Cardiovasc Surg. 2022;164(6):1980–90.

Mavroudis C. Congenitally corrected transposition of the great arteries. In: Mavroudis C, Backer CL, editors. Atlas of pediatric cardiac surgery. London: Springer; 2015. p. 211–24.

Mavroudis C, Dearani JA. Transposition of the great arteries. In: Mavroudis C, Dearani JA, editors. Atlas of adult congenital heart surgery. Cham: Springer; 2020.

Mavroudis C, Backer CL, Kohr LM, et al. Bidirectional Glenn shunt in association with congenital heart repairs: the 1(1/2) ventricular repair. Ann Thorac Surg. 1999;68:976–82.

Mavroudis C, Backer CL, Siegel A, Gevitz M. Revisiting the Baffes operation: its role in transposition of the great arteries. Ann Thorac Surg. 2014;97:373–7.

Mee RB. Severe right ventricular failure after Mustard or Senning operation. Two-stage repair: pulmonary artery banding and switch. J Thorac Cardiovasc Surg. 1986;92(3 Pt 1):385–90.

Mee RB. The double switch operation with accent on the Senning component. Semin Thorac Cardiovasc Surg Pediatr Card Surg Annu. 2005;8:57–65.

Metton O, Gaudin R, Ou P, et al. Early prophylactic pulmonary artery banding in isolated congenitally corrected transposition of the great arteries. Eur J Cardiothorac Surg. 2010;38:728–34.

Miller JR, Sebastian V, Eghtesady P. Management options for congenitally corrected transposition: which, when, and for whom? Semin Thorac Cardiovasc Surg Pediatr Card Surg Annu. 2022;25:38–47.

Monckeberg JG. Zur Entwicklungsgeschichte des Atrioventrikularsystems. Verhand Deutsch Path Gesell. 1913;16:228–49.

Morell VO, Jacobs JP, Quintessenza JA. Aortic translocation in the management of transposition of the great arteries with ventricular septal defect and pulmonary stenosis: results and follow-up. Ann Thorac Surg. 2005;79:2089–93.

Myers PO, del Nido PJ, Geva T, et al. Impact of age and duration of banding on left ventricular preparation before anatomic repair for congenitally corrected transposition of the great arteries. Ann Thorac Surg. 2013;96:603–10.

Nikaidoh H. Nikaidoh procedure: a perspective. Eur J Cardiothorac Surg. 2016;50:1001–5.

Ohye RG, Si MS, Bove EL, Hirsch-Romano JC. Left ventricular retraining: theory and practice. Semin Thorac Cardiovasc Surg Pediatr Card Surg Annu. 2015;18:40–2.

Picard F, Tadros VX, Asgar AW. From tricuspid to double orifice morphology: percutaneous tricuspid regurgitation repair with the MitraClip device in congenitally corrected-transposition of great arteries. Catheter Cardiovasc Interv. 2017;90:432–6.

Prabhu S, Anderson B, Ward C, Karl T, Alphonso N. A simplified technique for interventional extracardiac Fontan. World J Pediatr Congenit Heart Surg. 2017;8:92–8.

Quaegebeur JM, Rohmer J, Ottenkamp J, et al. The arterial switch operation. An eight-year experience. J Thorac Cardiovasc Surg. 1986;92(3 Pt 1):361–84.

Sano T, Riesenfeld T, Karl TR, Wilkinson JL. Intermediate-term outcome after intracardiac repair of associated cardiac defects in patients with atrioventricular and ventriculoarterial discordance. Circulation. 1995;92(Suppl 9):II272–8.

Schiebler GL, Edwards JE, Burchell HB, Dushane JW, Ongley PA, Wood EH. Congenital corrected transposition of the great vessels: a study of 33 cases. Pediatrics. 1961;27(Suppl 5):849–88.

Sharma R, Talwar S, Marwah A, et al. Anatomic repair for congenitally corrected transposition of the great arteries. J Thorac Cardiovasc Surg. 2009;137:404–12.

Talwar S, Ahmed T, Saxena A, Kothari SS, Juneja R, Airan B. Morphology, surgical techniques, and outcomes in patients above 15 years undergoing surgery for congenitally corrected transposition of great arteries. World J Pediatr Congenit Heart Surg. 2013;43:271–7.

Talwar S, Bansal A, Choudhary SK, et al. Results of Fontan operation in patients with congenitally corrected transposition of great arteries. Interact Cardiovasc Thorac Surg. 2016;22:188–93.

Tam VKH, Erez E, Roten L, Muyskens S, Sebastian V, Tsao C, Nikaidoh H. Senning with aortic translocation and anatomic repair for congenitally corrected transposition. Ann Thorac Surg. 2021;111(5):1607–12.

Tateishi A, Kasahara S, Kawabata T, et al. The effect of pulmonary root translocation on the left ventricular outflow tract. Ann Thorac Surg. 2013;96:1469–71.

Termignon JL, Leca F, Vouhé PR, et al. "Classic" repair of congenitally corrected transposition and ventricular septal defect. Ann Thorac Surg. 1996;62:199–206.

Tocharoenchok T, Sriyoschati S, Tongcharoen P, Tantiwongkosri K, Subtaweesin T. Midterm results of anatomic repair in a subgroup of corrected transposition. Asian Cardiovasc Thorac Ann. 2016;24:428–34.

Unolt M, Putotto C, Silvestri LM, et al. Transposition of great arteries: new insights into the pathogenesis. Front Pediatr. 2013;6(1):11.

von Rokitansky CF. Die Defecte der Scheidwande des Herzens. Vienna: Wilhelm Braumuller; 1875. p. 81–6.

Waldo AL, Pacifico AD, Bargeron LM, James TN, Kirklin JW. Electrophysiological delineation of the specialized A-V conduction system in patients with corrected transposition of the great vessels and ventricular septal defect. Circulation. 1975;52:435–41.

Walmsley T. Transposition of the ventricles and the arterial stems. J Anat. 1931;65(Pt 4):528–40.

Wilkinson JL, Cochrane AD, Karl TR. Congenital heart surgery nomenclature and database project: corrected (discordant) transposition of the great arteries (and related malformations). Ann Thorac Surg. 2000;69(Suppl 4):S236–48.

Wissocque L, Mondésert B, Dubart AE. Late diagnosis of isolated congenitally corrected transposition of the great arteries in a 92-year old woman. Eur J Cardiothorac Surg. 2016;49:1524–5.

Yacoub MH, Radley-Smith R, Maclaurin R. Two-stage operation for anatomical correction of transposition of the great arteries with intact interventricular septum. Lancet. 1977;310:1275–8.

Yamagishi M, Shuntoh K, Matsushita T, et al. Half-turned truncal switch operation for complete transposition of the great arteries with ventricular septal defect and pulmonary stenosis. J Thorac Cardiovasc Surg. 2003;125:966–8.

Zartner PA, Schneider MB, Asfour B, Hraška V. Enhanced left ventricular training in corrected transposition of the great arteries by increasing the preload. Eur J Cardiothorac Surg. 2016;49:1571–6.

Complications Associated with Bidirectional Glenn, Fontan Operations, and Arrhythmia Surgery

Constantine Mavroudis and Carl L. Backer

Abstract

Surgeons who treat patients with single ventricle physiology are well acquainted with the short- term and long-term complications leading up to and following the Fontan operation. This chapter will discuss specific surgical complications with the bidirectional Glenn shunt, Fontan operation, and arrhythmia surgery. New illustrations are provided to overcome obstacles that the surgeon may encounter during the implementation of these procedures such as stenosis, clot formation, or air embolism.

Keywords

Congenital heart surgery · Bidirectional Glenn · Fontan operation · Arrhythmia surgery · 1½ ventricular repair · Single ventricle · Extracardiac Fontan · Complications · Outcomes

C. Mavroudis (✉)
Chief of Pediatric Cardiothoracic Surgery (Retired), Peyton Manning Children's Hospital, Indianapolis, IN, USA

Professor Emeritus of Surgery, Johns Hopkins University School of Medicine, Baltimore, MD, USA

C. L. Backer
Chief, Section of Pediatric Cardiothoracic Surgery, UK Healthcare Kentucky Children's Hospital, Lexington, KY, USA

Cardiothoracic Surgery, Cincinnati Children's Hospital Medical Center, Cincinnati, OH, USA

1 Bidirectional Glenn Shunt

The bidirectional shunt (superior vena cava [SVC]) to confluence of pulmonary arteries) is a variation of the classic Glenn Shunt which was initially developed to palliate patients with tetralogy of Fallot before the advent of cardiopulmonary bypass and total correction (Glenn and Patino 1954; Kopf et al. 1990). The natural progression from a classical Glenn shunt to a bidirectional Glenn (BDG) shunt was facilitated by the use of cardiopulmonary bypass and the idea that a bidirectional Glenn shunt can be employed as a staged procedure en route to orthoterminal correction (Fontan operation) (Hopkins et al. 1985; Bridges et al. 1990; Pridjian et al. 1993; Albanese et al. 1992; Hawkins et al. 1993; Kawashima et al. 1994). Occasionally it is used in patients with two ventricles or in patients with a small but functional right ventricle to volume unload the right ventricle (Zias et al. 2003; Ilbawi et al. 1989).

2 Complications Associated with the Bidirectional Glenn Shunt

The bidirectional Glenn procedure is performed to balance pulmonary and systemic blood flow through a shunt which allows systemic venous return to be partially bypassed directly to the pul-

C. L. Backer, C. Mavroudis (eds.), *Complications in Pediatric and Congenital Heart Surgery*,
https://doi.org/10.1007/978-3-032-02661-3_17

monary arteries while taking advantage of the generally low pulmonary vascular resistance. The mortality rate is generally less than 2% (Salik et al. 2022) with complications occurring in approximately 30% of patients. These include emergency cardiac catheterization (9%), new onset of neurologic deficit (9%), reoperation (6%), cardiac arrest (3%), and feeding difficulties that require fundoplication or gastrostomy tube placement (15%) (Salik et al. 2022). When patient characteristics are considered, the most common risk factors for postoperative complications are mitral stenosis, aortic atresia, female gender, and failure to thrive perioperatively. Cannulation problems involving the SVC, especially in smaller sized patients, can be challenging and can lead to cannula site stenosis and potential neurologic dysfunction. Perioperative blood loss can be problematic especially in patients less than 2 years of age. Resternotomy, which is required for most patients undergoing bidirectional Glenn, represents the highest risk of bleeding complications owing to mediastinal adhesions, unwanted cavitary entry, and aspirin use. Induction of arrhythmias, hypoxemia, and deep hypothermia cardiopulmonary bypass can exacerbate these risks. To avoid these complications, the usual measures must be implemented that will ensure immediate peripheral cardiopulmonary bypass, external cardioversion, and administration of blood products.

The bidirectional Glenn shunt is usually performed using aortobicaval cardiopulmonary bypass after the pulmonary artery has been extensively dissected. The stages of the operation are shown in Figs. 1, 2, 3, 4, 5, 6, 7 and 8. Each figure

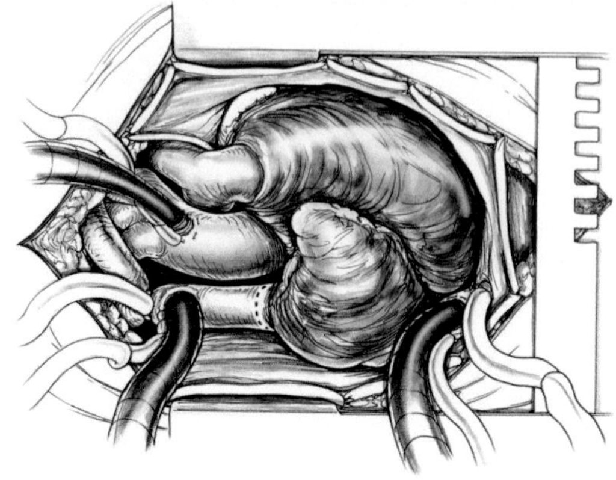

Fig. 1 Shows aortobicaval cardiopulmonary bypass being commenced. The dotted line shows the intended incision for caval transection. (With permission: Mavroudis 2015a)

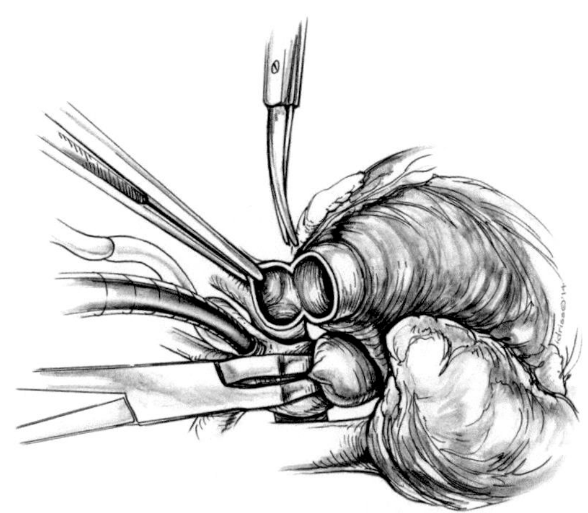

Fig. 2 When the pulmonary artery has not been detached from the heart at a prior operation, aortic cross-clamping and cardioplegic arrest is employed to prevent air embolism. (With permission: Mavroudis 2015a)

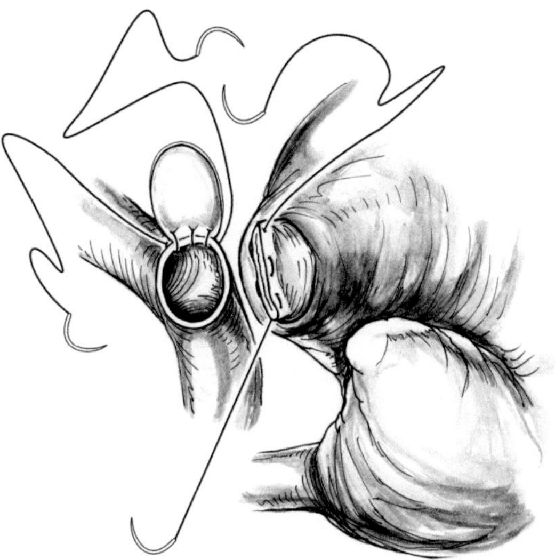

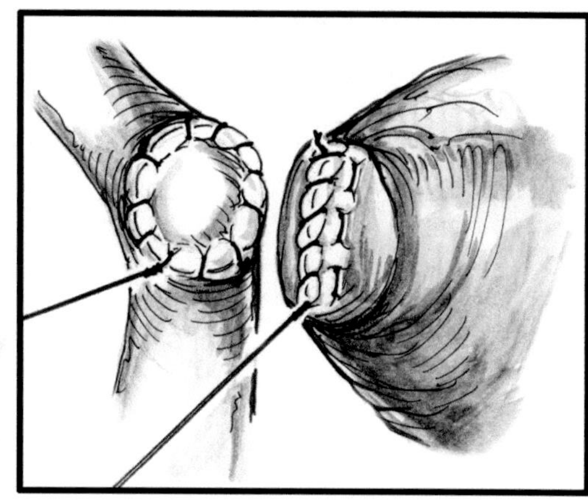

Fig. 3 Shows suture maneuvers while the pulmonary artery is transected. The pulmonary valve is sutured closed (not shown) and the proximal pulmonary artery is oversewn. The distal pulmonary artery is isolated using a pericardial or synthetic patch as noted in the inset. (With permission: Mavroudis 2015a)

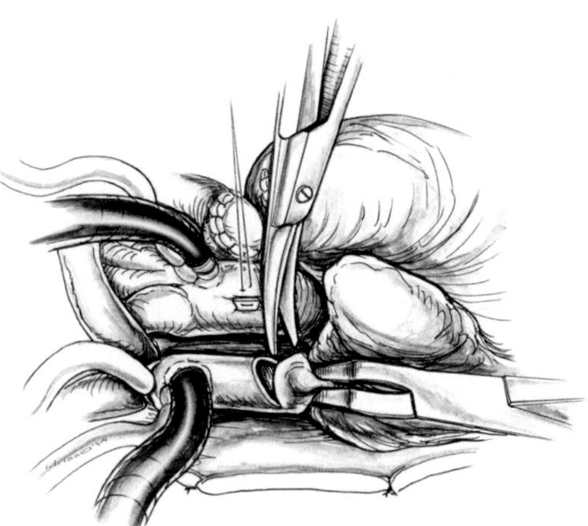

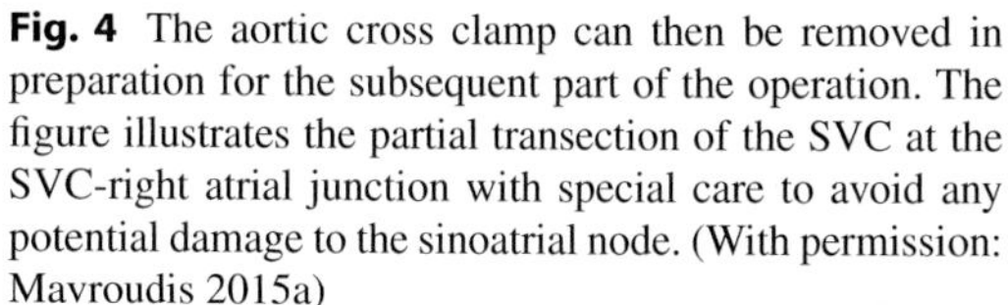

Fig. 4 The aortic cross clamp can then be removed in preparation for the subsequent part of the operation. The figure illustrates the partial transection of the SVC at the SVC-right atrial junction with special care to avoid any potential damage to the sinoatrial node. (With permission: Mavroudis 2015a)

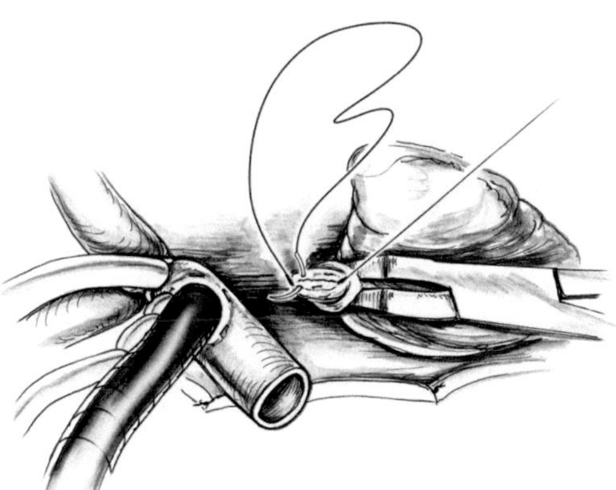

Fig. 5 Shows the superior vena caval tape being enforced, a vascular clamp placed on the cardiac end of the superior vena cava, and transection of the superior vena cava at the denoted site with oversewing of the cardiac portion of the superior vena cava. (With permission: Mavroudis 2015a)

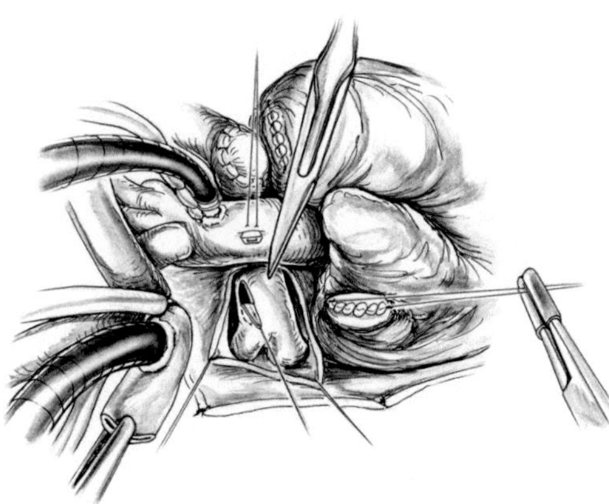

Fig. 6 Shows an incision in the superior portion of the right pulmonary artery in preparation for the SVC to pulmonary artery anastomosis. (With permission: Mavroudis 2015a)

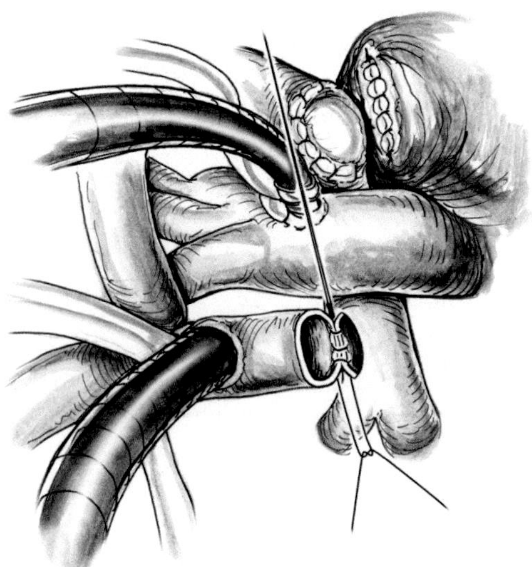

Fig. 7 Illustrates the SVC-Right Pulmonary Artery anastomosis in progress. We prefer interrupted sutures for the entire anastomosis while others perform the anastomosis with running suture technique for the posterior portion and interrupted suture technique for the anterior portion of the reconstruction. (With permission: Mavroudis 2015a)

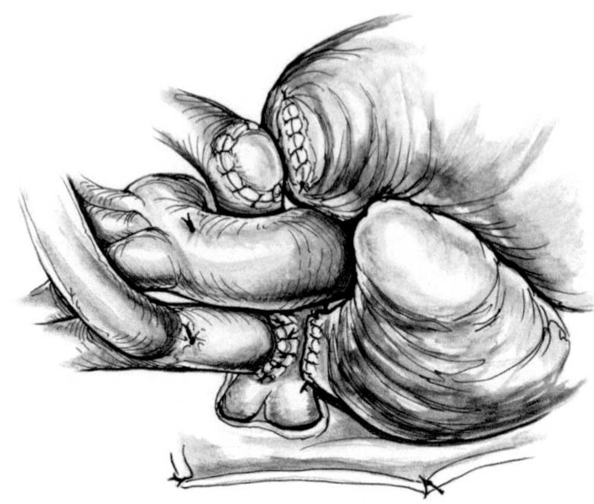

Fig. 8 Illustrates the completed bidirectional Glenn shunt and separation from cardiopulmonary bypass. (With permission: Mavroudis 2015a)

shows the multiple steps that allow for an uncomplicated operation free of anastomotic leaks, stenoses, and freedom from air embolism. Technical mishaps, failure to recognize stenoses, and failure to ligate the azygous vein can result in cyanosis, SVC hypertension or both. For instance, as noted herein, the SVC cannulation site can cause SVC stenosis as demonstrated in Fig. 9. Repair of this problem can be accomplished by suture takedown and transverse interrupted suture reapproximation (inset) or patch venoplasty using autologous pericardium (inset). Generally, this repair needs to be performed on cardiopulmonary bypass as noted in Fig. 9, inset. Another stenotic problem can become manifest owing to an unrecognized stricture of the main or left pulmonary artery. Figure 10 shows how the main pulmonary artery stenosis can be overlooked and the reparative measures that are taken to repair the problem. Another complication regarding the bidirectional Glenn shunt that presents late is a developed clot in the area between the supraval-

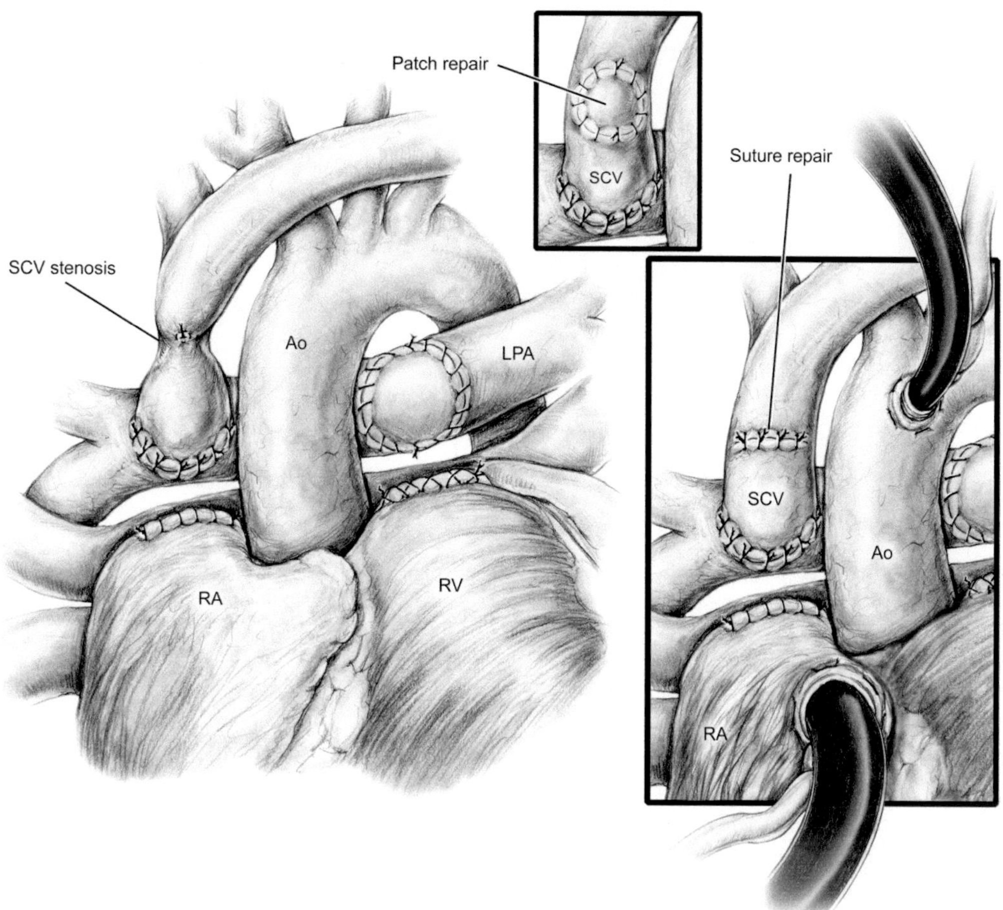

Fig. 9 Left panel shows the result of superior caval vein (SCV) purse-string stenosis which can occur from an initial large purse-string or a repaired SCV after disruption. The right lower inset shows a horizontal interrupted suture repair of the disrupted superior caval vein. The horizontal suture line will cause a shortening of the SCV, but not a longitudinal stenosis which will result in an unobstructed pathway. The upper inset shows pericardial patch repair of the SCV in the event that horizontal repair cannot be adequately performed. *Ao* aorta, *LPA* left pulmonary artery, *RA* right atrium, *RV* right ventricle, *SCV* superior caval vein

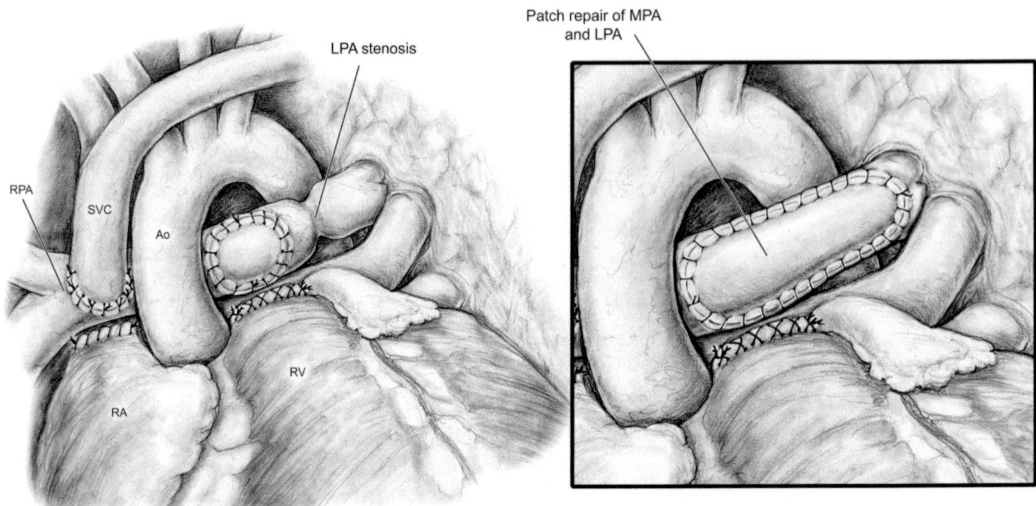

Fig. 10 Left panel shows the undiagnosed main pulmonary artery stenosis that can decrease pulmonary flow and result in cyanosis, Longitudinal incision across the stenosis and patch pulmonary artery arterioplasty as shown in the right panel can repair the problem and increase systemic saturation measurements. *Ao* aorta, *LPA* left pulmonary artery, *MPA* main pulmonary artery, *RA* right atrium, *RPA* right pulmonary artery, *RV* right ventricle, *SVC* superior vena cava

var ligation site and the pulmonary valve which was not oversewn. In other words, a clot develops in an area of stagnant blood flow causing clot formation and eventual embolization into the single ventricle pumping chamber and thence into the cerebral and myocardial circulations with resultant stroke and myocardial infarction. Figure 11 shows anatomically how a clot can form in the aforementioned condition. The best way to avoid this complication is to oversew the pulmonary valve and the supravalvar pulmonary artery trunk at the initial operation. In the case of an already developed clot in the supravalvar area, systemic anticoagulation therapy is indicated and removal of the clot during the subsequent completion Fontan operation.

After the completion of the BDG, the operating team must recognize that the pulmonary and systemic circulations are not separated and remain intermixed. Consequently, hypoxemia can occur due to suboptimal ventilation strategy or diminished pulmonary blood flow. In circumstances when oxygenation does not improve after optimization of volume status and ventilation strategy, collateral vessels from the upper body to the systemic circulation should be investigated. In many cases, these collateral vessels, if recognized, can be embolized before the operation. However, it is not uncommon that these vessels may require coil embolization in a persistently hypoxemic patient. Further to these considerations is early extubation which is recommended in these patients since spontaneous ventilation will augment cavopulmonary-cerebral circulation as long as PaO2and PaCO2 are optimized. A simple maneuver of elevating the head of the bed and maintaining the neck in a neutral position will enhance cerebral-venous drainage and enhance pulmonary blood flow.

Complications involving the bidirectional Glenn procedure can occur in the short term after the operation as well. Pleural effusions occur in about 9% of children that can prolong hospitalization. While the causes remain uncertain, increased left-to-right shunting from collaterals can be the cause in some cases. In longer postoperative circumstances, pulmonary arteriovenous (AV) fistulas can develop in children owing to the lack of hepatic venous circulation to the lungs on the first pass suggesting that a lack of hepatic factor may be a cause for pulmonary AV fistulas and systemic desaturation.

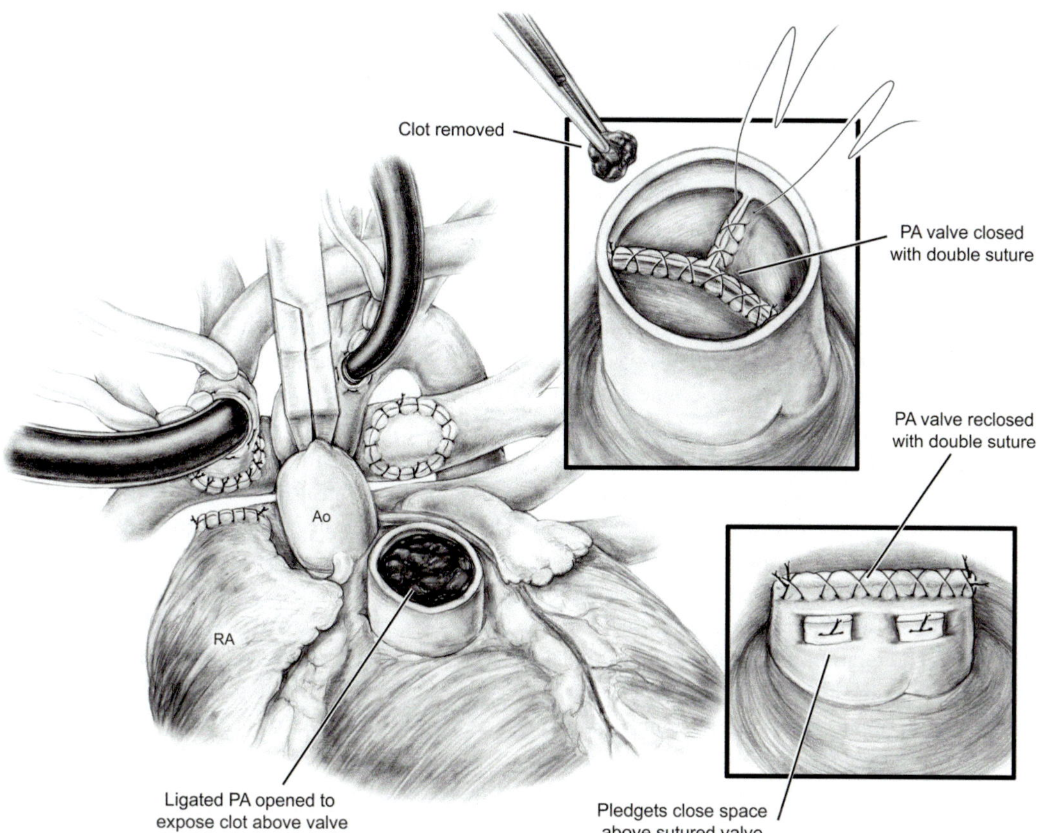

Fig. 11 Shows a developed clot upstream to the pulmonary valve which was not sutured closed and below the transection of the supravalvar pulmonary artery. This was initially performed to isolate the pulmonary artery in advance of orthoterminal connection. The problem with leaving the supravalvar portion of the circulation without an outlet is that a clot could form and be the nidus of movement into the single ventricle and form a systemic embolus resulting in stroke or coronary artery occlusion. The figure shows how this clot can be formed and how it can form the nidus of embolism. The upper inset shows a portion of clot being removed and oversewing of pulmonary valve. The lower inset demonstrates the closure of the pulmonary trunk with a running suture technique for the orifice and pledgetted sutures for the subpulmonary trunk. *Ao* aorta, *PA* pulmonary artery, *RA* right atrium

Over the long term, patients with a BDG shunt who are delayed towards the Fontan physiology can develop elevated venous pressures resulting in reduced pulmonary blood flow, impaired oxygenation, and inhibited cerebral venous drainage. The failing BDG physiology is frequently caused by AV valve regurgitation and decreased cardiac output. Jolley and associates documented seizures, cerebral hemorrhage, and embolic stroke as common complications in this population (Jolley et al. 2014). Extracorporeal membrane oxygenation (ECMO) support, when necessary is associated with renal injury, neurologic injury, and persistent acidosis leading to increased morbidity and mortality (Jolley et al. 2014; Allan et al. 2007). Treatments for these advanced complications are highly selective and may require valve repair, collateral embolization, or other treatable interventions before Fontan completion.

3 Fontan Operation and 1½ Ventricular Repair

3.1 Introduction

Since its introduction in 1968 by Francis Fontan and Guillermo Kreutzer (Fontan and Baudet 1971; Kreutzer et al. 1973; Mavroudis 2012), the Fontan operation has undergone many modifications. During the subsequent rapidly changing time period interposed venous pathway valves, right atrial to small subpulmonic connections and atriopulmonary connections were transitioned to the now accepted extracardiac venous-pulmonary artery connections with or without fenestration options. The standard pathway for orthoterminal (Fontan) palliation is determined by three distinct time periods that allow physiologic acclimation en route to low pulmonary vascular resistance, myocardial adaptation, and somatic growth. The first of these time periods is neonatal management of pulmonary artery flow which is optimized by systemic-to-pulmonary artery shunt, pulmonary artery band, or observation. The patient is closely followed to intervene in the event of interstage complications such as poor weight gain, cyanosis, or congestive heart failure (Wolff et al. 2014; Akintoye et al. 2019; Hansen et al. 2012; Simsic et al. 2005). These complications are best recognized early and treated appropriately with heightened observation, catheter intervention, or surgical procedures depending on the circumstances which can include shunt stenosis, pulmonary overcirculation, or pulmonary complications. These potential complications are discussed in chapter "Complications Associated with Palliative Operations". At approximately 6 months of age, depending on the circumstances, the second stage operation is performed which is systemic-to-pulmonary artery shunt takedown or pulmonary artery band takedown and a bidirectional Glenn shunt. This procedure optimizes the patient's single ventricle physiology by volume unloading resulting in favorable ventricular remodeling. The complications associated with this stage have been described previously in this chapter. At approximately 2 years of age, the Fontan operation is usually performed by either lateral tunnel or extracardiac techniques with or without atrial fenestration. Since the introduction of the atrial fenestration, some surgeons have used this obligatory right-to-left shunt in all cases; some use it selectively; others not at all (Lemler et al. 2002; Backer et al. 2011; Mavroudis et al. 1992; Daley et al. 2022; Toncu et al. 2020). Nowadays, most surgeons employ the fenestration selectively; especially in cases with borderline ventricular function, small pulmonary arteries, abundant aortopulmonary artery collaterals, and single lung physiology. The size and technique of the fenestration can be performed easily in the lateral tunnel Fontan operation, not so much for extracardiac Fontan connections (Sughimoto et al. 2017).

3.2 Complications Associated with Extracardiac Fontan Connections without Fenestration

Figures 12, 13, 14, 15, 16, 17 and 18 depict the important steps for the extracardiac, non-fenestrated Fontan operation in a patient with a prior bidirectional Glenn shunt. Some surgeons prefer to perform this operation without cardiopulmonary bypass using inferior vena cava (IVC) to right atrium temporary shunts and partial occluding clamps for the pulmonary artery

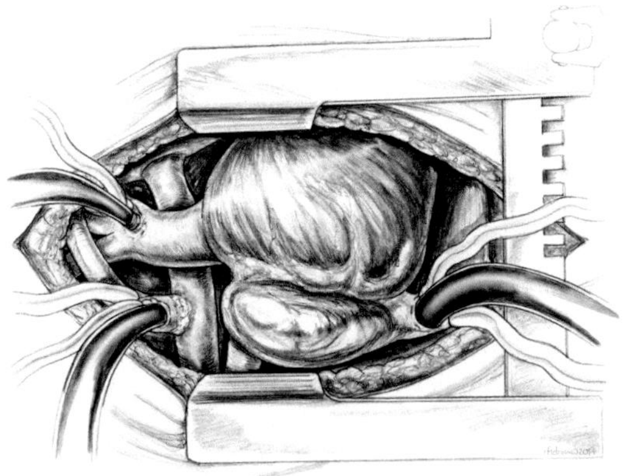

Fig. 12 Shows the standard cannulation techniques for the extracardiac Fontan operation. (With permission: Mavroudis 2015a)

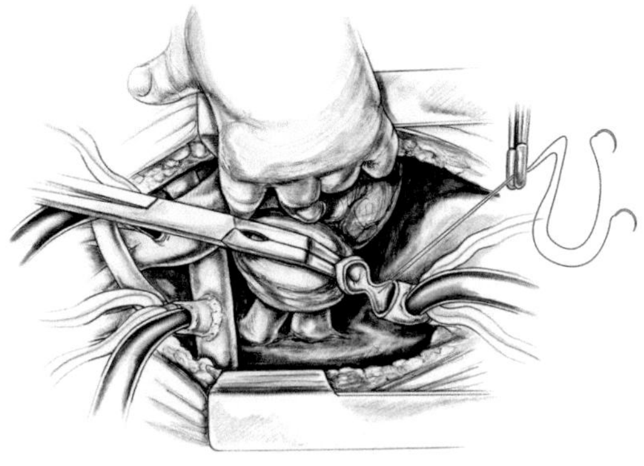

Fig. 13 Indicates inferior vena cava subtotal transection after the establishment of cardiopulmonary bypass and right atrial clamping across the inferior vena cava-right atrial junction. Care is taken to place a large vascular clamp across this junction well onto the right atrium with special care being taken to avoid injury to the right coronary artery and tricuspid valve before attempting to transect the inferior vena cava. This is an important maneuver since the operation is being performed in a beating nonworking heart. Clamp dislodgement will result in difficulty in performing the occlusive atrial suture line or worse, allow air to enter the cardiac chambers and result in a stroke or coronary embolus. Once the clamp is placed and secured, a suture is placed in the orifice of the inferior vena cava before the completion transection to assure exposure and prevent retraction below the diaphragm. (With permission: Mavroudis 2015b)

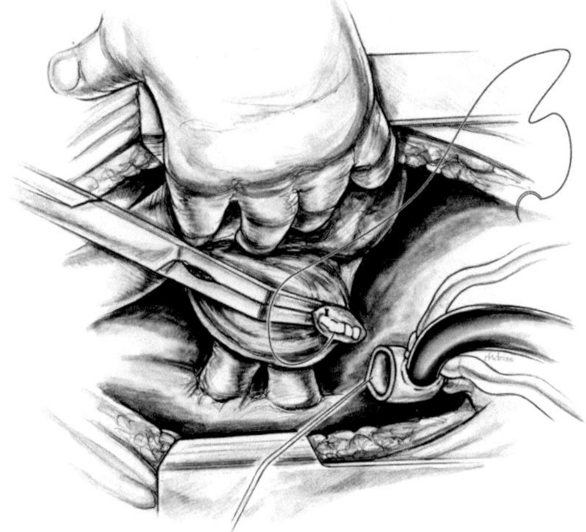

Fig. 15 Shows how the completion of the inferior vena cava transection is accomplished and the right atrium is closed with the clamp in place. A traction suture is placed on the inferior vena cava to prevent unwanted subdiaphragmatic retraction. (With permission: Mavroudis 2015b)

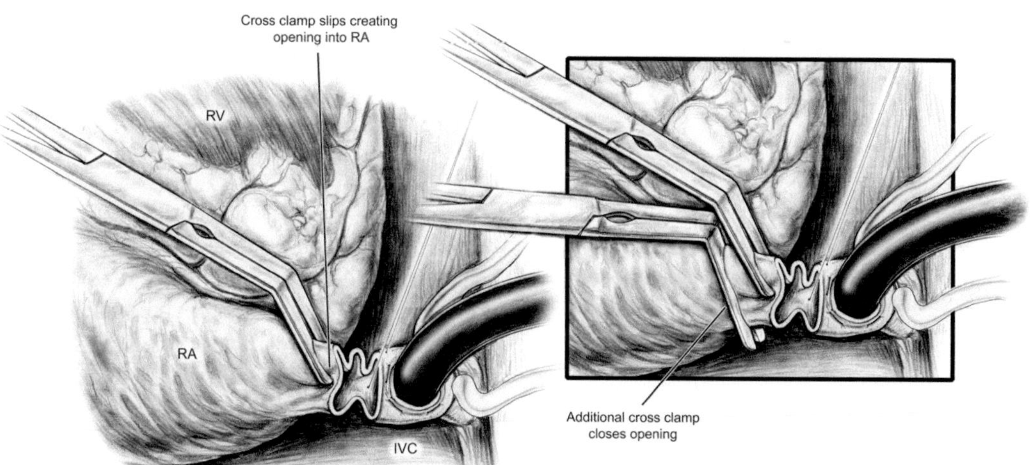

Fig. 14 Clamp dislodgment with chance of air embolism. The drawing shows how the cross clamp can slip and cause an unwanted opening in the right atrium which can result in air embolism. The inset shows how a supplemental clamp can be quickly placed to occlude the opening thereby allowing the anastomosis to proceed. A vent in the ascending aorta for air removal is prudent. (*IVC* inferior vena cava, *RA* right atrium, *RV* right ventricle)

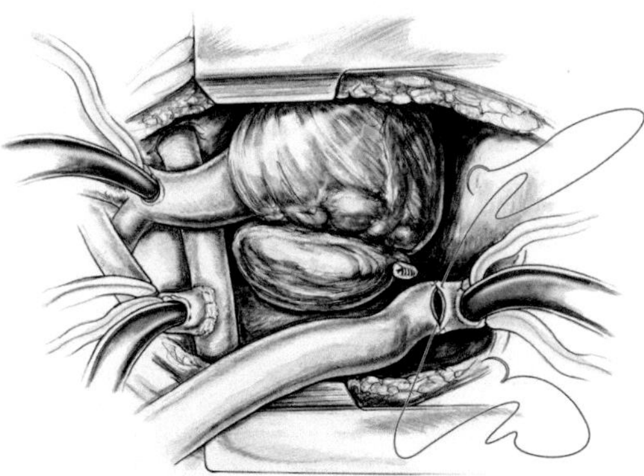

Fig. 16 Indicates how the right atrial clamp is removed and a PTFE graft (18 or 20 mm) is prepared and sutured end-to-end using running suture techniques into the inferior vena cava. (With permission: Mavroudis 2015b)

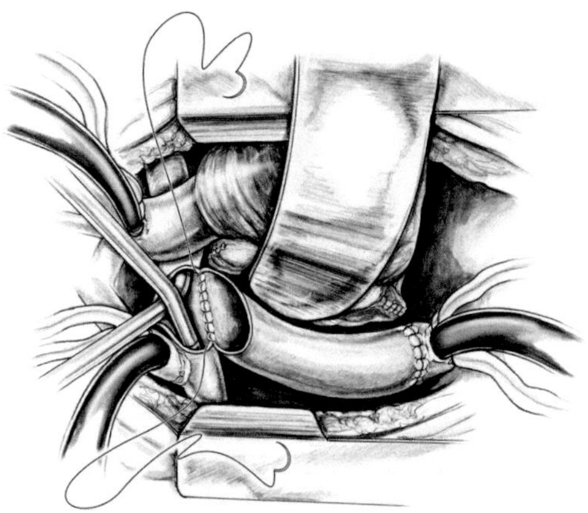

Fig. 17 The extracardiac conduit is now cut to size and on a bevel in preparation for the anastomosis to the inferior portion of the right pulmonary artery. The figure shows the anastomosis in progress to the pulmonary artery which is offset to the superior vena cava anastomosis to take advantage of the favorable flow and energy conservation characteristics that such connections afford. Care is taken to construct the conduit without tension and without redundancy to avoid any compromise in venous flow patterns. (With permission: Mavroudis 2015b)

(Mainwaring et al. 2014; Tam et al. 1999), but the majority choose to use standard aortobicaval cardiopulmonary bypass techniques without aortic cross-clamping (Stephens et al. 2021; Fuchigami et al. 2017). The technical complications that are associated with this operation are largely due to the extracardiac connection between the IVC and the inferior portion of the pulmonary artery. A

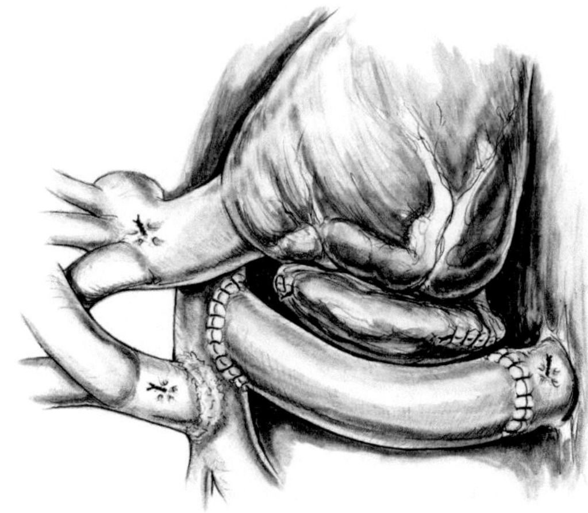

Fig. 18 Shows the completed reconstruction after separation from cardiopulmonary bypass. (With permission: Mavroudis 2015b)

very important complication is the possibility of clamp dislodgement at the right atrium where the IVC was transected. If the operation is being performed in the usual fashion, the heart is still beating without aortic cross-clamping and cardioplegic arrest. Clamp dislodgement has the potential for right and left atrial air entry with systemic air embolism causing stroke and myocardial damage. This situation requires immediate action. If ventricular fibrillation is present, the heart should be fibrillated during which time, the atrial clamp could be replaced, and air evacuation procedures could be implemented. This means an air vent in the ascending aorta and heart manipulation to remove any left ventricular air entrapment. Once the intracardiac air is purged, the heart can be defibrillated with continued attention to the progress of the operation. Figure 14 (left panel) shows partial dislodgement of the right atrial clamp which was placed to prevent air embolism en route to IVC transection and extracardiac Fontan completion. The inset of Fig. 14 shows how a supplemental clamp can be placed to stop the air embolism. Other intraoperative complications in the course of the extracardiac Fontan operation include problems with IVC retraction, venous pathway obstruction, and acute arrhythmias in the operating room. Vena cava retraction after transection in preparation for the Gore-Tex end-to-end anastomosis is a particularly vexing problem which is clearly a technical mishap that should be avoided. Nevertheless, it happens. A suture at the edge of the vena cava after transection will help, but not always. When this occurs, the surrounding tape has to be released and partial sucker bypass has to be instituted as shown in Figs. 73, 74 and 75 in the Fontan Conversion Section of this chapter. Once the Gore-Tex to IVC anastomosis is performed, the surrounding constricting tape can be reapplied, and the operation can proceed. Occasionally, difficulty with IVC cannulation causes a tear resulting in a larger than desired hole in the anterior wall of the IVC. This is also a vexing problem that requires attention since IVC stenosis caused by primary suture technique can cause postoperative stenosis. This is not always amenable to stent placement because of the close proximity of the hepatic venous tributaries which can be obstructed. It is better to repair the problem when recognized. This requires partial sucker bypass through the extracardiac Gortex tube, side-to-side interrupted suture anastomotic repair, or autologous pericardial patch repair of the IVC. The transverse Goretex incision to establish venous drainage by a suction catheter can be repaired later. The sequence of this repair technique is shown in Figs. 19 and 20. Acute arrhythmias during separation from cardiopulmonary bypass can also occur which will require intraoperative consultation from electrophysiology colleagues. Generally, the cause of this dilemma is atrial reentry tachycardia which is amenable to acute Amiodarone therapy. Clearly, atrial and ventricular temporary pacemaker wires should be placed. The operating team in close consultation can decide whether permanent epicardial wires should be placed in the event that pacemaker therapy is elected in the postoperative period. The permanent epicardial wires can be placed in the rectus muscle area which can obviate a resternotomy assuming that pacemaker therapy is elected. Acute hemodynamic problems can also occur in the process of separation from cardiopulmonary bypass. High venous pressure may indicate excess collateral flow which is best treated in the catheterization laboratory by targeted embolization. Other problems can be AV valve regurgitation, unrecognized venous pathway stenosis, and pulmonary artery obstruction. The operating room team is wise to consider all of these problems during visual inspection, trans-

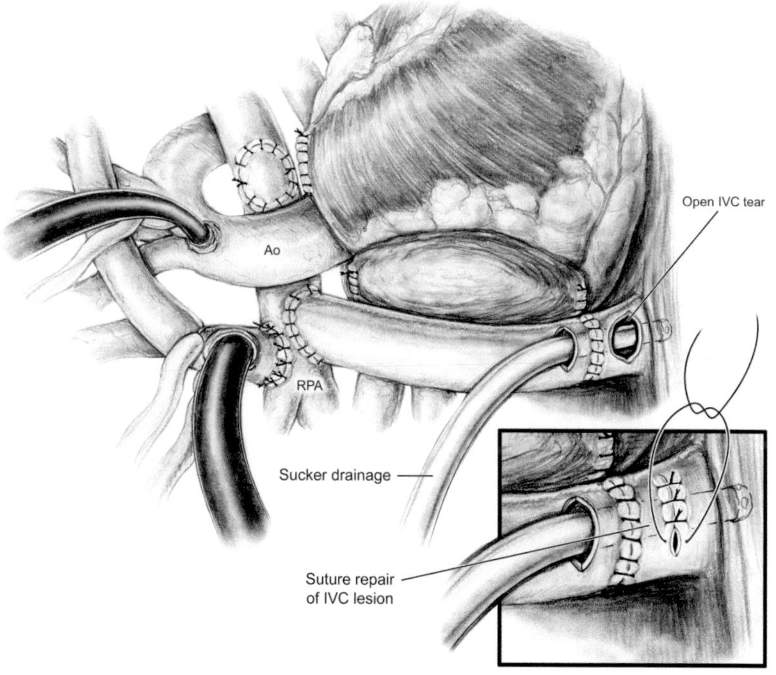

Fig. 19 Shows the large hole in the inferior vena cava which is controlled by sucker bypass through the Goretex tube to visualize the hole. The inset shows how the inferior vena cava can be repaired with transverse interrupted suture technique. (*Ao* aorta, *IVC* inferior vena cava)

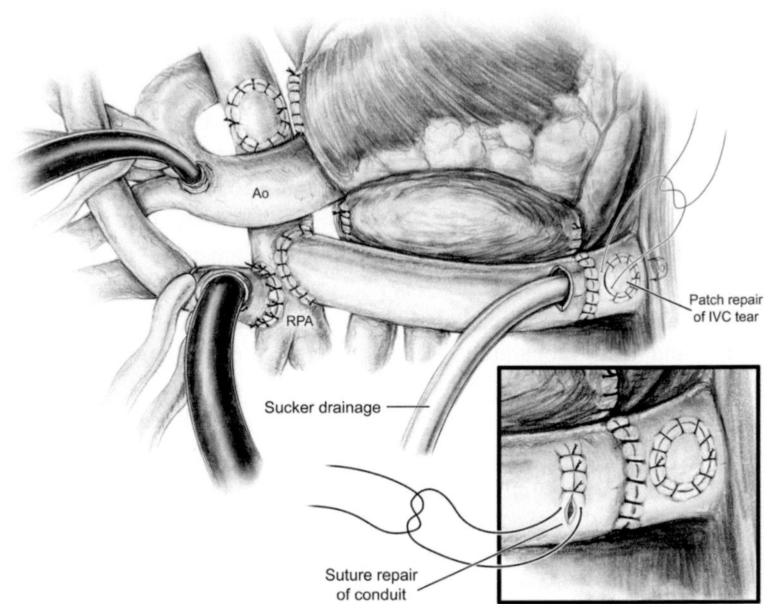

Fig. 20 Shows the patch venoplasty of the inferior vena cava in progress with a drainage tube through the Goretex graft to establish a blood free exposure while performing the operation. The inset shows the completed venoplasty with closure of the Gortex tube closure. (*Ao* aorta; *IVC* inferior vena cava, *RPA* right pulmonary artery)

esophageal echocardiography (TEE), and direct pressure measurements if warranted.

Long-term outcomes of the Fontan operation have been reported (Marcelletti et al. 1990; Masuda et al. 1998; Dabal et al. 2014; Nakano et al. 2015; d'Udekem et al. 2014; Pundi et al. 2015) with excellent results. Complications associated with the Fontan operation will be discussed further in this chapter in association with Fontan conversion, cardiac transplantation, valve repair, and aneurysm resolution.

3.3 Extracardiac Fontan Operation with Fenestration

Creating a fenestration in association with an extracardiac conduit, despite its implied simplicity, requires strategies to avoid air entry to the left side of the Fontan circulation. One method to perform this part of the operation is to employ the use of aortic cross-clamping and cardioplegic arrest. The antecedent technical requirements to use this technique involve a more extensive aortic dissection simply to apply the cross-clamp which can risk neoaortic or coronary artery injury. In addition, a period of myocardial ischemia is required which is not necessary for the extracardiac conduit placement. Nevertheless, this technique is probably the best way to perform the fenestration without the possibility of introducing air into the left side, assuming that all the air maneuvers are performed diligently. On the other hand, aortic cross-clamping and cardioplegic arrest can be avoided if partial occluding clamps are used on the atrium with careful anastomotic techniques. However, this method is more difficult and increases the chances of unwanted air entry into the left side. Figure 21 shows the result of side-to-side anastomosis at the midportion of the extracardiac conduit to the right atrium. This anastomosis is difficult to construct and predict due to the varying thickness of the atrial wall. The thicker the atrial wall, the more difficult it is to evaluate the actual size of the anastomosis and therefore the degree of the right-to-left shunt. A more accurate technique to accomplish a fenestration is shown in Fig. 22. A measured hole is made in the conduit after placement of a partial occluding clamp while a much larger hole is made in the right atrium at the level of the fenestration under a partial occluding clamp. The wall of the incised atrium is then sutured around the orifice of the fenestration without placing the sutures into the orifice. In this manner, the actual size of the fenestration is maintained. An alternative method to achieve a fenestration is the use of an interposed, sized polytetrafluoroethylene (PTFE) graft between the extracardiac conduit and the atrium

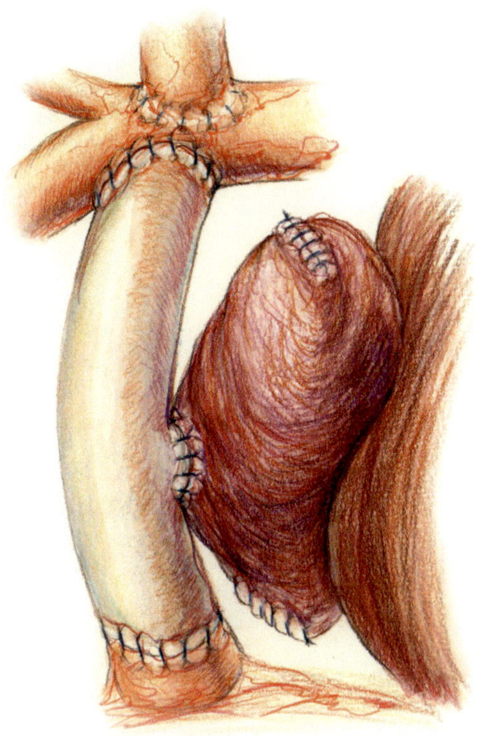

Fig. 21 Shows the result of a direct side-to-side mid-right atrial wall-to-side of the extracardiac conduit anastomosis that was performed after the completion of the Fontan operation. All the air maneuvers have been accomplished to remove any air from the extracardiac conduit. The direct side to side anastomosis using partial occluding clamps on both the right atrium and the extracardiac conduit is required for the anastomosis which relies on exact fenestration measurements for both structures. The accurate anastomosis is challenged by thickness of the right atrial wall and difficulty with suture placement owing to the confined area between clamps. The results can be inaccurate size of the desired shunt and in some cases, fenestration occlusion. (With permission: Mavroudis 2015b)

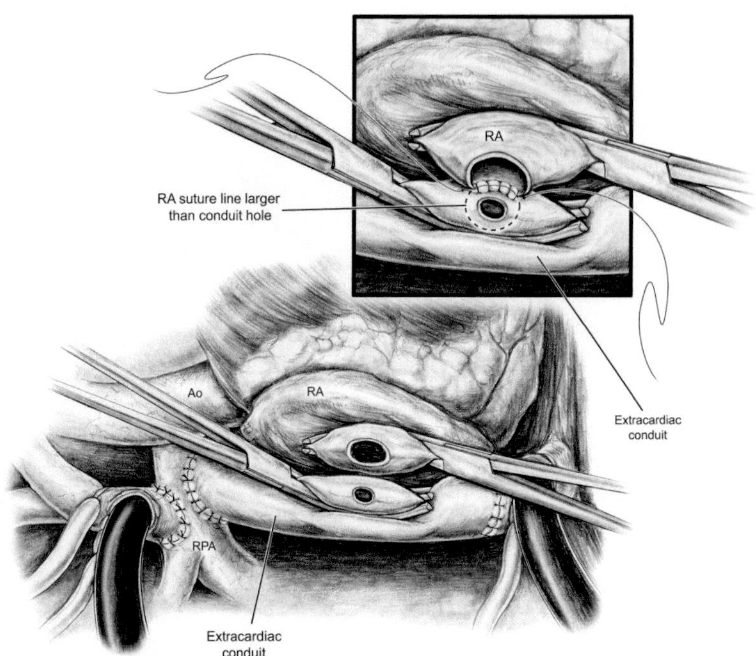

Fig. 22 Shows how the partial occluding clamps are placed on the side of the right atrium and the side of the extracardiac tube for the purpose of making an enlarged hole in the atrium to suture to the side of the Goretex graft which has been prepared by a measured hole to accurately size the desired anatomic and physiologic right to left shunt. The inset shows the progress of the side-to-side anastomosis. The hole in the atria wall is large enough to create a side-to-side anastomosis on the periphery of the measured hole in the extracardiac conduit. (Ao, aorta; RA, right atrium)

as noted in Fig. 23. Another technique which requires aortic cross-clamping and cardioplegic arrest is to perform a side-to-side anastomosis with the extracardiac conduit and a portion of the IVC as noted in Fig. 24. The most effective reconstruction is the one with which the surgeon is most comfortable and most experienced. We have used the technique as noted in Fig. 22 and mildly favor the side-to-side anastomosis although there may be indications for any of the methods described herein.

The common potential complication for all of these fenestration techniques is unwanted and unremoved cavitary air which can cause cerebral and myocardial air embolism. If a side-to-side anastomosis is elected, it is imperative that the air

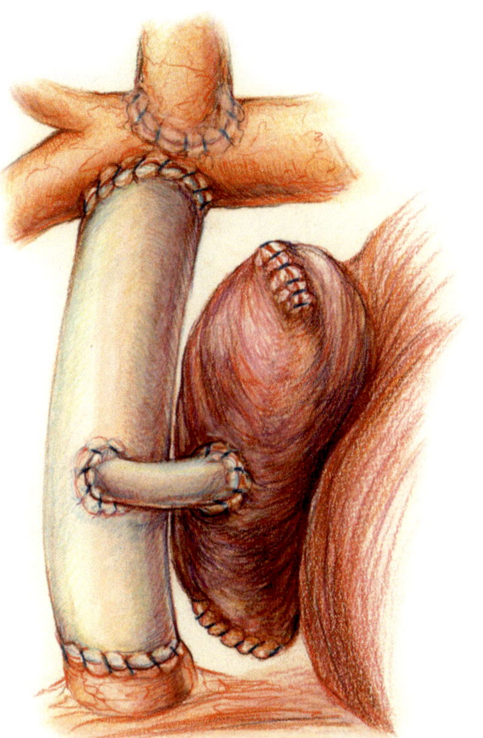

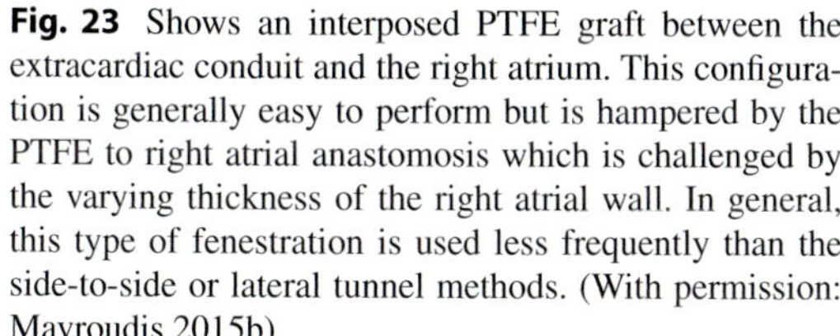

Fig. 23 Shows an interposed PTFE graft between the extracardiac conduit and the right atrium. This configuration is generally easy to perform but is hampered by the PTFE to right atrial anastomosis which is challenged by the varying thickness of the right atrial wall. In general, this type of fenestration is used less frequently than the side-to-side or lateral tunnel methods. (With permission: Mavroudis 2015b)

within the extracardiac conduit be removed before the partial occluding clamp is removed. When the anastomosis is completed, it is wise to place an aortic vent after the clamps are removed. TEE will also help to identify any remaining sequestered cavitary air, which can be removed by an ascending aortic vent.

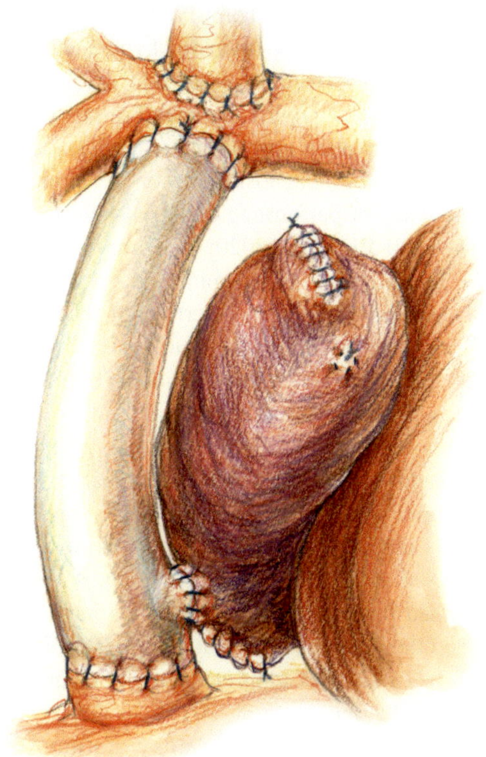

Fig. 24 Shows the fenestration that is performed by suturing a portion of the cardiac portion of the inferior vena cava-right atrial area. This anastomosis is difficult to perform without a cross clamp and cardioplegic arrest due to anatomic considerations that limit the placement of a partial occluding clamp to avoid air embolus. Nevertheless, this method could be used since the atrium in this location is more consistently thin which allows for a more predictive anastomosis. (With permission: Mavroudis 2015b)

3.4 Lateral Tunnel Fontan Operation with or Without Fenestration

In the present era, the lateral tunnel Fontan operation is generally performed for those patients who have had previous hemi-Fontan type second stage palliation, most often for hypoplastic left heart syndrome (Douglas et al. 1999). Some surgeons choose to employ the lateral tunnel for all Fontan completion operations, regardless of the single ventricle diagnosis, due to the ease and consistency of performing the atrial fenestration (Daley and d'Udekem 2020; Weixler et al. 2020). The incidence of arrhythmia development has played a pivotal role in determining whether a lateral tunnel or an extracardiac conduit will be used for the Fontan completion. Preliminary reports have shown that the lateral tunnel Fontan operation has more atrial arrhythmias likely due to the added suture load to create the baffle when compared with the extracardiac Fontan operation which requires no baffle and therefore no increased atrial suture load. However, it should be noted that no prospective studies have confirmed these results (Daley and d'Udekem 2020; Hirsch et al. 2007; Carins et al. 2016; Stephenson et al. 2010; Ben Ali et al. 2019). At the present time, while there is a bias towards performing the extracardiac Fontan, the choice between the extracardiac Fontan or lateral tunnel Fontan with or without fenestrations, respectively is dependent on the experience of the operating team. Figures 25, 26, 27, 28 and 29 show the progression of the lateral tunnel fenestrated Fontan procedure in a patient who had an antecedent hemi-Fontan procedure which involves pulmonary artery augmentation and amalgamation with the SVC coupled with an atrial baffle to maintain a division between the hemi-Fontan reconstruction and the right atrium. This has the same physiology as the bidirectional Glenn shunt, but anatomically offers a larger atrial to pulmonary artery orifice in preparation for the lateral tunnel Fontan connection. The mid-term results however have not shown improved survival (Edelson et al. 2020). Removal of the baffle between the pulmonary artery-superior vena cava amalgamation and the right atrium is shown in Fig. 25.

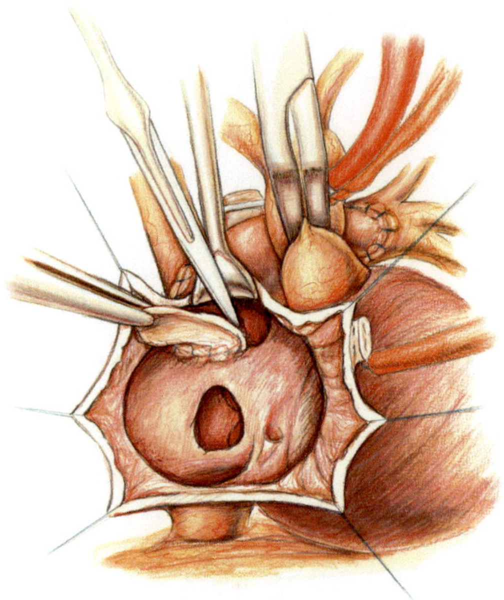

Fig. 25 Shows aortic cannulation and application of the aortic cross clamp with antegrade cardioplegia (not shown). Also not shown are the caval drainage catheters. The baffle that was placed to ensure superior vena cava flow to the right and left pulmonary arteries is now being resected in preparation for the lateral tunnel placement. Proponents of this type of Fontan completion point to the ease of creating the lateral tunnel with or without accompanying fenestrations. (With permission: Mavroudis 2015b)

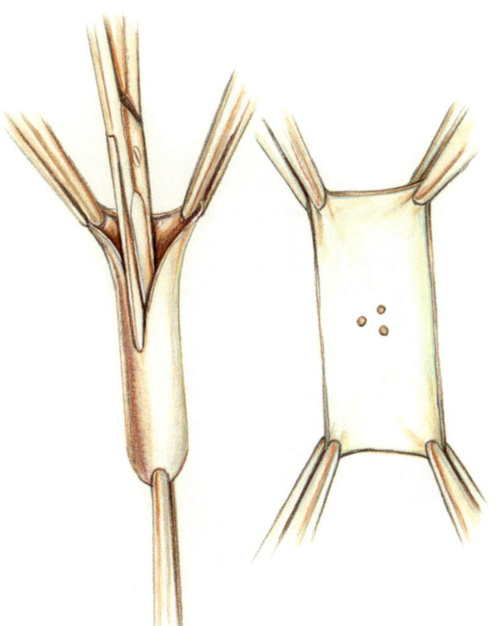

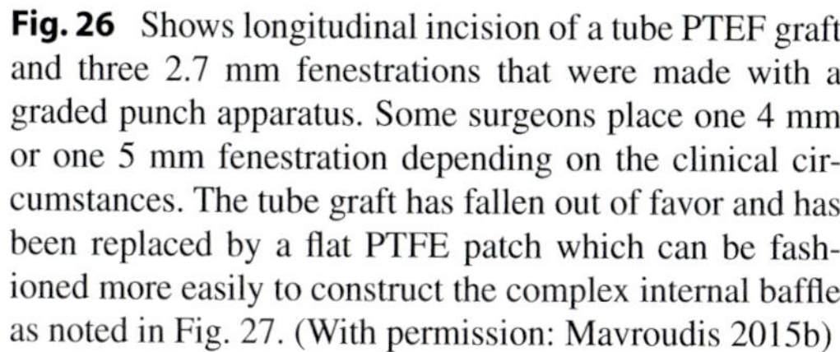

Fig. 26 Shows longitudinal incision of a tube PTEF graft and three 2.7 mm fenestrations that were made with a graded punch apparatus. Some surgeons place one 4 mm or one 5 mm fenestration depending on the clinical circumstances. The tube graft has fallen out of favor and has been replaced by a flat PTFE patch which can be fashioned more easily to construct the complex internal baffle as noted in Fig. 27. (With permission: Mavroudis 2015b)

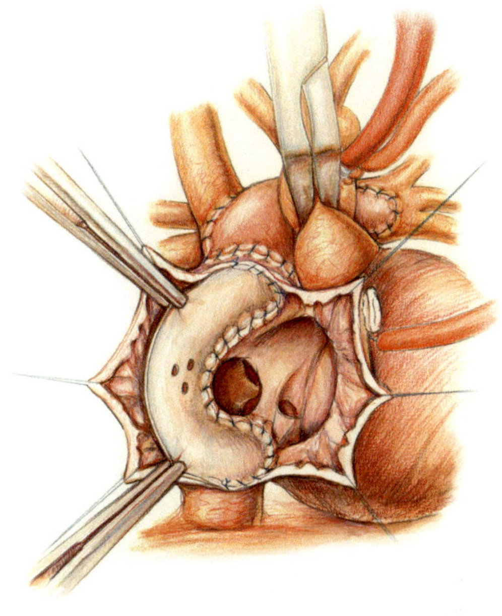

Fig. 27 Shows the fenestrated lateral tunnel in place. The important parts of this reconstruction are the maintenance of the internal caliber of the lateral tunnel to avoid stenosis, maintenance of an adequate atrial septal defect to ensure unobstructed flow between the atria, and attempts to keep the suture line away from the sinoatrial node for preservation of sinus rhythm. (With permission: Mavroudis 2015b)

After the removal of the baffle, the only parts of the operation that remain is construction of the lateral tunnel and atrial closure. Proponents of this type of procedure point to the simplicity of the operation; however, it requires a large suture load to construct the lateral tunnel which places the patient at risk for atrial arrhythmias (Backer et al. 2011). Like most choices in surgery, there are advantages and disadvantages to every binary decision. In the case of the lateral tunnel construction, the fenestration is easily performed and reproducible as noted in Figs. 26, 27 and 28. There is however a larger portion of the divided right atrium that is subject to increased venous pressure which is clearly associated with Fontan physiology. Theoretically, this portion of the right atrium is subject to dilatation and possible arrhythmia development. Already, there are data to support the idea that extracardiac connections have less arrhythmias than do lateral tunnel con-

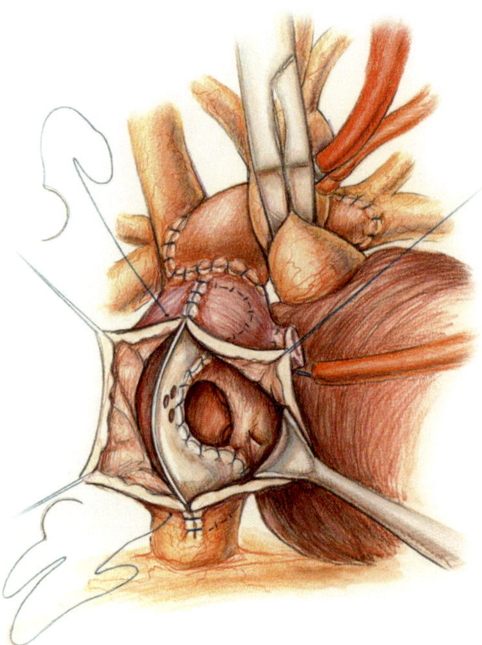

Fig. 28 Shows the atriorrhaphy in progress which is accomplished by suturing the lateral atrial wall, the anterior atrial wall and the PTFE graft into one suture line. (With permission: Mavroudis 2015b)

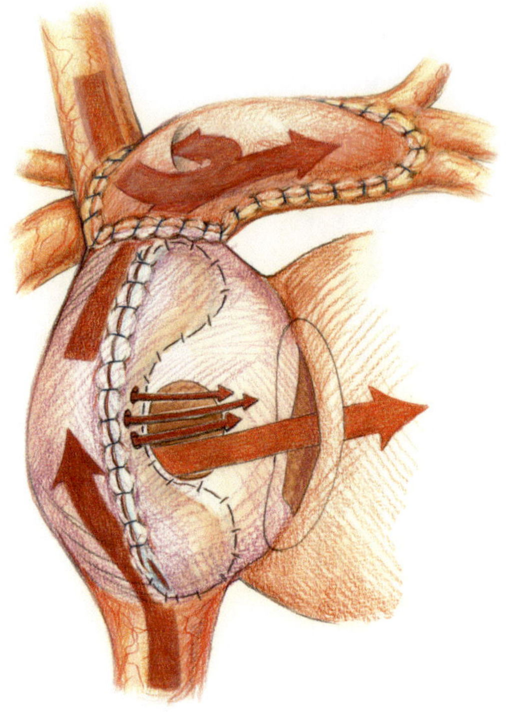

Fig. 29 Demonstrates the completed operation with the large arrow indicating the path of the pulmonary venous return from the pulmonary veins, through the atrial septal defect, and into the right ventricle. The smaller arrows signify the right to left flow through the fenestrations into the common atrium. (With permission: Mavroudis 2015b)

nections (Backer et al. 2011). Figure 29 shows the completed fenestrated lateral tunnel Fontan procedure which is employed for patients with a prior hemi-Fontan connection.

When a bidirectional Glenn shunt and not the hemi-Fontan reconstruction is used for the completion Fontan operation, the reconstruction for the lateral tunnel and IVC pathway to the right pulmonary artery is notably different as shown in Fig. 30. This type of lateral tunnel subjects less atrial wall to the increased venous pressure of the Fontan circulation. No studies, however, have compared the various types of lateral tunnel configurations and therefore the comparative incidence of arrhythmia development is largely unknown.

Further to the historical efforts to create the most effective and easy to perform fenestrated Fontan procedure, Jonas and associates (Sinha et al. 2013; Jonas 2011) introduced intracardiac/extracardiac Fontan modification that allows a simplified method to implement an accurately sized fenestration as noted in Fig. 31. The difficulty with this reconstruction is the intracavitary surface area of the PTFE graft which is subject to clot formation (Attard et al. 2018; Viswanathan 2016; Deshaies et al. 2019). This is the reason

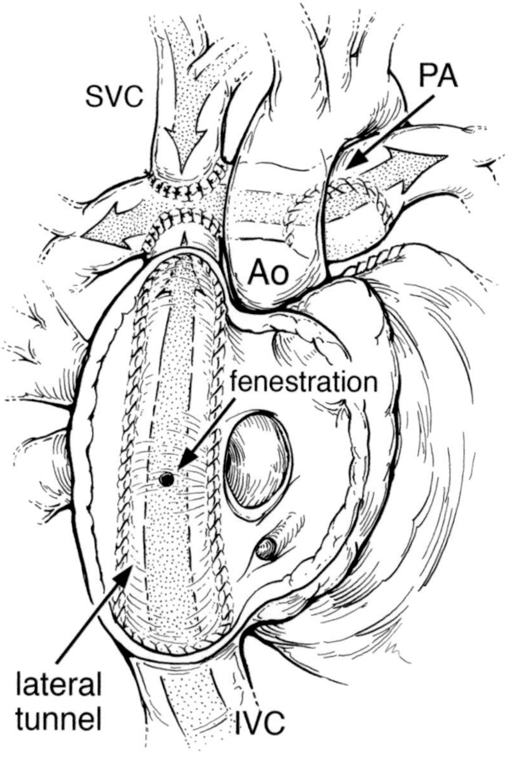

Fig. 30 The PTFE lateral tunnel reconstruction is more direct and does not need to be directed to the dome of the right atrium that was reconfigured for the hemi-Fontan reconstruction. The lateral tunnel is therefore more "lateral" and depends on the cardiac end of the superior vena cava to shunt blood flow to the right pulmonary artery as noted in the figure. Some surgeons note that the orifice of the cardiac end of the superior vena cava is smaller than the orifice of the inferior vena cava. This has not proven to be a clinical problem, however. There are circumstances where the cardiac end of the superior vena cava is indeed too small such as the condition of bilateral superior vena cavae. Under these circumstances, the cardiac end of the superior vena cava must be enlarged. This may threaten the sinoatrial node which is a concern for any incision that is performed in this area. In this case, a 4–5 mm single fenestration is accomplished. *Ao, aortic; IVC, inferior vena cava; PA, pulmonary artery; SVC, superior vena cava.* (With permission: Mavroudis 2015b)

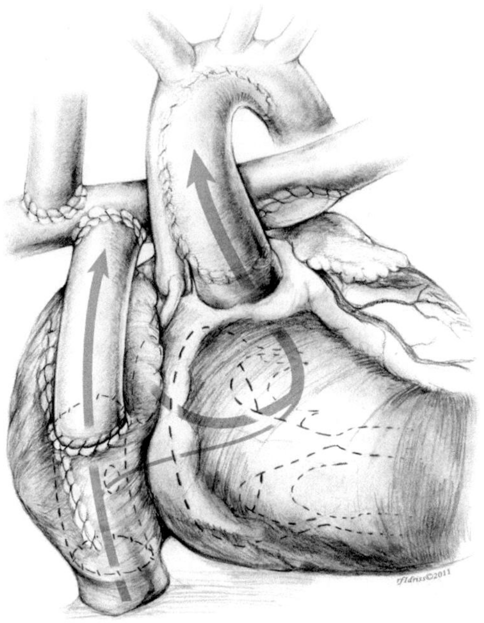

Fig. 31 In an effort to better standardize the fenestration size and maintain the benefits of an extracardiac Fontan operation, Jonas (Sinha et al. 2013; Jonas 2011) introduced the intracardiac/extracardiac repair which is noted in the figure. The operation is performed under aortobicaval cardiopulmonary bypass, aortic cross clamping, and cardioplegic arrest. A large PTFE graft (18–20 mm) is sutured to the orifice of the inferior vena cava. A fenestration is performed by a measured punch device in the graft that will remain within the atrium. The graft then is fashioned to emerge from the atrium and course in an extracardiac fashion to the inferior portion of the right pulmonary artery where it is anastomosed to complete the Fontan reconstruction. The large and small arrows indicate the blood flow of the pulmonary venous return and shunted right to left atrial flow, respectively. Some surgeons have expressed concern with this arrangement citing the possibility of systemic emboli from the intra-atrial portion of the PTFE graft. Anticoagulation is recommended if this procedure is to be used. (With permission: Mavroudis 2015b)

why anticoagulation is recommended (Jonas 2011). As with the other methods of fenestration, the answer to which is the best technique, is fleeting and will await an organized prospective study.

3.5 Long-Term Complications of the Fontan Procedure

Long-term complications associated with the Fontan procedure result in exercise intolerance and ventricular failure which are principally related to elevated systemic venous pressure, concomitant lesions such as valve pathology, venous pathway obstructions, and thromboembolic events (Udink Ten Cate et al. 2016; John et al. 2014; Rathgeber et al. 2020; Daniels et al. 2017; Bartz et al. 2006; Rogers et al. 2012; Lasa et al. 2014; Egbe et al. 2016; Yu et al. 2013; Ohuchi et al. 2013; Kodama et al. 2019; Bulic et al. 2017; Latus et al. 2013; Averin et al. 2018; Terashi et al. 2019; Starr et al. 1943). These physiologic abnormalities can cause right atrial dilatation, arrhythmias, protein losing enteropathy, pulmonary arteriovenous malformation, esophageal varices, and ascites (Udink Ten Cate et al. 2016; John et al. 2014; Rathgeber et al. 2020; Daniels et al. 2017; Bartz et al. 2006; Rogers et al. 2012; Lasa et al. 2014; Egbe et al. 2016; Yu et al. 2013; Ohuchi et al. 2013; Kodama et al. 2019; Bulic et al. 2017; Latus et al. 2013; Averin et al. 2018; Terashi et al. 2019; Starr et al. 1943). A thorough and comprehensive review of these problems is beyond the scope of this chapter; however, it is worthwhile to assess the surgical aspects of the Fontan operation and the potential problems that could contribute to these long-term complications. While these complications are invariably related to long-term Fontan patients, many of these issues can be ameliorated during the Fontan operation which can establish the most favorable conditions for long-term complication-free survival.

At the original Fontan operation it is best to make sure that the pulmonary arteries have no stenoses, and if necessary, they must be repaired with patch arterioplasty. The course and caliber of the lateral tunnel construction should be at least the caliber of the IVC with equal dimensions through the cardiac end of the SVC and into the pulmonary artery. In the case of the extracardiac Fontan, the size of the extracardiac conduit should be at least an 18 mm graft and preferably a 20–22 mm graft without any stenoses of the conduit to pulmonary artery connection (Cetta and Burkhart 2018). In adults undergoing a Fontan conversion a 24-mm graft is often used (Mavroudis et al. 1999a). Atrioventricular valve regurgitation or stenosis can have a major effect on pulmonary venous pressure which transfers to increased pulmonary artery resistance igniting the cascade which are noted herein. Atrioventricular valve repair has been successfully reported in patients undergoing a Fontan procedure (Sallehuddin et al. 2004; Podzolkov et al. 2015) and should be performed in association with the initial Fontan operation if needed. Oftentimes, operative repair can be performed at the time of the bidirectional Glenn procedure en route to orthoterminal palliation (Sinha et al. 2021). Concomitant arrhythmia surgery should also be considered if preoperative transcatheter ablative therapy was not successful. Other associated lesions that oftentimes require concomitant repair include aortic aneurysms, ligation of pulmonary arteriovenous collateral arteries, and existing venous obstructions such as cannulation sites in the superior and inferior caval veins. All of these repairs are considered in this chapter and in this textbook and should be applied whenever the initial Fontan operation is being planned and executed (Kim et al. 2016; Sumitomo et al. 2022; Sakamoto et al. 2014; Niwa 2018).

3.6 The 1½ Ventricular Repair

The 1½ ventricular repair was introduced as a corrective strategy to incorporate a small subpulmonic ventricle into the pulmonary circulation (Björk et al. 1979; Kreutzer et al. 1988; Henry and Danielson 1974; Van Arsdell et al. 1996; De Leval et al. 1985; Hanley et al. 1993; Muster et al. 1993; Alvarado et al. 1993; Gentles et al. 1994; Miyaji et al. 1995; Clapp et al. 1997; Reddy et al. 1997a; Ilbawi et al. 1990, 1989;

Billingsley et al. 1989; Anderson and Ho 1998; Van Arsdell et al. 1998). This was based on the idea that even a small amount of pulsatile flow into the pulmonary arterial bed is preferable to the laminar flow pattern that is defined by orthoterminal correction and Fontan physiology (Muster et al. 1993; Anderson and Ho 1998; Van Arsdell et al. 1998; Angelini et al. 1998; Freedom et al. 1998; Shumacker 1963). Early sentinel reports showed that separation of the pulmonary and systemic circulations could be accomplished in patients with small or poorly functioning pulmonary ventricles by intracardiac repair and diversion of a portion of the systemic venous return by a SVC to right pulmonary artery cavopulmonary anastomosis (classic Glenn shunt) (Shumacker 1963; Robicsek et al. 1956, Robicsek et al. 1991). This amalgamation of procedures allowed the small, volume unloaded pulmonary ventricle to function more efficiently in relation to its size and decreased ventricular preload. The disadvantage of this anatomic and physiological strategy became apparent with the discovery of pulmonary arteriovenous fistulas on the side of the Glenn anastomosis (Cloutier et al. 1985; Marianeschi et al. 1998). The origin of these fistulas has been ascribed to the lack of pulsatile flow and perhaps more importantly, because of the lack of direct visceral venous return, which contains, what has been described as "hepatic factor" (Muster et al. 1993; Clapp et al. 1997; Marianeschi et al. 1998; Krowka and Cortese 1990). More recently, clinical data and current scientific understanding leads to the possible role of miRNA, which inhibits vascular endothelial growth factor (VEGF) synthesis as a pathogenic mechanism for the development of pulmonary arteriovenous malformations (Vettukattil 2017). The concept of applying a bidirectional Glenn shunt in association with intracardiac correction for a small pulmonary ventricle was introduced by Billingsley and associates (Billingsley et al. 1989) in 1982.

This systemic venous in-parallel connection has been shown (Muster et al. 1993) to function by influencing both systolic and diastolic bilateral pulmonary artery blood flow. During systole IVC return which contains hepatic factor is pumped to both pulmonary arteries by pulmonary ventricular contraction. During diastole, the superior vena cava flow is delivered to both pulmonary arteries by venous pressure and laminar flow. In a scientific inquiry, we have performed selected intraoperative and postoperative hemodynamic studies, which allowed us to expand the use of the 1½ ventricular operation to a wider spectrum of congenital heart defects (Zias et al. 2003; Ilbawi et al. 1989). Recent studies have underscored the benefits of the 1½ ventricular repair based on short- and long-term clinical results (Marcelletti and Iorio 1998; Talwar et al. 2018).

The concept of the 1½ ventricular repair was expanded and presently is an integral part of a number of congenital heart repairs that can be defined by four categories as shown in Figs. 32, 33, 34 and 35. The most successful use of this strategy is described as Group A patients and is applied to those with small but functioning right ventricles with distinct inlet, body, and outlet anatomic characteristics as illustrated in Fig. 32 . There is however more to consider than only the bidirectional shunt; namely, that the right ventricular volume should be 40% of normal or more. In addition, while some surgeons create or leave an atrial fenestration, the right-sided bypass; a.k.a., the bidirectional Glenn shunt, precludes the need for this strategy, ensuring 100% or near 100% systemic oxygen saturation.

Group B 1½ ventricular patients as shown in Fig. 33 represent those with a poorly functional right ventricle as exists in some patients with advanced Ebstein anomaly of the tricuspid valve. The idea, as noted in Group A patients, is to unload the right ventricle, which can shift the Starling curve to the left thereby improving function and achieving the goals of the 1½ ventricular repair. The potential hemodynamic complications of such a strategy are the amount of tricuspid regurgitation and the pulmonary stenosis/regurgitation. Both of these valvar problems can mitigate against the forward flow of right ventricular output. The operating team must determine the best method of incorporating the poorly functional right ventricle into the circulation which may include tricuspid valve repair and pul-

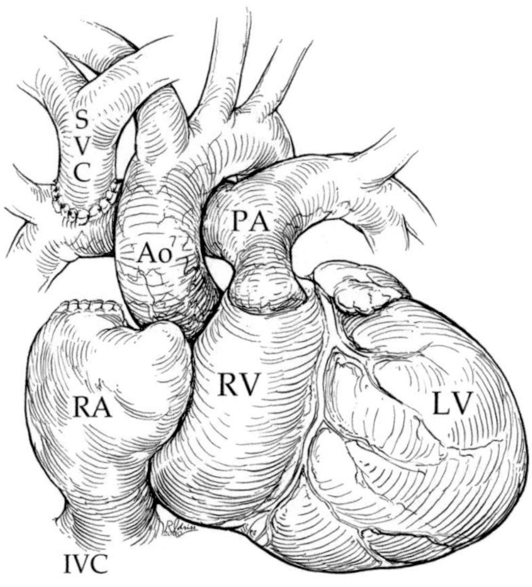

Fig. 32 The 1½ ventricular repair as depicted in this illustration is used for patients with small but functional right ventricles such as pulmonary atresia or pulmonary stenosis with intact ventricular septum with small but developed inlet, body, and outlet portions of the right ventricle. The completed operation is shown with the bidirectional Glenn at the superior portion of the right pulmonary artery (classic position), the cardiac end of the superior vena cava oversewn. *Ao, aorta; IVC, inferior vena cava; LV, left ventricle; PA, pulmonary artery; RA, right atrium; RV, right ventricle; SVC, superior vena cava).* (With permission: Mavroudis 2015b)

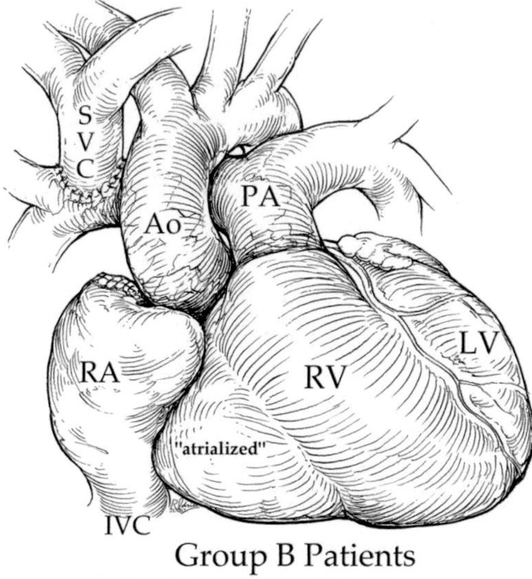

Fig. 33 Shows 1½ ventricular repair for Group B patients, namely those with a poorly functional right ventricle in association with advanced Ebstein anomaly of the tricuspid valve. The same idea as for Group A patients is applied for this group of patients, namely, to unload the right ventricle and allow a better hemodynamic situation for improvement of right ventricular function. Hemodynamic complications using this strategy relate to the extent to which tricuspid regurgitation and pulmonary stenosis/regurgitation affect the forward flow of right atrial to right ventricular flow. Practical wisdom and clinical experience will determine whether the application of tricuspid valve repair and pulmonary outflow tract repair in this setting will improve the circulation of the 1½ ventricular repair. *Ao* aorta, *IVC* inferior vena cava, *LV* left ventricle, *PA* pulmonary artery, *RA* right atrium, *RV* right ventricle, *SVC* superior vena cava. (With permission: Mavroudis 2015b)

monary outflow tract reparative techniques (Guzeltas et al. 2021). The operative experience of the program performing these operations will weigh heavily in the planning and execution of this complex situation (Malhotra et al. 2018).

Operative complications associated with this complex operation for Ebstein anomaly with a poorly functional right ventricle are related to the tricuspid cone repair and the technical problems relating to the bidirectional Glenn operation which have been noted herein. Intraoperative TEE will guide the operating team to perform immediate return to cardiopulmonary bypass to adjust the tricuspid valve repair and to add an atrial fenestration assuming that the right atrial pressure is high.

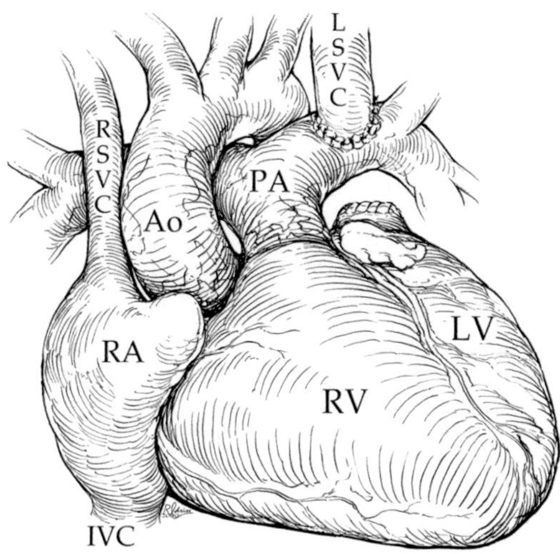

Fig. 34 Shows the 1½ ventricular repair as applied to patients with a left superior vena cava that drained to the dome of the left atrium causing cyanosis. Intra-atrial baffles are prone to obstruction and arrhythmias and as a result this strategy was applied to allow left superior vena cava flow without ligation. The hemodynamic result is favorable unless there is a left pulmonary artery stenosis distal to the entry of the superior vena cava pulmonary artery anastomosis. This results in intractable headaches and systemic venous hypertension. Care must be taken with this anastomosis which tends to be difficult owing to the location, oftentimes well into the left side of the mediastinum. *Ao* aorta, *IVC* inferior vena cava, *LSVC* left superior vena cava, *LV* left ventricle, *PA* pulmonary artery, *RA* right atrium, *RSVC* right superior vena cava, *RV* right ventricle. (With permission: Mavroudis 2015b)

Figure 34 shows application of the bidirectional Glenn shunt for repair of left SVC anomalous drainage into the dome of the left atrium resulting in cyanosis (Group C patients). As noted in Fig. 34 legend, the anomalous left SVC can be anastomosed to the left pulmonary artery. This solution has been advanced because of the long distance between the left SVC and the right-sided anatomic targets for proper diversion. The bidirectional Glenn shunt to treat this anomaly has its disadvantages, however. The possibility of resultant venous hypertension and acquired severe headaches make this solution potentially unsatisfactory as shown in Fig. 35. Intra-atrial tunneling techniques have been used to correct left SVC drainage to the left atrium in patients without atrial isomerism and with no connecting vein. While these techniques have been successful in the short term (van Son et al. 1998; Zhao et al. 2010), extracardiac solutions have been reported with success (Chihara et al. 2012; Erek et al. 2016) without the risks of acquired baffle leaks, baffle stenoses, and arrhythmias. Reddy and associates (Reddy et al. 1997b) have offered other solutions which involve interposed grafts as well as the bidirectional Glenn shunt option. Figure 36 shows the alternative solutions to the anomalous left SVC which include direct anastomosis to the right SVC and the interposed graft to the right atrial appendage or right superior vena cava.

A very intriguing application of the 1½ ventricular repair is in patients with congenitally corrected transposition of the great arteries (ccTGA) as shown in Fig. 37 (Group D patients). This strategy is discussed and illustrated in chapter “Complications Associated with Repair of Congenitally Corrected Transposition of the Great Arteries” as a part of the discussion for patients with ccTGA and associated lesions which include the presence or absence of ventricular septal defect (VSD) and pulmonary stenosis (PS). The 1½ ventricular option is appropriate for the rare patient with ccTGA, small VSD and significant PS which is repeated herein because of the obvious fit with the other diagnostic modalities which are candidates for this therapy. So, the bottom line for inclusion in this chapter is the application of the bidirectional Glenn shunt and 1½ ventricular repair and not so

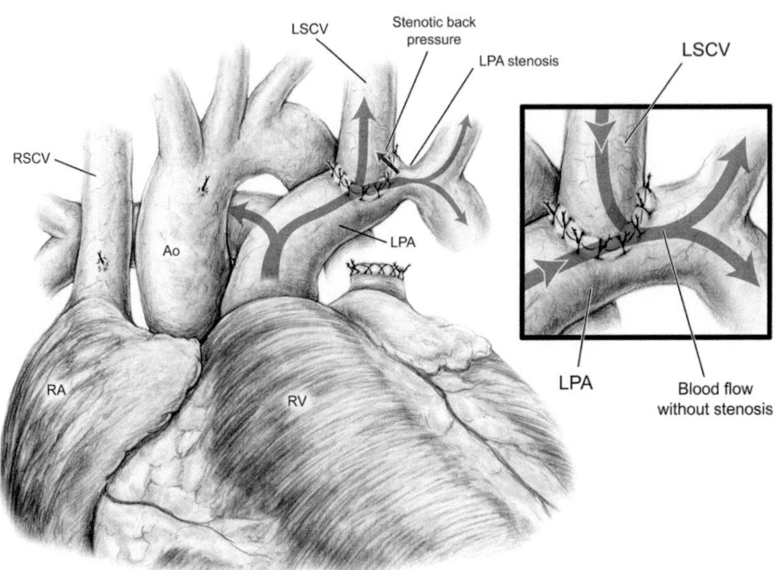

Fig. 35 Shows the abnormal flow characteristics of a bidirectional Glenn shunt and distal left pulmonary artery stenosis which results in systemic venous hypertension and severe headaches. The big arrow shows preferable proximal pulmonary artery flow into the left-sided Glenn shunt (Left SVC). The smaller arrow shows the remaining flow to the distal pulmonary artery owing to the distal pulmonary artery stenosis. The inset shows how the flow patterns are expected when there is no distal right pulmonary artery stenosis. *Ao* aorta, *LPA* left pulmonary artery, *LSCV* left superior caval vein, *RA* right atrium, *RSCV* right superior caval vein, *RV* right ventricle

much the diagnostic criteria of ccTGA and the other various options for surgical correction. The idea of 1½ ventricular repair for this entity is to construct a physiologic repair (right ventricle to aortic continuity) without having to perform the more extensive repair requiring an atrial baffle procedure, an enlargement of the VSD with intraventricular baffling, and right ventricular to pulmonary artery conduit. The complications of this type of biventricular and physiologic reconstruction are noteworthy and include potential coronary artery problems, baffle complications, conduit changes over time, and atrial arrhythmias. This 1½ ventricular repair is less complex but has the long-term problem of systemic right ventricular failure which can be mitigated by a higher left ventricular pressure which is inherent in the conduct of the operation (Zias et al. 2003; Ilbawi et al. 1989; Mavroudis et al. 1999b; Liu et al. 2022; Cabrelle et al. 2021) The operation is performed by VSD closure if present, pulmonary artery valvotomy/subpulmonic resection, and right atrial unloading by the BDG shunt. This maneuver lowers the developed pressure in the left ventricle to sub-systemic levels for optimal coronary artery flow and helps to stabilize the position of the interventricular septum which will prevent right ventricular distention. This in turn helps to avoid tricuspid regurgitation on the basis of papillary muscle stretching. This strategy is not new. Left ventricular training using pulmonary artery banding after failed atrial baffle operations with tricuspid regurgitation has been shown to cause a shift in the interventricular septum due to the higher left ventricular pressure which results in less tricuspid regurgitation (Myers et al. 2013; Winlaw et al. 2005; Erek et al. 2012). While the strategy for the 1½ ventricular repair for this rare set of patients is sound, the 20–25-year follow-up regarding this approach is yet to be determined.

Another indication for the 1½ ventricular repair can be applied to patients with ccTGA who are undergoing the double switch operation when the surgeon feels that the atrial baffle is too complex to include the SVC flow. Under these cir-

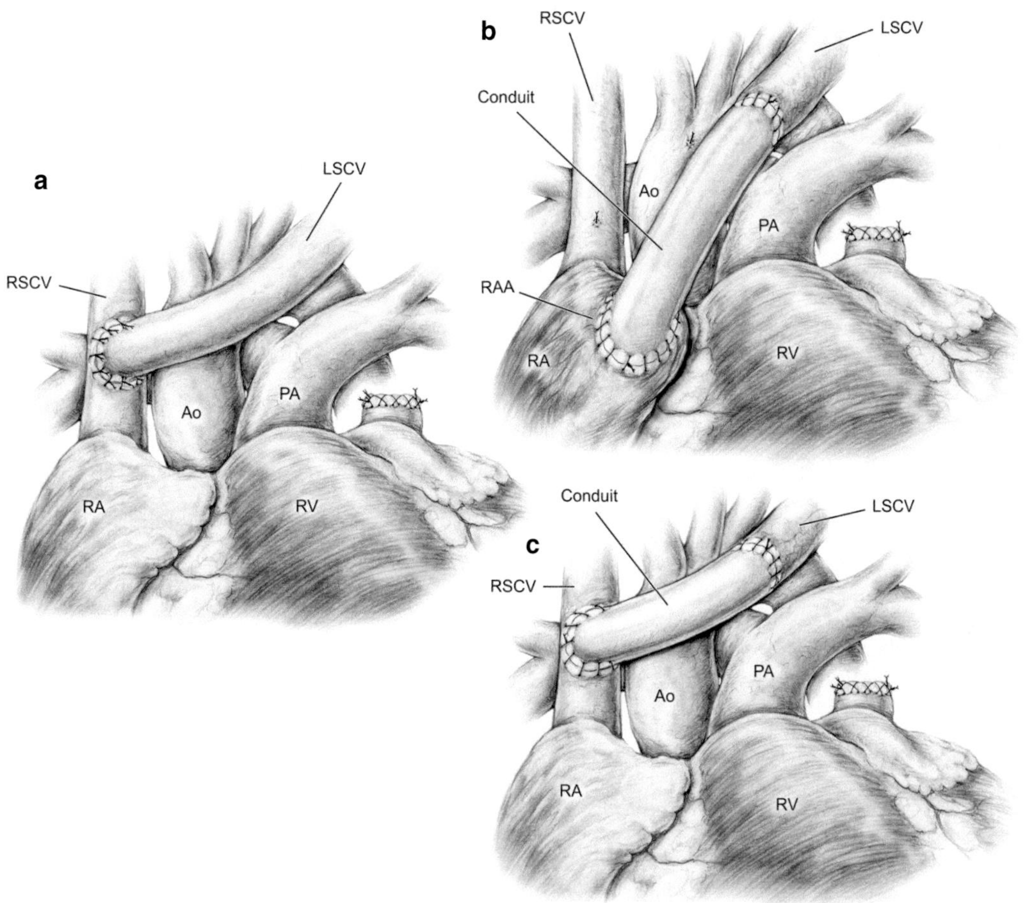

Fig. 36 Other extracardiac solutions to the anomalous left superior vena cava which include direct anastomosis to the right superior vena cava (**a**), and the interposed graft to the right atrial appendage (**b**), or right superior vena cava (**c**). *Ao* aorta, *LPA* left pulmonary artery, *LSCV* left superior caval vein, *PA* pulmonary artery, *RA* right atrium, *RAA* right atrial appendage, *RSCV* right superior caval vein, *RV* right ventricle

cumstances, a pericardial baffle is constructed to direct IVC flow to the tricuspid valve and right ventricle which is to become the pulmonary ventricle after the arterial switch operation. The superior vena cava flow problem is resolved by a BDG shunt thereby completing the 1½ ventricular repair. This reconstruction has the benefit of simplifying the atrial baffle, decreasing the chances of an atrial baffle leak or stenosis, and avoiding the risk of sinoatrial node injury since the intra-atrial suture load is basically cut in half with concentration in areas when the sinoatrial node is not at risk (Malhotra et al. 2011). The options and potential complications for repair of the common types of ccTGA are reviewed in chapter "Complications Associated with Repair of Congenitally Corrected Transposition of the Great Arteries".

It should surprise no one that occasionally operations which have been performed early in life become problematic in later life due to missed diagnoses, right ventricular growth, and misapplied operations. There have been reports of patients who underwent atriopulmonary Fontan operations for tricuspid atresia with eventual development of protein losing enteropathy. Usually, this complication is attended by right atrial hypertension, arrhythmias, and pathway obstructions. Fontan conversion under these circumstances is generally contraindicated due to

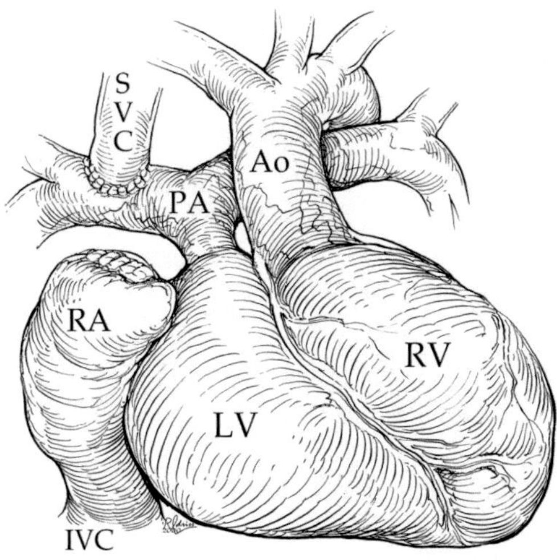

Fig. 37 Shows the completed bidirectional Glenn shunt which was performed in a patient with ccTGA, small VSD, and pulmonary stenosis. The double switch operations, namely (1) arterial switch, VSD closure, and atrial baffle operation and (2) Left ventricular to aortic tunneling, right ventricular to pulmonary artery conduit, and atrial baffle operation are not appropriate for this anatomic configuration owing to pulmonary stenosis which rules out the arterial switch operation and small VSD which rules out the atrial baffle-Rastelli operation. The idea of this 1 ½ ventricular repair is to perform a pulmonary stenosis repair by valvar incision or subvalvar resection, close the small VSD, and create the bidirectional Glenn shunt. By unloading the left ventricle, the pressure will be still high but should be sub-systemic which will optimize coronary flow characteristics. In addition, the increased left ventricular pressure will help to maintain the position of the interventricular septum which in turn will help to prevent right ventricular papillary muscle stretching and preserve tricuspid valve competency. *Ao* aorta, *IVC* inferior vena cava, *LV* left ventricle, *PA* pulmonary artery, *RA* right atrium, *RV* right ventricle, *SVC* superior vena cava. (With permission: Mavroudis 2015b)

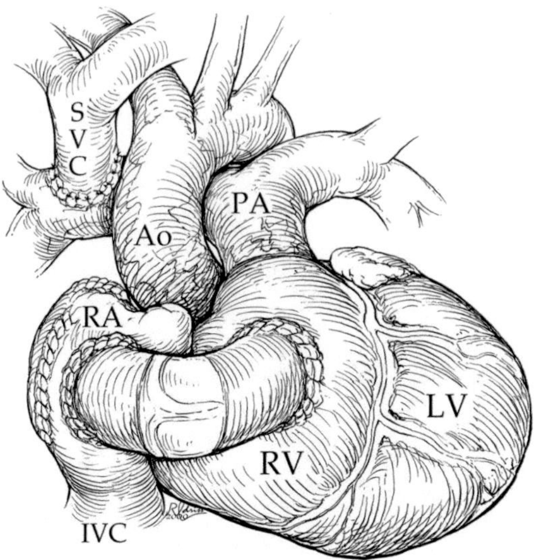

Fig. 38 Shows a 1½ ventricular repair that was performed in a patient with a prior artriopulmonary Fontan for tricuspid atresia and who developed protein losing enteropathy. During the patient evaluation, it was found that the right ventricle had grown to a size greater than 40% of the expected normal right ventricular volume. The patient underwent Fontan takedown, pulmonary artery reconnection, and a right atrial to right ventricular valved conduit which improved hemodynamics and led to resolution of protein losing enteropathy. *Ao* aorta, *IVC* inferior vena cava, *LV* left ventricle, *PA* pulmonary artery, *RA* right atrium, *RV* right ventricle, *SVC* superior vena cava. (With permission: Mavroudis 2015b)

protein losing enteropathy (Backer and Mavroudis 2019). Most clinicians would refer a patient like this for cardiac transplantation. However, occasionally, the right ventricle grows to levels above 40% of predicted normal right ventricular size. Interestingly, there have been reports of a 1½ ventricular repair in patients with atriopulmonary Fontan operations for tricuspid atresia who experienced right ventricular growth (Ono et al. 2016a). During maturation, they became candidates for right atrial to right ventricular conduit placement and reinstitution of right ventricle to pulmonary artery continuity in association with a bidirectional Glenn shunt (Fig. 38). The result was a lower right atrial pressure and pulsatile pulmonary artery blood flow. These are rare cases but should be considered when favorable hemodynamic and anatomic characteristics are identified.

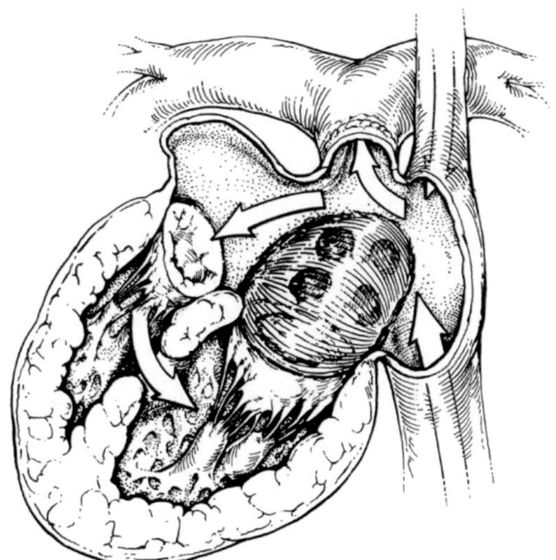

Fig. 39 Shows a coronal view of a patient who had repair of what was thought to be dextrocardia, tricuspid atresia, and no VSD by atriopulmonary Fontan and pulmonary venous baffle repair to the mitral valve/left ventricle. The patient developed a decrease in functional class and upon further evaluation resulted in a change of diagnosis to dextrocardia, crisscross heart, tricuspid stenosis, VSD, severe pulmonary artery stenosis, normally related great arteries, baffle stenosis, cyanosis, and atrial reentry tachycardia. The updated anatomic configuration and the previous repair are noted in the drawing. The arrows show systemic venous cardiac return with circulation to the pulmonary artery, the small tricuspid valve, and through the extant VSD resulting in cyanosis. (With permission: Mavroudis 2015b)

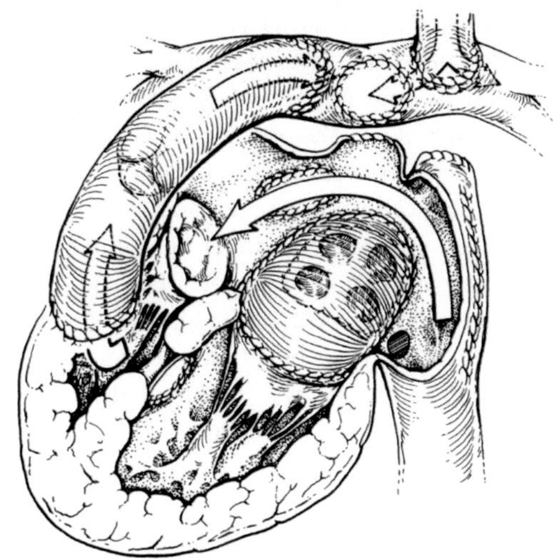

Fig. 40 Shows the result of the 1½ ventricular repair which involved VSD closure, pulmonary venous baffle augmentation, modified right-sided maze procedure, right ventricular to pulmonary artery valved conduit and a bidirectional Glenn. The arrows trace systemic venous return and pathway through the repaired heart and the bidirectional Glenn shunt. (With permission: Mavroudis 2015b)

Another clinical scenario, likely unique in character and scope, is noted in Figs. 39 and 40. Figure 39 shows the artist's coronal view of the resultant anatomy, physiology, and operative result in a patient who had an atriopulmonary Fontan operation for presumed dextrocardia, tricuspid atresia, and no VSD. Due to decreasing functional status, the patient underwent reassessment and was found to have dextrocardia, crisscross heart, tricuspid stenosis, VSD, severe pulmonary artery stenosis, normally related great arteries, baffle stenosis, cyanosis, and atrial reentry tachycardia. Figure 40 shows the operative repair by VSD closure, baffle augmentation, modified right-sided maze procedure, right ventricular to pulmonary artery valved conduit and a BDG shunt thereby completing the 1½ ventricular repair in this very complex patient.

4 Fontan Conversion and Arrhythmia Surgery

Medical and surgical management of patients with failing Fontan circulation has evolved over the past decade owing to focused scientific and clinical inquiry that have addressed the problems of the obligatory high venous pressure that characterizes this unique physiology. This singular physiologic aberration of high systemic venous pressure has resulted in protein losing enteropathy, plastic bronchitis, liver failure, liver cancer, atrial arrhythmias, pathway obstructions, valvar insufficiency, aneurysm formation, ventricular dysfunction, and decreased functional class (Mazza et al. 2021). Furthermore, these manifest complications become more significant and more likely as the patient ages. Consequently, it should be expected that most, if not all, patients with Fontan physiology will require therapeutic interventions which may include intense medical therapy, pacemaker placement, Fontan conversion, and eventually, cardiac transplantation (Mavroudis et al. 2008; Pundi et al. 2016).

To this end, we introduced the Fontan conversion operation in 1994 (Mavroudis et al. 1998) for patients with failing Fontan physiology and atrial arrhythmias. The operation is characterized by surgical conversion from atriopulmonary Fontan connections to extracardiac vena cava to pulmonary artery connections, arrhythmia surgery, and pacemaker placement (Deal et al. 2000; Mavroudis et al. 2002, 2003; Deal et al. 2002, 2003). Over the years of surgical application and retrospective study, we found that patients responded best to this therapeutic modality when there was preservation of ventricular function and absence of protein losing enteropathy (Backer and Mavroudis 2019). The long-term outcomes of this operation resulted in improved functional status, resolution of debilitating arrhythmias, repaired pathway obstructions, repaired valves, repaired aneurysms, and delayed cardiac transplantation. And, when statistical analysis is considered, this operation has been largely successful by our group and many other groups worldwide which have documented similar results (Hoashi et al. 2020; Terada et al. 2014). During the development and implementation of this operation, we have been confronted with many impediments that were resolved intraoperatively. These techniques are reviewed and explored in this chapter with reference to avoiding and/or treating potential complications as they occur.

Most of the drawings in this chapter are from the *Atlas of Pediatric Cardiac Surgery* (Mavroudis and Backer 2015) and *Atlas of Adult Congenital Heart Surgery* (Mavroudis and Dearani 2019). It did not seem appropriate or wise for Rachid Idriss, the illustrator, to redraw figures that showed the anatomy brilliantly in the first place. The prose has been altered to fit the conditions of the adult with congenital heart disease. New drawings have been introduced to highlight the potential complications that may be encountered during the conduct of the operations.

4.1 General Principles

Every invasive operation starts with an incision. In every case, Fontan conversion requires resternotomy which is attended by numerous potential complications relating to unwanted cavitary entry, hemorrhage, air embolus, and hemodynamic compromise that can quickly result in cardiovascular collapse. Cardiac output in the Fontan patient is driven by adequate venous pressure and volume delivery to the pulmonary circulation. Any instability during resternotomy, even if effectively controlled, can result in renal failure, ventricular dysfunction, and ischemic brain injury. To obviate these problems, some preoperative conditions should be considered. Patients with giant right atria which adheres to the underside of the sternum may require peripheral cannulation and partial bypass before resternotomy. Femoral cannulation has its own set of potential complications, however. If femoral cannulation is indeed employed, every effort should be made to convert to aortobicaval cannulation with femoral vessel repair to avoid the problems of limb ischemia, swelling, and compartment syndrome. Once successful mediastinal reentry is accomplished, strategic and careful dissection is performed to ensure hemostasis and comprehensive exposure for proper execution of the operation. It is wise to assess the circulation during this time by hemodynamic evaluation which should include serum lactate levels, hematocrit measurements, and maintenance of effective blood pressure. TEE evaluation of ventricular performance is also effective. Any circulatory aberrations that are discovered may signal early commencement of cardiopulmonary bypass during which time the rest of the dissection can be accomplished. This maneuver however prolongs the extent of cardiopulmonary bypass time and all the associated problems thereto pertaining (Mavroudis et al. 2003). The operating team must therefore use this strategy selectively and with the proper deserving considerations.

During the cardiac dissection, both thoracic cavities must be entered followed by lysis of pulmonary adhesions. This will control chest wall bleeding from adhesion takedown and enable effective tube thoracostomy during the closing stages of the operation. Comprehensive takedown of pulmonary chest wall adhesions is not easy. The adhesions can be deep in the chest cavity and oftentimes are associated with significant bleeding. This part of the operation should be performed with optimal exposure which is usually facilitated by self-retaining mammary retractors. Once comprehensive dissection is accomplished, aortobicaval cardiopulmonary bypass is instituted with slow systemic cooling to the desired systemic temperature, usually 32⁰ C for most cases or 28⁰ C if associated lesions will require repair. At this point during the conduct of the operation, the surgical team must execute the preoperative plan so that all the parts of the operation are performed in the proper sequence. Every patient will require a period of aortic cross-clamping and cardioplegic arrest, if for no other reason than to perform the atrial septectomy and maze procedure. Other considerations include valve repair, pathway revisions, aneurysm resection, pulmonary artery augmentation, and left sided maze procedures. The following are some of the characteristics of the Fontan conversion operation with regard to the anatomic substrate and type of arrhythmia surgery.

4.2 Uncomplicated Fontan Conversion with Modified Right Atrial Maze Procedure and Epicardial Pacemaker Lead Placement

The conduct of the uncomplicated Fontan conversion with modified right atrial maze procedure and epicardial pacemaker implantation is summarized in Figs. 41, 42, 43, 44, 45, 46, 47 and 48. The most important mishaps to avoid, besides

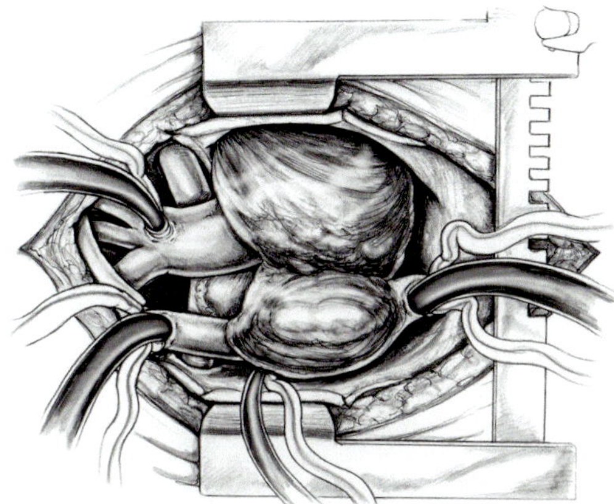

Fig. 41 Shows the cannulation technique for Fontan conversion using aortobicaval cardiopulmonary bypass with left ventricular venting through the right superior pulmonary vein in a patient with tricuspid atresia and extant atriopulmonary Fontan. (With Permission: Mavroudis 2015c)

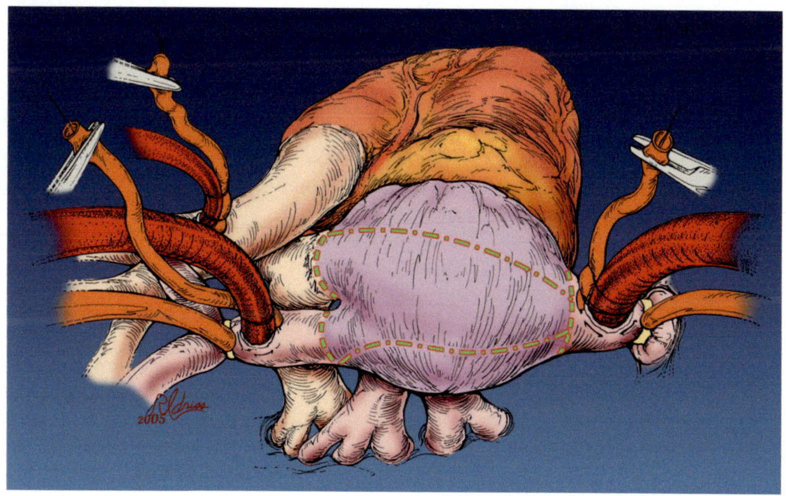

Fig. 42 Shows the extent of the right atrial wall resection that includes a significant part of the right atrial free wall. This maneuver is a significant part of the arrhythmia surgical procedure since it is instrumental in removing scarred myocardial tissue which could be responsible for atrial reentry circuits. (With Permission: Mavroudis 2015c)

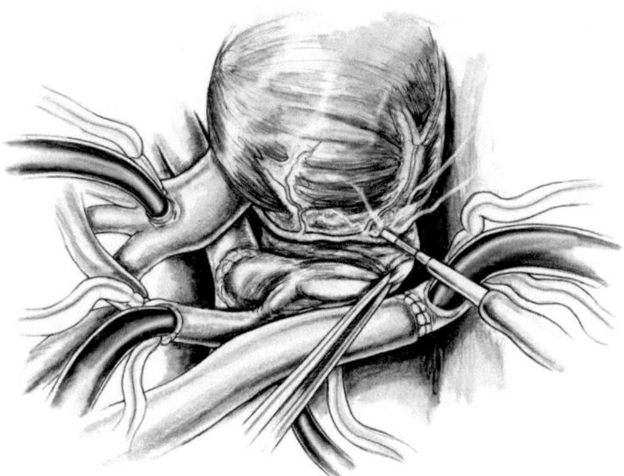

Fig. 43 Shows dissection of the atrioventricular groove to facilitate right atrial wall reduction and provide an unscarred location for right atrial pacemaker lead placement. Also shown is the first intracardiac part of the operation which involves inferior vena cava transection and separation from the right atrium and end to end anastomosis with a PTFE tube graft (24 mm). This part of the operation can be performed in a beating heart as long as there is no atrial communication to the left side of the heart, which is usually the case. (With Permission: Mavroudis 2015c)

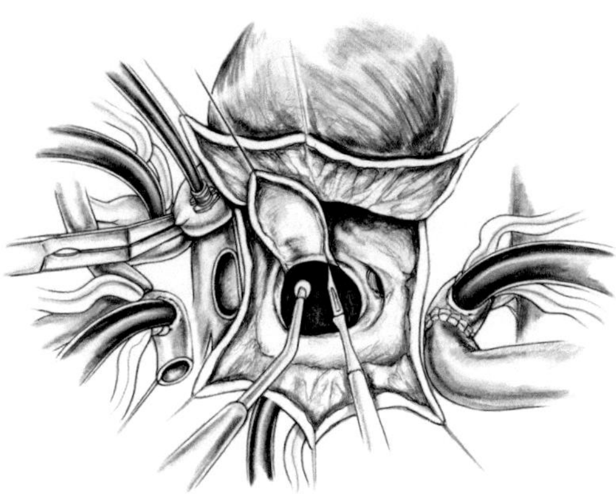

Fig. 44 The aorta is then cross clamped, administration of antegrade cardioplegia is accomplished and the superior vena cava is transected at the cavo-atrial junction as shown in the figure. An atriotomy is subsequently accomplished to connect the orifices of the superior and inferior vena cavae as shown in the figure. This allows exposure of the entire right atrium and facilitates atriopulmonary disconnection and septum primum resection as noted. (With Permission: Mavroudis 2015c)

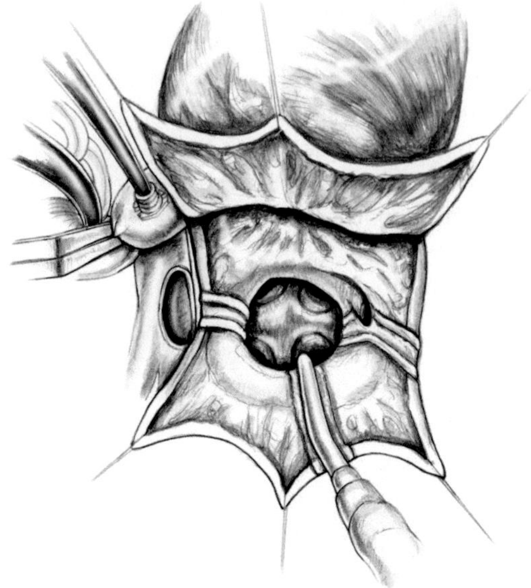

Fig. 45 Shows the completion of the modified right atrial maze procedure which entails cryoablation lesions to connect the coronary sinus with the cut edge of the inferior vena cava, to connect the coronary sinus with the atrial septal defect (ASD), to connect the ASD with the posterior atrial flap across the crista terminalis, and a lesion to connect the base of the resected atrial septum and the ASD. (With Permission: Mavroudis 2015c)

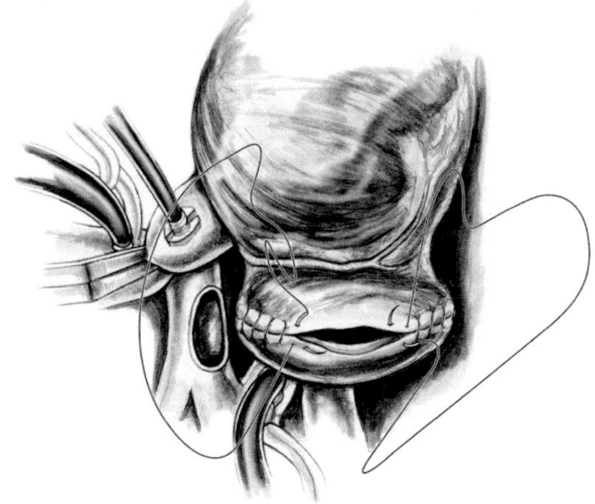

Fig. 46 A large atrial resection is undertaken to accomplish a right atrial wall reduction and the atrium is closed without regard to the sinoatrial node using running suture technique as shown in the figure. The sinoatrial node in these patients is often dysfunctional. Our intention is to use atrial pacing after the operation which will limit the occurrence of premature atrial contractions and therefore limit episodes of atrial reentry tachycardia. (With Permission: Mavroudis 2015c)

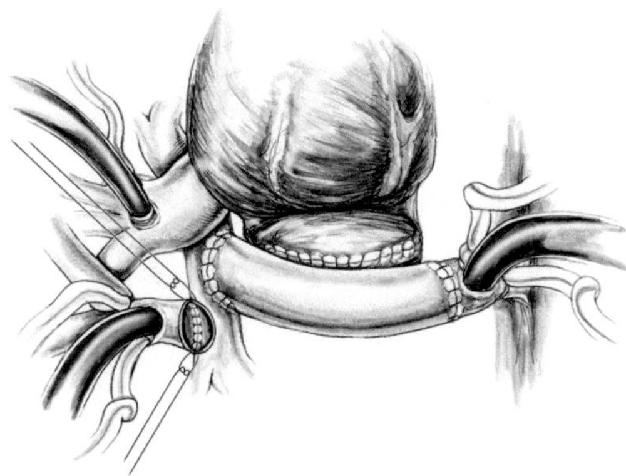

Fig. 47 The cross clamp can now be removed after all the air maneuvers are accomplished and the patient can be rewarmed. During this stage the extracardiac PTFE conduit is cut to size and on a bevel. It is then anastomosed to the inferior portion of the right pulmonary artery to ensure an anatomic offset with the superior vena cava as shown in the figure. This is followed by the superior cavopulmonary anastomosis which is performed using interrupted suture technique. (With Permission: Mavroudis 2015c)

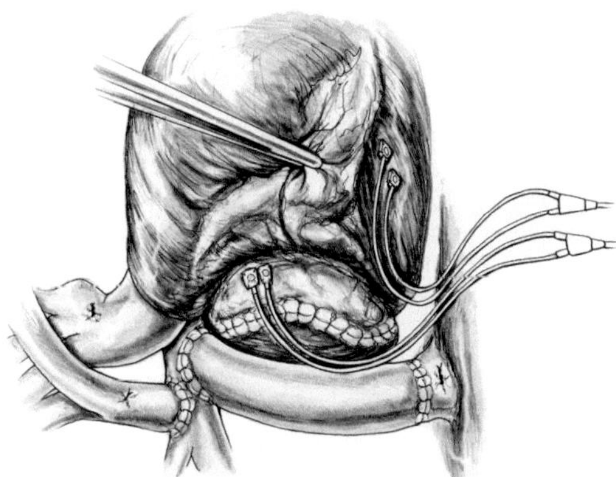

Fig. 48 After the patient is ventilated and separated from cardiopulmonary bypass, the Protamine is administered, and all bleeding is controlled. At this time, bipolar, steroid-eluting, epicardial leads are placed on the surface of the atrium and ventricle and tested for sensing and pacing as shown in the figure. The pacemaker is programmed for AAI function. A good sign for efficacy is if the patient is in nodal rhythm and responds to atrial pacing yielding a paced sinus rhythm. The operation is concluded by ensuring careful hemostasis which may take hours to achieve. It cannot be emphasized enough how important this part of the operation is. (With Permission: Mavroudis 2015c)

resternotomy and comprehensive dissection involve the management of the right atrioventricular groove dissection, right atrial wall resection, and placement of cryoablation lesions. Figure 42 shows the extensive resection lines of the right atrial wall in association with Fontan conversion. The resection is large to include the areas of scarring which are substrates for the subsequent development of atrial reentry tachycardia. In order to achieve a large resection and to have enough residual atrial wall left for atrial closure, the right atrioventricular groove is dissected as shown in Fig. 43. This maneuver is also performed to identify unscarred tissue for atrial lead placement. Most of the time, the atrioventricular groove is readily dissected by scar tissue separation which can be performed by low setting electrocautery lysis of adhesions. Clearly, the course of the right coronary artery is to be respected. During the dissection, the two most important objectives are to find unscarred atrial tissue for the atrial pacemaker lead and to mobilize enough atrial tissue for untethered closure after the scarred atrial wall resection as noted in Fig. 42. The course of the right coronary artery need not be identified unless the dissection is forthcoming without hemorrhage. Any venous bleeding should end the dissection so as not to cause atrial perforation or coronary artery injury. In the event of atrial perforation, the surgeon should take care in the repair to avoid any kinking or perforation of the right coronary artery. Any injury of the right coronary artery whether it be small or large, should trigger aortic cross-clamping, cardioplegic arrest and primary suture repair using interrupted suture technique or autologous pericardial/PTFE patch repair as described in chapter "Complications Associated with Repair of Congenital and Acquired Coronary Artery Anomalies". The cryoablation part of the operation is performed after the atrial septum is resected with special care to avoid injury to the underlying mitral valve and conduction system. Figure 45 indicates the recommended location of the cryoablation sites for the right- sided maze procedure. In some cases, with tricuspid atresia, a "tricuspid dimple" can be identified which is an embryologic remnant of the tricuspid valve (Thoele et al. 1991). It is tempting to place a cryoablation lesion between the coronary sinus and the "tricuspid dimple" thinking that this is an area of slow conduction and should be ablated to prevent postoperative atrial reentry tachycardia. More often than not, this unrecommended lesion will cause heart block and it should be avoided. The subsequent hemodynamic parts of the operation are described in the legends and are subject to the usual maneuvers of comprehensive cavitary air removal and cautious separation from cardiopulmonary bypass. Placement of atrial and ventricular leads is another matter entirely. This is difficult, can take time, and requires great attention to detail for optimal results. The challenge is not so much technical as it is for the search to find epicardial sites that will yield appropriate electrophysiologic parameters and allow proper pacemaker function without energy drainage (Fig. 48). If not performed properly, the patient may need to be returned to the operating room for pacemaker revision.

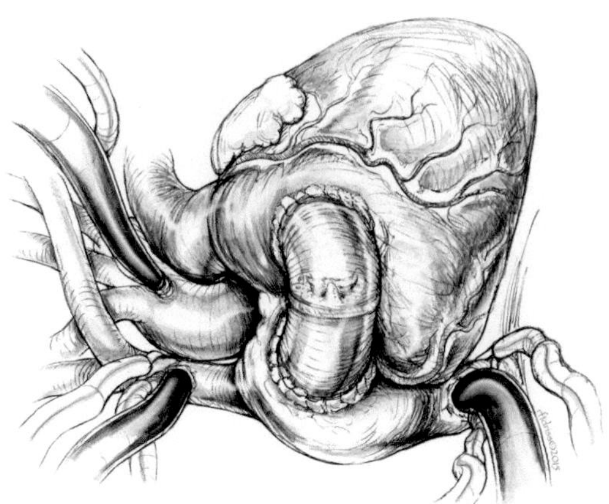

Fig. 49 The Bjork Modification was introduced to take advantage of a thick right atrium which could function as an auxiliary pump and a good-sized right ventricle that could help with the pulmonary circulation. While many reports have shown that this modification can result in improved exercise tolerance as long as the right ventricle is large enough to create pulsatile flow, other reports have documented gradual stenosis of the right atrial to ventricular conduit which results in poor function. In this illustrated case, the figure shows institution of aortobicaval cardiopulmonary bypass in a patient with tricuspid atresia who underwent previous right atrial-to-right ventricular Bjork modification Fontan operation. Note that the right atrial to right ventricular conduit was valved. Note also that the valve became sclerotic in the open position since almost immediately after it was placed it assumed a constantly open position relating to non-pulsatile laminar flow patterns from the right atrium to the right ventricle. (With Permission: Mavroudis 2015c)

4.3 Takedown of Right Atrial-to-Right Ventricular Bjork Modification

The Bjork Modification (Björk et al. 1979) as reviewed in the Fig. 49 legend was introduced to augment the circulatory pattern that propels the systemic venous return to the pulmonary arteries. The idea was to interpose a valved conduit between the thickened right atrium which was thought to have some pumping ability and the small right ventricle that could pump blood to the pulmonary arteries without back flow to the atrium on account of the interposed valve that would prevent regurgitation. This was the idea, and it was a good one. Ono and associates (Ono et al. 2016b) showed that as long as the right ventricle was large enough to deliver pulsatile flow to the pulmonary arteries, patients' exercise performance improved. This idea was reported by Hopkins and associates (Hopkins et al. 2019) who supported the concept of converting Fontan-Björk to 1.5- or 2-ventricle circulation.

However, other clinical reports have shown that complications can occur in the mid- and long-term application of this modification (Huang et al. 2011; Lemmer et al. 1983). The flow through the valved conduit was oftentimes laminar which caused the interposed homograft valve to sclerose in the open position oftentimes causing stenosis. The result was right atrial dilatation, atrial reentry tachycardia, and decreased functional class. In order to improve the Bjork modification, a non-valved conduit between the right atrium and small right ventricle has been proposed to avoid the development of sclerosis of the interposed homograft that defined the original

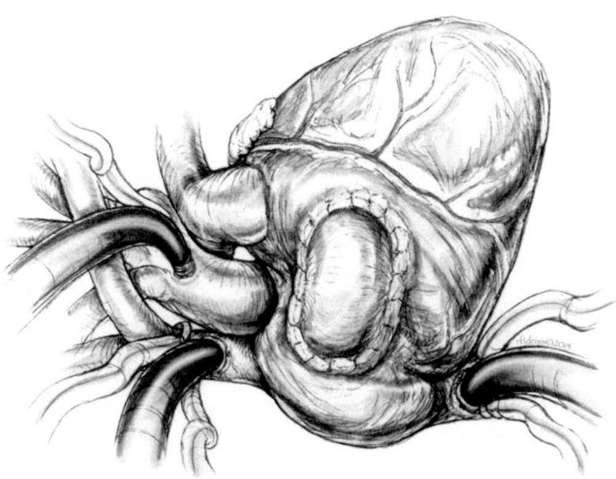

Fig. 50 Some surgeons used non-valved right atrial to right ventricular connections either with a tube graft or with right atrial flaps that were augmented with pericardial patches as shown in the figure. Whichever the case, these conduit pathways are removed very carefully to avoid injury to the pulmonary valve which was usually intact, and the course of the right coronary artery which was situated posterior to the course of the conduit connection. (With Permission: Mavroudis 2015c)

Bjork modification (Fig. 50). The purpose of this discussion is not so much to decide whether the Bork modification is better than the extracardiac Fontan operation or vice versa. The purpose is how to perform Fontan conversion for these patients while recognizing the potential complications. Figures 51, 52, 53, 54, 55 and 56 shows the progression of Fontan conversion for these patients. As discussed earlier in this chapter, the atrioventricular groove needs to be dissected very carefully as shown in Figs. 52 and 53, to prevent unwanted atrial wall perforation and right coronary artery injury. Once the right atrial to right ventricular conduit is removed, the dilemma arises in the question, "What do we do with the right ventricle?" If the pulmonary artery is disconnected and proximally oversewn such as what is done for total cavopulmonary artery connection, then the right ventricle has to be patched, thereby not allowing an outflow for the thebesian accumulated flow. This problem results in right ventricular distention, calcification, and interventricular septal shift towards the left ventricle

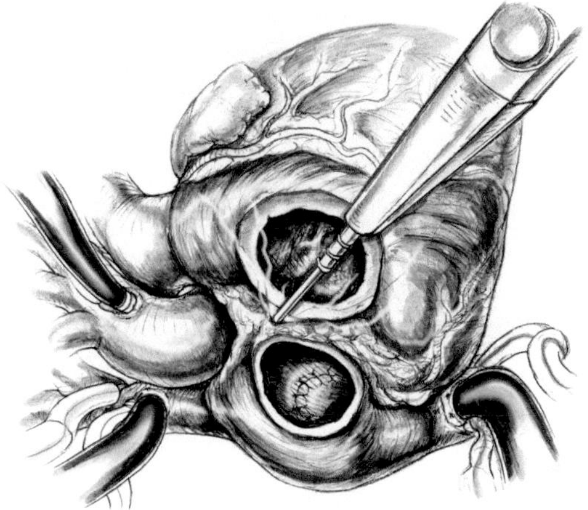

Fig. 51 Shows electrocautery dissection of the atrioventricular groove where lies the course of the coronary artery. This part of the operation requires careful attention to the right coronary artery, the ascending aorta, and the right atrial free wall. The dissection is started near the ascending aorta and extended inferiorly. (With Permission: Mavroudis 2015c)

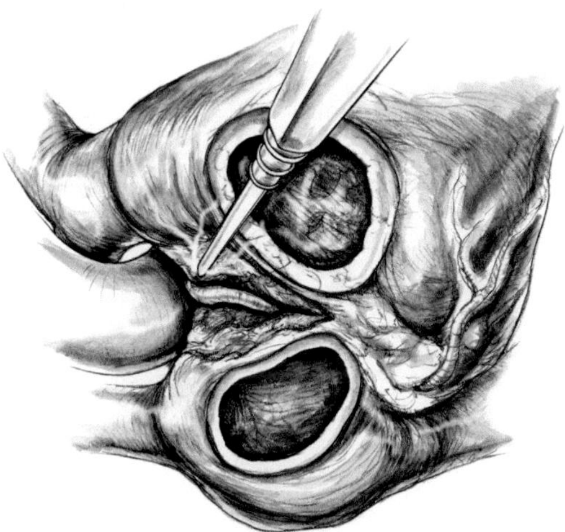

Fig. 52 Depicts the dissection at the midpoint as the course of the right coronary artery is exposed. It is not necessary to actually identify the right coronary artery. The reason to perform this dissection is twofold. First, it uncovers unscarred atrial tissue which can be an excellent implantation destination for the atrial pacemaker leads. The second reason is to gain enough atrial length for a more thorough atrial resection in association with the right-sided modified maze procedure. (With Permission: Mavroudis et al. 2007)

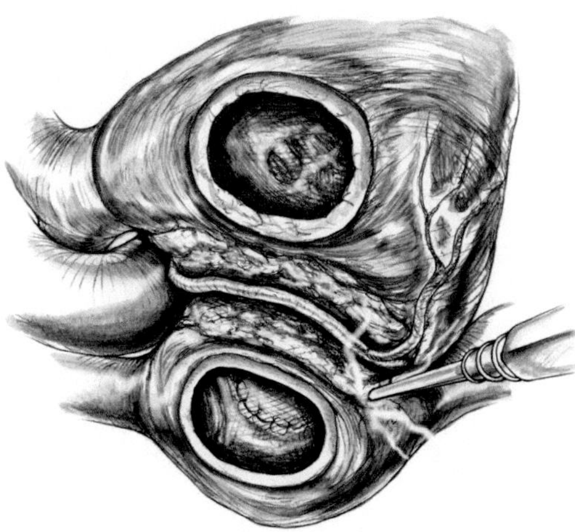

Fig. 53 Shows the completed resection. If the surgeon finds excessive bleeding with this part of the operation, it can be abandoned for fear of unwanted right coronary artery entry which will require immediate operative intervention by cardioplegic arrest and patch arterioplasty. (With Permission: Mavroudis et al. 2007)

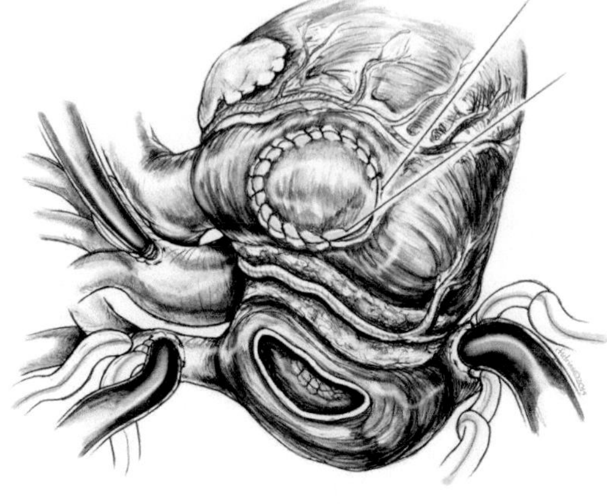

Fig. 55 We have found that the best management scheme is to leave the right ventricular to pulmonary artery continuity intact and patch the right ventricle as shown in the figure. The amount of thebesian flow into the right ventricular chamber is limited and does not result in enough developed pressure to interfere with the low-pressure Fontan physiology. (With Permission: Mavroudis 2015c)

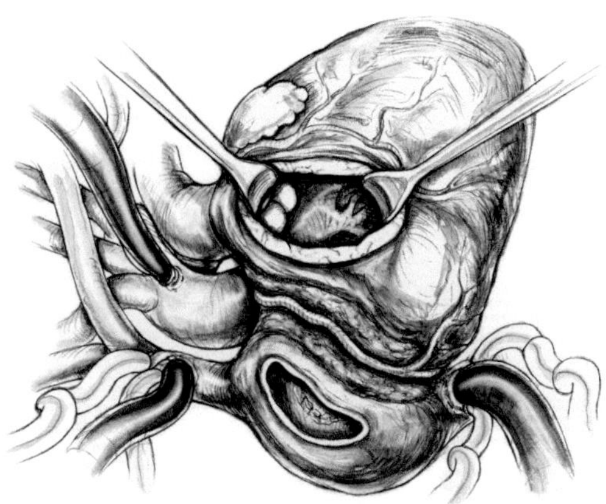

Fig. 54 Shows retraction of the right ventricle into which the Bjork modification was anastomosed and taken down. Notice that the pulmonary valve is present and has not been disconnected; also note that the valve appears to be trileaflet and competent. The ventricle is about 30% the size of the normal right ventricle. The dilemma is what to do with this chamber? Disconnecting the pulmonary artery as is usually performed for any Fontan operation together with right ventricular patching will leave a relatively large chamber with no outlet. This will result in stagnant thebesian blood flow, which will accumulate, cause ventricular distention over time and negatively impact the function of the left ventricle. We have seen this very situation of left ventricular dysfunction in a referred patient who was treated this way. Because of the calcification and the potential complications that would attend an operation, nothing could be done. (With Permission: Mavroudis 2015c)

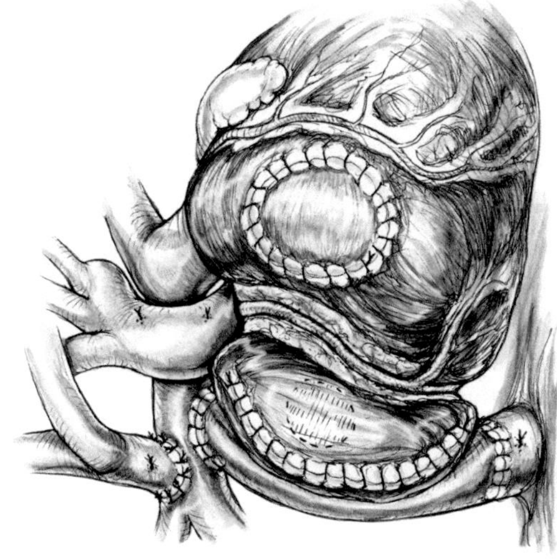

Fig. 56 Once the ventricular patch is accomplished, aortic cross clamping is performed and cardioplegic arrest is assured. The septum primum is resected (not shown); a reduction right atrioplasty is accomplished; and a modified right-sided maze procedure is performed (not shown). The right atriorrhaphy is accomplished while all the air maneuvers are performed, and the cross clamp is removed as shown in the figure. The patient is then weaned from cardiopulmonary bypass and the pacemaker leads are placed (not shown). The dotted lines in the right atrium signify the open atrial communication. (With Permission: Mavroudis 2015c)

causing systemic ventricular dysfunction. Clearly, this is not a good outcome. Better to leave the right ventricle to pulmonary artery intact and patch the right ventricle which will allow thebesian outflow egress and provide a modicum of pulsatile flow to the pulmonary circulation which has been shown to be beneficial (Kalia et al. 2021) (Fig. 55 and 56). Not shown in this series of drawings is atrial septectomy, the right-sided maze procedure, and epicardial pacemaker placement.

4.4 Fontan Conversion When There Are Discontinuous Pulmonary Arteries: Glenn Shunt to the Right Pulmonary Artery; Atriopulmonary Connection to the Left Pulmonary Artery

Early in the development of staged orthoterminal palliation (Fontan operation), a pre-Fontan Glenn shunt was performed en route to completion Fontan which was defined as the right classic Glenn procedure and a right atrial to left pulmonary artery connection. This idea was the beginning of the staged approach to extracardiac connections that are used nowadays. These discordant connections resulted in the development of right-sided pulmonary arteriovenous malformation due to the lack of hepatic factor to the right pulmonary circulation. This situation and recent discoveries describing hepatic factor are discussed in the previous section on the bidirectional Glenn shunt. As noted, these patients oftentimes present with cyanosis and atrial reentry tachycardia that makes them good candidates for Fontan conversion and pulmonary artery reconnection. During our early experience with these reparative techniques, we used aortic homografts to connect the two pulmonary arteries and establish the total extracardiac Fontan reconstruction as noted in Fig. 57. The aortic homograft has favorable sewing and hemostatic characteristics and is naturally configured for the anatomic repair as noted. The long-term impediments for this reconstruction are that homograft grafts induce the induction of preformed antibodies which can adversely affect immunosuppressive protocols in the event of eventual cardiac transplantation. We subsequently changed our protocol to use PTFE grafts for pulmonary artery reconnection as shown in Fig. 58. The complications associated with PTFE reconstruction are bleeding and size discrepancies during the course of the operation. Proper suture technique and accurate measurements will obviate these complications which will lead to a favorable reconstruction.

4.5 Pulmonary Atresia with Intact Ventricular Septum After Atriopulmonary Fontan and Right Ventricular Growth

Patients with pulmonary atresia and intact ventricular septum are selected at birth based on tricuspid valve size and the presence or absence of tripart right ventricular anatomy; namely, inlet, body, and outlet development. Those with adequate right ventricles can be prepared for eventual biventricular repair; those with smaller ventricles (approximately 30%–50% of normal size) can undergo 1½ ventricular repair, while those with very small ventricles are prepared for staged orthoterminal palliation. Some patients diagnosed with pulmonary atresia and intact ventricular septum who had atriopulmonary Fontan procedures develop enlarged right ventricular cavities resulting in significant tricuspid regurgitation and increased right atrial pressure. This situation impacts unfavorably on Fontan

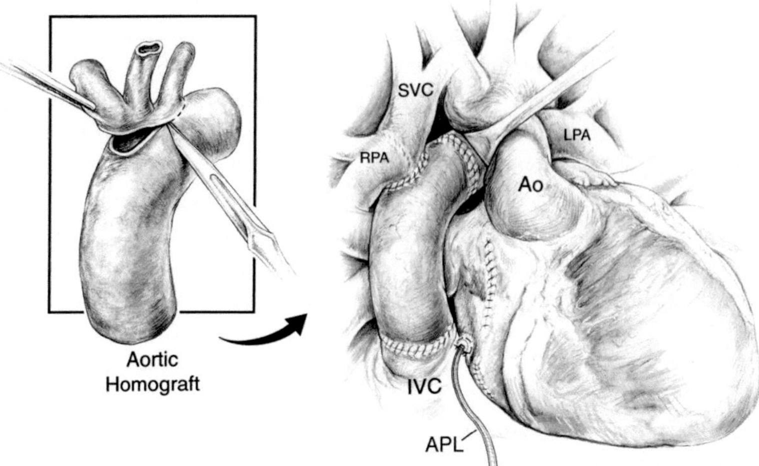

Fig. 57 In the days before the obligatory second stage bidirectional Glenn shunt en route to the Fontan operation, some surgeons performed a second stage right Glenn shunt and systemic to pulmonary artery shunt to the left pulmonary artery en route to Fontan connections that included the classic right Glenn shunt and a right atrial to left pulmonary artery connection. These connections obviously left the pulmonary arteries disconnected and established the substrate for right-sided pulmonary arteriovenous malformation owing to the lack of hepatic factor to the right pulmonary circulation. These patients often present with cyanosis and atrial reentry tachycardia that requires Fontan conversion and pulmonary artery reconnection. During our early experience with these patients, we reasoned that we would use aortic homografts to accomplish the reconnection since the homograft material is easy to sew and affords better hemostasis and anastomotic leeway than PTFE as shown in the figure. The long-term difficulty with this approach is that homograft material induces preformed antibodies which can adversely affect immunosuppressive protocols in the event of eventual cardiac transplantation. We therefore changed our protocol to use PTFE grafts for pulmonary artery reconnection as shown in Fig. 58 which was adapted from the Pediatric Atlas). *Ao* aorta, *APL* antiitachycardia pacemaker lead, *IVC* inferior vena cava, *LPA* left pulmonary artery, *RPA* right pulmonary artery, *SVC* superior vena cava

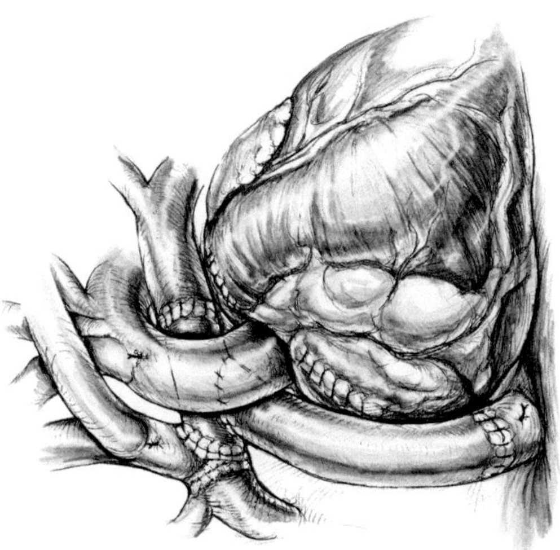

Fig. 58 Shows right and left pulmonary artery reconnection after the original Fontan procedure which involved a classic right-sided Glenn procedure in conjunction with atrial to left pulmonary artery connection thereby leaving the pulmonary arteries disconnected. This resulted in right-sided pulmonary arteriovenous malformation owing to the lack of hepatic factor to the right pulmonary circulation. The figure shows PTFE graft reconnection of the right and left pulmonary arteries, preservation of the Glenn circuit, and extracardiac PTFE connection between the inferior vena cava and the reconstructed main pulmonary artery. (With Permission: Mavroudis 2015c)

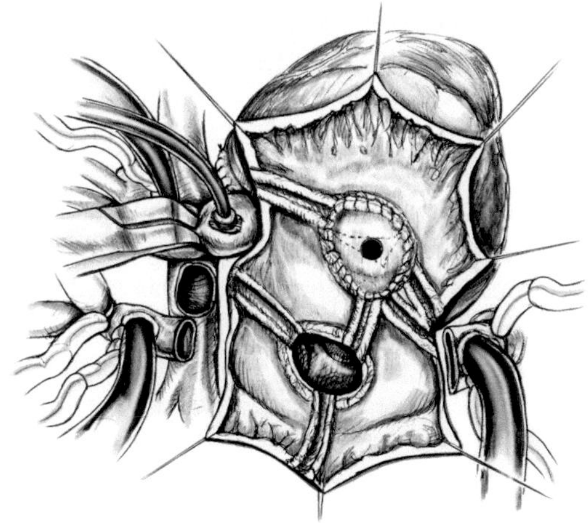

Fig. 59 For those patients with a pulmonary atresia and intact ventricular septum who have small ventricles, the best chance for long term survival has been preparations that lead to the Fontan operation. In the initial experience with this strategy, some surgeons performed atriopulmonary connections and intentionally caused tricuspid regurgitation to prevent right ventricular dilatation. The strategy did not take into consideration that this small ventricle could eventually grow and generate substantial pressure during systole. Such a condition results in tricuspid regurgitation, elevated right atrial pressure, right atrial dilatation, atrial reentry tachycardia and eventual failure of the Fontan circulation. We have solved these problems with a right-sided modified maze procedure as noted in the figure and with a fenestrated patch over the orifice of the tricuspid valve. The fenestrated patch functions to limit the entry of blood into the right ventricular chamber during diastole and thus decreases the preload of the right ventricle thereby decreasing the developed pressure in that chamber. As a result, during systole the developed pressure is lower and does not affect the Fontan circulation. This strategy was borrowed from Starnes's application of such a fenestrated patch for neonatal patients with severe Ebstein anomaly of the tricuspid valve. The resultant hemodynamics are favorable to the systemic venous pathway which along with the maze procedure improves the patient's hemodynamics and clinical function. (With Permission: Mavroudis 2015c)

physiology resulting in atrial arrhythmias and debilitating systemic complications previously described. Further descriptions of this aberrant circulation and repair techniques are noted in Fig. 59 and the legend thereto pertaining.

Complications relating to this operation involve injury to the AV node and size of the fenestration that is used to patch the tricuspid valve orifice. Misapplied cryoablation lesions as well as suture proximity to the AV node can result in heart block. The PTFE fenestration is a strategic part of the operation and should be assessed properly. We have used a 4-mm fenestration for this part of the operation; however, the size should be assessed based on patient size. The function of the fenestrated patch is to limit blood entry into the right ventricular chamber during diastole. This results in decreased preload of the right ventricle which decreases the developed cavitary pressure. Consequently, the developed pressure during systole is lower and does not unfavorably affect the Fontan circulation. This hemodynamic strategy is based on Starnes's application of such a fenestrated patch for neonatal patients with severe Ebstein anomaly of the tricuspid valve (Starnes et al. 1991). The resultant hemodynamic improvements are favorable to the systemic venous pathway which along with the maze procedure enhances the patient's hemodynamics and clinical functional status.

4.6 Takedown of Tricuspid Valve Isolation for Right-Sided Maze Procedure

After success with orthoterminal palliation (Fontan operation) for tricuspid atresia, more complex forms of functionally single ventricle were treated by this strategy. As was predicted, various anatomical substrates required individual creative solutions. Those patients with double inlet left ventricle, tricuspid stenosis, heterotaxy syndrome, and other complex lesions required right AV valve isolation in order to create separation of the pulmonary and systemic circulations by right atrial to pulmonary artery connection. This strategy involved those patients who had a functioning left AV valve. A patch was placed to cover the right AV valve which would isolate the right atrium thereby making an obligatory conduit into the main pulmonary artery resulting in an atriopulmonary Fontan connection. The patch was placed around the coronary sinus to avoid heart block as noted in Fig. 60. Patients with this operative anatomy develop atrial tachycardia and various forms of venous pathway obstruction which makes them candidates for Fontan conversion. Figures 60, 61, 62, 63 and 64 show the progression of Fontan conversion by management of the AV patch, arrhythmia surgery, and extracardiac connections. The objectives of Fontan conversion in this particular group of patients is to

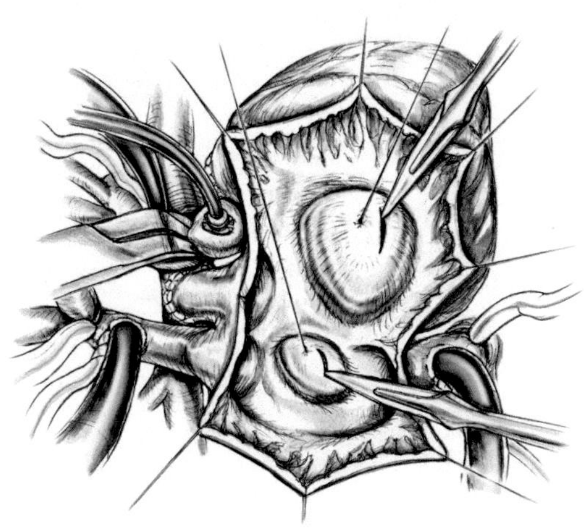

Fig. 61 The strategy for removal of the ASD patch is clear since after the extracardiac Fontan, the right atrium will need an exit pathway for the thebesian blood flow. The strategy for the right-sided atrioventricular valve patch removal is to perform a comprehensive modified maze procedure since one of the landmarks for the operation is the coronary sinus which is below the patch and not amenable to cryoablation. The figure therefore shows aortic cross clamping and cardioplegic arrest with the initial phases of patch removal of the two structures. (With Permission: Mavroudis 2015c)

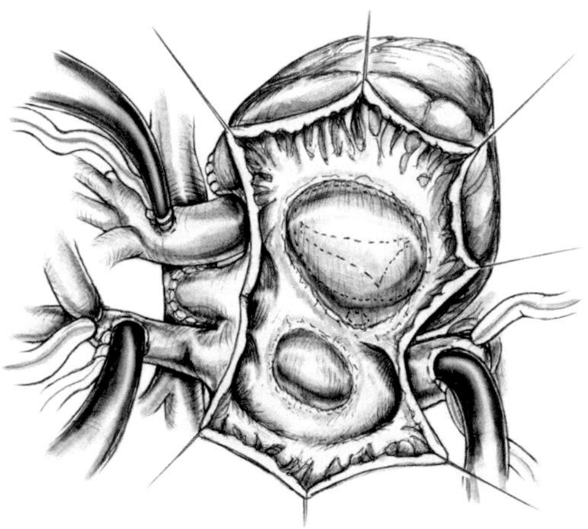

Fig. 60 Shows aortobicaval cardiopulmonary bypass with right atrial exposure in a patient who underwent atrial septal defect closure, right atrioventricular valve isolation (along with the coronary sinus), and atriopulmonary Fontan. (With Permission: Mavroudis 2015c)

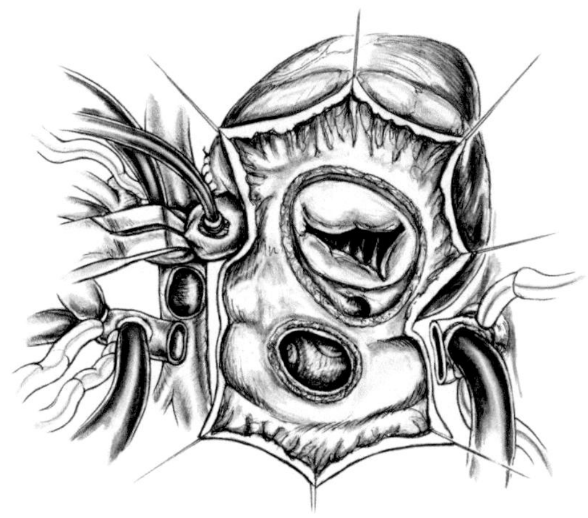

Fig. 62 Shows the patches removed with identification of the coronary sinus near the right- sided AV valve which in this case is the tricuspid valve. Care is taken during the patch removal above the atrioventricular valve not to injure the leaflets. (With Permission: Mavroudis 2015c)

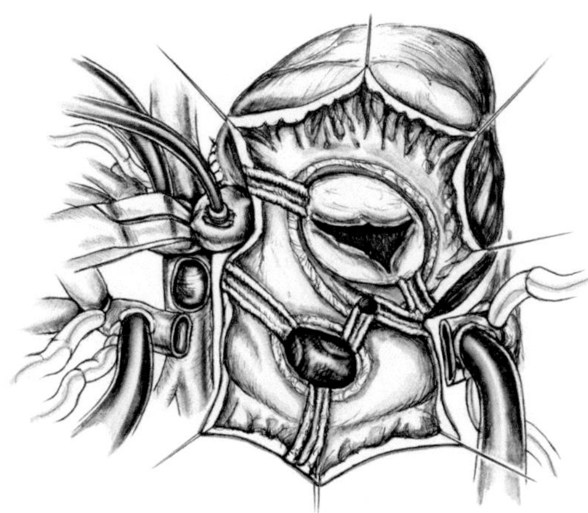

Fig. 63 The cryoablation lesions that have been described for the modified right-sided maze procedure for Fontan conversion are noted in the figure. As has been described in the other drawings and associated prose, the cryoablation lesions need to be placed away from the atrioventricular node to avoid acquired heart block. (With Permission: Mavroudis 2015c)

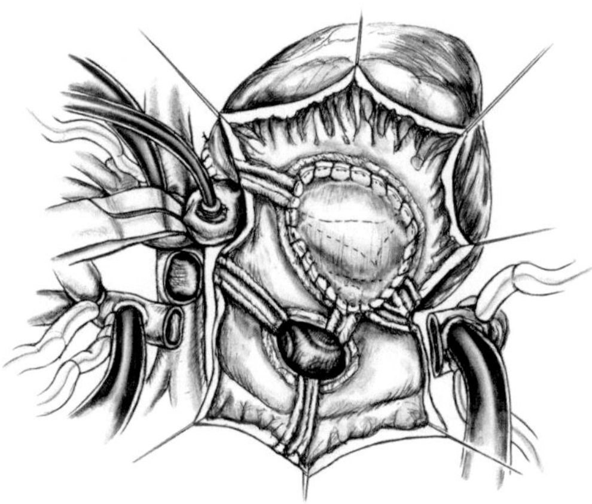

Fig. 64 Once the lesions are performed with respect to the coronary sinus, the valve annulus can be covered with another PTFE patch as noted in the figure. Alternatively, the patch can be omitted if it can be demonstrated that the right-sided valve is competent. (With Permission: Mavroudis 2015c)

perform a right-sided modified maze procedure and extracardiac connections for incessant atrial tachycardia. So, why take down the right-sided AV patch? Since the coronary sinus is on the other side of the patch, the cryoablation line connecting the IVC and the coronary sinus cannot be adequately performed. And since the area of slow conduction extends to the orifice of the coronary sinus, it is important to include this area in the cryoablation lesion set. So, the patch is removed and the coronary sinus to IVC lesion can be performed which is followed by a new patch that is placed over the AV valve. Alternatively, if the valve is found to be competent by bulb syringe testing, the patch can be omitted since the resultant orthoterminal connections will be extracardiac in nature.

Complications associated with this procedure center around avoidance of cryoablation induced heart block and miscalculation of right-sided AV valve competency which may result in unwanted regurgitation and higher Fontan pressures. Better to replace the patch when valve competency is not assured.

4.7 Left Atrial Venous Pathway Obstruction After Fontan Conversion in Functionally Single Right Ventricle Anatomy

Our initial experience with Fontan conversion was mostly applied to those patients with tricuspid atresia. Because these patients had gigantic atria and multiple areas of fibrotic scarring, we resected large portions of the atrial wall which did not impact on the venous return or cavitary flow patterns. Simply put, if there was enough atria for cavitary closure without tension, the hemodynamic effects were satisfied since the venous circuits were extracardiac and the pulmonary venous return was to the left atrium with connection to the left ventricle through the mitral valve. This is not the case for those patients with functionally single ventricle whose ventricle is anteriorly situated. In these circumstances, the pulmonary venous flow must pass through the atrial septal defect en route to the right-sided ventricle. The pathway therefore has to be large enough to accommodate the flow. Figure 65 shows the classic exposure for Fontan conversion in a patient with functionally single right ventricle and preexisting atriopulmonary Fontan. In this case, overzealous right atrial wall resection

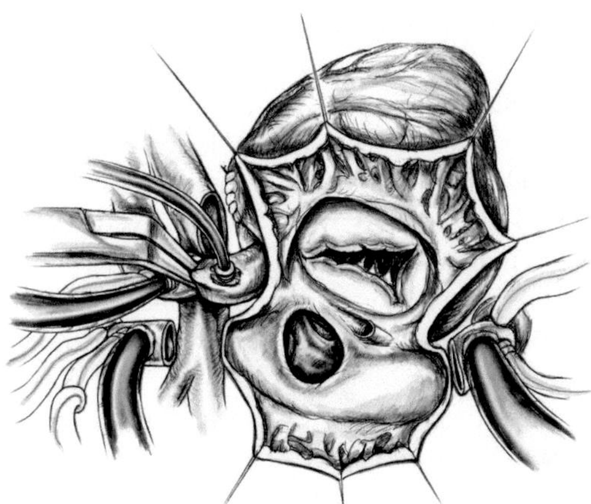

Fig. 65 Shows aortobicaval cardiopulmonary bypass, aortic cross clamping, cardioplegic arrest, and right atrial exposure in a patient with functionally single right ventricle and mitral atresia undergoing Fontan Conversion with extracardiac connections. After the reconstruction, this patient underwent transesophageal echocardiography (TEE) which showed significant turbulence in the pathway from the left atrium, through the ASD and into the right ventricle. (With Permission: Mavroudis 2015c)

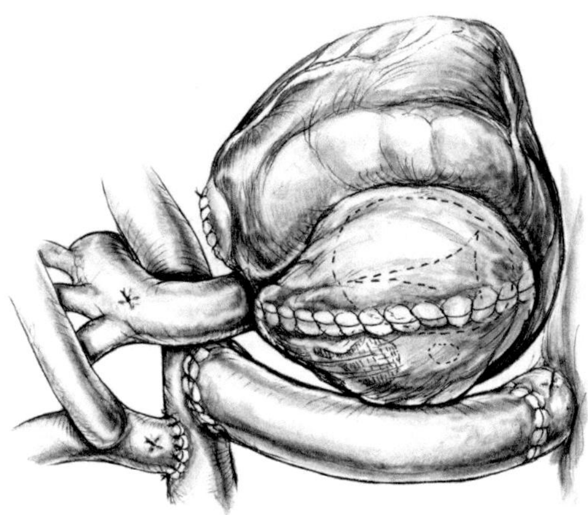

Fig. 66 Shows how an over extensive right atrial wall reduction can negatively impact the flow pattern originating in the left atrium en route to the right ventricle. Such a condition can cause pulmonary edema, elevated right systemic venous pressure and Fontan failure. The solution to this problem is immediate reinstitution of cardiopulmonary bypass, aortic cross clamping, cardioplegic arrest and right atrial wall augmentation using a PTFE patch as noted in Fig. 67. (With Permission: Mavroudis 2015c)

resulted in a stenosed pulmonary vein to right ventricular pathway as noted in Fig. 66. This is clearly a technical complication caused by the

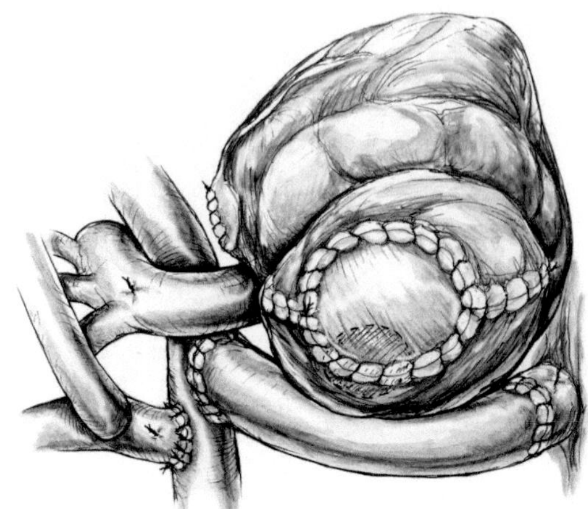

Fig. 67 The resultant TEE showed normal laminar flow throughout the Fontan connections. (With Permission: Mavroudis 2015c)

extensive atrial wall resection which was identified by TEE. This situation requires immediate intervention by return to cardiopulmonary bypass, aortic cross-clamping, cardioplegic arrest, and patch augmentation of the right atrial wall which is depicted in Fig. 67. The resultant flow patterns after the redo operation as defined by TEE analysis were normal. This potential occurrence emphasizes the important role of intraoperative TEE which must be respected and acted upon.

4.8 Distended Left Superior Vena Cava Obstructing the Left Pulmonary Veins

A left superior vena cava in association with any congenital heart diagnosis is a challenge with regard to cannulation during reparative surgery, a dilemma when the vena cava drains into the left atrium, and certainly a problem when total cavopulmonary artery reconstruction is necessary en route to orthoterminal palliation (Fontan operation). Complications regarding management of this entity include unwanted resultant distal left pulmonary artery during bidirectional Glenn anastomosis, kinking of the translocated left superior vena cava to the right superior vena cava, and the unanticipated consequences of left

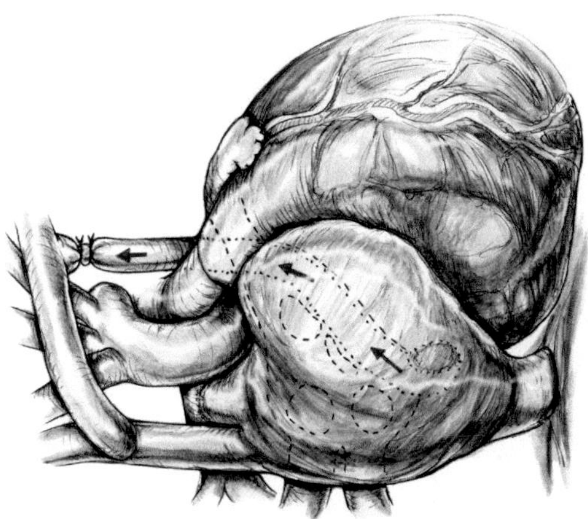

Fig. 68 A left superior vena cava (SVC) should alert any clinician to the possibility of systemic venous anomalies that could impact on the execution of any corrective congenital heart operation. Nowadays, bilateral SVCs in patients with functionally single ventricle physiology are managed by bilateral bidirectional Glenn shunts en route to Fontan completion at a later date. Previous to this era, the left SVC was ligated, especially if it was small, to prepare the patient for atriopulmonary Fontan connections. While this strategy has been successful in most patients, rarely a left SVC will have congenital or acquired coronary ostial atresia thereby causing the myocardial venous flow to drain normally into the brachiocephalic vein in a retrograde fashion. Ligating the left SVC in the presence of ostial atresia of the coronary sinus os, as shown in the figure will cause obstruction to coronary sinus flow, dilatation of the intracardiac portion of the coronary sinus chamber, and eventual left pulmonary vein obstruction as noted in a patient who had left SVC ligation as shown in the figure. The dashed lines show the course of the coronary sinus which is enlarged and compressing on the outflow of the left pulmonary vein. (With Permission: Mavroudis 2015c)

SVC ligation in preparation for the atriopulmonary Fontan procedure when there is orifice atresia of the coronary sinus (Hoashi et al. 2020). The latter problem can result in localized pulmonary venous obstruction owing to intracavitary coronary sinus pathway dilation owing to lack of coronary venous outflow as shown in Fig. 68. The original intent of left superior vena cava ligation was to prepare the patient for atriopulmonary Fontan without the problem of dealing with this pesky venous pathway. The reasoning was that the right SVC would adapt to the increased venous flow through collateral development.

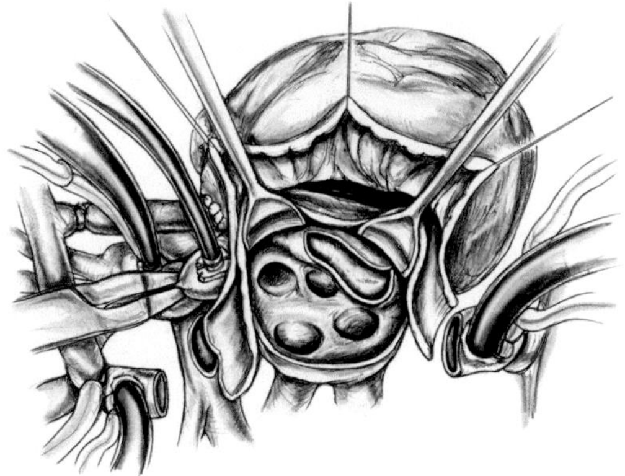

Fig. 69 This problem as defined in Fig. 68 was recognized and solved by Fontan conversion and intracardiac unroofing of the coronary sinus. The figure shows how the coronary sinus pathway was decompressed which allowed unobstructed thebesian flow into the cardiac chamber. The pulmonary venous pathway obstruction was treated successfully with this intervention. (With Permission: Mavroudis 2015c)

Occasionally, there is atresia of the coronary sinus os which directs coronary venous flow through the coronary sinus pathway with drainage into the extant venous structures. Under these anatomic circumstances, left SVC ligation will cause coronary sinus pathway dilatation and obstruction of the nearby left pulmonary veins, also shown in Fig. 68. This problem needs to be recognized preoperatively and treated by coronary sinus pathway unroofing in association with Fontan conversion as noted in Fig. 69.

4.9 "Dropped Atrial Septum" for Atriopulmonary Fontan

The "Dropped Atrial Septum" as shown in Fig. 70 is mostly included in this discussion to highlight some variations of the Fontan operation that have historical significance in addition to which are retroaortic atriopulmonary connections, antero-aortic atriopulmonary connections, and atrio-right ventricular connections (Bjork modification) (Mavroudis et al. 2007). Each of these modifications have unique characteristics and problems owing to systemic venous pathway

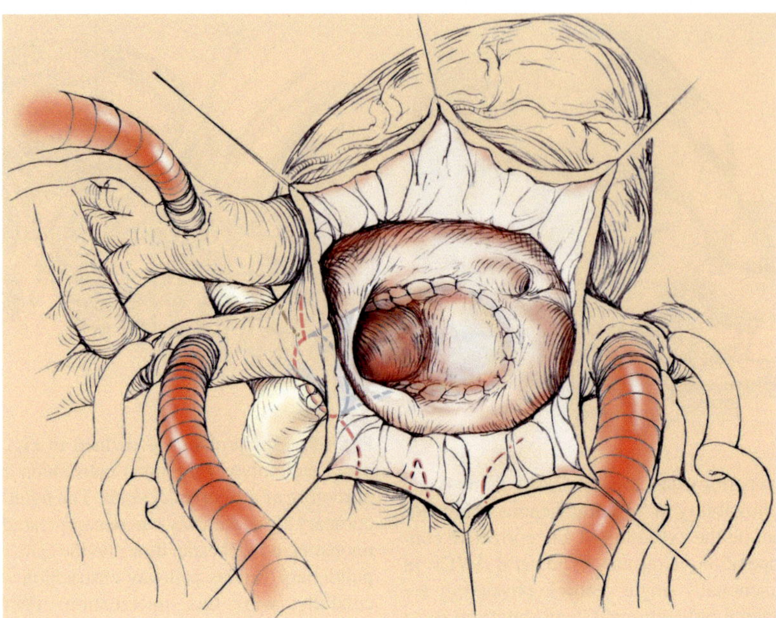

Fig. 70 Some surgeons postulated that a more direct anastomosis between the right atrium and pulmonary artery would result in better hemodynamic properties; hence the introduction of the "dropped atrial septum" as noted in the figure. Basically, the superior edge of the septum primum is disconnected, the dome of the left atrium is incised, and a patch is formed to connect the incised septum primum into the left atrium. This way the atriopulmonary anastomosis is deemed to be more favorably aligned. The long term complications of this arrangement are a series of suture lines in the left atrium which can result in areas of slow conduction and atrial reentry tachycardia. (With Permission: Mavroudis 2015c)

obstructions, atrial suture load leading to arrhythmias, and cavitary dilatation. The atriopulmonary connection using the "Dropped Atrial Septum" technique obligatorily requires a left atrial dome incision and an atrial suture line to construct the presumed favorable connection. In the event of atrial arrhythmias and decreased functional class, a Fontan conversion may establish improved venous pathways and treatment for the atrial arrhythmias. Because of the left atrial suture lines and the probability of areas of slow conduction in this area, a biatrial maze procedure is recommended during pathway takedown and Fontan conversion to extracardiac connections (Fig. 71). The complications associated with this procedure are standard for Fontan conversion that have been enumerated. Bleeding complications are noteworthy since the left atrial patch repair tends to be posteriorly located. Attention to this potential problem will obviate bleeding complications.

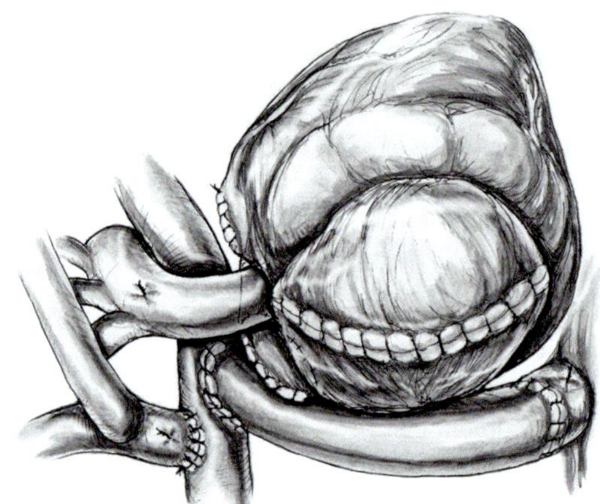

Fig. 71 The electrophysiologic solution is to take down the anastomosis, perform right and left atrial maze procedures and augment the dome of the left atrium with a PTFE patch as noted in the figure. A ghost suture line is noted in the dome of the left atrium near the extracardiac tube and right atrial suture line. (With Permission: Mavroudis 2015c)

4.10 Cannulation Technique for Right Atrial Clot

Right atrial clots in association with failing atriopulmonary Fontan circulation are problematic not only for the presence of the clot but also for the associated hemodynamic problems leading to localized thrombosis (Marcelletti et al. 2000). The operating team should also be cognizant that atrial clot formation can occur after attempted preoperative transcatheter arrhythmia ablation. Intraoperative TEE should be carefully interpreted for clot formation, the management of atrial cannulation, and the conduct of cardiopulmonary bypass as noted in Fig. 72.

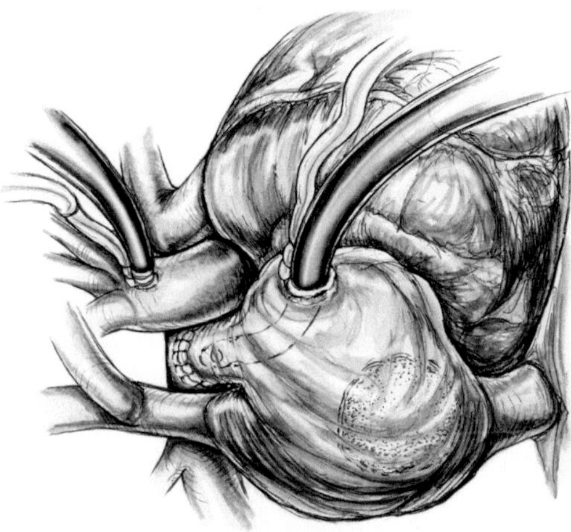

Fig. 72 Some patients with failed Fontan physiology develop clots in the large right atrium owing to poor cardiac output and decreased forward flow. Proper management of cardiopulmonary bypass is essential to prevent untoward events. For instance, when the right atrium is large and doesn't allow easy access to the inferior vena cava for cannulation, a right atrial catheter can be placed to initiate cardiopulmonary bypass and cardiac decompression which will allow easy inferior vena cava cannulation which can be followed by right atrial decannulation. A clot in the right atrium during attempted cardiopulmonary bypass and cardiac decompression could embolize to the single atrial catheter, cause obstruction, and result in interruption of cardiopulmonary bypass, a period of hypoperfusion and possible renal and hepatic failure after the operation. It is wise to locate the right atrial clot by echocardiography and place the temporary right atrial catheter away from the clot and near the atriopulmonary connection as noted in the figure. (With Permission: Mavroudis 2015c)

4.11 Maneuvers to Retrieve Inferior Vena Cava Retraction During Extracardiac Fontan Reconstruction

Retraction of the IVC and dislodgement of the established drainage system is a very frustrating and unsatisfying experience that makes one pledge to never let it happen again. Every surgeon has a preventive solution to this problem. We have found that strategic suture placement in two locations during the transection of the inferior vena cave en route to cavo-PTFE graft anastomosis works well. Others have incised the IVC to include some atrial wall which will increase the size of the PTFE graft placement as well as an insurance maneuver to prevent IVC retraction. Whatever the precautionary procedures, invariably this complication occurs. Figures 73, 74 and 75 identify the problem and show the steps towards resolution. Care must be taken to identify any tears in the cannulation site which may require patch augmentation. This is not an easy complication to resolve, especially since other

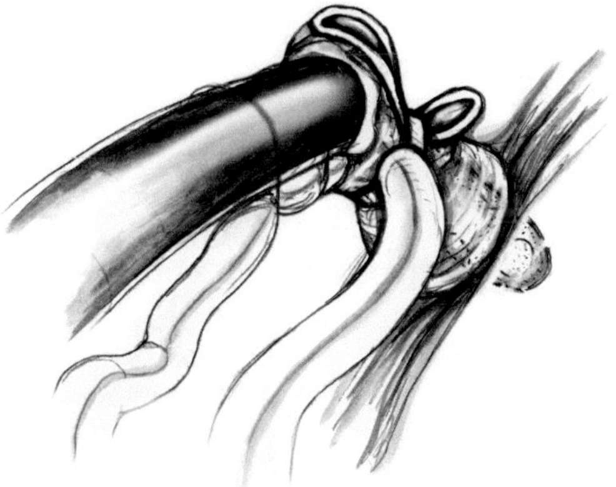

Fig. 73 Surgeons who routinely perform extracardiac Fontan connections have developed methods to prevent inferior vena cava (IVC) retraction during the extracardiac PTFE anastomosis. We offer a method to retrieve the retracted IVC. The figure shows the retracted IVC. The IVC orifice is trapped by the sling. IVC retrieval by readjusting the sling will invariably cause IVC disruption resulting in a torn IVC well below the diaphragm. Figures 74 and 75 show the management scheme. (With Permission: Mavroudis 2015c)

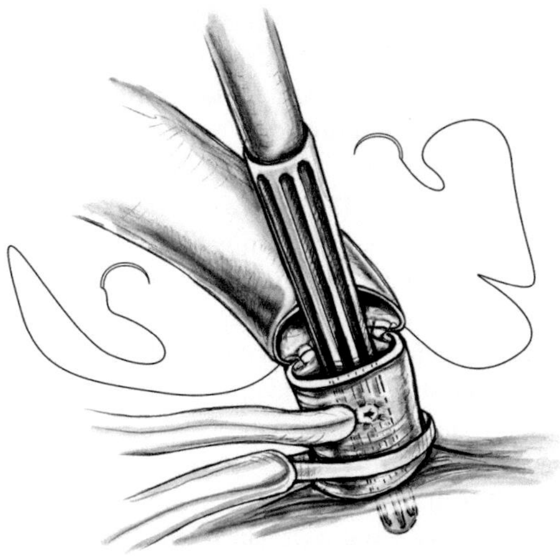

Fig. 74 The best way to manage the situation of inferior vena cava (IVC) retraction is to loosen the sling, remove the IVC cannula, and insert a pump sucker into the orifice of the IVC while performing the IVC to PTFE anastomosis as shown in the figure. (With Permission: Mavroudis 2015c)

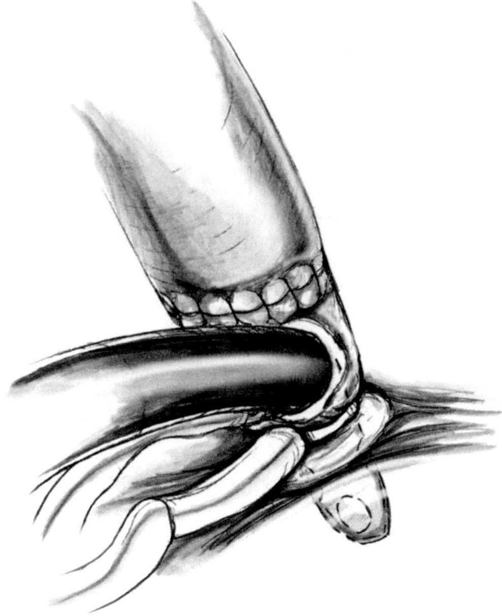

Fig. 75 As shown in the figure, once the anastomosis is completed, the inferior vena cava catheter can be replaced with subsequent sling enforcement and progression with the operation. (With Permission: Mavroudis 2015c)

associated problems can arise. Better to take one's time, plan a reasonable solution, and execute the repair with minimal chances of complications.

4.12 Valve Repair Strategies for Fontan Conversion Patients with Atrioventricular Valve Regurgitation

Fontan conversion often requires repair or replacement of AV valves owing to regurgitation. Since most of these regurgitant valves tend to be dilated, valve sparing strategies that involve cleft closures, reduction techniques, and leaflet repairs are often successful. Figure 76 illustrates anterior

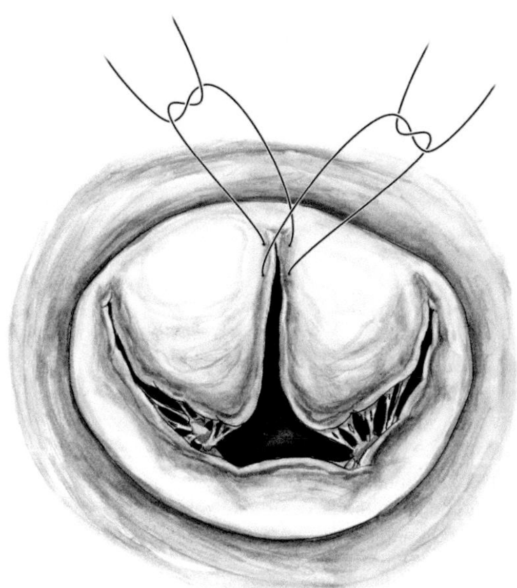

Fig. 76 Shows a cleft (zone of apposition) in the anterior leaflet of a dilated mitral valve in a patient with tricuspid atresia. It is well known that mitral valves in patients with tricuspid atresia are abnormal. In this case, the cleft is being closed with interrupted suture technique. In the case of a larger or older patient who is not subject to further somatic growth, a mitral ring (not shown) can be added to the repair which will decrease the size of the annulus and support the repair. In addition, pledgetted mattress sutures (not shown) can be used to avoid leaflet tears. (With Permission: Mavroudis 2015c)

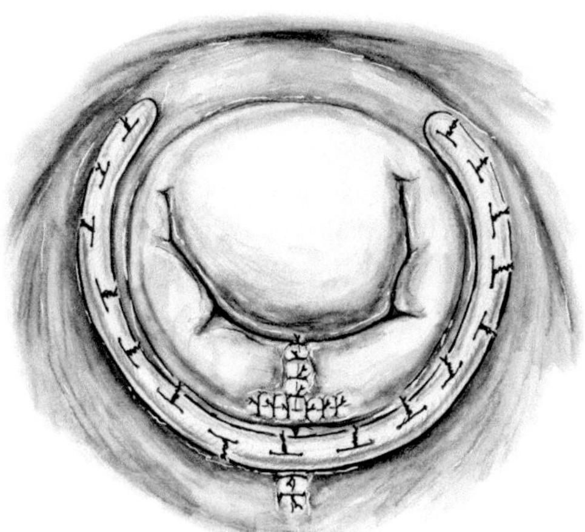

Fig. 77 Carpentier mitral repair techniques have been adopted for congenital heart repairs involving the left and right atrioventricular valves. The figure shows an early version of the Carpentier annuloplasty which involves posterior leaflet middle scallop resection, posterior reduction annuloplasty, and a mitral ring. Nowadays, sliding annuloplasty techniques are employed to preserve as much of the posterior leaflet as possible. See chapter "Complications Associated with Mitral Valve Surgery for Congenital Anomalies and Degenerative Diseases" for more extensive repair solutions

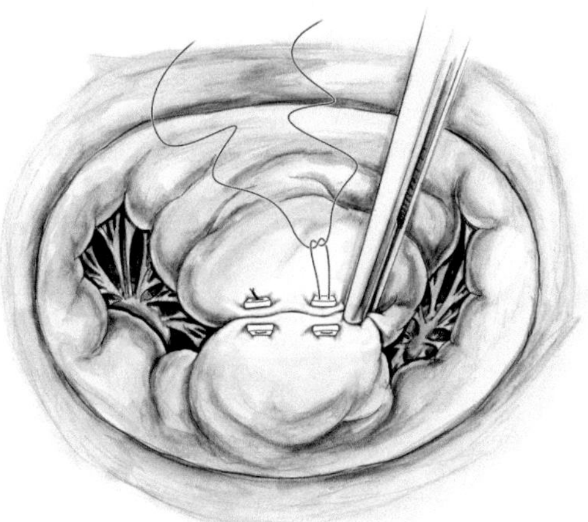

Fig. 78 The Alfieri stitch or side to side repair, as it has come to be called, is a very simple method for mitral and tricuspid valve repair that is performed by suturing the opposing leaflets at the most prolapsed area and thereby transforming the valve into a double orifice valve with better anatomic and physiological characteristics. Pledgetted sutures are recommended for the side-to-side reconstruction to avoid disruption and failure of the repair. Shown in the figure is a mitral valve with an Alfieri stitch in the midpoint of the anterior and posterior leaflets which is supported by a circular mitral ring. Tricuspid valves can be repaired in this manner as well (not shown), especially if one of the leaflets is very prolapsed and is not easily amenable to other repair options such as chordal shortening

leaflet cleft (zone of apposition) closure. Depending on the leaflet integrity and strength, the surgeon may want to use pledgetted mattress sutures to accomplish the cleft closure and render the valve competent.

Patients with functionally single left ventricle may have mitral regurgitation (Yang et al. 2021). These patients are amenable to Carpentier techniques as noted in Fig. 77. Modern day annuloplasty techniques include variations of this repair to include sliding annuloplasty and chordal repairs as noted in chapter "Complications Associated with Mitral Valve Surgery for Congenital Anomalies and Degenerative Diseases".

In addition to reduction annuloplasty and cleft closures is the use of the Alfieri stitch which is gaining popularity because of its simplicity, efficiency, and effectiveness (see chapter "Complications Associated with Mitral Valve Surgery for Congenital Anomalies and Degenerative Diseases"). Figure 78 illustrates the Alfieri stitch technique which can be used for significantly prolapsed leaflets. The idea is to attach the anterior leaflet to the posterior leaflet in the area of prolapse which will form a double orifice competent valve. Another method of performing

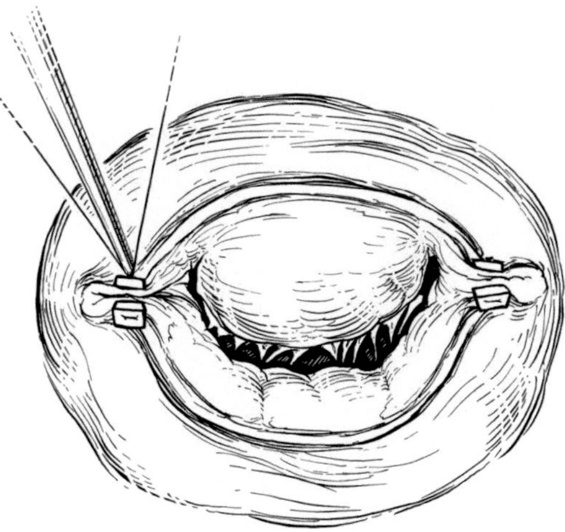

Fig. 79 Named annular reduction procedure can also be applied for dilated mitral valves as shown in the figure. (With Permission: Mavroudis 2015c)

an expedient annular reduction valve repair is noted in Fig. 79, the particulars of which are noted in chapter "Complications Associated with Mitral Valve Surgery for Congenital Anomalies and Degenerative Diseases". The attractive part of this technique is the ease and reproducible favorable results when considering a long operation involving multiple repair strategies and long cross-clamp times.

When other atrioventricular anatomic substrates are considered, the most advantageous repair for any given patient with right- or left-sided regurgitation is highly dependent on the operating surgeon, the type of valve, and the experience of the center.

4.13 Therapeutic Ablation Sets for Right- and Left-Sided Maze Procedures

Fontan conversion is defined by performance of extracardiac connections, arrhythmia surgery, repair of associated lesions, and pacemaker implantation. This operation is performed in patients with varying anatomic substrates with different landmarks that affect the arrhythmia ablation technique required for a successful outcome. For example, patients with tricuspid atresia do not have a tricuspid valve; those with heterotaxy syndrome do not have a coronary sinus (right atrial isomerism) and often have a common AV valve which complicates the performance of the arrhythmia operation. Other considerations include direct atrial entry of the hepatic veins, juxtaposition of the atrial appendages, left SVC draining into the left atrium, and displaced AV node all of which can impact the anatomic application of cryoablation lesions in order to avoid arrhythmia recurrence. Figures 80, 81, 82, 83, 84 and 85 show the particular lesion sets for the different anatomic substrates that are described. The complications associated with application of these lesion sets center around potential injury to the AV node. Oftentimes, injury to the AV node occurs with the extensive right atrial wall resection. The atrial pacemaker will take over sinoatrial node function under the circumstances of injury to the node. Our experience has shown that atrial pacing is more favorable than counting on the sinoatrial node which oftentimes is non-functional (Mavroudis and Deal 2016).

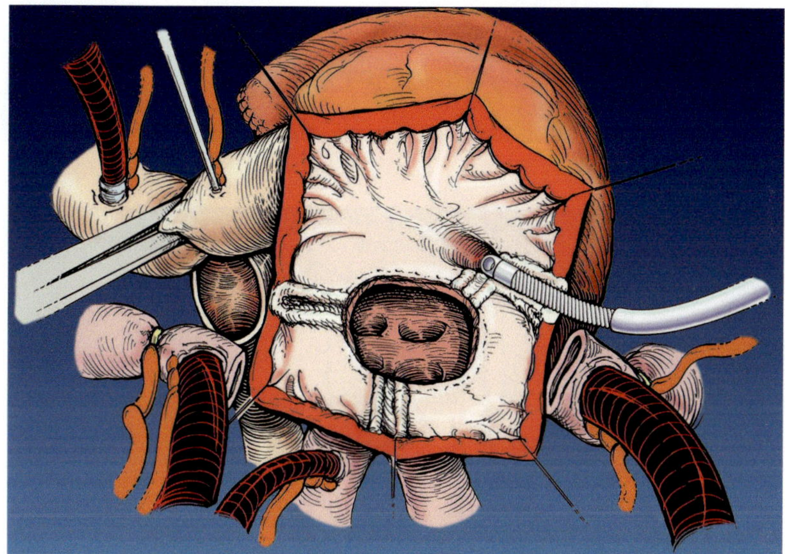

Fig. 80 Cryoablation lesions for the modified right-sided maze procedure as applied for tricuspid atresia are noted in the figure. Since there is no tricuspid valve, no lesion can be placed from the os of the inferior vena cava (IVC) to the tricuspid annulus. Sometimes there is a forme fruste of a tricuspid valve which can be identified as an underdeveloped atrioventricular valve or a "dimple" of a valve (not shown). The conduction system is very close to these underdeveloped structures; efforts to apply a cryoablation lesion from the IVC to this structure will result in heart block and is not recommended. The four cryoablation lesions that are shown have efficacy and can be applied safely without regard to atrioventricular node injury. (With permission: Mavroudis et al. 2001)

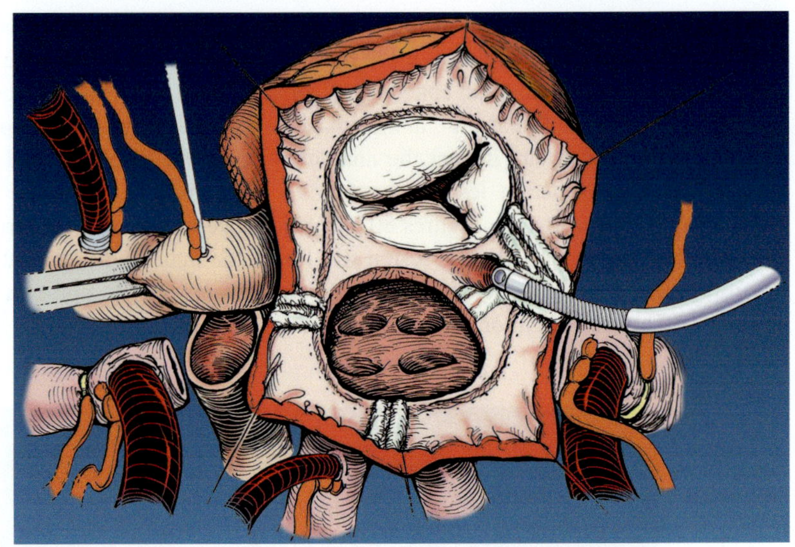

Fig. 81 Shows the cryoablation lesions for the modified right-sided maze procedure in a patient with mitral atresia. The tricuspid valve and the associated structures are normally related and as such the five cryoablation lesions can be placed as noted. (With permission: Mavroudis et al. 2001)

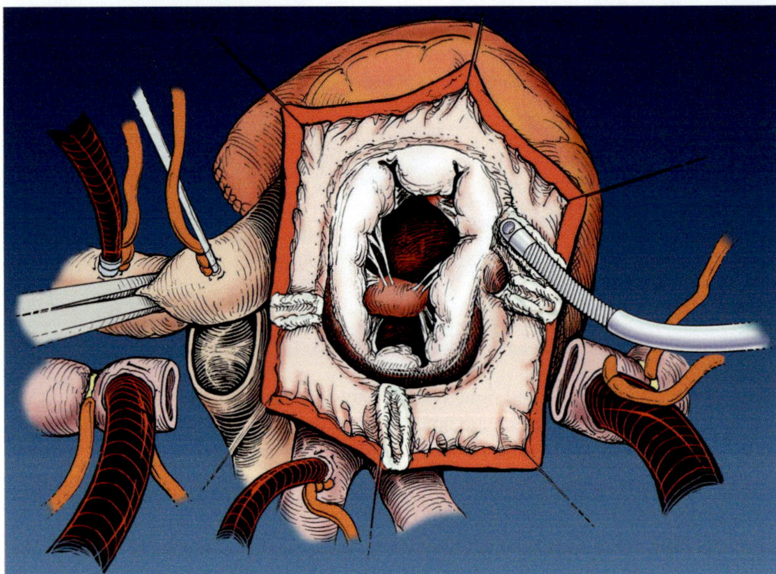

Fig. 82 Cryoablation lesions for patients undergoing Fontan conversion with unbalanced atrioventricular valve are more challenging owing to the fact that heterotaxy could be encountered with absence of the coronary sinus. In addition, the atrioventricular node and conduction system is displaced closer to the coronary sinus and common annulus. The recommended lesions for such a patient with a present coronary sinus are noted in the figure. If there is no coronary sinus, we recommend eliminating the lesion between the inferior vena cava and coronary sinus for obvious reasons. (With permission: Mavroudis et al. 2001)

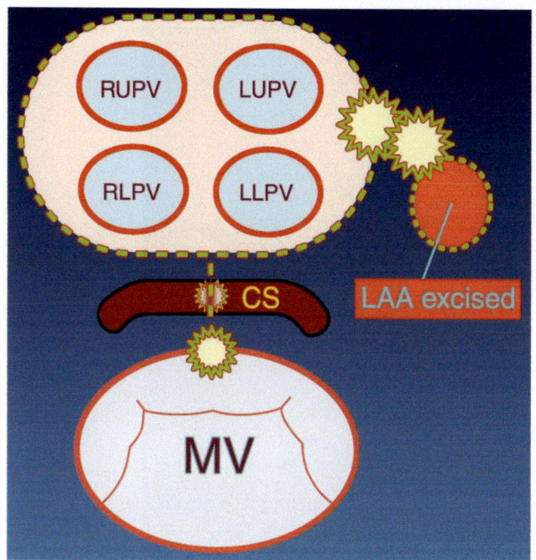

Fig. 83 The Cox maze III procedure requires left atrial lesions that have been shown to eliminate atrial fibrillation in most cases. The figure is a cartoon that demonstrates the lesions that are necessary to complete the procedure. Notice that there is a lesion that encircles the confluence of the pulmonary veins, a lesion that extends from the confluence of the pulmonary veins to the left atrial appendage, which is to be amputated, and a lesion extending from the confluence of the pulmonary veins to the posterior mitral valve annulus. This particular lesion is shown extending to the middle scallop of the posterior leaflet. Most surgeons have advocated applying this lesion to the P3 scallop to better align with the lesion that is placed on the epicardial surface of the heart directly on the coronary sinus. This lesion is better demonstrated in Fig. 84 which shows the cryoablation probe being placed on the epicardial surface of the coronary sinus which *aligns* with the P3 lesion which was placed within the left atrium. *CS* coronary sinus, *LAA* left atrial appendage, *LLPV* left lower pulmonary vein, *LUPV* left upper pulmonary vein, *MV* mitral valve, *RLPV* right lower pulmonary valve, *RUPV* right upper pulmonary vein. (With permission: Mavroudis et al. 2001)

4.14 Arrhythmia Surgery and Pacemaker Placement Not Associated with Fontan Conversion

We have published our experience with patients undergoing arrhythmia surgery not associated with Fontan conversion (Mavroudis et al. 2003). We reasoned that these lesion sets and indications for use in prophylactic situations will be discussed in the chapters associated with these operations such as reoperative tetralogy repair, cone procedure for Ebstein anomaly, and late presentation of atrial septal defects, among others.

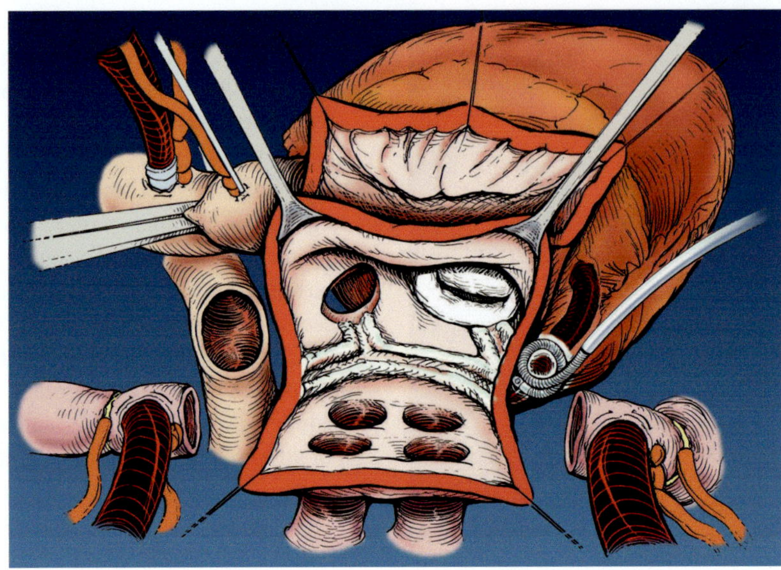

Fig. 84 Shows the continuation of fig. 83 which demonstrates the cryoablation probe being placed on the epicardial surface of the coronary sinus which aligns with the P3 lesion which was placed within the left atrium. This eliminates the isthmus area of slow conduction which can result in recurrence of atrial fibrillation. In particular, this drawing shows the left- sided maze procedure being performed with a "cut and sew" technique for the right side of the left atrium and cryoablation lesions for the rest of the procedure. More recently, we have been employing cryoablation for the left atrial isolation of the pulmonary veins. The procedure is less lengthy and just as effective. (With permission: Mavroudis et al. 2001)

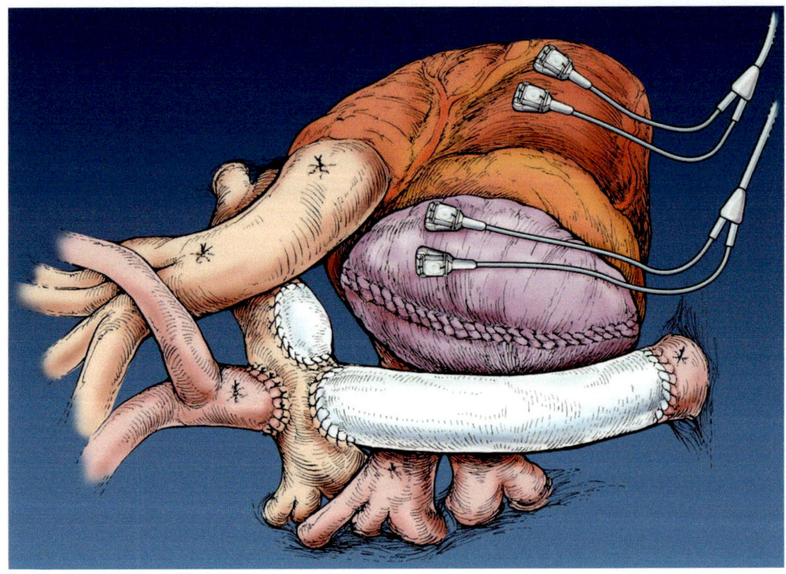

Fig. 85 Shows the completed Fontan conversion with the atrial and ventricular bipolar, steroid eluting, epicardial leads that are connected to a dual chamber, atrioventricular, antitachycardia pacemaker. (With permission: Backer et al. 2006)

References

Akintoye E, Miranda WR, Veldtman GR, Connolly HM, Egbe AC. National trends in Fontan operation and in-hospital outcomes in the USA. Heart. 2019;105(9):708–14.

Albanese SB, Carotti A, Di Donato RM, et al. Bidirectional cavopulmonary anastomosis in patients under two years of age. J Thorac Cardiovasc Surg. 1992;104:904–9.

Allan CK, Thiagarajan RR, del Nido PJ, Roth SJ, Almodovar MC, Laussen PC. Indication for initiation of mechanical circulatory support impacts survival of infants with shunted single-ventricle circulation supported with extracorporeal membrane oxygenation. J Thorac Cardiovasc Surg. 2007;133:660–7.

Alvarado O, Sreeram N, McKay R, Boyd IM. Cavopulmonary connection in repair of atrioventricular septal defect with small right ventricle. Ann Thorac Surg. 1993;55(3):729–36.

Anderson RH, Ho SY. Pathologic substrates for 1½ ventricular repair. Ann Thorac Surg. 1998;66(2):673–7.

Angelini A, Frescura C, Stellin G, Thiene G. Cavopulmonary anastomosis in staging toward Fontan operation: pathologic substrates. Ann Thorac Surg. 1998;66(2):659–63.

Attard C, Huang J, Monagle P, Ignjatovic V. Pathophysiology of thrombosis and anticoagulation post Fontan surgery. Thromb Res. 2018;172:204–13.

Averin K, Byrnes JW, Benscoter DT, Whiteside W, DeSena H, Hirsch R, et al. Life-threatening airway bleeding after palliation of single ventricle congenital heart disease. Heart. 2018;104:254–60.

Backer CL, Mavroudis C. 149 Fontan conversions. Methodist Debakey Cardiovasc J. 2019;15(2):105–10.

Backer CL, Deal BJ, Mavroudis C, Franklin WH, Stewart RD. Conversion of the failed Fontan circulation. Cardiol Young. 2006;16(Suppl 1):85–91.

Backer CL, Deal BJ, Kaushal S, Russell HM, Tsao S, Mavroudis C. Extracardiac versus intra-atrial lateral tunnel Fontan: extracardiac is better. Semin Thorac Cardiovasc Surg Pediatr Card Surg Annu. 2011;14(1):4–10.

Bartz PJ, Driscoll DJ, Dearani JA, Puga FJ, Danielson GK, O'Leary PW, et al. Early and late results of the modified Fontan operation for heterotaxy syndrome 30 years of experience in 142 patients. J Am Coll Cardiol. 2006;48(11):2301–5.

Ben Ali W, Bouhout I, Khairy P, Bouchard D, Poirier N. Extracardiac versus lateral tunnel Fontan: a meta-analysis of long-term results. Ann Thorac Surg. 2019;107(3):837–43.

Billingsley AM, Laks H, Boyce SW, George B, Santulli T, Williams RG. Definitive repair in patients with pulmonary atresia and intact ventricular septum. J Thorac Cardiovasc Surg. 1989;97(5):746–54.

Björk VO, Olin CL, Bjarke BB, Thorén CA. Right atrial-right ventricular anastomosis for correction of tricuspid atresia. J Thorac Cardiovasc Surg. 1979;77(3):452–8.

Bridges ND, Jonas RA, Mayer JE, Flanagan MF, Keane JF, Castañeda AR. Bidirectional cavopulmonary anastomosis as interim palliation for high-risk Fontan candidates. Circulation. 1990;82:170–6.

Bulic A, Zimmerman FJ, Ceresnak SR, Shetty I, Motonaga KS, Freter A, et al. Ventricular pacing in single ventricles-A bad combination. Heart Rhythm. 2017;14(6):853–7.

Cabrelle G, Castaldi B, Vedovelli L, Gregori D, Vida VL, Padalino MA. Long-term experience with the one-and-a-half ventricle repair for simple and complex congenital heart defects. Eur J Cardiothorac Surg. 2021;59(1):244–52.

Carins TA, Shi WY, Iyengar AJ, Nisbet A, Forsdick V, Zannino D, Gentles T, Radford DJ, Justo R, Celermajer DS, Bullock A, Winlaw D, Wheaton G, Grigg L, d'Udekem Y. Long-term outcomes after first-onset arrhythmia in Fontan physiology. J Thorac Cardiovasc Surg. 2016;152(5):1355–1363.e1.

Cetta F, Burkhart HM. The Fontan extracardiac conduit: one size does not fit all. Transl Pediatr. 2018;7(3):233–4.

Chihara S, Yasunaga H, Todo K. Anastomosis of left to right superior vena cava for repair of unroofed coronary sinus. Gen Thorac Cardiovasc Surg. 2012;60(4):244–6.

Clapp SK, Tantengco MV, Walters HL III, Lobdell KW, Hakimi M. Bidirectional cavopulmonary anastomosis with intracardiac repair. Ann Thorac Surg. 1997;63(3):746–50.

Cloutier A, Ash JM, Smallhorn JF, Williams WG, Trusler GA, Rowe RD, et al. Abnormal distribution of pulmonary blood flow after the Glenn shunt or Fontan procedure: risk of development of arteriovenous fistulae. Circulation. 1985;72(3):471–9.

Dabal RJ, Kirklin JK, Kukreja M, Brown RN, Cleveland DC, Eddins MC, Lau Y. The modern Fontan operation shows no increase in mortality out to 20 years: a new paradigm. J Thorac Cardiovasc Surg. 2014;148(6):2517–23.

Daley M, d'Udekem Y. The optimal Fontan operation: lateral tunnel or extracardiac conduit? J Thorac Cardiovasc Surg. 2020;162(6):1825–34.

Daley M, Buratto E, King G, Grigg L, Iyengar A, Alphonso N, Bullock A, Celermajer DS, Ayer J, Robertson T, d'Udekem Y, Konstantinov IE. Impact of Fontan fenestration on long-term outcomes: a propensity score-matched analysis. J Am Heart Assoc. 2022;11(11):e026087. https://doi.org/10.1161/JAHA.122.026087.

Daniels CJ, Bradley EA, Landzberg MJ, Aboulhosn J, Beekman RH, Book W, et al. Fontan-associated liver disease: proceedings form the American College of Cardiology stakeholders meeting. J Am Coll Cardiol. 2017;70(25):3173–94.

De Leval M, Bull C, Hopkins R, Rees P, Deanfield J, Taylor JF, et al. Decision making in the definitive repair of the heart with a small right ventricle. Circulation. 1985;72(Suppl 2):52–60.

Deal BJ, Mavroudis C, Backer CL, Johnsrude CL. New directions in surgical therapy of arrhythmias. Pediatr Cardiol. 2000;21(6):576–83.
Deal BJ, Mavroudis C, Backer CL, Buck SH, Johnsrude CL. Comparison of anatomic isthmus block with the modified right atrial maze procedure for late atrial tachycardia in Fontan patients. Circulation. 2002;106(5):575–9.
Deal BJ, Mavroudis C, Backer CL. Beyond Fontan conversion: surgical therapy of arrhythmias including patients with associated complex congenital heart disease. Ann Thorac Surg. 2003;76(2):542–54.
Deshaies C, Hamilton RM, Shohoudi A, Trottier H, Poirier N, Aboulhosn J, et al. Alliance for adult research in congenital cardiology (AARCC). Thromboembolic risk after atriopulmonary, lateral tunnel, and Extracardiac conduit Fontan surgery. J Am Coll Cardiol. 2019;74(8):1071–81.
Douglas WI, Goldberg CS, Mosca RS, Law IH, Bove EL. Hemi-Fontan procedure for hypoplastic left heart syndrome: outcome and suitability for Fontan. Ann Thorac Surg. 1999;68(4):1361–8.
d'Udekem Y, Iyengar AJ, Galati JC, Forsdick V, Weintraub RG, Wheaton GR, Bullock A, Justo RN, Grigg LE, Sholler GF, Hope S, Radford DJ, Gentles TL, Celermajer DS, Winlaw DS. Redefining expectations of long-term survival after the Fontan procedure: twenty-five years of follow-up from the entire population of Australia and New Zealand. Circulation. 2014;130(11 Suppl 1):S32–8.
Edelson JB, Ravishankar C, Griffis H, Zhang X, Faerber J, Gardner MM, Naim MY, Macsio CE, Glatz AC, Goldberg DJ. A comparison of bidirectional Glenn vs. hemi-Fontan procedure: an analysis of the single ventricle reconstruction trial public use dataset. Pediatr Cardiol. 2020;41(6):1166–72.
Egbe AC, Connolly HM, McLeod CJ, Ammash NM, Niaz T, Yogeswaran V, et al. Thrombotic and embolic complications associated with atrial arrhythmia after Fontan operation: role of prophylactic therapy. J Am Coll Cardiol. 2016;68(12):1312–9.
Erek E, Abud B, Oz K, Güzeltas A. Preservation of systemic tricuspid valve function by pulmonary conduit banding in a patient with corrected transposition of the great arteries. Interact Cardiovasc Thorac Surg. 2012;15(2):332–4.
Erek E, Aydin S, Suzan D. Right atrial flap repair for left superior vena cava draining into left atrium. Thorac Cardiovasc Surg. 2016;64(1):59–61.
Fontan F, Baudet E. Surgical repair of tricuspid atresia. Thorax. 1971;26(3):240–8.
Freedom RM, Nykanen D, Benson LN. The physiology of the bidirectional cavopulmonary connection. Ann Thorac Surg. 1998;66(2):664–7.
Fuchigami T, Nagashima M, Hiramatsu T, Matsumura G, Tateishi M, Masuda N, Yamazaki K. Long-term follow-up of Fontan completion in adults and adolescents. J Card Surg. 2017;32(7):436–42.
Gentles TL, Keane JF, Jonas RA, Marx GE, Mayer JE. Surgical alternatives to the Fontan procedure incorporating a hypoplastic right ventricle. Circulation. 1994;90(Suppl 2):1–6.
Glenn WW, Patino JF. Circulatory by-pass of the right heart. I. Preliminary observations on the direct delivery of vena caval blood into the pulmonary arterial circulation; azygos vein-pulmonary artery shunt. Yale J Biol Med. 1954;27(3):147–51. PMID: 13226952; PMCID: PMC2599414
Guzeltas A, Ugan Atik S, Tanidir I. Transcatheter pulmonary valve implantation in tetralogy of Fallot and Ebstein's anomaly with one and a half ventricular repair. Cardiol Young. 2021;31(4):658–60.
Hanley FL, Sade RM, Blackstone EH, Kirklin JW, Freedom RM, Nanda NC. Outcomes in neonatal pulmonary atresia with intact ventricular septum: a multi-institutional study. J Thorac Cardiovasc Surg. 1993;105:406–27.
Hansen JH, Furck AK, Petko C, Buchholz-Berdau R, Voges I, Scheewe J, Rickers C, Kramer HH. Use of surveillance criteria reduces interstage mortality after the Norwood operation for hypoplastic left heart syndrome. Eur J Cardiothorac Surg. 2012;41(5):1013–8.
Hawkins JA, Shaddy RE, Day RW, Sturtevant JE, Orsmond GS, McGough EC. Midterm results after bidirectional cavopulmonary shunts. Ann Thorac Surg. 1993;56:833–7.
Henry JN, Danielson GK. Successful "correction" of tricuspid atresia: results of a detailed anatomical study. Surg Forum. 1974;25:163–5.
Hirsch JC, Ohye RG, Devaney EJ, Goldberg CS, Bove EL. The lateral tunnel Fontan procedure for hypoplastic left heart syndrome: results of 100 consecutive patients. Pediatr Cardiol. 2007;28(6):426–32.
Hoashi T, Shimada M, Imai K, et al. Long-term therapeutic effect of Fontan conversion with an extracardiac conduit. Eur J Cardiothorac Surg. 2020;57(5):951–7.
Hopkins RA, Armstrong BE, Serwer GA, Peterson RJ, Oldham HN. Physiologic rationale for a bidirectional cavopulmonary shunt. J Thorac Cardiovasc Surg. 1985;90:391–8.
Hopkins KA, Brown JW, Darragh RK, Kay WA. Converting Fontan-Björk to 1.5- or 2-ventricle circulation. Ann Thorac Surg. 2019;107(4):e259–61. https://doi.org/10.1016/j.athoracsur.2018.07.097.
Huang C, Gao L, Zhao T, Xu X, Yang Y. Modified Bjork procedure for tricuspid atresia with pulmonary hypertension. J Card Surg. 2011;26(6):657–9.
Ilbawi MN, Idriss FS, DeLeon SY, Kucich VA, Muster AJ, Paul MH, et al. When should the hypoplastic right ventricle be used in a Fontan operation? An experimental and clinical correlation. Ann Thorac Surg. 1989;47:533–8.
Ilbawi MN, Idriss FS, DeLeon SY, Kurich VA, Muster AJ, Paul MH, et al. When should the hypoplastic right ventricle be used in a Fontan operation? An experimental and clinical correlation. Ann Thorac Surg. 1989;47(4):533–8.
Ilbawi MN, DeLeon SY, Backer CL, Duffy CE, Muster AJ, Zales VR, et al. An alternative approach to the surgical management of physiologically corrected trans-

position with VSD and pulmonary stenosis or atresia. J Thorac Cardiovasc Surg. 1990;100(3):410–5.

John AS, Johnson JA, Khan M, Driscoll DJ, Warnes CA, Cetta F. Clinical outcomes and improved survival in patients with protein-losing enteropathy after the Fontan operation. J Am Coll Cardiol. 2014;64(1):54–62.

Jolley M, Thiagarajan RR, Barrett CS, Salvin JW, Cooper DS, Rycus PT, Teele SA. Extracorporeal membrane oxygenation in patients undergoing superior cavopulmonary anastomosis. J Thorac Cardiovasc Surg. 2014;148(4):1512–8.

Jonas RA. The intra/extracardiac conduit fenestrated Fontan. Semin Thorac Cardiovasc Surg Pediatr Card Surg Annu. 2011;14(1):11–8.

Kalia K, Walker-Smith P, Ordoñez MV, Barlatay FG, Chen Q, Weaver H, et al. Does maintenance of pulmonary blood flow pulsatility at the time of the Fontan operation improve hemodynamic outcome in functionally univentricular hearts? Pediatr Cardiol. 2021;42(5):1180–9.

Kawashima Y, Matsuki O, Yagihara T, Matsuda H. Total cavopulmonary shunt operation. Semin Thorac Cardiovasc Surg. 1994;6:17–20.

Kim YY, Rathod RH, Gauvreau K, Keenan EM, Del Nido P, Geva T. Factors associated with severe aortic dilation in patients with Fontan palliation. Heart. 2016;103(4):280–6.

Kodama Y, Kuraoka A, Ishikawa Y, Nakamura M, Ushinohama H, Sagawa K, et al. Outcome of patients with functional single ventricular heart after pacemaker implantation: what makes it poor, and what can we do? Heart Rhythm. 2019;16(12):1870–4.

Kopf GS, Laks H, Stansel HC, Hellenbrand WE, Kleinman CS, Talner NS. Thirty-year follow-up of superior vena cava-pulmonary artery (Glenn) shunts. J Thorac Cardiovasc Surg. 1990;100(5):662–71.

Kreutzer G, Galíndez E, Bono H, De Palma C, Laura JP. An operation for the correction of tricuspid atresia. J Thorac Cardiovasc Surg. 1973;66(4):613–21.

Kreutzer GO, Allaria AE, Schlichter AJ, Roman MI, Capelli H, Berri GG, et al. A comparative long-term follow-up of the results of anterior and posterior approaches in bypassing the rudimentary right ventricle in patients with tricuspid atresia. Int J Cardiol. 1988;19(2):167–79.

Krowka JM, Cortese DA. Hepatopulmonary syndrome: an evolving perspective in the era of liver transplantation. Hepatology. 1990;11(1):138–42.

Lasa JJ, Glatz AC, Daga A, Shah M. Prevalence of arrhythmias late after the Fontan operation. Am J Cardiol. 2014;113(7):1184–8.

Latus H, Gummel K, Diederichs T, Bauer A, Rupp S, Kerst G, et al. Aortopulmonary collateral flow is related to pulmonary artery size and affects ventricular dimensions in patients after the Fontan procedure. PLoS One. 2013;8(11):e81684. https://doi.org/10.1371/journal.pone.0081684.

Lemler MS, Scott WA, Leonard SR, Stromberg D, Ramaciotti C. Fenestration improves clinical outcome of the Fontan procedure: a prospective, randomized study. Circulation. 2002;105(2):207–12.

Lemmer JH, Coran AG, Behrendt DM, Heidelberger KP, Stern AM. Liver fibrosis (cardiac cirrhosis) five years after modified Fontan operation for tricuspid atresia. J Thorac Cardiovasc Surg. 1983;86(5):757–60.

Liu R, Pang K, Rui L, Zhang B, Wang C, Li S. Congenitally corrected transposition with left ventricular outflow obstruction and cardiac malposition: one-and-a-half ventricular repair vs. Fontan pathway? Front Cardiovasc Med. 2022;17(9):938118. https://doi.org/10.3389/fcvm.2022.938118. PMID: 36324751; PMCID: PMC9618694

Mainwaring RD, Reddy VM, Hanley FL. Completion of the three-stage Fontan pathway without cardiopulmonary bypass. World J Pediatr Congenit Heart Surg. 2014;5(3):427–33.

Malhotra SP, Reddy VM, Qiu M, Pirolli TJ, Barboza L, Reinhartz O, Hanley FL. The hemi-mustard/bidirectional Glenn atrial switch procedure in the double-switch operation for congenitally corrected transposition of the great arteries: rationale and midterm results. J Thorac Cardiovasc Surg. 2011;141(1):162–70.

Malhotra A, Agrawal V, Patel K, Shah M, Sharma K, Sharma P, et al. Ebstein's anomaly: "the one and a half ventricle heart". Braz J Cardiovasc Surg. 2018;33(4):353–61.

Marcelletti CF, Iorio FS. Workshop on one and one-half ventricular repairs. Ann Thorac Surg. 1998;66(2):613–92.

Marcelletti C, Corno A, Giannico S, Marino B. Inferior vena cava-pulmonary artery extracardiac conduit. A new form of right heart bypass. J Thorac Cardiovasc Surg. 1990;100(2):228–32.

Marcelletti CF, Hanley FL, Mavroudis C, McElhinney DB, Abella RF, Marianeschi SM, et al. Revision of previous Fontan connections to total extracardiac cavopulmonary anastomosis: a multicenter experience. J Thorac Cardiovasc Surg. 2000;119(2):340–6.

Marianeschi SM, McElhinney DB, Reddy VM. Pulmonary arteriovenous malformations in and out of the setting of congenital heart disease. Ann Thorac Surg. 1998;66(2):688–91.

Masuda M, Kado H, Shiokawa Y, Fukae K, Suzuki M, Murakami E, Yasui H. Clinical results of the staged Fontan procedure in high-risk patients. Ann Thorac Surg. 1998;65(6):1721–5.

Mavroudis C. A tribute to Francis Fontan, MD and Guillermo Kreutzer, MD. World J Pediatr Congenit Heart Surg. 2012;3:156–8.

Mavroudis C. Palliation techniques. In: Mavroudis C, Backer C, editors. Atlas of pediatric cardiac surgery. London: Springer; 2015a.

Mavroudis C. Fontan Operation and 1½ Ventricular Repair. In: Mavroudis C, Backer CL, editors. Atlas of pediatric cardiac surgery. London: Springer; 2015b.

Mavroudis C. Fontan conversion and arrhythmia surgery. In: Mavroudis C, Backer CL, editors. Atlas of pediatric cardiac surgery. London: Springer; 2015c.

Mavroudis C, Backer CL, editors. Atlas of pediatric cardiac surgery. 1st ed. London: Springer; 2015.

Mavroudis C, Deal BJ. Prophylactic arrhythmia surgery in association with congenital heart disease. Transl Pediatr. 2016;5(3):148–59.

Mavroudis C, Dearani J, editors. Atlas of adult congenital heart surgery. 1st ed. London: Springer; 2019.

Mavroudis C, Zales VR, Backer CL, Muster AJ, Latson LA. Fenestrated Fontan with delayed catheter closure. Effects of volume loading and baffle fenestration on cardiac index and oxygen delivery. Circulation. 1992;86(Suppl 5):II85–92.

Mavroudis C, Backer CL, Deal BJ, Johnsrude CL. Fontan conversion to cavopulmonary connection and arrhythmia circuit cryoablation. J Thorac Cardiovasc Surg. 1998;115(3):547–56.

Mavroudis C, Deal BJ, Backer CL, Johnsrude CL. The favorable impact of arrhythmia surgery on total cavopulmonary artery Fontan conversion. Semin Thorac Cardiovasc Surg Pediatr Card Surg Annu. 1999a;2:143–56.

Mavroudis C, Backer CL, Kohr LM, Deal BJ, Stinios J, Muster AJ, et al. Bidirectional Glenn shunt in association with congenital heart repairs: the 1½ ventricular repair. Ann Thorac Surg. 1999b;68(3):976–82.

Mavroudis C, Backer CL, Deal BJ, Johnsrude C, Strasburger J. Total cavopulmonary conversion and maze procedure for patients with failure of the Fontan operation. J Thorac Cardiovasc Surg. 2001;122(5):863–71.

Mavroudis C, Deal BJ, Backer CL. The beneficial effects of total cavopulmonary conversion and arrhythmia surgery for the failed Fontan. Semin Thorac Cardiovasc Surg Pediatr Card Surg Annu. 2002;5:12–24.

Mavroudis C, Deal BJ, Backer CL. Arrhythmia surgery in association with complex congenital heart repairs excluding patients with Fontan conversion. Semin Thorac Cardiovasc Surg Pediatr Card Surg Annu. 2003;6:33–50.

Mavroudis C, Backer CL, Deal BJ, Stewart RD, Franklin WH, Tsao S, et al. Evolving anatomic and electrophysiologic considerations associated with Fontan conversion. Semin Thorac Cardiovasc Surg Pediatr Card Surg Annu. 2007:136–45.

Mavroudis C, Backer CL, Deal BJ. Late reoperations for Fontan patients: state of the art invited review. Eur J Cardiothorac Surg. 2008;34(5):1034–40.

Mazza GA, Gribaudo E, Agnoletti G. The pathophysiology and complications of Fontan circulation. Acta Biomed. 2021;92(5):e2021260. https://doi.org/10.23750/abm.v92i5.10893.

Miyaji K, Shimada M, Sekiguchi A, Ishizawa A, Isoda T, Tsunemoto M. Pulmonary atresia with intact ventricular septum: long-term results of "one and a half ventricular repair". Ann Thorac Surg. 1995;60(6):1762–4.

Muster AJ, Zales VR, Ilbawi MN, Backer CL, Duffy CE, Mavroudis C. Biventricular repair of hypoplastic right ventricle assisted by pulsatile bidirectional cavopulmonary anastomosis. J Thorac Cardiovasc Surg. 1993;105:112–9.

Myers PO, del Nido PJ, Geva T, Bautista-Hernandez V, Chen P, Mayer JE Jr, et al. Impact of age and duration of banding on left ventricular preparation before anatomic repair for congenitally corrected transposition of the great arteries. Ann Thorac Surg. 2013;96(2):603–10.

Nakano T, Kado H, Tatewaki H, et al. Results of extracardiac conduit total cavopulmonary connection in 500 patients. Eur J Cardiothorac Surg. 2015;48(6):825–32.

Niwa K. Aortic dilatation in complex congenital heart disease. Cardiovasc Diagn Ther. 2018;8(6):725–38.

Ohuchi H, Yasuda K, Miyazaki A, Kitano M, Sakaguchi H, Yazaki S, et al. Haemodynamic characteristics before and after the onset of protein losing enteropathy in patients after the Fontan operation. Eur J Cardiothorac Surg. 2013;43(3):e49–57. https://doi.org/10.1093/ejcts/ezs714.

Ono M, Vogt M, Cleuziou J, Kasnar-Samprec J, Burri M, Strbad M, et al. Improved exercise performance in patients with tricuspid atresia after the Fontan-Björk modification with pulsatile systolic pulmonary flow. Ann Thorac Surg. 2016a;101(3):1012–9.

Ono M, Vogt M, Cleuziou J, Kasnar-Samprec J, Burri M, Strbad M, et al. Improved exercise performance in patients with tricuspid atresia after the Fontan-Björk modification with pulsatile systolic pulmonary flow. Ann Thorac Surg. 2016b;101(3):1012–9.

Podzolkov VP, Chiaureli MR, Yurlov IA, Zelenikin MM, Kovalev DV, Dontsova VI, et al. Results of Fontan operation in patients with atrioventricular valve regurgitation. Eur J Cardiothorac Surg. 2015;48(2):308–15.

Pridjian AK, Mendelsohn AM, Lupinetti FM, et al. Usefulness of the bidirectional Glenn procedure as staged reconstruction for the functional single ventricle. Am J Cardiol. 1993;71:959–62.

Pundi KN, Johnson JN, Dearani JA, Pundi KN, Li Z, Hinck CA, Dahl SH, Cannon BC, O'Leary PW, Driscoll DJ, Cetta F. 40-year follow-up after the Fontan operation: long-term outcomes of 1,052 patients. J Am Coll Cardiol. 2015;66(15):1700–10.

Pundi KN, Pundi K, Driscoll DJ, Dearani JA, Li Z, Dahl SH, et al. Heart transplantation after Fontan: results from a surgical Fontan cohort. Pediatr Transplant. 2016;20(8):1087–92.

Rathgeber SL, Guttman OR, Lee AF, Voss C, Hemphill NM, Schreiber RA, et al. Fontan-associated liver disease: Spectrum of disease in children and adolescents. J Am Heart Assoc. 2020;9(1):e012529. https://doi.org/10.1161/JAHA.119.012529.

Reddy VM, Liddicoat JR, McElhinney DB, Brook MM, van Son JAM, Hanley FL. Biventricular repair of lesions with straddling tricuspid valves using techniques of cordal translocation and realignment. Cardiol Young. 1997a;7(2):147–52.

Reddy VM, McElhinney DB, Hanley FL. Correction of left superior vena cava draining to the left atrium using extracardiac techniques. Ann Thorac Surg. 1997b;63(6):1800–2.

Robicsek F, Temesvari A, Kadar RL. A new method for the treatment of congenital heart disease associ-

ated with impaired pulmonary circulation. Acta Med Scand. 1956;154(2):151–61.
Robicsek F, Riopel DA, Robicsek LK. Long-term results after cavopulmonary anastomosis. J Thorac Cardiovasc Surg. 1991;101(4):740–3.
Rogers LS, Glatz AC, Ravishankar C, Spray TL, Nicolson SC, Rychik J, et al. 18 years of the Fontan operation at a single institution: results from 771 consecutive patients. J Am Coll Cardiol. 2012;60(11):1018–25.
Sakamoto I, Takemoto M, Nagao M, Yamamura K, Hiasa K, Sunagawa K. Giant pulsatile coronary aneurysms associated with pulmonary atresia with an intact ventricular septum after a Fontan procedure. Circulation. 2014;130(14):e121–3. https://doi.org/10.1161/CIRCULATIONAHA.114.009631.
Salik I, Mehta B, Ambati S. Bidirectional Glenn procedure or Hemi-Fontan. In: StatPearls [Internet]. Treasure Island: StatPearls Publishing; 2022.
Sallehuddin A, Bulbul Z, Otero F, Al Dhafiri K, Al-Halees Z. Repair of atrioventricular valve regurgitation in the modified Fontan operation. Eur J Cardiothorac Surg. 2004;26(1):54–9.
Shumacker HB. Discussion of Reed WA, Kittle CF, Heilbrunn A. Superior vena cava-pulmonary artery anastomosis. Arch Surg. 1963;86:101.
Simsic J, Bradley S, Stroud M, et al. Risk factors for interstage death after the Norwood procedure. Pediatr Cardiol. 2005;26:400–3.
Sinha P, Zurakowski D, He D, Yerebakan C, Freedenberg V, Moak JP, Jonas RA. Intra/extracardiac fenestrated modification leads to lower incidence of arrhythmias after the Fontan operation. J Thorac Cardiovasc Surg. 2013;145(3):678–82.
Sinha R, Altin HF, McCracken C, Well A, Rosenblum J, Kanter K, et al. Effect of atrioventricular valve repair on multistage palliation results of single-ventricle defects. Ann Thorac Surg. 2021;111(2):662–70.
Starnes VA, Pitlick PT, Bernstein D, Griffin ML, Choy M, Shumway NE. Ebstein's anomaly appearing in the neonate. A new surgical approach. J Thorac Cardiovasc Surg. 1991;101(6):1082–7.
Starr L, Jeffers WA, Meade RH. The absence of conspicuous increments of venous pressure after severe damage to the right ventricle of the dog, with a discussion of the relation between clinical congestive failure and heart disease. Am Heart J. 1943;26:291–301.
Stephens EH, Talwar AA, Devlin PJ, Eltayeb O, Mongé MC, Tsao S, Backer CL. 24-year results of nonfenestrated extracardiac Fontan including Fontan conversions. Ann Thorac Surg. 2021;112(2):619–25.
Stephenson EA, Lu M, Berul CI, Etheridge SP, Idriss SF, Margossian R, Reed JH, Prakash A, Sleeper LA, Vetter VL, Blaufox AD, Pediatric Heart Network Investigators. Arrhythmias in a contemporary Fontan cohort: prevalence and clinical associations in a multicenter cross-sectional study. J Am Coll Cardiol. 2010;56(11):890–6.
Sughimoto K, Asakura Y, Brizard CP, Liang F, Fujiwara T, Miyaji K, Liu H. Impact of the location of the fenestration on Fontan circulation haemodynamics: a three-dimensional, computational model study. Cardiol Young. 2017;27(7):1289–94.
Sumitomo NF, Tamura M, Asano S, Yuasa E, Oyanagi T, Inoue M, et al. Successful preoperative partial splenic artery and aneurysm embolization for thrombocytopenia associated with failed Fontan circulation. Int Heart J. 2022;63(5):984–8.
Talwar S, Siddharth B, Choudhary SK, Airan B. One and half ventricle repair: rationale, indications, and results. Indian J Thorac Cardiovasc Surg. 2018;34(3):370–80.
Tam VK, Miller BE, Murphy K. Modified Fontan without use of cardiopulmonary bypass. Ann Thorac Surg. 1999;68(5):1698–703.
Terada T, Sakurai H, Nonaka T, et al. (2014) surgical outcome of Fontan conversion and arrhythmia surgery: need a pacemaker? Asian Cardiovasc Thorac Ann. 2014;22(6):682–6.
Terashi E, Kodama Y, Kuraoka A, Ishikawa Y, Nakamura M, Sagawa K, et al. Usefulness of liver stiffness on ultrasound shear-wave Elastography for the evaluation of central venous pressure in children with heart diseases. Circ J. 2019;83(6):1338–41.
Thoele DG, Ursell PC, Ho SY, Smith A, Bowman FO, Gersony WM, et al. Atrial morphologic features in tricuspid atresia. J Thorac Cardiovasc Surg. 1991;102(4):606–10.
Toncu A, Rădulescu CR, Dorobanţu D, Stoica Ş. Does routine fenestration improve early and late postoperative outcomes in patients undergoing Fontan palliation? Interact Cardiovasc Thorac Surg. 2020;30(5):773–9.
Udink Ten Cate FE, Hannes T, Germund I, Khalil M, Huntgeburth M, Apitz C, et al. Towards a proposal for a universal diagnostic definition of protein-losing enteropathy in Fontan patients: a systematic review. Heart. 2016;102(14):1115–9.
Van Arsdell GS, Williams WG, Maser CM, Streitenberger KS, Rebeyka IM, Coles GJ, et al. Superior vena cava to pulmonary artery anastomosis: an adjunct to biventricular repair. J Thorac Cardiovasc Surg. 1996;112:1143–9.
Van Arsdell GS, Williams WG, Freedom RM. A practical approach to 11/2 ventricle repairs. Ann Thorac Surg. 1998;66(2):678–80.
van Son JA, Black MD, Haas GS, Falk V, Hambsch J, Onnasch JF, et al. Extracardiac repair versus intracardiac baffle repair of complex unroofed coronary sinus. Thorac Cardiovasc Surg. 1998;46(6):371–4.
Vettukattil JJ. Is the hepatic factor a miRNA that maintains the integrity of pulmonary microvasculature by inhibiting the vascular endothelial growth factor? Curr Cardiol Rev. 2017;13(3):244–50.
Viswanathan S. Thromboembolism and anticoagulation after Fontan surgery. Ann Pediatr Cardiol. 2016;9(3):236–40.
Weixler VHM, Zurakowski D, Kheir J, Guariento A, Kaza AK, Baird CW, et al. Fontan with lateral tunnel is associated with improved survival compared with extracardiac conduit. J Thorac Cardiovasc Surg. 2020;159:1480–91.

Winlaw DS, McGuirk SP, Balmer C, Langley SM, Griselli M, Stümper O, et al. Intention-to-treat analysis of pulmonary artery banding in conditions with a morphological right ventricle in the systemic circulation with a view to anatomic biventricular repair. Circulation. 2005;111(4):405–11.

Wolff D, van Melle JP, Ebels T, Hillege H, van Slooten YJ, Berger RM. Trends in mortality (1975–2011) after one- and two-stage Fontan surgery, including bidirectional Glenn through Fontan completion. Eur J Cardiothorac Surg. 2014;45(4):602–9.

Yang Y, Feng Z, Ma K, Zhang S, Zhang B, Qi L, et al. Long-term results of concomitant atrioventricular valve intervention and the Fontan operation. Eur J Cardiothorac Surg. 2021;59(4):832–8.

Yu JJ, Yun TJ, Yun SC, Im YM, Lee SC, Shin HJ, et al. Low pulmonary vascular compliance predisposes post-Fontan patients to protein-losing enteropathy. Int J Cardiol. 2013;165(3):454–7.

Zhao T, Yang Y, Wu Z, Yang J. Surgical repair for anomalous drainage of left superior vena cava to left atrium. Zhong nan da xue xue bao. Yi xue ban. 2010;35(4):374–766. Chinese. https://doi.org/10.3969/j.issn.1672-7347.2010.04.016.

Zias EA, Mavroudis C, Cook KE, Makarewicz AJ, Backer CL, Hernandez JM. The effect of pulmonary circulation hemodynamics on right ventricular unloading via the bidirectional Glenn shunt: implications for congenitally corrected transposition repair. Semin Thorac Cardiovasc Surg Pediatr Card Surg Annu. 2003;6:27–32.

Complications Associated with Mechanical Circulatory Support for Pediatric and Congenital Heart Surgery

Ahmet Bilgili, Omar M. Sharaf, Zane Borenstein, Robert Hoffberger, Giles J. Peek, Mark S. Bleiweis, and Jeffrey P. Jacobs

Abstract

This chapter will describe complications associated with mechanical circulatory support (MCS) for pediatric and congenital heart surgery. This chapter will be divided into the following five sections:

- Section 1: Physiological Complications Associated with Extracorporeal Membrane Oxygenation
- Section 2: Circuit Complications Associated with Extracorporeal Membrane Oxygenation
- Section 3: Physiological Complications Associated with Ventricular Assist Device Support
- Section 4: Circuit Complications Associated with Ventricular Assist Device Support
- Section 5: Future Research

Keywords

Congenital heart disease · Congenital heart surgery · Extracorporeal membrane oxygenation · Ventricular assist device · Hemolysis · Cannulation · Coagulation · Pediatric

A. Bilgili · O. M. Sharaf · Z. Borenstein
R. Hoffberger · G. J. Peek · M. S. Bleiweis
J. P. Jacobs (✉)
Congenital Heart Center, Division of Cardiovascular Surgery, Department of Surgery, University of Florida, Gainesville, FL, USA
e-mail: JeffreyJacobs@ufl.edu

1 Physiological Complications Associated with Extracorporeal Membrane Oxygenation

1.1 Bleeding and Hemolysis

Due to a significant increase in the use of extracorporeal membrane oxygenation (ECMO) in pediatric patients over the past decade, the clinical application and management of ECMO have notably improved within a short timeframe. However, the incidence of hemostatic complications, such as bleeding and hemolysis, remains high among children supported with ECMO (Barbaro et al. 2017; Drop et al. 2021; Dalton et al. 2017). It is a fact that these hemostatic complications contribute to increased morbidity and mortality in patients supported with ECMO, with most hemostatic complications occurring within the first 2 weeks after initiation of ECMO support (Dalton et al. 2017). A prospective multicenter observational cohort study of pediatric ECMO patients revealed that bleeding occurred in 70.2% of the cohort and was independently associated with a higher daily risk of mortality (Dalton et al.

C. L. Backer, C. Mavroudis (eds.), *Complications in Pediatric and Congenital Heart Surgery*,
https://doi.org/10.1007/978-3-032-02661-3_18

2017). Additionally, data from larger databases, like the Extracorporeal Life Support Organization (ELSO) registry, indicate that bleeding is a prevalent issue, affecting up to 28.5% of pediatric ECMO patients (Barbaro et al. 2017).

Hemolysis caused by mechanical trauma and complement activation during ECMO also remains a significant problem in the pediatric population (Annich et al. 2000; Lou et al. 2014), with a multi-institutional cohort study involving 216 pediatric patients supported with ECMO reporting that 98.9% experienced hemolysis and 43.5% experienced severe hemolysis based on plasma free hemoglobin (PFH) levels (Dalton et al. 2018). Additionally, the prevalence of hemolysis is still largely unknown due to a lack of measurement and reporting of PFH levels at most centers (Betrus et al. 2007).

Hemostatic complications in ECMO patients arise from a combination of circuit-related and systemic factors, both of which disrupt the delicate balance of the hemostatic system. Various factors contribute to this imbalance, including:

- anticoagulation therapy,
- cannulation and circuit-related issues,
- underlying coagulation disorders,
- an immature coagulation system in neonates and infants, and
- infections.

However, the primary cause of this shift in the hemostatic balance can be attributed to the activation and increased production of thrombin, as a result of continuous contact between circulating blood and the foreign surfaces of the extracorporeal circuit (Drop et al. 2020; Murphy et al. 2015). Thrombin production triggers the activation of other factors in the coagulation pathway, leading to enhanced fibrin production and platelet activation, ultimately promoting a prothrombotic state (Penk et al. 2019). Consequently, this alteration of hemostatic balance disrupts the normal coagulation cascade and increases the risks of both clotting and bleeding.

Moreover, systemic anticoagulation is necessary in patients supported with ECMO to prevent thrombotic complications and maintain the integrity of the ECMO circuit. However, achieving the appropriate balance of anticoagulation is challenging, as excessive anticoagulation can result in bleeding, while insufficient anticoagulation can lead to clot formation. Anticoagulants increase the susceptibility of patients to bleeding complications, especially those patients with disseminated intravascular coagulation (DIC) and infection. Traditionally, unfractionated heparin (UFH) is used for anticoagulation in patients supported with ECMO, although recently, the use of bivalirudin for anticoagulation in patients supported with ECMO has become increasingly common. In patients supported with ECMO after surgery, anticoagulation to manage and prevent thrombotic risks is typically started in the postoperative period after bleeding has subsided.

Heparin prevents clotting by binding to the plasma glycoprotein antithrombin, inducing a conformational change that makes antithrombin an efficient inactivator of coagulation factors. Therefore, UFH inhibits thrombin (factor IIa). UFH binds to endothelial cells and other plasma proteins, apart from antithrombin, contributing to the variability in heparin's anticoagulant response among patients, making heparin response unpredictable (Raffini 2017). Mechanistically, UFH functions by inactivating free thrombin and preventing the formation of fibrin as well as by preventing thrombin-induced activation of platelets and factors V, VIII, and XI (Neunert et al. 2022). However, due to patient variability, the use of anticoagulants can potentially lead to heparin-induced thrombocytopenia and exacerbate bleeding susceptibility (Vakil et al. 2012).

On another note, the risk factors associated with hemolysis are multifactorial, although reports on these factors have been inconsistent. However, studies show that it is important to consider pump-related factors such as pump speed, venous inlet pressure, and oxygenator type, as well as patient-related parameters, such as high hemoglobin levels, as potential risk factors (Lou et al. 2014; Dalton et al. 2018; Steinhorn et al. 1989; Gbadegesin et al. 2009).

Traditionally, UFH has been the primary anticoagulant used in pediatric patients supported with ECMO. UFH's longstanding use in conjunction with MCS, lack of better alternatives, and quick reversal with protamine sulfate have made it a preferred choice. However, UFH has its drawbacks; particularly in terms of its variable binding and unpredictable response. Furthermore, the wide variation in anticoagulant strategies and management among different ECMO centers has led to significant discrepancies in UFH-related data, making it challenging to draw conclusive findings regarding UFH strategy (Bembea et al. 2013). Until 2018, UFH was predominantly utilized in most centers. However, since then, there has been a notable increase in the use of direct thrombin inhibitors (DTIs), specifically bivalirudin (Angiomax) and argatroban (Neunert et al. 2022). It is commonly thought that DTIs, especially bivalirudin, offer distinct advantages over UFH. For example, bivalirudin can inhibit both circulating and clot-bound thrombin without binding to other circulating plasma proteins. These advantages provide greater predictability of its activity and support thrombolysis. However, unlike UFH, there is currently no specific reversal agent available for bivalirudin. Furthermore, in certain situations where a prolonged half-life is advantageous, such as stasis, UFH may still be considered a better alternative. Nevertheless, the literature regarding the use of bivalirudin in MCS, specifically ECMO, is expanding (Sanfilippo et al. 2017). Comparative studies conducted in adults have shown no significant difference in rates of complication between UFH and bivalirudin (Pieri et al. 2013; Ranucci et al. 2011). Additionally, Ranucci and colleagues have reported that bivalirudin offers a more favorable coagulation profile, reduced bleeding, and fewer allogeneic transfusions when compared with UFH (Ranucci et al. 2011). Regardless, anticoagulation strategy is extremely patient-specific and an interdisciplinary team of surgeons, hematologists, cardiologists, and ECMO specialists must come together to decide upon the best anticoagulative strategy to pursue. The use of bivalirudin is clearly increasing and may potentially decrease complications of bleeding and clotting during prolonged MCS.

1.2 Stroke

Studies have indicated that after experiencing acute neurologic injury while on ECMO, only 36% of children survive until they are discharged from the hospital, with 6–13% experiencing severe neurologic disability (Hervey-Jumper et al. 2011; Hanekamp et al. 2006; Nijhuis-van der Sanden et al. 2009). An additional 9–26% of children may encounter relatively milder challenges, such as motor difficulties or cognitive delays (Hanekamp et al. 2006; Nijhuis-van der Sanden et al. 2009). The incidence of stroke in pediatric ECMO patients has been the subject of inconsistent reports, with rates ranging from 5% to 27.7% (Hervey-Jumper et al. 2011; Pinto et al. 2017). However, a recent comprehensive analysis of the National Inpatient Sample database conducted by Ezetendu and colleagues shed light on the rates, outcomes, and trends of stroke in pediatric patients supported with ECMO. Among a population of 28,695 pediatric ECMO patients, 10.4% had experienced a stroke. Of these cases, 49% were hemorrhagic, 43% were ischemic, and 8% were a combination of both types (Ezetendu et al. 2022). Ischemic stroke in particular can have a profound impact on a child's quality of life, leaving them with long-term neurological deficits and increasing the prevalence of other complications (Hervey-Jumper et al. 2011; Felling et al. 2020). Moreover, Ezetendu and colleagues found the frequency of stroke was significantly higher in patients between the ages of 1–18 years compared with those under 1 year, with no notable differences based on gender or ethnicity (Ezetendu et al. 2022). Importantly, patients with stroke while on ECMO had higher rates of mortality compared with those without stroke (46.6% vs. 40.8%, $p < 0.001$) (Ezetendu et al. 2022). Patients with stroke while on ECMO also exhibited a significantly higher frequency of cardiac comorbidities, including hypertension, cardiac arrest, myocarditis, congenital heart disease, acute kidney injury, ventricular assist device use, heart failure, and cardiomyopathy (Ezetendu et al. 2022). Nevertheless, the brain in children, and especially neonates and infants, has a remarkable ability to recover from stroke; this "neuroplasticity of youth" provides hope and the rationale to continue the pursuit of recovery in many neonates, infants, and children.

In any case, a dynamic interaction of multiple variable disposes supported patients to cerebrovascular accidents (CVA); these variables include:

- the ECMO support and procedure itself,
- pediatric physiology, and
- anticoagulation therapy.

Most notably, the exposure of blood to the extracorporeal circuit incites the coagulation cascade, in turn creating a prothrombic environment that eases clot and emboli formation. Additionally, pro-coagulant factors related to cardiopulmonary bypass and decreased cardiac output preceding cannulation have also been shown to exacerbate neurologic injury in the pediatric ECMO population (Werho et al. 2015). One must also consider that the unique physiology of pediatric patients further contributes to their increased stroke risk. Children have developing cerebral blood vessels that may be more susceptible to injury or ischemia. The coagulation mechanisms, arterial structure, and neurological systems in children exhibit distinct characteristics, and each of these factors significantly impacts their response to medical intervention. More specifically, the immaturity of the coagulation system in children, and especially in neonates and infants, impacts the balance between clotting and bleeding; consequently, it is no surprise that children undergoing invasive procedures like ECMO cannulation and support are disproportionately impacted by cerebrovascular complications (Bowers et al. 2011). Studies have shown that the ECMO cannulation itself can also directly contribute to the risk of stroke—insertion of cannulas into large blood vessels can disrupt normal blood flow and lead to the formation of clots by triggering inflammatory and prothrombic responses (Besser and Klein 2010). It is important to consider that most children requiring ECMO already have severe cardiac or respiratory illnesses, which in turn predisposes them to the development of blood clots or emboli that may directly travel to the brain. Paradoxically, the use of anticoagulation therapy during ECMO to prevent clotting can also often result in bleeding complications, including hemorrhagic stroke (Ezetendu et al. 2022). Both the need for anticoagulation during ECMO and undergoing hypoxic ischemic events before initiating ECMO have also been shown to be large contributory factors to the development of adverse neurological outcomes (Ezetendu et al. 2022). Thus, it is important to titrate an optimal balance between anticoagulation treatment and subsequent bleeding related complications. Furthermore, the duration of ECMO support plays a role, with prolonged exposure to ECMO increasing the cumulative risk of cerebrovascular complications (Said et al. 2020). Overall, the increased risk of stroke in pediatric ECMO patients is a complex interplay of multiple variables:

- underlying medical conditions,
- the ECMO procedure itself,
- the unique physiology of children, and
- the duration of ECMO support.

Understanding and mitigating these risk factors is essential in managing pediatric patients on ECMO and minimizing the occurrence and impact of cerebrovascular incidents.

Consequently, researchers are actively investigating the underlying mechanisms of stroke in ECMO patients, particularly in pediatrics, with the aim of developing targeted interventions. This research includes exploring novel monitoring techniques such as cerebral oximetry and continuous electroencephalogram (EEG) to gather comprehensive data in at-risk intensive care unit (ICU) populations (Sekhon et al. 2019; Cho et al. 2020; Lorusso et al. 2017). Additionally, the evaluation of quantitative EEG and cerebrovascular autoregulation software is being pursued for rapid interpretation of continuous data (Doerrfuss et al. 2020; Rivera-Lara et al. 2019). The emergence of plasma biomarkers for brain injury shows promise for real-time, non-invasive assessment of acute neurologic injury (Bembea et al. 2015). Recognizing the importance of post-ECMO functional outcome assessments, efforts are being made to establish standardized measures of outcome through collaboration among professional societies and research networks (Said et al. 2020). This collaboration aims to enhance our understanding of risk factors, prognostic markers, and opportunities for intervention. The establishment of large-scale multicenter studies and data registries is also underway to gather comprehensive data on stroke incidence and outcomes, enabling more robust conclusions. Furthermore, advancements in ECMO technology, such as surface modifications of the ECMO circuit, are being pursued to minimize pro-inflammatory and pro-thrombotic effects, potentially reducing the risk of ischemic embolic stroke and intracranial hemorrhage (Lafç et al. 2014). The future direction of research is centered around several critical domains designed to enhance neurodevelopmental outcomes in pediatric ECMO patients:

- improving neurologic monitoring,
- standardizing outcome assessments,
- optimizing anticoagulative strategies, and
- implementing early neuroprotective interventions.

1.3 Infection

Infection presents a significant challenge in patients supported with ECMO, primarily related to various factors associated with the patient and the circuit itself (Bizzarro et al. 2011; Meyer et al. 1995; Douglass et al. 1996). Studies based on the Extracorporeal Life Support Organization (ELSO) registry have reported a prevalence of infection ranging from 11.7% to 20.8% in supported patients, with a rate of 15.4 infections per 1000 ECMO days (Bizzarro et al. 2011). Coagulase-negative staphylococcus, Candida, and Pseudomonas species are commonly identified perpetrators of ECMO-related bacterial infections. The incidence of infection in ECMO supported patients in the current literature ranges from 10% to 21% in adult cohorts and 3–33% in pediatric cohorts, with bloodstream infections and pneumonia being the most common types in children (Bizzarro et al. 2011; Biffi et al. 2017; Cashen et al. 2018; Castagnola et al. 2018; Cheng et al. 2014a). More specifically, the prevalence of blood stream infections has been reported to be between 6% and 18% in the pediatric ECMO population (Biffi et al. 2017). Additionally, neonates generally have a lower risk of infection compared with older children who receive ECMO in a pediatric ICU (Cashen et al. 2018). Single institutional retrospective cohort studies have reported higher mortality and increased days of mechanical ventilation in those with acquired infections during support than those without (Bizzarro et al. 2011; Castagnola et al. 2018; O'Neill et al. 2001; Kaczala et al. 2009; Schutze and Heulitt 1995) A site of common bacterial entry occurs during the cannulation of large blood vessels which breaches barrier protection; furthermore, a greater number of procedures for ECMO cannula placement has been found to be independently associated with increased risk of acquired infection during the duration of support (Cashen et al. 2018). Clinical signs of infection in ECMO patients are challenging to diagnose due to several factors:

- non-specificity,
- artificial control of respiratory rate and temperature, and
- ECMO-related factors that can mask infectious symptoms.

Definitive diagnosis relies on microbiological cultures, which can take up to 48–72 h for analysis, further complicating reported rates of infection. Consequently, studies have speculated that under-reporting of presumed "contaminants" (such as coagulase-negative staphylococci, which are frequently considered as contaminants and therefore not reported by many centers although coagulase-negative staphylococci may be pathogenic) occurs in the ELSO registry, diluting down database-centered study results (Kaczala et al. 2009). The true incidence of blood stream infections may therefore actually be higher than previously reported (Kaczala et al. 2009).

Mechanistically, in pediatric patients on ECMO, routes of infection are similar to those in adults, but may be influenced by the unique characteristics of pediatric physiology and the specific challenges associated with ECMO support. More specifically, most patients on ECMO have several life-sustaining indwelling catheters, including arterial and venous cannulas, which provide access to the patient's circulation. These catheters can serve as a potential source of infection, either through direct contamination during insertion or subsequent colonization of the catheter surfaces by microorganisms; additionally, catheter-related bloodstream infections (CRBSI) are also of significant concern (Montgomery et al. 2000). Pediatric ECMO patients often undergo frequent invasive procedures, such as:

- blood sampling,
- central line access, or
- surgical interventions.

Each invasive procedure increases the risk of introducing pathogens into the bloodstream or other sites of the body of the patient, potentially leading to infections (Biffi et al. 2017). Additionally, MCS can cause alterations in the immune response, such as activation of inflammatory pathways and modulation of immune cell function. These changes can disrupt the normal defense mechanisms against infections, making pediatric ECMO patients more susceptible to microbial invasion (Millar et al. 2016). Moreover, biofilms that develop on the surfaces of ECMO circuits, oxygenators, and cannulas can provide a protective environment for microorganisms, allowing them to resist host immune defenses and antimicrobial treatments. In fact, biofilms have been reported to be the most common cause of nosocomial septicemia and CRBSI (Donlan 2011). It is also important to note that pathogens can be transmitted through improper hand hygiene, contaminated equipment, or inadequate cleaning practices, leading to healthcare-associated infections. Therefore, it is critical to adhere to common sense hygiene practices, as children on ECMO are already critically ill and immunocompromised, increasing their susceptibility to infection in a healthcare-associated environment.

Unfortunately, limited research and evidence exist about how to prevent infections occurring during and after ECMO support. Institutional antibiotic protocols vary, with survey results of questionnaires given to ELSO members reporting that 50%–68% of respondents administer antibiotic prophylaxis to their patients supported with ECMO, and more broadly, 42% of ECMO centers systematically administer antibiotics to all their patients supported with ECMO (Kao et al. 2011; Glater-Welt et al. 2016). However, no trials or observational studies are available that assess the effectiveness of these protocols of antibiotic prophylaxis, and surprisingly, prior administration of antibiotic therapy has not been associated with a lower risk of complications (Hsu et al. 2009). Thus, it is critical to maintain antimicrobial stewardship, because concern exists that there can be pharmacokinetic alterations of antibiotics while treating patients on ECMO. If these antibiotics are altered, they can be counterproductive to patients (Biffi et al. 2017). Recommendations from the ELSO Infectious Disease Task Force suggest that ECMO patients should be treated like common ICU patients, with a protected central line for hyperalimentation; however, there is no known specific treatment for ECMO-derived infections—due to the variety of bacteria involved and the variable responses of individual patients. In any case, common sense measures should always be taken, such as

- adhering to strict aseptic technique during procedures,
- regular surveillance for infections,
- judicious use of antibiotics, and
- routine monitoring and maintenance of ECMO circuits and catheters to prevent biofilm formation.

Multidisciplinary teams involving surgeons, infectious disease specialists, ECMO specialists, and critical care physicians should collaborate to implement strategies aimed at reducing rates of infection and improving outcomes of patients.

2 Circuit Complications Associated with Extracorporeal Membrane Oxygenation

2.1 Circuit Thrombosis

Understanding the management of circuit thrombosis in an ECMO circuit is critical to improving patient complications related to clotting and bleeding. Clotting-related problems play a significant role in equipment malfunctions, often requiring interventions like the replacement of circuits or oxygenators. Unfortunately, limited studies exist on the sources of circuit thrombosis in pediatric ECMO. However, in a single institution study out of Emory University, specifics related to circuit thrombosis were investigated (Hastings et al. 2017). Thrombus formation was found to be present in 94% of circuits, with an uneven distribution within the various components of the ECMO circuit. Most thrombi were located at the tubing-connector junctions (TCJ) and in the oxygenator. Interestingly, no clots were present on the free tubing surface. Histology and composition of the clots varied with the location of the clots, with TCJ clots being fibrin-rich, coiled, and mobile, whereas oxygenator clots appeared as nonadherent, expanded structures on the premembrane (Hastings et al. 2017). Moreover, in the diagnosis of thrombi formation, decreased pump flow rate should be a clear indicator of potential pump thrombosis. If access inefficiency and mean arterial pressure induced increased pressure afterload are ruled out, circuit thrombosis should be considered as the primary culprit of decreased pump flow rate. Diagnosis of where the pump thrombosis has occurred can be detected based on various pressure changes: (Mason et al. 2022).

- Firstly, an obstruction between the drainage cannula and pump inlet would result in drainage pressures becoming more negative than baseline.
- Secondly, obstruction to blood flow within the membrane lung itself would result in pre- and postmembrane differential increases.
- Thirdly, an obstruction between the membrane lung and return cannula would result in similar increases in premembrane and postmembrane pressures.

Identifying the location of thrombus formation, such as TCJs and the oxygenator, and recognizing specific clot characteristics, can aid in diagnosis and guide appropriate interventions. Monitoring changes in pump flow rate and pressure differentials can further assist in identifying the location of thrombosis within the circuit. In summary, more research related to preventative measures of circuit thrombosis needs to be undertaken and preventative guidelines should be followed. Regardless, having diagnostic awareness can help to reduce the incidence of circuit thrombosis and related patient complications.

2.2 Air in the Circuit

Fortunately, air entering the extracorporeal life support (ECLS) circuit or causing a systemic air embolism is a rare occurrence, reported to have an incidence between 1.4% and 4.6% (Barbaro et al. 2017; Kumar et al. 2019; Timpa et al. 2011). However, the quantity and location of air entry greatly influence outcomes, with significant risks of fatality when a large amount of air enters and interrupts blood flow. Immediate separation from ECMO is crucial to prevent catastrophic air embolism. Therefore, there is no room for error when it comes to air in the circuit, necessitating consistent implementation of preventative strategies. It is crucial to recognize that this complication is largely avoidable. Implementing prevention strategies is critical to ensure air-related complications are minimized; such preventative strategies include:

- limiting access points on the negative pressure side of the circuit,
- meticulous attention to circuit priming,
- cautious handling of central lines,
- utilization of air detection alarms, and
- careful technique when operating stopcocks.

While there is only one existing protocolized management of air in the ECMO circuit from a consecutive cohort, albeit not in a pediatric population, this protocol provides valuable guidelines for addressing air in the circuit based on the presence or absence of arterial air (Chan et al. 2022). Most modern ECLS systems are equipped with integrated bubble detectors, serving as an initial indicator of air in the circuit. Configuring the user-adjustable sensor before the membrane lung enables early detection and intervention by healthcare providers. ECLS systems can also be configured to trigger alarms and stop pumps upon air detection. However, it is important to consider different configurations for veno-arterial (V-A) versus veno-venous (V-V) ECMO, because V-V ECMO patients may tolerate small amounts of air better than pump stoppage (Mason et al. 2022). Determining the location of air within the circuit is crucial, and a thorough end-to-end check of the circuit should be conducted to diagnose the source of the air and prevent recurrence. Various techniques can be employed to remove air, depending on its location, such as:

- aspiration through a pigtail or stopcock,
- passive diffusion through a port,
- clamping and replacing tubing, or
- removing the pump head.

Proactive measures and comprehensive institutional protocols aimed at preventing air entry into the ECLS circuit are of paramount importance due to the potential fatality of systemic air embolism. Vigilance, effective detection mechanisms, and swift removal techniques must be undertaken to ensure patient safety in managing air-related complications.

2.3 Console or Power Failure

The ECMO console plays a vital role in controlling and monitoring the entire ECMO system, encompassing pump function, gas exchange, and alarm systems. Any failure in the console or power supply can result in an immediate loss of flow in ECMO support, emphasizing the need for prompt recognition and response to prevent harm to the patient. While ELSO guidelines recommend connecting the console to an emergency backup power source, it is important to acknowledge that power failures can still occur due to various sporadic causes (Gajkowski et al. 2022). Managing this complication requires preparedness and adherence to established protocols. Depending on the ECMO system, alternative options may be available, such as using a hand crank to manually operate the pump or utilizing a backup second motor or console.

In cases of pump failure, guidelines for pump management can be applied, including: (Mossadegh 2017).

- clamping the cannulas to prevent retrograde blood flow,
- reducing the RPM to zero,
- transferring the pump head to the backup motor,
- initiating the backup pump either manually or electronically, and
- subsequently removing the clamps on the admission and reinfusion cannulas.

Ensuring that all members of the team are proficient in performing these measures, initiating the backup pump is of critical importance. Ongoing training and continuous education should be provided to the entire team, keeping them updated on the latest protocols and procedures. By following these guidelines and maintaining a well-prepared and educated team, the management of console or power failure during ECMO can be effectively addressed.

2.4 Circuit Disruption

Circuit disruption in ECMO refers to a situation where the blood is exposed to atmospheric pressure due to a loss of integrity in any component of the circuit. Various factors exist that can contribute to circuit disruption, including:

- tubing disconnection,
- careless application of tubing clamps, and
- stopcock or pigtail defects.

The effect of circuit disruption depends on whether it occurs in the positive pressure side or the negative pressure side of the circuit. Positive pressure breaches can lead to blood loss, while negative pressure breaches pose the risk of air entrainment (Mason et al. 2022; Ryu and Park 2018). However, these issues can be easily prevented by conducting a thorough circuit check, assessing plugs, fluid connectors, alarms, and the overall integrity of the circuit. If circuit disruption does occur and the breach is significant, it can result in the stoppage of the pump. Regardless of the type or size of the breach, any circuit disruption is a critical situation that requires immediate attention. It can lead to inadequate oxygenation and perfusion, blood loss, and the risk of air entrainment. Therefore, prompt intervention and resolution are crucial to ensuring the safety and well-being of the patient.

2.5 Membrane Lung Dysfunction

The membrane lung (ML) serves as a gas exchange device, facilitating the transfer of oxygen from the external gas supply to the blood and removing carbon dioxide from the blood. Problems related to ML dysfunction stem from its role in the ECMO circuit. The non-biological surface of the ML activates inflammatory and coagulation pathways, resulting in thrombus formation and hematologic abnormalities, which can lead to mechanical obstruction and systemic coagulopathy (Dornia et al. 2014; Doyle and Hunt 2018; Lubnow et al. 2014). Furthermore, the accumulation of moisture in the gas phase and the buildup of protein and cellular debris in the blood phase can contribute to impaired gas exchange (Lehle et al. 2008). However, problems associated with the ML tend to be more subtle than other circuit complications, making the decision to exchange a ML complex (Mason et al. 2022). Zakhary and colleagues suggest an algorithmic and physiological approach to tackling ML dysfunction: (Zakhary et al. 2020).

- First, identify the cause of dysfunction based on one of three reasons: the hematologic profile, pressure monitoring, or ML gas transfer.
- Then, based on physiological and ML parameters, decide whether to consider ML or circuit exchange.

Alarming parameters should prompt evaluation of the ML; such alarming parameters include:

- an increasing pressure drop across the ML divided by the blood flow rate (ΔP/BFR),
- ML with maximal membrane lung oxygen uptake ($V'O_2$) < 100–150 mL/min, or
- persistent partial pressure of post-ML CO2 ($P_{Post\text{-}MLCO2}$) greater than 40 mmHg.

However, these are general guidelines to follow, and the urgency of ML replacement should be based on the rapidity of ML dysfunction and the condition of the patient.

2.6 Inadvertent Decannulation

Life-threatening mechanical complications during ECMO support are rare, unpredictable, and sometimes unpreventable. In pediatric ECMO, cannulas are typically inserted into large blood vessels such as the carotid artery, internal jugular vein, or femoral artery and vein (Jensen et al. 2022). These cannulas are firmly secured, sutured, and anchored in place to prevent accidental removal. However, despite taking precautions, inadvertent decannulation can occur due to various reasons, including:

- physical activity,
- accidental manipulation, and
- equipment-related issues.

Unfortunately, inadvertent decannulation has been shown to be one of the most common life-threatening mechanical complications during ECMO, often occurring when patients are mildly sedated or engaged in active rehabilitation (Kim et al. 2021). Inadvertent or accidental decannulation happens when the cannula is partially or completely dislodged from the vessel. This can result in two potential scenarios, both of which can lead to significant blood loss from the cannulation site: (Mason et al. 2022).

- Firstly, if the return cannula is affected, rapid blood loss can occur.
- Secondly, if the drainage cannula is displaced, air embolism or interrupted blood flow may occur.

These complications require urgent attention, and the immediate response should be to clamp the circuit near the patient and call for assistance. Manual pressure should be emergently applied to any area of active bleeding. In all cases, life support interventions must be initiated promptly, while a separate team diligently troubleshoots the ECMO circuit.

2.7 Gas Supply Interruption

Gas supply interruption can have severe consequences if left unaddressed, leading to abrupt deterioration of the patient. An important indicator of gas exchange is the assessment of color difference between pre- and post-ML blood (Mason et al. 2022). If both appear dark red, it suggests that no gas exchange is taking place in the membrane. As aforementioned, ML dysfunction typically manifests as a gradual decline in gas exchange efficiency. Therefore, an abrupt change indicates that interruption of the gas supply is likely the cause. The assessment process is relatively straightforward, involving tracing the gas supply line from the ML to the source (whether it is a hospital supply line or an external source like a compressed oxygen cylinder) to identify the problem. Prompt measures should be taken to diagnose and resolve the issue. Gas supply interruption is a preventable circuit complication, and it is essential to implement a rigorous and continuous checklist to ensure the integrity of the gas supply line and sources.

3 Physiological Complications Associated with Ventricular Assist Device Support

3.1 Bleeding and Hemolysis

While Ventricular Assist Devices (VADs) can be life-saving, supported pediatric patients face significant challenges related to hemocompatibility and adverse events, including bleeding, hemolysis, and thrombosis. Due to the increased use of VADs, managing these complications with current antithrombosis agents remains an ongoing concern and priority in pediatric patients on VAD support.

Bleeding complications in pediatric VAD patients are one of the most frequent early adverse events for children supported with temporary devices, with one study utilizing the Pediatric Interagency Registry for Mechanical Circulatory Support (Pedimacs) reporting bleeding in 29% of patients (n = 63) (Lorts et al. 2018). Additional retrospective studies and meta-analyses have reported major bleeding occurring in more than a third of pediatric patients supported with VADs (Huang et al. 2018, 2019) Known factors associated with bleeding complications are: (Ghbeis et al. 2021).

- the lack of a standardized approach to anticoagulation and antiplatelet dosing in children,
- surgical techniques,
- poor wound healing, and
- developmental hemostasis in children.

Additionally, the mechanical components of the VAD, including cannulas and pumps, can cause damage to blood vessels, leading to device-related bleeding. Moreover, pediatric patients may experience gastrointestinal bleeding while supported with VAD, which can be caused by factors like stress-related mucosal injury, medication side effects, or clotting abnormalities (Romano et al. 2017).

Hemolysis is another complication associated with pediatric VADs. The turbulent flow and shear stress within the VAD can damage red blood cells, causing their rupture and the release of hemoglobin into the bloodstream (Yen et al. 2014; Alexy et al. 2022). This hemolytic process can result in anemia, jaundice, and other symptoms associated with the release of hemoglobin. In severe cases, hemolysis can lead to kidney injury and renal dysfunction. Most, if not all, patients supported with VADs are run with an initial course of anticoagulants such as heparin or bivalirudin, and while this anticoagulation is necessary to prevent clotting within the device, anticoagulation therapy itself poses an increased risk of bleeding. Studies have indicated that most bleeding events and thromboembolisms occur while patients are on unfractionated heparin, or making the transition between heparin and warfarin (Huang et al. 2019).

Different anticoagulants, such as heparin, warfarin, and direct oral anticoagulants (DOACs), work through various mechanisms to inhibit clot formation (Loyaga-Rendon et al. 2021; Heestermans et al. 2022). Heparin enhances antithrombin III's activity to neutralize clotting factors, warfarin interferes with the production of clotting factors in the liver, and DOACs directly target specific factors involved in the clotting cascade. However, balancing the need for anticoagulation with the risk of bleeding is a challenge. Excessive anticoagulation can increase bleeding tendencies, while inadequate anticoagulation may lead to clot formation. Thus, close monitoring of laboratory parameters are essential to ensure the appropriate anticoagulation effect and mitigate bleeding risks in pediatric VAD patients, such laboratory parameters and assays include:

- prothrombin time (PT),
- activated partial thromboplastin clotting time (PTT),
- platelet count,
- international normalized ratio (INR),
- thromboelastography (TEG), and
- rotational thromboelastometry.

One must also consider that no outside material can be fundamentally considered biologically inert; and thus, VADs interactions with circulating blood will have ramifications to the coagulation system in any case.

Furthermore, the management of anticoagulant therapy in pediatric VAD patients requires a multidisciplinary approach. Healthcare professionals must carefully individualize dosages and monitor patients for signs of bleeding or clotting complications. The choice of anticoagulant and its subsequent protocol should consider the patient's condition, age, weight, and device characteristics. Regular evaluation and adjustments are necessary to maintain a delicate balance between preventing clot formation within the VAD and minimizing the risk of bleeding complications. With close monitoring and individualized management, healthcare teams can optimize anticoagulation therapy in pediatric VAD patients, ensuring the device's function while minimizing risks of bleeding.

To offer an example, our institutional anticoagulation protocol and surgical techniques for pulsatile paracorporeal VAD (Berlin EXCOR [Berlin Heart, Inc., Berlin, Germany]) insertion and support at University of Florida have been extensively discussed in the literature (Bleiweis et al. 2022, 2023). Our strategy for anticoagulation involves a phased approach to anticoagulation after VAD insertion, with certain considerations for specific patient groups:

- Bivalirudin: Bivalirudin is initiated on postoperative day 1. During hours 24–72, bivalirudin is titrated to a PTT of 50–70. After 72 h, bivalirudin is titrated to a PTT of 70–100.
- Aspirin: For patients with a systemic-to-pulmonary artery shunt, aspirin is started on the initial night of VAD insertion at a dose of 5 mg/kg/day (divided into 2 daily doses), and aspirin is increased each week until a dose of 30 mg/kg/day is reached by week 4. For patients without a systemic-to-pulmonary artery shunt, aspirin is started on day 5 after VAD implantation at a dose of 5 mg/kg/day (divided into 2 daily doses), and aspirin is increased each week until a dose of 30 mg/kg/day is reached by week 4.
- Dipyridamole: Dipyridamole is started on week 5 after VAD implantation at a dose of 2.5 mg/kg/day, and dipyridamole is increased twice each week until a dose of 15 mg/kg/day is reached by week 6.
- Omega-3 fatty acid: Omega-3 fatty acid is typically started at 3–4 months after VAD implantation.

Of note, with the above protocol, initially, we do not administer any anticoagulation for the first 24 h after VAD insertion in patients without a systemic-to-pulmonary artery shunt; however, in patients with a systemic-to-pulmonary artery shunt, aspirin is started on the initial night of VAD insertion at a dose of 5 mg/kg/day (divided into 2 daily doses).

This University of Florida approach for anticoagulation during Berlin Heart support represents an example of a successful anticoagulation protocol for patients supported with VAD. While our approach has been successful, it is important to note that different institutions employ alternative anticoagulation strategies (Raffini 2017; Drews et al. 2007). For example, the Edmonton Anticoagulation and Platelet Inhibition Protocol has demonstrated positive outcomes. This protocol incorporates prior experience with pediatric VADs and takes into account developmental hemostasis. The Edmonton Anticoagulation and Platelet Inhibition Protocol includes a comprehensive evaluation of coagulation assays such as PTT, anti-factor Xa (anti-Xa) levels, TEG, and TEG with platelet mapping (Steiner et al. 2016).

Regardless, the prevention and management of bleeding and hemolysis complications in pediatric VAD patients requires an individualized approach. Cardiac surgeons, pediatric cardiologists, hematologists, critical care specialists, anesthesiologists, dedicated nurses, perfusionists, physical therapists, and occupational therapists should all collaborate to optimize patient care. This collaboration includes careful management of anticoagulation therapy to balance the need for prevention of clotting while minimizing the risk of bleeding. Adjusting pump settings to minimize shear stress can help reduce hemolysis. Transfusion of blood products may be necessary to address anemia resulting from bleeding or hemolysis. Close monitoring of laboratory parameters is crucial to detect and address complications early. It is essential for pediatric VAD patients to receive specialized care from a multidisciplinary team of experienced healthcare professionals who are knowledgeable about managing these devices in children. By employing these strategies and providing comprehensive care, healthcare teams can effectively mitigate the complications of bleeding and hemolysis associated with VADs in pediatric patients.

In the future, pediatric VAD patients may benefit from additional advances in multiple domains: (Ghbeis et al. 2021).

- advanced hemostatic monitoring techniques,
- individualized anticoagulation regimens based on patient characteristics and pharmacogenomic testing,
- targeted anticoagulation therapies,
- improved biocompatible surfaces and coatings for VADs,
- refinements in surgical techniques and device design, and
- enhanced education and training for healthcare professionals.

These advancements aim to achieve multiple objectives:

- provide real-time monitoring of hemostasis,
- personalize anticoagulation therapy,
- develop targeted anticoagulant agents,
- improve VAD biocompatibility,
- optimize surgical procedures, and
- enhance the knowledge and skills of healthcare teams.

3.2 Stroke

Neurologic complications and CVAs are frequently and strongly linked to mortality in pediatric patients receiving VAD support (Almond et al. 2013). However, as described above in the ECMO section of this chapter, the brain in children, and especially neonates and infants, has a remarkable ability to recover from stroke; this "neuroplasticity of youth" provides hope and the rationale to continue the pursuit of recovery in many neonates, infants, and children. It is important to understand that some discrepancies exist in the literature as it pertains to the incidence of stroke in cohorts of patients supported with VADs. For example, in the patient cohort used to justify the approval of the Berlin Heart EXCOR system by the Food and Drug Administration (FDA) of the United States of America, the incidence of neurologic events was 29% (Almond et al. 2013; Rosenthal et al. 2016, 2017; Stein et al. 2016). In a larger cohort of 662 patients derived from the Pedimacs registry, a CVA incidence of less than 11% was reported and significant associations with mortality were highlighted, with a hazard ratio of 4.7 (Niebler et al. 2021). Altogether, stroke appears to be a prevalent complication as it relates to pediatric VAD patients and regardless of incidence, the relationship with mortality is clear—if a patient experiences a CVA, they are more likely to die before transplant (Niebler et al. 2021). However, it is also important to consider a study conducted by Thangappan and colleagues that found if a patient is successfully bridged to transplant on a VAD, then similar survival outcomes are observed in patients regardless of the presence or absence of a prior stroke (Thangappan et al. 2022). Furthermore, demographically, a study conducted by the Advanced Cardiac Therapies Improving Outcomes Network (ACTION), revealed that approximately half of the pediatric patients who experienced strokes while on VAD were 1 year of age or younger and/or had congenital heart disease. Additionally, most strokes were reported to be ischemic in nature, associated with paracorporeal VADs, and occurred within the first 30 days after implantation (Peng et al. 2022). A s such, there appears to be a vital period following implantation when a patient is the most susceptible to a CVA, and understanding the underlining causative mechanisms are critical to preventing occurrence.

To elaborate, VADs are commonly associated with both thrombotic and hemorrhagic complications. These complications play direct roles in systemic bleeding, intracranial hemorrhage, and thromboembolic stroke and have been shown extensively in the adult literature (Parikh et al. 2016). It is important to note however, that these complications are not limited to adult patients, as pediatric patients receiving VAD support are oftentimes equally if not more susceptible. While it is challenging to pinpoint the precise pathology of each patient's CVA, notable similarities exist among different cohorts of patients. Oftentimes, strokes arise because of VAD-related complications and/or the use of therapeutic anticoagulation medication:

- One potential and common cause is thromboembolism, where abnormal blood flow patterns caused by the VAD can lead to the formation of blood clots within the device or blood vessels. More specifically, mechanical complications or malfunctions of the VAD, such as clotting within the device or inadequate regulation of blood flow, can contribute to clot formation (Eckman and John 2012). These clots can subsequently travel to the brain, triggering a CVA. While non-contrast computed tomography (CT) is better at identifying hemorrhagic CVA, ischemic CVA can be visualized as an area of hypodensity, representing cytotoxic edema (Fig. 1).
- Regarding anticoagulants, the administration of these medications in VAD patients to prevent clotting can increase the risk of bleeding,

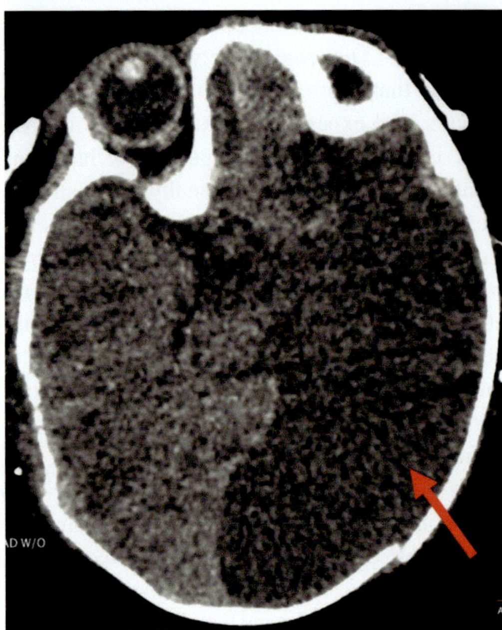

Fig. 1 Non-contrast computed tomography with large territory ischemic stroke in left middle cerebral artery and posterior cerebral artery territories

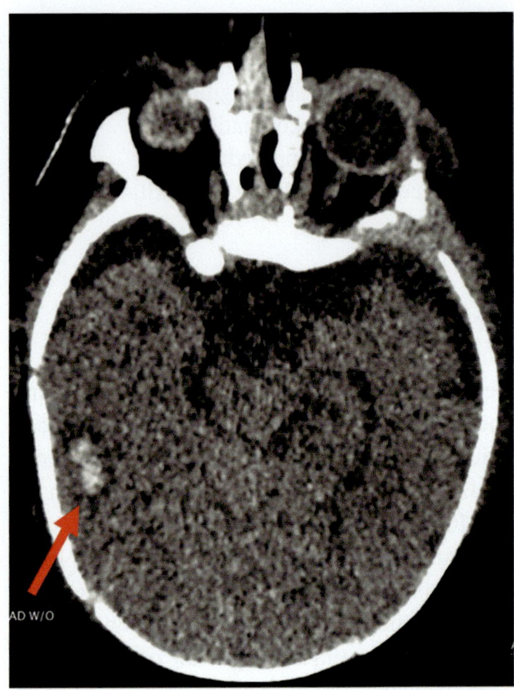

Fig. 2 Non-contrast computed tomography with focal acute parenchymal hemorrhage in right temporo-occipital region

potentially resulting in hemorrhage-related strokes (Boehme et al. 2015). On non-contrast CT, hemorrhagic CVA appears as a bright white density, representing blood (Fig. 2).

Additionally, underlying cardiovascular conditions, particularly congenital heart disease commonly observed in pediatric VAD patients, can predispose patients to strokes by disrupting normal blood flow or heightening the risk of clot formation. Individual patient factors, such as age, overall health status, and genetic predispositions, may also further increase risk. Younger patients, especially infants, may be more susceptible due to their developing vascular system and unique physiological characteristics. Efforts are being made to minimize the occurrence of strokes in pediatric VAD patients through ongoing research and advancements in VAD technology, surgical techniques, and anticoagulation strategies (Ghbeis et al. 2021). These advancements aim to improve blood flow patterns, reduce the risk of clot formation, and optimize patient-specific care to mitigate the occurrence of CVA.

3.3 Infection

In children, infectious complications associated with VAD are a prevalent adverse event. Retrospective and prospective studies have reported infection rates ranging from 40% to 63% during VAD support (Almond et al. 2013; Rosenthal et al. 2016; Fraser et al. 2012; Fragasso et al. 2011). Specifically focusing on the Berlin Heart EXCOR system, two studies have highlighted infection rates of 1.5–5.4 infections per 100 VAD days and revealed an association between thromboembolic events and infection (Almond et al. 2013; Fragasso et al. 2011). An analysis comparing continuous-flow VAD outcomes in children and adults reported infection rates of 1.12 infections per patient-year in children, with non-device-related infections being predominant (Cabrera et al. 2013). Analysis of the Pedimacs registry involving 135 patients identified a total of 263 adverse events, with 19.8% attributed to infection (Rosenthal et al. 2016). In another analysis of the Pedimacs registry, Auerbach and colleagues found that infections accounted for 17% (96 of 564) of reported adverse events, with the most common infection types being non-device infection, sepsis, external pump component infection, and internal pump component infection, respectively. Additionally, most reported infections were bacterial in nature. Patient survival was significantly poorer in those who experienced a first infectious adverse event compared with those without an infectious event, with varying impacts based on device type (no significant difference observed in the pulsatile group, while patients with continuous-flow devices had significantly worse survival) (Auerbach et al. 2018). Infections, although not as impactful on mortality as stroke or bleeding complications, have been reported to be directly related to patient death, albeit at low rates. For example, Cabrera and colleagues reported 3 deaths that were directly related to infections that occurred in a cohort of 51 patients during VAD support (Cabrera et al. 2013). Other studies (Fragasso et al. 2011) have elucidated that in patients supported with VAD, the presence of an infected VAD had no impact on survival; however, when compared with noninfected patients supported with VAD, patients with healthcare-associated infections (HAIs) supported with VAD had:

- a longer mechanical support period,
- a longer length of ICU stay,
- a longer length of hospital stay, and
- increased healthcare costs.

Thus, the literature points out that infection related complications are prevalent but fortunately play a smaller role in directly causing mortality (in comparison with bleeding and stroke) in pediatric cohorts supported with VADs. Nevertheless, understanding the role of infection in pediatric VAD patients and defining causative factors is critical.

Moreover, VAD implantation exposes parts of the body and the bloodstream to foreign chemicals, air, and bioactive organisms, opening the door to acquired infection (Qu et al. 2021). Broadly speaking, VAD-associated infections can be divided into three categories: (Nienaber et al. 2013; Hannan et al. 2011).

- VAD-specific,
- VAD-related, and
- non-VAD infections.

Infections associated with VAD can be caused by:

- bacteria,
- viruses,
- fungi, and
- protozoa.

These infections can manifest in different locations, each characterized by distinct features; (Qu et al. 2021).

- Localized non-device infections involve an entire organ system or region without evidence of systemic involvement. They are confined and do not directly contact the blood-device interface.
- External pump component infections occur when the skin, tissue cultures surrounding the drive-line, or the tissue around the external pump housing become infected.
- Internal pump component infections, also known as inflow or outflow tract infections, occur when the surfaces of the VAD that come into contact with the blood become infected. These infections involve the VAD itself and can lead to significant complications.
- Additionally, sepsis infections occur when there is evidence of systemic involvement, often indicated by positive blood cultures and hypotension. Sepsis can arise as a result of infection spreading from any of the aforementioned locations or due to contamination during the implantation procedure.

Given the exposure of the body and bloodstream to foreign substances (and potentially organisms) during VAD implantation, the risk of infection is a significant concern. The types and locations of infections can vary, ranging from localized non-device infections to external and internal pump component infections, as well as sepsis (Qu et al. 2021). Careful monitoring, appropriate infection prevention strategies, and prompt management of infections are all crucial to minimize the risk and impact of infections in VAD patients.

A multitude of guidelines and protocols exist to prevent VAD-specific infections, and preventing infection in pediatric VAD implantation is crucial for successful outcomes. Firstly, it is critical to understand that the different materials of the drivelines can play a large role in attracting microorganisms and thus lead to infection. Although there is limited research comparing different materials of drivelines as predictors of driveline infections, other implantable device studies have pinpointed that the biomaterial itself is one of the key determinants of device-related infections (Pascual 2002; Lopez-Lopez et al. 1991; Qu et al. 2020). Several measures can be taken to minimize the risk of infection: (Qu et al. 2021; Mattner et al. 2007; Cannon et al. 2012).

- Adhering to strict aseptic technique, including thorough hand hygiene and wearing sterile attire, helps maintain a sterile field during any invasive procedure.
- Administering preoperative prophylactic antibiotics based on local guidelines can reduce the risk of surgical site infections.
- Proper skin preparation using antiseptic solutions such as chlorhexidine gluconate or povidone-iodine.
- Minimizing micro-trauma at the driveline exit site, which serves as a vulnerable point for microbial entry.
- Reducing the risk of microbial contamination during the postimplantation stage.
- Careful selection of the surgical site, considering tissue perfusion and minimizing contamination risk.
- Implementing rigorous catheter care protocols, including regular dressing changes and proper handling.
- Providing healthcare providers regularly updated training on VAD related infection prevention and management.
- Regular surveillance and monitoring of the VAD site for signs of infection.
- Patient and caregiver education about hygiene practices and recognizing infection signs, empowering them to actively participate in prevention (Mattner et al. 2007; Cannon et al. 2012).

Ultimately, these measures can collectively contribute to minimizing the risk of infection in pediatric VAD implantation and prevent unnecessary infection.

4 Circuit Complications Associated with Ventricular Assist Device Support

4.1 Pump Thrombosis

Pump thrombosis is a serious and potentially life-threatening complication that can occur in children with implanted VADs. Thrombotic complications are common in VAD patients and can arise from various factors. Patient systemic inflammation following VAD implantation amplifies susceptibility to thrombotic events (Connors 2015). The interaction between artificial surfaces of the device and high shear stress is a major contributor, activating endothelial cells, platelets, and white blood cells, leading to thrombotic events (Ghbeis et al. 2021). Other factors such as turbulence at anastomotic sites and device-generated heat can also contribute to thrombotic complications. Pump thrombosis starts when fibrin thrombi form around stagnant blood or when platelet thrombi form in areas of turbulence, leading to local coagulation of blood; such thrombosis imposes an increased risk of morbidity and mortality, with device thrombosis reported in 18% of pediatric patients using paracorporeal pulsatile devices (Hetzer et al. 1998). Specifically, the rate of pump thrombotic events was 3.7 per 1000 patient-days for the Berlin Heart EXCOR VAD and 13.7 per 1000 patient-days for centrifugal-flow VAD support (Tume et al. 2019). A multicenter study using the Pedimacs registry reported an 11% pump thrombosis rate in children using the HeartWare device (O'Connor et al. 2020). While the incidence as reported in the literature of pump thrombosis in children is relatively low, its impact on health and quality of life can be significant. Early detection and intervention are crucial for successful treatment, as delayed treatment can lead to irreversible damage to the heart, brain, and other organs. In the setting of implantable (non-paracorporeal) VADs, symptoms such as shortness of breath, chest pain, fatigue, and low blood pressure are clear warning signs, and accessible diagnostic tests like echocardiography and magnetic resonance imaging (MRI) help confirm the diagnosis. Treatment typically involves anticoagulation or surgical removal and device replacement. Intravenous thrombotic agents, such as fibrinolytics and glycoprotein IIb/IIIa inhibitors, may also be used (Rimsans et al. 2017). Preventing pump thrombosis requires excellence in multiple domains: (Connors 2015; Hetzer et al. 1998).

- careful patient selection,
- appropriate device sizing and placement,
- regular monitoring,
- adjustment of anticoagulant therapy, and
- optimization of underlying conditions like anemia and infections.

By implementing these preventive measures, the risk of pump thrombosis can be effectively minimized.

4.2 Console or Power Failure

Console or power failure in pediatric VADs, although extremely uncommon, is a critical concern. However, there are limited analyses regarding power failure in pediatric VADs. To offer some context, a retrospective analysis of device malfunction in patients supported with left ventricular assist device (LVAD) reported device malfunction occurring at an incidence of roughly 3.73 per 1000 patient-days in the Heartmate II, and it was found that controller failure and battery failure accounted for 30% and 20% of all device malfunctions, respectively, albeit in adult patients (Kormos et al. 2017). A pediatric specific analysis of the Pedimacs registry evaluated data from 30 hospitals that implanted 508 devices in 423 patients who were younger than 19 years of age between September 19, 2012, and December 31, 2017. This analysis found that the incidence of early device malfunction (within 3 months) was 20% and the incidence of late device malfunction (beyond 3 months) was 7%, although type of malfunction was not specified (Morales et al. 2019). However, only one death in this patient cohort was attributed to device malfunction; it is likely that a majority of these device malfunctions are not console or power failure derived. Regardless, VADs are fundamentally machines and as such they have the possibility of failure. Even with systems of protocolized protection and constant maintenance, devices fail and humans make errors. Pediatric VAD console or power failure can lead to sudden interruptions in MCS, jeopardizing patient safety. Preventive measures such as regular maintenance and inspections of the VAD system, including the console and backup power sources, are vital (Reagor 2012). Institutions should have protocols in place for immediate response and backup plans, utilizing uninterruptible power supply systems or battery backups. Healthcare providers must be well-trained in recognizing and managing console or power failure, and regular drills can enhance their preparedness. Prompt action, including switching to backup power and assessing the clinical status of the patient, is crucial during such events. Ensuring a swift and effective response minimizes potential harm to the patient and maintains circulatory support until the issue is resolved.

4.3 Pulsatile Versus Continuous-Flow Ventricular Assist Device

The nature of how fluid is pushed through space is what defines the difference between a pulsatile versus continuous-flow VAD, and as such, complications can be specific to each device type. Pulsatile-flow VADs (PF-VAD) mimic the natural pulsatile flow of the heart, while continuous-flow VADs (CF-VAD) provide a constant flow of blood.

Pulsatile flow involves a pump within the VAD that is programmed to expand and engulf a set amount of volume, and the pump then uses positive displacement to move blood to the periphery. The pump has a cavity that expands to receive a set amount of volume, and the pump eventually contracts to displace that volume to the aorta and circulate blood around the body. Pulsatile flow more closely resembles native cardiac output, offering pulsatile end-organ perfusion (Loor and Gonzalez-Stawinski 2012). PF-VADs are often preferred in smaller children or those with complex congenital heart disease (Bleiweis et al. 2023). The Berlin Heart (Berlin EXCOR [Berlin Heart, Inc., Berlin, Germany]) is a pulsatile paracorporeal VAD that is commonly used in neonates, infants, and smaller children [https://www.berlinheart.com/].

VADs that use continuous flow are characterized by centrifugal or axial flow pumps propelled by a magnet-controlled central rotor. Continuous-flow LVADs typically deliver a non-pulsatile stream of blood from the left ventricle (LV) to the systemic circulation. The magnets are activated by changes in current detected by coils within the pump, leading to precise blood flow. Some CF-VADs are paracorporeal while others are implantable (Loor and Gonzalez-Stawinski 2012). Implantable CF-VADs are commonly used in older children, adolescents, and adults (Cheng et al. 2014b). Paracorporeal CF-VADs include the PediMag (Abbott, Pleasanton, California) and CentriMag (Abbott, Pleasanton, California) [https://www.cardiovascular.abbott/content/dam/cv/cardiovascular/hcp/products/heart-failure/centrimag/documents/hf-centrimag-pedimag-pumps-spec-sheet.pdf]. Meanwhile, the HeartMate 3 (Abbott, Pleasanton, California) is an implantable CF-VAD. [https://www.cardiovascular.abbott/us/en/hcp/products/heart-failure/left-ventricular-assist-devices/heartmate-3/about.html].

The Medtronic HeartWare Ventricular Assist Device (HVAD) System (HeartWare International Inc., Medtronic, Framingham, Massachusetts) is another example of an implantable CF-VAD; however, the HeartWare HVAD is no longer available. On June 3, 2021, Medtronic stopped the sale and distribution of the HeartWare Ventricular Assist Device (HVAD) system given the increased risk of mortality and neurological adverse events in patients using the device, and a malfunction where the device may fail to restart. [https://www.fda.gov/medical-devices/cardiovascular-devices/medtronic-heartware-ventricular-assist-device-hvad-system].

Complications will vary between PF-VADs and CF-VADs, and there have been conflicting reports regarding when to use which device in certain populations of pediatric patients, with institutional recommendations and preferences varying. At the University of Florida, in small patients, and especially small patients with functionally univentricular circulation supported with single ventricle-ventricular assist device (sVAD) (Figs. 3 and 4), we prefer PF-VADs rather than CF-VADs (Bleiweis et al. 2023), because we believe that:

- pulsatile VAD is more physiologic,
- pulsatile VAD is easier to manage,
- the management of patients on pulsatile VAD is more intuitive to the healthcare team,
- pulsatile VAD is associated with decreased risk of pulmonary overcirculation, and
- pulsatile VAD is associated with improved renal function.

Other groups, however, have regarded CF-VAD as superior to PF-VAD for isolated systemic ventricular support (Horne et al. 2015). It is worth noting that the field of pediatric VADs continues to evolve, and ongoing research aims to further optimize VAD technology and outcomes. Hybrid devices that combine elements of both pulsatile and continuous-flow mechanisms are also being explored (Lichtenstein et al. 2021; Throckmorton et al. 2021).

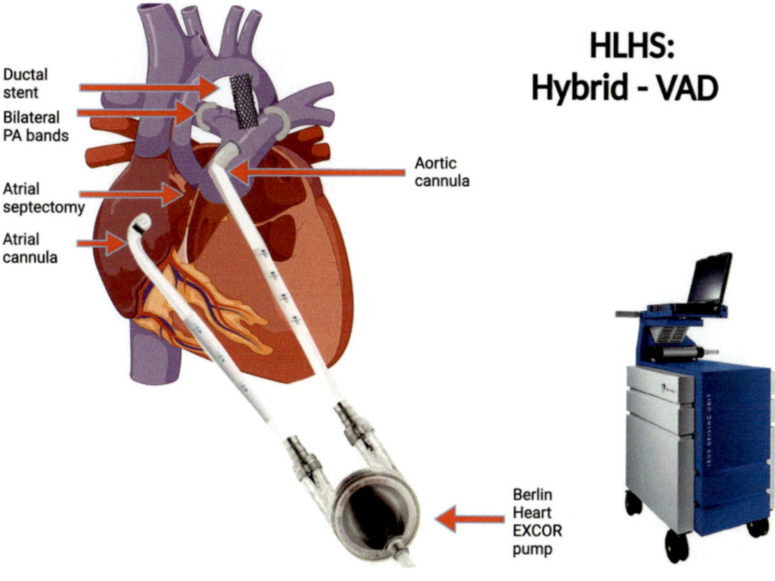

Fig. 3 Hybrid + single ventricle-ventricular assist device approach for patients with functionally univentricular ductal-dependent systemic circulation. *HLHS* hypoplastic left heart syndrome, *PA* pulmonary artery, *VAD* ventricular assist device

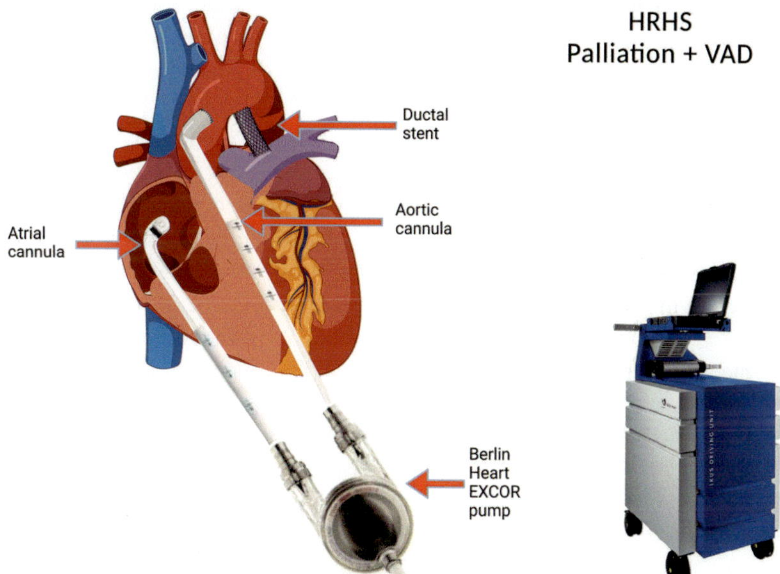

Fig. 4 Palliation + single ventricle-ventricular assist device approach for patients with functionally univentricular ductal-dependent pulmonary circulation. *HRHS* hypoplastic right heart syndrome, *VAD* ventricular assist device

4.4 Ventricular Assist Device Pump Exchanges

Berlin Heart VAD pump exchanges do not necessarily represent a complication experienced by the patient because Berlin Heart VAD pump exchanges may be performed at the bedside in the ICU for a variety of indications including upsizing the pump secondary to the growth of the patient. Berlin Heart VAD pump exchanges may also be performed in the setting of other complications, including stroke and sepsis. One large study reported 46 device exchanges among 48 VAD-supported pediatric patients (Fraser et al. 2012). The most common indication for VAD exchange is the identification of visible pump deposits, although these pump exchanges serve different purposes based on the indication for exchange (Maeda et al. 2018). When visible pump deposits are identified, device exchange may be performed to reduce the risk of a thromboembolic event. In the setting of stroke, pump exchange may be performed as a precautionary measure even if no device thrombi are identified. Pump exchanges can also be performed for benign reasons. For example, patients requiring an upgrade in device size secondary to growth may undergo pump exchange.

Protocols for evaluating devices and for performing device exchange differ by institution (Fraser et al. 2012; Maeda et al. 2018; Hetzer et al. 2006; Schweiger et al. 2013). Generally, most institutions have a protocol for periodically examining the pump for thrombi. At one institution, Maeda and colleagues reported a protocol of visually assessing the device hourly in the ICU and every 4 h on the acute care floor, with increasing frequency of assessment of the VAD in the setting of any of the following issues: (Maeda et al. 2018).

- infection,
- bleeding,
- subtherapeutic anticoagulation, and
- incomplete ejection.

Visual assessment should include assessment of the following components:

- the inflow and outflow valves,
- the inflow and outflow cannulas, and
- the pump body.

The inflow and outflow valves should especially be carefully assessed. In one study of 67 Berlin Heart VAD pump exchanges, 73% of deposits were located in the outflow valve and 22% were located in the inflow valve (Maeda et al. 2018). Other key findings from that study included that smaller pumps (compared with larger pumps) and right ventricular assist devices (compared with LVADs) required increased frequency of exchange. Importantly, no studies have identified an association between the frequency of pump exchange and incidence of stroke (Fraser et al. 2012; Hetzer et al. 2006; Schweiger et al. 2013). It is a fact that pump exchanges

- can be performed at the bedside without sedation (or with minimal sedation),
- can be performed with low risk, and
- may potentially improve the outcomes of these patients.

5 Future Research

5.1 Long-Term Neurodevelopmental Outcomes

Some research has been conducted on the long-term neurodevelopmental outcomes of children who have undergone ECMO and/or VAD support. However, the results obtained from these studies have been inconsistent. For instance, one study focused on children under the age of 6 years who were supported with a Berlin Heart paracorporeal VAD through the Complex Pediatric Therapies Follow-up Program (CPTFP) (VanderPluym et al. 2017). This study revealed that 75% of the patients had radiographic evidence of brain injury at some point before, during, or after VAD implantation. Additionally, neurologic physical examinations were abnormal in 62.5% of the children during follow-up (VanderPluym et al. 2017). A comparison between VAD patients with normal neurologic physical examinations and those with abnormal neurologic physical examinations showed significantly lower intelligence quotient (IQ), Visual-Motor Integration (VMI), and Adaptive Behavior Assessment System-II (ABAS-II) scores in the latter group. This finding suggests that abnormal neurologic physical examinations following VAD implantation increase the risk of lower intelligence, stroke, and other brain injuries (VanderPluym et al. 2017). However, it is important to note that this study only examined a small cohort of children under the age of 6 (n = 16) (VanderPluym et al. 2017).

Another study focused on pediatric heart transplant recipients who required VAD support as a bridge to transplantation (n = 9). This study assessed intellectual functioning, memory, processing speed, and perceptual reasoning and comprehension. This study reported that 78% of the children performed in the average range of other children their age who had undergone direct cardiac transplantation without VAD support (Stein et al. 2013).

Another comprehensive study examined pediatric VAD patients 8 years of age or older who had been on VAD support until heart transplantation. This study concluded that 40% of these patients received a psychiatric diagnosis, mainly consisting of adjustment and mood disorders. Additionally, it was found that the need for VAD support was independently associated with psychiatric diagnosis and antidepressant therapy in this database derived cohort (Diaz et al. 2020).

Long-term effects of VAD implantation on the psychological functioning of children have also been studied, but similar to the studies of short-term neurodevelopmental outcomes, the results have been inconsistent and based on small cohorts of patients. Some studies report that up to 62.5% of patients experience psychiatric symptoms at 1- and 6-months post-VAD implantation follow-up (n = 5), while other case studies have reported improvements in psychological functioning following VAD implantation (n = 3) (Ozbaran et al. 2012, 2015). Overall, the development of short-term and long-term psychiatric disorders following VAD implantation is a complex issue. There appears to be a relationship between patient neurodevelopment, psychological function, and VAD implantation; however, more comprehensive research analyzing larger cohorts of patients is needed to address the existing inconsistencies in available data.

Future directions in neurodevelopmental testing following VAD implantation in pediatric patients should focus on addressing existing gaps in knowledge and providing comprehensive insights; these directions include:

- conducting long-term follow-up studies to assess persistence of deficits or improvements over time,
- enrolling larger cohorts to enhance statistical power and generalizability,
- examining neurodevelopmental outcomes across different age groups,
- examining neurodevelopmental outcomes across different types of VAD (e.g., PF-VADs versus CF-VADs and implantable VADs versus paracorporeal VADs),
- incorporating neuroimaging techniques to identify structural and functional brain changes,
- investigating the influence of psychosocial factors on outcomes,
- conducting intervention trials to explore effectiveness of early interventions,
- implementing longitudinal study designs to track developmental trajectories, and
- assessing the impact of VAD support on neurodevelopment.

Additionally, utilizing a consistent battery of comprehensive neurocognitive assessments to evaluate various domains is key to reliable and standardized findings; such domains include:

- intelligence,
- memory,
- attention,
- executive functions, and
- academic achievement.

This strategy will provide a more detailed understanding of the specific neurocognitive profiles associated with VAD implantation and support. By pursuing these directions, researchers can deepen their understanding and develop targeted interventions to optimize long-term neurocognitive and psychosocial functioning in pediatric VAD patients.

5.2 Neurodevelopmental Testing

The following five common tests are typically used that assess various domains of neurodevelopment in pediatric patients: (StatPearls 2023; Marino et al. 2010; Frandsen and Higginson 1951; Basnet et al. 2015).

- Bayley-IV Test,
- Pediatric Cardiac Quality of Life Inventory (PCQLI),
- Stanford-Binet Test (SB-5),
- Wechsler Intelligence Scale for Children (WISC-V), and
- Woodcock-Johnson III Test (WJ-III NU ACH).

The main focus of all tests is on assessing cognitive and intellectual functioning. However, the Bayley-IV Test and PCQLI cover the widest range of domains. Both tests evaluate physical, emotional, and social functioning. In addition, the Bayley-IV Test assesses cognitive functioning and language, while the PCQLI also includes assessment of academic development. While most of these tests can be administered to any patient within the specified age range, the PCQLI is specifically designed for children who have undergone cardiac surgery, making the PCQLI a more tailored test in that context. All tests require professional administration, and most have a cost of over $1000 per test. The Bayley-IV Test is available at a lower cost of $343 if the assessment of social, emotional, and behavioral development is omitted. The WJ-III NU ACH is the least expensive test but focuses primarily on cognition and academic functioning.

Furthermore, determining the most ideal test to use in future research depends on the specific research goals, target population, and the domains of neurodevelopment being examined. However, the Bayley-IV Test and the PCQLI appear to be the most comprehensive in assessing multiple domains of neurodevelopment in pediatric patients, although they are not without limitations.

The Bayley-IV Test is suitable for a wide range of neurodevelopmental assessments; this test evaluates:

- cognitive functioning,
- language,
- physical functioning,
- emotional functioning, and
- social functioning.

The Bayley-IV Test is commonly used in early childhood and can provide valuable insights into the overall developmental profile of young children. However, it cannot assess neurodevelopment beyond 42 months of age (StatPearls 2023).

As a focused alternative, the PCQLI is specifically designed for children who have undergone cardiac surgery, emphasizing testing of physical, emotional, social, and academic development (Marino et al. 2010). As such, we recommend that if the research involves pediatric patients who have received VAD implants or undergone cardiac procedures, the PCQLI may be better suited for assessing the specific challenges and outcomes associated with these interventions. Ultimately, the choice of test will depend on the specific research questions, the target population, and the desired domains of neurodevelopment to be evaluated. Clinicians and researchers should carefully consider the strengths and limitations of each test and select the test that aligns best with their clinical and research objectives. Additionally, consulting with experts in the field of pediatric neurodevelopmental assessment can provide valuable guidance in selecting the most appropriate test for specific clinical objectives or study design.

5.3 Implantable Devices

A clear need exists to improve ventricular assist device (VAD) support options for pediatric patients, and especially those with complex functionally univentricular circulation and those with primary diastolic dysfunction (PDD). These patients traditionally have poor outcomes when using pulsatile VAD support with the Berlin Heart. Survival rates for patients with these conditions are reported to be 42% and 50% for functionally univentricular patients and patients with PDD, respectively (Peng et al. 2019; Weinstein et al. 2014; Su and Menteer 2017). At the University of Florida, we have developed a novel approach to supporting functionally univentricular patients with paracorporeal sVAD; (Bleiweis et al. 2022, 2023) our results with paracorporeal sVAD are promising for this challenging subset of patients (Bleiweis et al. 2022, 2023).

Such advances, as well as the development of new implantable devices, will greatly impact the therapeutic options for pediatric patients requiring MCS. Technological improvements in pump design, refined surgical techniques, and improved patient management have significantly contributed to increased rates of survival of patients supported with VAD (Burki and Adachi 2017; Shaffer et al. 2021). These factors are the main driving forces behind improving patient outcomes. A focus on developing devices that can reduce stroke, nonsurgical bleeding, and infection will be crucial in the next decade of improving MCS technology. Moreover, a focus on developing smaller implantable VADs suitable for younger and smaller patients is critical.

Advancements in VAD technology designed for adults, such as smaller and more efficient implantable devices like the HeartMate 3 VAD, also have a significant impact on the pediatric population. The HeartMate 3 VAD, a fully magnetically levitated centrifugal-flow LVAD, has gained popularity among larger pediatric patients and those with congenital heart disease, due to its implantability, ergonomic size, and low incidence of mortality and adverse events (Peng et al. 2019; Mehra et al. 2019). In a multicenter registry analysis of the HeartMate 3 in pediatric patients and patients with congenital heart disease (n = 35), there was only one reported death on device, and all patients who underwent cardiac transplantation had no posttransplant mortality. Notably, there were no episodes of stroke or thrombosis (O'Connor et al. 2020). This experience provides an optimistic outlook on the future of pediatric VADs that focuses on reducing device related and postoperative complications.

Ongoing clinical trials, like the Pump for Kids, Infants, and Neonates (PumpKIN) trial, evaluating the investigational Jarvik 2015 VAD in pediatric patients with heart failure, could potentially offer promising results. The Jarvik 2015 VAD is the first and currently the only implantable CF-VAD specifically designed for small children. While we await the results of the PumpKIN trial, compassionate use cases of patients supported with the Jarvik 2015 VAD and associated outcomes have been reported, demonstrating the feasibility of the Jarvik 2015 VAD for pediatric patients. In a small sample of two patients under the age of 13 months, successful cardiac transplantation was achieved with the use of the Jarvik 2015 VAD as a bridge to transplantation (Spinner et al. 2021).

Promising advancements in totally implantable VADs can also lead to generalized improvements in MCS. The implementation of thermal energy transfer system (TETS) technology into MCS has resulted in lower incidences of device-related infections compared to MCS devices with external components. However, the clinical instances of TETS, such as AbioCor and LionHEAT LVAD, did not achieve satisfactory long-term rates of survival (Slaughter and Myers 2010; Mehta et al. 2001; Dowling et al. 2004).

Finally, significant progress has been made in surgical techniques, particularly in less invasive approaches to accessing the heart and performing off-pump procedures. These advancements offer multiple potential advantages, including: (Shaffer et al. 2021).

- minimizing scar tissue formation for future surgeries,
- reducing systemic inflammation,
- decreasing surgical trauma and bleeding during and after the operation,
- lowering the risk of complications in the sternal wound,
- improving cosmetic outcomes, and
- potentially reducing the occurrence of right ventricular failure following surgery.

In summary, advancements in MCS offer promising prospects for improving outcomes in pediatric patients with complex heart conditions, through the development of new implantable devices, technological enhancements, refined surgical techniques, and improved patient management.

5.4 Enhanced Biocompatibility

The human body is not naturally adapted to function flawlessly with the assistance of machines, and heavily relying on immunosuppressive medication, while appropriate for transplantation of other organs, has its limitations in terms of VAD and ECMO compatibility. The materials and substances used in these devices do not inherently interact harmoniously with the cells, tissues, and organs of the body, and it takes time for the body to adjust to such sudden surgical interventions. A major issue that arises with VAD and ECMO is the immune response of the body to foreign objects, leading to excessive inflammation and an increased risk of blood clot formation, which can cause various additional complications. This immune response is one of the primary causes of failure in cardiac biomaterials (Weng et al. 2012).

When developing cardiac medical devices, extensive research and processes of development take place, considering various factors, including: (Alipour et al. 2022).

- biocompatibility,
- mechanical properties,
- toxicity,
- infection prevention,
- surface properties,
- degradability, and
- cost.

Biocompatibility is typically prioritized as the foundational criterion in device design, aiming to balance the response of the human body, while ensuring device functionality. Surface modification, through the immobilization of bioactive molecules, is commonly employed to enhance biocompatibility and reduce the risk of infections (Nie et al. 2016; Yang et al. 2018; Kazemzadeh-Narbat et al. 2021). Surface modifications are viewed as a promising approach to achieve the next generation of cardiac medical devices without significantly altering their design (Coronel-Meneses et al. 2023). However, future research is crucial in exploring novel materials and surface modifications. Additionally, emphasis must also be placed on the following opportunities:

- improving hemocompatibility to minimize blood damage and clot formation,
- mitigating immune activation and inflammation,
- assessing long-term biocompatibility effects, and
- exploring personalized approaches based on patient-specific factors.

These efforts will play a pivotal role in improving ECMO technology and advancing highly biocompatible pediatric VADs.

5.5 Xenotransplantation

Xenotransplantation, the process of transplanting organs from one species to another, has been experimented with and researched for multiple decades. Currently, waitlist mortality for neonates, infants, and children awaiting heart transplantation is among the highest in solid organ transplantation (Zafar et al. 2015). Xenotransplantation has the potential to vastly reduce the shortage of access to critically needed organ grafts. Due to advances in gene editing, hearts from pigs optimal for xenotransplantation have kept nonhuman primates alive for up to 9 months (Mohiuddin et al. 2022). However, this complicated and intricate process requires additional research and testing to become a reliable method readily available to be used at hospitals around the world. Within neonates and infants with congenital heart disease, heart xenotransplantation could be a viable option, but there is still a large gap between theoretical implementation and practice (Konstantinov et al. 2022).

Historically, instances of human xenotransplantation began in 1984, when the first operation was performed by Dr. Leonard Bailey, on an infant who received a baboon heart that kept her alive for 21 days. This operation paved the path for both clinical cardiac transplantation in neonates and infants and the coming decades of research and devotion to understanding the science of xenotransplantation (Wadiwala et al. 2022). Recent xenograft clinical trials have offered compelling results. On January 7, 2022, at University of Maryland, a 57-year-old man received a 10G-pig xenoheart. Remarkably, following transplant, the xenograft functioned immediately and ECMO was severed after a few days (Rothblatt 2022). The patient survived for 2 months after which his status started to decline, and he passed away from multiorgan failure (Carrier et al. 2022). Xenotransplantation has come a long way, but there is still work to be done before optimal outcomes can be achieved.

References

Alexy T, Detterich J, Connes P, et al. Physical properties of blood and their relationship to clinical conditions. Front Physiol. 2022;13:906768. https://doi.org/10.3389/fphys.2022.906768.

Alipour S, Taromian F, Ghomi ER, Zare M, Singh S, Ramakrishna S. Nitinol: from historical milestones to functional properties and biomedical applications. Proc Inst Mech Eng H. 2022;236(11):1595–612. https://doi.org/10.1177/09544119221123176.

Almond CS, Morales DL, Blackstone EH, et al. Berlin heart EXCOR pediatric ventricular assist device for bridge to heart transplantation in US children. Circulation. 2013;127(16):1702–11. https://doi.org/10.1161/CIRCULATIONAHA.112.000685.

Annich GM, Meinhardt JP, Mowery KA, et al. Reduced platelet activation and thrombosis in extracorporeal circuits coated with nitric oxide release polymers. Crit Care Med. 2000;28(4):915–20. https://doi.org/10.1097/00003246-200004000-00001.

Auerbach SR, Richmond ME, Schumacher KR, et al. Infectious complications of ventricular assist device use in children in the United States: data from the pediatric interagency registry for mechanical circulatory support (Pedimacs). J Heart Lung Transplant. 2018;37(1):46–53. https://doi.org/10.1016/j.healun.2017.09.013.

Barbaro RP, Paden ML, Guner YS, et al. Pediatric extracorporeal life support organization registry international report 2016. ASAIO J. 2017;63(4):456–63. https://doi.org/10.1097/MAT.0000000000000603.

Basnet P, Noggle CA, Dean RS. Neurocognitive problems in children and adolescents with depression using the CHC theory and the WJ-III. Appl Neuropsychol Child. 2015;4(4):257–65. https://doi.org/10.1080/21622965.2014.908124.

Bembea MM, Annich G, Rycus P, Oldenburg G, Berkowitz I, Pronovost P. Variability in anticoagulation management of patients on extracorporeal membrane oxygenation: an international survey. Pediatr Crit Care Med. 2013;14(2):e77–84. https://doi.org/10.1097/PCC.0b013e31827127e4.

Bembea MM, Rizkalla N, Freedy J, et al. Plasma biomarkers of brain injury as diagnostic tools and outcome predictors after extracorporeal membrane oxygenation. Crit Care Med. 2015;43(10):2202–11. https://doi.org/10.1097/CCM.0000000000001145.

Besser MW, Klein AA. The coagulopathy of cardiopulmonary bypass. Crit Rev Clin Lab Sci Theor Decis. 2010;47(5–6):197–212. https://doi.org/10.3109/10408363.2010.549291.

Betrus C, Remenapp R, Charpie J, et al. Enhanced hemolysis in pediatric patients requiring extracorporeal membrane oxygenation and continuous renal replacement therapy. Ann Thorac Cardiovasc Surg. 2007;13(6):378–83.

Biffi S, Di Bella S, Scaravilli V, et al. Infections during extracorporeal membrane oxygenation: epidemiology, risk factors, pathogenesis and prevention. Int J Antimicrob Agents. 2017;50(1):9–16. https://doi.org/10.1016/j.ijantimicag.2017.02.025.

Bizzarro MJ, Conrad SA, Kaufman DA, Rycus P. Extracorporeal life support organization task force on infections EtMO. Infections acquired during extracorporeal membrane oxygenation in neonates, children, and adults. Pediatr Crit Care Med. 2011;12(3):277–81. https://doi.org/10.1097/PCC.0b013e3181e28894.

Bleiweis MS, Fudge JC, Peek GJ, et al. Ventricular assist device support in neonates and infants with a failing functionally univentricular circulation. JTCVS Tech. 2022;13:194–204. https://doi.org/10.1016/j.xjtc.2021.09.056.

Bleiweis MS, Stukov Y, Philip J, et al. Analysis of 82 children supported with pulsatile paracorporeal ventricular assist device: comparison of patients with biventricular versus univentricular circulation. Semin Thorac Cardiovasc Surg. 2023;35(2):367–76. https://doi.org/10.1053/j.semtcvs.2022.05.002.

Boehme AK, Pamboukian SV, George JF, et al. Predictors of thromboembolic events in patients with ventricular assist device. ASAIO J. 2015;61(6):640–7. https://doi.org/10.1097/MAT.0000000000000284.

Bowers KJ, Deveber GA, Ferriero DM, Roach ES, Vexler ZS, Maria BL. Cerebrovascular disease in children: recent advances in diagnosis and management. J Child Neurol. 2011;26(9):1074–100. https://doi.org/10.1177/0883073811413585.

Burki S, Adachi I. Pediatric ventricular assist devices: current challenges and future prospects. Vasc Health Risk Manag. 2017;13:177–85. https://doi.org/10.2147/VHRM.S82379.

Cabrera AG, Khan MS, Morales DL, et al. Infectious complications and outcomes in children supported with left ventricular assist devices. J Heart Lung Transplant. 2013;32(5):518–24. https://doi.org/10.1016/j.healun.2013.02.002.

Cannon A, Elliott T, Ballew C, et al. Variability in infection control measures for the percutaneous lead among programs implanting long-term ventricular assist devices in the United States. Prog Transplant. 2012;22(4):351–9. https://doi.org/10.7182/pit2012612.

Carrier AN, Verma A, Mohiuddin M, et al. Xenotransplantation: a new era. Front Immunol. 2022;13:900594. https://doi.org/10.3389/fimmu.2022.900594.

Cashen K, Reeder R, Dalton HJ, et al. Acquired infection during neonatal and pediatric extracorporeal membrane oxygenation. Perfusion. 2018;33(6):472–82. https://doi.org/10.1177/0267659118766436.

Castagnola E, Gargiullo L, Loy A, et al. Epidemiology of infectious complications during extracorporeal membrane oxygenation in children: a single-center experience in 46 runs. Pediatr Infect Dis J. 2018;37(7):624–6. https://doi.org/10.1097/INF.0000000000001873.

Chan KM, Wan WTP, Ling L, So JMC, Wong CHL, Tam SBS. Management of circuit air in extracorporeal membrane oxygenation: a single center experience. ASAIO J. 2022;68(3):e39–43. https://doi.org/10.1097/MAT.0000000000001494.

Cheng R, Hachamovitch R, Kittleson M, et al. Complications of extracorporeal membrane oxygenation for treatment of cardiogenic shock and cardiac arrest: a meta-analysis of 1,866 adult patients. Ann Thorac Surg. 2014a;97(2):610–6. https://doi.org/10.1016/j.athoracsur.2013.09.008.

Cheng A, Williamitis CA, Slaughter MS. Comparison of continuous-flow and pulsatile-flow left ventricular assist devices: is there an advantage to pulsatility? Ann Cardiothorac Surg. 2014b;3(6):573–81. https://doi.org/10.3978/j.issn.2225-319X.2014.08.24.

Cho SM, Ziai W, Mayasi Y, et al. Noninvasive neurological monitoring in extracorporeal membrane oxygenation. ASAIO J. 2020;66(4):388–93. https://doi.org/10.1097/MAT.0000000000001013.

Connors JM. Anticoagulation management of left ventricular assist devices. Am J Hematol. 2015;90(2):175–8. https://doi.org/10.1002/ajh.23836.

Coronel-Meneses D, Sánchez-Trasviña C, Ratera I, Mayolo-Deloisa K. Strategies for surface coatings of implantable cardiac medical devices. Front Bioeng Biotechnol. 2023;11:1173260. https://doi.org/10.3389/fbioe.2023.1173260.

Dalton HJ, Reeder R, Garcia-Filion P, et al. Factors associated with bleeding and thrombosis in children receiving extracorporeal membrane oxygenation. Am J Respir Crit Care Med. 2017;196(6):762–71. https://doi.org/10.1164/rccm.201609-1945OC.

Dalton HJ, Cashen K, Reeder RW, et al. Hemolysis during pediatric extracorporeal membrane oxygenation: associations with circuitry, complications, and mortality. Pediatr Crit Care Med. 2018;19(11):1067–76. https://doi.org/10.1097/PCC.0000000000001709.

Diaz I, Thurm C, Hall M, et al. Disorders of adjustment, mood, and anxiety in children and adolescents undergoing heart transplantation and the Association of Ventricular Assist Device Support. J Pediatr. 2020;217:20–24.e1. https://doi.org/10.1016/j.jpeds.2019.10.022.

Doerrfuss JI, Kilic T, Ahmadi M, Holtkamp M, Weber JE. Quantitative and qualitative EEG as a prediction tool for outcome and complications in acute stroke patients. Clin EEG Neurosci. 2020;51(2):121–9. https://doi.org/10.1177/1550059419875916.

Donlan RM. Biofilm elimination on intravascular catheters: important considerations for the infectious disease practitioner. Clin Infect Dis. 2011;52(8):1038–45. https://doi.org/10.1093/cid/cir077.

Dornia C, Philipp A, Bauer S, et al. Analysis of thrombotic deposits in extracorporeal membrane oxygenators by multidetector computed tomography. ASAIO J. 2014;60(6):652–6. https://doi.org/10.1097/MAT.0000000000000133.

Douglass BH, Keenan AL, Purohit DM. Bacterial and fungal infection in neonates undergoing venoarterial extracorporeal membrane oxygenation: an analysis of the registry data of the extracorporeal life support organization. Artif Organs. 1996;20(3):202–8. https://doi.org/10.1111/j.1525-1594.1996.tb04428.x.

Dowling RD, Gray LA, Etoch SW, et al. Initial experience with the AbioCor implantable replacement heart system. J Thorac Cardiovasc Surg. 2004;127(1):131–41. https://doi.org/10.1016/j.jtcvs.2003.07.023.

Doyle AJ, Hunt BJ. Current understanding of how extracorporeal membrane oxygenators activate haemostasis and other blood components. Front Med (Lausanne). 2018;5:352. https://doi.org/10.3389/fmed.2018.00352.

Drews T, Stiller B, Hübler M, Weng Y, Berger F, Hetzer R. Coagulation management in pediatric mechanical circulatory support. ASAIO J. 2007;53(5):640–5. https://doi.org/10.1097/MAT.0b013e3181492929.

Drop JGF, Wildschut ED, Gunput STG, de Hoog M, van Ommen CH. Challenges in maintaining the hemostatic balance in children undergoing extracorporeal membrane oxygenation: a systematic literature review. Front Pediatr. 2020;8:612467. https://doi.org/10.3389/fped.2020.612467.

Drop JG, Erdem Ö, Wildschut ED, et al. Use of rotational thromboelastometry to predict hemostatic complications in pediatric patients undergoing extracorporeal membrane oxygenation: A retrospective cohort study. Res Pract Thromb Haemost. 2021;5(5):e12553. https://doi.org/10.1002/rth2.12553.

Eckman PM, John R. Bleeding and thrombosis in patients with continuous-flow ventricular assist devices. Circulation. 2012;125(24):3038–47. https://doi.org/10.1161/CIRCULATIONAHA.111.040246.

Ezetendu C, Baloglu O, Othman HF, Nandakumar V, Latifi S, Aly H. Stroke in pediatric ECMO patients: analysis of the National Inpatient Sample (NIS) database. Pediatr Res. 2022;92(3):754–61. https://doi.org/10.1038/s41390-022-02088-7.

Felling RJ, Rafay MF, Bernard TJ, et al. Predicting recovery and outcome after pediatric stroke: results from the international pediatric stroke study. Ann Neurol. 2020;87(6):840–52. https://doi.org/10.1002/ana.25718.

Fragasso T, Ricci Z, Grutter G, et al. Incidence of healthcare-associated infections in a pediatric population with an extracorporeal ventricular assist device.

Artif Organs. 2011;35(11):1110–4. https://doi.org/10.1111/j.1525-1594.2011.01389.x.

Frandsen AN, Higginson JB. The Stanford-Binet and the Wechsler intelligence scale for children. J Consult Psychol. 1951;15(3):236–8. https://doi.org/10.1037/h0059816.

Fraser CD, Jaquiss RD, Rosenthal DN, et al. Prospective trial of a pediatric ventricular assist device. N Engl J Med. 2012;367(6):532–41. https://doi.org/10.1056/NEJMoa1014164.

Gajkowski EF, Herrera G, Hatton L, Velia Antonini M, Vercaemst L, Cooley E. ELSO guidelines for adult and pediatric extracorporeal membrane oxygenation circuits. ASAIO J. 2022;68(2):133–52. https://doi.org/10.1097/MAT.0000000000001630.

Gbadegesin R, Zhao S, Charpie J, Brophy PD, Smoyer WE, Lin JJ. Significance of hemolysis on extracorporeal life support after cardiac surgery in children. Pediatr Nephrol. 2009;24(3):589–95. https://doi.org/10.1007/s00467-008-1047-z.

Ghbeis MB, Vander Pluym CJ, Thiagarajan RR. Hemostatic challenges in pediatric critical care medicine-hemostatic balance in VAD. Front Pediatr. 2021;9:625–32. https://doi.org/10.3389/fped.2021.625632.

Glater-Welt LB, Schneider JB, Zinger MM, Rosen L, Sweberg TM. Nosocomial bloodstream infections in patients receiving extracorporeal life support: variability in prevention practices: a survey of the extracorporeal life support organization members. J Intensive Care Med. 2016;31(10):654–69. https://doi.org/10.1177/0885066615571540.

Hanekamp MN, Mazer P, van der Cammen-van Zijp MH, et al. Follow-up of newborns treated with extracorporeal membrane oxygenation: a nationwide evaluation at 5 years of age. Crit Care. 2006;10(5):R127. https://doi.org/10.1186/cc5039.

Hannan MM, Husain S, Mattner F, et al. Working formulation for the standardization of definitions of infections in patients using ventricular assist devices. J Heart Lung Transplant. 2011;30(4):375–84. https://doi.org/10.1016/j.healun.2011.01.717.

Hastings SM, Ku DN, Wagoner S, Maher KO, Deshpande S. Sources of circuit thrombosis in pediatric extracorporeal membrane oxygenation. ASAIO J. 2017;63(1):86–92. https://doi.org/10.1097/MAT.0000000000000444.

Heestermans M, Poenou G, Hamzeh-Cognasse H, Cognasse F, Bertoletti L. Anticoagulants: a short history, their mechanism of action, pharmacology, and indications. Cells. 2022;11(20) https://doi.org/10.3390/cells11203214.

Hervey-Jumper SL, Annich GM, Yancon AR, Garton HJ, Muraszko KM, Maher CO. Neurological complications of extracorporeal membrane oxygenation in children. J Neurosurg Pediatr. 2011;7(4):338–44. https://doi.org/10.3171/2011.1.PEDS10443.

Hetzer R, Loebe M, Potapov EV, et al. Circulatory support with pneumatic paracorporeal ventricular assist device in infants and children. Ann Thorac Surg. 1998;66(5):1498–506. https://doi.org/10.1016/s0003-4975(98)00914-x.

Hetzer R, Potapov EV, Stiller B, et al. Improvement in survival after mechanical circulatory support with pneumatic pulsatile ventricular assist devices in pediatric patients. Ann Thorac Surg. 2006;82(3):917–24.; discussion 924-5. https://doi.org/10.1016/j.athoracsur.2006.03.065.

Horne D, Conway J, Rebeyka IM, Buchholz H. Mechanical circulatory support in univentricular hearts: current management. Semin Thorac Cardiovasc Surg Pediatr Card Surg Annu. 2015;18(1):17–24. https://doi.org/10.1053/j.pcsu.2015.02.002.

Hsu MS, Chiu KM, Huang YT, Kao KL, Chu SH, Liao CH. Risk factors for nosocomial infection during extracorporeal membrane oxygenation. J Hosp Infect. 2009;73(3):210–6. https://doi.org/10.1016/j.jhin.2009.07.016.

Huang JY, Monagle P, Massicotte MP, VanderPluym CJ. Antithrombotic therapies in children on durable ventricular assist devices: a literature review. Thromb Res. 2018;172:194–203. https://doi.org/10.1016/j.thromres.2018.02.145.

Huang JY, Ignjatovic V, Sheridan BJ, et al. Bleeding and thrombotic events occur early in children on durable ventricular assist devices. Thromb Res. 2019;173:65–70. https://doi.org/10.1016/j.thromres.2018.11.019.

Jensen AR, Davis C, Gray BW. Cannulation and decannulation techniques for neonatal ECMO. In: Seminars in fetal and neonatal medicine, vol. 27(6). WB Saunders; 2022. p. 101404.

Kaczala GW, Paulus SC, Al-Dajani N, et al. Bloodstream infections in pediatric ECLS: usefulness of daily blood culture monitoring and predictive value of biological markers. The British Columbia experience. Pediatr Surg Int. 2009;25(2):169–73. https://doi.org/10.1007/s00383-008-2299-1.

Kao LS, Fleming GM, Escamilla RJ, Lew DF, Lally KP. Antimicrobial prophylaxis and infection surveillance in extracorporeal membrane oxygenation patients: a multi-institutional survey of practice patterns. ASAIO J. 2011;57(3):231–8. https://doi.org/10.1097/MAT.0b013e31820d19ab.

Kazemzadeh-Narbat M, Cheng H, Chabok R, et al. Strategies for antimicrobial peptide coatings on medical devices: a review and regulatory science perspective. Crit Rev Biotechnol. 2021;41(1):94–120. https://doi.org/10.1080/07388551.2020.1828810.

Kim DH, Cho WH, Son J, Lee SK, Yeo HJ. Catastrophic mechanical complications of extracorporeal membrane oxygenation. ASAIO J. 2021;67(9):1000–5. https://doi.org/10.1097/MAT.0000000000001354.

Konstantinov IE, Cooper DKC, Adachi I, et al. Consensus statement on heart xenotransplantation in children: toward clinical translation. J Thorac Cardiovasc Surg. 2022; https://doi.org/10.1016/j.jtcvs.2022.09.001.

Kormos RL, McCall M, Althouse A, et al. Left ventricular assist device malfunctions: it is more than just the pump. Circulation. 2017;136(18):1714–25. https://doi.org/10.1161/CIRCULATIONAHA.117.027360.

Kumar A, Keshavamurthy S, Abraham JG, Toyoda Y. Massive air embolism caused by a central venous catheter during extracorporeal membrane oxygenation. J Extra Corpor Technol. 2019;51(1):9–11.

Lafç G, Budak AB, Yener A, Cicek OF. Use of extracorporeal membrane oxygenation in adults. Heart Lung Circ. 2014;23(1):10–23. https://doi.org/10.1016/j.hlc.2013.08.009.

Lehle K, Philipp A, Gleich O, et al. Efficiency in extracorporeal membrane oxygenation-cellular deposits on polymethylpentene membranes increase resistance to blood flow and reduce gas exchange capacity. ASAIO J. 2008;54(6):612–7. https://doi.org/10.1097/MAT.0b013e318186a807.

Lichtenstein KM, Tunuguntla HP, Peng DM, Buchholz H, Conway J. Pediatric ventricular assist device registries: update and perspectives in the era of miniaturized continuous-flow pumps. Ann Cardiothorac Surg. 2021;10(3):329–38. https://doi.org/10.21037/acs-2020-cfmcs-18.

Loor G, Gonzalez-Stawinski G. Pulsatile vs. continuous flow in ventricular assist device therapy. Best Pract Res Clin Anaesthesiol. 2012;26(2):105–15. https://doi.org/10.1016/j.bpa.2012.03.004.

Lopez-Lopez G, Pascual A, Perea EJ. Effect of plastic catheter material on bacterial adherence and viability. J Med Microbiol. 1991;34(6):349–53. https://doi.org/10.1099/00222615-34-6-349.

Lorts A, Eghtesady P, Mehegan M, et al. Outcomes of children supported with devices labeled as “temporary” or short term: a report from the pediatric interagency registry for mechanical circulatory support. J Heart Lung Transplant. 2018;37(1):54–60. https://doi.org/10.1016/j.healun.2017.10.023.

Lorusso R, Taccone FS, Belliato M, et al. Brain monitoring in adult and pediatric ECMO patients: the importance of early and late assessments. Minerva Anestesiol. 2017;83(10):1061–74. https://doi.org/10.23736/S0375-9393.17.11911-5.

Lou S, MacLaren G, Best D, Delzoppo C, Butt W. Hemolysis in pediatric patients receiving centrifugal-pump extracorporeal membrane oxygenation: prevalence, risk factors, and outcomes. Crit Care Med. 2014;42(5):1213–20. https://doi.org/10.1097/CCM.0000000000000128.

Loyaga-Rendon RY, Kazui T, Acharya D. Antiplatelet and anticoagulation strategies for left ventricular assist devices. Ann Transl Med. 2021;9(6):521. https://doi.org/10.21037/atm-20-4849.

Lubnow M, Philipp A, Foltan M, et al. Technical complications during veno-venous extracorporeal membrane oxygenation and their relevance predicting a system-exchange--retrospective analysis of 265 cases. PLoS One. 2014;9(12):e112316. https://doi.org/10.1371/journal.pone.0112316.

Maeda K, Almond C, Hollander SA, et al. Characteristics of deposits and pump exchange in the Berlin heart EXCOR ventricular assist device: experience with 67 cases. Pediatr Transplant. 2018;22(4):e13181. https://doi.org/10.1111/petr.13181.

Marino BS, Tomlinson RS, Wernovsky G, et al. Validation of the pediatric cardiac quality of life inventory. Pediatrics. 2010;126(3):498–508. https://doi.org/10.1542/peds.2009-2973.

Mason PE, Velia Antonini M, Agerstrand CL, Filip De Somer M, Vercaemst L. (2022) Chapter 7: Circuit malfunction and crisis management. In: Brogan TV, Lequier L, Lorusso R, MacLaren G, Peek GJ, (eds). Extracorporeal life support: the ELSO red book. 6 Extracorporeal Life Support Organization; 113–122.

Mattner F, Chaberny IF, Mattner L, Gastmeier P, Tessmann R, Strüber M. Infection control measures and surveillance of patients with ventricular assist devices. Anaesthesist. 2007;56(5):429–36. https://doi.org/10.1007/s00101-007-1155-3.

Mehra MR, Uriel N, Naka Y, et al. A fully magnetically levitated left ventricular assist device—final report. N Engl J Med. 2019;380(17):1618–27. https://doi.org/10.1056/NEJMoa1900486.

Mehta SM, Pae WE, Rosenberg G, et al. The LionHeart LVD-2000: a completely implanted left ventricular assist device for chronic circulatory support. Ann Thorac Surg. 2001;71(Suppl 3):S156–61.; discussion S183-4. https://doi.org/10.1016/s0003-4975(00)02641-2.

Meyer DM, Jessen ME, Eberhart RC. Neonatal extracorporeal membrane oxygenation complicated by sepsis. Extracorporeal life support organization. Ann Thorac Surg. 1995;59(4):975–80. https://doi.org/10.1016/0003-4975(95)00044-l.

Millar JE, Fanning JP, McDonald CI, McAuley DF, Fraser JF. The inflammatory response to extracorporeal membrane oxygenation (ECMO): a review of the pathophysiology. Crit Care. 2016;20(1):387. https://doi.org/10.1186/s13054-016-1570-4.

Mohiuddin MM, Goerlich CE, Singh AK, et al. Progressive genetic modifications of porcine cardiac xenografts extend survival to 9 months. Xenotransplantation. 2022;29(3):e12744. https://doi.org/10.1111/xen.12744.

Montgomery VL, Strotman JM, Ross MP. Impact of multiple organ system dysfunction and nosocomial infections on survival of children treated with extracorporeal membrane oxygenation after heart surgery. Crit Care Med. 2000;28(2):526–31. https://doi.org/10.1097/00003246-200002000-00040.

Morales DLS, Rossano JW, VanderPluym C, et al. Third annual pediatric interagency registry for mechanical circulatory support (pedimacs) report: Preimplant characteristics and outcomes. Ann Thorac Surg. 2019;107(4):993–1004. https://doi.org/10.1016/j.athoracsur.2019.01.038.

Mossadegh C. Monitoring the ECMO. nursing care and ECMO. Cham: Springer; 2017. p. 45–70.

Murphy DA, Hockings LE, Andrews RK, et al. Extracorporeal membrane oxygenation-hemostatic complications. Transfus Med Rev. 2015;29(2):90–101. https://doi.org/10.1016/j.tmrv.2014.12.001.

Neunert C, Chitlur M, van Ommen CH. The changing landscape of anticoagulation in pediatric extracorporeal membrane oxygenation: use of the direct thrombin inhibitors. Front Med (Lausanne). 2022;9:887199. https://doi.org/10.3389/fmed.2022.887199.

Nie B, Ao H, Zhou J, Tang T, Yue B. Biofunctionalization of titanium with bacitracin immobilization shows potential for anti-bacteria, osteogenesis and reduction of macrophage inflammation. Colloids Surf B Biointerfaces. 2016;145:728–39. https://doi.org/10.1016/j.colsurfb.2016.05.089.

Niebler RA, Amdani S, Blume B, et al. Stroke in pediatric ventricular assist device patients-a pedimacs registry analysis. J Heart Lung Transplant. 2021;40(7):662–70. https://doi.org/10.1016/j.healun.2021.03.008.

Nienaber J, Wilhelm MP, Sohail MR. Current concepts in the diagnosis and management of left ventricular assist device infections. Expert Rev Anti-Infect Ther. 2013;11(2):201–10. https://doi.org/10.1586/eri.12.163.

Nijhuis-van der Sanden MW, van der Cammen-van Zijp MH, Janssen AJ, et al. Motor performance in five-year-old extracorporeal membrane oxygenation survivors: a population-based study. Crit Care. 2009;13(2):R47. https://doi.org/10.1186/cc7770.

O'Connor MJ, Lorts A, Davies RR, et al. Early experience with the HeartMate 3 continuous-flow ventricular assist device in pediatric patients and patients with congenital heart disease: a multicenter registry analysis. J Heart Lung Transplant. 2020;39(6):573–9. https://doi.org/10.1016/j.healun.2020.02.007.

O'Neill JM, Schutze GE, Heulitt MJ, Simpson PM, Taylor BJ. Nosocomial infections during extracorporeal membrane oxygenation. Intensive Care Med. 2001;27(8):1247–53. https://doi.org/10.1007/s001340101029.

Ozbaran B, Kose S, Yagdi T, et al. Psychiatric evaluation of children and adolescents with left ventricular assist devices. Psychosom Med. 2012;74(5):554–8. https://doi.org/10.1097/PSY.0b013e318258853a.

Ozbaran M, Yagdi T, Engin C, et al. New era of pediatric ventricular assist devices: let us go to school. Pediatr Transplant. 2015;19(1):82–6. https://doi.org/10.1111/petr.12399.

Parikh NS, Cool J, Karas MG, Boehme AK, Kamel H. Stroke risk and mortality in patients with ventricular assist devices. Stroke. 2016;47(11):2702–6. https://doi.org/10.1161/STROKEAHA.116.014049.

Pascual A. Pathogenesis of catheter-related infections: lessons for new designs. Clin Microbiol Infect. 2002;8(5):256–64. https://doi.org/10.1046/j.1469-0691.2002.00418.x.

Peng DM, Koehl DA, Cantor RS, et al. Outcomes of children with congenital heart disease implanted with ventricular assist devices: an analysis of the pediatric interagency registry for mechanical circulatory support (Pedimacs). J Heart Lung Transplant. 2019;38(4):420–30. https://doi.org/10.1016/j.healun.2018.10.008.

Peng DM, Shezad MF, Lorts A, et al. Decreased risk of strokes in children with ventricular assist devices within ACTION. Pediatr Cardiol. 2022;43(6):1379–82. https://doi.org/10.1007/s00246-022-02863-7.

Penk JS, Reddy S, Polito A, et al. Bleeding and thrombosis with pediatric extracorporeal life support: a roadmap for management, research, and the future from the pediatric cardiac Intensive Care Society: part 1. Pediatr Crit Care Med. 2019;20(11):1027–33. https://doi.org/10.1097/PCC.0000000000002054.

Pieri M, Agracheva N, Bonaveglio E, et al. Bivalirudin versus heparin as an anticoagulant during extracorporeal membrane oxygenation: a case-control study. J Cardiothorac Vasc Anesth. 2013;27(1):30–4. https://doi.org/10.1053/j.jvca.2012.07.019.

Pinto VL, Pruthi S, Westrick AC, Shannon CN, Bridges BC, Le TM. Brain magnetic resonance imaging findings in pediatric patients post extracorporeal membrane oxygenation. ASAIO J. 2017;63(6):810–4. https://doi.org/10.1097/MAT.0000000000000580.

Qu Y, Li Y, Cameron DR, et al. Hyperosmotic infusion and oxidized surfaces are essential for biofilm formation of *Staphylococcus capitis* From the Neonatal Intensive Care Unit. Front Microbiol. 2020;11:920. https://doi.org/10.3389/fmicb.2020.00920.

Qu Y, Peleg AY, McGiffin D. Ventricular assist device-specific infections. J Clin Med. 2021;10(3):453. https://doi.org/10.3390/jcm10030453.

Raffini L. Anticoagulation with VADs and ECMO: walking the tightrope. Hematology Am Soc Hematol Educ Program. 2017;1:674–80. https://doi.org/10.1182/asheducation-2017.1.674.

Ranucci M, Ballotta A, Kandil H, et al. Bivalirudin-based versus conventional heparin anticoagulation for postcardiotomy extracorporeal membrane oxygenation. Crit Care. 2011;15(6):R275. https://doi.org/10.1186/cc10556.

Reagor JA. Ventricular assist device malfunction: sometimes it is a zebra. J Extra Corpor Technol. 2012;44(3):155–9.

Rimsans J, Sylvester KW, Connors JM. Direct thrombin inhibitor for LVAD thrombosis: a closer look. Clin Appl Thromb Hemost. 2017;23(5):405–9. https://doi.org/10.1177/1076029616672583.

Rivera-Lara L, Geocadin R, Zorrilla-Vaca A, et al. Optimizing mean arterial pressure in acutely comatose patients using cerebral autoregulation multimodal monitoring with near-infrared spectroscopy. Crit Care Med. 2019;47(10):1409–15. https://doi.org/10.1097/CCM.0000000000003908.

Romano C, Oliva S, Martellossi S, et al. Pediatric gastrointestinal bleeding: perspectives from the Italian society of pediatric gastroenterology. World J Gastroenterol. 2017;23(8):1328–37. https://doi.org/10.3748/wjg.v23.i8.1328.

Rosenthal DN, Almond CS, Jaquiss RD, et al. Adverse events in children implanted with ventricular assist devices in the United States: data from the pediatric interagency registry for mechanical circulatory support (PediMACS). J Heart Lung Transplant. 2016;35(5):569–77. https://doi.org/10.1016/j.healun.2016.03.005.

Rosenthal DN, Lancaster CA, McElhinney DB, et al. Impact of a modified anti-thrombotic guideline on stroke in children supported with a pediatric ventricular assist device. J Heart Lung Transplant. 2017;36(11):1250–7. https://doi.org/10.1016/j.healun.2017.05.020.

Rothblatt M. Commentary on achievement of first life-saving xenoheart transplant. Xenotransplantation. 2022;29(3):e12746. https://doi.org/10.1111/xen.12746.

Ryu SM, Park SM. Unexpected complication during extracorporeal membrane oxygenation support: ventilator associated systemic air embolism. World J Clin Cases. 2018;6(9):274–8. https://doi.org/10.12998/wjcc.v6.i9.274.

Said AS, Guilliams KP, Bembea MM. Neurological monitoring and complications of pediatric extracorporeal membrane oxygenation support. Pediatr Neurol. 2020;108:3139. https://doi.org/10.1016/j.pediatrneurol.2020.03.014.

Sanfilippo F, Asmussen S, Maybauer DM, et al. Bivalirudin for alternative anticoagulation in extracorporeal membrane oxygenation: a systematic review. J Intensive Care Med. 2017;32(5):312–9. https://doi.org/10.1177/0885066616656333.

Schutze GE, Heulitt MJ. Infections during extracorporeal life support. J Pediatr Surg. 1995;30(6):809–12. https://doi.org/10.1016/0022-3468(95)90753-x.

Schweiger M, Schrempf J, Sereinigg M, et al. Complication profile of the Berlin heart EXCOR biventricular support in children. Artif Organs. 2013;37(8):730–5. https://doi.org/10.1111/aor.12062.

Sekhon MS, Gooderham P, Menon DK, et al. The burden of brain hypoxia and optimal mean arterial pressure in patients with hypoxic ischemic brain injury after cardiac arrest. Crit Care Med. 2019;47(7):960–9. https://doi.org/10.1097/CCM.0000000000003745.

Shaffer A, Cogswell R, John R. Future developments in left ventricular assist device therapy. J Thorac Cardiovasc Surg. 2021;162(2):605–11. https://doi.org/10.1016/j.jtcvs.2020.07.125.

Slaughter MS, Myers TJ. Transcutaneous energy transmission for mechanical circulatory support systems: history, current status, and future prospects. J Card Surg. 2010;25(4):484–9. https://doi.org/10.1111/j.1540-8191.2010.01074.x.

Spinner JA, Tunuguntla HP, Tume SC, et al. "Compassionate" cases of the Jarvik 2015 ventricular assist device. ASAIO J. 2021;67(9):1036–43. https://doi.org/10.1097/MAT.0000000000001351.

StatPearls. 2023. https://www.ncbi.nlm.nih.gov/books/NBK557518/ Accessed 10/2/2025.

Stein ML, Bruno JL, Konopacki KL, Kesler S, Reinhartz O, Rosenthal D. Cognitive outcomes in pediatric heart transplant recipients bridged to transplantation with ventricular assist devices. J Heart Lung Transplant. 2013;32(2):212–20. https://doi.org/10.1016/j.healun.2012.11.006.

Stein ML, Dao DT, Doan LN, et al. Ventricular assist devices in a contemporary pediatric cohort: morbidity, functional recovery, and survival. J Heart Lung Transplant. 2016;35(1):92–8. https://doi.org/10.1016/j.healun.2015.06.006.

Steiner ME, Bomgaars LR, Massicotte MP, Investigators BHEPVIs. Antithrombotic therapy in a prospective trial of a pediatric ventricular assist device. ASAIO J. 2016;62(6):719–27. https://doi.org/10.1097/MAT.0000000000000434.

Steinhorn RH, Isham-Schopf B, Smith C, Green TP. Hemolysis during long-term extracorporeal membrane oxygenation. J Pediatr. 1989;115(4):625–30. https://doi.org/10.1016/s0022-3476(89)80299-9.

Su JA, Menteer J. Outcomes of Berlin heart EXCOR. Pediatr Transplant. 21. 2017;(8) https://doi.org/10.1111/petr.13048.

Thangappan K, Haney LC, Riggs K, et al. Children who stroke on VAD support: when is it safe to transplant and what are their outcomes? Artif Organs. 2022;46(7):1389–98. https://doi.org/10.1111/aor.14194.

Throckmorton A, Garven E, Hirschhorn M, Day S, Stevens R, Tchantchaleishvili V. Forward-thinking design solutions for mechanical circulatory support: multifunctional hybrid continuous-flow ventricular assist device technology. Ann Cardiothorac Surg. 2021;10(3):383–5. https://doi.org/10.21037/acs-2020-cfmcs-14.

Timpa JG, O'Meara C, McILwain RB, Dabal RJ, Alten JA. Massive systemic air embolism during extracorporeal membrane oxygenation support of a neonate with acute respiratory distress syndrome after cardiac surgery. J Extra Corpor Technol. 2011;43(2):86–8.

Tume SC, Conway J, Ryan KR, Philip J, Fortkiewicz JM, Murray J. Developments in pediatric ventricular assist device support. World J Pediatr Congenit Heart Surg. 2019;10(6):759–68. https://doi.org/10.1177/2150135119880890.

Vakil NH, Kanaan AO, Donovan JL. Heparin-induced thrombocytopenia in the pediatric population: a review of current literature. J Pediatr Pharmacol Ther. 2012;17(1):12–30. https://doi.org/10.5863/1551-6776-17.1.12.

VanderPluym JH, Robertson CM, Joffe AR, et al. Neurologic, neurocognitive, and functional outcomes in children under 6 years treated with the Berlin heart Excor ventricular assist device. ASAIO J. 2017;63(2):207–15. https://doi.org/10.1097/MAT.0000000000000462.

Wadiwala IJ, Garg P, Yazji JH, et al. Evolution of xenotransplantation as an alternative to shortage of donors in heart transplantation. Cureus. 2022;14(6):e26284. https://doi.org/10.7759/cureus.26284.

Weinstein S, Bello R, Pizarro C, et al. The use of the Berlin heart EXCOR in patients with functional single ventricle. J Thorac Cardiovasc Surg.

2014;147(2):697–704.; discussion 704-5. https://doi.org/10.1016/j.jtcvs.2013.10.030.

Weng Y, Chen J, Tu Q, Li Q, Maitz MF, Huang N. Biomimetic modification of metallic cardiovascular biomaterials: from function mimicking to endothelialization in vivo. Interface Focus. 2012;2(3):356–65. https://doi.org/10.1098/rsfs.2011.0126.

Werho DK, Pasquali SK, Yu S, et al. Epidemiology of stroke in pediatric cardiac surgical patients supported with extracorporeal membrane oxygenation. Ann Thorac Surg. 2015;100(5):1751–7. https://doi.org/10.1016/j.athoracsur.2015.06.020.

Yang M, Jiang P, Ge Y, et al. Dopamine self-polymerized along with hydroxyapatite onto the preactivated titanium percutaneous implants surface to promote human gingival fibroblast behavior and antimicrobial activity for biological sealing. J Biomater Appl. 2018;32(8):1071–82. https://doi.org/10.1177/0885328217749963.

Yen JH, Chen SF, Chern MK, Lu PC. The effect of turbulent viscous shear stress on red blood cell hemolysis. J Artif Organs. 2014;17(2):178–85. https://doi.org/10.1007/s10047-014-0755-3.

Zafar F, Castleberry C, Khan MS, et al. Pediatric heart transplant waiting list mortality in the era of ventricular assist devices. J Heart Lung Transplant. 2015;34(1):82–8. https://doi.org/10.1016/j.healun.2014.09.018.

Zakhary B, Vercaemst L, Mason P, Antonini MV, Lorusso R, Brodie D. How I approach membrane lung dysfunction in patients receiving ECMO. Crit Care. 2020;24(1):671. https://doi.org/10.1186/s13054-020-03388-2.

Complications Associated with Repair of Ebstein Anomaly of the Tricuspid Valve

Elizabeth H. Stephens and Joseph A. Dearani

Abstract

Surgical repair of Ebstein anomaly, and in particular the tricuspid valve are accomplished via median sternotomy with aortic and bicaval cannulation. Complications associated with Ebstein anomaly include incomplete delamination and/or residual tethering, papillary muscle injury, fenestration of the free wall, and inadvertent ligation of the right coronary artery. The focus of this chapter is potential complications related to Ebstein repair, how to avoid such complications, and how to address them.

Keywords

Ebstein anomaly · Tricuspid valve · Congenital heart surgery · Cone technique · Valve replacement

E. H. Stephens (✉)
Department of Cardiovascular Surgery, Mayo Clinic, Rochester, MN, USA
e-mail: Stephens.Elizabeth@mayo.edu

J. A. Dearani
Department of Cardiovascular Surgery, Mayo Clinic, Rochester, MN, USA

Mayo Clinic College of Medicine, Rochester, MN, USA

1 Introduction

Ebstein anomaly is a rare congenital heart defect occurring in <1% of patients with congenital heart disease, but it accounts for 40% of all congenital malformations of the tricuspid valve (Perloff 1994; Keith et al. 1958; Fyler et al. 1980). It is characterized by lack of tricuspid valve delamination accompanied by an underlying right ventricular myopathy. First described by Dr. Wilhelm Ebstein in 1866, (Ebstein 1866) the anomaly did not receive significant attention until the mid-1900s. The first tricuspid valve replacement for Ebstein anomaly was reported by Barnard and Schire in 1962, (Barnard and Schrire 1963) shortly followed by Cartwright and colleagues in 1964 (Cartwright et al. 1964). Surgical strategies have evolved with increasing effort to preserve the native valve. The earliest repairs focused on a "mono-cusp" reconstruction, such as those by Carpentier and Danielson, that utilized the anterior leaflet and its redundancy to create a competent valve with coaptation against the ventricular septum or diminutive septal leaflet (Carpentier et al. 1988; Danielson et al. 1979). Da Silva introduced the "cone" technique in which he mobilized all available leaflet tissue, connected segments side-to-side thereby creating a "cone" of circumferential leaflet tissue. This "cone" is re-anchored at the true tricuspid annulus. This results in a more anatomic correction, since leaflet tissue coapts with leaflet tissue with

C. L. Backer, C. Mavroudis (eds.), *Complications in Pediatric and Congenital Heart Surgery*,
https://doi.org/10.1007/978-3-032-02661-3_19

the hinge point at the true annulus, but commissures are absent (da Silva and da Silva 2012). When there is inadequate native leaflet tissue, autologous pericardium is used to augment the cone circumference allowing an adequately-sized cone to be created and occasionally to augment leaflet height. Since the cone reattachment is at the true annulus, the size of the functional right ventricle (RV) is increased. This more anatomic repair has undergone a number of modifications as described by Dearani (2020).

Contemporary Ebstein repair is defined as: (1) tricuspid valve repair (or replacement), (2) closure vs subtotal closure of patent foramen ovale/atrial septal defect, (3) plication of atrialized right ventricle, and (4) right reduction atrioplasty. Concomitant procedures performed selectively include bidirectional cavopulmonary anastomosis and anti-arrhythmia surgery.

The focus of this chapter is potential complications related to Ebstein repair, including how to avoid such complications and how to address them.

2 Preoperative Evaluation

Preoperative evaluation and patient selection are critical to the successful care of these patients. Certain findings on preoperative testing may direct the patient toward a certain pathway and are important in counseling the family.

Routine preoperative imaging includes transthoracic echocardiography for valve analysis and evaluation of right and left ventricular (LV) function, and magnetic resonance imaging for right and left ventricular size and function. The importance of a thorough preoperative transthoracic echocardiogram (TEE) to gauge the feasibility of tricuspid valve repair cannot be overemphasized. All views are important, but the four-chamber view is particularly helpful to the surgeon because it shows the following important anatomical features:

- size and mobility of the anterior leaflet, and the points of muscular and fibrous attachments (i.e., tethering) to RV free wall and ventricular septum that would be consistent with “failure of delamination.”
- presence of a septal leaflet. Importantly, the presence of some septal leaflet with a degree of mobility is essential if a cone type of anatomic repair is being considered.
- size of the atrialized right ventricle. The combination of echocardiography and magnetic resonance imaging provides the necessary anatomical information about atrialization of the right ventricle. The atrialized segment is most often located along the inferior wall and is represented by areas of dyskinesis (as opposed to akinesis) during systolic contraction. From a surgical standpoint, the atrialized RV is smooth, thinned and is marked by the absence of muscular trabeculations. When atrialization is present, internal plication of this tissue is performed from the most distal point of atrialization (typically around the mid-apical ventricular level) up to and slightly across the atrioventricular groove, to exclude this dyskinetic segment of ventricle.
- presence of any atrial or ventricular level shunts.
- size of the functional right ventricle (i.e., the right ventricular cavity beyond the functional orifice of the valve).
- position of the ventricular septum. When there is marked right ventricular enlargement, the ventricular septum is displaced toward the left ventricle. In the short-axis view, the left ventricle is D-shaped (instead of circular) when the RV is severely enlarged. Sometimes the ventricular septal displacement toward the left ventricle can be so substantial that there may be mild to moderate left ventricular outflow tract obstruction.
- presence of left ventricular noncompaction.
- systolic function of both the left and right ventricles. Of note, the LV function can be challenging to assess in patients with significant bowing of the ventricular septum into the LV and underfilling of the LV. For assessment, attention should be focused on the contractility of the free wall portions of the left ventricle.

Pulmonary regurgitation should be assessed, as some patients may need a bidirectional cavopulmonary anastomosis with cone repair, in which case significant pulmonary regurgitation would need to be addressed.

The presence of concomitant cardiac anomalies such as patent arterial duct and pulmonary stenosis or atresia can also be obtained from the echocardiographic images.

Arrhythmias associated with Ebstein anomaly include Wolff-Parkinson-White syndrome (i.e., accessory conduction pathway[s]), atrial fibrillation/flutter and atrioventricular nodal reentry tachycardia. Electrophysiology (EP) evaluation is an important component. For children, if there is no history of palpitations (atrial fibrillation or flutter) and no preexcitation evident on electrocardiography, an EP study is rarely performed at our institution (Wackel et al. 2018). If there is concern or evidence of arrhythmia, a formal EP consultation is obtained, and a diagnostic/therapeutic EP study is performed. Generally, it is preferred that the patient is >15 kg, but EP studies at smaller body sizes are feasible, although these studies carry higher risk. Almost all adult patients undergo preoperative electrophysiological study to assess for the presence of atrial tachyarrhythmias, which most often include atrial fibrillation or flutter.

Other arrhythmias associated with Ebstein anomaly include atrioventricular nodal reentry tachycardia and ventricular tachycardia. Atrial tachyarrhythmias are generally treated with maze lesions at the time of surgery (cavotricuspid isthmus, right atrial or left atrial, or biatrial). Atrioventricular nodal reentry tachycardia and accessory conduction pathways are generally diagnosed and treated with percutaneous radiofrequency ablation during the preoperative EP study.

In the above evaluation, certain pearls of wisdom are worth noting. Patients with severe RV dilation or significant RV systolic dysfunction preoperatively may benefit from RV unloading with a bidirectional Glenn. While an atrial level fenestration provides additional preload to the LV in a low cardiac output state, it does not effectively unload the dysfunctional RV and does result in some degree of arterial desaturation. In an adult or any patient where there is concern about elevated pulmonary artery pressures or elevated left ventricular end diastolic pressure (LVEDP), preoperative hemodynamic catheterization is essential to determine the feasibility of either a bidirectional Glenn or an atrial level fenestration.

The age of the patient is also important in consideration of who may most benefit from a cone repair (or other technique of tricuspid repair) as opposed to a valve replacement. In our practice, *valve repair* can be successfully performed in 98%–99% of children and in 80% of adults. In general, older patients (>60 years of age), the presence of mild-moderate pulmonary hypertension or severe tricuspid annular dilation (>6 cm), massive RV dilation, and mildly depressed left ventricular systolic function, valve replacement is usually preferred.

Another important consideration is surgeon experience with Ebstein repair. Given the rarity of the anomaly combined with wide anatomic variability of Ebstein anomaly, strong consideration should be given to referral to a center of excellence with Ebstein repair; this pertains to patients of all ages—from the neonate to the adult. The recent analysis of the Society of Thoracic Surgeons (STS) data revealed an average of 1–2 patients per center annually, and a 27% operative mortality for neonates with Ebstein anomaly undergoing surgical intervention, compared with 9% in infants (Holst et al. 2018). While not discussed in detail in the context of this chapter, the decision between biventricular repair and single ventricle pathway is difficult and also requires program experience and expertise (Knott-Craig et al. 2012; Starnes et al. 1991).

In the rare instance when there is significant LV dysfunction, heart transplantation is usually preferred.

3 Surgical Procedure and Potential Complications: Cone Repair

The steps and techniques involved in a cone repair have been covered in detail in other venues (da Silva and da Silva 2012; Dearani and Mavroudis 2020). Briefly, cardiopulmonary bypass is instituted via aortic and bicaval cannulation, and aortic occlusion with cardioplegia is required for intracardiac repair. For cone repair, the anterior leaflet is incised at the level of the annulus, allowing thorough examination for tethered segments and complete mobilization (incision and excision of tethering points) is performed. The proximal edge of the displaced septal leaflet is mobilized off the ventricular septum and mobilized in a similar fashion. Side-to-side approximations of leaflet tissue are performed to create a cone of native tissue. When inadequate native tissue is present this is augmented with a triangular-shaped piece of untreated autologous pericardium. The cone then is reattached at the level of the true annulus; in the area of conduction tissue the suture line runs caudal (just below) to the area of conduction. In contrast, in the setting of valve replacement in Ebstein anomaly, annular sutures are placed cephalad (atrial side) to the conduction tissue for valve replacement.

3.1 Incomplete Surgical Delamination

One of the most important steps is ensuring that native leaflets have been sufficiently delaminated, and all tethered segments are released (Fig. 1). While some areas of tethering can be identified with the leaflet still attached at the annulus, incising the leaflet off the annulus allows a more thorough examination, as some points of tethering are challenging to identify until the valve is "flipped" and the ventricular side is fully examined. Chordal support of the leaflet leading edges is preserved to the anterior free wall and ventricular septum; however, chordal support to the inferior wall is divided (much of which may be atrialized). Incomplete delamination and/or residual tethering is a common cause of tricuspid regurgitation after repair since leaflet mobility into the inlet that results in leaflet-to-leaflet coaptation is restricted.

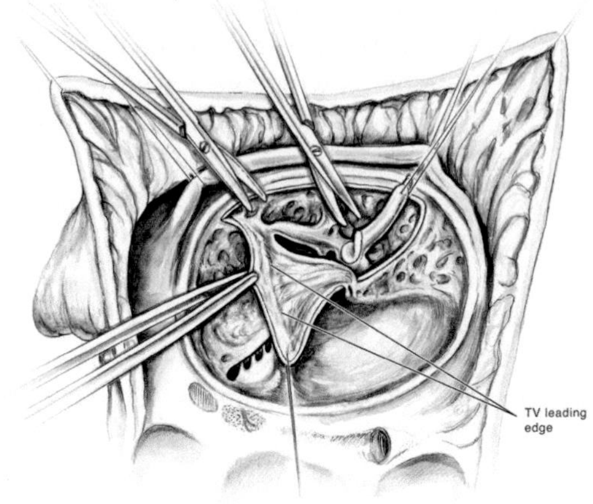

Fig. 1 Surgical division of these abnormal muscular and fibrous attachments is clearly demonstrated. The surgeon should have a mental image that there should be no attachments between the body of the anterior and inferior leaflets and the free wall of the right ventricle. The only attachments that persist after complete surgical mobilization (i.e., surgical delamination) are the chordal attachments to the leading edge of the anterior and inferior leaflets. This is the most challenging and intimidating portion of the procedure and the reason for the difficult learning curve. The common mistake is failure to divide *all* attachments; the consequence of a single residual attachment is tethering of that leaflet and the inability of the leaflet to float into the ventricular inlet to coapt with surrounding leaflet tissue to attain competence of the valve. *TV* tricuspid valve. (With permission: Dearani and Mavroudis 2020)

3.2 Papillary Muscle Injury

In the process of mobilizing the leaflets, it is common to release portions of the papillary muscle(s) *fusion* to the free wall. This may involve incising between the papillary muscle and free wall down to the base of the papillary muscle. Care should be taken to retain adequate muscle at the base of the papillary muscle both for structural stability and maintenance of its blood supply. Should the papillary muscle inadvertently become transected, various options may be possible including anchoring the papillary to a neighboring papillary muscle with pledgetted suture, or to a portion of the ventricular septum or RV free wall. Alternatively, Gore-Tex artificial chords can be applied, particularly if somatic growth is complete. Care should be taken not to change the height/length of the papillary muscle as that may distort the valve and coaptation.

3.3 Right Ventricular Fenestration

The right ventricular walls and ventricular septum in patients with Ebstein anomaly are typically thin. During delamination of the anterior leaflet (or inferior leaflet if present), retraction of the leaflet tissue or papillary muscle(s) during surgical delamination can result in inadvertent fenestration of the free wall, (i.e., creating a "buttonhole"). Free wall fenestration can be repaired by direct suture. This should be done from the outside in order to avoid inadvertent coronary artery injury with suture repair. Similarly, septal leaflet mobilization can result in the creation of an iatrogenic ventricular septal defect (VSD). If small, this VSD fenestration can be reapproximated by direct suture, but care must be taken to ensure bites are in sturdy tissue bordering the defect itself. Larger defects require patch repair.

3.4 Inadequate Leaflet Height

The construction of the "cone" is unique to each patient based on the available native tissue, its configuration, and quality. One potential pitfall related to creation of the cone is inadequate leaflet height; (i.e., the distance between the leading edge of the leaflet and the annulus). In general, it is preferable to have this distance to be similar circumferentially—the leading edges all at the same level. Deciphering whether the height of different portions of the cone will be adequate is a subjective decision after analyzing the coaptation of the different portions of the cone and is highly dependent on surgeon experience. There needs to be sufficient height between the portions of leaflet coaptation to prevent regurgitation. Deficient height can be addressed by an ellipse of untreated autologous pericardium in the belly of the anterior leaflet or septal leaflet.

3.5 Inadequate Leaflet Tissue

The constructed cone must have sufficient circumference at both the annular level and at the distal aspect of the cone. It is essential that the orifice at the distal cone is adequate since there are no longer any commissures around the valve orifice. An insufficient cone circumference will result in a stenotic valve. Ideally, the z-score at the distal orifice should be zero. This is especially important if autologous pericardium has been used since it does get slightly thicker over time and can increase the gradient through the valve. Clearly, it is advantageous to diagnose the deficiency in tissue prior to completion of the cone. A Hegar dilator can be used to assess adequate circumference throughout the height of the cone prior to reattachment of the cone. If inadequate, this can be rectified by using a triangle of autologous pericardium to augment the cone circumference. The three sides of the triangle are anastomosed to the mobilized edge of the septal leaflet, medial edge of the anterior leaflet, and ventricular septum/inferior annulus, respectively.

3.6 Coronary Compromise

The markedly dilated annulus is down-sized during the repair to accommodate the neotricuspid valve orifice that should be more normally sized. It is important to not compromise the right coronary artery with aggressive annular plication maneuvers inferiorly or close to the coronary sinus (Fig. 2). This can result in kinking (or ligation) of the right coronary artery if annular reduction occurs along the free wall of the annulus, or compromise to the posterior descending or posterolateral coronary artery when adjacent to the coronary sinus, (i.e., at the crux of the heart). To minimize this complication, several smaller

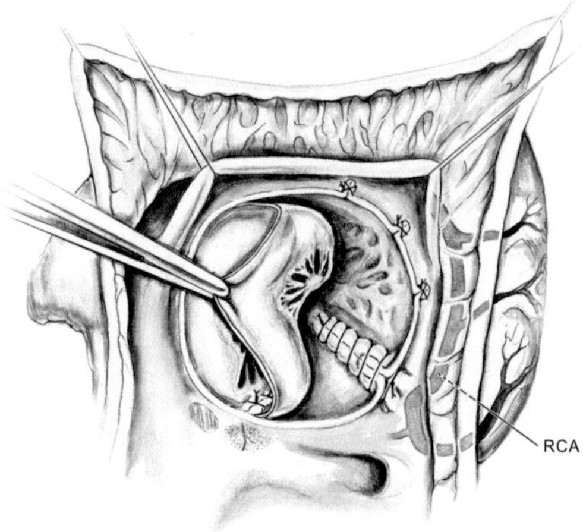

Fig. 2 Plication sutures are spaced evenly around the anterior and inferior annulus until the true tricuspid valve annulus matches the smaller size of the newly reconstructed tricuspid valve. These intermittent, localized plications are preferred so that kinking or injuring the right coronary artery is avoided. (With permission: Dearani and Mavroudis 2020)

eccentric annuloplasty sutures are placed evenly around the annulus.

The second area of potential coronary compromise is with plication of the atrialized RV. It is important to emphasize that the plication must be confined to the inferior RV free wall. Since plication is usually done internally and focuses on the smooth, non-trabeculated portion of the inferior wall, there is a tendency for the suture line to drift too close to the ventricular septum which is also smooth and non-trabeculated. If the plication suture line starts to include the ventricular septum, then the posterior descending coronary artery will be compromised. It is essential to periodically examine the external surface of the heart when the plication suture line is being performed to be sure coronary arteries are not distorted or ligated. Ventricular arrhythmias at the time of separation from cardiopulmonary bypass and after elimination of left heart air indicates coronary compromise until proven otherwise. The culprit lesion is most often right coronary artery kinking from excessive annular reduction in one location or deep bites with the atrialized right ventricular plication suture line resulting in kinking or ligation of the posterior descending or posterolateral coronary artery. TEE typically shows a regional wall abnormality in the inferior wall of the *left* ventricle and (more than expected) RV systolic dysfunction than anticipated from correction of tricuspid repair alone. Treatment requires suture line revision around the area of concern. In an adult, coronary artery bypass grafting to the distal right coronary artery or posterior descending coronary artery can also be performed.

3.7 Cleft and Commissure Closure

While cleft and commissure closure are standard in creating the cone of tissue, care should be taken to not be overzealous as too many such closures, particularly at the distal cone, will limit the effective orifice and result in valve stenosis. Unlike a normal tricuspid valve that has commissures allowing inflow, a cone repair does not have commissures in the same manner, so the inflow (and effective orifice) is the diameter of the *distal* aspect of the cone (Fig. 3a, b).

Consequently, one should note that the distal portion of the cone must be of adequate diameter (normal z score) for laminar flow. Postbypass TEE should focus on the mean gradient at the distal aspect of the cone, not the gradient at the level of the true tricuspid valve annulus, which is always larger. Documentation of the hemoglobin, heart rate, and the flow characteristics on TEE (i.e., laminar vs turbulent) are all factored into the decision-making as to whether significant tricuspid stenosis is present. Ideally, the mean gradient should be <5 mmHg.

3.8 Sebening Stitch Dehiscence

The original Sebening stitch involved suture fixation of the anterior papillary muscle to the ventricular septum and was most useful in a neonate undergoing a mono-cusp repair. In a neonate, this distance is small enough (RV is usually not severely dilated) that dehiscence is unlikely. However, as the child gets older and the RV dilates, the distance becomes more substantial

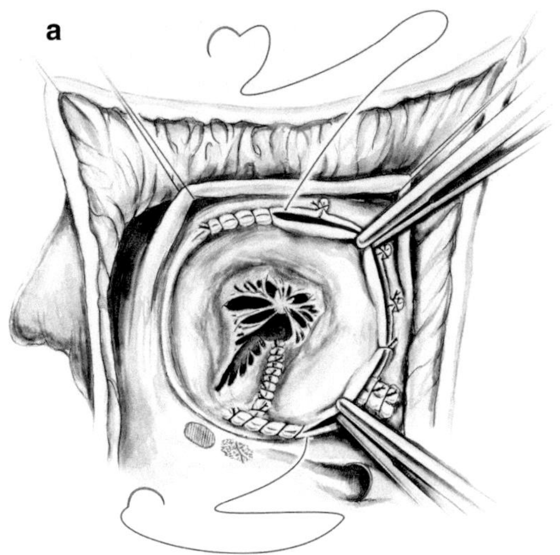

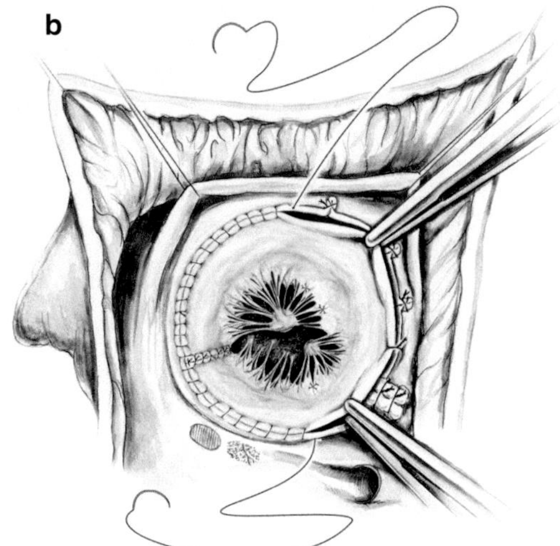

Fig. 3 Demonstration of an ideal cone result with adequate distal cone diameter and evenly spaced annuloplasty sutures. Note in (**a**) a commissure has been retained whereas in (**b**) one has not. Generally, we would prefer obliterating the commissures so long as the distal cone diameter is adequate, but if there is concern regarding distal diameter it is best to retain the commissure. This figure additionally demonstrates how the neotricuspid valve reconstruction is reattached to the true tricuspid valve annulus. This generally begins inferiorly and anteriorly, with the suture line meeting at approximately 1–2 o'clock at the annulus. Most importantly, the suture line for the septal leaflet reattachment is shifted to the ventricular side of the conduction tissue to avoid injury. (With permission: Dearani and Mavroudis 2020)

and direct anastomosis of the anterior papillary muscle(s) to the ventricular septum typically results in too much tension and subsequent dehiscence.

The modified Sebening stitch described by us can include one of the following: (1) mobilization of the anterior papillary muscle and mobilization of a corresponding major septal papillary muscle (when present) with approximation of the heads of these muscles, (2) placement of Gore-Tex artificial chords from a ventricular septal trabeculation up to the head of the anterior papillary muscle that is secured in a manner similar to artificial chords but with the attachment to the papillary muscle as opposed to the leading edge of the anterior leaflet. While previously we had completely approximated the papillary muscles (Fig. 4a), we now commonly secure this stitch with a 10-mm Hegar dilator between the chords in a child and a 14–16 mm Hegar dilator in an adult (Fig. 4b). The modified Sebening stitch maneuver effectively brings the leading edges of the anterior and septal leaflets together without excess tension. There should be no dimple in the anterior right ventricular free wall in the beating heart at the completion of the procedure if it has been done properly.

3.9 Inadequate Leading Edge Support

At times there may be lack of chordal support along areas of the anterior leaflet that can lead to prolapse with inadequate coaptation and resultant regurgitation. In general, this is avoided with a deeper cone reconstruction. However, there are instances when leaflet prolapse occurs and artificial chordal support or chordal transfer can correct this. Artificial cords are generally avoided in children. However, if there is inadequate chordal support to the leading edge resulting in residual regurgitation, neochordae can be utilized. For this Gore-Tex suture (6-O in pediatrics, 5-O in adults) are secured in trabeculations in ventricular septum toward the RV apex. The anterior pap-

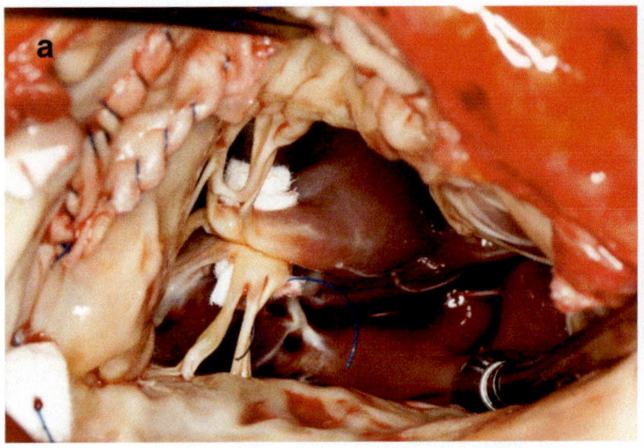

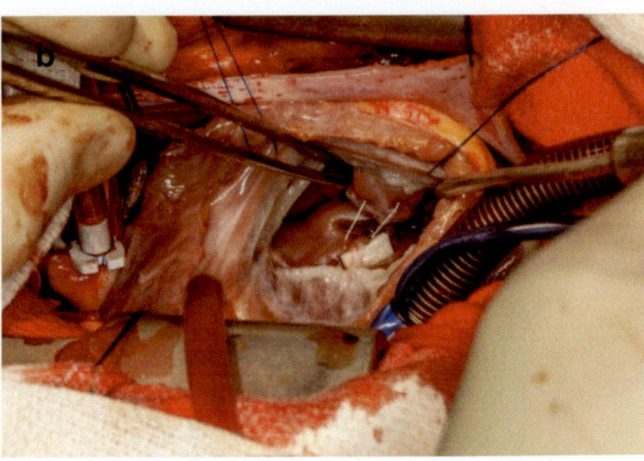

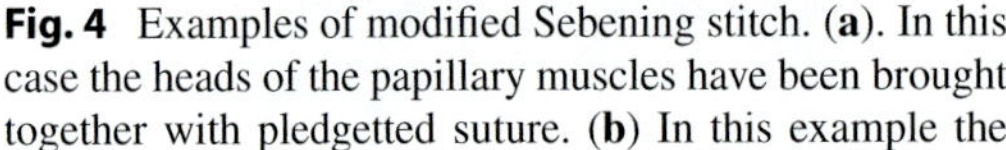

Fig. 4 Examples of modified Sebening stitch. (**a**). In this case the heads of the papillary muscles have been brought together with pledgetted suture. (**b**) In this example the chord has been brought from a ventricular septal trabeculation to the head of the anterior papillary muscle and tied over a Hegar dilator

illary muscles are not used for anchoring as appropriating chordae length is very challenging to determine in a flaccid heart. Furthermore, as the right ventricle remodels with correction of tricuspid regurgitation, the chord length may be too long or too short at that time. Consequently, chordal length and anchoring the chords into the ventricular septum is more predictable and pulls the anterior leaflet toward the septal leaflet and ventricular septum optimizing coaptation. These pledgetted sutures are passed through the trabeculations and then passed through a sturdy portion of the leading edge twice. The length is adjusted based on assessment with saline insufflation and then the sutures are tied.

3.10 Reinforcement Maneuvers

The inferior annulus tends to be under the most tension, is the site most likely to dilate, and is the site that is at the highest risk for repair dehiscence. We commonly reinforce this area either with pledgetted sutures or a short inferior, annular pericardial strip. In patients in whom the annulus is adult-size, annuloplasty bands are used to reinforce the repair (Fig. 5). Annuloplasty band size is typically 26 or 28 mm in an adult.

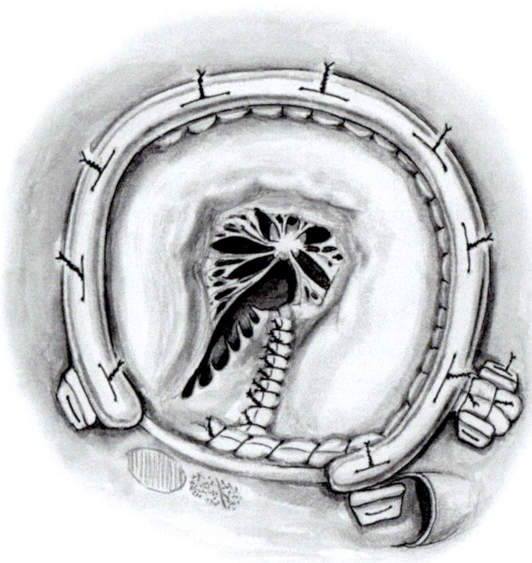

Fig. 5 Note reinforcement of the inferior corner, that tends to be under increased tension. Dehiscence in this area would result in the appearance of a periprosthetic leak on echocardiography. If this inferior plication is too aggressive the coronary artery can be compromised. (With permission: Dearani and Mavroudis 2020)

3.11 Conduction Tissue

To preserve the conduction tissue, the annular suture line for the reattachment of the cone is caudal (toward the apex) to the conduction system (Fig. 3).

3.12 Right Ventricular Plication

Certain aspects of the plication of the atrialized portion of the right ventricle require particular attention (Fig. 6). This muscle is very thin, and the plication suture line is internal and confined to the endocardium (not full thickness) in order to avoid inadvertent injury to coronary arteries. After performing the first layer of plication, we examine the epicardial surface of the inferior wall of the RV to ensure there is no coronary kinking/ligation; the right coronary artery and posterior descending artery being most at risk. Additionally, the suture line should not drift onto the ventricular septum itself to avoid injury to the posterior descending coronary artery. Sutures in trabeculated right ventricular myocardium should also be avoided to optimize ventricular systolic function and minimize potential ventricular arrhythmias. The plication suture line is continued beyond the true annulus onto the right atrium itself. This helps reduce the dilated annulus to help match the smaller and more normally sized neotricuspid valve reconstruction. Lastly, the apex of the suture line on the atrial side should be completely obliterated to avoid a persistent blind pouch that will result in a hematoma along the inferior RV free wall.

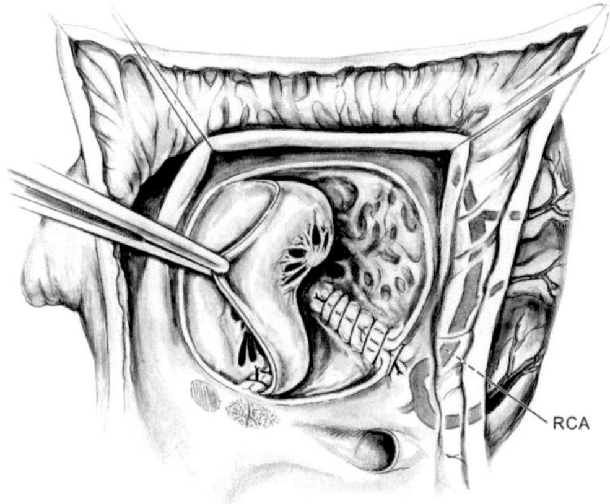

Fig. 6 An internal plication is performed with two continuous running layers of monofilament suture, beginning distally at a point where the smooth, atrialized portion of the right ventricle begins and extends across the annulus and into the right atrium as shown in the figure. The suture line is performed from the apical portion of the right ventricle up across the atrioventricular groove, taking care not to compromise the right coronary artery. Anteriorly, the transition zone between trabeculated and smooth myocardium marks the suture line. The left aspect of the suture line must remain within the free wall of the right ventricle. There is a temptation to have the suture line drift into the ventricular septum because it, too, is relatively smooth. It is important to avoid this mistake; the posterior descending coronary artery is very vulnerable to injury, as all these muscular structures are quite thin. The suture line generally extends across the atrioventricular groove so that the true tricuspid valve annulus is reduced in size with the plication process. It is equally important not to narrow the true tricuspid valve annulus excessively in this inferior location because of the susceptibility to right coronary artery distortion. After these suture lines are completed, the external surface of the heart is inspected to confirm that the right coronary artery and its branches have not been compromised. (With permission: Dearani and Mavroudis 2020)

3.13 Right Atrial Reduction

Right atrial reduction is routinely performed, taking care to not resect too close to the atrioventricular groove, and avoiding suture placement in the crista terminalis with atriotomy closure, which can increase the risk of atrial arrhythmias.

4 Surgical Procedure and Potential Complications: Valve Replacement

4.1 Prosthetic Valve Sizing

In general, large prosthetic valves can be utilized in Ebstein anomaly because of significant annular dilation. Complications related to valve replacement center around coronary artery injury or heart block. Since septal leaflet tissue is typically absent or severely displaced below the true annulus, the position of the prosthesis is usually to the atrial side of the true annulus. This is in contrast to tricuspid valve replacement for acquired heart disease where suture placement is in native leaflet tissue.

In Ebstein anomaly, correct suture placement inferiorly is along the atrial septum leaving the conduction tissue (marked by a small vein in fat tissue) to the ventricular side of the prosthesis.

Anteriorly the suture line is located where the smooth and trabeculated portions of the right atrium meet each other; this is cephalad to the course of the right coronary artery. With this strategy the conduction tissue is avoided, and right coronary artery injury is avoided. It is important to emphasize that suture placement along the ventricular septum to anchor the prosthesis should be avoided since it will almost certainly result in coronary artery injury at the level of the coronary sinus due to posterolateral or posterior descending coronary artery injury.

In general, when valve replacement is performed, a porcine (as opposed to pericardial) bioprosthesis is preferred given good durability and greater pliability of the porcine leaflets in the setting of the low right atrial pressure and presence of poor RV systolic function. This combination can result in poor leaflet movement, particularly in a large prosthesis. Since the conduction tissue will be below the level of the prosthesis, it is important to position the bioprosthetic valve so that the recess between 2 struts straddles the conduction tissue. Specifically, avoid a strut of the bioprosthesis sitting directly on top of the conduction tissue that can result in heart block.

In the occasional circumstance where a concomitant bidirectional cavopulmonary anastomosis is being performed, it is important to downsize the prosthesis slightly since venous return is reduced so that all leaflets open and close normally. Warfarin anticoagulation is typically used postoperatively for 3 months when bioprosthetic valve replacement has been performed. In addition, bioprosthetic valve replacement facilitates future percutaneous valve-in-valve replacement by interventional cardiology. Mechanical valves are generally avoided in Ebstein anomaly because of poor disc motion and potential thrombosis even in the setting of adequate INR.

5 Surgical Procedure and Potential Complications: Arrhythmia Surgery

Arrhythmia surgery is commonly performed in the setting of surgery for patients with Ebstein anomaly. Cryoablation procedures are generally preferred. However, in the setting of Ebstein anomaly, annular and RV free wall tissues are markedly thin, and care should be taken to not allow a prolonged freeze across the annulus or in the vicinity of coronary arteries since this can inadvertently injure the right coronary artery resulting in a coronary stenosis that will not be apparent until weeks or months later. Additionally, attention should be paid to the probe position laterally, relative to the pericardium and phrenic nerve, in order to avoid potential phrenic nerve injury.

6 Ebstein Anomaly Repair Completion and Chest Closure

After intracardiac repair, we do an aggressive right reduction atrioplasty and obliterate or amputate the tip of the right atrial appendage. If recurrent tricuspid regurgitation occurs in the future, progressive right atrial dilation can be substantial, resulting in the dilated right atrial appendage being directly posterior to the sternum. This can result in right atrial injury at the time of future resternotomy.

Pericardial effusions are not uncommon particularly if warfarin anticoagulation is being used in the short term and when there has been a large plication of the atrialized right ventricle and reduction atrioplasty, We routinely perform a right-sided pericardiectomy down to 2 cm anterior to the phrenic nerve allowing the mediastinal space to communicate with the right pleural space in order to minimize the potential complication of large pericardial effusion or pericardial tamponade.

7 Postoperative Management

Standard medical management at the time of separation from cardiopulmonary bypass includes pharmacologic support with epinephrine and milrinone, maintaining a low right atrial pressure (< 10 mmHg), and a heart rate of 100–120 beats per minute. This strategy helps support RV systolic dysfunction, which is always present, and decreases diastolic filling time to minimize excess stretch on the numerous suture lines present. This strategy also results in some degree of metabolic acidosis that is due in part to relative hypovolemia and tachycardia. This lactic acidosis generally resolves in the first 12 h. We aim to extubate patients either in the operating room or the afternoon of surgery, before the lactic acidosis plateaus, as this reduces RV afterload and may be helpful to the dysfunctional right ventricle.

Low cardiac output from RV failure is manifested by poor urine output and persistent metabolic acidosis as well as some hemodynamic instability. If this were to occur, an echocardiogram is performed, and poor RV systolic function is treated with return to the operating room to perform a bidirectional cavopulmonary anastomosis. Of note, this decision is not governed by the appearance of RV function by echocardiogram, as many patients have moderately or severely decreased RV function especially after a competent valve is created. For most of these patients, hemodynamics are satisfactory, and the patient is weaned slowly from inotropic support over a period of 48–72 h. In selected situations when RV function is quite poor (but hemodynamics are good) or the patient lives at a high altitude, sildenafil therapy is used for 4–6 weeks.

References

Barnard CN, Schrire V. Surgical correction of Ebstein's malformation with prosthetic tricuspid valve. Surgery. 1963;54:302–8.

Carpentier A, Chauvaud S, Mace L, Relland J, Mihaileanu S, Marino JP, Abry B, Guibourt P. A new reconstructive operation for Ebstein's anomaly of the tricuspid valve. J Thorac Cardiovasc Surg. 1988;96(1):92–101.

Cartwright RS, Smeloff EA, Cayler GG, Fong WY, Huntley AC, Blake JR, McFall RA. Total correction of Ebstein's anomaly by means of Triscuspid replacement. J Thorac Cardiovasc Surg. 1964;47:755–61.

da Silva JP, da Silva LF. Ebstein's anomaly of the tricuspid valve: the cone repair. Semin Thorac Cardiovasc Surg Pediatr Card Surg Annu. 2012;15(1):38–45.

Danielson GK, Maloney JD, Devloo RA. Surgical repair of Ebstein's anomaly. Mayo Clinic Proc. 1979;54(3):185–92.

Dearani JA. Ebstein repair: how I do it. JTCVS Tech. 2020;3:269–76.

Dearani JA, Mavroudis C. Ebstein anomaly. In: Mavroudis C, Dearani JA, editors. Atlas of adult congenital heart surgery. Cham: Springer; 2020. p. 337–43.

Ebstein W. Ueber einen sehr seltenen Fall von Insufficienz der Valvula tricuspidalis, bedingt durch eine angeborene hochgradige Missbiuldung derselben. Arch Anat Physiol Wissensch Med. 1866:238–54.

Fyler DC, et al. Report of the New England regional infant cardiac program. Pediatrics. 1980;65(2 Pt 2):375–461.

Holst KA, Dearani JA, Said SM, Davies RR, Pizarro C, Knott-Craig C, Kumar TKS, Starnes VA, Kumar SR, Pasquali SK, Thibault DP, Meza JM, Hill KD, Chiswell K, Jacobs JP, Jacobs ML. Surgical management and outcomes of Ebstein anomaly in neonates and infants: a society of thoracic surgeons congenital heart surgery database analysis. Ann Thorac Surg. 2018;106(3):785–91.

Keith JD, Rowe RD, Vlad P. Heart disease in infancy and childhood. New York: Macmillan; 1958.

Knott-Craig CJ, Goldberg SP, Ballweg JA, Boston US. Surgical decision making in neonatal Ebstein's anomaly: an algorithmic approach based on 48 consecutive neonates. World J Pediatr Congenit Heart Surg. 2012;3(1):16–20.

Perloff J. The clinical recognition of congenital heart disease. 4th ed. Philadelphia: WB Saunders; 1994. 797 pp

Starnes VA, Pitlick PT, Bernstein D, Griffin ML, Choy M, Shumway NE. Ebstein's anomaly appearing in the neonate. A new surgical approach. J Thorac Cardiovasc Surg. 1991;101(6):1082–7.

Wackel P, Cannon B, Dearani J, Sessions K, Holst K, Johnson J, Cetta F. Arrhythmia after cone repair for Ebstein anomaly: the Mayo Clinic experience in 143 young patients. Congenit Heart Dis. 2018;13(1):26–30.

Complications Associated with Operations to Repair Left Ventricular Outflow Tract Obstruction

Elizabeth H. Stephens and Joseph A. Dearani

Abstract

Left ventricular outflow tract obstruction is a general term that includes all the obstructive lesions affecting the left ventricle, aortic valve, and the aortic arch. Many patients who require intervention during childhood may also require reintervention later in life for residual or recurrent lesions. Each disease entity has associated reparative operations and this chapter focuses on potential pitfalls and complications related to the surgical management of these conditions and how they can be prevented or rectified.

Keywords

Left ventricular outflow tract obstruction · Subaortic membrane · Tunnel subaortic stenosis · Hypertrophic obstructive cardiomyopathy · Aortic stenosis · Supravalvar stenosis

E. H. Stephens (✉)
Department of Cardiovascular Surgery, Mayo Clinic, Rochester, MN, USA
e-mail: Stephens.Elizabeth@mayo.edu

J. A. Dearani
Department of Cardiovascular Surgery, Mayo Clinic, Rochester, MN, USA

Mayo Clinic College of Medicine, Rochester, MN, USA

1 Introduction

Left ventricular outflow tract obstruction (LVOTO) includes all obstructive lesions affecting the outflow from the left ventricle, thereby including obstruction within the left ventricle and at the level of the aortic valve. Aortic coarctation and hypoplastic arch are addressed elsewhere in the textbook, while etiologies in this chapter include subaortic membrane, tunnel subaortic stenosis, hypertrophic obstructive cardiomyopathy (HCM), aortic stenosis, and supravalvar stenosis. Many of these patients require intervention during childhood but may also require reintervention later in life for residual or recurrent lesions. Each disease entity has associated reparative operations and this chapter focuses on potential pitfalls and complications related to the surgical management of these conditions and how they can be prevented or rectified.

Fixed obstruction in the LVOT (below the aortic valve) includes membranous subaortic stenosis and muscular "tunnel" subaortic stenosis. Fixed obstruction at the level of the aortic valve or below the aortic valve is not responsive to medical therapy (DeCampli and Pourmoghadam 2023). *Dynamic* LVOT obstruction includes obstructive hypertrophic cardiomyopathy, accompanied by systolic anterior motion (SAM) of the mitral valve, and the degree of obstruction that can be reduced with medical therapy, (e.g., beta or calcium channel blocker therapy).

C. L. Backer, C. Mavroudis (eds.), *Complications in Pediatric and Congenital Heart Surgery*,
https://doi.org/10.1007/978-3-032-02661-3_20

Fixed subaortic stenosis (i.e., fibrous membrane) can be mistaken for obstructive HCM (Anderson et al. 2015). The important difference between this lesion and obstructive HCM is the presence of "fixed" obstruction and the absence of SAM in most patients. The fibrous membrane of subaortic stenosis is often circumferential and extends around the subaortic area involving the septum, free wall, anterior mitral valve leaflet, and frequently the hinge point and underside of the aortic valve cusps. Some degree of aortic valve regurgitation may be present due to encroachment of the membrane onto the ventricular aspect of the aortic valve with impaired cusp mobility; this should be a clue that it is membranous subaortic stenosis and not obstructive HCM. While friction lesions can be evident in obstructive HCM, they do not extend onto the aortic valve. Treatment is transaortic membrane resection with or without limited septal myectomy, as detailed below. In contrast to patients with obstructive HCM who have a low risk of recurrent obstruction following extended septal myectomy (<5%), reoperation for recurrent subaortic stenosis is reported in 10%–15%, with higher recurrence risk at younger age of first intervention (Dodge-Khatami et al. 2008).

2 Membranous Subaortic Stenosis

Membranous subaortic stenosis is commonly due to a fibrous membrane, often circumferential, but most evident on the ventricular septum. Membrane extension occurs onto the posterolateral left ventricular free wall and onto the anterior leaflet of the mitral valve. Encroachment of the membrane onto the ventricular aspect of the aortic valve cusps is common. This may result in some degree of aortic regurgitation. Occasionally the LVOT is hypoplastic. In contrast to obstructive HCM, the ventricular septum is not usually severely hypertrophied. Treatment is *enucleation and excision* of the membrane via aortotomy (Hirata et al. 2009). This involves "peeling" the membrane off the ventricular septum. When this is done properly, the fibrous peel also includes the portion that extends onto the anterior leaflet of the mitral valve and posterolateral free wall and the specimen is nearly a complete circle. Membrane encroachment onto the aortic valve is common; careful peeling of the aortic valve cusps is done separately to minimize potential cusp injury. The decision to perform a concomitant, limited septal myectomy is individualized depending on septal thickness and surgeon experience (Stephens et al. 2020).

3 Anatomic Considerations and Potential Complications

1. *Heart block* occurs from trauma or direct injury to the conduction tissue below the commissure between the right noncusps. In general, the membrane is usually just below this level. The importance of "peeling" instead of "cutting" cannot be overemphasized. If concomitant septal myectomy is being performed, beginning the resection at the nadir of the right cusp, and extending leftward toward the mitral valve is proper technique being mindful of septal thickness to avoid iatrogenic ventricular septal defect (VSD). A left bundle branch block is not uncommon after a properly performed septal myectomy. If heart block occurs, the decision to proceed with epicardial vs transvenous permanent pacing is individualized.
2. *Aortic valve injury* may occur with enucleation of the membrane off the ventricular

aspect of the cusps. All cusps may have membrane involvement. A plane can often be established and then peel begins at the level of the annulus and proceeds upward toward the leading edge of the cusp. If injury is going to occur, it typically occurs within the belly of the cusp that can be quite thin after membrane removal. If resistance is encountered when removing the fibrous peel, careful cutting of the membrane flush with the cusp with a scissors leaving some residual membrane behind on the cusp is preferred to avoid cusp fenestration. The presence of fibrous peel across the annulus can restrict cusp motion and contribute to aortic regurgitation; removal of the fibrous peel at that level improves cusp excursion and often results in an improvement in aortic regurgitation. Treatment of aortic valve injury most commonly includes closure of the defect with autologous pericardium and fine interrupted sutures to minimize distortion of the aortic cusp. Rarely, a slit-like injury to the cusp can be closed by direct suture(s). If aortic valve injury is complex, aortic valve replacement is necessary.

3. *Mitral valve injury* may also occur with fibrous peel removal. Injury can include anterior leaflet fenestration, which is rare provided the membrane is peeled off the leaflet; specifically, a knife should not be used in this area since it is easy to inadvertently cut the leaflet. An additional complication can include chordal disruption when the membrane is being teased out of the chordae. Again, sharp dissection should be avoided and when resistance to membrane removal is encountered; instead, careful cutting of the fibrous tissue flush with the subvalvar apparatus using scissors is recommended. In the event of mitral valve injury, defects in the anterior leaflet are closed by either direct suture or patch repair depending on the size of the defect. Care must be taken to avoid distortion of the anterior leaflet. If chordal disruption occurs, treatment consists of either Gore-Tex artificial chordae or chordal transfer from posterior to anterior leaflet.
4. *Ventricular septal defect* is rare with enucleation of the membrane. VSD is more likely to occur when concomitant septal myectomy is being performed. In contrast to hypertrophic cardiomyopathy, the ventricular septum is often near normal thickness (<14 mm in an adult). If iatrogenic VSD occurs, repair can be difficult. The VSD usually occurs in the outlet septum and exposure is generally preferred through a high right ventriculotomy. This allows "freshening up" the edges of the VSD (the muscle border of the VSD is fragile and denuded from the myectomy) which inevitably makes the VSD a bit larger and then patch repair is performed. In rare circumstances, a small VSD can be closed through the aortotomy but should be done with caution since injury to the aortic valve can occur, particularly if the aortic annulus is small.

4 Tunnel Subaortic Stenosis

In contrast to membranous subaortic stenosis where the membrane is "peeled" out of the LVOT, treatment of tunnel subaortic stenosis that is secondary to a hypoplastic LVOT involves a modified Konno procedure (i.e., iatrogenic creation of an outlet VSD with subsequent patch closure and preservation of the normal-sized native aortic valve). If muscular hypertrophy of the septum is a key contributor to the inadequate LVOT, a septal myectomy may provide adequate enlargement (Jonas 2002).

5 Modified Konno Procedure

The modified Konno allows enlargement of the subvalvar portion of the LVOT while maintaining the patient's native aortic valve. Certain technical caveats are worth noting, including that the right ventricular (RV) incision can be either transverse or vertical, whereas the incision is always vertical in a Konno procedure. The authors' preference for a modified Konno is a small vertical incision directed toward the aortic valve (like a Konno right ventriculotomy), since this optimizes and centers the exposure for the septal incision that will be performed as a mirror image just below the ventriculotomy. If a transverse incision is performed, it is essential that the assistant does not aggressively retract and tear the ventriculotomy into the left anterior descending artery. It is helpful to place a stitch at the lateral aspect of the transverse incision that can protect and be a constant reminder to avoid excessive retraction. The papillary muscle of Lancisi on the ventricular septum that supports the tricuspid valve is noted through the right ventriculotomy and is preserved when the septal incision is being performed. The septal incision extends leftward of the papillary muscle of Lancisi and apically beyond the level of tunnel subaortic stenosis, usually to the bases of the papillary muscles. Additional VSD resection (myectomy) along the left side of the septotomy is performed to further augment the size of the hypoplastic left ventricular outflow tract. Septal resection along the right side of the septotomy is avoided to minimize heart block. The surgically created VSD is then closed with an oval-shaped patch. The upper extent of the patch that is adjacent to the aortic valve annulus is reinforced with pledgeted mattress sutures that are seated in the right aortic sinus just above the annulus of the right aortic cusp but well below the right coronary artery (RCA). These mattress sutures extend out onto the right side of the ventricular septum and are anchored to the top of the patch. This maneuver is helpful since there may be minimal muscular tissue present at the basal extent of the ventricular septotomy for patch securement and can reduce the possibility of patch dehiscence. The technique of VSD closure can be performed with interrupted pledgeted mattress sutures (authors' preference) or continuous suture. The right ventriculotomy may be closed primarily or with a small oval-shaped pericardial patch if there is significant right ventricular hypertrophy.

6 Anatomic Considerations and Potential Complications

1. *Aortic valve injury*. The septal incision must get close to the aortic valve to minimize residual LVOT obstruction at the base of the heart. Consequently, it is easy to injure the aortic valve. To help prevent this, we place a suture via the aortotomy at the nadir of the right coronary cusp and exit the ventricular septum as visualized from the right ventriculotomy (Fig. 1) (Stephens et al. 2020). This marking suture is the "stopping point" for the upper end of the septal incision. This essential suture marks the upper extent of the ventricular septal incision and accomplishes two things: first, provides a marker to avoid potential iatrogenic injury of the aortic valve when the upper extent of the septal incision is being performed and second, allows maximal enlargement of the uppermost aspect of the basal septum to minimize residual obstruction immediately below the aortic valve. The lower end of the septal incision is generally at the level of the papillary muscles (Fig. 2) (Stephens et al. 2020). Additionally, this septal incision can be made with a Hegar dilator across the aortic annulus that also serves to protect the mitral valve.

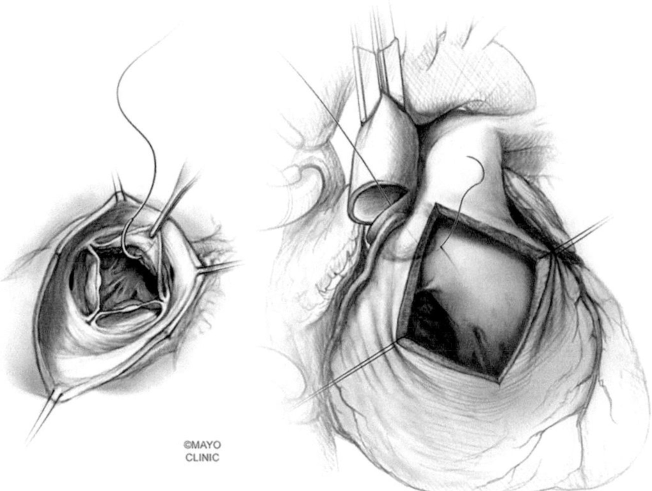

Fig. 1 An oblique aortotomy down toward the noncoronary sinus and a high right ventriculotomy that is directed toward the aortic is performed as shown. The papillary muscle of Lancisi on the ventricular septum that supports the tricuspid valve is noted through the right ventriculotomy. A marking suture is placed from the aortic root through the ventricular septum just beneath the center of the aortic annulus at the nadir of the right coronary cusp. This suture exits through the right side of the ventricular septum and comes out the right ventriculotomy. This suture marks the upper extent of the ventricular septal incision to avoid potential iatrogenic injury of the aortic valve. (With permission: Stephens et al. 2020)

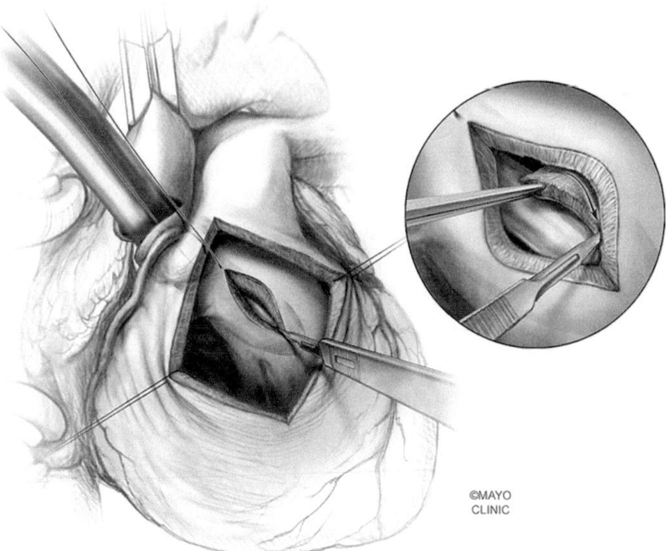

Fig. 2 A Hegar dilator is passed across the aortic annulus and into the left ventricular cavity. The Hegar dilator functions to protect the mitral valve and subvalvar apparatus and guides the septal incision. A #15 or #10 blade (depending on patient age and septal thickness) is inserted into the ventricular septum beginning at the marking suture in the ventricular septum just below the aortic valve and is extended apically using the Hegar dilator as a guide. Beginning the incision close to the aortic valve is important to minimize persistent residual obstruction just beneath the aortic valve. The septal incision extends apically beyond the level of tunnel subaortic stenosis. The inset demonstrates additional left-sided septal resection (myectomy) to further augment the size of the hypoplastic left ventricular outflow tract. (With permission: Stephens et al. 2020)

7 Ross and Ross-Konno Operations

The Ross operation is a complex operation that requires attention to anatomic details to minimize complications (Ross 1967).

8 Anatomic Considerations and Potential Complications

1. *Autograft harvest.* Autograft harvest must not injure the pulmonary valve, the left main coronary posteriorly, left anterior descending laterally, and the first septal perforator. Additionally, ample conus beneath the annulus must be retained for the aortic annular anastomosis.
2. *Autograft distortion.* Implantation should be performed in a manner that preserves alignment of the autograft commissures with the native aortic valve commissures. In the setting of a bicuspid or unicuspid valve in which three symmetric commissural posts are not present, alignment should begin by focusing on the position of the left-non and left-right to preserve a vacant sinus location for left coronary implantation that typically occurs low in the sinus. The decision to use interrupted sutures or continuous suture is generally surgeon preference. Interrupted *simple* suture technique may be preferred since it minimizes annular distortion, but it does take considerably more time. If a running stitch is used, particular care must be made to avoid autograft distortion as well as a purse-string effect, which can narrow and/or distort the annulus. Horizontal mattress sutures should be avoided since eversion of the autograft annulus can result in distortion of the autograft annulus and result in aortic regurgitation. This is especially more likely if the muscle bar below the autograft annulus is small.
3. *Annular reinforcement.* Various techniques can be applied and range from a Dacron collar around the proximal annulus to preserving the entire native aortic root that is wrapped around the autograft. In general, prosthetic material is avoided when somatic growth is incomplete.
4. *Autograft support.* When somatic growth is complete, placement of the autograft into a Valsalva graft has been preferred by some surgeons. Sizing of the graft is achieved with measurement of the autograft annulus. The distal suture line is placed at the top of the Valsalva graft. Technical issues of importance include adequate orifices within the graft for coronary button reimplantation, preventing coronary compromise from the rigid graft. A hematoma can form between the graft and autograft in the area of the noncoronary sinus and distort the autograft. To prevent this a hole in the graft is created to allow evacuation of blood/hematoma formation in this area. Once the autograft has been sutured proximally and distally within the Valsalva graft, implantation of the supported autograft can be with either simple, interrupted sutures, or a continuous suture line. There is generally no concern about a purse string effect with continuous suture given the presence of mild rigidity provided by the Dacron graft.
5. *Proximal/Distal autograft support.* In general, the distal autograft is already supported with the inclusion technique described above in #4. However, if the annulus was supported by a Dacron collar, the distal autograft should be trimmed to close the commissures and an ascending aortic Dacron graft is used. In all techniques the autograft should be kept as short as possible. In general, graft size is matched to the size of the original main pulmonary artery prior to procurement. It is important to not oversize the distal graft to avoid "splaying" of the commissures that can lead to aortic regurgitation. Without a rigid sewing ring as in a prosthesis, the autograft can easily be distorted resulting in autograft regurgitation. Attention must be paid to implant the autograft maintaining its native shape and geometry. While some surgeons perform this suture line with a running continuous suture, simple interrupted sutures can be helpful to ensure the autograft is

implanted symmetrically and geometry is maintained.

6. *LVOT pseudoaneurysm/aneurysm.* This is most likely to occur when a Konno incision is performed. While some surgeons maintain a tongue of right ventricular outflow tract (RVOT) muscle on the autograft at the time of autograft procurement and use this muscle to fill in the surgically created VSD, others believe that this "thinner" RVOT muscle is susceptible to aneurysm formation in the setting of systemic pressure (Shahid et al. 1999). An alternative is to patch the Konno incision with prosthetic patch material (Dacron, Gore-Tex, or bovine pericardium) and anchor the proximal autograft to the prosthetic patch. Finally, it is important to trim most of the proximal autograft muscle prior to implantation so the native annular suture line is close to the autograft annulus, (i.e., do not leave a large bar of [thin] muscle between the two).
7. *Coronary ischemia.* Issues with coronary artery button implantation can lead to coronary ischemia. First, both coronaries should be adequately mobilized to allow a tension-free implantation. This is particularly important in the setting of prior cardiac surgery when scar tissue is invariably present. Also, the RCA often requires a more generous mobilization out onto the RVOT. The autograft should be positioned in such a way that the left coronary button lies lower in the center of one of the sinuses of the autograft and the RCA typically is positioned higher in the right sinus. Some surgeons buttress this coronary anastomosis with native tissue (aorta, pericardium) or felt material. As in other root surgery, the coronary arteries must not be under tension, but also not be mobilized to the extent that kinking can occur. Ventricular arrhythmias coming off pump (once air has been excluded), are highly concerning for a coronary problem and regional wall motion abnormalities are not always present.
8. *Residual VSD.* When a ventriculotomy has been performed in a Ross-Konno, care must be taken to securely close the ventriculotomy, as this muscular suture line will be under systemic pressure. There are many VSD closure techniques utilized. It is the authors' approach to use interrupted pledgeted mattress sutures (pledgets on LV side) and a second continuous suture line on the RV side.
9. *Heart block.* Injury to the conduction system can occur by either direct injury to the membranous septum with annular suture placement, ventricular septal muscle resection (i.e., during myectomy), or with ventricular septal incision during a Ross-Konno. In general, any septal incisions should not veer to the right of the nadir of the right coronary cusp. While incisions that begin at the nadir of the right cusp may cause a left bundle branch block, it rarely causes complete heart block. In the setting of a standard Konno incision, the incision aims to be between the commissure between the left-right cusps and the ostium of the RCA. Care is taken to not injure the pulmonary valve that is in close proximity. In the setting of Ross-Konno, the septal incision can be even further leftward, but not beyond the left-non commissure (Fig. 3) (Dearani and Mavroudis 2020). since the procured autograft is already out of the way.
10. *Pulmonary artery stenosis.* In general, it is desirable to oversize the pulmonary homograft during the Ross procedure since homograft failure is usually a combination of stenosis and regurgitation. When performing the distal pulmonary homograft suture line, care must be taken to not narrow the proximal right or left pulmonary artery. To this end, during the anastomosis pulmonary homograft tissue excess is "donated" to the corners of the branch pulmonary arteries (i.e., sutures are close together on the pulmonary artery and wider on the pulmonary homograft) to help prevent stenosis.
11. *Coronary injury.* During the proximal homograft suture line, care must be taken to achieve adequate bites of RVOT myocardium posteriorly and laterally without com-

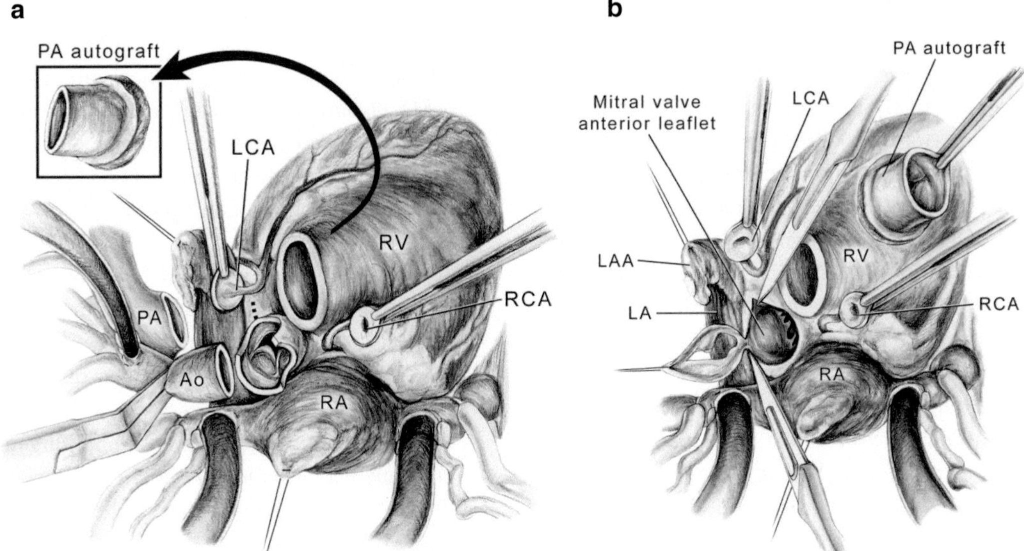

Fig. 3 (Left). The dotted line on this diagram demonstrates the location under the left main coronary button that can be incised to enlarge the aortic root. (Right) In this diagram the completed incision is shown. *Ao* aorta, *LA* left atrium, *LAA* left atrial appendage, *LCA* left coronary artery, *PA* pulmonary artery, *RA* right atrium, *RCA* right coronary artery, *RV* right ventricle. (With permission: Dearani and Mavroudis 2020)

promising the left main, first septal perforator, and left anterior descending, all of which are in close proximity.

9 Konno-Rastan

The Konno-Rastan, commonly referred to as the Konno, is utilized when the left ventricular outflow tract diameter is inadequate and the aortic valve also requires replacement, in this case when a prosthetic is used (in contrast to autograft in a Ross or Ross-Konno operation). These are patients whose anatomy does not allow for simple posterior annular enlargement accompanying a valve replacement (Griffeth et al. 2024).

10 Anatomic Considerations and Potential Complications

1. *Konno incision and right ventriculotomy.* In this case, the incision in the right ventricle is vertical and is aimed toward the center of the aortic annulus. It does not need to extend very far into the RV, (i.e., it is a high small ventriculotomy). The incision across the aortic annulus is then performed into the ventricular septum and is slightly to the left of the nadir of the right sinus (Fig. 4) (Dearani and Mavroudis 2020). It is important to not get too close to the commissure between the left and right cusps since the pulmonary valve is right there ("kissing commissures"). This contrasts with the Ross-Konno when the incision can be further leftward since the pulmonary valve has already been procured. Similarly, chordal attachments of the tricuspid valve can also be at risk on the right side of the ventriculotomy.
2. *Pulmonary valve.* As described above, it is important to be mindful of the pulmonary valve when making the septal incision. When reconstructing the ventricular septal defect, it is common for the surgeon to use the same patch that is folded back to close the right ventriculotomy. It is important to preserve sufficient muscle adjacent to the pulmonary valve to facilitate this. Finally, while the Konno allows generous LVOT enlargement and placement of almost any size aortic pros-

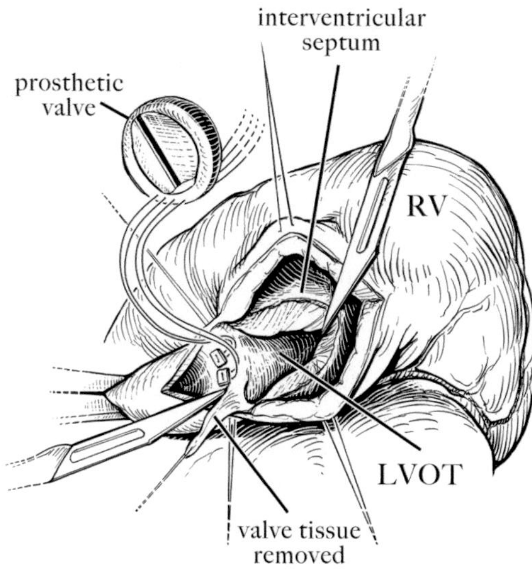

Fig. 4 Demonstration of the incision made across the aortic annulus into the ventricular septum, respecting the conduction system. This incision is continued to allow an adequate left ventricular outflow tract. Care must be made not to disrupt tricuspid valve chordal attachments or to get too close to the pulmonary valve. Also note the right ventriculotomy is relatively high. *LVOT* left ventricular outflow tract, *RV* right ventricle. (With permission: Dearani and Mavroudis 2020)

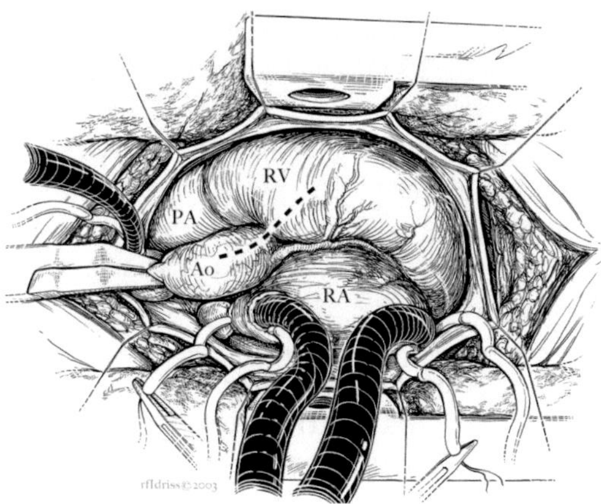

Fig. 5 Demonstration of the proximity of the right coronary artery to the incision. This must be adequately distant from the right coronary to allow for the future suture lines. *Ao* aorta, *PA* pulmonary artery, *RA* right atrium, *RV* right ventricle. (With permission: Dearani and Mavroudis 2020)

thesis, it is possible to oversize the aortic prosthesis which can then distort the native pulmonary valve. This should be avoided.

3. *Tricuspid valve*. While uncommon to directly injure the tricuspid valve, it is not uncommon for the geometry of the tricuspid valve to be distorted given both a septal incision and a right ventriculotomy that all result in some RV systolic dysfunction. As a result, it is the routine practice of the authors to empirically perform a suture annuloplasty of the tricuspid valve in all such cases.
4. *Coronary ischemia*. Coronary ischemia can occur from multiple aspects of this operation. While the ventricular and aortic incisions are designed to give adequate room for the right coronary artery, the suture line of the reconstruction almost always ends up being near the right coronary ostium and can be easily compromised, particularly when it is alongside a rigid prosthesis (Fig. 5) (Dearani and Mavroudis 2020). In this situation, the threshold to remove the RCA and mobilize it as in a button during a root replacement should be low.
5. *Mitral valve injury*. Injury to the mitral valve should be rare during a Konno procedure but can occur during the Konno incision. It is important to retract the mitral valve posteriorly (away from the ventricular septum) when incising into the septum. The same principle applies when concomitant myectomy is being performed.
6. *Residual VSD*. See above under Ross Konno.
7. *Right ventricular outflow tract (RVOT) obstruction or aneurysm*. The proper sizing of both the LVOT patch and RVOT patch is important. With the LV pressurized, the patch of the ventricular septum will bow into the RVOT. This must be sized appropriately to accommodate a good-sized aortic prosthesis (do not oversize) and concomitantly the RVOT patch sized to allow for this billowing into the RVOT. An RVOT patch that is too small will lead to RVOT obstruction. If insufficient bites are made in the RVOT patch or in the RVOT muscle border, a pseudoaneurysm or true aneurysm can develop. This can be particularly challenging since an aneurysm is located anteriorly and can become adherent to the underside of the sternum complicating a

subsequent reoperation. It is important to anchor the RVOT patch at the level of the aortic prosthesis to avoid the appearance of an RVOT aneurysm sitting above the ascending aorta (beyond the plane of the aortic prosthesis).

8. *Heart block.* See above in Ross Konno.

11 Septal Myectomy for Obstructive Hypertrophic Cardiomyopathy

Septal myectomy effectively relieves LVOT obstruction and cardiac symptoms in both adults and children with obstructive hypertrophic cardiomyopathy (Griffeth et al. 2023). Obstruction can occur at the basal level, the mid-ventricular level, or a combination of both. In general, with basal left ventricular outflow tract obstruction, there is SAM of the mitral valve and some degree of SAM-mediated mitral regurgitation. In contrast, mid-ventricular obstruction is usually not associated with SAM of the mitral valve since the point of obstruction is below the chords and anterior leaflet and between the papillary muscles and the septum.

12 Preoperative Evaluation

While this chapter focuses mostly on technical complications, there are some preoperative issues that are relevant and are discussed here. Preoperative work-up includes echocardiography and cardiac magnetic resonance imaging (Saikrishnan et al. 2014). These document the degree of obstruction, delineates the anatomy responsible for the obstruction as well as where the point of obstruction begins, and provides information on septal thickness and degree of mitral regurgitation. Additional anatomical issues include the presence of abnormal/additional mitral and/or papillary muscle attachments, and length of anterior leaflet, etc. It is also important to be aware that patients may have a low resting gradient but a significant provokable gradient causing considerable symptoms. This can be investigated with stress echo or a cardiac catheterization with provocative maneuvers when clarification is needed.

Also important is an understanding of the degree of diastolic dysfunction, especially if significant symptoms are present but in the setting of a low/minimal gradient. For patients with high pulmonary artery pressures and left-sided filling pressures, a high resting LVOT gradient is reassuring. However, for those with high pulmonary artery pressures and left-sided filling pressures who have minimal gradient, especially those without a provokable gradient, substantial diastolic dysfunction is likely present and myectomy will not be helpful since symptoms are likely related to the diastolic disease.

A second caveat is regarding surgical approach(es). Generally, a transaortic approach is used for basal LVOT obstruction with SAM, and this approach can also access some degree of mid-ventricular obstruction depending on the size of the aortic annulus. In the situation of isolated mid ventricular obstruction without SAM, the approach is via left ventriculotomy. A combined transaortic and transapical approach is used for a combination of basal and mid-ventricular obstruction (Pelliccia et al. 2020). Early mortality in experienced hands in either situation is low (1%) in adults with no comorbidities and symptomatic improvement is predictable. Late survival is improved compared with the natural history of unoperated patients with symptomatic obstructive HCM (Theodoro et al. 1996).

Transaortic landmarks are shown in Fig. 6 (Stephens et al. 2020).

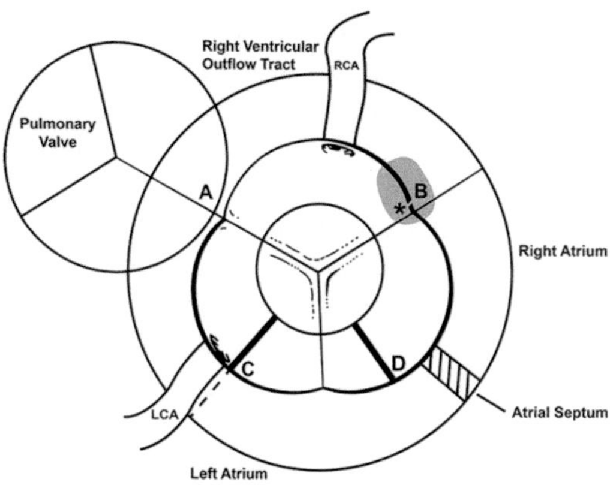

Fig. 6 Important anatomic landmarks with a transaortic approach. (**a**) Left–right coronary commissure, (**b**) right-noncoronary commissure, (**c** and **d**) mark the medial and lateral borders of the anterior mitral leaflet. Ventricular septum is between (**a**) and (**b**). Posterolateral free wall is between (**a**) and (**c**). *Marks membranous septum and conduction tissue with gray shading indicating tissue to be preserved. *RCA* indicates right coronary artery, *LCA* left coronary artery. (With permission: Stephens et al. 2020)

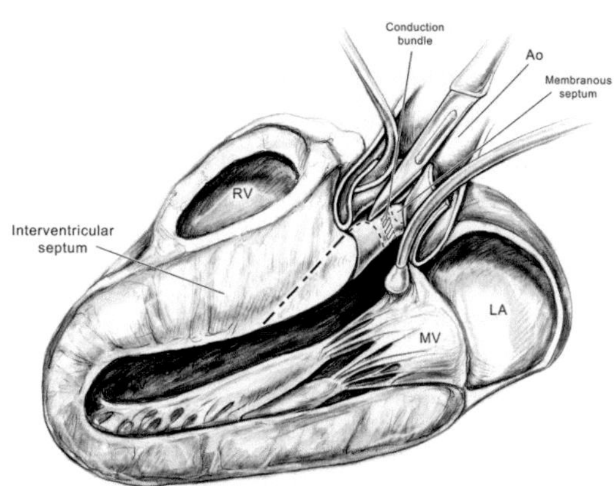

Fig. 7 Demonstration of the angle and extent of resection required. In this case the resection ends across from the midportion of the papillary muscles. Careful examination of preoperative imaging helps inform the needed extent of resection. *Ao* aorta, *LA* left atrium, *MV* mitral valve, *RV* right ventricle. (With permission: Dearani and Mavroudis 2020)

13 Anatomic Considerations and Potential Complications

13.1 Transaortic Extended Left Ventricular Septal Myectomy

1. *Inadequate muscle resection.* The primary cause of "recurrent" obstruction is residual obstruction due to inadequacy of the original resection (Fig. 7) (Dearani and Mavroudis 2020). The resection is often not distal enough, (i.e., apical extent of the myectomy is inadequate). We strongly recommend using direct, simultaneous pressure measurement of the distal LV cavity and the aorta before and after the myectomy confirming adequacy of the myectomy. This also includes inducing a premature ventricular contraction and the use of pharmacologic provocation (isoproterenol) when the gradient is <30 mmHg. This is the most accurate way to determine a residual gradient (or lack thereof) and the most sensitive method for ensuring no residual obstruction. Generally, further resection is performed if the gradient is greater than 15–20 mmHg or if there is SAM of the anterior leaflet of the mitral valve on transesophageal echocardiogram (TEE) off cardiopulmonary bypass (CPB). Many patients with sizable gradients on transthoracic echocardiogram (TTE) will not demonstrate gradients under anesthesia and isoproterenol is used in those circumstances (Elesber et al. 2008).
2. *Aortic valve injury and right coronary artery ostial injury.* While exposure is essential to safely perform the myectomy, this exposure and the process of the myectomy itself places the aortic valve at risk. For retraction, we use a vein retractor in the right coronary sinus; this retraction must be gentle and not deviate into the commissural posts or inadvertently injure the RCA ostium itself (retraction is lateral parallel to the operating table, not upward). An alternative for retraction is a flat aortic valve retractor that can cover the right cusp since the right coronary cusp is at risk both as the blade is brought in and out of the LVOT, but also the base of the cusp is at risk if the trough extends too close to or actually involves injury to the cusp itself. Caution is advised with placing a vein retractor below the annulus since the curve of the vein retractor can cut into the thinned and denuded ventricular septum and cause an iatrogenic VSD immediately beneath the annulus. The non-

coronary cusp is at risk with retraction of the aortic annulus and mitral valve rightward. When performing the aortotomy, we create a hockey-stick shaped incision that extends into the noncoronary cusp. If this aortotomy extends too close to the aortic annulus, then retraction ends up being against the noncoronary cusp as opposed to retraction against the aortic wall. It is most helpful to have two assistants using handheld retractors that can constantly be adjusted and repositioned as opposed to rigid retractors that are mounted against the sternotomy retractor since repositioning occurs frequently and continuously throughout the procedure. The primary surgeon must pay close attention to the position of these retractors while also focusing on the myectomy. Key in any of these circumstances is immediate recognition of the injury. Fortunately, most of these can be repaired and rarely, valve replacement is necessary.

3. *Mitral valve injury*. An important step in the procedure is to examine the mitral apparatus for any abnormal attachments to the septum or posterolateral free wall, or anomalous/accessory papillary muscles that could also contribute to LVOTO. These attachments tether the mitral valve into the LVOT. Abnormal attachments and anomalous or accessory papillary muscles should be examined to ensure that they are not providing vital support for the mitral valve (i.e., not attached to the leaflet leading edge) and often can be excised when they do not support the leading edge of the anterior leaflet. In these instances, a vital support may mistakenly be cut resulting in an unsupported segment of the mitral valve (usually anterior leaflet). Another instance of potential mitral valve injury is during the septal resection itself. Attention must be paid that the mitral valve is retracted rightward and away from the septum. If mitral valve injury occurs, it is usually an injury of the anterior leaflet or the subvalvar apparatus. Fenestrations in the anterior leaflet can usually be repaired via the aortotomy. However, injury to the subvalvar apparatus requires proper visualization and examination of the mitral valve via left atriotomy. The mitral valve is usually reparable but may require replacement if major injury has occurred. If mitral valve replacement is required, it is important to excise the anterior leaflet to avoid residual SAM which could happen particularly if inadequate septal resection occurred. This contrasts with mitral valve replacement for ischemic heart disease where it is desirable to maintain the subvalvar apparatus.
4. *Iatrogenic ventricular septal defect (VSD)*. When the myectomy is continued too deep, an iatrogenic VSD may be created. This is particularly at risk when the septum is not very thick, or when a sponge stick is used pushing the septum into view. Caution is advised to avoid concomitant sponge stick exposure in combination with the use of a nerve hook to also pull the septum posteriorly and upward toward the surgeon; this can make it easier to "buttonhole" the septum. We routinely assess for an iatrogenic VSD by temporarily occluding the venous bypass line while visualizing the septum and watching for blood coming across the septum. If a VSD is created, conversion is made to bicaval cannulation and exposure to repair is generally via right ventriculotomy. The defect is visualized, and the edges are freshened up (this makes the VSD larger) to make a sturdier border since the muscular edges are often friable and denuded from the myectomy. Patch closure is preferred using interrupted pledgeted sutures. The importance of visualizing the VSD border precisely cannot be overemphasized since the location of the VSD is usually in the trabeculated portion of the septum making residual VSD more likely.
5. *Coronary-cameral fistula*. During the myectomy resection of a small branch of a coronary artery may be seen occasionally and should be cauterized if noted. However, this may not be seen until post-bypass TEE imaging. When this is the case, it is essential to

confirm that it is not a VSD since the two can be confused. These small coronary cameral fistulae have not been shown to cause heart failure and should be left alone.

6. *Heart block*. This complication should be <2% when myectomy is performed in experienced centers. A properly performed myectomy usually results in a left bundle branch block. Circumstances when it may be more likely include preoperative right bundle branch block. In this situation, it is helpful for the myectomy to start slightly leftward of the nadir of the right cusp (as opposed to the exact nadir). As the trough extends more distally (Fig. 8) (Dearani and Mavroudis 2020), this incision can drift more rightward as it will be past the conduction tissue. More aggressive resection leftward along the free wall (to the left of the dotted line by the knife in Fig. 8) can also be performed to minimize residual obstruction.

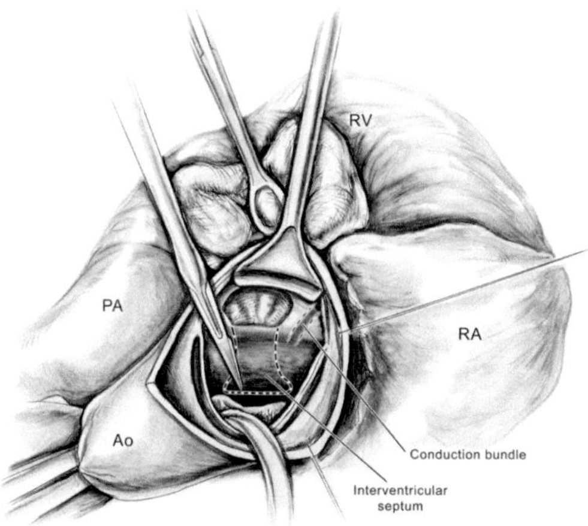

Fig. 8 Demonstration of the apical extension of the myectomy. This extension finishes well below the area of mitral septal contact. As the incision extends more apically, it can angle more rightward without injuring the conduction bundle (indicated with dotted line). The dotted box indicates the interventricular septum; to the left of that is the ventricular free wall and limited resection can be done there with preoperative imaging informing the width of that tissue, which can be substantially thinner than the septum. *Ao* aorta, *PA* pulmonary artery, *RA* right atrium, *RV* right ventricle. (With permission: Dearani and Mavroudis 2020)

7. *Pre-existing ICD/PPM leads*. For patients with pre-existing transvenous leads in the heart, particular care should be taken not to dislodge them during atrial cannulation. Prior to cannulation, palpation of the right atrium and right atrial appendage can help guide where the purse string should be placed, and cannula threaded. These leads should also be tested at the end of the case to ensure they still work appropriately. If moderate or more tricuspid regurgitation is present, tricuspid repair is advised. Finally, if a patent foramen ovale (PFO) is present it should be closed to minimize potential paradoxical embolism.

13.2 Transapical Septal Myectomy

In general, the apical ventriculotomy is small and (in an adult) typically 1.5–2 cm lateral and parallel to the left anterior descending (LAD) artery. It begins in the LV apical "dimple." Two-thirds of the incision is on the anterior wall and 1/3 on the posterior wall (Fig. 9). Figure 10 shows key structures and their relationship in a transapical approach (Dearani and Mavroudis 2020).

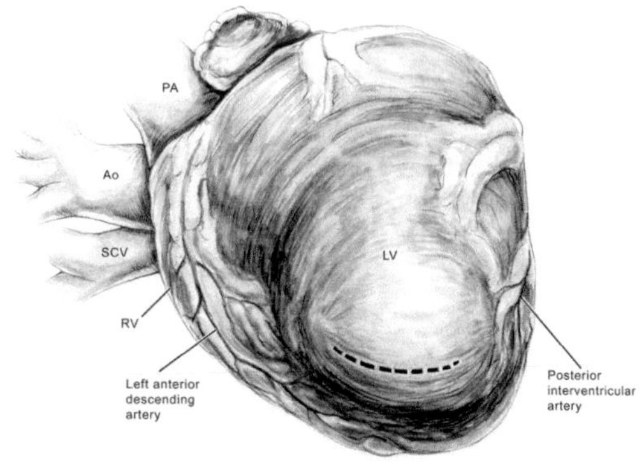

Fig. 9 Demonstration of the apical incision allowing adequate distance from the left anterior descending to allow deep bites to secure the ventriculotomy at completion without injuring the left anterior descending. Approximately 2/3 of the incision is on the anterior wall and 1/3 posterior. *Ao* aorta, *LV* left ventricle, *PA* pulmonary artery, *RV* right ventricle, *SCV* superior caval vein. (With permission: Dearani and Mavroudis 2020)

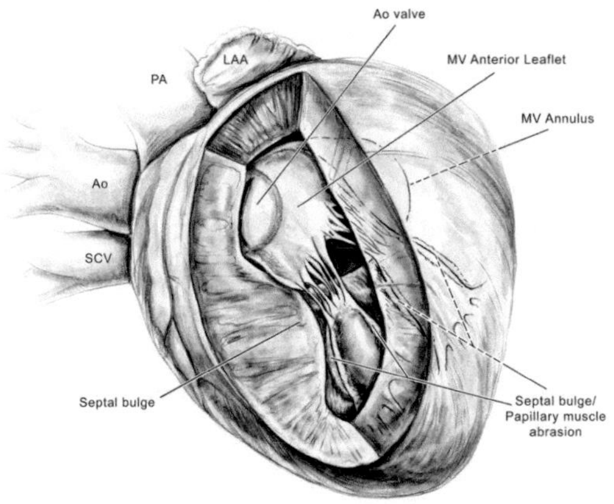

Fig. 10 Demonstration of key structures and landmarks when performing a transseptal myectomy as shown in a coronal view. The septal bulge and its contact with the papillary muscle is key to note. Mitral valve (MV) apparatus is also shown as well as Aortic (Ao) valve. *Ao* aorta, *LAA* left atrial appendage, *MV* mitral valve, *PA* pulmonary artery, *SCV* superior caval vein. (With permission: Dearani and Mavroudis 2020)

1. *Papillary muscle injury*. In HCM the papillary muscles are often apically displaced. Therefore, care should be taken when performing the apical incision to locate the bases of the papillary muscles once the cavity is opened and before continuing the incision. The papillary muscles always arise from the free wall, not the septum. Once the ventriculotomy is made, a retractor is placed into the LV and the mitral valve (papillary muscles, chords, and anterior leaflet) are retracted laterally, (i.e., away from the septum). Hypertrophied papillary muscles can be carefully shaved but it is essential to perform an even shaving and avoid cutting into the center of the papillary muscle that would disrupt its blood supply. Maintaining adequate tissue at the base of the papillary muscle is also essential to maintain integrity of the entire muscle. Should the papillary muscle be inadvertently transected, reimplantation can be attempted but mitral valve replacement is most likely needed. As mentioned earlier, if mitral valve replacement is required, excision of the anterior leaflet and some papillary muscle resection is desirable to optimize space (and eliminate any gradient) in the LV cavity. Systolic function of the LV is usually normal or above normal so there is little concern about adversely affecting LV ejection fraction.
2. *Ventriculotomy Dehiscence or Aneurysm Formation*. Secure closure of the ventriculotomy can be challenging particularly in older patients in whom tissue quality is more fragile. Resection of myocardium should be avoided along the apical incision. Ventriculotomy closure is generally performed in two layers over large felt strips with generous bites at least a centimeter back from the edge and extended slightly beyond the ends of the incision. If coming off bypass and there is bleeding around the ventriculotomy, the threshold for resuming bypass with cardioplegic arrest should be low to properly revise the closure. Aneurysm formation has not been encountered in the authors' experience. There is a small group of patients that may have a pre-existing LV apical aneurysm. When this is the case, the apical incision is more easily performed. Resection of the aneurysm sac prior to ventriculotomy closure (but retaining a small border to facilitate closure) in the same manner as described above is preferred. We have not seen ventricular arrythmias with apical incisions to date.

14 Repair of Supravalvar Aortic Stenosis

Multiple techniques have been described for the repair of supravalvar aortic stenosis. Those include the single patch (McGoon et al. 1961), Doty (two-patch) (Doty et al. 1977), Brom (three-patch) (Brom 1988), and autologous/Myers technique (Myers et al. 1993). There are several complications that can be seen with these repair types that are relevant across techniques. These patients are also at higher risk for coronary ischemia and arrest with induction of anesthesia. Consequently, precautionary protocols with surgical backup are common in experienced centers.

15 Anatomic Considerations and Potential Complications

1. *Coronary ischemia or injury*. While preoperative imaging should evaluate for ostial stenosis and potential coronary ischemia, this detail is not always well visualized on imaging even when present. During the operation each coronary should be carefully examined for any ostial compromise and fibrotic ridges carefully excised. Coronary ischemia can also occur secondary to distortion or compromise of the coronary ostia during the patching procedure(s) (Fig. 11) (Dearani and Mavroudis 2020). Additionally, initial exposure can be challenging given the frequently very narrow aortic lumen at the level of the sinotubular junction. Surgeons should also be cognizant of aortotomy location since the coronaries may arise higher on the ascending aorta (above the sinotubular junction).
2. *Aortic cannulation complications*. These patients commonly have very thickened aortas, which can make aortic cannulation more difficult. The aorta must be deeply incised to reach the lumen but avoiding "back walling" the aorta with the blade. Importantly, the actual aortic lumen can be very narrow.
3. *Aortic valve injury*. During patch augmentation care must be taken to allow sufficient room to perform the suture line without injuring or distorting the aortic cusps along the annulus and adjacent to the commissures. Also, retraction must be gentle. While exposure in these cases can be challenging due to the excess of fibrous tissue and supravalvar ridge, the aortic cusps usually are not fibrotic and remain thin and may be at risk for traction injury.

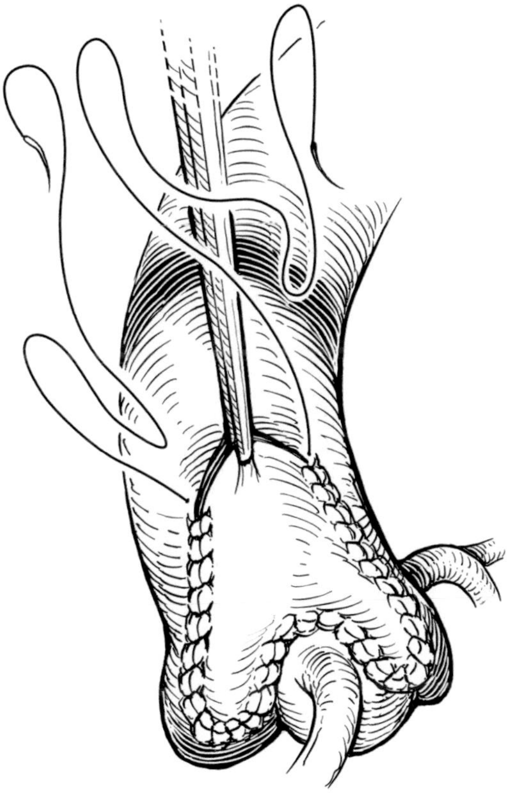

Fig. 11 Demonstration of the proximity of the coronary ostia, in this case shown in the context of the Doty technique. (With permission: Dearani and Mavroudis 2020)

References

Anderson MJ, Arruda-Olson A, Gersh B, Geske J. Subaortic membrane mimicking hypertrophic cardiomyopathy. BMJ Case Rep. 2015;4:bcr2015212321. https://doi.org/10.1136/bcr-2015-212321.

Brom AG. Obstruction of the left ventricular outflow tract. In: Khonsari S, editor. Cardiac surgery: safeguards and pitfalls in operative technique. Rockville: Aspen Publishers; 1988. p. 276–80.

Dearani JA, Mavroudis C. Left ventricular outflow tract obstruction in the adult. In: Mavroudis C, Dearani JA, editors. Atlas of adult congenital heart surgery. Cham: Springer; 2020. p. 271–304.

DeCampli WH, Pourmoghadam KK. Left ventricular outflow tract obstruction. In: Mavroudis C, Backer CL, editors. Pediatric cardiac surgery. 5th ed. West Sussex: Wiley-Blackwell; 2023. p. 669–703.

Dodge-Khatami A, Schmid M, Rousson V, Fasnacht M, Doell C, Bauersfeld U, Prêtre R. Risk factors for reoperation after relief of congenital subaortic stenosis. Eur J Cardiothorac Surg. 2008;33(5):885–9.

Doty DB, Polansky DB, Jenson CB. Supravalvular aortic stenosis. Repair by extended aortoplasty. J Thorac Cardiovasc Surg. 1977;74:362–71.

Elesber A, Nishimura RA, Rihal CS, Ommen SR, Schaff HV, Holmes DR Jr. Utility of isoproterenol to provoke outflow tract gradients in patients with hypertrophic cardiomyopathy. Am J Cardiol. 2008;101(4):516–20.

Griffeth EM, Dearani JA, Schaff HV, Johnson JN, Ackerman MJ, Bos JM, et al. Septal myectomy outcomes in children and adolescents with obstructive hypertrophic cardiomyopathy. Ann Thorac Surg. 2023;116(3):499–507.

Griffeth EM, Dearani JA, Hassler KR, Todd A, Johnson JN, Miranda WR, Stephens EH. Late outcomes of Konno-Rastan and modified Konno for left ventricular outflow tract obstruction. Ann Thorac Surg. 2024;117(5):973–81.

Hirata Y, Chen JM, Quaegebeur JM, Mosca RS. The role of enucleation with or without septal myectomy for discrete subaortic stenosis. J Thorac Cardiovasc Surg. 2009;137(5):1168–72.

Jonas RA. Modified Konno procedure for tunnel subaortic stenosis. Oper Tech Thorac Cardiovasc Surg. 2002;7:176–80.

McGoon DC, Mankin HT, Vlad P, Kirklin J. The surgical treatment of supravalvular aortic stenosis. J Thorac Cardiovasc Surg. 1961;41:125–33.

Myers JL, Waldhausen JA, Cyran SE, Gleason MM, Weber HS, Baylen BG. Results of surgical repair of congenital supravalvular aortic stenosis. J Thorac Cardiovasc Surg. 1993;105:281–8.

Pelliccia F, Alfieri O, Calabrò P, Cecchi F, Ferrazzi P, Gragnano F, Kaski JP, Limongelli G, Maron M, Rapezzi C, Seggewiss H, Yacoub MH, Olivotto I. Multidisciplinary evaluation and management of obstructive hypertrophic cardiomyopathy in 2020: towards the HCM heart team. Int J Cardiol. 2020;304:86–92.

Ross DN. Replacement of aortic and mitral valves with a pulmonary autograft. Lancet. 1967;2(7523):956–8.

Saikrishnan N, Kumar G, Sawaya FJ, Lerakis S, Yoganathan AP. Accurate assessment of aortic stenosis: a review of diagnostic modalities and hemodynamics. Circulation. 2014;129:244–53.

Shahid MS, Al-Halees Z, Khan SM, Pieters FA. Aneurysms complicating pulmonary autograft procedure for aortic valve replacement. Ann Thorac Surg. 1999;68(5):1842–3.

Stephens EH, Dearani JA, Johnson JN, Ackerman MJ, Ommen SR, Schaff HV. The surgeon's view of the left ventricular outflow tract in congenital heart surgery. World J Pediatr Congenit Heart Surg. 2020;11(5):595–610.

Theodoro DA, Danielson GK, Feldt RH, Anderson BJ. Hypertrophic obstructive cardiomyopathy in pediatric patients: results of surgical treatment. J Thorac Cardiovasc Surg. 1996;112(6):1589–99.

Complications Associated with the Norwood Operation

Awais Ashfaq and David L. S. Morales

Abstract

Hypoplastic left heart syndrome (HLHS) is a constellation of congenital cardiac anomalies characterized by hypoplasia or absence of the left ventricle and severe hypoplasia of the ascending aorta. The first successful palliation of HLHS was reported by Norwood and colleagues in 1981. This chapter will review the steps of the Norwood operation and examine complications that can occur during the conduct of this palliative procedure.

Keywords

Congenital heart surgery · Hypoplastic left heart syndrome · Norwood · Palliation · Outcomes · Complications

1 Introduction

Hypoplastic left heart syndrome (HLHS) is the most common form of single ventricle congenital heart defects in the United States (Morris et al. 1990). The incidence is 1.6–3.6 in 10, 000 in the United States and HLHS represents 2%–3% of all cases of congenital heart disease (CHD) (Greenwood et al. 1975; Connor and Thiagarajan 2007; Grossfeld et al. 2019). Despite the low incidence of HLHS overall, it is still responsible for a high percentage of mortality due to CHD (Fruitman 2000; Ohman et al. 2019). HLHS is responsible for 25%–40% of neonatal cardiac deaths (Yabrodi and Mastropietro 2017; Talner 1980; Samanek et al. 1989).

Hypoplastic left heart syndrome is a spectrum of CHD characterized by significant hypoplasia or atresia of the mitral and aortic valves with underdevelopment of the left ventricle, normally related great vessels, and hypoplasia of the ascending aorta and arch (Tchervenkov et al. 2000; Gobergs et al. 2016). Clinically the anatomical diagnosis is distinguished by the status of the mitral and the aortic valves (hypoplasia versus atresia). At one end of the spectrum is HLHS with mitral atresia and aortic atresia (MA-AA) which is usually associated with a severely hypoplastic left ventricular cavity and on the other end is mitral stenosis and aortic stenosis (MS-AS) where the left ventricle is usually larger in size. In between the two there is the mitral stenosis aortic atresia subtype (Tchervenkov et al. 2000). Advances in surgical and medical management have resulted in improvement in survival (Brosig et al. 2013; Frommelt et al. 2007; Ghanayem et al. 2004; Tweddell et al. 2002). Despite that, the mortality for HLHS remains high even with optimal medical management (Norwood et al. 1983).

A. Ashfaq (✉) · D. L. S. Morales
Heart Institute, Department of Cardiothoracic Surgery, Cincinnati Children's Hospital Medical Center, University of Cincinnati College of Medicine, Cincinnati, OH, USA
e-mail: awais.ashfaq@cchmc.org

C. L. Backer, C. Mavroudis (eds.), *Complications in Pediatric and Congenital Heart Surgery*,
https://doi.org/10.1007/978-3-032-02661-3_21

Norwood and colleagues reported the first successful palliation of hypoplastic left heart syndrome in 1983 (Norwood et al. 1983). Today, there are several surgical strategies for stage I palliation, including the right-ventricle-to-pulmonary artery conduit (Sano) modification, the so-called hybrid procedure (ductal stenting and branch pulmonary artery banding), and perhaps the most widely adopted, the Norwood procedure with an innominate artery-to-pulmonary artery (Blalock-Taussig-Thomas) shunt (Sano et al. 2003; Akintuerk et al. 2002).

Regardless of the surgical approach, neonatal palliation of the hypoplastic left heart requires relief of systemic outflow obstruction, provision of unobstructed coronary blood flow, creation of a nonrestrictive atrial septal communication, and limitation of excessive pulmonary blood flow.

2 Basic Anatomy

HLHS combines multiple entities with characteristic anatomic and physiologic features characterized by variable degrees of left ventricular hypoplasia and underdevelopment. Most broadly HLHS is a syndrome with a dominant right ventricle and systemic outflow obstruction that is not amenable to biventricular repair.

2.1 Hypoplasia of the Left Ventricle to Aortic Connection

The spectrum of HLHS includes aortic atresia with mitral atresia, aortic atresia with mitral stenosis and critical aortic stenosis with mitral stenosis. Among patients undergoing the Norwood procedure, aortic atresia with mitral atresia is the most common phenotype seen in 36%–46% of patients. Aortic atresia and mitral stenosis is seen in 23%–26% of patients and aortic stenosis with mitral stenosis is seen in 20%–29% of patients (Stasik et al. 2006; Mahle et al. 2000). Among patients receiving stage I palliation, the mean ascending aortic diameter was 3.3 mm and up to 55% had an ascending aorta that measures <2 mm (Ghanayem et al. 2003). Further distally, coarctation of the aorta is a common occurrence in more than 80% of the patients (Elzenga and Gittenberger-de Groot 1985; Machii and Becker 1995).

2.2 The Left Atrium and Atrial Septum

The left atrium is usually small although there can be hypertrophy of the left atrial walls, the foramen ovale is usually patent; however, in up to one-tenth of patients, the atrial septum will be intact (Glatz et al. 2007). In some of these patients with an intact foramen ovale there will be an outflow of the left atrium through the presence of a so-called levo-atrial cardinal vein or because of a fenestration of the walls of the coronary sinus (Hellmund et al. 2017). If no left atrial outflow exists this will result in an increase in left atrial pressure producing increased left atrial hypertrophy, along with changes in the lungs, including arterialization of the pulmonary veins and lymphangiectasia, with a "cobblestone" appearance of the pulmonary surfaces seen at autopsy and a nutmeg appearance by fetal magnetic resonance imaging (MRI) (Saul et al. 2016). These are ominous prognostic features.

2.3 The Tricuspid Valve

Among the tricuspid valve abnormalities, tricuspid valve dysplasia is common in HLHS and occurs in up to 50% of cases with mitral stenosis (Stamm et al. 1997; Ho and Stamm 2004). Tricuspid regurgitation is a very important prognostic factor in HLHS (King et al. 2019). A small septal leaflet and anterior leaflet prolapse is associated with the development of tricuspid valve regurgitation (TR) (Takahashi et al. 2009). Frequently encountered abnormalities are leaflet dysplasia and leaflet prolapse that alter the valve geometry resulting in malcoaptation (Tsang and Raja 2012; Ohye et al. 2004; Honjo et al. 2011).

Leaflet tethering can result in restricted leaflet motion, deficient coaptation and regurgitation. Tethering can also occur as a consequence of lateral displacement of the anterior papillary muscle due to the abnormal geometry and dilation of a single right ventricle in HLHS (Takahashi et al. 2009). Abnormal chordae tendinae, including elongation, deficiency, or inadequate attachment, are pathologic findings that result in TR as well.

2.4 The Ventricle

In patients with mitral atresia, the left ventricle is severely hypoplastic and is no more than a slit in the posteroinferior ventricular mass. There are varying degrees of left ventricular hypoplasia in aortic stenosis. The right ventricle is usually both enlarged and hypertrophied. The right ventricle folds around the hypoplastic left ventricular apex. This may impact the tricuspid valve anatomy and function by affecting the geometry of the inlet portion of the right ventricle and the subvalvar apparatus.

2.5 The Coronary Arteries

Coronary artery abnormalities are rare but can have important consequences on outcomes. Despite the origin of the coronaries from the hypoplastic aortic root, the coronary ostia and the proximal coronaries are typically normal (Lloyd et al. 1986). Abnormal origin of the left coronary artery from the right pulmonary artery has been reported and represents a challenging diagnostic dilemma. Preoperative imaging as well as surgical repair can have a substantial effect on surgical outcomes (Baffa et al. 1992). In patients with mitral stenosis and aortic atresia, ventriculo-coronary connections between the hypertensive left ventricle and the epicardial coronaries have been documented (Baffa et al. 1992; Nathan et al. 2012). This group of patients have a higher mortality after the Norwood procedure (Nathan et al. 2012).

3 Norwood Procedure with an Innominate Artery to Pulmonary Artery Shunt

Surgery is typically scheduled electively approximately 2–5 days after presentation. Initial arterial cannulation is via a synthetic expanded polytetrafluorethylene (ePTFE) graft anastomosed end-to-side to the innominate artery. This graft will ultimately become the innominate artery-to-pulmonary artery shunt. We cool the patient to a bladder temperature of 18–20 °C over at least 30 min with a pH-stat perfusion strategy for cooling. The hematocrit is maintained above 25%. We routinely use continuous cerebral perfusion to minimize the period of deep hypothermic circulatory arrest. Flow is maintained to the innominate artery at a rate of 20–30 mL/kg/min, and near-infrared spectroscopy is used to assist in achieving adequate perfusion. Modified ultrafiltration is used routinely after separation from cardiopulmonary bypass. Postoperative management is facilitated by the routine use of an oximetric catheter and 2-site near-infrared spectroscopy that has been previously described.

3.1 General Steps of the Operation

After a median sternotomy, vascular structures, including innominate vein, brachiocephalic vessels, ascending aorta, main pulmonary artery, arch and ductus arteriosus are mobilized (Tweddell 2005) (Fig. 1). Arterial cannulation is performed by suturing an ePTFE graft end-to-side on the innominate artery destined to become the systemic-to-pulmonary artery shunt. It is brought up and cut in a beveled manner as shown (Fig. 2a–c).

Additional purse string sutures are placed for right atrial cannulation, and one in the right atrial free wall for a vent that will be placed in the right ventricle. With initiation of cardiopulmonary bypass, the branch pulmonary arteries are snared and the patient is cooled over 30 min to a bladder temperature of less than 20 °C. The vent is use-

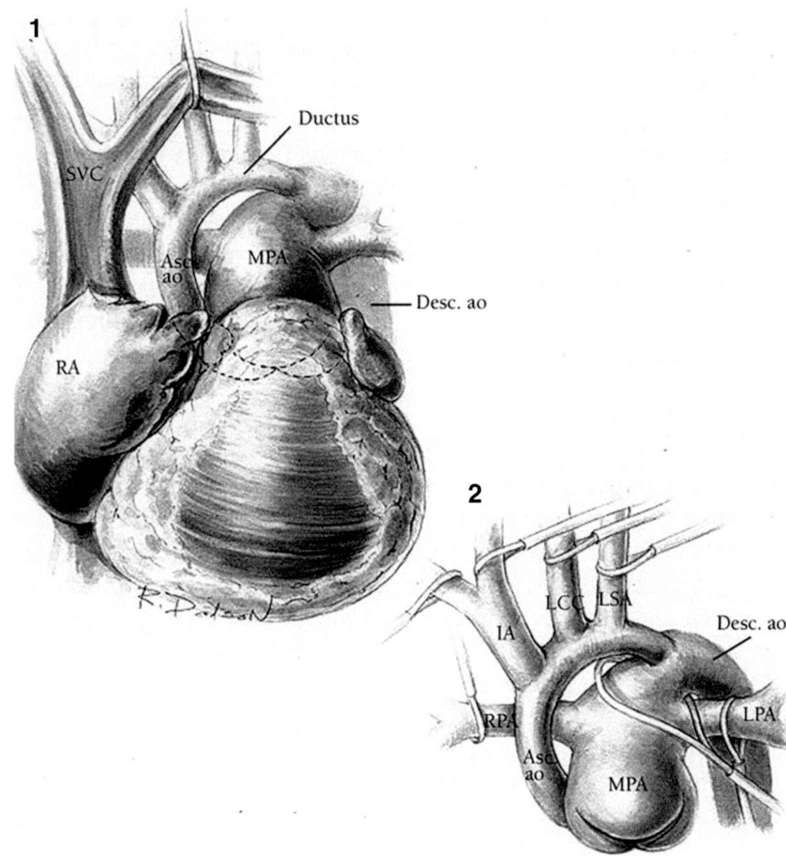

Fig. 1 (1) The innominate vein is mobilized after median sternotomy to facilitate exposure of the brachiocephalic vessels. (2) The brachiocephalic vessels are fully mobilized. The ascending aorta is separated from the main pulmonary artery, and the arch and ductus arteriosus are also mobilized. The branch pulmonary arteries are mobilized to their first branches. (With permission Tweddell 2005). *Asc ao* ascending aorta, *Desc ao* descending aorta, *IA* innominate artery, *LCC* left common carotid artery, *LPA* left pulmonary artery, *LSA* left subclavian artery, *MPA* main pulmonary artery, *RA* right atrium, *RPA* right pulmonary artery, *SVC* superior vena cava

ful in preventing ventricular distension as contractions become less effective with hypothermia.

After cooling the patient for approximately 10 min, the ductus is snared, and the main pulmonary artery is divided just proximal to the takeoff of the branch pulmonary arteries. We have not noticed significant entrainment of air into the venous cannula that the vent cannot handle. Alternatively, the proximal pulmonary artery can be controlled with a Cooley carotid clamp. The distal pulmonary artery confluence is patched with pulmonary homograft. After this, the proximal descending aorta is mobilized ensuring the safety of the recurrent nerve (Tweddell 2005) (Fig. 3). Once adequate temperature has been achieved, circulatory arrest is established and cardioplegia is delivered via a side arm on the arterial cannula. During this procedure, the venous cannula is removed and an atrial septectomy is performed. Once completed, antegrade cerebral perfusion is initiated by controlling the origin of the innominate artery, the left common carotid artery, and left subclavian artery. A descending thoracic aortic clamp is then placed and the aortic isthmus and ductus arteriosus divided with a generous excision of ductal tissue (Tweddell 2005) (Fig. 4).

The undersurface of the aortic arch is then incised beginning at the open aortic isthmus and extending proximally down the ascending aorta (Fig. 5a). A cutback is made in the pulmonary root at the site of implantation of the ascending aorta. Another cutback is made into the left posterolateral descending thoracic aorta. The opened distal arch is interdigitated into the cutback in the proximal descending aorta. This allows enough distal dissection beyond the coarctation tissue to use good aortic tissue for reconstruction (Fig. 5b). The clamp on the descending thoracic aorta assists with pulling it up and approximating it to the distal arch (Tweddell 2005) (Fig. 6a, b) that

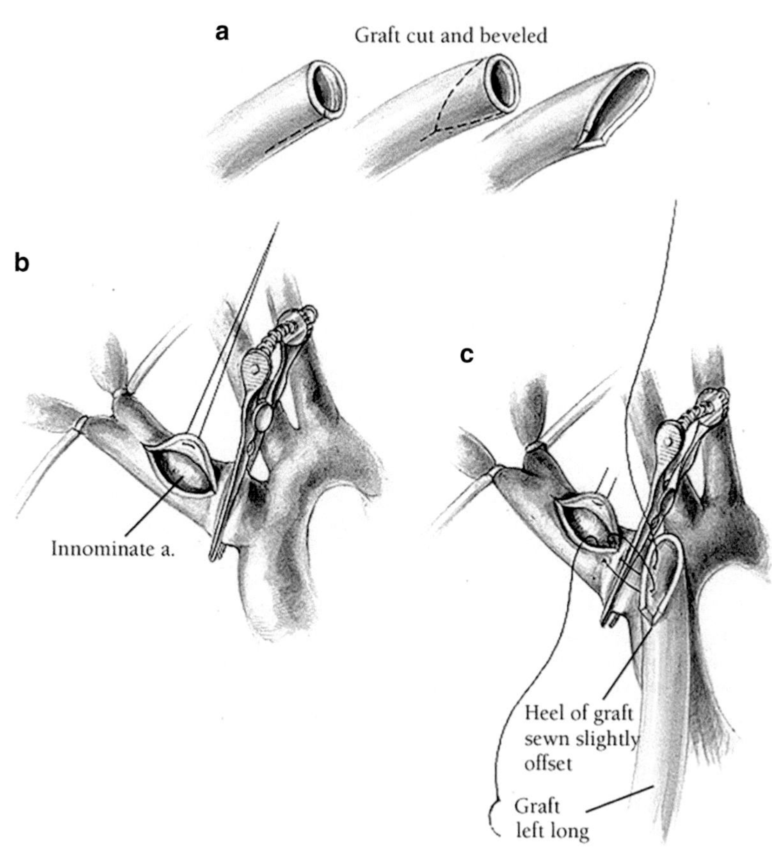

Fig. 2 (**a**, **b**, **c**) The innominate artery is isolated by tightening snares around the right subclavian artery and right carotid artery. A PTFE graft, which will become the systemic-to-pulmonary artery shunt is used initially for arterial cannulation, brought up and cut in a beveled manner as shown. This results in a large "cobra head" connection between the proximal graft and the innominate artery. The anastomosis of the graft to the innominate artery is slightly offset to achieve a more vertical orientation of the innominate artery-to-pulmonary artery shunt. (With permission Tweddell 2005). *PTFE* Polytetrafluoroethylene

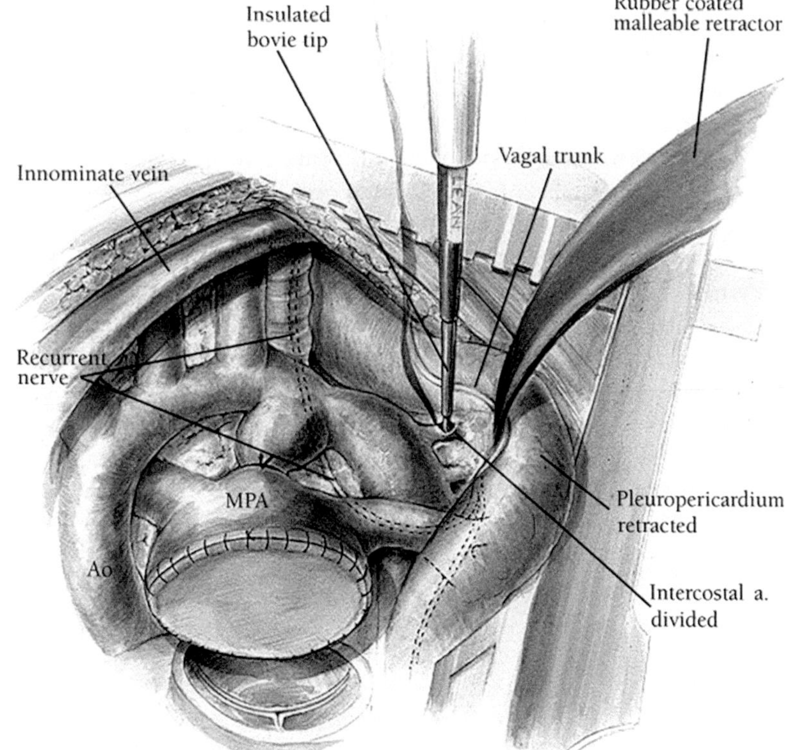

Fig. 3 The ductus arteriosus is ligated, and the proximal descending aorta is mobilized. An insulated malleable retractor is used to retract the pericardium and pleura. An insulated cautery is used at low settings (10%) to divide the first 2 or 3 sets of intercostal branches and in some cases a bipolar cautery may be used. The use of an insulated retractor and cautery tip minimizes the risk of recurrent nerve injury. (With permission Tweddell 2005). *Ao* aorta, *MPA* main pulmonary artery

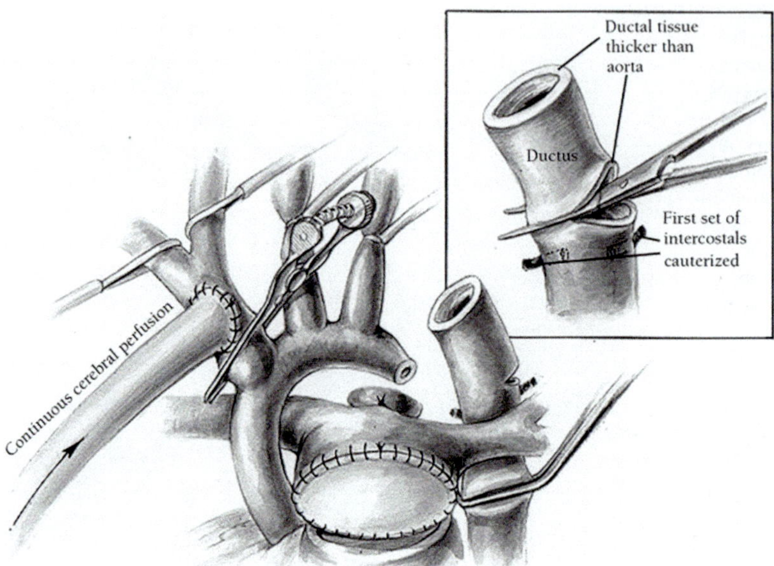

Fig. 4 All residual ductal tissue is excised from the descending thoracic aorta. Two indicators are used to ensure that the ductal tissue is completely excised. First, the arterial duct is thicker walled and the texture more friable than the true descending aorta. Excision is continued until a thin-walled, normal-textured artery is encountered. Second, the excision is continued to within 2–3 mm of the first set of intercostal branches; because the intercostals arise from the descending thoracic aorta and not the ductus arteriosus, this will further ensure complete excision of the ductal tissue. (With permission Tweddell 2005)

facilitates interdigitating and decreasing the tension on the anastomosis while suturing. A pulmonary homograft branch patch is used for completion of the arch reconstruction and creation of the neo-ascending aorta (Tweddell 2005) (Fig. 7a–d).

After reconstruction of the arch, ascending aorta, and completion of the Damus-Kaye-Stansel anastomosis, the arterial cannula is transferred from the ePTFE graft to the neoaortic root. Air is evacuated from the neoaortic root and arch. This can be accomplished by tightening the snares on the right common carotid artery and right subclavian arteries and giving some turns on the arterial cannula while evacuating any residual air through the Gore-Tex graft. After deairing, the patient is placed in the Trendelenburg position, the clamp on the descending aorta is removed, cardiopulmonary bypass is resumed, snares on the brachiocephalic vessels are released, and rewarming is initiated.

The central pulmonary confluence is mobilized to the right side of the ascending aorta. The ePTFE graft is trimmed to a length of about 10 mm, and an anastomosis is constructed between the graft and the pulmonary artery (Fig. 8) (Tweddell 2005). The central position of the shunt helps to promote equivalent growth of the branch pulmonary arteries. After rewarming the patient to a bladder temperature greater than 35 °C, inotropic support is initiated, the vent is removed, and mechanical ventilation is resumed. If after several minutes hemodynamics remain satisfactory, modified ultrafiltration is commenced, the cannulae removed, and protamine is administered.

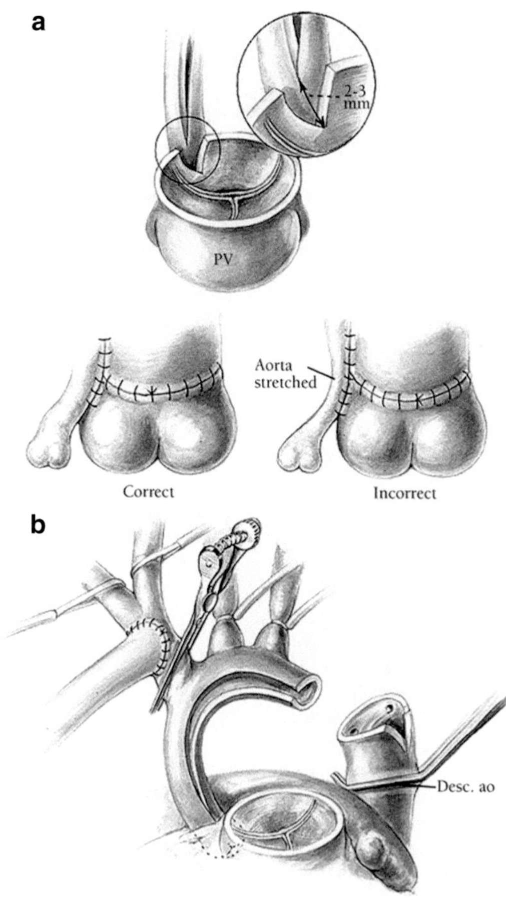

Fig. 5 (**a**, **b**) The undersurface of the aortic arch is incised beginning at the open aortic isthmus and extending proximally down the ascending aorta**.** Great care must be taken with the diminutive ascending aorta to avoid spiraling posteriorly on the ascending aorta. The incision must end precisely at the kissing point between the ascending aorta and the pulmonary root. A cutback is made in the pulmonary root at the site of implantation of the ascending aorta. This cutback is in the posterior sinus of Valsalva just leftward of the commissure between the right and posterior sinus of Valsalva of the pulmonary valve. It is also important to end the aortic incision 2–3 mm cephalad to the level of the pulmonary root cutback. The opened distal arch is interdigitated into the cutback in the proximal descending aorta. This allows enough distal dissection beyond the coarctation tissue to use good aortic tissue for reconstruction. (With permission Tweddell 2005). *Desc ao* descending aorta, *PV* pulmonary valve

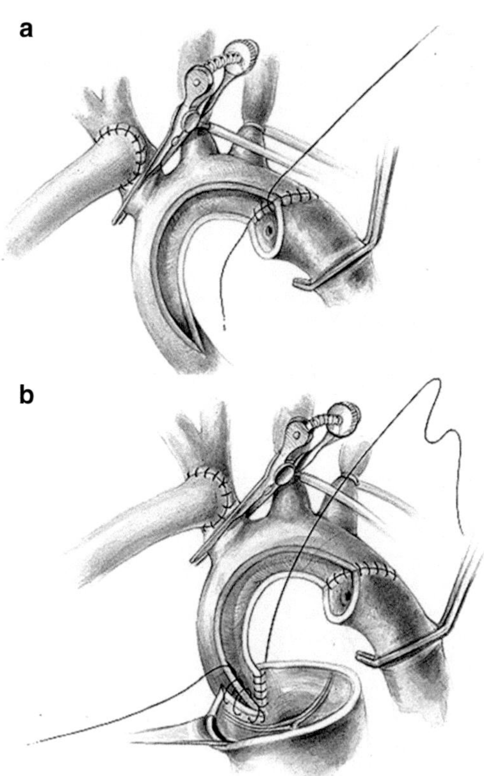

Fig. 6 (**a**, **b**) Mobilization of proximal descending aorta is necessary to permit the reconstruction of the distal aortic arch. The opened distal arch is interdigitated into the cutback in the proximal descending aorta. The clamp on the descending thoracic aorta assists with pulling it up and approximating it to the distal arch. A cutback is made in the pulmonary root at the site of implantation of the ascending aorta. Another cutback is made into the left posterolateral descending thoracic aorta. (With permission Tweddell 2005)

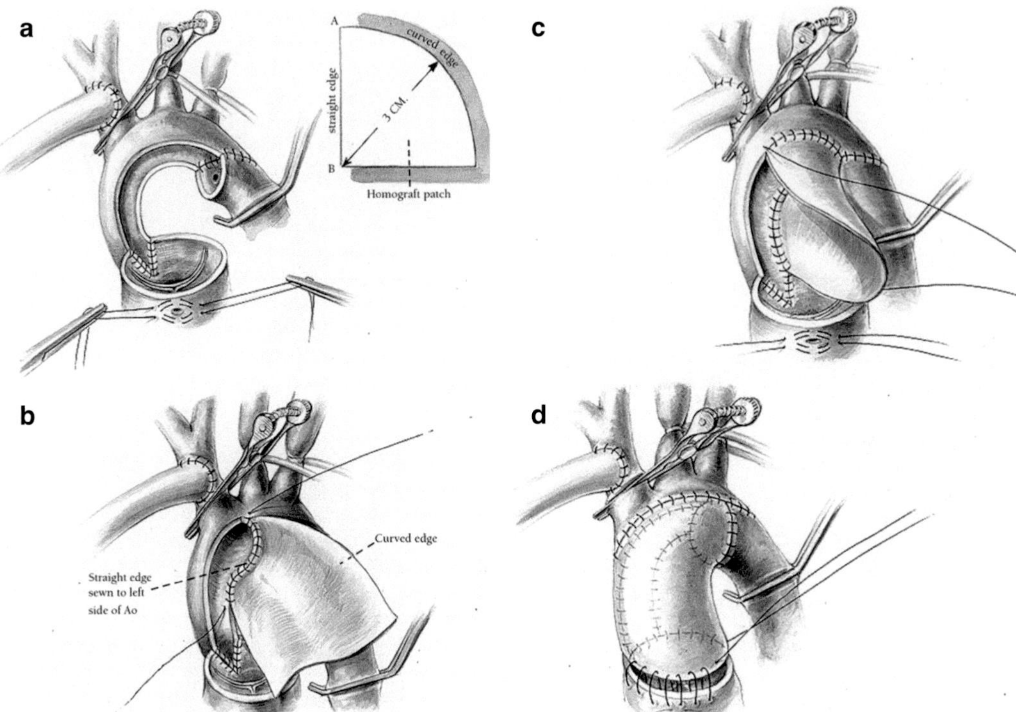

Fig. 7 (**a–d**) A pulmonary homograft patch is used for completion of the arch reconstruction and creation of the neo-ascending aorta. This patch is a quarter circle with a radius of 3 cm. The straight edge of the circle from 12 o'clock to the center is sewn down the left edge of the ascending aorta. The curved edge is sewn to the right edge of the ascending aorta. When the junction of the ascending aorta and pulmonary root is reached, excess patch is trimmed, and the proximal connection between the patch and the pulmonary root is completed. (With permission Tweddell 2005)

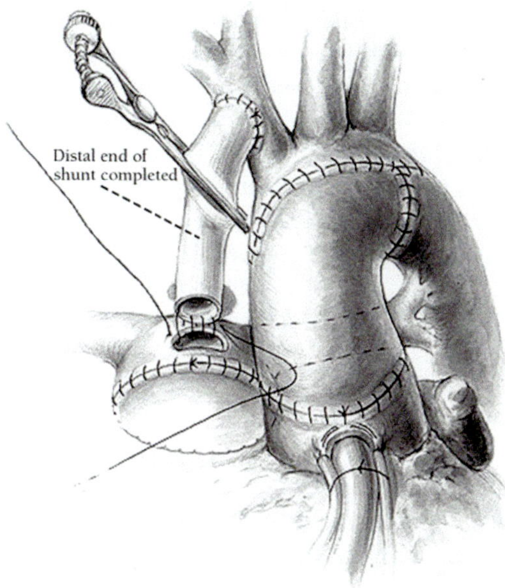

Fig. 8 After reconstruction of the arch, ascending aorta, and completion of the Damus-Kaye-Stansel anastomosis, the arterial cannula is transferred from the Gore-Tex graft to the neoaortic root. The central pulmonary confluence (distal main pulmonary artery) is moved to the right side of the ascending aorta. An arteriotomy is made in the central pulmonary artery confluence close to the patch suture line. The PTFE graft is trimmed to an adequate length, and an anastomosis is constructed between the graft and the pulmonary artery. The central position of the shunt helps to promote equivalent growth of the branch pulmonary arteries. (With permission Tweddell 2005)

3.2 Anatomical Innominate Artery to Pulmonary Shunt Complications

It is important to bevel the graft used to become the systemic-to-pulmonary artery shunt. This results in a large "cobra head" connection between the proximal graft and the innominate artery. For patients under 3.5 kg, we generally use a 3.0-mm graft, and for patients greater than 3.5 kg, we commonly use a 3.5-mm graft. Rarely, larger grafts are used for larger patients or those who present late (>2 weeks of age). The anastomosis of the graft to the innominate artery is slightly offset to achieve a more vertical orientation of the innominate artery-to-pulmonary artery shunt (Fig. 2). In addition, it is imperative to keep the length as straight as possible and not have the shunt too long as that may become prone to some stasis and thrombus formation in the postoperative period.

3.3 Complications Related to Damus-Kaye-Stansel Anastomosis and Arch Reconstruction

As shown in Fig. 5, A, great care must be taken with the diminutive ascending aorta to avoid spiraling posteriorly when making the cutback incision from the arch towards the proximal aorta.

This cutback is in the posterior sinus of Valsalva just leftward of the commissure between the right and posterior sinus of Valsalva of the pulmonary valve. It is also important to end the aortic incision 2–3 mm cephalad to the level of the pulmonary root cutback (Fig. 5a). This results in a small degree of redundancy in the proximal ascending aorta and ensures a patulous nonstenotic connection between the aortic root and the pulmonary root. If the ascending aorta is incised too far proximally, a short segment of the ascending aorta will be left, and stretching of this narrow caliber vessel will result in stenosis and coronary insufficiency.

Adequate mobilization as mentioned earlier is also imperative as shown in Fig. 6a. The surgeons must pay attention to go beyond the first set of intercostal spaces and widely mobilize the descending aorta. We generally have also done an aggressive coarctectomy to make sure the suture lines are on the native aortic tissue to prevent recoarctation.

The patch used for arch reconstruction is usually a quarter circle with a radius of 3 cm although there are several variations of how the patch is reconstructed by different surgeons. The straight edge of the circle from 12 o'clock to the center is sewn down the left edge of the ascending aorta (Fig. 7a). The curved edge is sewn to the right edge of the ascending aorta (Fig. 7b). There are several variations of fashioning the patch such as a "shark fin" configuration or using a hemi-homograft and using the curve of the graft to mimic the arch curve. When the junction of the ascending aorta and pulmonary root is reached, the excess patch is trimmed, and the proximal connection between the patch and the pulmonary root is completed (Fig. 7c, d).

3.4 Complications Related to Recoarctation

All residual ductal tissue is excised from the descending thoracic aorta (Fig. 4). Two indicators are used to ensure that the ductal tissue is completely excised. First, the arterial duct has a thicker wall and the texture is more friable than the true descending aorta. Excision is continued until a thin-walled, normally-textured artery is encountered. Second, the excision is continued to within 2–3 mm of the first set of intercostal branches because the intercostals arise from the descending thoracic aorta and not the ductus arteriosus. This will further ensure complete excision of the ductal tissue and prevent recoarctation.

3.5 Complications Related to Nerve Injury

An insulated malleable retractor is used to retract the pericardium and pleura (Fig. 3). An insulated cautery is used at low settings (10%) to divide the first 2 or 3 sets of intercostal branches. The use of an insulated retractor and cautery tip minimizes the risk of recurrent nerve injury, which can be the source of respiratory and feeding difficulties. We have also started using bipolar cautery to minimize the further thermal spread that can happen. Since this takes a little longer, we make an effort to complete the arch and descending aortic dissection before commencing antegrade cerebral perfusion.

3.6 Complications Related to Hemodynamic Issues

Should hemodynamics prove unsatisfactory after weaning from cardiopulmonary bypass, residual lesions must be sought out and corrected. It is rare to have residual arch obstruction or a restrictive atrial septal defect, and therefore most problems are related to overall ventricular function or problems with the systemic-to-pulmonary artery shunt. We generally aim for an SaO_2 of at least 75%, and in the face of unacceptably low SaO_2, upsizing of the shunt should be considered. Arterial saturations greater than 90% are tolerable, unless there is evidence of decreased systemic perfusion as indicated by low SvO_2 or a diastolic pressure of less than 30 mm Hg, in which case downsizing or "banding" of the shunt may be necessary.

4 Norwood Procedure with a Right Ventricle-to-Pulmonary Artery Shunt

As shown in Fig. 9 (Tweddell et al. 2012) while the pulmonary root is open, a small right-angle clamp is directed across the valve taking care not

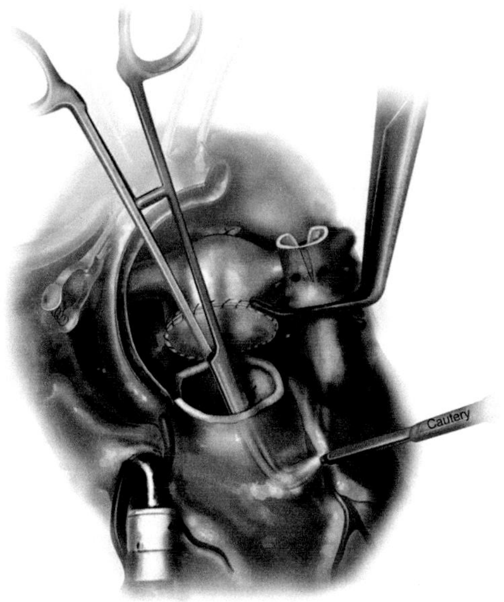

Fig. 9 While the pulmonary root is open, a small right-angle clamp is directed across the valve. A site for the proximal RV-PA conduit is identified at least 1 cm below the nadir of the pulmonary valve cusp and well away from any large epicardial coronary arteries. This site is marked with the electrocautery. (With permission Tweddell et al. 2012)

to damage the leaflets. A site for the proximal right ventricle-to-pulmonary artery (RV-PA) conduit is identified at least 1 cm below the nadir of the pulmonary valve cusp and well away from any large epicardial coronary arteries. This site is marked with the electrocautery and opened. It is generally not required to resect muscle but in some instances, there may be additional muscle that may obstruct proximal RV-PA conduit and we generally incise that.

4.1 Complications Related to Construction of the Right Ventricle to Pulmonary Artery Conduit

A ringed ePTFE graft is brought up and one end is cut flush with the external ring (Fig. 10a). A marking pen is used to mark the third ring from the end. This corresponds to the thickness of the RV free wall and ensures that only a millimeter or two of the graft protrudes into the RV cavity. If too long a portion of the graft is placed within the RV cavity, the conduit can contact the opposite wall of the ventricle, resulting in obstruction.

A stab incision is made in the RV free wall at the previously identified site for the proximal RV-PA conduit connection (Fig. 10b). No muscle resection is usually necessary. The graft is then inserted across the RV free wall into the RV cavity. The ringed Gore-Tex tube graft is positioned so that the third ring from the end is flush with the epicardium (Fig. 10c). This ensures that only a millimeter or two of the graft protrudes into the RV cavity. Two 6-0 Prolene purse-string sutures are used to tighten the epicardium around the proximal conduit. No additional fixation sutures are used. The distal conduit is positioned to the right of the neo-ascending aorta (Fig. 10d) (Tweddell et al. 2012). The branch pulmonary arteries are fully mobilized to their first order branches, similar to the mobilization used for an arterial switch operation, and this allows the central pulmonary artery to be positioned to the right of the neo-ascending aorta. An arteriotomy is made in the pulmonary artery patch and the distal RV-PA connection is completed with 7-0 Prolene. We have currently adopted only a purse string suture to "dunk" the distal RV-PA conduit rather than an end-side anastomosis and have noticed minimal bleeding from that suture line.

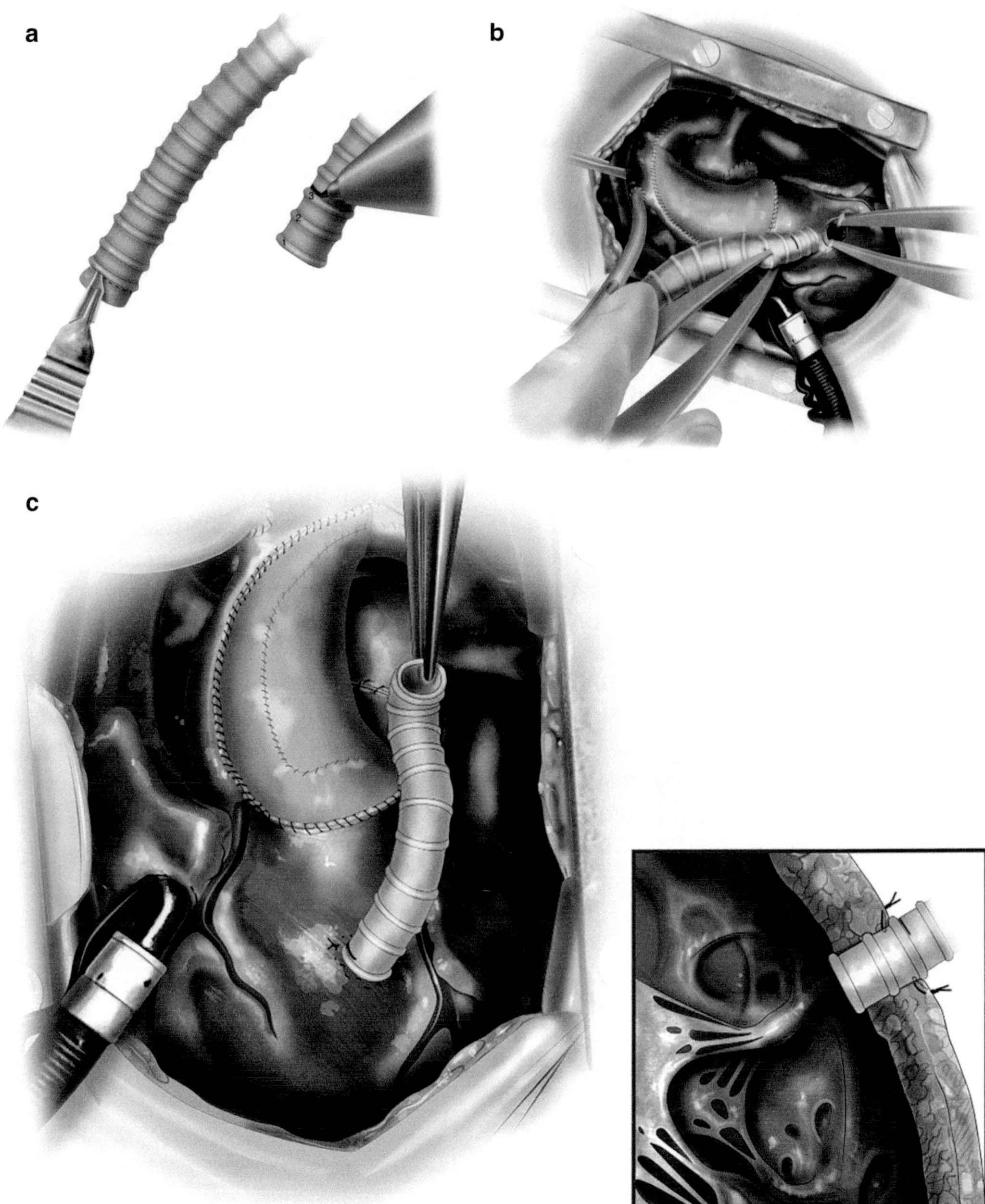

Fig. 10 (**a**) A ringed PTFE graft is brought up and one end is cut flush with the external ring. A marking pen is used to mark the third ring from the end. (**b**) A stab incision is made in the RV free wall at the previously identified site. No muscle resection is usually necessary. (**c**) The third ring from the end is flush with the epicardium. This ensures that only a millimeter or two of the graft protrudes into the RV cavity. Two 6-0 Prolene purse-strings are used to tighten the epicardium around the proximal conduit. (**d**) The conduit is usually positioned to the right of the neo-ascending aorta. The branch pulmonary arteries are fully mobilized and this allows the central pulmonary artery to be positioned to the right of the neo-ascending aorta. An arteriotomy is made in the pulmonary artery patch and the distal RV-PA connection is completed. (With permission Tweddell et al. 2012)

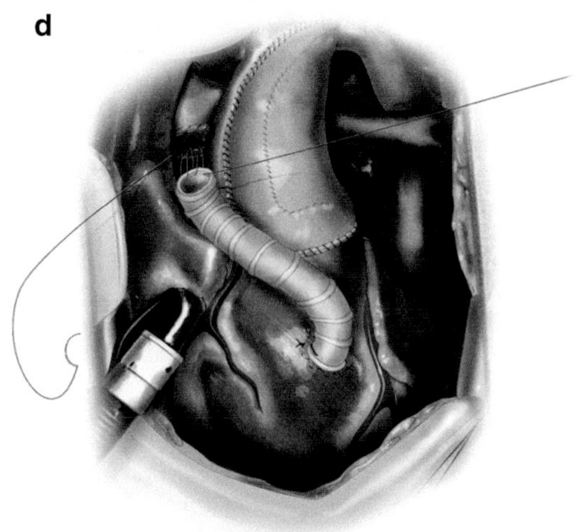

Fig. 21.10 (continued)

5 Conclusion

Complications associated with the Norwood procedure can frequently challenge the surgical team. Attention to detail, anatomic considerations, and spatial planning can help to identify problems during the operation and allow the team to institute reparative techniques to arrive at an excellent outcome.

References

Akintuerk H, Michel-Behnke I, Valeske K, et al. Stenting of the arterial duct and banding of the pulmonary arteries: basis for combined Norwood stage I and II repair in hypoplastic left heart. Circulation. 2002;105:1099–103.

Baffa JM, Chen SL, Guttenberg ME, Norwood WI, Weinberg PM. Coronary artery abnormalities and right ventricular histology in hypoplastic left heart syndrome. J Am Coll Cardiol. 1992;20:350–8.

Brosig C, Mussatto K, Hoffman G, et al. Neurodevelopmental outcomes for children with hypoplastic left heart syndrome at the age of 5 years. Pediatr Cardiol. 2013;34:1597–604.

Connor JA, Thiagarajan R. Hypoplastic left heart syndrome. Orphanet J Rare Dis. 2007;2:23. https://doi.org/10.1186/1750-1172-2-23.

Elzenga NJ, Gittenberger-de Groot AC. Coarctation and related aortic arch anomalies in hypoplastic left heart syndrome. Int J Cardiol. 1985;8:379–93.

Frommelt PC, Sheridan DC, Mussatto KA, et al. Effect of shunt type on echocardiographic indices after initial palliations for hypoplastic left heart syndrome: Blalock-Taussig shunt versus right ventricle-pulmonary artery conduit. J Am Soc Echocardiogr. 2007;20:1364–73.

Fruitman DS. Hypoplastic left heart syndrome: prognosis and management options. Paediatr Child Health. 2000;5:219–25.

Ghanayem NS, Hoffman GM, Mussatto KA, et al. Home surveillance program prevents interstage mortality after the Norwood procedure. J Thorac Cardiovasc Surg. 2003;126:1367–77.

Ghanayem NS, Cava JR, Jaquiss RD, Tweddell JS. Home monitoring of infants after stage one palliation for hypoplastic left heart syndrome. Semin Thorac Cardiovasc Surg Ped Card Surg Annu. 2004;7:32–8.

Glatz JA, Tabbutt S, Gaynor JW, et al. Hypoplastic left heart syndrome with atrial level restriction in the era of prenatal diagnosis. Ann Thorac Surg. 2007;84:1633–8.

Gobergs R, Salputra E, Lubaua I. Hypoplastic left heart syndrome: a review. Acta Med Litu. 2016;23:86–98.

Greenwood RD, Rosenthal A, Parisi L, Fyler DC, Nadas AS. Extracardiac abnormalities in infants with congenital heart disease. Pediatrics. 1975;55:485–92.

Grossfeld P, Nie S, Lin L, Wang L, Anderson RH. Hypoplastic left heart syndrome: a new paradigm for an old disease? J Cardiovasc Dev Dis. 2019;6(1):10. https://doi.org/10.3390/jcdd6010010.

Hellmund A, Berg C, Herberg U, Geipel A, Kempe A, Gembruch U. Levoatrial cardinal vein in a series of five prenatal cases with hypoplastic left heart syndrome and intact atrial septum. Ultraschall Med. 2017;38:206–11.

Ho SY, Stamm C. Tricuspid valve in hypoplastic left heart syndrome. J Thorac Cardiovasc Surg. 2004;128:329; author reply 329–330.

Honjo O, Atlin CR, Mertens L, et al. Atrioventricular valve repair in patients with functional single-ventricle physiology: impact of ventricular and valve function and morphology on survival and reintervention. J Thorac Cardiovasc Surg. 2011;142:326–335.e2.

King G, Ayer J, Celermajer D, et al. Atrioventricular valve failure in Fontan palliation. J Am Coll Cardiol. 2019;73:810–22.

Lloyd TR, Evans TC, Marvin WJ Jr. Morphologic determinants of coronary blood flow in the hypoplastic left heart syndrome. Am Heart J. 1986;112:666–71.

Machii M, Becker AE. Nature of coarctation in hypoplastic left heart syndrome. Ann Thorac Surg. 1995;59:1491–4.

Mahle WT, Spray TL, Wernovsky G, Gaynor JW, Clark BJ 3rd. Survival after reconstructive surgery for hypoplastic left heart syndrome: a 15-year experience from a single institution. Circulation. 2000;102:III136–41.

Morris CD, Outcalt J, Menashe VD. Hypoplastic left heart syndrome: natural history in a geographically defined population. Pediatrics. 1990;85:977–83.

Nathan M, Williamson AK, Mayer JE, Bacha EA, Juraszek AL. Mortality in hypoplastic left heart syndrome: review of 216 autopsy cases of aortic atresia with attention to coronary artery disease. J Thorac Cardiovasc Surg. 2012;144:1301–6.

Norwood WI, Lang P, Hansen DD. Physiologic repair of aortic atresia- hypoplastic left heart syndrome. N Engl J Med. 1983;308:23–6.

Ohman A, El-Segaier M, Bergman G, et al. Changing epidemiology of hypoplastic left heart syndrome: results of a National Swedish Cohort Study. J Am Heart Assoc. 2019;8(2):e010893. https://doi.org/10.1161/JAHA.118.010893.

Ohye RG, Gomez CA, Goldberg CS, Graves HL, Devaney EJ, Bove EL. Tricuspid valve repair in hypoplastic left heart syndrome. J Thorac Cardiovasc Surg. 2004;127:465–72.

Samanek M, Slavik Z, Zborilova B, Hrobonova V, Voriskova M, Skovranek J. Prevalence, treatment, and outcome of heart disease in live-born children: a prospective analysis of 91,823 live-born children. Pediatr Cardiol. 1989;10:205–11.

Sano S, Ishino K, Kawada M, et al. Right ventricle-pulmonary artery shunt in first-stage palliation of hypoplastic left heart syndrome. J Thorac Cardiovasc Surg. 2003;126:504–9.

Saul D, Degenhardt K, Iyoob SD, et al. Hypoplastic left heart syndrome and the nutmeg lung pattern in utero: a cause and effect relationship or prognostic indicator? Pediatr Radiol. 2016;46:483–9.

Stamm C, Anderson RH, Ho SY. The morphologically tricuspid valve in hypoplastic left heart syndrome. Eur J Cardiothorac Surg. 1997;12:587–92.

Stasik CN, Gelehrter S, Goldberg CS, Bove EL, Devaney EJ, Ohye RG. Current outcomes and risk factors for the Norwood procedure. J Thorac Cardiovasc Surg. 2006;131:412–7.

Takahashi K, Inage A, Rebeyka IM, et al. Real-time 3-dimensional echocardiography provides new insight into mechanisms of tricuspid valve regurgitation in patients with hypoplastic left heart syndrome. Circulation. 2009;120:1091–8.

Talner CN. Report of the New England regional infant cardiac program. Pediatrics. 1980;65:375–461.

Tchervenkov CI, Jacobs ML, Tahta SA. Congenital heart surgery nomenclature and database project: hypoplastic left heart syndrome. Ann Thorac Surg. 2000;69:S170–9.

Tsang VT, Raja SG. Tricuspid valve repair in single ventricle: timing and techniques. Semin Thorac Cardiovasc Surg Pediatr Card Surg Annu. 2012;15:61–8.

Tweddell JS. The Norwood procedure with an innominate artery-to-pulmonary artery shunt. Oper Tech Thorac Cardiovasc Surg. 2005;10(2):123–40.

Tweddell JS, Hoffman GM, Mussatto KA, et al. Improved survival of patients undergoing palliation of hypoplastic left heart syndrome: lessons learned from 115 consecutive patients. Circulation. 2002;106:I82–189.

Tweddell JS, Mitchell ME, Woods RK, Spray TL, Quintessenza JA. Construction of the right ventricle-to-pulmonary artery conduit in the Norwood: the "Dunk" technique. Oper Tech Thorac Cardiovasc Surg. 2012;17(2):81–98.

Yabrodi M, Mastropietro CW. Hypoplastic left heart syndrome: from comfort care to long-term survival. Pediatr Res. 2017;81:142–9.

Complications Associated with Repair of Aortico-Left Ventricular Tunnel

Constantine Mavroudis

Abstract

Aortico-left ventricular (Ao-LV) tunnel is a rare congenital anomaly that results in a communication between the ascending aorta and the LV. The clinical presentation is characterized by congestive heart failure and dilation of the ascending aorta within the first year of life due to significant regurgitation. There is considerable morphology variability which may affect the aortic valve and the right ventricular outflow tract. Prenatal diagnosis is not always contributory, and echocardiography remains the optimal imaging modality. Computed tomography is useful for surgical planning. Surgical intervention is usually indicated and typically involves patch aortoplasty. Following surgical repair, prognosis is good although long-term risk factors include progressive aortic regurgitation and ascending aortic dilatation.

Keywords

Aortic-left ventricular tunnel · Prenatal · Congenital heart defect · Aortic disease · Non-valvular aortic regurgitation · Coronary artery anomaly · Aneurysm · Outflow tract obstruction · Patch aortoplasty · Transcatheter closure

1 Introduction

Aortico-left ventricular (Ao-LV) tunnel is a rare congenital heart malformation that is characterized by a communication between the ascending aorta and the LV. Incidence is estimated at 1 in 1000 infants born with congenital heart disease (Martins et al. 2004). The first description of this entity was by Levy and colleagues who reported three cases of aortico-left ventricular tunnel in

C. Mavroudis (✉)
Chief of Pediatric Cardiothoracic Surgery (Retired), Peyton Manning Children's Hospital, Indianapolis, IN, USA

Professor Emeritus of Surgery, Johns Hopkins University School of Medicine, Baltimore, MD, USA

C. L. Backer, C. Mavroudis (eds.), *Complications in Pediatric and Congenital Heart Surgery*, https://doi.org/10.1007/978-3-032-02661-3_22

1963 (Levy et al. 1963). In most cases, patients with aortico-LV tunnel present with symptoms of congestive heart failure, dilation of the ascending aorta, and a diastolic murmur within the first year of life. Rarely will a patient present in later life with complicated aortic valve endocarditis (Xu et al. 2015) or Takayasu's arteritis (Sui et al. 2022).

In general, following uncomplicated surgical repair, the prognosis is good. Lifelong follow-up is recommended for the possibility of progressive aortic regurgitation in some patients.

2 Pathophysiology and Anatomy

Aortico-left ventricular tunnel is characterized by an abnormal, paravalvular, endothelialized communication between the ascending aorta and the left ventricle that creates bidirectional blood flow from the aorta to the left ventricle. In particular, the paravalvular aortico-LV tunnel typically originates from an aortic orifice cephalad and upstream to the sinotubular junction adjacent to the right coronary cusp and follows a descending pathway along the aortopulmonary window before entering the fibrous trigone of the left ventricle directly below the left-right commissure of the aortic valve. The majority of cases involving aortic-LV tunnel arise from the right coronary sinus; origin from the left coronary sinus is exceedingly rare (Hermann and Fuller 2023; Michielon et al. 1998; Hovaguimiam et al. 1988; Grant et al. 1985).

In a postmortem study of 37 patients, Morgan and associates reported the anatomic characteristics of the variants of aortico-LV tunnel, namely that the aortic opening was found to be above the right coronary artery (RCA) ostium in 14 (38%) of the patients, below the RCA in 9 (25%) and at the level of the RCA in 6 (16%) (Morgan and Mazur 1963). Aortic origins arising from the left coronary sinus (Ono et al. 2008; Nezafati et al. 2010; Zhu et al. 2014) and the noncoronary sinus (Song et al. 2015) have also been described. Additionally, the main coronary arteries may arise directly from the tunnel (Bautista-Hernandez et al. 2010; Gundel et al. 2010). The epicardial anatomy in patients with Ao-LV tunnel is characterized by a visible and pulsatile bulge along the anterolateral margin of the aorta. This represents the fibromuscular tunnel wall that lies in direct histologic continuity with the aorta. The posterior wall is comprised of the true aortic wall; the inferomedial aspect or the floor of the tunnel is comprised of the right ventricular outflow tract (RVOT) muscle (Ho et al. 1998). Classification of Ao-LV tunnel has been offered by Hovaguimian and associates. Their nomenclature describes four types and is characterized by: those with a slit-like aortic orifice with no valvular distortion (type I, Fig. 1); those with a larger, oval-shaped aortic orifice with an aneurysmal extracardiac component with or without valvular distortion (type II; Fig. 2); those with an oval aortic orifice and an aneurysmal septal (intracardiac) component with or without right ventricular outflow tract obstruction (type III; Fig. 3); and those with a combination of type II and III (classified as type IV; Fig. 4) (Hovaguimiam et al. 1988).

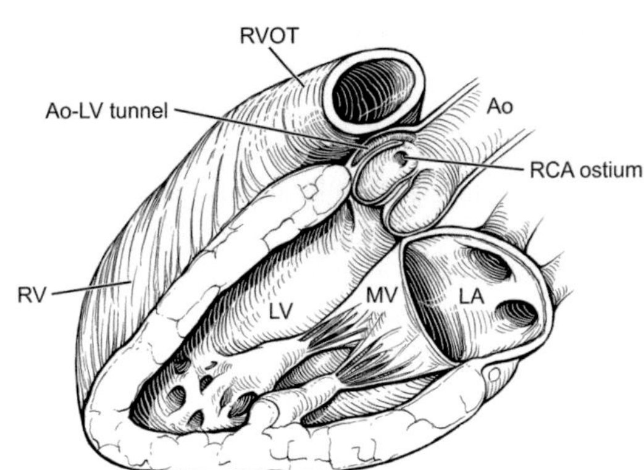

Fig. 1 Operative epicardial findings are characterized by a visible bulge along the anterolateral aspect of the aorta, which represents the fibromuscular tunnel wall that lies in direct histologic continuity with the aorta. The posterior wall contains the true aortic wall with the inferomedial aspect or the floor of the tunnel involving the muscle of the right ventricular outflow tract. There are four accepted types of Aortico-left ventricular tunnel which are noted in Figs. 1, 2, 3 and 4. Figure 1 shows Type I defect which is defined as an anomaly with a slit-like aortic orifice with no valvular distortion. *Ao* aorta, *LA* left atrium, *LV* left ventricle, *MV* mitral valve, *RCA* right coronary artery, *RV* right ventricle, *RVOT* right ventricular outflow tract. (With permission Shum-Tim and Tchervenov 2003)

Extracardiac aneurysm

Fig. 2 Type II defects are those with a larger, oval-shaped aortic orifice with an aneurysmal extracardiac component with or without valvular distortion. (With permission Shum-Tim and Tchervenov 2003)

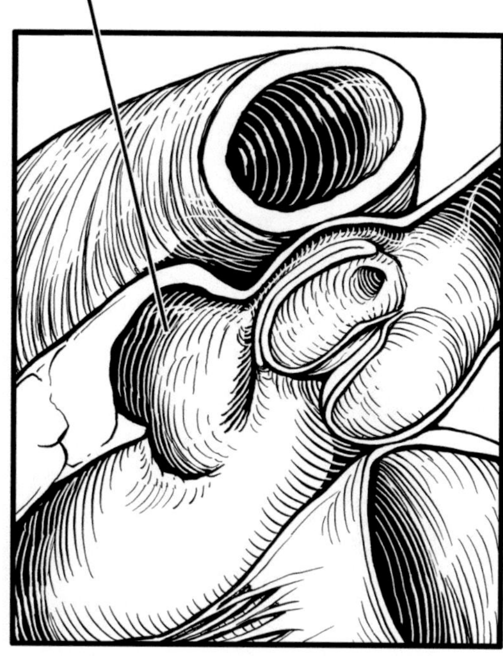

Fig. 3 Type III defects are those with an oval aortic orifice and an aneurysmal septal (intracardiac) component with or without right ventricular outflow tract obstruction. (With permission Shum-Tim and Tchervenov 2003)

As is so often the case, nomenclature schemes tend to have amendments and clarifications. Ho and associates (Ho et al. 1998) performed a careful analysis of several pathologic specimens and suggested that the Ao-LV tunnels never engage or cross the interventricular septum, but rather course inferiorly in the fibrofatty plane between the aortic root and the subpulmonary infundibulum to enter the LV outflow tract in the adjacent subcommissural triangle below the right and left valvular cusps just superficial to the intracardiac myocardium and superiorly adjacent to the actual aortic-ventricular junction. These are important findings with relevant anatomic details, pathophysiologic considerations and therapeutic implications. Clinicians must be aware and be mindful of the etiology of aortic valvular insufficiency as well as coronary flow, particularly when the right coronary artery arises within the tunnel. Such variants will necessitate adjustment to the surgical procedure to avoid the complications of myocardial ischemia and aortic regurgitation.

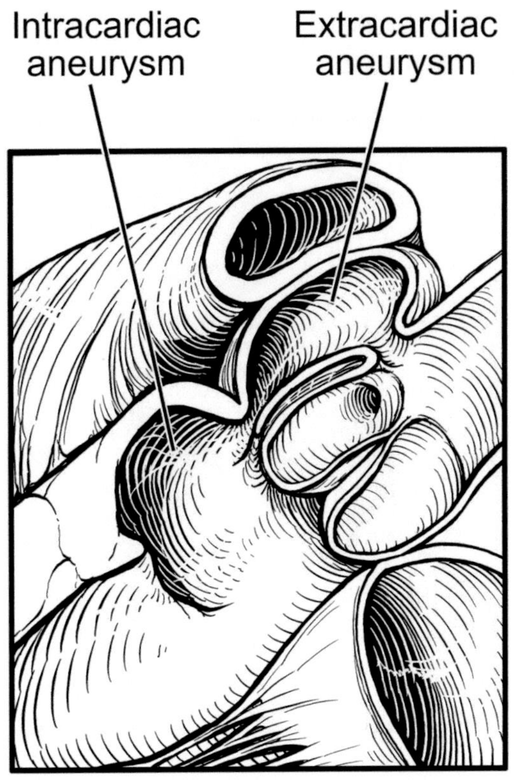

Fig. 4 Type IV defects as shown in the figure are those with a combination of type II and III defects. (With permission Shum-Tim and Tchervenov 2003)

3 Pathogenesis

The exact pathogenesis of aortico-left ventricular tunnel formation is not known. It has been proposed that possible etiologies include in-utero rupture of a sinus of Valsalva aneurysm (Michielon et al. 1998; Shum-Tim and Tchervenkov 2003; Myers and Mehta 2000; Sousa-Uva et al. 1996), degeneration of the true aortic wall analogous to in-utero cystic medial necrosis (Turley et al. 1982), dissection of an aberrant or anomalous coronary artery (Martins et al. 2004), and malformation of the bulbus cordis (Martins et al. 2004; Michielon et al. 1998; Llorens et al. 1982). The bulbus cordis develops into components of both the subpulmonary infundibulum and the aortic vestibule and comprises the anatomic area through which the developing coronary arteries move to attach to the sinus segment. Abnormal development of the bulbus cordis may account for the association between aortic-LV tunnel and valvular pulmonary stenosis, valvular aortic stenosis, and proximal coronary artery anomalies (Llorens et al. 1982). Aortico-LV tunnel typically originates from an aortic orifice cephalad to the sinus segment of the aorta and it is thus unlikely that a rupture of a sinus of Valsalva aneurysm could account for the typical appearance of this anomaly. Alternatively, Myers and associates maintain that sinus aneurysm rupture occurs only in the rare instance of aortic to right ventricle fistulization (Myers and Mehta 2000). While Myers' suggestion is an attractive hypothesis, Vargas and associates (1998) clearly document an aortic origin of an aortic-right ventricular tunnel cephalad to the left sinotubular junction which would make antecedent sinus rupture equally unlikely. The actual etiology remains elusive.

4 Presentation and Diagnosis

Severity of symptoms in patients with Ao-LV tunnel will determine the size of the tunnel and the age of presentation. It follows then that neonatal and infant presentation denotates a large Ao-LV tunnel with severe left ventricular volume overload. Accurate prenatal diagnosis of aortico-LV tunnel has been challenging and only documented in abbreviated case reports. In the first clinical report, prenatal diagnoses were correct in only one of four presumed cases (Vargas et al. 1998). In the second report, the diagnosis was correct in two of three cases (Michielon et al. 1998). Subsequent reports have been published which documented 1–2 cases each (Cook et al. 1995; Grab et al. 2000; Napoleone et al. 2001; Singh et al. 2011; Smith et al. 2016). A synopsis of the collective results showed that several fetuses were electively aborted and only three prenatally diagnosed patients survived until correction. The earliest survivor amongst these cases was detected at 28 weeks gestation. In general, prenatal echocardiography demonstrated preserved cardiac architecture and chambers which were associated with valvular aortic insufficiency and/or stenosis, dysplastic valve leaflets, and severe LV hypertrophy and dilatation. In addition, an identifiable paravalvular tunnel with regurgitant diastolic flow could be identified in three cases. Overall survival was rare in this group of patients and may represent the most severe end of the clinical spectrum. Postmortem examination of these affected hearts confirmed significant pathologic findings which included extensive myocardial fibrosis and severe aortic valve dysplasia.

Postnatal diagnosis of Ao-LV tunnel can be performed readily and accurately. Predictably, clinical severity is dependent on the amount of regurgitant paravalvular flow and the hemodynamic impact of associated coexistent anomalies such as valvular aortic regurgitation, aortic stenosis, pulmonary stenosis, and subpulmonary right ventricular outflow tract obstruction. Differential diagnosis includes ventricular septal defect with aortic insufficiency, ruptured sinus of Valsalva aneurysm, coronary artery fistula and tetralogy of Fallot with absent pulmonary valve syndrome. Physical examination is characterized by "to and fro" systolic and diastolic murmurs with a wide pulse pressure and bounding peripheral pulses. Right ventricular outflow tract obstruction can occur owing to valvar pulmonary stenosis or aneurysmal dilation of the intracardiac portion of the Ao-LV tunnel. Chronic volume overload often results in LV hypertrophy, LV dilatation, and diminished ventricular function.

In the majority of cases, echocardiography can result in a comprehensive diagnosis. In particular, color flow Doppler can differentiate the direction of blood flow in the aortic root and the tunnel. Paravalvular aorto-ventricular communication with regurgitant diastolic flow confirms the diagnosis. Demonstration of aortic insufficiency in a neonate should raise suspicion of an aortic-LV tunnel. Further diagnostic modalities such as cardiac catheterization and cardiac magnetic resonance imaging (MRI) are reserved for evaluating spatial relationships between coronary artery anatomy and the Ao-LV Tunnel (Hsu et al. 2007).

5 Complete Repair of Ao-LV Tunnel and Associated Complications

Surgical correction has been the preferred method of therapeutic intervention with some notable corollaries. While medical management alone is deemed to be ineffective, rare patients have presented late in life without previous surgical treatment (Ando et al. 2004). Interestingly, spontaneous closure of Ao-LV tunnel has been reported which begs the question of whether small asymptomatic lesions could be serially observed with endocarditis prophylaxis as indicated (Martins et al. 2004). As noted herein, there have been successful reports documenting the use of percutaneous devices to close the tunnel. The long-term results of this approach have not been assessed (Chessa et al. 2000; Vijayalakshmi et al. 2004; Thomas et al. 2013).

Surgical closure of the Ao-LV tunnel is indicated at the time of diagnosis in the majority of cases. Surgical options include direct closure, patch aortoplasty, or with combined patch closure of the aortic and the ventricular opening. Long-term durable outcomes have been achieved by direct aortic closure as the only intervention (Martins et al. 2004). However, if this technique is to be used without a patch, it is more likely to be applicable to the Type I Ao-LV tunnel with a slit-like orifice. Pathologic examination of autopsy specimens suggest that the ventricular orifice is not surrounded by firm muscular margins and in some cases may not be amenable to direct closure (Ho et al. 1998).

The intraoperative course of the reparative operation begins with transesophageal echocardiography which is useful to delineate the course of the tunnel, aortic valvular competence, as well as the left ventricular outflow tract and right ventricular outflow tract. Median sternotomy is the

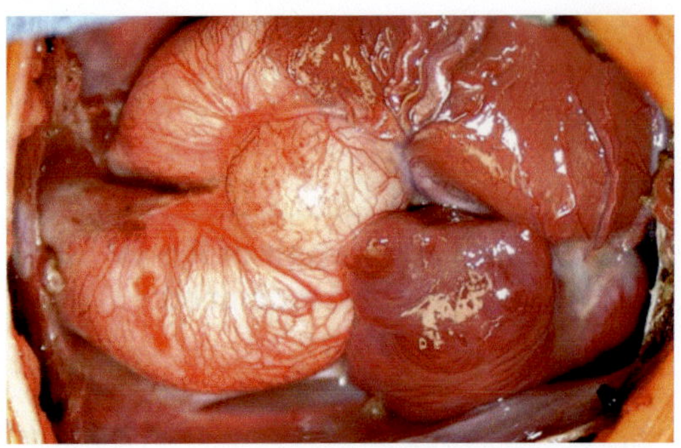

Fig. 5 Intraoperative photograph of Type II Aortico-LV Tunnel demonstrating large aortic wall aneurysm of the tunnel. (With Permission Herrmann and Fuller 2023)

rule for operative exposure with aortobicaval cannulation, left ventricular venting, as well as preparations for antegrade and retrograde cardioplegic arrest. Epicardial inspection will often reveal an aortic bulge demonstrating a Type II Ao-LV tunnel as noted in Fig. 5. The hemodynamic elements characteristic of Ao-LV tunnel are demonstrated in Fig. 6 which emphasizes the "to and fro" flow patterns by the large arrows and the lateral developed pressure sites as noted by the smaller arrows.

After appropriate cannulation, cardiopulmonary bypass is commenced with moderate cooling (28–32 °C) all the while being attentive to the development of ventricular fibrillation which should trigger immediate cross-clamping with antegrade and retrograde cardioplegia. Figure 7 demonstrates the operative exposure after cardioplegic arrest and aortic transection.

In most cases, the orifice of the tunnel is located above the origin of the right coronary artery as noted in the figure. Figure 8 demonstrates the large and oval shaped opening of the Ao-LV tunnel. The aortic valve is shown directly posterior which is stenotic. The generally accepted operative procedure in all cases of Ao-LV tunnel is patch aortoplasty to avoid aortic valve distortion and to effect a tension-free closure resulting in long-term favorable outcomes (Napoleone et al. 2001; Weldner et al. 1996; Kathare et al. 2015). A conscientious examination of the aortic and ventricular orifices of the tunnel internally through the aortic valve or through the aortic bulge should be performed to

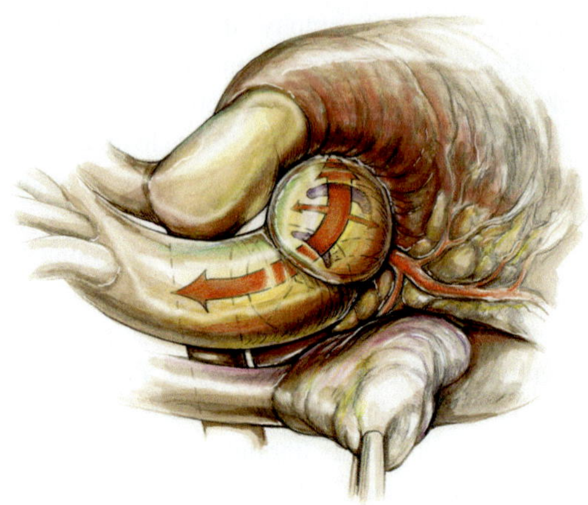

Fig. 6 Operative exposure for patients with Aortico-left ventricular tunnel is through a median sternotomy and standard aortobicaval cardiopulmonary bypass with mild cooling, left ventricular venting and a combination of antegrade and retrograde cardioplegia. The topical anatomy and echocardiographic findings will determine whether to use one or two patches for the repair. The coronary artery is usually not involved, but special care is taken not to constrict the orifice with the suture technique used to close the tunnel. Those patients with extracardiac or intracardiac aneurysmal dilatation will require two patches for repair. The figure shows a Type II extracardiac aneurysm with the "to and fro" flow characteristics of a Ao-LV tunnel as demonstrated by the arrows. The tunnel is depicted as being above the right coronary sinus and above or downstream of the right coronary orifice. (With permission Mavroudis 2015)

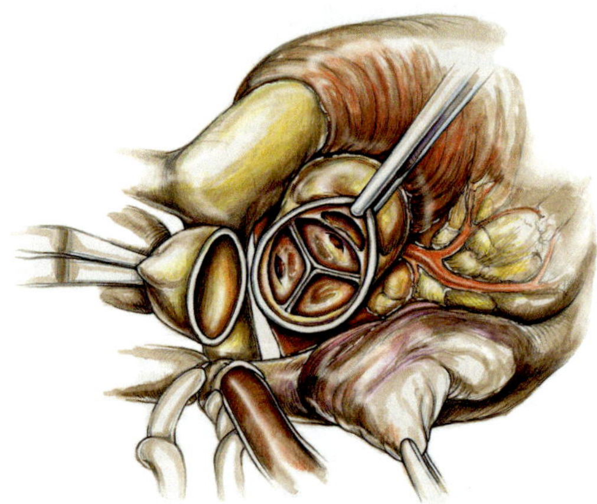

Fig. 7 After aortobicaval cardiopulmonary bypass and cardioplegic arrest (antegrade and retrograde techniques) are established, the aorta is sub-totally or totally transected to maximally display the anatomy as noted in the figure. Note that the tunnel is situated above the orifice of the right coronary artery. Care must be taken to confirm both pathways, the coronary course, and the Ao-LV tunnel. (With permission Mavroudis 2015)

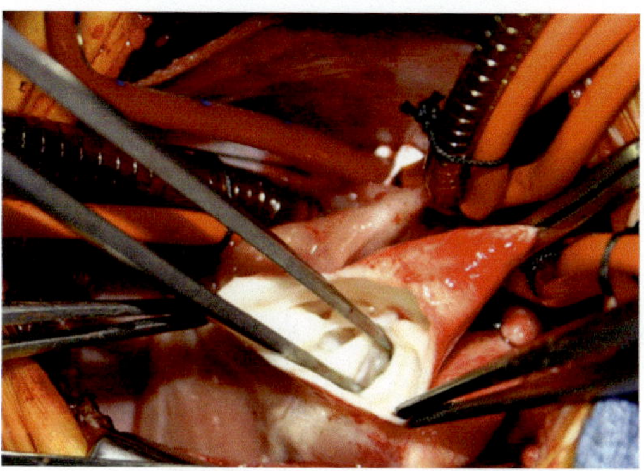

Fig. 8 Intraoperative photograph of Type II Aortico-LV Tunnel demonstrating oval opening (with forceps passing through the Ao-LV Tunnel) and aortic valve directly posterior. Note that the aortic valve shows central stenosis and commissural fusion. (With Permission Herrmann and Fuller 2023)

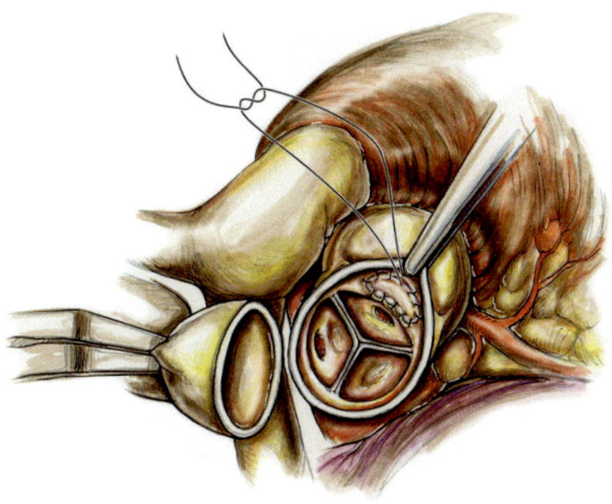

Fig. 9 shows how a piece of autologous pericardium or PTFE patch is used to close the tunnel using running suture technique. Care is taken to confirm the unobstructed course of the right coronary artery after the patch is placed. (With permission Mavroudis 2015)

determine if an additional ventricular patch should prove to be necessary. The aortic patch closure should be a complication free procedure; however, two important situations must be kept in mind to avoid hemodynamic problems. Firstly, the patch closure must be performed carefully to avoid distortion of the left-right aortic valve commissure because the tunnel orifice is usually located just above the right sinotubular junction as noted in Fig. 9. Secondly, the transaortic patch can be placed too closely to the right coronary artery orifice or in fact cover the orifice completely. Clearly, this will result in coronary artery hypoperfusion and myocardial ischemia. Figure 10 left panel (a) demonstrates the anatomic configuration of the Ao-LV tunnel with close proximity to the orifice of the right coronary artery. The black arrow signifies the regurgitant flow pattern from the aorta to the left ventricle. Figure 10 inset (b) shows the unwanted closure of both the orifice of the right coronary artery and the Ao-LV tunnel orifice. Obviously, this will result in myocardial ischemia. Being covered by the transaortic patch. Figure 10 inset (c) shows the corrected patch placement after takedown of the unwanted patch. The ventricular end of the Ao-LV tunnel can be approached by a longitudinal incision of the external or internal aneurysm as noted in Fig. 11. The location of the ventricular end of the tunnel that occupies the space within the left-right interleaflet triangle requires careful attention during patch closure to avoid distortion of the right coronary leaflet. While this area is anatomically distant from the noncoronary-right coronary interleaflet triangle, anterior extensions of the left bundle branch may be jeopardized by sutures placed through the ventricular wall. This has led some surgeons to close the ventricular orifice through the incised tunnel (Hovaguimiam et al. 1988; Ho et al. 1998). Figure 12 shows the completed repair with aortic reanastomosis and linear closure of the external aneurysmal bulge.

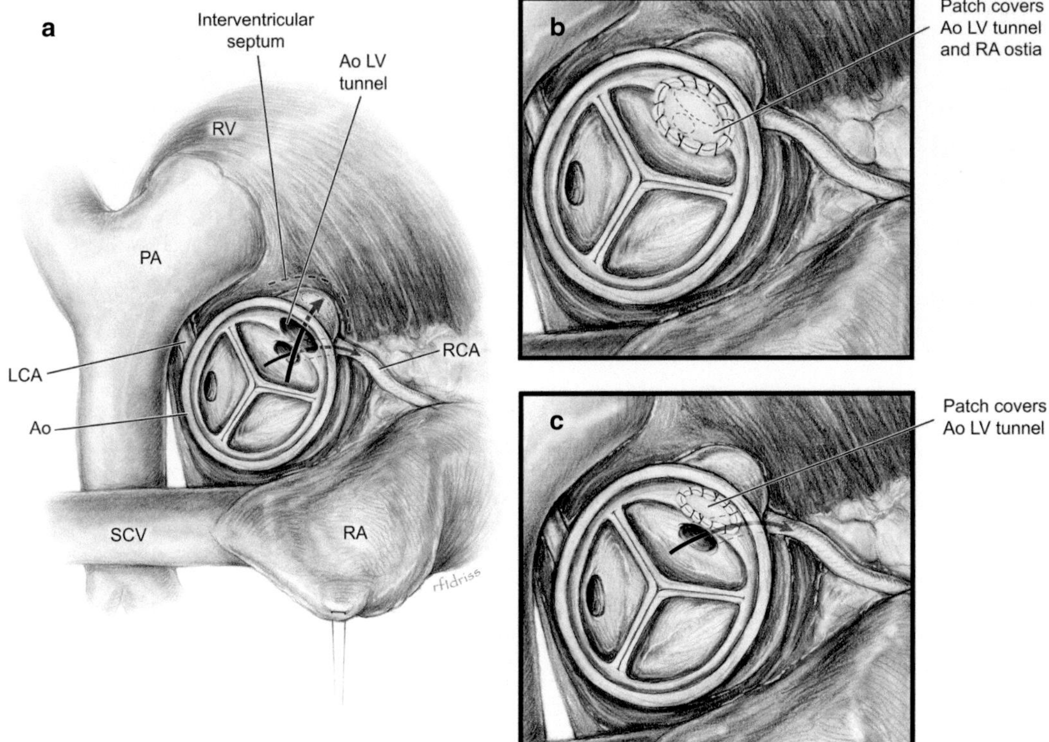

Fig. 10 (**a**) Shows the close distance between the right coronary artery orifice and the Ao-LV tunnel (ghosted view) with the black arrow showing the regurgitant flow into the left ventricle. The inset (**b**) shows unwanted patch closure of both the Ao-LV tunnel and the orifice of the right coronary artery thereby causing right coronary artery obstruction and myocardial ischemia. The inset (**c**) shows the proper placement of the patch to occlude the tunnel and spare the orifice of the RCA. *Ao* aorta, *Ao-LV* aortico-left ventricle, *LCA* left coronary artery, *PA* pulmonary artery, *RA* right atrium, *RCA* right coronary artery, *RV* right ventricle, *SCV* superior caval vein

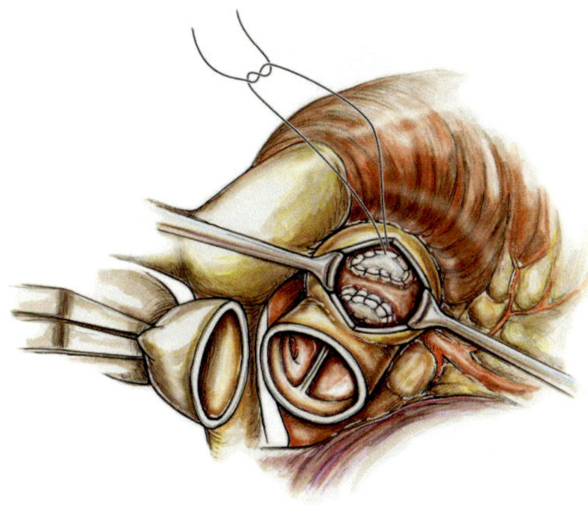

Fig. 11 A second patch is usually required for Type II defects. A longitudinal incision is made in the ventricular aneurysm as shown in the figure. The ventricular orifice of the Ao-LV tunnel is visualized and closed with another patch of autologous pericardium or PTFE. It is at this point that the right ventricular outflow tract can be judged to be obstructed or non-obstructed. In general, repairing the Ao-LV tunnel in this manner will relieve the RVOT obstruction, assuming that it is present. Subpulmonary valve right ventricular outflow tract patch augmentation is another alternative. (With permission Mavroudis 2015)

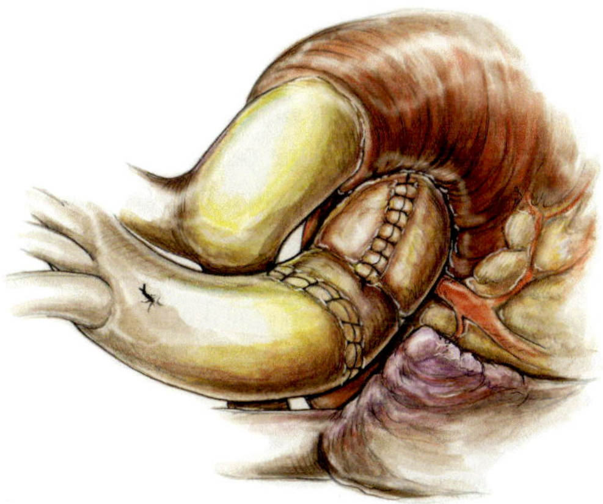

Fig. 12 The ventricular aneurysm can be closed, the aortic anastomosis can be performed, and the patient can be separated from cardiopulmonary bypass as noted in the figure. Transesophageal echocardiography can determine the adequacy of the repair in the event that a return to cardiopulmonary bypass and re-repair is necessary. The beneficial results of this operative procedure are immediate and long-lasting. (With permission Mavroudis 2015)

In very rare cases, the right coronary artery arises from within the Ao-LV tunnel making the relatively straightforward patch repair much more complicated and at risk for myocardial ischemia. Such a case with severe aortic regurgitation was reported by Gundel and associates (2010) who described the diagnosis and operative management. Figures 13 and 14 show the relevant anatomy as depicted by MRI. The authors described their experience in the following citation,

> Because of severe aortic regurgitation, an operation was indicated. On surgery, a severely dilated AoV was identified. The right coronary cusp was displaced toward the ALVT, causing central valvar incompetence. The RCA originated from the ALVT. Only selective injection into the left anterior descending artery disclosed the LV orifice of

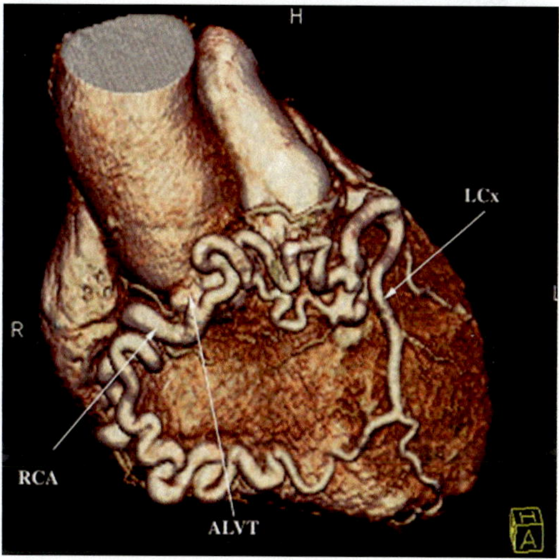

Fig. 13 Origin of the right coronary artery (RCA) from the Ao-Left ventricular tunnel (ALVT). Collaterals from the left coronary artery to the RCA. Multislice computed tomography confirmed the catheter findings which are shown in Fig. 14 and showed the blind aortic end of the ALVT. The ventricular end was traversing the infundibular septum just beneath the AoV. The RCA originated directly from the tunnel as shown in Fig. 14. Myocardial scintigraphy was normal. *LCx* Left circumflex, *RCA* right coronary artery, *ALVT* aortico-left ventricular tunnel, *R* Right, *H* Head. (With permission Gundel et al. 2010)

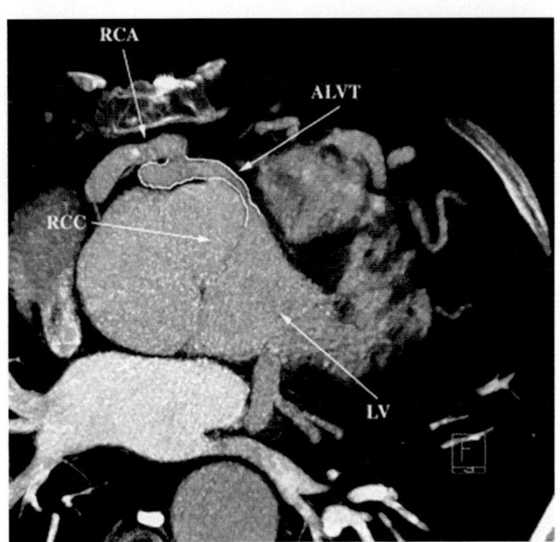

Fig. 14 ALVT located anteriorly and laterally to the right coronary cusp with origin of the RCA. *RCA* Right coronary artery, *RCC* right coronary cusp, *ALVT* aortico-left ventricular tunnel, *LV* left vent. (With permission Gundel et al. 2010)

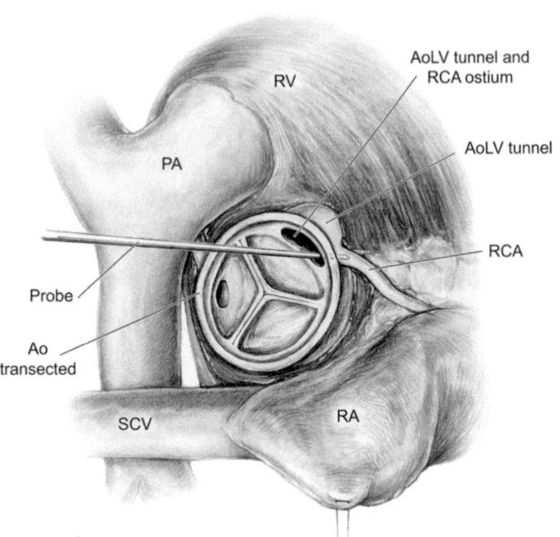

Fig. 15 shows a transaortic view of the right coronary artery arising from the Ao-LV tunnel adjacent to the course of the tunnel. The identification and distinction between the coronary artery and the tunnel requires gentle probing and antecedent evaluation by transesophageal echocardiography and magnetic resonance imaging. The featured view shows the probe into the coronary artery to identify the vessel in order to exclude the orifice for the reparative procedure. *Ao* aorta, *LV* left ventricle, *PA* pulmonary artery, *RA* right atrium, *RCA* right coronary artery, *RV* right ventricle, *SCV* superior caval vein

> the ALVT. The AoV could not be preserved and was replaced by a biological prosthesis (Carpentier-Edwards Perimount Magna 31 mm, Edwards Lifesciences, Irvine, Calif). On implantation of the valve, the tunnel was closed. An end-to-side anastomosis of the right internal thoracic artery to the RCA was performed. The patient made an uneventful recovery. Myocardial scintigraphy showed no myocardial perfusion defects. Angiography demonstrated patency of the bypass and significantly less flow through the collaterals to the RCA. LV function had recovered on echocardiography (LV end-diastolic dimension of 45 mm, shortening fraction of 30% (Gundel et al. 2010)).

Figure 15 shows the dilemma of encountering tunnel origin of the RCA. The transaortic view depicts the proximity of the RCA origin with the Ao-LV tunnel with a dilator into the orifice of the right coronary artery. It is important to carefully identify the coronary artery and the continuation of the tunnel by gentle dilator probing and plan the patch repair of the tunnel while preserving the orifice of the coronary artery. Figure 16 illustrates in two drawings an unwanted patching of both the tunnel and the orifice of the coronary artery. Figure 16 left panel shows how an unwanted closure of the Ao-LV tunnel can be performed if the preoperative diagnosis and anatomic identification are not accurate. Figure 16 right panel shows how the problem can be corrected by a well-placed patch that will occlude the Ao-LV tunnel and enhance RCA flow. If the orifice of the RCA is unamenable to patch repair, especially in older patients, the Ao-LV tunnel can be closed to incorporate both the tunnel and the RCA while adding an internal mammary bypass graft to the proximal RCA as performed in the case presentation by Gundel and associates (2010).

Regardless of initial technique, patients should be followed for life due to the possibility of progressive aortic regurgitation. Approximately 50% of patients with Ao-LV tunnel eventually require aortic valve replacement (Weldner et al. 1996). The clinical evidence suggests that early repair may prevent late consequences of chronic volume overload, premature deterioration of the valve leaflets secondary to turbulent flow and subsequent dilatation of the aortic annulus and ascend-

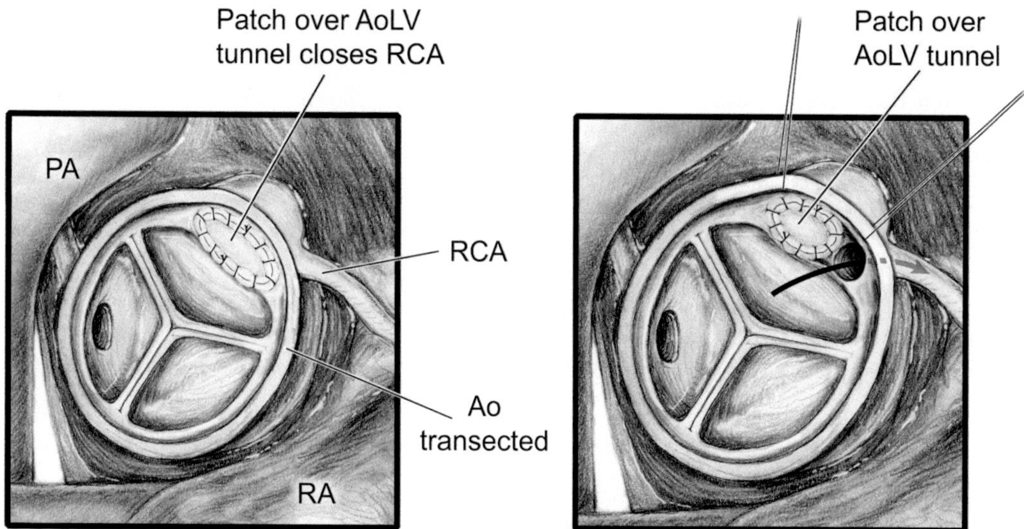

Fig. 16 Left panel shows the unwanted closure of the tunnel orifice at the proximal aortic orifice that includes closure of both the tunnel and the coronary artery. The right panel shows the correct patch repair of the Ao-LV tunnel while sparing the orifice of the right coronary artery which arises from the aneurysmal course of the Ao-LV tunnel. The arrow shows the proper unobstructed blood flow into the right coronary artery. *Ao* aorta, *LV* left ventricle, *PA* pulmonary artery, *RA* right atrium, *RCA* right coronary artery

ing aorta (Shum-Tim and Tchervenkov 2003; Llorens et al. 1982; Weldner et al. 1996; Kathare et al. 2015). In addition, there is likely further theoretical advantage to closure of the ventricular orifice by buttressing the right-left commissure and supporting the lateral margin of the right coronary cusp left unsupported by the ventricular tunnel opening (Ho et al. 1998; Shum-Tim and Tchervenkov 2003).

6 Conclusion

Aortico-LV tunnel is a rare cardiac malformation of unclear etiology that presents with signs and symptoms of aortic regurgitation. Accurate diagnosis will elucidate associated coronary artery and valve anatomy which will determine the best technique of surgical repair. Advances in diagnostic echocardiography and CT angiography may facilitate earlier detection, and percutaneous devices may eventually result in an alternative treatment strategy. Short-term prognosis is excellent, although some patients may eventually require valve replacement because of progressive valvular regurgitation.

References

Ando M, Igari T, Ando S, et al. Repair of the aortico-left ventricular tunnel originating from the right aortic sinus with severe aortic valve regurgitation. Ann Thorac Surg. 2004;10:47–50.

Bautista-Hernandez V, Portela F, Marcos-Alonso S, Rueda F. Pericardial single-patch repair of right coronary artery from aorto-left ventricular tunnel. Pediatr Cardiol. 2010;31:714–6.

Chessa M, Chaudhari M, DeGiovanni J. Aorto-left ventricular tunnel: transcatheter closure suing an Amplatzer duct occluder device. Am J Cardiol. 2000;86:253–4.

Cook A, Fagg N, Ho S, et al. Echocardiographic-anatomical correlations in aorto-left ventricular tunnel. Br Heart J 1995. 1995;74:443–8.

Grab D, Paulus W, Terinde R. Prenatal diagnosis of an aortico-left ventricular tunnel. Ultrasound Obstet Gynecol. 2000;15:435–8.

Grant P, Abrams L, DeGiovanni J, et al. Aortico-left ventricular tunnel arising from the left aortic sinus. Am J Cardiol. 1985;55(13 Pt 1):1657–8.

Gundel F, Hendrich E, Horndasch M, Fratz S, Gildein HP, Mebus S, Eicken A, Mayr N, Hess J, Kaemmerer H. A rare coronary artery anomaly: origin of the right coronary artery from an aortico-left ventricular tunnel. J Thorac Cardiovasc Surg. 2010;139(2):e8–9.

Hermann JL, Fuller S. Aortico-left ventricular tunnel. In: Mavroudis C, Backer CL, editors. Pediatric cardiac surgery. 5th ed. London: Wiley-Blackwell Inc; 2023. p. 743–8.

Ho S, Muiago M, Cook A, et al. Surgical anatomy of aorto-left ventricular tunnel. Ann Thorac Surg. 1998;65:509–14.

Hovaguimiam H, Cobanoglu A, Starr A. Aortico-left ventricular tunnel: a clinical review and new surgical classification. Ann Thorac Surg. 1988;45:106–12.

Hsu JH, Wu DK, Chen YF, et al. Virtual intraluminal evaluation of aortico-left ventricular tunnel by multislice computed tomography. Int J Cardiol. 2007;116:266–8.

Kathare P, Subramanyam RG, Dash TK, et al. Diagnosis and management of aorto-left ventricular tunnel. Ann Pediatr Cardiol. 2015;8:103–7.

Levy MJ, Lillehei CW, Anderson RC, Amplatz K, Edwards JE. Aortico-left ventricular tunnel. Circulation. 1963;27(4):841–53.

Llorens R, Arcas R, Herreros J, et al. Aortico-left ventricular tunnel: a case report and review of the literature. Tex Heart Inst J. 1982;9:169–75.

Martins J, Sherwood M, Mayer J, et al. Aortico-left ventricular tunnel: 35-year experience. J Am Coll Cardiol. 2004;44:446–50.

Mavroudis C. Aortico–left ventricular tunnel. In: Mavroudis C, Backer CL, editors. Atlas of pediatric cardiac surgery. Springer: London; 2015. p. 305–9.

Michielon G, Sorbara C, Casrotto D. Repair of aortico-left ventricular tunnel originating from the left aortic sinus. Ann Thorac Surg. 1998;65:1780–3.

Morgan T, Mazur H. Congenital aneurysm of aortic root with fistula to the left ventricle: a case report with autopsy findings. Circulation. 1963;28:589–94.

Myers JL, Mehta SM. Congenital heart surgery nomenclature and database project: aortico-left ventricular tunnel. Ann Thorac Surg. 2000;69(4 Suppl):S164–9.

Napoleone C, Gargiulo G, Pierangeli A. Aortico-left ventricular tunnel: two new cases with a long-term follow-up. Ital Heart J. 2001;2:624–6.

Nezafati MH, Maleki MH, Javan H, Zirak N. Repair of aorto-left ventricular tunnel arising from the left sinus of Valsalva. J Card Surg. 2010;25:345–6.

Ono M, Goerler H, Boethig D, Breymann T. Surgical repair of aortico-left ventricular tunnel arising from the left aortic sinus. Interact Cardiovasc Thorac Surg. 2008;7:510–1.

Shum-Tim D, Tchervenkov C. Aortico-left ventricular tunnel. In: Mavroudis C, Backer CL, editors. Pediatric cardiac surgery. 3rd ed. St. Louis: Mosby; 2003. p. 575–9.

Singh A, Reinhardt Z, Desai T, Rasiah SV. Case series of antenatally diagnosed aortico-left ventricular tunnel. Pediatr Cardiol. 2011;32:822–5.

Smith BM, Cochran CD, Owens ST. Aortico-left ventricular tunnel and left ventricular non-compaction: a case series. Cardiol Young. 2016;26:382–5.

Song L, Jin J, Tao L. Surgical correction of an aortico-left ventricular tunnel originating from the left aortic sinus with a left coronary artery anomaly. J Card Surg. 2015;30:108–10.

Sousa-Uva M, Touchot A, Fermont L, et al. Aortico-left ventricular tunnel in fetuses and infants. Ann Thorac Surg. 1996;61:1805–10.

Sui R, Zhong J, Zi J, Wang A. Surgical repair of an aortico-left ventricular tunnel with Takayasu's arteritis. J Cardiothorac Surg. 2022;17(1):12.

Thomas E, Maskari S, Farqani A. Percutaneous device closure of aortico-left ventricular tunnel using Amplatzer vascular plug III. Cardiol Young. 2013;23:755–8.

Turley K, Silverman N, Teitel D, et al. Repair of aortico-left ventricular tunnel in the neonate: surgical, anatomic and echocardiographic considerations. Circulation. 1982;65:1015–20.

Vargas FJ, Molina A, Martinez JC, et al. Aortico-right ventricular tunnel. Ann Thorac Surg. 1998;66:1793–5.

Vijayalakshmi IB, Chitra N, Prabhu Deva AN. Use of an Amplatzer duct occluder for closing an aortico-left ventricular tunnel in a case of noncompaction of the left ventricle. Pediatr Cardiol. 2004;25:77–9.

Weldner PDR, Taylor JFN, et al. An alternative method for repair of aortico-left ventricular tunnel associated with severe aortic stenosis presenting in a newborn. Eur J Cardiothorac Surg. 1996;10:380–2.

Xu SS, Shi KH, Sha JM, Xie X. Surgical repair of an aortico-left ventricular tunnel with acute infective endocarditis. Ann Thorac Cardiovasc Surg. 2015;21(1):81–3.

Zhu J, Jiang Z, Huang J, Wu S, Mei J. Aortico-left ventricular tunnel arising from the noncoronary sinus associated with a ventricular septal defect. Ann Thorac Surg. 2014;98:e135–7.

Complications Associated with Mitral Valve Surgery for Congenital Anomalies and Degenerative Diseases

Constantine Mavroudis and Joseph A. Dearani

Abstract

Congenital abnormalities of the mitral valve may involve one or more components of the valve and may result in stenotic or regurgitant lesions. Mitral valve congenital anomalies can be found in infants, children, and adults. Stenotic lesions can be characterized as supravalvar (encircling rings), annular hypoplasia, valvar restrictions, and subvalvar conditions. Congenital regurgitant lesions can be characterized as annular dilatation, valvar deficiencies, chordal abnormalities, and papillary muscle anomalies. Operative techniques for mitral valve intervention are usually performed by median sternotomy, standard or mini right thoracotomy, or robotic technology. Complications associated with these specialized approaches for mitral valve repair will be discussed in this chapter.

C. Mavroudis (✉)
Chief of Pediatric Cardiothoracic Surgery (Retired), Peyton Manning Children's Hospital, Indianapolis, IN, USA

Professor Emeritus of Surgery, Johns Hopkins University School of Medicine, Baltimore, MD, USA

J. A. Dearani
Department of Cardiovascular Surgery, Mayo Clinic, Rochester, MN, USA

Mayo Clinic College of Medicine, Rochester, MN, USA

Keywords

Congenital mitral valve disease · Degenerative mitral disease · Marfan syndrome · Loeys-Dietz syndrome

1 Introduction

The mitral valve is an atrioventricular valve that guards the inlet into the left ventricle whether it be a systemic ventricle or pulmonary ventricle (Muresian 2009; Séguéla et al. 2011; Federici et al. 2010). Congenital abnormalities of the mitral valve are differentiated into regurgitant and stenotic lesions that can be diagnosed in infants, children, and adults (Choi and Emani 2023; Dearani and Mavroudis 2020; Frank et al. 1998; Zias et al. 1998; Creech Jr. et al. 1962; Yeong et al. 2015; Van Praagh et al. 2003; Ota et al. 2010; Zalzstein et al. 2004; Marino et al. 2009; Fraisse et al. 2001; Lange et al. 2007; Cabrera et al. 2015; Johnson et al. 2015; McElhinney et al. 2005; Ruiz 2005; Fuller and Spray 2009; Alghamdi et al. 2011; Schidlow et al. 2015; Yakub et al. 2013; Artrip et al. 2012; Takahashi et al. 2014; Evans et al. 2013; Oda et al. 2013; Minami et al. 2005; Vricella et al. 2017; Ohye 2012; Delmo Walter et al. 2016; Waikittipong 2015). Oftentimes, mitral stenosis is found in association with hypoplasia of other left sided structures including left ventricle, aor-

C. L. Backer, C. Mavroudis (eds.), *Complications in Pediatric and Congenital Heart Surgery*,
https://doi.org/10.1007/978-3-032-02661-3_23

tic valve, aortic arch and coarctation (Muresian 2009; Séguéla et al. 2011; Federici et al. 2010; Choi and Emani 2023; Dearani and Mavroudis 2020; Frank et al. 1998; Zias et al. 1998; Creech Jr. et al. 1962; Yeong et al. 2015; Van Praagh et al. 2003; Ota et al. 2010; Zalzstein et al. 2004; Marino et al. 2009; Fraisse et al. 2001; Lange et al. 2007; Cabrera et al. 2015; Johnson et al. 2015; McElhinney et al. 2005; Ruiz 2005; Fuller and Spray 2009; Alghamdi et al. 2011; Schidlow et al. 2015; Yakub et al. 2013; Artrip et al. 2012; Takahashi et al. 2014; Evans et al. 2013; Oda et al. 2013; Minami et al. 2005; Vricella et al. 2017; Ohye 2012; Delmo Walter et al. 2016; Waikittipong 2015). In addition, there are associated abnormalities of common atrioventricular valve in patients with unbalanced or balanced complete atrioventricular canal defect which may result in stenosis or regurgitation. These valves are called right or left atrioventricular valves to differentiate them from patients with true tricuspid and mitral valves and are discussed in chapter "Complications Associated with Repair of Atrioventricular Septal Defect". Acquired mitral regurgitant and stenotic lesions include endocarditis, rheumatic heart disease, ischemic injury, and traumatic injury to the mitral valve (Frank et al. 1998; Skoularigis et al. 1994; Kalangos 2012; Remenyi et al. 2013; Selamet Tierney et al. 2008). This chapter, however, will center less on the acquired lesions and more on congenital and degenerative stenotic and regurgitant lesions of the mitral valve. Operative techniques will be emphasized as they have appeared in the *Atlas of Adult Congenital Heart Surgery* (Dearani and Mavroudis 2020) with additional discussion highlighting operative complications and the resolutions thereto pertaining.

Historical surgical management of mitral valve disease in children preceded the open-heart surgery era with the treatment of rheumatic heart disease and mitral stenosis. Cutler, in 1923 performed closed heart surgery on an 11-year-old female with mitral stenosis. Open heart techniques followed with visual repair of congenital mitral stenosis by Starkey in 1959, Creech in 1962, and Young in 1964. It remained for Carpentier in 1976 to devise a surgically oriented classification of congenital lesions of the mitral valve. He proposed a systematic approach to surgical management of congenital mitral valve disease. The introduction and improvement of echocardiographic techniques allowed newer techniques for mitral valve repair and replacement to be developed with excellent results (Choi and Emani 2023; Kanter et al. 2011; Adatia et al. 1997; Myers et al. 2013, 2015; Brown et al. 2006, 2012; Emani et al. 2016; Madriago et al. 2016; Arunamata et al. 2015; Weill et al. 2015; Stellin et al. 2010; Vida et al. 2016; Talwar et al. 2005; Liberman et al. 2016; Ando and Takahashi 2016; Kalfa et al. 2014; Hetzer et al. 2008; Yakub et al. 2016; Oppido et al. 2008; Rajesh et al. 2014; Caldarone et al. 2001; van Doorn et al. 2000; Gunther et al. 2000; Alexiou et al. 2001; Becher and Anderson 1982).

As noted, congenital mitral abnormalities can be found in infants, children, and adults. In the adult population most congenital heart abnormalities of the mitral valve that require surgery are regurgitant lesions. Adult patients with congenital mitral stenosis who require treatment are often associated with Shone's complex, rheumatic valve disease, or occasionally atrioventricular septal defect (AVSD). Because the left-sided valve in patients with atrioventricular septal defect is materially different from the mitral valve, it is generally referred to as the "left atrioventricular" valve, although many authors refer to this valve as the mitral valve to simplify the nomenclature (Galusko et al. 2022). Additional controversies with atrioventricular septal defects is the term "zone of apposition" which many clinicians term "cleft." This chapter will mostly refer to the structures in atrioventricular septal defect as "left atrioventricular valve" and "zone of apposition" as a cleft with some exceptions.

Congenital anomalies of the mitral valve may include the supravalvar area, annulus, leaflets or the subvalvar anatomy. These lesions result in stenosis, regurgitation, or a combination of both. Classification and nomenclature for these lesions is not straightforward because of the varied anatomic conditions that can cause hemodynamic aberrations. Surgeons and anatomists have employed a segmental approach. For stenotic lesions, the characteristics are supravalvar (encircling rings), annular hypoplasia, valvar or leaflet restrictions, and subvalvar pathoanatomic conditions. Congenital regurgitant lesions are not as common in infants and children. They are characterized as annular dilation, valvar deficiencies, chordal abnormalities, and papillary muscle anomalies (Séguéla et al. 2011; Federici et al. 2010; Dearani and Mavroudis 2020; Zias et al. 1998; Ota et al. 2010; Lange et al. 2007; Yakub et al. 2013).

Innovative diagnostic imaging and improved surgical techniques have allowed clinicians to achieve reproducible and excellent clinical outcomes, resulting in valve repair for regurgitant lesions for most adult patients instead of valve replacement.

When considering etiologic factors for degenerative mitral regurgitation in older age groups, mitral valve prolapse is the most common causative agent, brought about by fibroblastic deficiency (lack of connective tissue) which leads to chordal rupture or elongation. In younger aged groups, more common etiologies involve severe myxomatous degeneration of the mitral valve defined by gross redundancy of the anterior leaflet, the posterior leaflet, and the chordal apparatus (Barlow's valve). Other causes of mitral regurgitation include infective endocarditis (see chapter "Complications Associated with Repair of Congenitally Corrected Transposition of the Great Arteries"), connective tissue disorders (e.g., Marfan, Loeys-Dietz, and other connective tissue disorders), rheumatic heart disease, and radiation heart disease. The definition of severe mitral regurgitation includes an Effective Regurgitant Orifice (ERO) of >0.40 cm^2, regurgitant volume ≥60 mL, and regurgitant fraction ≥50% (Dearani and Mavroudis 2020; Ohye 2012).

The natural history of mitral regurgitation (MR) is multifactorial and not easily predictable. This situation has been attended by a management spectrum that has ranged from conservative medical management which leads to valve repair or valve replacement depending upon the severity of MR, patient age, and comorbidities (Mick et al. 2015). In the early era of surgical management of the mitral valve, it became clear that mitral repair techniques were superior to mitral valve replacement for a variety of obvious reasons which include hemodynamic advantages, elimination of anticoagulation strategies in most cases, and a lesser incidence of endocarditis (Shuhaiber and Anderson 2007). Early multivariate analyses comparing outcomes of mitral replacement with mitral repair for degenerative diseases showed significant survival benefits for mitral valve repair over replacement at 5 and 10 years (83% vs 69% and 68% vs 52% respectively). This study (Seese et al. 2020) and others like it (Lazam et al. 2017; Farivar and Fernandez 2012), enhanced the shift away from valve replacement to valve repair whenever possible.

With regard to the anatomic and physiologic aberrations that these patients' experience over a lifetime of multiple operations and or medical management without therapy, it is important to note that many of these patients develop a combination of mitral stenosis and regurgitation. These patients are likely to require mitral valve replacement; the techniques and complications of which are discussed at the end of this chapter.

2 Surgical Approach and General Principles

While the focus of this book and chapters is the recognition and management of surgical complications, it is important to review the basic principles of surgical repairs which are highlighted in our previous text on *Atlas of Adult Congenital Heart Surgery* and paraphrased in the upcoming paragraphs (Dearani and Mavroudis 2020). A discussion of surgical complications will be additive with new drawings and new prose.

Operative exposure for mitral valve intervention is usually performed by a number of techniques and include median sternotomy, standard or mini right thoracotomy, or robotic technology (Dearani and Mavroudis 2020) depending on the circumstances and patient preference. In centers with expertise, all of these techniques have been attended with excellent results (Dearani and Mavroudis 2020). When median sternotomy is elected, standard aortic and bicaval cannulation with normothermic or hypothermic cardiopulmonary bypass and aortic occlusion with antegrade and/or retrograde cardioplegia is performed. The mitral valve is approached by left atrial exposure through the interatrial groove or the transseptal approach through a right atriotomy. Both are effective and depend to a large extent on other associated repairs that may be necessary. Exposure of the mitral valve is facilitated by left atrial dilation which is almost always present.

When the surgical approach is performed by mini right thoracotomy or by robot-assisted methods, the cannulation strategy requires some adjustment and includes femoral artery and vein cannulation (via cut down) and percutaneous superior vena cava cannulation via the right internal jugular vein. Under the circumstances that a less invasive approach is used, one of two strategies can be implemented. The first is aortic occlusion using a customized clamp placed through the right lateral chest wall, cardioplegic arrest and an ascending aortic tack vent placement to decompress the left ventricle. The second adjustment is the use of an endo-balloon device which will occlude the ascending aorta while antegrade cardioplegia is administered. Valve exposure is established by left atriotomy. Regardless of the incision, the same mitral repair is performed. Limited exposure is no excuse or reason to accept an inferior repair.

Complications associated with these specialized approaches for mitral valve repair are centered around the alternative cannulation methods which can cause poor venous drainage, interruption of antegrade cardioplegic administration (especially using the endo-balloon method), difficulty in establishing retrograde cardioplegia, and managing anomalous systemic venous return such as left superior vena cava (Grossi et al. 2002; Carpentier et al. 1976).

3 Normal Mitral Valve Anatomy, Relationships, and Classification

The anatomic characteristics of the normal mitral valve is comprised of a complex anatomic structure which is defined by an annulus, leaflets, chordae tendineae, and papillary muscles. Mitral valve function is dependent on the structural integrity of its components and the contractility of the left ventricle. Figure 1 is a cross-sectional artist's rendition of the heart which shows the mitral valve and its anatomic relationships. Based on the descriptions by Carpentier and associates (Carpentier et al. 1976; Chauvaud et al. 1998; Abdul and Chowdhury 2022), there are two classification systems for congenital mitral lesions. These classifications define the different lesion sets by leaflet motion, deformed annulus, cleft leaflets, agenesis, commissural fusion, chordal shortening/elongation, and subvalvar apparatus anatomy. Figure 2 shows the differences between the normal atrioventricular valve anatomy and the valvar anatomy associated with atrioventricular septal defect (AVSD). These subsets will be defined further and combined with traditional methods for treatment. Complications will be discussed.

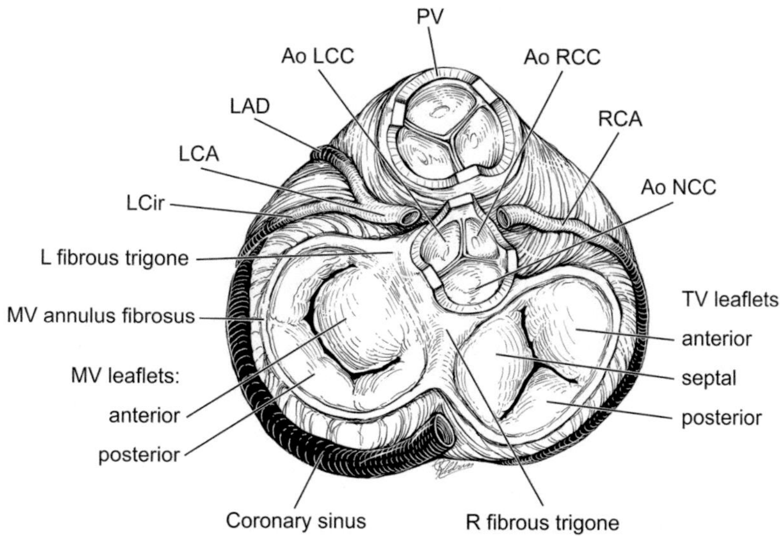

Fig. 1 Shows how a fibrous annulus divides the left atrium from the left ventricle. The leaflets are attached to the annulus; important adjacent structures are noted. The mitral valve annulus projects along the left atrioventricular sulcus; it is fixed medially to the central cardiac skeleton at the aortic root. The mitral valve is a bileaflet structure and is further defined by two well-delineated commissures in the anterolateral and posteromedial positions. The posterior (mural) leaflet is longer and narrower than the anterior leaflet and is generally divided into three scallops. The anterior (septal) leaflet is larger and wider than the posterior leaflet and is shaped like a trapezoid. Each leaflet has a more proximal clear zone and a thicker basal zone at the region of attachment to the annulus. The chordae tendineae arise from two papillary muscles that are attached to the anterolateral and posteromedial ventricular free wall. The posterior descending coronary artery supplies the posterior papillary muscle; the circumflex coronary artery supplies the anterolateral papillary muscle. Each of the papillary muscles supports chordae tendineae from both leaflets. The papillary muscle anatomy varies considerably between individuals, but always arises from the free wall and never from the ventricular septum. Some are broad-based, others are fingerlike; still others are broad-based and have fingerlike characteristics. In patients with normal cardiac anatomy, there is generally an offset between the hinge point of the mitral and tricuspid valves; the hinge point of the tricuspid valve is slightly lower than the mitral valve. The conduction tissue is adjacent to the membranous septum and is located at the apex of the triangle of Koch. (With permission Lamberti and Mitruka 2003). *Ao* aorta, *LAD* left anterior descending coronary artery, *LCA* left coronary artery, *LCC* left coronary artery cusp, *LCir* left circumflex coronary artery, *MV* mitral valve, *NCC* noncoronary cusp, *PV* pulmonary valve, *RCA* right coronary artery, *RCC* right coronary cusp, *TV* tricuspid valve

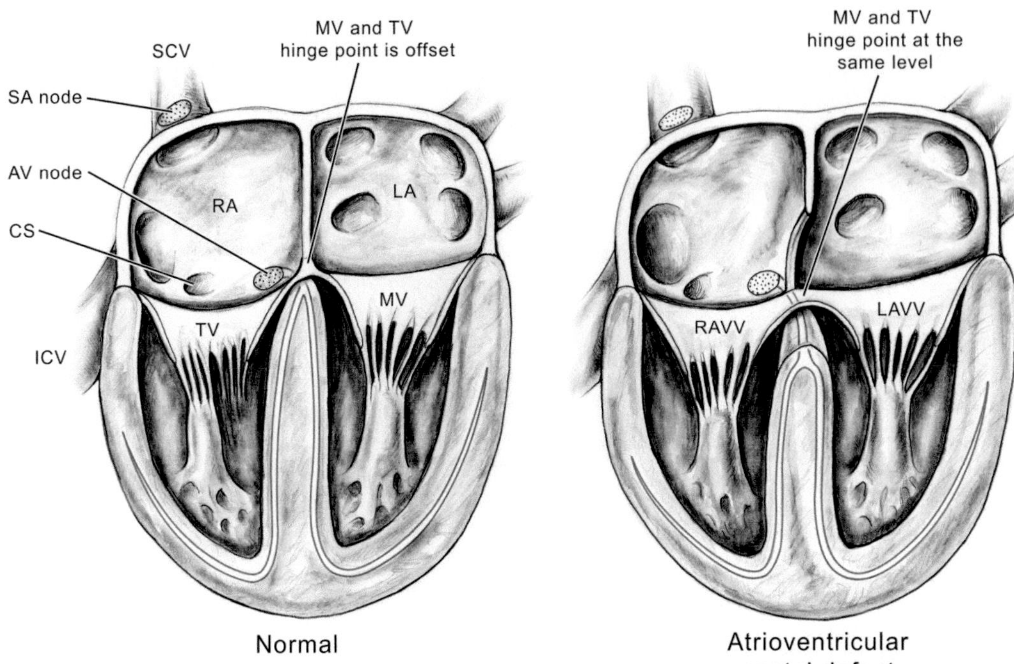

Fig. 2 Shows the contrast between patients with normal atrioventricular valve anatomy and AVSD. The common atrioventricular valve has a hinge point that lies in the same plane for both the mitral and tricuspid valves and the conduction tissue is displaced inferiorly and is located closer to the coronary sinus. (With permission Dearani and Mavroudis 2020). *AV* atrioventricular, *CS* coronary sinus, *ICV* inferior caval vein, *LA* left atrium, *LAVV* left atrioventricular valve, *MV* mitral valve, *RA* right atrium, *RAVV* right atrioventricular valve, *SA* sinoatrial, *SCV* superior caval vein, *TV* tricuspid valve

4 Stenotic and Combined Stenotic/Regurgitant Lesions

4.1 Supravalvar and Intravalvar Mitral Rings

Supravalvar mitral stenosis is characterized by a circular restrictive fibrous membrane that is connected and continuous with the mitral valve annulus. The thick fibrous membrane is typically attached at the level of the annulus or just above it. The fibrous membrane typically has a single central opening that is usually ovoid in configuration and conforms to the shape of the mitral valve annulus. In general, the size of the opening is directly proportional to the grade of obstruction and the severity of symptoms. While the inference is that the underlying mitral valve structure is normal, this is not always the case. The valve may be functionally normal, but more often, the valve is small and may have abnormal anatomic characteristics in some cases. From the diagnostic point of view, supravalvar mitral stenosis should be differentiated from and not confused with cor triatriatum. On one hand, while the fibrous membrane associated with cor triatriatum separates the atrium into two chambers, the atrial appendage originates downstream from the membrane in this anatomic entity. On the other hand, the left atrial appendage is located upstream from a supravalvar ring.

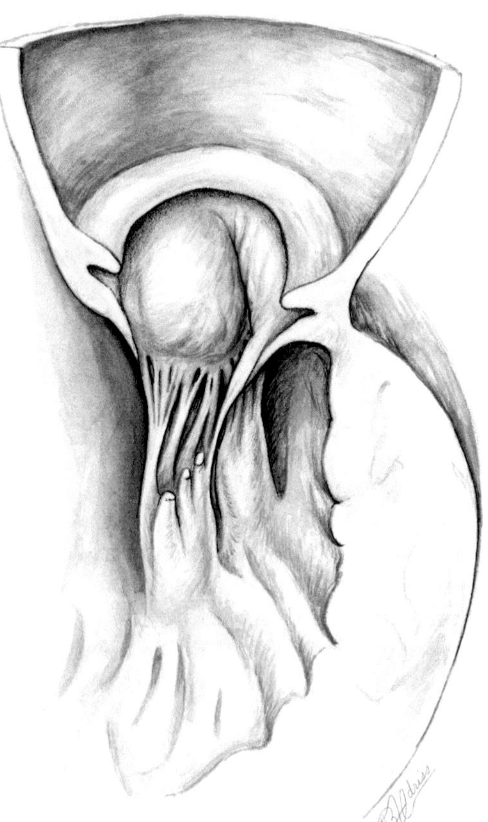

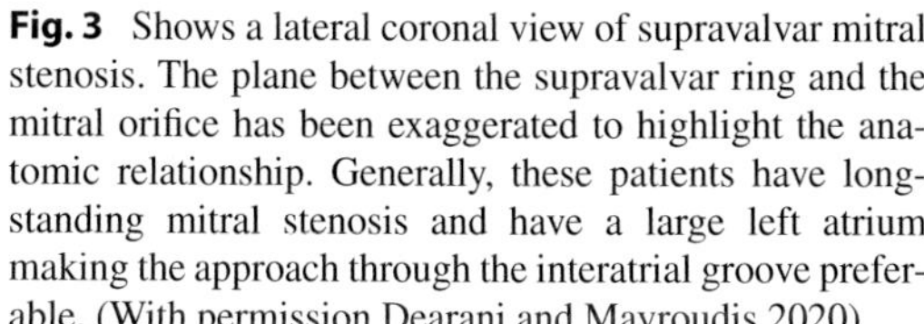

Fig. 3 Shows a lateral coronal view of supravalvar mitral stenosis. The plane between the supravalvar ring and the mitral orifice has been exaggerated to highlight the anatomic relationship. Generally, these patients have long-standing mitral stenosis and have a large left atrium making the approach through the interatrial groove preferable. (With permission Dearani and Mavroudis 2020)

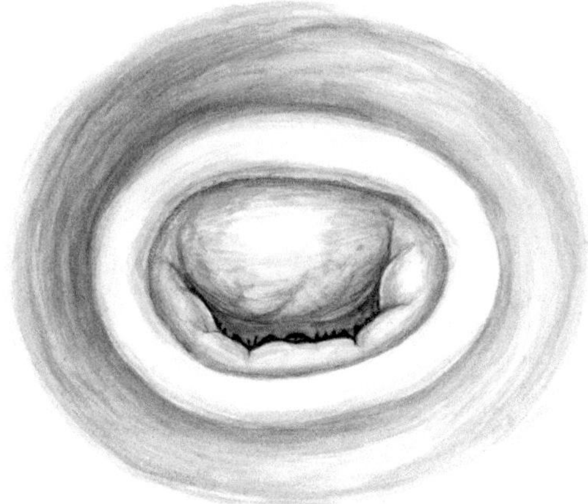

Fig. 4 The key to proper exposure is to employ a large left atrial incision with traction annular sutures to bring the annulus into the operative field for the membrane excision as shown in the figure. (With permission Dearani and Mavroudis 2020)

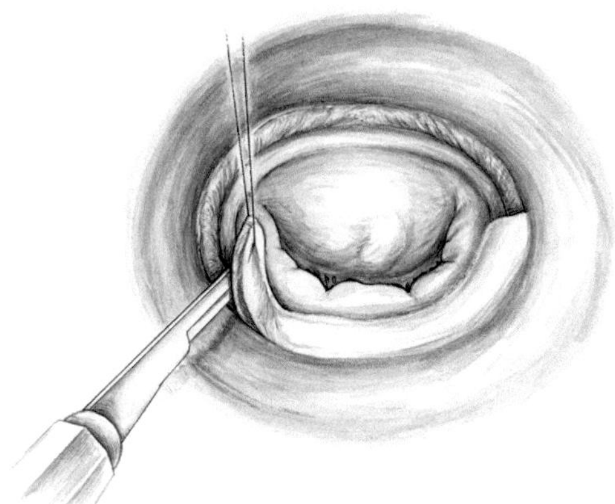

Fig. 5 Shows how a Beaver blade is employed to find the dissection plane between the fibrous ring and the annulus using endarterectomy techniques. The dissection plane can be developed much like removal (i.e., enucleation) of a subvalvar aortic ridge. Careful and deliberate dissection will effectively remove the fibrous ring without injury to the underlying mitral annulus. (With permission Dearani and Mavroudis 2020)

Figures 3, 4, 5 and 6 show the anatomic details of supravalvar mitral fibrous ring resection using endarterectomy techniques with special attention to avoid deep dissection and trans-epicardial perforation. Figure 7 left panel illustrates the unwanted transatrial tear through the epicardial surface resulting in a hole at the atrioventricular

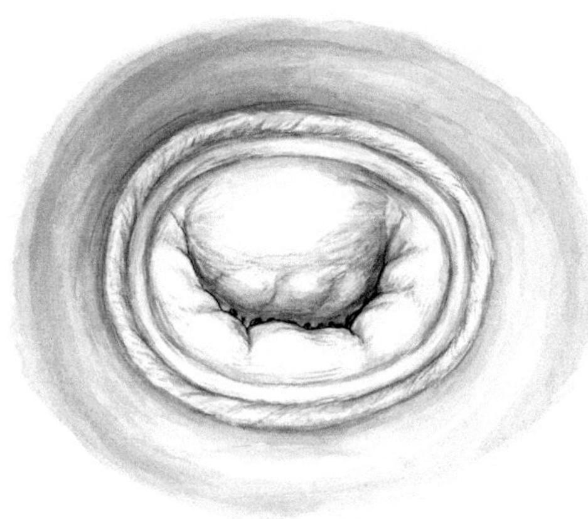

Fig. 6 Shows the result of supravalvar excision. With complete excision of the ring, the restricted motion of the leaflets is alleviated resulting in a much larger mitral orifice. The mitral valve can then be tested for competence with a cold saline injection into the left ventricle. The atrium is closed with proper de-airing of the left heart, and the cross-clamp is removed. After separation from cardiopulmonary bypass, transesophageal echocardiography is used for valve analysis. (With permission Dearani and Mavroudis 2020)

groove. The right panel shows how the transatrial repair can be accomplished by pericardial patch augmentation to include the mitral annulus and the left atrium away from the course of the circumflex coronary artery, which traverses in the atrioventricular groove.

In some anatomic variants, the fibrous ring may be located within the leaflets of the mitral valve and result in an intravalvar obstructive ring as shown in Fig. 8. The principles for resection are the same as for the supravalvar ring except that the underlying structure to which the membrane is attached is the valve leaflet and not the mitral annulus or the left atrial wall. This makes the resection more tenuous during the resection which can easily result in injury and perforation to the valve leaflet. Figure 9 left panel shows an unwanted trans-leaflet injury to the mitral valve during the resection process. While careful endarterectomy techniques are used, injury to the valve can still occur. The repair method can range

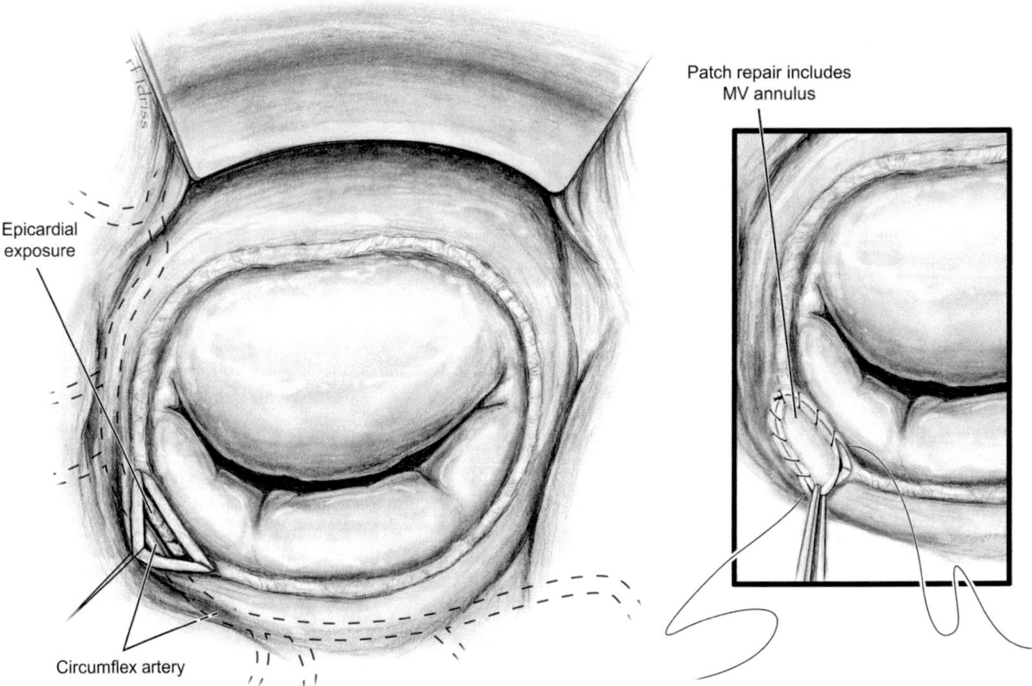

Fig. 7 Shows an unwanted transatrial excursion to the epicardial surface during the removal of the mitral supravalvar circular fibrous ring (left panel). The most important part of this complication is recognition which requires patch repair of the hole as noted (right panel). The surgeon must be mindful of the course of the circumflex coronary artery which traverses along the atrioventricular ridge. Repair is best performed by suture placement in the true mitral annulus and the wall of the left atrium away from the course of the coronary artery. *MV* mitral valve

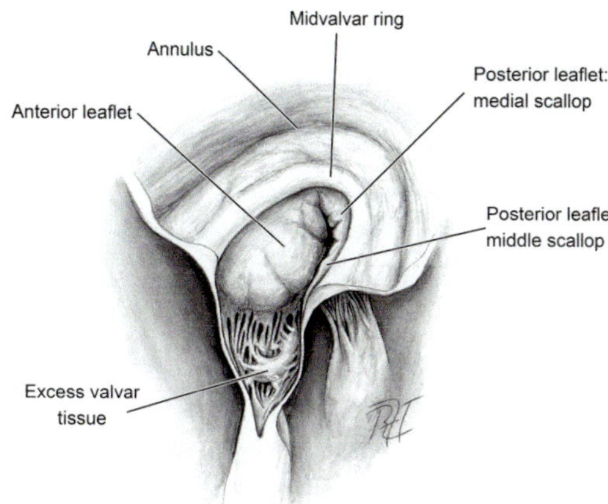

Fig. 8 Occasionally, the mitral valve ring will be situated within the body of the mitral valve as shown in the figure. Under these circumstances, the valve is approached and exposed in the same manner as for supravalvar stenosis. The dissection plane is developed using endarterectomy techniques and the fibrous ring is carefully dissected from the surrounding valvar tissue with special care not to cause injury to the underlying valve. In the event that unwanted mitral leaflet perforation complicates the excision, a piece of bovine pericardium can be used to repair the leaflet perforation. Ordinarily, the orifice of the mitral valve can be enlarged significantly. When the subvalvar papillary muscle structure is also stenotic, carefully calculated papillary muscle incisions between the chordae can be accomplished to allow further mobility of the leaflets to maximize inflow to the body of the left ventricle. (With permission Dearani and Mavroudis 2020)

from simple interrupted suture techniques to pericardial patch leaflet repair/augmentation to preserve the mitral competency as noted in the right panel of Fig. 9.

4.2 Double Orifice Mitral Valve

Double orifice mitral valve (DOMV), first described by Greenfield in 1872 (Linka et al. 2000; Sherlock et al. 2011), is a rare congenital cardiac anomaly of the subvalvar mitral valve affecting the chordae tendineae and papillary muscles. The defining characteristic consists of an accessory bridge of fibrous tissue, which partially or completely separates the mitral valve into two orifices as shown in Figs. 10 and 11. The relative size of the orifices is balanced in only 15% of cases. The anatomic and functional features of the mitral leaflets are essentially normal in most cases, but they can be regurgitant or stenotic. DOMV rarely occurs as an isolated anomaly and is generally associated with other cardiac anomalies which include atrioventricular septal defects, coarctation of the aorta, bicuspid aortic valve, sinus venosus atrial septal defect, ventricular septal defect, patent ductus arteriosus, hypoplastic left heart syndrome, double orifice tricuspid valve, tetralogy of Fallot, and Ebstein anomaly.

Recent advances with mitral valve repair not involving DOMV include "edge to edge" repair or "double orifice repair", as described by Alfieri (Belluschi et al. 2020; Duan and Gao 2014), which is achieved by surgical correction of a mitral valve prolapse where the free edge of the middle portion of the prolapsing anterior or posterior leaflet is anchored to the facing edge of the opposite leaflet. It is very interesting that an ana-

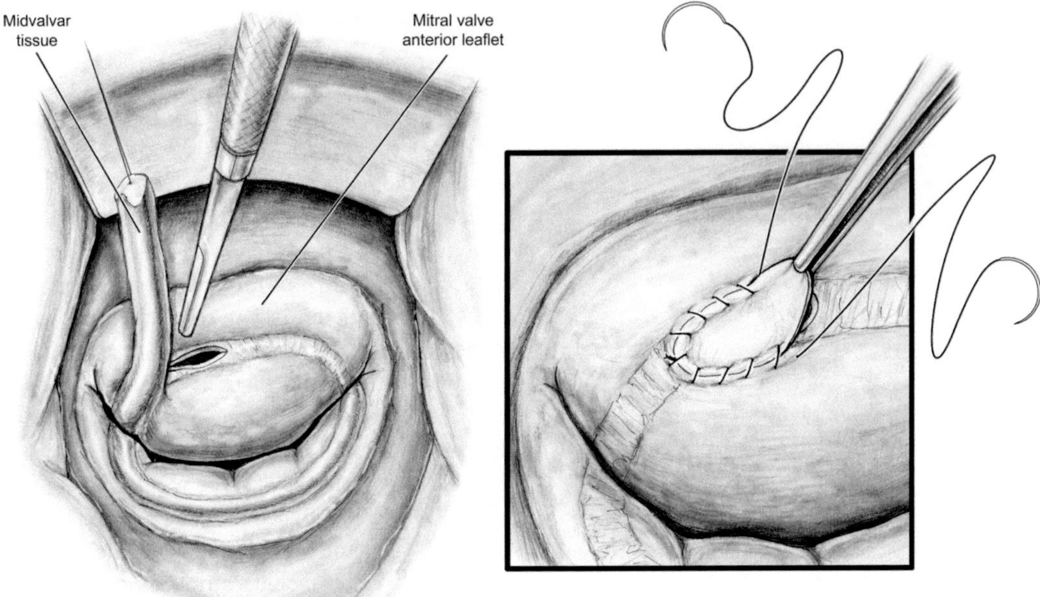

Fig. 9 Left panel shows an unwanted transleaflet injury to the mitral valve during the removal of the intraleaflet mitral ring. The method of this intraleaflet ring removal is similar to endarterectomy techniques that are used for vascular stenoses. This therapeutic reference is appropriate since the leaflet is quite thin and can easily be injured resulting in a transleaflet perforation and hole. The right panel shows pericardial patch leaflet repair which should be instrumental in preserving mitral valve function

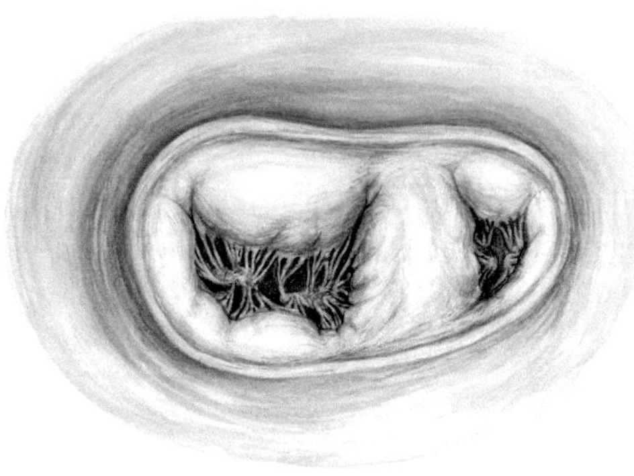

Fig. 10 Double orifice mitral valve is an anatomic abnormality in which there are two reasonably formed inlets into the left ventricle. The figure shows a left atrial superior view of the double orifice mitral valve. In general, one orifice is larger than the other which can be difficult to identify without a careful inspection and heightened awareness. (With permission Dearani and Mavroudis 2020)

tomic variation of nature would lead to an anatomic repair performed by humans. Nevertheless, there are some pathophysiologic problems with DOMV which may need to be addressed. For instance, a cleft involving one portion of the DOMV, usually the dominant orifice, can cause regurgitation as noted in the left panel of Fig. 12. Repair of the cleft or zone of apposition (Alghamdi et al. 2010) can be performed by cleft closure using interrupted sutures as shown in the right panel of Fig. 12. The trouble with this seemingly easy and innocuous repair of left AV valve regurgitation is the possibility of creating left AV valve stenosis. This dilemma is encountered during repair of some forms of intermediate or complete atrioventricular septal defect. There are no rules to govern this problem except what some

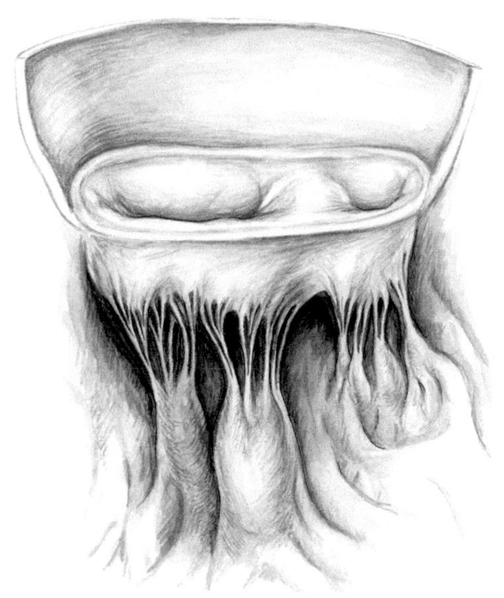

Fig. 11 Shows the same atrioventricular valve in a coronal view. Typically, the smaller of the two orifices is rightward while the larger orifice is leftward as seen by the surgeon across from the left atrium. The degree of stenosis is variable and effective orifice enlarging operations have not been reported. The most important tenet when approaching this valve is not to cut the isthmus between the two orifices. This results in severe regurgitation that cannot be repaired due to lack of subtended supporting chordae tendineae in the middle of the valve. The best approach to a stenotic double orifice valve is to look for and treat any secondary causes of stenosis such as papillary muscle obstructive lesions. Sometimes a cleft will be present in the anterior leaflet of the larger orifice. Experience and judgement will determine whether the cleft should be closed depending on the amount of resultant stenosis if the cleft is closed or the amount of regurgitation if the cleft is unrepaired. (With permission Dearani and Mavroudis 2020)

might call, "experience" or "wisdom" which on the face of it does nothing to explain, educate, or advise the reader. If the surgeon encounters a DOMV with regurgitation that is caused by a cleft in the dominant orifice, then it is reasonable to close the cleft and instill cold saline to float the leaflets and check for repair status. One could measure both leaflets with gauged dilators and estimate the size necessary to form a nonstenotic valve. In the end, chamber closure, separation from cardiopulmonary bypass, and transesophageal echocardiography (TEE) inquiry will allow the surgical team to make an assessment and end the operation or re-explore with the intention of taking down the repair either completely or partially and trust that the decreased amount of residual regurgitation and absence of stenosis will allow for a better clinical outcome, growth, and eventual further attention to the valve at another operation.

Some DOMV valves are so stenotic and regurgitant that some might find it tempting to incise the accessory valvar bridge and use valvar reparative techniques to attempt a repair. Radical repair of the DOMV, however, has a very poor outcome. The aim of surgical treatment of double orifice mitral valve is to correct abnormal mitral valve function and to repair all associated defects. A functionally normal double orifice mitral valve may be left intact even when the accompanying lesions are repaired, assuming that the resultant hemodynamic conditions of the DOMV are favorable.

4.3 Mitral Valve Hypoplasia and Arcade (Hammock) and Parachute Mitral Valve

Mitral valve anomalies associated with hypoplasia, Arcade (Hammock) valve, and Parachute Mitral valve oftentimes are overlapping structures with elements of some associated with the other (Fraisse et al. 2001). To offer a more distinct anatomical description, Parachute Mitral valve is a congenital abnormality of the mitral

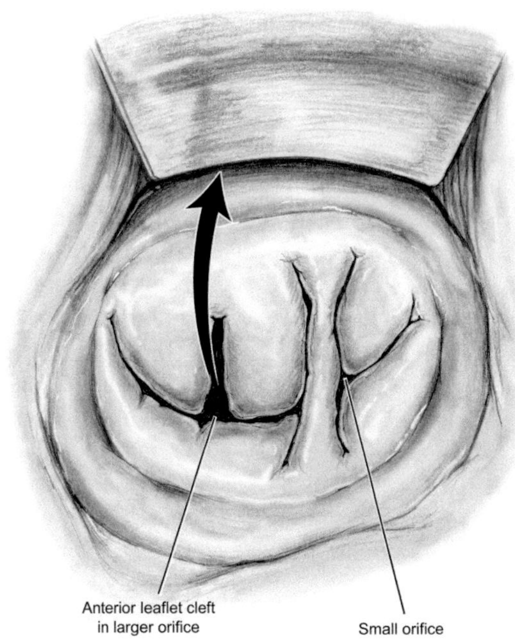

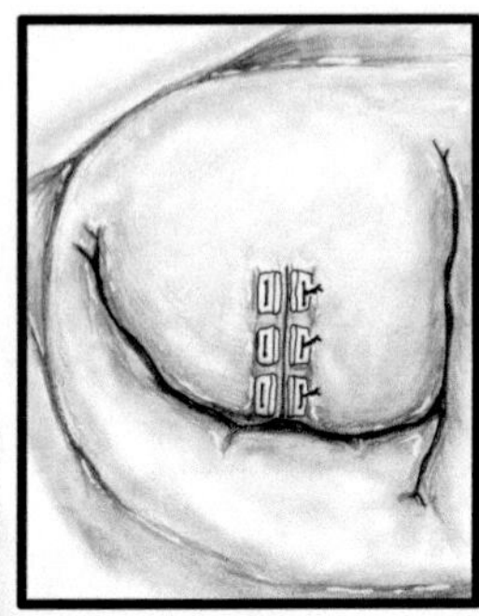

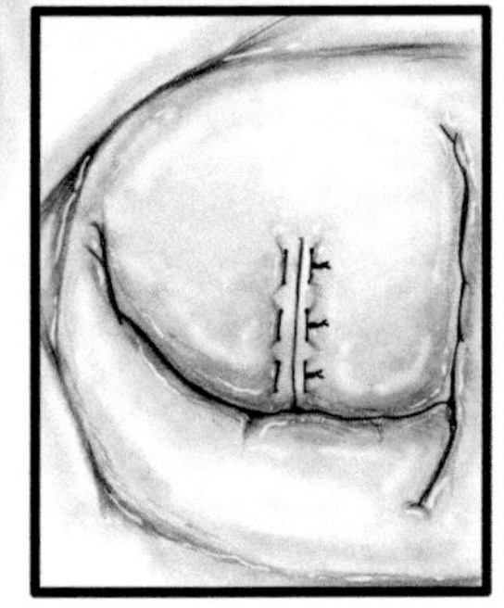

Fig. 12 Left panel shows a cleft in the left side of the double orifice mitral valve through which shows the regurgitant jet depicted by the arrow. The right panel shows the repair using pericardial pledgeted sutures in the upper portion of the illustration and interrupted sutures without pledgets in the lower portion of the illustration

valve in which all chordal attachments from both anterior and posterior leaflets merge onto a single papillary muscle within the left ventricular cavity. Figure 13 shows the description of Parachute Mitral Valve and how Hammock Mitral Valve share similar characteristics. A related and defining shared abnormality is the closely spaced papillary muscles, or multiple papillary muscle fusion, in which distinct papillary muscles can be identified. These single papillary muscle fusions result in impaired excursion of leaflet edges causing mitral stenosis. In those cases, in which there is a single papillary muscle or two distinct papillary muscles, abnormal fusion can occur with attachment to the left ventricular free wall resulting in leaflet edge tethering which can cause both mitral stenosis and regurgitation. In the majority of cases, papillary muscles are thickened with attachments to the free wall resulting in bridging muscles or complete fusion. This important anatomical description will help the surgeon with the proper incisional techniques that can offer a solution to the stenotic pattern of this anomaly, which will be discussed in the ensuing paragraphs. Other characteristics of these anomalies are important as well. For instance, shortened primary chordae tendinea in association with hypertrophied immobile papillary muscles can restrict the mobility of the mitral leaflets in a fixed position. Unfortunately, this constellation of abnormalities contributes to both stenosis as it limits opening of the valve leaflets, as well as regurgitation if it prevents leaflet edges from coapting during systole. Repair of this entity will require careful incision of papillary muscle attachments with the hope that the shortened chordae will be mobilized enough to allow freedom from stenosis and regurgitation (Choi and Emani 2023; Dearani and Mavroudis 2020; Zias et al. 1998; Waikittipong 2015; Caldarone et al. 2001).

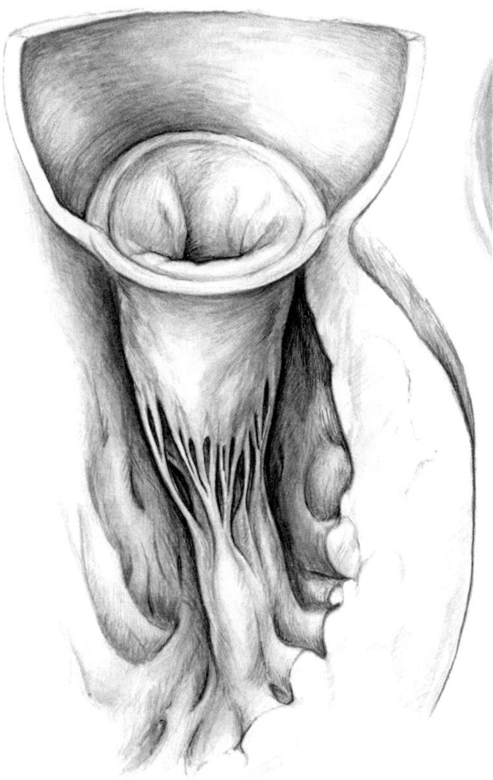

Fig. 13 Shows a coronal atrioventricular view of a parachute mitral valve which has similar characteristics of an arcade or hammock mitral valve. When mitral valve stenosis and annular hypoplasia are associated with an inadequately sized left ventricle, the patient is generally treated along the single ventricle pathway en route to a Fontan circulation. A hypoplastic valve and annulus can occasionally be associated with a functionally adequate-sized left ventricle, especially if a ventricular septal defect is present. The hypoplastic valve may appear quite similar to a normal mitral valve in so far that there are two leaflets with corresponding chordae tendineae that appear appropriate. The leaflets are generally mobile with non-fused commissures. Alternatively, the leaflets are thickened, and the commissures are fused. These valves can be associated with thickened, short, and inadequate chordae tendineae with poorly developed interchordal spaces. If the chordae are shortened, a funnel-like appearance may occur. Most often these characteristics match up very well with what most anatomists call an "arcade" mitral valve. The anterior and posterior group of papillary muscles joins together and fuses with the entire leading edge of the leaflet without the presence of well-formed chordae. Only one papillary muscle may participate in the arcade in some cases. The arcade mitral configuration can produce mitral stenosis or regurgitation, or a mixed lesion. It may also be associated with a parachute valve. In general, therapy is aimed at incising the elongated and shortened papillary muscle that is responsible for the central obstructing orifice and making fenestrations in the existing valve leaflets. (With permission Dearani and Mavroudis 2020)

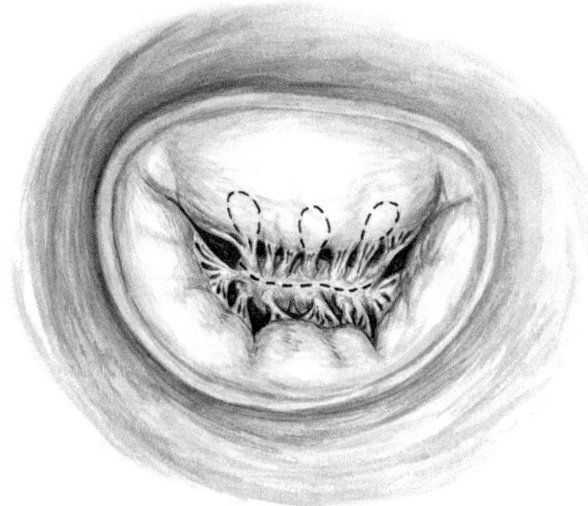

Fig. 14 Shows a left atrial view of a stenotic parachute valve which has similar anatomic characteristics as an arcade/hammock mitral valve. The dashed line at the papillary muscles is the area that can be incised with care being taken to avoid injury to the chordal attachments and avulsion of the papillary muscles. The curved dashed lines represent areas within the anterior mitral valve leaflet where fenestrations can be made to enlarge the inlet of the left ventricle. These excisions are more complicated than meets the eye. The fenestrations cannot be made too far towards the annulus since there will be a moiety of coaptation during systole and mitral valve closure. Better to make the papillary muscle incision first; then infuse cold saline with a bulb syringe and accurately estimate the coaptation site between the anterior and posterior leaflets and make sure that any applied fenestrations of the anterior leaflet do not extend past the coaptation site. (With permission Dearani and Mavroudis 2020)

In cases of abnormal secondary and tertiary chordae, extensive tethering due to chordal attachments from hypertrophied or foreshortened secondary chordae can result in leaflet immobility. In particular, hypertrophied tertiary chordal attachments to the left ventricular wall may occur concomitantly with papillary muscle fusion and restrict leaflet motion during systole and diastole. These abnormalities frequently coexist with shortened primary chordae (Choi and Emani 2023; Dearani and Mavroudis 2020; Zias et al. 1998; Waikittipong 2015; Caldarone et al. 2001).

Hammock Valve is a distinct form of chordal anomalies and has been referred to as "arcade", "funnel", or, as noted, "hammock" mitral valve and further explained in Fig. 14. These descriptions and terminology illustrate the characteristics of this valve which entails obliteration of

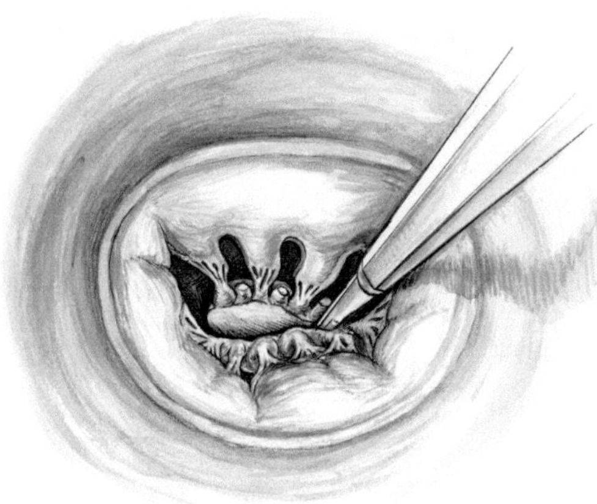

Fig. 15 Once the appropriate incisions and fenestrations are performed, the valve orifice can be measured with dilators. The predictive adequacy of the valvuloplasty can be evaluated by comparison with standard measurements of normal mitral valves for somatic size. The mitral valve competence can be assessed by a saline filled bulb syringe. The most important advice and technical "pearls" from one surgeon to another is to "establish excellent exposure with retraction sutures in the annulus, measure 10 times, and cut once." Incision into the papillary muscle must be made accurately, deliberately, and centrally to avoid papillary muscle avulsion and to maintain chordal attachments. These valve repair techniques are applied in childhood when surgery is most often performed for mitral stenosis. It is rare that these procedures are successfully performed in a "redo" setting when it has been done earlier in childhood. Leaflets are often thickened, restricted and calcified in adulthood and valve excision with prosthetic replacement is the more common course of action. (With permission Dearani and Mavroudis 2020)

interchordal spaces by the presence of a membrane that extends from the leaflet edges to the level of the papillary muscles. The interchordal membrane appears like and has the consistency of leaflet tissue which creates the appearance of a "hammock" which can be characterized by echocardiography and visual appearance (Waikittipong 2015; Caldarone et al. 2001; Hung et al. 1997). The repair of Hammock valve is rather complex and can involve papillary muscle incision and separation as well as intentional leaflet fenestration to enlarge the mitral valve orifice. Figures 14 and 15 show the techniques that can be applied to create a stenotic free valve. However, overzealous incisions and fenestrations can cause valve disruption as noted in Fig. 16. In the case of excessive incisions and excisions of the valve leaflets, primary suture closure or patch augmentation of the center of the involved leaflet will free the valve excursion and allow central coaptation as noted in the right panel. In addition, the transected chordal attachment can be reattached to the papillary muscle, also noted in the right panel.

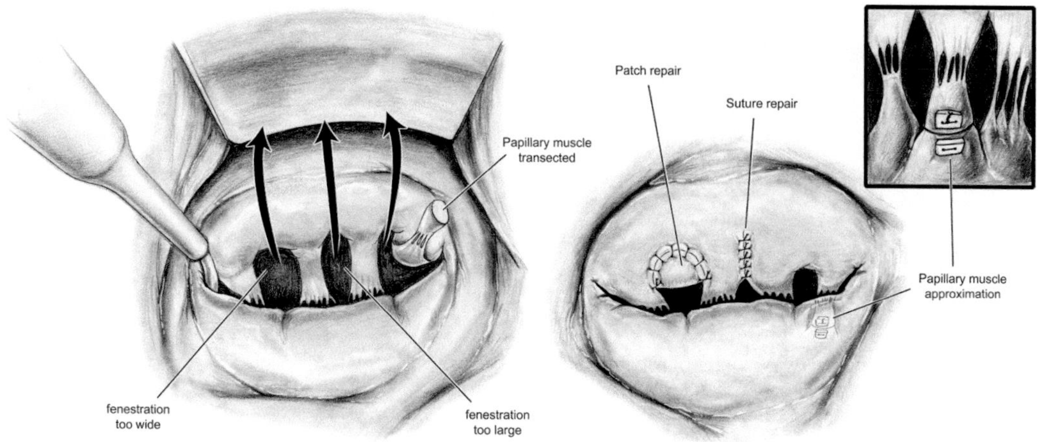

Fig. 16 Left panel shows a bulb syringe cold saline inflation of the left ventricle which is intended to test the repaired valve for competency. The most important part of this maneuver is to ascertain that the incisions that were made in the anterior leaflet were not too large as to cause poor coaptation and leakage through incised/excised portions of the valve and to determine if the chordal attachments to the edge of the valve leaflet were not transected. The left panel shows overly incised and excised portions of the anterior leaflet which resulted in central regurgitation shown by the three arrows during bulb syringe cold saline inflation. In addition, a chordal attachment to the papillary muscle is shown to be transected. These unwanted maneuvers can be repaired as noted in the right panel by suture placement in the areas of unwanted incision, patch augmentation of the leaflet body to allow central coaptation, and reattachment of the severed chordal attachments to the papillary muscle as shown in the inset

5 Regurgitant Lesions

Congenital mitral regurgitation can be associated with many of the aforementioned abnormalities of mitral valve stenosis. Primary regurgitant lesions, however, include annular dilatation as well as degenerative diseases that result in chordal elongation and leaflet anomalies.

Ventricular dilatation from whatever cause such as cardiomyopathy, and aortic regurgitation can also cause mitral regurgitation as a secondary manifestation. Another example includes functional mitral regurgitation which can occur in association with an anomalous left coronary artery arising from the pulmonary artery due to decreased myocardial oxygen delivery and poor ventricular function. Further to these descriptions is the common atrioventricular valve which is not a true mitral valve but functionally acts as a left atrioventricular valve and can be found in patients with AVSD and is often associated with regurgitation of the left atrioventricular orifice. This can be caused by annular dilatation or a cleft (zone of apposition) of the anterior leaflet. This is often the case in the adult with undiagnosed partial AVSD. Double-orifice mitral valve which was discussed in the previous section (Figs. 10, 11 and 12) can also be associated with AVSD with a cleft in the larger of the two orifices. This anomalous configuration may or may not be associated with regurgitation.

Young patients with Marfan syndrome or other connective tissue disorders can present with important mitral regurgitation due to abnormal mitral valves with billowing leaflets, elongated chordae, and dilated annuli. Other forms of degenerative mitral disease include those with Barlow's valve (Fig. 17) which is characterized by excess valvar tissue involving both the anterior and posterior leaflets which are subject to chordal elongation, chordal rupture, and annular dilatation. These valves can be repaired using valvular-annular reduction techniques as well as artificial chord insertion which will be illustrated in the following section.

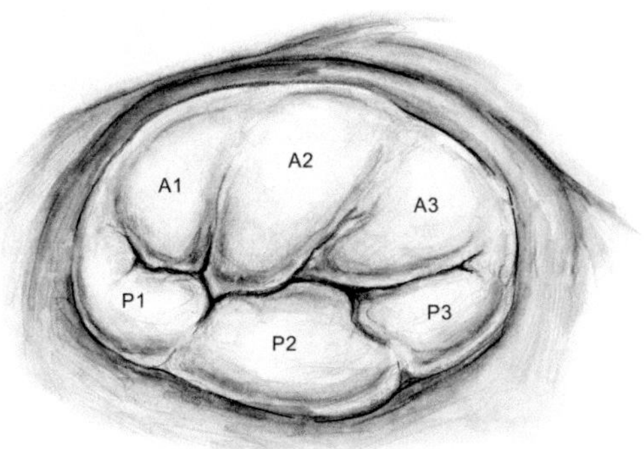

Fig. 17 Mitral valve prolapse due to degenerative disease is characterized by excess valvar tissue involving the posterior or anterior leaflet, elongated or ruptured chordae and annular dilation. Barlow's valve is illustrated in the figure and represents severe redundancy and thickening of both anterior and posterior leaflets. (With permission Dearani and Mavroudis 2020)

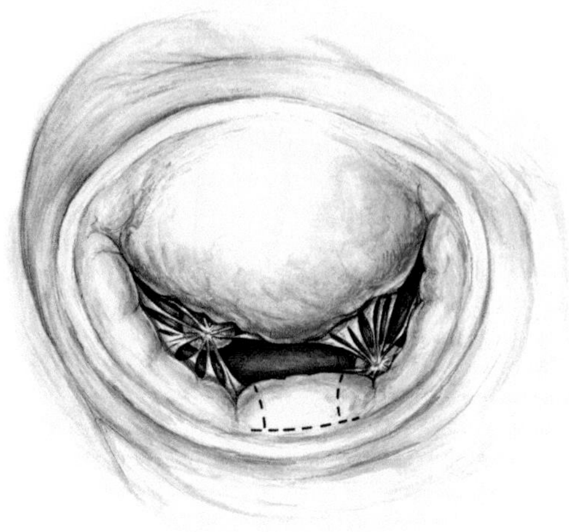

Fig. 18 Shows the beginning of the Carpentier posterior leaflet quadrangular resection annular reduction technique with a supportive annular ring. The figure illustrates the regurgitant mitral valve due to annular dilation. The dotted lines depict the valvar incision for the proposed posterior leaflet quadrangular resection. (With permission Dearani and Mavroudis 2020)

5.1 Repair of Mitral Regurgitation Due to Annular Dilation or Leaflet Prolapse/Flail

Repair of mitral regurgitation due to annular dilation has undergone many changes from the introduction of posterior leaflet quadrangular resection, annular reduction, and supporting annular rings by Carpentier. In adults, annular bands are used liberally to reduce annular size and stabilize the repair. Figures 18, 19, 20, 21 and 22 show the progression of steps that are taken to perform the classic repair using posterior annuloplasty with physiologic and complete rings as noted in Figs. 21 and 22.

One of the dilemmas associated with reduction posterior annuloplasty using a supportive ring is an unanticipated resultant localized area of regurgitation as judged by bulb syringe saline infusion. This situation is shown in Fig. 22 indicating a completed repair and unanticipated leaking at the 3:00 o'clock position. Assuming that the leak is not extensive, a localized edge-to-edge suture repair in this location as shown in Fig. 23 can decrease or eliminate the amount of regurgitation. However, depending on the amount of valve tissue required to execute a localized edge-to-edge repair, the resultant repair may prove to be stenotic. Like so many situations and resolutions which are not definitive, practical wisdom will play a part in determining the "way out" of this dilemma. Some surgeons will prefer to accept a small amount of localized regurgitation and separate from cardiopulmonary bypass and evaluate the valve by TEE. Others prefer to have as perfect as a repair as possible before separation from cardiopulmonary bypass. The best solution to such a case is to perform conscientious preoperative and intraoperative assessment of the mitral valve annulus, chords, and papillary muscle anatomy. This will lead to a properly planned operation which may include chordal shortening, papillary muscle incisions, and annular reduction. As discussed, mitral valve repair for congenital and degenerative conditions will require a combination of reparative techniques. And it should be noted that annular reduction operations may allow repair of mitral regurgitation, there is always the possibility of recurrent regurgitation.

Hung and associates (Hung et al. 1999) have highlighted studies that have "demonstrated the MR can persist or recur after ring annuloplasty, consistent with clinical observations (Calafiore

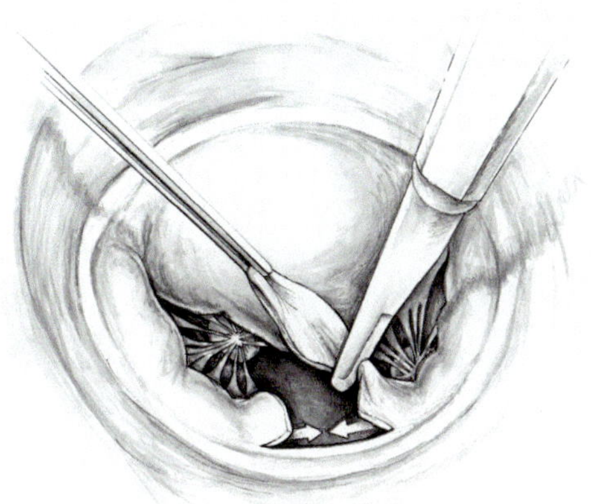

Fig. 19 Shows the quadrangular resection in progress and the completed linear incisions (arrows) that were performed in anticipation of the sliding valvuloplasty. The quadrangular resection involves the middle (P2) scallop of the mitral valve posterior leaflet. The resection is carefully performed to remove the middle scallop up to the supporting chordae of the right (P3) and left (P1) scallops which will support the valve during systole and prevent regurgitation. Once the sliding incisions are made, a posterior reduction annuloplasty can be performed as noted in Fig. 20. (With permission Dearani and Mavroudis 2020)

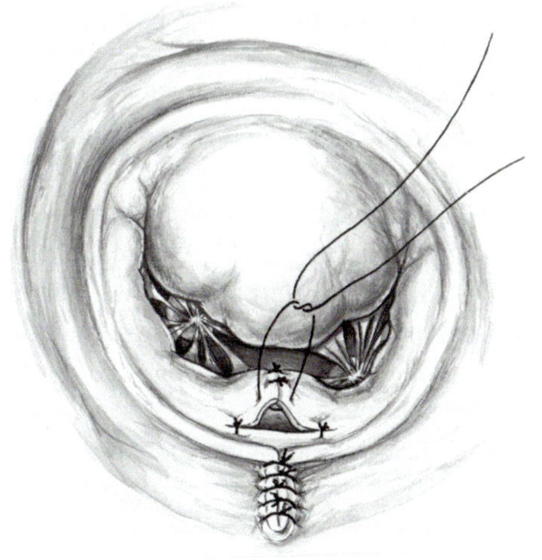

Fig. 20 Illustrates the individual sutures which can be reinforced with pledgets (not shown) depending on the size of the patient. Once the reduction annuloplasty is performed, the remaining posterior leaflets can be brought into apposition and closed thereby forming a new posterior leaflet which has annular and chordal support. (With permission Dearani and Mavroudis 2020)

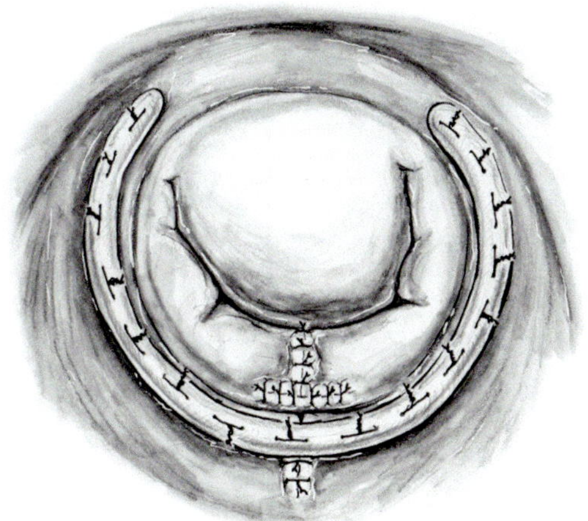

Fig. 21 Shows the completed repair with a supporting posterior annuloplasty band. The band is meant to support the annuloplasty and prevent dehiscence. In general, each end of the ring should be anchored in the left and right fibrous trigones. Not shown in this series of figures is the complete annular ring which encompasses and supports the entire annulus. (With permission Dearani and Mavroudis 2020)

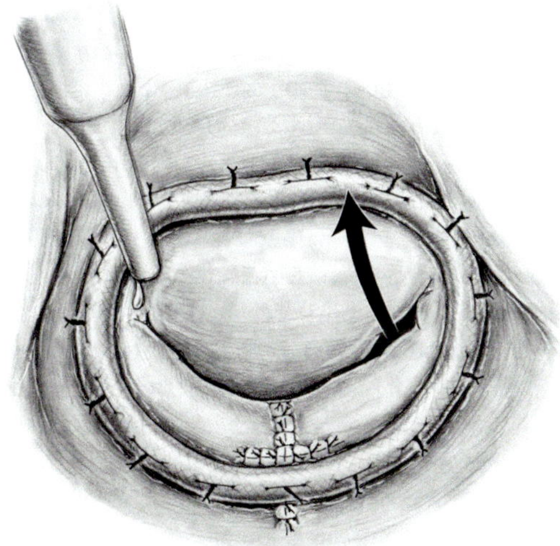

Fig. 22 Shows the completed mitral ring in place with a leak that was induced by a bulb syringe cold saline infusion

et al. 2001; Lachmann et al. 2001; Tahta et al. 2002; Spinale 1999). Given the fundamental mechanism of mitral leaflet tethering, ring annuloplasty addresses only the annular end and does

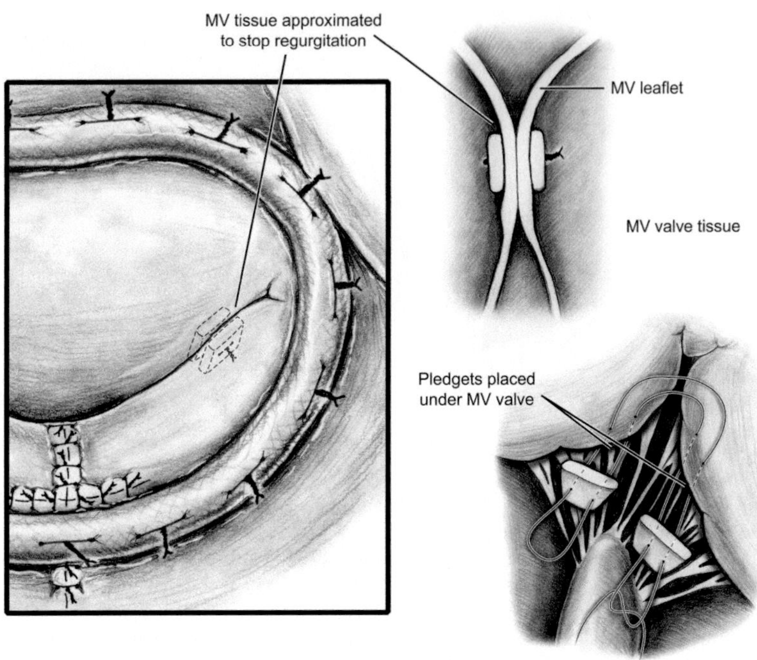

Fig. 23 The leak is repaired by interrupted sutures at the site of leakage with pledgets and knots on the ventricular side of the coaptation site as demonstrated in the corresponding figs. *MV* mitral valve

not directly address tethering by the remodeled ventricle. Remodeling is progressive (Garrido and Oz 2002; Moainie et al. 2002; Hein et al. 2003; Udelson et al. 2003) so that initial annular compensation for ventricular dilatation may not be durable." In the preoperative setting the surgical team will need to assess the origin of the recurrent leak and perhaps assign the leak to chordal abnormalities which may require a different method of mitral repair. To complete this analysis and discussion, persistent mitral regurgitation after ring annuloplasty requires careful attention to the operative circumstances, which includes amount of persistent regurgitation, degree of ventricular dysfunction, and whether the patient can tolerate another course of cardiopulmonary bypass and cross-clamp time.

Another clinical dilemma regarding mitral valve repair or replacement is the post repair attempted separation from cardiopulmonary bypass resulting in ventricular dysfunction, localized posterior wall motion abnormalities, and electrocardiographic evidence of ST-T elevations indicating acute myocardial injury in progress (Aubert et al. 2008). The acute observer will conclude that the circumflex coronary artery might have been occluded or injured by deep annular suture placement during the repair or replacement. Figure 24 shows the result of coronary artery compression after mitral repair and balloon dilatation with stent placement in the catheterization laboratory, In this case (Hiltrop et al. 2017), the artery was successfully opened; however, the patient suffered a myocardial infarction possibly due to the period that it took to close the chest, get the patient to the catheterization laboratory and perform the stent placement. Some surgeons might consider acting on the ischemic situation on the basis of probable cause, namely that the ischemic episode is caused by circumflex coronary artery stenosis/occlusion due to the deep suture placement from the mitral intervention. The choice is reoperation including cross-clamp time to redo the mitral repair/replacement (which is preferable in the younger patient) (Fig. 25 left panel) or coronary artery bypass to the obtuse marginal coronary artery using a vein graft (Fig. 25, right panel). These two proposed solutions allow the surgeon to perform an operation while still in the operating room and intervene in a timely manner which might avoid myocardial infarction (Paparella et al. 2022; Jebara et al. 1993). The obvious problem with this proposed solution is the uncertainty of the

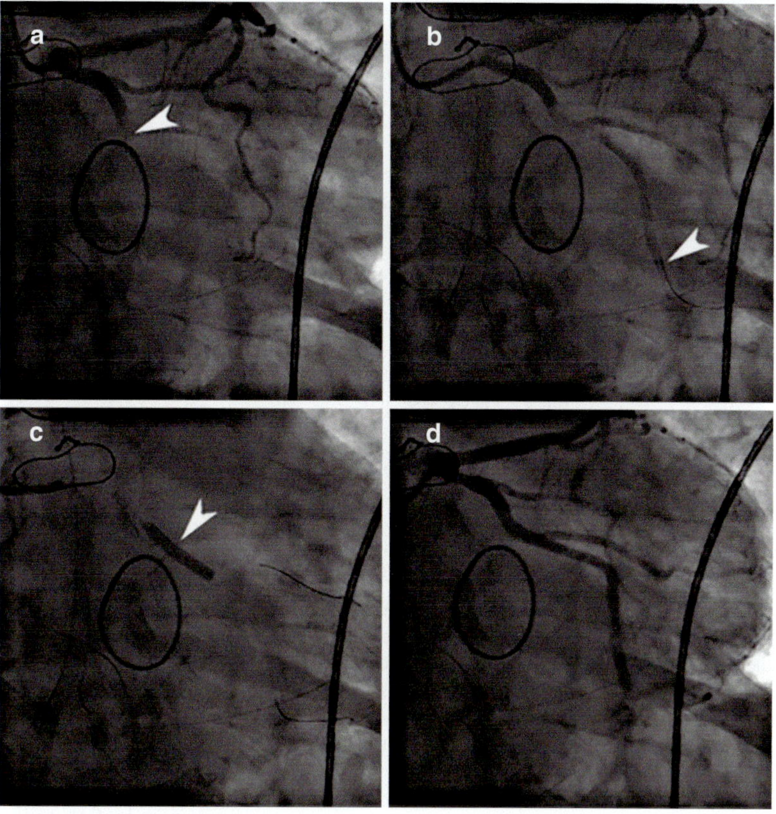

Fig. 24 Arteriogram showing the occlusion of the circumflex coronary artery. (With permission Aubert et al. 2008)

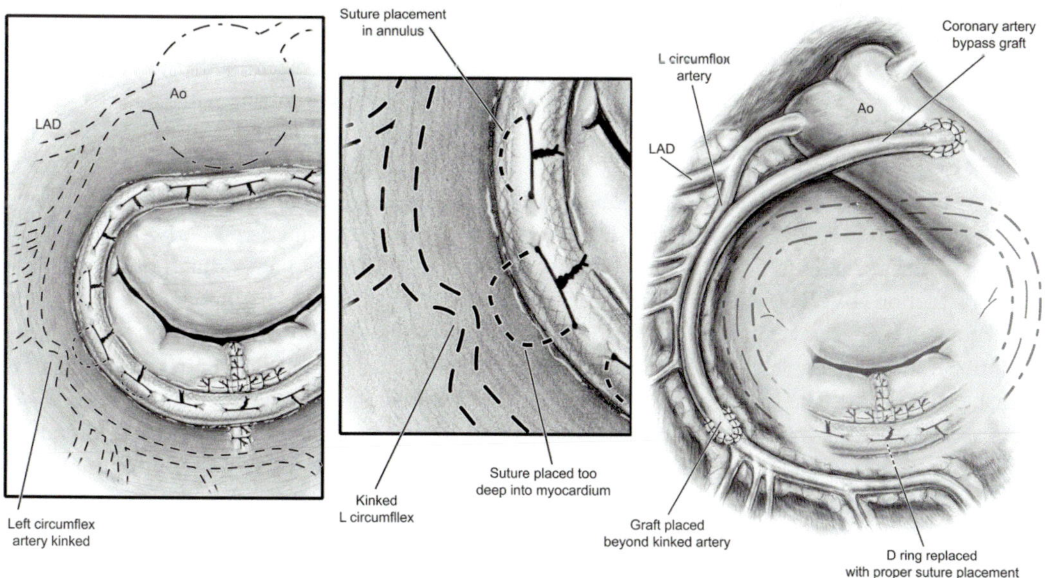

Fig. 25 Shows the cause and repair of an entrapped circumflex coronary artery after mitral ring placement. The left panel shows the ghosted circumflex coronary artery being kinked by a deeply placed annular suture to anchor the mitral ring. The suture was placed through the mitral annulus towards the atrioventricular groove and close to the course of the coronary artery. The middle panel demonstrates more clearly how the malplaced suture causes angulation of the extant coronary artery and therefore poor perfusion. The right panel shows the two methods of repairing this problem, namely to replace the mitral ring and/or to perform a coronary bypass distal to the area of coronary artery kinking. *Ao* aorta, *LAD* left anterior descending

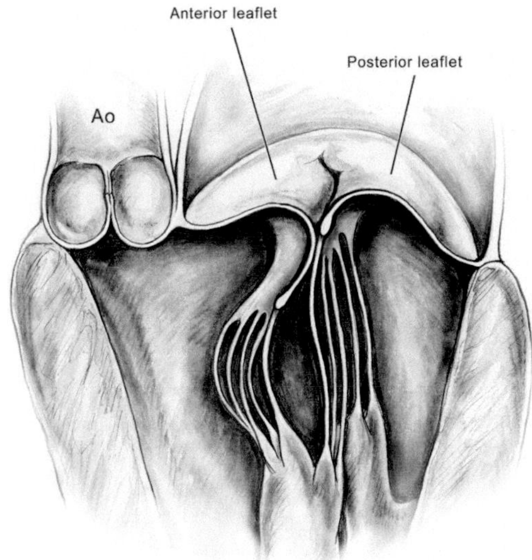

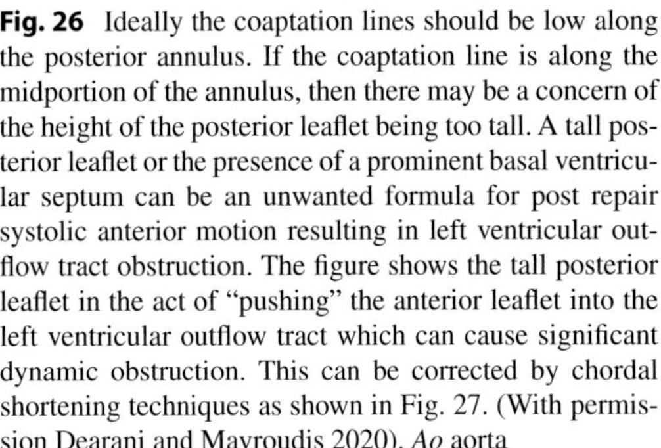
Fig. 26 Ideally the coaptation lines should be low along the posterior annulus. If the coaptation line is along the midportion of the annulus, then there may be a concern of the height of the posterior leaflet being too tall. A tall posterior leaflet or the presence of a prominent basal ventricular septum can be an unwanted formula for post repair systolic anterior motion resulting in left ventricular outflow tract obstruction. The figure shows the tall posterior leaflet in the act of "pushing" the anterior leaflet into the left ventricular outflow tract which can cause significant dynamic obstruction. This can be corrected by chordal shortening techniques as shown in Fig. 27. (With permission Dearani and Mavroudis 2020). *Ao* aorta

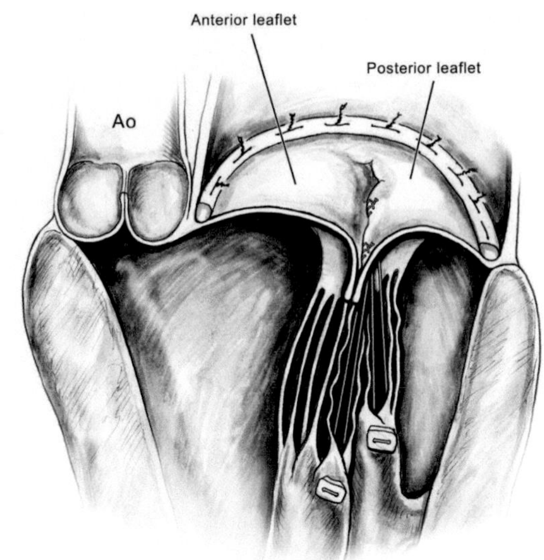

Fig. 27 Shows the technique of chordal shortening by placing Gore-Tex artificial chords to the posterior leaflet that "tethers" the posterior leaflet further into the ventricle and restricts its ability to ride higher. (With permission Dearani and Mavroudis 2020). *Ao* aorta

situation and the reliance on "probable cause" without diagnostic angiography.

Another complication involving ring annuloplasty is post repair Systolic Anterior Motion {SAM) which causes left ventricular outflow tract obstruction (LVOTO) as defined in Fig. 26. This problem was discovered early on during the evolution of ring annuloplasty (Cohen et al. 1992; Manabe et al. 2018). The idea that this complication can be treated by posterior leaflet intervention and not anterior leaflet intervention was not initially intuitive but proved to be appropriate based on careful echocardiographic evaluation (Donzeau-Gouge et al. 1979). Figure 27 shows one resolution to this problem by posterior leaflet chordal shortening which will "tether" the posterior leaflet enough to restrict the motion of the posterior leaflet without causing regurgitation and prevent the pushing effect on the anterior leaflet into the LVOT as described in Fig. 26.

Figure 28 emphasizes another physiologic and anatomic parameter that will lead to SAM, namely that an undersized ring will have the effect of pushing all of the leaflet tissue into the left ventricular outflow tract (Donzeau-Gouge et al. 1979). If the ring is properly sized and still results in SAM, the high riding posterior leaflet can be corrected with an elliptical excision of the posterior leaflet body which effectively reduces its height and prevents the anterior leaflet apparatus from leaning into the left ventricular outflow tract (Donzeau-Gouge et al. 1979). The proposed solution to the high riding posterior mitral leaflet from the left atrial aspect is shown in Fig. 28. Further to this illustrative analysis is shown in Fig. 29 which highlights the bulging of the anterior leaflet apparatus into the left ventricular outflow tract which is the source of SAM and

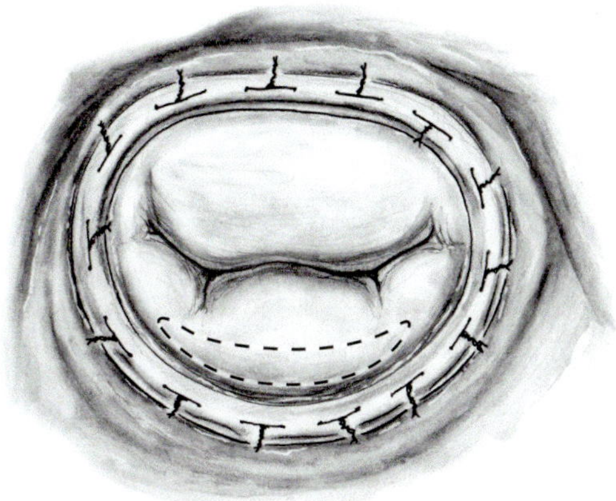

Fig. 28 When a ring is applied it is important not to undersize it as this will also contribute to SAM by pushing all of the leaflet tissue into the left ventricular outflow tract. Alternatively, the high riding posterior leaflet can be corrected with an elliptical resection of the body of the posterior leaflet to effectively reduce its height. The figure shows the atrial view of the prominent posterior leaflet after mitral ring repair. The prominent posterior leaflet is emphasized with a dashed line indicating the extent of planned leaflet excision. (With permission Dearani and Mavroudis 2020)

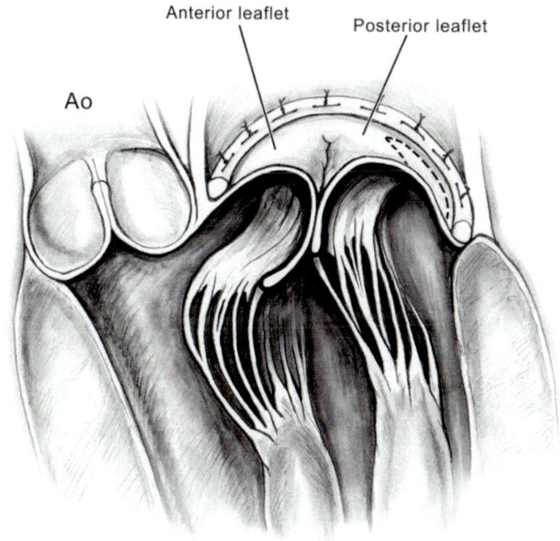

Fig. 29 Shows the corresponding coronal view after ring placement with anterior leaflet apparatus being pushed into the left ventricular outflow tract by the action of the posterior leaflet. The dashed line in the posterior leaflet indicates the area where the leaflet reduction valvuloplasty is planned. (With permission Dearani and Mavroudis 2020). *Ao* aorta

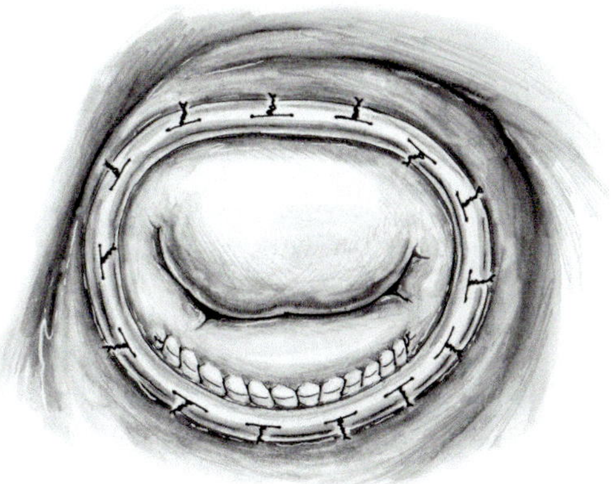

Fig. 30 The repair of this condition which is shown in Fig. 26 is noted in this figure which demonstrate the linear suture line in the posterior leaflet after focal resection and reconstruction. (With permission Dearani and Mavroudis 2020)

LVOTO. Also shown in the figure is the dashed line indicating the area of posterior leaflet focal resection which will prevent the bulging of the anterior leaflet into the outflow tract. The focal posterior leaflet resection and reanastomosis as noted from a left atrial view is shown in Fig. 30. A coronal view of the same repair is shown in Fig. 31 which emphasizes the curative effect that posterior leaflet focal resection can have with regard to SAM.

5.2 Repair of Mitral Regurgitation Due to Annular Dilation by Eccentric Annuloplasty

Figures 32 and 33 illustrate the reduction annuloplasty technique attributed to Wooler (Hetzer et al. 2008) and reported by others (Mavroudis and Deal 2016). This repair has advantages in so far that it is quick, easy to perform, and effective as long as the other parts of the mitral apparatus are not hampered by elongated chordae or papillary muscle fusion. This type of mitral repair, assuming that the other parts of the mitral apparatus are normal, can be used when it is performed in association

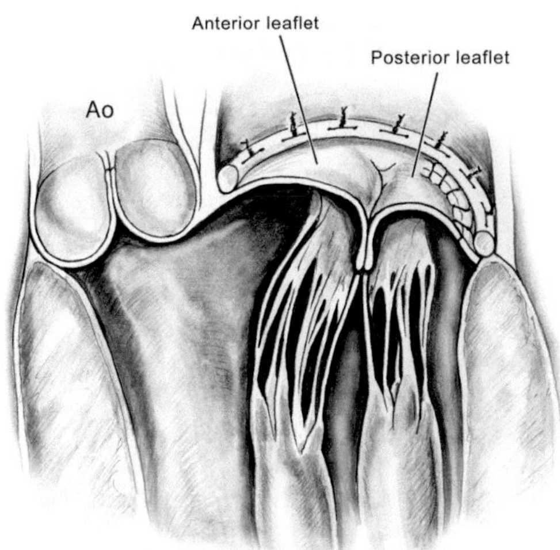

Fig. 31 Illustrates the coronal view showing how posterior leaflet focal resection can restrict unwanted action on the anterior leaflet thereby relieving left ventricular outflow tract obstruction. (With permission Dearani and Mavroudis 2020). *Ao* aorta

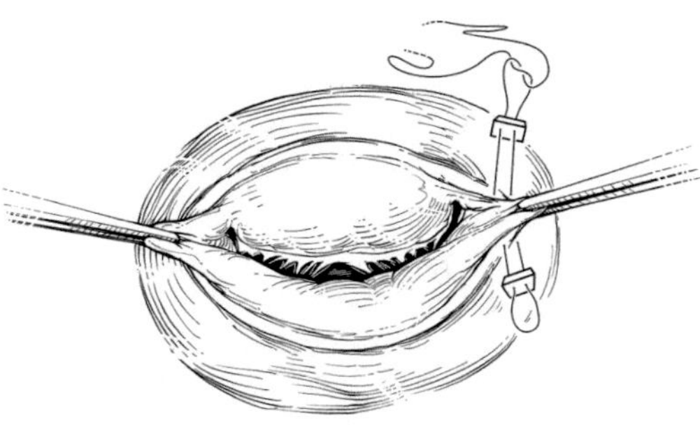

Fig. 32 Variations of the segmental annuloplasty technique have been described by Wooler and many others (Hetzer et al. 2008). The principles are similar to the Carpentier technique, namely that a reduction annuloplasty procedure will better approximate the mitral leaflets rendering them competent. The surgical approach is the same as previously noted for the other mitral procedures. The figure shows a pledgeted mattress suture of nonabsorbable suture material being placed. The sutures are located along the mitral annulus at the commissures. The length and number of sutures determines the degree of annular reduction. Obviously, the purpose of the sutures is to reduce the posterior annulus without disturbing leaflet coaptation. (With permission Dearani and Mavroudis 2020)

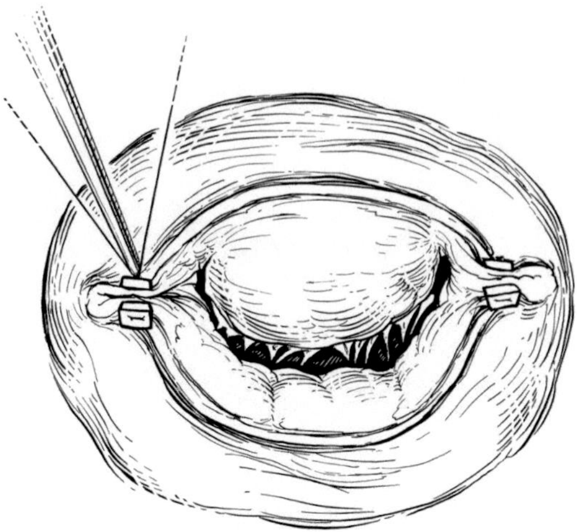

Fig. 33 Shows the completed annular reduction procedure. The orifice can now be calibrated with sized dilators and the valve can be assessed by a saline injection into the left ventricle. The benefit of this technique is that additional sutures can be placed as needed. Occasionally, the annular plication distorts the leaflet coaptation requiring re-repair, which can be performed without difficulty since no incisions were made in the valve apparatus. (With permission Dearani and Mavroudis 2020)

with more complex repairs such as Fontan Conversion (Oc et al. 2005), multiple valve repairs, or aortic aneurysm interventions where an extended cross-clamp time is encountered. Other advantages include the ability to add pledgeted sutures for better leaflet apposition and to remove them as well without the problems of leaflet injury since the leaflets are not incised or locally resected. Acute complications associated with Eccentric Annuloplasty are therefore few with the unusual exception of leaflet injury during suture placement. In most cases, leaflet injuries can be managed by local suture repair or patch valvuloplasty. Long term complications involve progression of the valvar and subvalvar disease and not generally due to secondary annular dilatation, which is in keeping with the proposed application of this operation for patients with principally annular disease and not valvar or subvalvar disease.

5.3 Repair of Mitral Regurgitation by the "Edge-to-Edge" Valvuloplasty Technique

Figure 34 shows the essential advantages and operative description of the "Edge-to-Edge" or "Alfieri Stitch" (Belluschi et al. 2020; Duan and Gao 2014). This type of repair is optimally used when annular dilation and valve prolapse are coexistent. The operation is performed by placing pledgeted mattress sutures at the midportions of the anterior and posterior leaflets (A2-P2 apposition) as shown in Fig. 34.

Interestingly, the repair establishes a double orifice mitral valve by creating a leaflet bridge thereby decreasing the amount of prolapse and regurgitation. If a bulb syringe evaluation shows residual regurgitation, a reduction annuloplasty can be performed using the eccentric annuloplasty technique. This approach is preferable to adding a reduction annuloplasty ring to the repair since a banded annuloplasty in combination with an edge-to-edge repair may result in iatrogenic mitral stenosis. Others, however, have reported good results with a banded annuloplasty and edge-to-edge repair (De Bonis and Alfieri 2010). The cautious surgeon can view the situation and make a wise intraoperative decision based on the mitral inflow measurements. As noted, some surgeons use the edge-to-edge repair as a primary procedure (Ibrahim et al. 2014); others use it as a rescue procedure when all else has failed. We have found that the edge-to-edge repair has merit and we don't hesitate to use it as a primary intervention, particularly when there exists both annular dilatation and significant prolapse due to elongated chords in patients with degenerative disease of the mitral valve. In addition, the simplicity of this procedure is attractive in cases where an anticipated long cross-clamp time will require expeditious repairs especially in patients undergoing Fontan conversion or a multivalve procedure. Even so, complications can occur which involve suture disruption of the edge-to-edge repair by failure to use pledgeted sutures. Figure 35 shows how suture disruption can occur and the resolution of the problem using pledgeted sutures. In older patients, Teflon pledgets can be used. In younger patients, pericardial pledgets can be used to avoid the mass element that Teflon pledgeted sutures might impart.

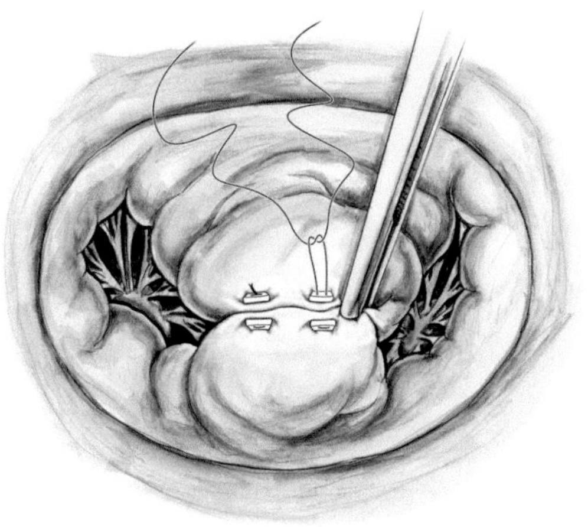

Fig. 34 When annular dilation and valve prolapse are concurrently present, another option for valve repair is the edge-to-edge valvuloplasty, i.e., the "Alfieri Stitch." A pledgeted mattress suture is placed in the midportion of the anterior mitral leaflet and connected to the midportion of the posterior leaflet (i.e., A2-P2 approximation) as shown in the figure. This mattress suture establishes a bridge between the leaflets and creates a double orifice mitral valve. The suture prevents leaflet prolapse which generally is the main cause of the regurgitation. In addition, if a reduction annuloplasty is needed, an eccentric annuloplasty may be preferable since a banded annuloplasty in combination with an edge-to-edge repair may result in iatrogenic mitral stenosis. Some surgeons use this technique as a primary procedure; others use it as a "bail out" procedure when all else has failed. Our experience with this technique has been positive; we don't hesitate to use this procedure as a primary intervention, particularly when there is substantial annular dilation or in situations where an anticipated long cross-clamp time will require expeditious repairs especially in situations of a redo Fontan operation or multi-valve procedure. (With permission Dearani and Mavroudis 2020)

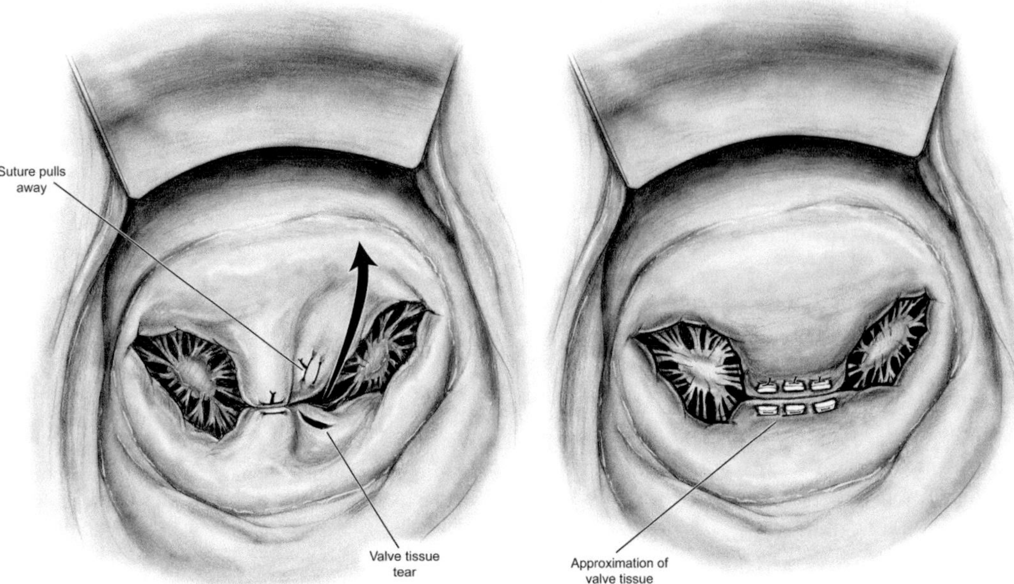

Fig. 35 Left panel demonstrates edge-to-edge repair without pledgets with disruption of one of the nonpledgeted sutures. The right panel shows re-repair with pericardial pledgets

5.4 Repair of Left-Sided Atrioventricular Valve Regurgitation

Although technically and anatomically not a mitral valve, the left-sided atrioventricular valve associated with partial and complete AVSD may require attention either primarily or secondarily after initial repair for left-sided AV valve regurgitation or stenosis. A detailed description of primary and secondary operations for the complications of AVSD is noted in chapter "Complications Associated with Repair of Atrioventricular Septal Defect".

5.5 Chordal Transfer and Chordal Replacement Techniques

Chordal transfer and chordal replacement techniques have been developed for patients with flail or unsupported anterior leaflets which are associated with Marfan or other connective tissue syndromes, atrioventricular valve anomalies with ventricle, injured or rupture chords as well as congenital absence of chordal attachments (Gillinov and Cosgrove 2004). The particular characteristics of chordal transfer are noted in Figs. 36, 37 and 38. In general, chordal transfer can be accomplished with any leaflet scallop but usually involves transfer of the posterior leaflet (typically P2) to the underside of an unsupported anterior leaflet (typically A2). The optimal outcome of this maneuver is dependent on the leaflets not being too bulky and when the cause is an isolated flail segment of the anterior leaflet. A triangular or quadrangular incision and mobilization of the P2 leaflet while maintaining an intact subvalvar apparatus to the papillary muscle is the first step towards leaflet translocation to the disrupted anterior leaflet. Figures 37 and 38 show this translocation in both left atrial and corresponding coronal views.

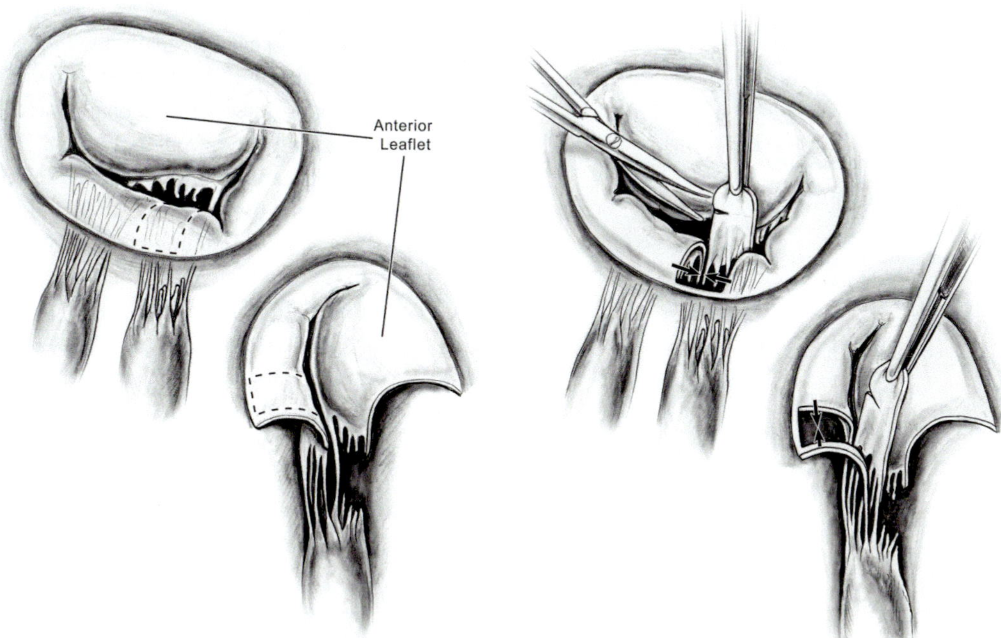

Fig. 36 The most common indications for application of chordal transfer or replacement techniques are for patients with flail or unsupported anterior leaflet, Marfan or other connective tissue syndromes, atrioventricular valve anomalies associated with single ventricle, and injured, ruptured, or congenital absence of chordal attachments. Chordal transfer can be performed with any scallop but typically involves the incision and transfer of the posterior leaflet (usually P2) to the underside of an unsupported anterior leaflet (usually A2). This is ideal when the leaflets are not too bulky and the cause is an isolated flail segment of the anterior leaflet. A triangular or quadrangular resection of P2 leaflet while maintaining an intact subvalvar apparatus to the papillary muscle is performed The figure shows left atrial and corresponding coronal views of an A2 anterior mitral valve chordal rupture. The dashed lines of the atrial view show the proposed quadrangular incision which correct the anterior leaflet rupture/prolapse. (With permission Dearani and Mavroudis 2020)

Fig. 37 Demonstrates atrial and coronal views of the P2 quadrangular mobilization with intact cords to the papillary muscle. The transfer to the ruptured anterior leaflet is anticipated. (With permission Dearani and Mavroudis 2020)

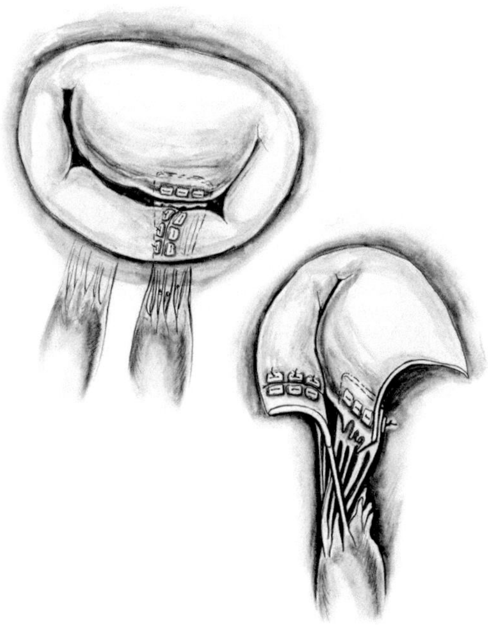

Fig. 38 The P2 leaflet is then transferred (rotated) and sutured to the underside of the flailed A2 segment with 3 monofilament sutures as shown in the figure. The defect in the posterior leaflet at the P2 scallop is reapproximated with two layers of 3-0 or 4-0 monofilament suture. The repair is supported with a posterior annuloplasty ring as described previously. In general, we avoid chordal transfer in the setting of a Barlow's valve, which is typically very bulky with thickened, redundant leaflets. Adding more bulk to a pre-existing thickened anterior leaflet can result in dynamic left ventricular outflow tract obstruction, particularly if the posterior annuloplasty is too tight. In the situation of a Barlow's valve, posterior leaflet resection in combination with artificial Gore-Tex (PTFE) chords to the anterior leaflet is our preference. (With permission Dearani and Mavroudis 2020)

Complications associated with this repair are generally ascribed to suture disruption and recurrent mitral regurgitation. This potential outcome can be avoided by the use of pledgeted sutures, either Teflon or pericardial, to bolster the repair as noted in Figs. 37 and 38. The length of the subleaflet apparatus is generally optimal for translocation (Di Mauro et al. 2022) and need not be a concern such as the placement of artificial chords. Intraoperative TEE can help guide the team whether immediate operation will be required to make adjustments to the repair.

When chordal transfer is thought to be suboptimal such as in the case of a bulky and thickened Barlow's valve, an unsupported anterior leaflet (A2 most commonly) can be repaired with placement of PTFE artificial chordae as shown in Fig. 39. The particular operative characteristics of the operation are reviewed in Fig. 38. The operation is complex and exacting since the artificial chords must be properly measured and tied in place without undue cinching caused by overzealous knot tying which may alter the previously determined chordal height. Other potential complications are associated with artificial chord papillary muscle attachment which optimally requires pledgeted sutures (shown in the figures) and proper assessment of papillary muscle strength to avoid repair disruption (Kluin et al. 2017). The long-term results have been supportive of this technique (Santana Filho et al. 2009).

6 Post-repair Assessment

Transesophageal echocardiographic evaluation of the mitral repair is routinely performed which will allow immediate reoperation should the outcome be suboptimal. When mitral valve repair has been satisfactorily performed, the result should show trivial residual mitral regurgitation and no mitral stenosis. Preferably, the mean gradient across the repaired mitral valve should be <5 mmHg as measured by echocardiographic Doppler techniques. Acceptable outcomes are based on the amount of residual mitral regurgitation, the difficulty of the repair, and the possibility of a successful re-repair. Mild residual mitral regurgitation is considered an acceptable result, especially if the leaflets are dysplastic, if there is anterior leaflet pathology, or if the valve repair was deemed to be technically challenging. In general, we do not accept moderate mitral regurgitation except under extraordinary circumstances and typically would resume cardiopulmonary bypass and re-repair to try and lessen the degree of regurgitation, particularly if the mechanism of regurgitation can be easily corrected. A mild regurgitant jet needs to be carefully evaluated by TEE to determine the extent to which the jet is striking the prosthetic ring. Hemodynamic jets which are in close proximity

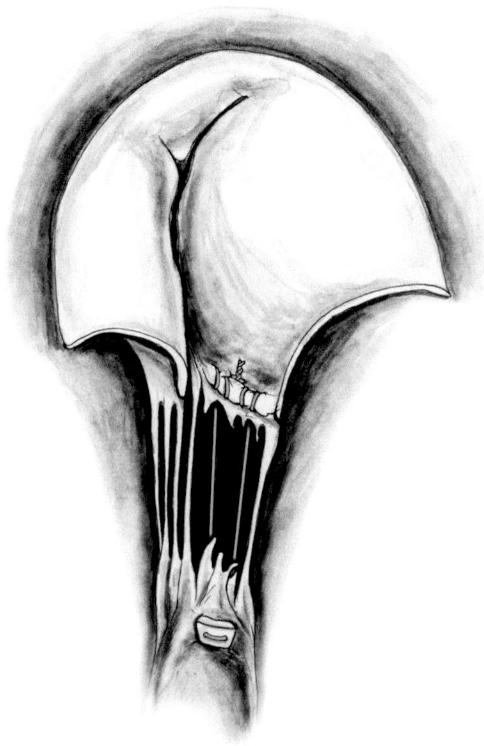

Fig. 39 Alternatively, an unsupported anterior leaflet (A2 most commonly) can be repaired with placement of PTFE artificial chordae as shown in the figure. This is achieved by using a double-armed 4-0 PTFE suture with a felt pledget. The limb of each needle is brought through the head of one of the papillary muscles (and not tied). Each needle is then brought through the leading edge of the unsupported segment of the anterior leaflet twice. The edge of the anterior leaflet is then placed in the plane of the mitral annulus; placing the suture through the leading edge twice facilitates and maintains the position of the leaflet in the desired location during LV saline injection. If the anterior leaflet needs to be repositioned (inward or outward) it can be done so without difficulty; the sutures can then be tied when valve competence has been achieved. We typically use a second double armed suture that is brought through the other papillary muscle and through the leading edge twice in the same manner. The valve is examined with left ventricular saline injection to determine competence. If the anterior leaflet is still too redundant or too tethered, then it is repositioned accordingly. Once the proper position of the leaflet is achieved, then the second Gore-Tex sutures are tied being careful not to alter the optimized leaflet position. The repair is then supplemented with a posterior annuloplasty band. In the setting of a Barlow's valve, our preferred valve repair often consists of a posterior (P2) quadrangular leaflet resection *and* placement of PTFE chordae to the anterior leaflet followed by posterior band annuloplasty as described. (With permission Dearani and Mavroudis 2020)

to unincorporated prosthetic material have been associated with persistent hemolysis. Consequently, when it is clear that the residual jet is hitting the prosthetic ring, even if it is a mild jet, we have a low threshold to resume cardiopulmonary bypass and revise the mitral valve repair to avoid the potential consequences of hemolysis. Other sources of treatable complications include atrioventricular disruption, focal ventricular wall motion abnormalities caused by coronary entrapment (discussed in Figs. 23 and 24), and residual atrial septal defect in the case where the left atrium is approached through the atrial septum.

7 Mitral Valve Replacement

Mitral valve replacement for patients with congenital abnormalities of the mitral valve has been performed judiciously since the preference for mitral valve repair in a growing child is clearly optimal. The prospect, however, of multiple reparative operations makes mitral valve replacement more appealing assuming that patient age and development are favorable. It is common for patients with mitral valve pathology to present with one or more prior mitral repair procedures; oftentimes beginning in childhood. Even so, mitral valve repair continues to be preferred in this relatively younger adult population. However, successful outcomes of repeated repairs is often not possible because of the combination of both stenosis and regurgitation. Under these circumstances, the better option is valve replacement to reduce the cumulative number of operations over the course of a lifetime. When mitral valve replacement becomes necessary, the choice to use a mechanical vs a biological valve is individualized. Technical issues to be considered are reviewed below.

Preoperative evaluation through transthoracic (routinely) and transesophageal (selectively) echocardiography is essential to understand valve anatomy including leaflet, chordal, and papillary muscle structures. Furthermore, the anatomy of the left ventricular outflow tract can be evaluated to assess the amount of potential outflow tract obstruction, especially for patients with Shone complex and AVSD. Deficiency of the inlet septum and the hinge point of the mitral and tricuspid valves at the same level results in the narrowed left ventricular outflow tract. Mitral valve replacement in these patients can result in left ventricular outflow tract obstruction if the prosthesis is not positioned properly. Figure 40 shows how a mitral valve prosthesis is placed in a patient with left AV Valve regurgitation to avoid left ventricular outflow tract obstruction and heart block.

Preservation of the native mitral valve apparatus including the leaflets and subvalvar apparatus in association with prosthesis replacement has been universally accepted to maintain left ventricular geometry and corresponding left ventricular systolic function. This procedural dictum can generally be applied to adults with acquired lesions. However, when mitral valve replacement is being considered for patients with congenital lesions, the process of maintaining the mitral apparatus can be very challenging owing to acquired valvar calcification, leaflet rigidity, and restricted valvar mobility. Moreover, in patients with a double orifice mitral valve, parachute mitral valve or AVSD, significant mitral stenosis may be present, which will require complete or near complete valve excision prior to replacing the mitral valve. The important part of mitral valve apparatus resection is to perform it judiciously; too overzealous of a resection can result in acute (intraoperative) or remote (postoperative) ventricular disruption; too superficial a resection of the subvalvar mitral apparatus could result in prosthetic mitral leaflet interference which can cause both prosthetic valve regurgitation and/or stenosis. Optimally, we prefer to excise the mitral leaflets while maintaining a rim of residual leaflet tissue which will facilitate subsequent suture placement. Since many of these patients have a small mitral annulus, several techniques have been developed to facilitate placement of a properly sized prosthesis so as to avoid annular-somatic disproportion. These techniques are the following: a), placement of pledgeted mattress sutures with the pledgets on the ventricular side of the annulus, b), drifting the posterior suture line away from the annulus and onto the left atrium, and c) placement of the anterior sutures through the atrial septum from the right atrial side (Dearani and Mavroudis 2020). These aforementioned procedures are more often applied in patients with AVSD where the anterior leaflet is so calcified (in part related to a calcified VSD patch) that it is not possible to place sutures in the residual rim anterior leaflet. This maneuver can also be helpful when the left ventricular outflow tract is small since it optimizes the prosthe-

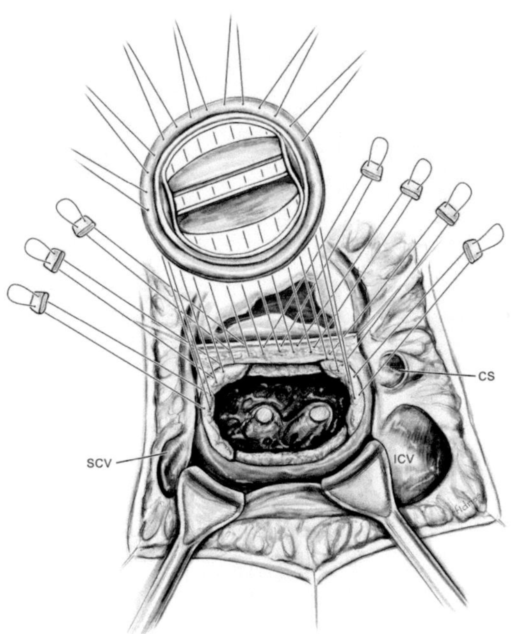

Fig. 40 Shows how the pledgeted sutures are placed through the top of the existing ventricular septal defect patch and posteriorly at the posterior leaflet valvar tissue intentionally left for the valve replacement. Care is taken not to injure the right atrioventricular valve (AV) which is in close proximity to the left AV valve. The prosthetic valve is shown using a hovering technique with the sutures placed into the sewing ring. The valve can then be lowered into the intended implanting site using the pledgetted sutures. It is wise to include simultaneous left atrial appendectomy and a prophylactic left-sided maze procedure to mitigate against the future possibility of atrial fibrillation and left atrial clot formation (see Chapter "Complications Associated with Repair of Tetralogy of Fallot"). Once the valve repair or replacement is performed, a left ventricular vent is placed, the atrial septum is repaired either primarily or with another patch, and the right atrium is closed. All the air maneuvers are performed, and the cross-clamp can be removed. Sinus rhythm can be expected with favorable postoperative hemodynamic results. (With permission Dearani and Mavroudis 2020). *SCV* superior caval vein

sis being (further) away from the left ventricular outflow tract and "in the left atrium" so as to avoid left ventricular outflow tract obstruction (Dearani and Mavroudis 2020). As noted, it is important to remember that many of these patients have a history of many prior operations making the use of a low-profile mechanical valve the prosthesis of choice in the greater majority of cases. In most circumstances, a low profile bileaflet mechanical prosthesis is preferred because it minimizes the development of left ventricular outflow tract obstruction and reduces the cumulative number of operations over the course of a lifetime. The complications associated with a stented bioprosthesis mitral replacement are noteworthy and include the disadvantages of a), creating left ventricular outflow tract obstruction from the struts of the prosthesis, b), smaller effective orifice when compared with a similar sized mechanical valve, and c), additional reoperations can be very difficult when the struts have scarred into the ventricular free wall and surrounding structures (Dearani and Mavroudis 2020). When considering all the issues involved with mitral valve replacement in patients who have had previous operations, the benefit of a low profile bileaflet mechanical prosthesis seems obvious. Associated operations with mitral valve replacement are closure of the left atrial appendage to prevent clot accumulation and stroke and the application of the maze procedure which is individualized based on the history of arrhythmias and underlying heart rate. The indications for these associated procedures are discussed in chapter "Complications Associated with Bidirectional Glenn, Fontan Operations, and Arrhythmia Surgery".

References

Abdul R, Chowdhury YS. Double orifice mitral valve. In: StatPearls [Internet]. Treasure Island: StatPearls Publishing; 2022. Double Orifice Mitral Valve—StatPearls—NCBI Bookshelf (nih.gov). Accessed 25 Feb 2024.

Adatia I, Moore PM, Jonas RA, Colan SD, Lock JE, Keane JF. Clinical course and hemodynamic observations after supraannular mitral valve replacement in infants and children. J Am Coll Cardiol. 1997;29:1089–94.

Alexiou C, Galogavrou M, Chen Q, McDonald A, Salmon AP, Keeton BK, Haw MP, Monro JL. Mitral valve replacement with mechanical prostheses in children: improved operative risk and survival. Eur J Cardiothorac Surg. 2001;20:105–13.

Alghamdi, et al. Surgical management of congenital mitral stenosis. Oper Tech Thorac Cardiovasc Surg. 2010;15:273–81.

Alghamdi AA, Yanagawa B, Singh SK, Horton A, Al-Radi OO, Caldarone CA. Balancing stenosis and regurgitation during mitral valve surgery in pediatric patients. Ann Thorac Surg. 2011;92:680–4.

Ando M, Takahashi Y. Durability of mitral valve repair performed before the age of 5 years. Circ J. 2016;80:124–9.

Artrip JH, Rumball EM, Finucane K. Repair of left atrioventricular valve cleft defects with patch augmentation. Ann Thorac Surg. 2012;93:2081–3.

Arunamata A, Selamet Tierney ES, Tacy TA, Punn R. Echocardiographic measures associated with early postsurgical myocardial dysfunction in pediatric patients with mitral valve regurgitation. J Am Soc Echocardiogr. 2015;28:284–93.

Aubert S, Barthélémy O, Landi M, Acar C. Circumflex coronary artery injury following mitral annuloplasty treated by emergency angioplasty. Eur J Cardiothorac Surg. 2008;34(4):922–4.

Becher AE, Anderson RH. Atrioventricular septal defects. What's in a name? J Thorac Cardiovasc Surg. 1982;83:461–9.

Belluschi I, Buzzatti N, Castiglioni A, Alfieri O, De Bonis M. The Alfieri's edge-to-edge technique for mitral valve repair: from a historical milestone of cardiac surgery to the origin of the transcatheter era. Mini-invasive. Surgery. 2020;4:58. https://doi.org/10.20517/2574-1225.2020.48. Accessed 25 Feb 2024.

Brown JW, Ruzmetov M, Rodefeld MD, Turrentine MW. Mitral valve replacement with Ross II technique: initial experience. Ann Thorac Surg. 2006;81:502–8.

Brown JW, Fiore AC, Ruzmetov M, Eltayeb O, Rodefeld MD, Turrentine MW. Evolution of mitral valve replacement in children: a 40-year experience. Ann Thorac Surg. 2012;93:626–33.

Cabrera AG, Chen DW, Pignatelli RH, Khan MS, Jeewa A, Mery CM, McKenzie ED, Fraser CD Jr. Outcomes of anomalous left coronary artery from pulmonary artery repair: beyond normal function. Ann Thorac Surg. 2015;99:1342–7.

Calafiore AM, Gallina S, DiMauro M, Gaeta F, Iaco AL, D'Allesandro S, Mazzei V, Di Giammarco G. Mitral valve procedure in dilated cardiomyopathy: repair or replacement. Ann Thorac Surg. 2001;71:1146–52.

Caldarone CA, Raghuveer G, Hills CB, Atkins DL, Burns TL, Behrendt DM, Moller JH. Long-term survival after mitral valve replacement in children aged <5 years: a multi-institutional study. Circulation. 2001;104:I143–7.

Carpentier A, Branchini B, Cour JC, Asfaou E, Villani M, Deloche A, et al. Congenital malformations of the mitral valve in children. J Thorac Cardiovasc Surg. 1976;72:854–66.

Chauvaud S, Fuzellier JF, Houel R, Berrebi A, Mihaileanu S, Carpentier A. Reconstructive surgery in congenital mitral valve insufficiency (Carpentier's techniques). J Thorac Cardiovasc Surg. 1998;115:84–93.

Choi PS, Emani SM. Congenital anomalies of the mitral valve. In: Mavroudis C, Backer CL, editors. Pediatric cardiac surgery. 5th ed. Oxford: Wiley-Blackwell; 2023.

Cohen DJ, Norris LP, Montemayor IE, O'Rourke RA, Zabalgoitia M. Systolic anterior motion of the chordal apparatus after mitral ring insertion. Am Heart J. 1992;124(3):666–70.

Creech O Jr, Ledbetter MK, Reemtsma K. Congenital mitral insufficiency with cleft posterior leaflet. Circulation. 1962;25:390–4.

De Bonis M, Alfieri O. The edge-to-edge technique for mitral valve repair. HSR Proc Intensive Care Cardiovasc Anesth. 2010;2(1):7–17.

Dearani JA, Mavroudis C. Mitral valve repair for congenital lesions. In: Dearani JA, Mavroudis C, editors. Atlas of adult congenital cardiac surgery. Cham: Springer; 2020.

Delmo Walter EM, Javier M, Hetzer R. Repair of parachute and hammock valve in infants and children: early and late outcomes. Semin Thorac Cardiovasc Surg. 2016;28:448–59.

Di Mauro M, Bonalumi G, Giambuzzi I, Messi P, Cargoni M, Paparella D, Lorusso R, Calafiore AM. Mitral valve repair with artificial chords: tips and tricks. J Card Surg. 2022;37(12):4081–7.

Donzeau-Gouge GP, Bical O, Daussy M, Vanetti A, Daumet P. Traitement de l'insuffisance mitrale par annuloplastie de Wooler-Reed. Résultats lointains [Treatment of mitral insufficiency by Wooler-Reed annuloplasty. Remote results]. Arch Mal Coeur Vaiss. 1979;72(2):182–91.

Duan QJ, Gao Z. Mitral valve repair for double-orifice mitral valve. Heart Lung Circ. 2014;23:e267–9.

Emani SM, Piekarski BL, Zurakowski D, Baird CA, Marshall AC, Lock JE, Del Nido PJ. Concept of an expandable cardiac valve for surgical implantation in infants and children. J Thorac Cardiovasc Surg. 2016;152:1514–23.

Evans CF, DeFilippi CR, Shang E, Griffith BP, Gammie JS. Fresh autologous pericardium for leaflet perforation repair in mitral valve infective endocarditis. J Heart Valve Dis. 2013;22:560–6.

Farivar RS, Fernandez JD. Use of axillary cannulation for simultaneous endo-occlusion and antegrade perfusion during minimally invasive surgery. Innovations (Phila). 2012;7:201–3.

Federici D, Palmerini E, Lisi M, Centola L, Chiavarelli M, Mondillo S. Congenital mitral disease: anomalous mitral arcade in a young man. Ann Thorac Surg. 2010;89:629–31.

Fraisse A, del Nido PJ, Gaudart J, Geva T. Echocardiographic characteristics and outcome of straddling mitral valve. J Am Coll Cardiol. 2001;38:819–26.

Frank MW, Mavroudis C, Backer CL, Rocchini AP. Repair of mitral valve and subaortic mycotic aneurysm in a child with endocarditis. Ann Thorac Surg. 1998;65:1788–90.

Fuller S, Spray TL. How I manage mitral stenosis in the neonate and infant. Semin Thorac Cardiovasc Surg Pediatr Card Surg Annu. 2009;2009:87–93.

Galusko V, Sekar B, Ricci F, Wong K, Bhattacharyya S, Mullen M, Gallina S, Ionescu A, Khanji MY. Mitral regurgitation management: a systematic review of clinical practice guidelines and recommendations. Eur Heart J Qual Care Clin Outcomes. 2022;17(8):481–95.

Garrido MJ, Oz MC. New surgical treatments for heart failure. Curr Cardiol Rep. 2002;4:233–7.

Gillinov AM, Cosgrove DM. Chordal transfer for repair of anterior leaflet prolapse. Semin Thorac Cardiovasc Surg. 2004;16(2):169–73.

Grossi EA, Galloway AC, LaPietra A, Ribakove GH, Ursomanno P, Delianides J, Culliford AT, Bizekis C, Esposito RA, Baumann FG, Kanchuger MS, Colvin SB. Minimally invasive mitral valve surgery: a 6-year experience with 714 patients. Ann Thorac Surg. 2002;74:660–34.

Gunther T, Mazzitelli D, Schreiber C, Wottke M, Paek SU, Meisner H, Lange R. Mitral-valve replacement in children under 6 years of age. Eur J Cardiothorac Surg. 2000;17:426–30.

Hein S, Arnon E, Kostin S, Schonburg M, Elsasser A, Polyakova V, Bauer EP, Klovekorn WP, Schaper J. Progression from compensated hypertrophy to failure in the pressure-overloaded human heart: structural deterioration and compensatory mechanisms. Circulation. 2003;107:984–91.

Hetzer R, Delmo Walter EB, Hübler M, Alexi-Meskishvili V, Weng Y, Nagdyman N, Berger F. Modified surgical techniques and long-term outcome of mitral valve reconstruction in 111 children. Ann Thorac Surg. 2008;86(2):604–13.

Hiltrop N, Bennett J, Desmet W. Circumflex coronary artery injury after mitral valve surgery: a report of four cases and comprehensive review of the literature. Catheter Cardiovasc Interv. 2017;89(1):78–92.

Hung J, Papakostas L, Tahta SA, Hardy BG, Bollen BA, Duran CM, Levine RA. Mechanism of recurrent ischemic mitral regurgitation after annuloplasty: continued LV remodeling as a moving target. Circulation. 1997;110(11 Suppl 1):II85–90.

Hung J, Handschumacher MD, Rudski L, Chow CM, Guerrero JL, Levine RA. Persistence of ischemic mitral regurgitation despite annular ring reduction: mechanistic insights from 3D echocardiography. Circulation. 1999;100:73.

Ibrahim M, Rao C, Savvopoulou M, Casula R, Athanasiou T. Outcomes of mitral valve repair using artificial chordae. Eur J Cardiothorac Surg. 2014;45(4):593–601.

Jebara VA, Mihaileanu S, Acar C, Brizard C, Grare P, Latremouille C, Chauvaud S, Fabiani JN, Deloche A,

Carpentier A. Left ventricular outflow tract obstruction after mitral valve repair. Results of the sliding leaflet technique. Circulation. 1993;88(5 Pt 2):II30–4.

Johnson JT, Eckhauser AW, Pinto NM, Weng HY, Minich LL, Tani LY. Indications for intervention in asymptomatic children with chronic mitral regurgitation. Pediatr Cardiol. 2015;36:417–22.

Kalangos A. The rheumatic mitral valve and repair techniques in children. Semin Thorac Cardiovasc Surg Pediatr Card Surg Annu. 2012;15:80–7.

Kalfa D, Vergnat M, Ly M, Stos B, Lambert V, Baruteau A, Belli E. A standardized repair-oriented strategy for mitral insufficiency in infants and children: midterm functional outcomes and predictors of adverse events. J Thorac Cardiovasc Surg. 2014;148:1459–66.

Kanter KR, Kogon BE, Kirshbom PM. Supra-annular mitral valve replacement in children. Ann Thorac Surg. 2011;92:2221–9.

Kluin J, Sojak V, Koolbergen DR, Boon R, Bökenkamp R, Hazekamp MG. Fifteen years' experience with the use of artificial chords for valve reconstruction in children. Eur J Cardiothorac Surg. 2017;52(6):1155–60.

Lachmann J, Shirani J, Plestis KA, Frater RW, LeJemtel TH. Mitral ring annuloplasty: an incomplete correction of functional mitral regurgitation associated with left ventricular remodeling. Curr Cardiol Rep. 2001;3:241–6.

Lamberti JJ, Mitruka SN. Congenital anomalies of the mitral valve. In: Mavroudis C, Backer CL, editors. Pediatric cardiac surgery. 3rd ed. Philadelphia: Mosby, Inc; 2003.

Lange R, Vogt M, Horer J, Cleuziou J, Menzel A, Holper K, Hess J, Schreiber C. Long-term results of repair of anomalous origin of the left coronary artery from the pulmonary artery. Ann Thorac Surg. 2007;83:1463–71.

Lazam S, Vanoverschelde JL, Tribouilloy C, Mitral Regurgitation International Database) Investigators), et al. Twenty-year outcome after mitral repair versus replacement for severe degenerative mitral regurgitation: analysis of a large, prospective, multicenter, international registry. Circulation. 2017;135:410–22.

Liberman L, Silver ES, Chai PJ, Anderson BR. Incidence and characteristics of heart block after heart surgery in pediatric patients: a multicenter study. J Thorac Cardiovasc Surg. 2016;152:197–202.

Linka AZ, Fatio R, Attenhofer JC. Images in cardiology: double orifice mitral valve. Heart. 2000;84:244. https://doi.org/10.1136/heart.84.3.244.

Madriago EJ, Punn R, Geeter N, Silverman NH. Routine intra-operative trans-oesophageal echocardiography yields better outcomes in surgical repair of CHD. Cardiol Young. 2016;26:263–8.

Manabe S, Kasegawa H, Arai H, Takanashi S. Management of systolic anterior motion of the mitral valve: a mechanism-based approach. Gen Thorac Cardiovasc Surg. 2018;66(7):379–89.

Marino BS, Kruge LE, Cho CJ, Tomlinson RS, Shera D, Weinberg PM, Gaynor JW, Rychik J. Parachute mitral valve: morphologic descriptors, associated lesions, and outcomes after biventricular repair. J Thorac Cardiovasc Surg. 2009;137:385–93.

Mavroudis C, Deal BJ. Fontan conversion: literature review and lessons learned over 20 years. World J Pediatr Congenit Heart Surg. 2016;7(2):192–8.

McElhinney DB, Sherwood MC, Keane JF, del Nido PJ, Almond CS, Lock JE. Current management of severe congenital mitral stenosis: outcomes of transcatheter and surgical therapy in 108 infants and children. Circulation. 2005;112:707–14.

Mick SL, Keshavamurthy S, Gillinov AM. Mitral valve repair versus replacement. Ann Cardiothorac Surg. 2015;4:230–7.

Minami K, Kado H, Sai S, Tatewaki H, Shiokawa Y, Nakashima A, Fukae K, Hirose H. Midterm results of mitral valve repair with artificial chordae in children. J Thorac Cardiovasc Surg. 2005;129:336–42.

Moainie SL, Guy TS, Gorman JH 3rd, Plappert T, Jackson BM, St John-Sutton MG, Edmunds LH Jr, Gorman RC. Infarct restraint attenuates remodeling and reduces chronic ischemic mitral regurgitation after posterolateral infarction. Ann Thorac Surg. 2002;74:444–9.

Muresian H. The clinical anatomy of the mitral valve. Clin Anat. 2009;22:85–98.

Myers PO, del Nido PJ, McElhinney DB, Khalpey Z, Lock JE, Baird CW. Annulus upsizing for mitral valve re-replacement in children. J Thorac Cardiovasc Surg. 2013;146:347–51.

Myers PO, Baird CW, Del Nido PJ, Pigula FA, Lang N, Marx GR, Emani SM. Neonatal mitral valve repair in biventricular repair, single ventricle palliation, and secondary left ventricular recruitment: indications, techniques, and mid-term outcomes. Front Surg. 2015;2:59. https://doi.org/10.3389/fsurg.2015.00059.

Oc M, Doukas G, Alexiou C, Oc B, Hadjinikolaou L, Sosnowski AW, Spyt TJ. Edge-to-edge repair with mitral annuloplasty for Barlow's disease. Ann Thorac Surg. 2005;80(4):1315–8.

Oda S, Nakano T, Tatewaki H, Hinokiyama K, Machida D, Kado H. A 17-year experience with mitral valve repair with artificial chordae in infants and children. Eur J Cardiothorac Surg. 2013;44:44–5.

Ohye RG. Mitral regurgitation in congenital heart defects: surgical techniques for reconstruction. Semin Thorac Cardiovasc Surg Pediatr Card Surg Annu. 2012;15:75–9.

Oppido G, Davies B, McMullan DM, Cochrane AD, Cheung MM, d'Udekem Y, Brizard CP. Surgical treatment of congenital mitral valve disease: midterm results of a repair-oriented policy. J Thorac Cardiovasc Surg. 2008;135:1313–21.

Ota N, Fujimoto Y, Hirose K, Tosaka Y, Nakata T, Ide Y, Sakamoto K. Improving results of atrioventricular valve repair in challenging patients with heterotaxy syndrome. Cardiol Young. 2010;20:60–5.

Paparella D, Squiccimarro E, Di Mauro M, Katsavrias K, Calafiore AM. Acute iatrogenic complications after mitral valve repair. J Card Surg. 2022;37(12):4088–93.

Rajesh GN, Sajeer K, Nair A, Sajeev CG, Krishnan MN. Hammock mitral valve: a rare cause of congenital mitral regurgitation—a case report. Indian Heart J. 2014;66:370–1.

Remenyi B, Webb R, Gentles T, Russell P, Finucane K, Lee M, Wilson N. Improved long-term survival for rheumatic mitral valve repair compared to replacement in the young. World J Pediatr Congenit Heart Surg. 2013;4:155–64.

Ruiz CE. Transcatheter aortic valve implantation and mitral valve repair: state of the art. Pediatr Cardiol. 2005;26:289–94.

Santana Filho GP, Gomes OM, Oliveira GJ, Rodrigues D, Nogueira AC, Sales R, Pinheiro DB, Machado AC, Oliveira NG. Echocardiographic evaluation of patients undergoing mitral valve replacement with crossed papillopexy. Arq Bras Cardiol. 2009;93(2):92–6.

Schidlow DN, Zaidi A, Gauvreau K, Emani SM, Geva T. Echocardiographic characteristics of annulo-leaflet mitral ring. J Am Soc Echocardiogr. 2015;28:541–8.

Seese LM, Sultan I, Gleason TG, et al. Outcomes of mitral valve repair versus replacement in the elderly. Ann Thorac Surg. 2020;109(4):1202–9.

Séguéla PE, Houyel L, Acar P. Congenital malformations of the mitral valve. Arch Cardiovasc Dis. 2011;04:465–79.

Selamet Tierney ES, Pigula FA, Berul CI, Lock JE, del Nido PJ, McElhinney DB. Mitral valve replacement in infants and children 5 years of age or younger: evolution in practice and outcome over three decades with a focus on supra-annular prosthesis implantation. J Thorac Cardiovasc Surg. 2008;136:954–61.

Sherlock KE, Muthuswamy G, Basu R, Mitchell IM. The Alfieri stitch: the advantages for mitral valve repair in difficult circumstances. J Card Surg. 2011;26:475–7.

Shuhaiber J, Anderson RJ. Meta-analysis of clinical outcomes following surgical mitral valve repair or replacement. Eur J Cardiothorac Surg. 2007;31(2):267–75.

Skoularigis J, Sinovich V, Joubert G, Sareli P. Evaluation of the long-term results of mitral valve repair in 254 young patients with rheumatic mitral regurgitation. Circulation. 1994;90:II167–74.

Spinale FG. Novel approaches to retard ventricular remodeling in heart failure. Eur J Heart Fail. 1999;1:17–23.

Stellin G, Padalino MA, Vida VL, Boccuzzo G, Orru E, Biffanti R, Milanesi O, Mazzucco A. Surgical repair of congenital mitral valve malformations in infancy and childhood: a single-center 36-year experience. J Thorac Cardiovasc Surg. 2010;140:1238–44.

Tahta SA, Oury JH, Maxwell JM, Hiro SP, Duran CM. Outcome after mitral valve repair for functional ischemic mitral regurgitation. J Heart Valve Dis. 2002;11:11. Kurrelmeyer K, Kalra D, Bozkurt B, Wang F, Dibbs Z, Seta Y, Baumgarten G, Engle D, Sivasubramanian N, Mann DL. Cardiac remodeling as a consequence and cause of progressive heart failure. Clin Cardiol. 1998;21(12 Suppl 1):I14–I19.

Takahashi H, Kadowaki T, Maruo A, Yutaka O, Oshima Y. Mid-term results of mitral valve repair with autologous pericardium in pediatric patients. J Heart Valve Dis. 2014;23:302–9.

Talwar S, Rajesh MR, Subramanian A, Saxena A, Kumar AS. Mitral valve repair in children with rheumatic heart disease. J Thorac Cardiovasc Surg. 2005;129:875–9.

Udelson JE, Patten RD, Konstam MA. New concepts in post-infarction ventricular remodeling. Rev Cardiovasc Med. 2003;4(Suppl3):S3–S12.

van Doorn C, Yates R, Tsang V, deLeval M, Elliott M. Mitral valve replacement in children: mortality, morbidity, and haemodynamic status up to medium term follow up. Heart. 2000;84:636–42.

Van Praagh S, Porras D, Oppido G, Geva T, Van Praagh R. Cleft mitral valve without ostium primum defect: anatomic data and surgical considerations based on 41 cases. Ann Thorac Surg. 2003;75:1752–62.

Vida VL, Carrozzini M, Padalino M, Milanesi O, Stellin G. Surgical treatment of congenital mitral valve dysplasia. J Card Surg. 2016;31:352–6.

Vricella LA, Ravekes WA, Arbustini E, Jaquiss RD, Mavroudis C, Dietz HC, Jacobs ML, Hibino N, Cameron DE. Simplified mitral valve repair in pediatric patients with connective tissue disorders. J Thorac Cardiovasc Surg. 2017;153:399–403.

Waikittipong S. Mitral valve repair for rheumatic mitral regurgitation: mid-term results. Asian Cardiovasc Thorac Ann. 2015;23:658–64.

Weill O, Peyre M, Vergnat M, Cazavet A, Stos B, Belli E, Hascoet S, Acar P. Repeat mitral valve repair for haemolysis in children. Arch Cardiovasc Dis. 2015;108:118–21.

Yakub MA, Dillon J, Krishna Moorthy PS, Pau KK, Nordin MN. Is rheumatic aetiology a predictor of poor outcome in the current era of mitral valve repair? Contemporary long-term results of mitral valve repair in rheumatic heart disease. Eur J Cardiothorac Surg. 2013;44:673–81.

Yakub MA, Krishna Moorthy PS, Sivalingam S, Dillon J, Kong PK. Contemporary long-term outcomes of an aggressive approach to mitral valve repair in children: is it effective and durable for both congenital and acquired mitral valve lesions? Eur J Cardiothorac Surg. 2016;49:553–60.

Yeong M, Silbery M, Finucane K, Wilson NJ, Gentles TL. Mitral valve geometry in paediatric rheumatic mitral regurgitation. Pediatr Cardiol. 2015;36:827–34.

Zalzstein E, Hamilton R, Zucker N, Levitas A, Gross GJ. Presentation, natural history, and outcome in children and adolescents with double orifice mitral valve. Am J Cardiol. 2004;93:1067–9.

Zias E, Mavroudis C, Backer CL, Kohr LM, Gotteiner NL, Rocchini AP. Surgical repair of the congenitally malformed mitral valve in infants and children. Ann Thorac Surg. 1998;66:1551–9.

Complications Associated with Total Anomalous Pulmonary Venous Connection: Surgical Decision Making

Rachel D. Vanderlaan
and Christopher A. Caldarone

Abstract

Total anomalous pulmonary venous connection (TAPVC) constitutes a heterogeneous group of lesions in which all of the pulmonary veins are connected to the right atrium or its systemic venous tributaries. A concomitant right-to-left shunt, typically through an interatrial communication, is required for survival. Significant obstruction to pulmonary venous drainage results in pulmonary edema and cardiogenic shock which is rapidly lethal if untreated. Surgical results for the treatment of TAPVC have greatly improved over the last three decades, reducing operative mortality to less than 10% in most centers. The main complication resulting from surgical repair is the development of postrepair pulmonary vein stenosis (PR-PVS) which is associated with high morbidity and mortality.

Keywords

Total anomalous pulmonary venous connection · Pulmonary venous obstruction · Sutureless repair · Postrepair pulmonary vein stenosis · Anomalous pulmonary veins · Pediatric cardiac surgery

1 Embryology

The development of the pulmonary veins requires coordination of lung and cardiac development. The splanchnic plexus, develops around the lung buds and allows the drainage of blood into the anterior cardinal veins (the primordial superior vena cava, coronary sinus, and azygous vein) and into the umbilicovitelline veins, which develop into the portal system. A solitary pulmonary vein then develops and makes contact with the wall of the left atrium (Neill 1956; Douglas et al. 2011; van den Berg and Moorman 2011), after which it bifurcates and dilates. This process occurs with coordination of atrial septation from the right pulmonary vein ridge of the dorsal mesenchymal protrusion and coincides with involution of the pulmonary-to-systemic posterior aspect of the left atrial cavity.

Failure of all the pulmonary veins to divide from the splanchnic venous system and, possibly, a concomitant leftward displacement of the developing atrial septum is hypothesized to be

R. D. Vanderlaan (✉)
Division of Cardiac Surgery, University of Toronto, Toronto, ON, Canada

C. A. Caldarone
Texas Children's Hospital, Houston, TX, USA

C. L. Backer, C. Mavroudis (eds.), *Complications in Pediatric and Congenital Heart Surgery*,
https://doi.org/10.1007/978-3-032-02661-3_24

the primary defect in embryological development responsible for total anomalous pulmonary venous connection (TAPVC) (Neill 1956; Becker and Anderson 1981; Herlong et al. 2000; Kirshbom et al. 2003; Moorman et al. 2003). Therefore. supracardiac TAPVC results from failure of the pulmonary vein to separate from the right cardinal venous system, cardiac TAPVC is failure to separate from the left cardinal venous system and infracardiac TAPVC represents a failure of the pulmonary vein to separate from the umbilicovitelline system. Right atrial pulmonary vein connections seen in right atrial isomerism result from development of the atrial septum from the left pulmonary ridge and do not necessarily represent a failure in separation of the pulmonary vein from the splanchnic venous plexus (van den Berg and Moorman 2011).

2 Total Anomalous Pulmonary Venous Connection and Genetics

Total anomalous pulmonary venous connection is a rare disease that accounts for approximately 1.5% of all congenital heart disease (Correa-Villaseñor et al. 1991). Typically, anomalous pulmonary venous connections occur as sporadic isolated cases, and like most congenital heart disease, the etiology is likely multifactorial, with a complex interaction between environmental and genetic factors. TAPVC can present as an isolated malformation, but it can also be associated with syndromes such as cat eye syndrome, asplenia syndrome and Holt-Oram syndrome (Correa-Villaseñor et al. 1991). There are familial nonsyndromic cases reported in the literature, which support an autosomal dominant pattern of inheritance with variable penetrance and expression. Candidate genes include a *KDR*, *PDGFRA*, *ANKRD1* (Bleyl et al. 2006, 2010; Cinquetti et al. 2008), while alterations in Semaphorin 3d and retinoic acid signaling have also been associated with TAPVC in animal genetics (Degenhardt et al. 2013; Nash et al. 2015).

3 Classification

Total anomalous pulmonary venous connection classification is based on the level of connection of the anomalous connecting vein and the degree of obstruction (Krabill and Lucas Jr. 1995; Craig et al. 1957). In type 1 (supracardiac TAPVC), the common vein connects to structures above the heart (right superior vena cava, azygos vein, left superior vena cava, or innominate vein). In type 2 (cardiac TAPVC), the connecting vein is attached to cardiac structures (e.g., the right atrium or the coronary sinus). In type 3 (infracardiac TAPVC) the connection is situated below the diaphragm to the inferior vena cava/portal vein system. Type 4, (mixed TAPVC) represents a combination of the above conditions (Craig et al. 1957).

TAPVC can also be stratified by the presence/absence of obstruction to pulmonary venous drainage (Burroughs and Edwards 1960; Smith et al. 1961). Obstructions can be found at the level of the connecting vein, due to intrinsic narrowing or extrinsic compression, or at the level of the interatrial communication (Herlong et al. 2000).

4 Cardiac Anatomy and Associated Lesions

A communication between the systemic and the pulmonary venous return is necessary for survival after birth, and this is typically an interatrial communication. Atrial level shunts are typically of adequate size and the interatrial gradient is usually low (Delisle et al. 1976; Hastreiter et al. 1962). In the absence of atrial level shunt, ventricular septal defects, or a patent ductus arteriosus may rarely be associated with TAPVC as the sole source of shunting (Behrendt et al. 1972; Gathman and Nadas 1970).

In TAPVC there is an absence of the myocardial sleeve of smooth muscle within the wall of the pulmonary vein due to failure of the pulmonary vein to connect with the left atrium (Douglas et al. 2009). The left atrium is often small and associated with an underfilled left ventricle with enlarged right-sided heart structures (Mathew et al. 1977; Bove et al. 1975; Rosenquist et al. 1985; Haworth and Reid 1977).

Up to 90% of patients with heterotaxy and asplenia have TAPVC. Tetralogy of Fallot, double-outlet right ventricle, and interrupted aortic arch have also been reported as associated lesions (Delisle et al. 1976; Barratt-Boyes et al. 1971; DeLeon et al. 1987; James et al. 1994).

5 Natural History

The clinical presentation of TAPVC depends on two critical elements: the degree of obstruction to the pulmonary venous drainage and the degree of obstruction to the compensatory right-to-left shunt. Left untreated, the mortality of TAPVC is greater than 80% (Burroughs and Edwards 1960).

At one end of the spectrum, there are neonates with completely unobstructed circulation (typically supracardiac and cardiac types). These patients present with signs and symptoms of a large left-to-right shunt. Tachypnea and arterial desaturation are present to various degrees together with signs of right ventricular volume overload. If untreated, this condition can lead to congestive heart failure. Late sequelae include pulmonary edema, pulmonary hypertension, and cyanosis.

At the other end of the neonatal clinical spectrum are neonates with severe pulmonary venous flow obstruction. In these cases, the resulting pulmonary venous and pulmonary arterial hypertension produce severe acute pulmonary edema, right ventricular antegrade flow reduction due to the excessive afterload, extreme hypoxemia, and circulatory collapse. The presence of a restrictive atrial septal defect (ASD) results in reduced preload to the left ventricle, diminished systemic cardiac output, and severe cardiogenic shock. Obstructed TAPVC is rapidly lethal and requires swift action to correct.

6 Diagnosis

Neonates with an obstructed circulation become critically ill immediately after birth. They present with hypoxia and profound cyanosis, hypotension, and metabolic acidosis (James et al. 1994; Murphy and Greeley 1995). On the other hand, unobstructed TAPVC may be difficult to diagnose in the first few days of life because patients may have very mild cyanosis and the absence of a murmur. After a few months, infants may present with tachypnea, mild cyanosis, failure to thrive, and feeding difficulties. Hepatomegaly, venous congestion, and fine crackles on lung auscultation are possible in cases of noncompensated cardiac failure.

Keys to diagnosis are obtaining chest radiographs and echocardiography. Chest radiographs of unobstructed TAPVC show plethoric lungs and a large cardiac silhouette in unobstructed TAPVC, while obstructed neonatal TAPVC shows severe pulmonary edema in the presence of a normally sized and shape of the heart. In neonates, the reticular pattern of obstructed TAPVC may portend poor prognosis as there is secondary lymphangiectasia due to in utero obstruction.

Echocardiography is the primary diagnostic tool and demonstrates a distended right ventricle and a vascular confluence coupled with absent venous drainage to the left atrium. Doppler interrogation will demonstrate the presence of an accessory common vein or a dilated coronary sinus, and turbulent flow in the right atrium with a right-to-left shunt (Patel et al. 2005; Valsangiacomo et al. 2003a; Brown et al. 1998; Chin et al. 1987). Angiography is rarely preformed.

When echocardiography cannot clearly delineate the pulmonary veins, contrast-enhanced magnetic resonance angiography (MRA) or computed tomography (CTA) can be used to provide a complete anatomic diagnosis. In addition to anatomic detail, MRA can provide additional functional information regarding pulmonary flow patterns (Grosse-Wortmann et al. 2007). Both modalities provide excellent visualization of all pulmonary veins and other pulmonary-to-systemic venous connections (Valsangiacomo et al. 2003b). From a functional point of view, the amount of anomalous drainage and the resulting Qp/Qs can be calculated by using phase-contrast MRA (Grosse-Wortmann et al. 2007; Valsangiacomo et al. 2003b; Greil et al. 2002). This is particularly helpful in mixed TAPVC or complex cases of TAPVC.

7 Preoperative Management

Definitive management of TAPVC, both unobstructed and obstructed, is surgical repair. In patients with evidence of pulmonary venous obstruction, surgical repair is conducted promptly after diagnosis (Caldarone et al. 1998a, b). Patients with unobstructed TAPVC can be repaired in the neonatal period, with some centers electively repairing at 4–6 weeks of age. Medical management of unobstructed TAPVC is typically directed at congestive heart failure symptoms.

Medical maneuvers in patients with obstructed TAPVC have very limited efficacy and should not delay repair. Neonates with obstructed TAPVC often require intubation and hyperventilation with 100% oxygen to promote respiratory alkalosis. Correction of metabolic acidosis and inotropic support is required. Prostaglandin E1 can be infused to maintain patency of the ductus arteriosus. Medical efforts are minimally effective in correcting the hemodynamic and metabolic crisis and are limited to short-lived palliation until definitive repair.

8 Surgical Decision-Making: Preoperative Management of Obstructed TAPVC

In some centers, cardiac catheterization has been used in critically ill patients for diagnosis and percutaneous palliation of obstructed TAPVC. In rare cases, an isolated restrictive interatrial communication can be relieved with balloon septostomy. Use of percutaneous angioplasty and stenting of the obstructed common vein to palliate shock and improve preoperative optimization of the metabolic state (Fig. 1a, b) (Kyser et al. 2006; Lim et al. 2016) has gained some momentum particularly in obstructed supracardiac TAPVC. Decisions for stenting should be multidisciplinary, as stent placement too close to the pulmonary vein ostia can promote stenosis in the native pulmonary veins and require stent removal and potential pulmonary venoplasty at the time of definitive repair. Close surveillance is needed as repeated stenting for in-stent restenosis can be required. The use of extracorporeal membrane oxygenation (ECMO) has a role in obstructed TAPVC to rescue neonates in cardiorespiratory collapse and/or to stabilize them during a palliative procedure (Ishino et al. 1999). Some centers have reported favourable results using ECMO in the critically ill neonate as preparation for surgery (Stewart et al. 1996). ECMO complications such as bleeding, stroke, and infection may occur and add to the cumulative risk in obstructed TAPVC. In some instances, postoperative ECMO is used in patients with severe residual pulmonary hypertension (Seale et al. 2010; Khan et al. 2015). This is particularly true in patients with severe lung pathology resulting from intrauterine obstruction.

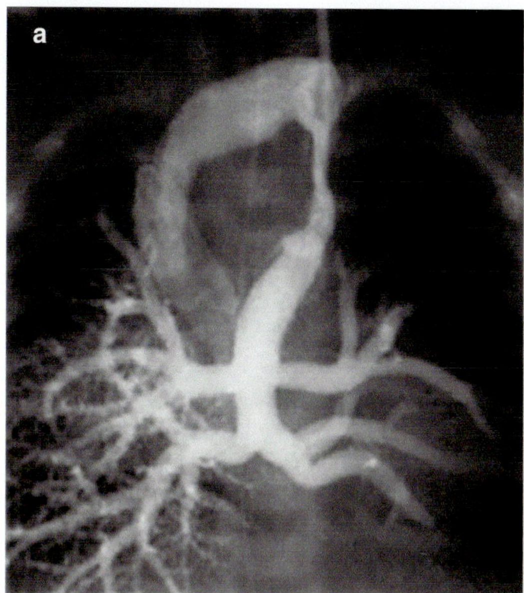

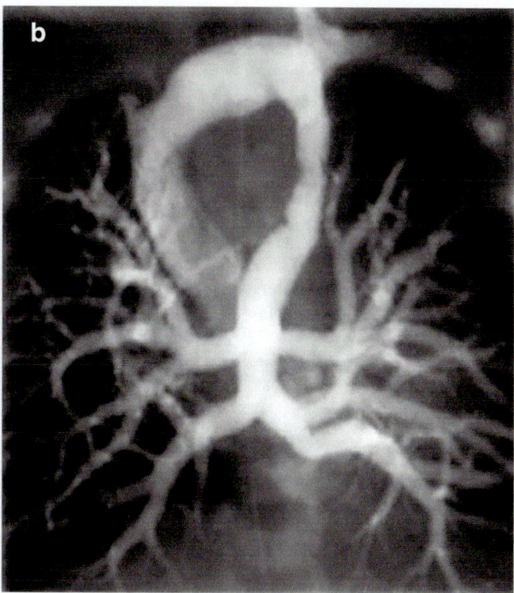

Fig. 1 Total anomalous pulmonary venous connection of supracardiac type to the innominate vein. (**a**) Both right and left pulmonary veins are unobstructed. The vertical vein, however, is severely stenotic at the junction with the innominate vein. (**b**) Emergency percutaneous stent dilation in a child with multiple comorbidities was performed with acceptable short-term result. Decision for vertical vein stenting should be a multidisciplinary approach and care must be taken to ensure the stent does not encroach on the individual pulmonary vein ostia, which can complicate subsequent surgical repair. (Courtesy of Dr Shi-Joon Yoo and Mr Omar Thabit. With permission Viola and Caldarone 2013)

9 Surgical Repair of TAPVC

To aid surgical planning, it is imperative to delineate the pulmonary venous anatomy and proximity of adjacent structures and concomitant congenital heart lesions. When echocardiography is not sufficient, stabilized patients should undergo a CTA or MRA.

Surgical repair of TAPVC is accomplished via sternotomy with aortic cannulation and bicaval cannulation. After initiation of cardiopulmonary bypass, the ductus arteriosus (if present) is ligated and divided. The patient is cooled to mild hypothermia (28–30 °C) to allow for periods of low-flow perfusion and to aid visualization. Some centers routinely use deep hypothermia (18–20 °C) to allow deep hypothermic circulatory arrest and ensure good visualization of the venous confluence. The aorta is cross-clamped and cardiac arrest induced with antegrade cardioplegia solution.

In supracardiac and infracardiac TAPVC repair (Figs. 2a–c and 3a–c), the heart is retracted to visualize the venous confluence. In infracardiac TAPVC, the confluence is typically a vertical Y-shaped configuration. A longitudinal incision is made in the pulmonary confluence and can be extended into the base of the vertical vein. It is imperative to create a large anastomosis between the pulmonary venous confluence and the left atrium. If the pulmonary venous confluence is small, incision into the pulmonary veins is mandatory to ensure a sufficiently large anastomosis. Cardiopulmonary bypass flow rates may need to be decreased temporarily to facilitate visualization and placement of the incision. Small cardiotomy suction cannulas can then be placed to aid visualization and perfusion flow rates restored. A counter incision is made in the left atrium, extending into the left atrial appendage to ensure a large anastomosis. The goal is to have the largest possible anastomosis and tissue on the pulmonary venous confluence that can be

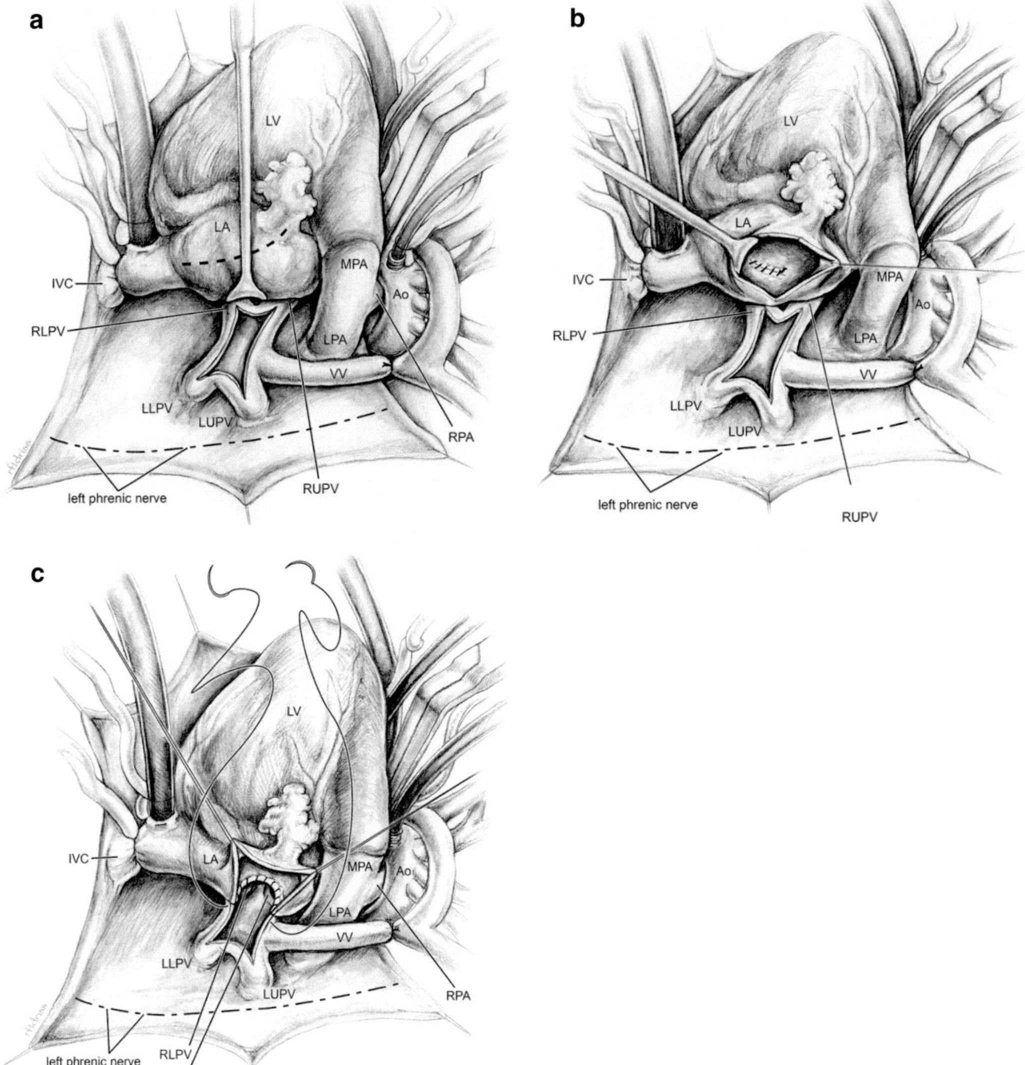

Fig. 2 Repair of supracardiac total anomalous pulmonary venous connection with the vertical vein (VV) connected to the innominate vein. (**a**) The vertical vein is ligated next to its connection to the innominate, due to its accessibility in this point. Care must be taken to ensure the phrenic nerve is not injured as it is in close proximity. The incision into the confluence must be large to maximize the anastomosis size and can be extended into each of the pulmonary veins to increase the length of the anastomosis. (**b**) A secundum atrial septal defect is closed through the left atriotomy. If the left atrium is quite diminutive, the atrial septum can be sifted. In cases of severe preoperative obstruction and risk factors for postrepair pulmonary vein stenosis, a patent foramen ovale may be left. (**c**) The anastomosis between the left atrium (LA) and the venous confluence is started rightward and continued leftward on the superior and inferior rims as the heart is returned to its anatomic position. The anastomosis must not distort the ostia of the pulmonary veins and should be large enough to provide unobstructed egress of pulmonary blood flow back to the atria. *Ao* aorta, *IVC* inferior vena cava, *LA* left atrium, *LLPV* left lower pulmonary vein, *LPA* left pulmonary artery, *LUPV* left upper pulmonary vein, *LV* left ventricle, *MPA* main pulmonary artery, *PA* pulmonary artery, *RLPV* right lower pulmonary vein, *RPA* right pulmonary artery, *RUPV* right upper pulmonary vein, *SVC* superior vena cava. (With permission Viola and Caldarone 2013)

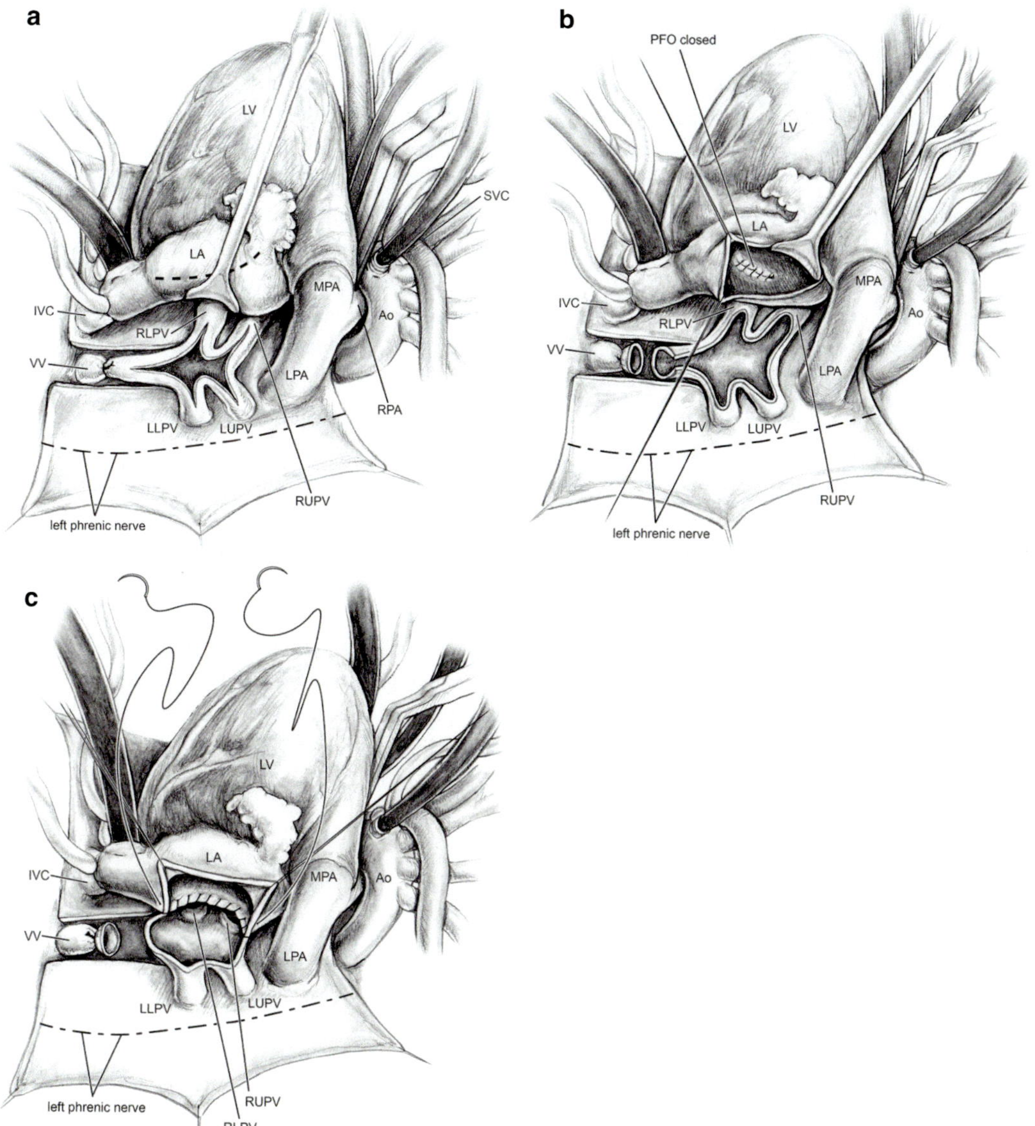

Fig. 3 Repair of cardiac total anomalous pulmonary venous connection with connecting vein (CV) to the coronary sinus (CS). (**a**) The CS is enlarged and the ostium of the CV is visualized near its ostium. A secundum atrial septal defect is retracted to permit visualization of the mitral valve (MV) in the left atrium. The pulmonary vein (PV) orifices are not present in the left atrium (LA). The CS is unroofed into the LA and the atrial septal defect thus enlarged (dotted lines). Care must be taken to avoid leaving residual atrial tissue that will obstruct pulmonary vein blood flow back to the right atrium. (**b**) The PV confluence is inspected through the unroofed CS and all four vein ostia are inspected. (**c**) The defect is then closed with a patch of autologous pericardium, leaving the unroofed CS draining to the reconstructed LA. *Ao* aorta, *IVC* inferior vena cava, *LA* left atrium, *LLPV* left lower pulmonary vein, *LUPV* left upper pulmonary vein, *LV* left ventricle, *PA* pulmonary artery, *RA* right atrium, *RLPV* right lower pulmonary vein, *RPA* right pulmonary artery, *RUPV* right upper pulmonary vein, *SVC* superior vena cava, *TV* tricuspid valve. (With permission Viola and Caldarone 2013)

judicially trimmed. Attention must be paid to avoid distortion of the ostium of the pulmonary veins. Through a right atriotomy, the interatrial communication is closed primarily or with a patch of autologous pericardium. If the left atrium is diminutive or the septum is close to the anastomosis, the atrial septum can be shifted rightwards to improve capacitance of the left atrium. In very sick patients with a high risk of postrepair pulmonary vein stenosis (PR-PVS), an atrial fenestration can be left to facilitate catheter procedures and postoperative management. Prior to closing the interatrial communication, the left atrial anastomosis can be inspected to ensure patency and not obvious redundant atrial tissue that may obstruct the anastomosis. The decision for vertical vein ligation will be discussed in a subsequent section.

In cardiac TAPVC repair (Fig. 4a–c), when the communicating vein is connected to the coronary sinus, access is obtained through a right atriotomy. The atrial septum between the ostium of the coronary sinus and the fossa ovalis is divided and the Thebesian valve removed, allowing visualization of the connecting vein. The coronary sinus is then unroofed towards the left atrium. Any obstructing tissue is resected. The resulting large interatrial defect is closed with a patch, leaving the coronary and the pulmonary venous drainage to the left of the reconstructed septum. In cases of TAPVC to the right atrium, the pulmonary drainage can be redirected into the left atrium with a baffle repair through the patent foramen ovale. Alternatively, the septum can be shifted to recreate the normal functional anatomic relationships (Tucker et al. 1976).

The most common pattern of mixed TAPVC is three veins to a posterior confluence and one separately connecting to the systemic venous system. Repair often involves an anastomosis between the left atrium and the confluence as described above and reimplantation of the fourth vein if possible. Single, unobstructed pulmonary veins can be left in situ to avoid postsurgical restenosis. These veins, if small, can be left without causing hemodynamic compromise or can be reimplanted when the patient is older (Imoto et al. 1998). CTA or MRA can help surgical planning for more complex arrangements.

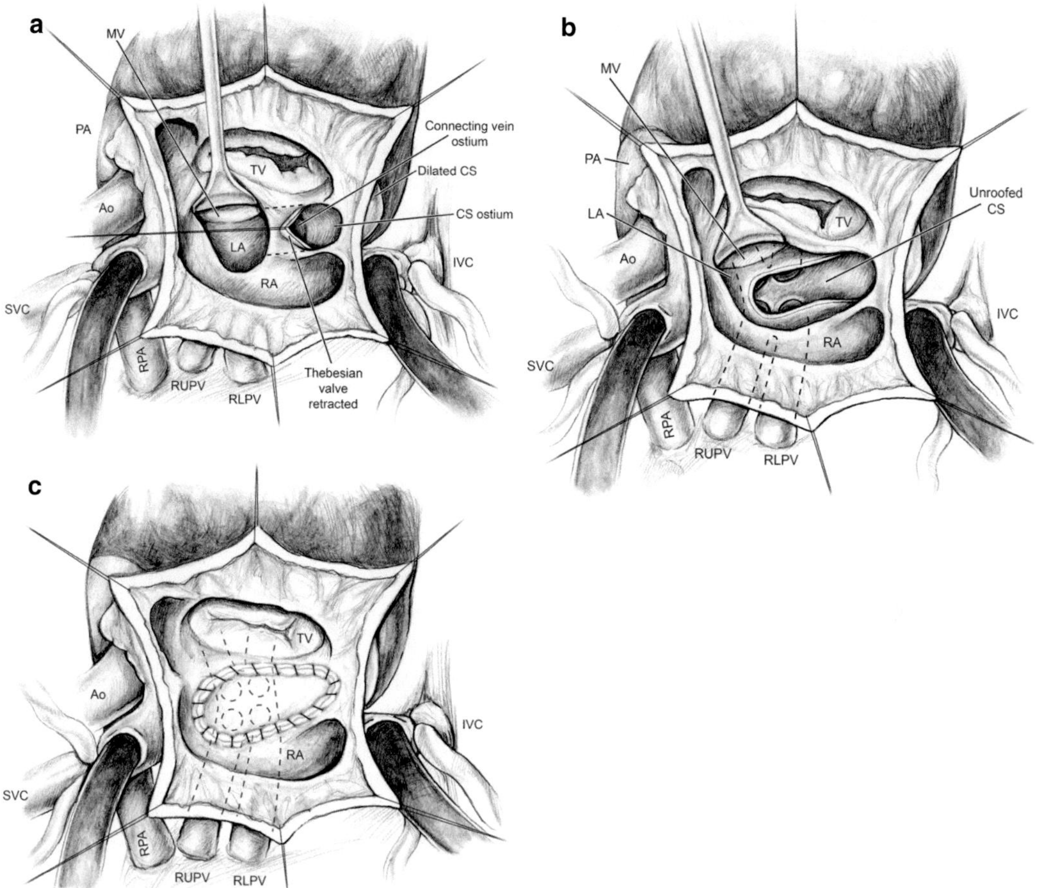

Fig. 4 Repair of infracardiac total anomalous pulmonary venous connection with ligation of the vertical vein (VV). (**a**) The VV is ligated at its emergence through the esophageal hiatus. Care must be taken to ensure no damage to surrounding structures. The confluence is opened widely to ensure maximal size of the anastomosis. The incision can be extended into the individual ostia if the confluence is diminutive. The left atrium is opened with an incision extending into the left atrial appendage (dotted line). Position of the incision in the left atrium should ensure no distortion of the confluence when the heart is returned to its normal position in the heart. Extension into the left atrial appendage will help maximize the anastomosis. (**b**) The atrial septal defect is closed via the atriotomy. The VV can be divided to increase the length of the anastomosis or alternatively, it can be incised down its length to increase the anastomosis length. (**c**) In a conventional repair technique, the anastomosis is directly to the wall of the pulmonary veins. *Ao* aorta, *IVC* inferior vena cava, *LA* left atrium, *LLPV* left lower pulmonary vein, *LPA* left pulmonary artery, *LUPV* left upper pulmonary vein, *LV* left ventricle, *MPA* main pulmonary artery, *PFO* patent foramen ovale, *RLPV* right lower pulmonary vein, *RPA* right pulmonary artery, *RUPV* right upper pulmonary vein, *SVC* superior vena cava. (With permission Viola and Caldarone 2013)

10 Surgical Decision-Making: Ligation of the Vertical Vein

Leaving the vertical vein open at the time of repair of TAPVC can result in an important left-to-right shunt (Cope et al. 1997; Caspi et al. 2001), while in some cases it may be of little hemodynamic consequences (Cheung et al. 2005), with many closing spontaneously. Importantly, leaving the vertical vein intact can allow for decompression of the small, noncompliant left atrium into the systemic venous system, and thereby diminish postoperative pulmonary venous hypertension (Caspi et al. 2001). Interventional device closure of an unligated vertical vein is a feasible alternative in those children who develop significant left-to-right shunts postoperatively (Devendran et al. 2013; Kobayashi et al. 2012).

The vertical communicating vein is ligated near its connection with the systemic venous connection to avoid tethering of the pulmonary vein ostia. Utilization of the vertical vein into the pulmonary venous confluence can help maximize a small confluence. The vertical communicating vein is ligated near its connection with the systemic venous connection to avoid tethering of the pulmonary vein ostia. Division of the vertical vein at the time of repair and utilization of the vertical vein tissue into the pulmonary venous confluence can help to increase the size of a small confluence. When ligating a supracardiac vertical vein near the innominate junction, it is imperative to identify the closely associated phrenic nerve to avoid injury at the time of ligation.

11 Complications Due to Inadequate Exposure

Exposure must be adequate to aid in construction of the pulmonary venous anastomosis and so utilization of moderate or deep hypothermia allows for low flow states that facilitate visualization. Poor exposure may result in potential distortion of the anastomosis, injury to adjacent structures and potentially contribute to longer cross-clamp times. Retraction by the assistant must be firm, but not excessive to prevent ventricular hematoma or injury to fragile tissues. Cephalad or lateral retraction of the heart to perform the anastomosis carries the potential for distortion of the atrium and confluence at the time of the repair and subsequent development of postoperative stenosis. One can use a marking pen for marking sutures to help guide counter incisions in the atrium to ensure proper alignment when the heart is returned to its proper position in the chest. Alternative approaches include performing the posterior anastomosis across the roof of the left atrium between the superior vena cava and the aortic root in cases of supracardiac TAPVC (Tucker et al. 1976). This maintains the normal position of the two chambers during the repair. Alternatively, the venous confluence behind the left atrium is accessed from the right following a leftward retraction of the heart. A transverse incision is conducted along the right atrium inferiorly through the Waterston groove and into the posterior wall of the left atrium. The pulmonary confluence is incised longitudinally between the pulmonary vein ostia directly posterior to the left atrial incision (Kumar et al. 2001). This approach offers excellent visualization of the confluence without significant distortion and avoids rightward retraction of the heart. This technique permits patch enlargement of the small left atrium.

12 Complications with Pulmonary Venous Anastomosis

Obstruction at the pulmonary-atrial anastomosis can occur in 5%–15% of TAPVC repairs. This can occur due to fibrous ridge formation at the suture line or due to redundant atrial tissue creating a ridge. Postrepair pulmonary vein stenosis typically refers to intraluminal obstruction of the individual veins and can be attributed to geometric distortion, external compression of the pulmonary veins and intrinsic patient factors.

To prevent fibrous anastomotic stenosis, some authors have advocated for the use of interrupted sutures or reabsorbable sutures with inconclusive data to support either technique. Independent of suture technique, redundant atrial tissue can be folded inward after completion of the anastomosis with flow acceleration across the anastomosis. If recognized early, reoperation with resection of the fibrous tissue or flap can be done without touching the individual veins. If the anastomosis itself is diminutive, then full revision is required.

There is evidence for using the sutureless repair in primary repair of TAPVC (Najm et al. 1998; Seale et al. 2013). The sutureless technique refers to anastomosis of the left atrium to the pericardial reflection on the venous confluence (Fig. 5a–c). This is in contrast to the conventional repair, whereby the anastomosis is directly to the wall of the pulmonary veins. The extension of the sutureless technique to a prophylactic strategy to prevent pulmonary vein stenosis after repair of TAPVC has been driven by optimism that maximizing confluence size and minimizing injury and distortion of the pulmonary veins would improve outcomes, particularly in high-risk patients (Zhang et al. 2016). Retrospective studies support the non-inferiority of the sutureless repair for prevention of PR-PVS during supracardiac, infracardiac, and mixed-type TAPVC repairs (Honjo et al. 2010; Yanagawa et al. 2011; Lo Rito et al. 2015). The sutureless technique is associated with decreased PR-PVS in patients considered high risk for PR-PVS due to preoperative pulmonary vein obstruction (Zhang et al. 2016). In addition, the sutureless repair has been used in high risk patients with diminutive pulmonary veins (i.e., TAPVC in right atrial isomerism) and univentricular physiology (Yun et al. 2005). The sutureless technique is an important tool to mitigate PR-PVS in high-risk patients.

Important rare complications of the sutureless technique include the formation of bronchiole-atrial fistula due to aggressive pulmonary vein incision into the lung parenchyma. This can be resolved by oversewing the divided bronchiole after identification with lung insufflation under direct visualization. Pleural disruption due to dissection out by the hilum is also possible. It can also be easy to exit the heart or vein with aggressive resection. Careful dissection and closure of any potential disruptions should decrease the occurrence of this rare complication.

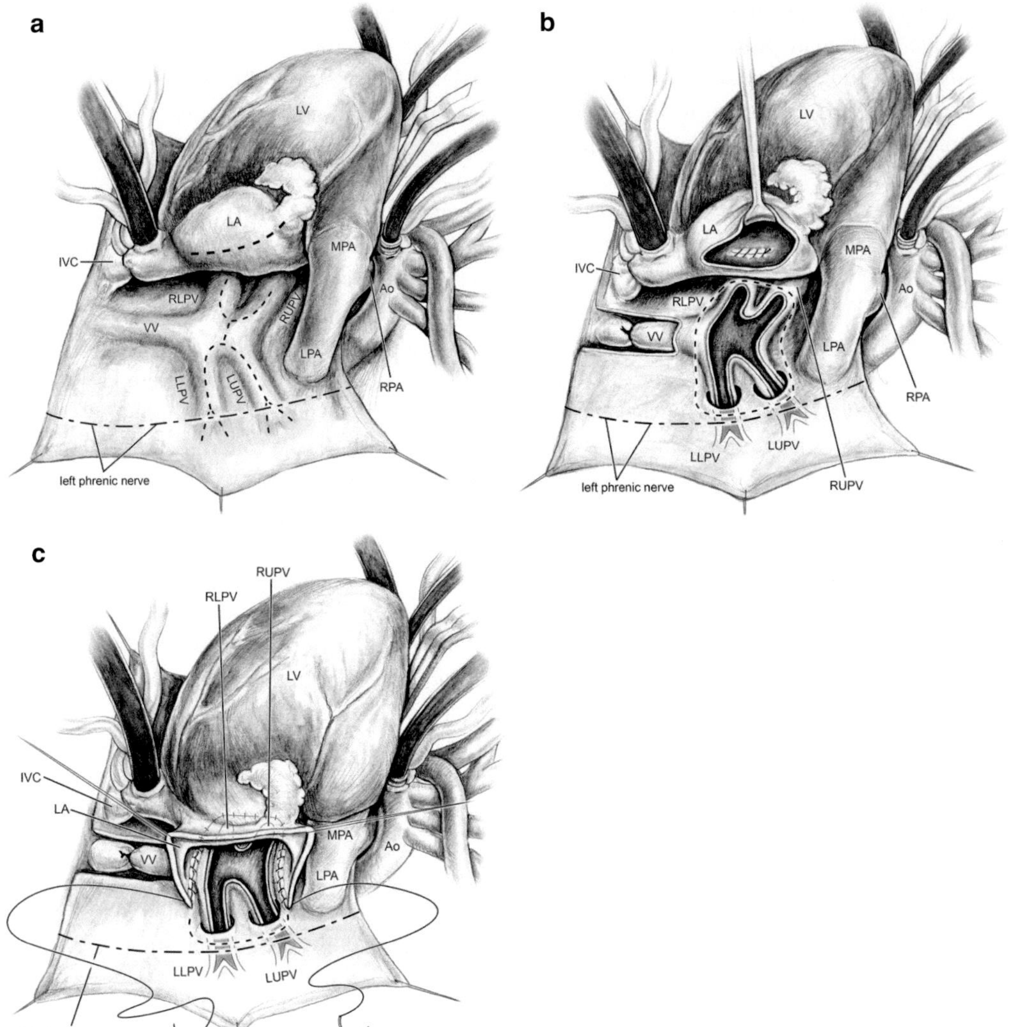

Fig. 5 Repair of infracardiac total anomalous pulmonary venous connection with a sutureless technique. (**a**) The venous confluence is retropericardial. The left atrium (LA) incision is extended into the appendage to create the widest possible opening. (**b**) The posterior pericardium is breached and the descending vertical vein (VV) ligated. It is important to ensure that the surgeon is some distance from the pulmonary venous confluence to avoid disruption of the pericardium over the venous confluence as this will be part of the anastomosis. The pulmonary veins are opened starting at the atrial junction and the incision is continued upstream into the pulmonary veins to maximize the anastomosis. (**c**) The atrial edge is sutured to the pericardium along the dotted line, as indicated, avoiding direct suturing of the veins. The anastomosis is conducted from left to right. *Ao* aorta, *IVC* inferior vena cava, *LA* left atrium, *LLPV* left lower pulmonary vein, *LUPV* left upper pulmonary vein, *LV* left ventricle, *MPA* main pulmonary artery, *RLPV* right lower pulmonary vein, *RPA* right pulmonary artery, *RUPV* right upper pulmonary vein, *SVC* superior vena cava. (With permission Viola and Caldarone 2013)

13 Complications Following TAPVC: Postrepair Pulmonary Vein Stenosis

The development of PR-PVS in TAPVC cohorts has been identified as an important risk factor impacting survival (Caldarone et al. 1998a; Seale et al. 2010; Karamlou et al. 2007). PR-PVS occurs in approximately 5%–15% of repaired TAPVC with increased incidence in those with obstructive TAPVC or hypoplastic pulmonary veins prior to repair (Seale et al. 2010; Jenkins et al. 1993). Progressive multivessel disease is associated with poor prognosis.

Surveillance in high-risk TAPVC populations is paramount for early detection of PR-PVS and potential early intervention (Hyde et al. 1999). Echocardiography may underestimate disease severity and so axial imaging (CTA or MRA) should be done when there is concern for stenosis. Lung perfusion scans are an alternative modality but will not provide the anatomical detail required for surgical planning. A dedicated PVS team or multidisciplinary team should review the patient to ensure catheter interventions, surgical options, and hybrid options (i.e., intraoperative stenting) are explored.

Many patients with PR-PVS require surgical intervention. Conventional repair of PVS, such as resection of the anastomotic endocardial fibrotic overgrowth, patch venoplasty with or without endarterectomy, as well as percutaneous stenting techniques are associated with a high incidence of recurrent stenosis (Caldarone et al. 1998b; Seale et al. 2013; Lacour-Gayet et al. 1999). An alternative to conventional repair is the sutureless technique which utilizes an atriopericardial anastomosis to allow for aggressive resection of stenosis while minimizing intimal injury and anatomical distortion at the veno-atrial junction (Najm et al. 1998; Yun et al. 2005; Lacour-Gayet et al. 1999).

In redo pulmonary vein surgery there is always a risk of phrenic nerve damage so careful dissection is required; this is particularly true in redo sutureless repairs. Once the patient is on bypass and the heart is arrested, the left atrium is incised along its posterior wall with the incision extending into the appendage to create the widest possible opening. The pulmonary veins are opened at the atrial junction and the incision is continued outwards opening up the secondary or tertiary branches. The pericardium is breached below the phrenic nerve to allow incision of the vein below the reflection of the mediastinal pleura at the hilum of the lung. All obstructing tissue is incised or resected. The atrial edge is sutured to the pericardium around the incised pulmonary veins avoiding the phrenic nerve. Drainage of pulmonary blood flow is then maintained by the pleura and adhesions inside the newly constructed atrium (Fig. 6) (Vanderlaan and Caldarone 2023).

Preoperative planning for surgical repair should involve axial imaging as it can point to anatomical reasons for the stenosis, a principle underlying the concept of the anatomically focused repair (Peng et al. 2016). This involves removing potential angulations or fulcrums to the pulmonary veins thereby removing a potential

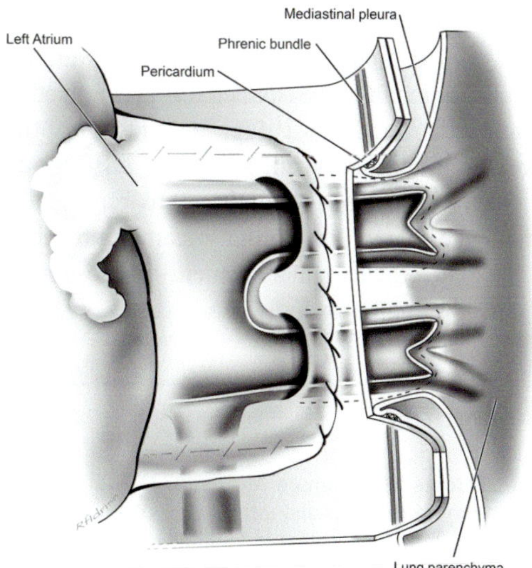

Fig. 6 Sutureless repair for PR-PVS. The pericardium is breached below the phrenic nerve to avoid damaging it and to allow the incision of the vein below the reflection of the mediastinal pleura at the hilum of the lung. Any obstruction is then incised or resected. The free edge of the left atrial wall is anastomosed to the pericardium below the phrenic bundle. The integrity of the mediastinal pleura and the presence of adhesions allow drainage of pulmonary venous blood inside the newly constructed atrium. (With permission Viola and Caldarone 2013)

nidus for restenosis. The affected pulmonary vein can be reimplanted in a more linear trajectory and may require patch material to augment the pulmonary vein. Release of tethering pericardium and shifting of the atrial septum may all help to improve long term patency using this approach.

With progressive recurrent restenosis of pulmonary veins, multidisciplinary teams can best manage the long-term trajectory of the patient and surgeons must work together with interventional cardiologists to maximize vein patency and pulmonary hypertension specialists to manage pre- and postrepair pulmonary hypertension and right heart failure. Medical therapies such as Gleevec and Sirolimus are used in select patients to ameliorate progressive disease or in-stent stenosis; however, results from larger multi-institutional studies are required to confirm which patients derive the most benefit. Early involvement of lung transplant teams and palliative care is also important for those with recurrent multi-vessel disease.

In summary, TAPVC represents a broad spectrum of anomalies that can be isolated or associated with complex cardiac anomalies. Surgical results for repair in the isolated form have steadily improved over the last three decades and offer good long-term survival. Recurrent diffuse pulmonary vein stenosis continues to represent a challenge. A multidisciplinary team approach is critical to effective management of those with aggressive multivessel disease.

References

Barratt-Boyes BG, Simpson M, Neutze JM. Intracardiac surgery in neonates and infants using deep hypothermia with surface cooling and limited cardiopulmonary bypass. Circulation. 1971;43(5 Suppl):I25–30.

Becker AE, Anderson RH. Anomalies of pulmonary veins. In: Pathology of congenital heart disease. 2nd ed. London: Butterworths; 1981.

Behrendt DM, Aberdeen E, Waterson DJ, et al. Total anomalous pulmonary venous drainage in infants. I. Clinical and hemodynamic findings, methods, and results of operation in 37 cases. Circulation. 1972;46:347–56.

Bleyl SB, Botto LD, Carey JC, et al. Analysis of a Scottish founder effect narrows the TAPVR-1 gene interval to chromosome 4q12. Am J Med Genet A. 2006;140(21):2368–73.

Bleyl SB, Saijoh Y, Bax NA, et al. Dysregulation of the PDGFRA gene causes inflow tract anomalies including TAPVR: integrating evidence from human genetics and model organisms. Hum Mol Genet. 2010;19:1286–2301.

Bove KE, Geiser EA, Meyer RA. The left ventricle in anomalous pulmonary venous return. Morphometric analysis of 36 fatal cases in infancy. Arch Pathol. 1975;99:522–8.

Brown VE, De Lange M, Dyar DA, et al. Echocardiographic spectrum of supracardiac total anomalous pulmonary venous connection. J Am Soc Echocardiogr. 1998;11:289–93.

Burroughs JT, Edwards JE. Total anomalous pulmonary venous connection. Am Heart J. 1960;59:913–31.

Caldarone CA, Najm HK, Kadletz M, et al. Surgical management of total anomalous pulmonary venous drainage: impact of coexisting cardiac anomalies. Ann Thorac Surg. 1998a;66:1521–6.

Caldarone CA, Najm HK, Kadletz M, et al. Relentless pulmonary vein stenosis after repair of total anomalous pulmonary venous drainage. Ann Thorac Surg. 1998b;66:1514–20.

Caspi J, Pettitt TW, Fontenot EE, et al. The beneficial hemodynamic effects of selective patent vertical vein following repair of obstructed total anomalous pulmonary venous drainage in infants. Eur J Cardiothorac Surg. 2001;20:830–4.

Cheung YF, Lun KS, Chau AK, Chiu CS. Fate of the unligated vertical vein after repair of supracardiac anomalous pulmonary venous connection. J Paediatr Child Health. 2005;41:361–4.

Chin AJ, Sanders SP, Sherman F, et al. Accuracy of subcostal two-dimensional echocardiography in prospective diagnosis of total anomalous pulmonary venous connection. Am Heart J. 1987;113:1153–9.

Cinquetti R, Badi I, Campione M, et al. Transcriptional deregulation and a missense mutation define ANKRD1 as a candidate gene for total anomalous pulmonary venous return. Hum Mutat. 2008;29:468–74.

Cope JT, Banks D, McDaniel NL, Shockey KS, Nolan SP, Kron IL. Is vertical vein ligation necessary in repair of total anomalous pulmonary venous connection? Ann Thorac Surg. 1997;64(1):23–9.

Correa-Villaseñor A, Ferencz C, et al. Total anomalous pulmonary venous return: familial and environmental factors. The Baltimore-Washington Infant Study Group. Teratology. 1991;44:415–28.

Craig JM, Darling RC, Rothney WB. Total pulmonary venous drainage into the right side of the heart; report of 17 autopsied cases not associated with other major cardiovascular anomalies. Lab Investig. 1957;6:44–64.

Degenhardt K, Singh MK, Aghajanian H, et al. Semaphorin 3d signaling defects are associated with anomalous pulmonary venous connections. Nat Med. 2013;19:760–5.

DeLeon SY, Gidding SS, Ilbawi MN, et al. Surgical management of infants with complex cardiac anomalies associated with reduced pulmonary blood flow and total anomalous pulmonary venous drainage. Ann Thorac Surg. 1987;43:207–11.

Delisle G, Ando M, Calder AL, et al. Total anomalous pulmonary venous connection: report of 93 autopsied cases with emphasis on diagnostic and surgical considerations. Am Heart J. 1976;91:99–122.

Devendran V, Wilson N, Jesudian V. Percutaneous closure of a large unligated vertical vein using the Amplatzer Vascular Plug II after supracardiac total anomalous pulmonary venous connection (TAPVC) repair. Pediatr Cardiol. 2013;34:1976–8.

Douglas YL, Jongbloed MR, den Hartog WC, et al. Pulmonary vein and atrial wall pathology in human total anomalous pulmonary venous connection. Int J Cardiol. 2009;134:302–12.

Douglas YL, Jongbloed MR, Deruiter MC, et al. Normal and abnormal development of pulmonary veins: state of the art and correlation with clinical entities. Int J Cardiol. 2011;147:13–24.

Gathman GE, Nadas AS. Total anomalous pulmonary venous connection: clinical and physiologic observations of 75 pediatric patients. Circulation. 1970;42:143–54.

Greil GF, Powell AJ, Gildein HP, et al. Gadolinium-enhanced three-dimensional magnetic resonance angiography of pulmonary and systemic venous anomalies. J Am Coll Cardiol. 2002;39:335–41.

Grosse-Wortmann L, Al-Otay A, Goo HW, et al. Anatomical and functional evaluation of pulmonary veins in children by magnetic resonance imaging. J Am Coll Cardiol. 2007;49:993–1002.

Hastreiter AR, Paul MH, Molthan ME, et al. Total anomalous pulmonary venous connection with severe pulmonary venous obstruction. A clinical entity. Circulation. 1962;25:916–28.

Haworth SG, Reid L. Structural study of pulmonary circulation and of heart in total anomalous pulmonary venous return in early infancy. Br Heart J. 1977;39:80–92.

Herlong JR, Jaggers JJ, Ungerleider RM. Congenital heart surgery nomenclature and database project: pulmonary venous anomalies. Ann Thorac Surg. 2000;69(4 Suppl):S56–69.

Honjo O, Atlin CR, Hamilton BC, et al. Primary sutureless repair for infants with mixed total anomalous pulmonary venous drainage. Ann Thorac Surg. 2010;90:862–8.

Hyde JA, Stümper O, Barth MJ, Wright JG, Silove ED, de Giovanni JV, Brawn WJ, Sethia B. Total anomalous pulmonary venous connection: outcome of surgical correction and management of recurrent venous obstruction. Eur J Cardiothorac Surg. 1999;15(6):735–41.

Imoto Y, Kado H, Asou T, et al. Mixed type of total anomalous pulmonary venous connection. Ann Thorac Surg. 1998;66:1394–7.

Ishino K, Alexi-Meskishvili V, Hetzer R. Preoperative extracorporeal membrane oxygenation in newborns with total anomalous pulmonary venous connection. Cardiovasc Surg. 1999;7:473–5.

James CL, Keeling JW, Smith NM, et al. Total anomalous pulmonary venous drainage associated with fatal outcome in infancy and early childhood: an autopsy study of 52 cases. Pediatr Pathol. 1994;14:665–78.

Jenkins KJ, Sanders SP, Orav EJ, Coleman EA, Mayer JE Jr, Colan SD. Individual pulmonary vein size and survival in infants with totally anomalous pulmonary venous connection. J Am Coll Cardiol. 1993;22(1):201–6.

Karamlou T, Gurofsky R, Al Sukhni E, et al. Factors associated with mortality and reoperation in 377 children with total anomalous pulmonary venous connection. Circulation. 2007;115:1591–8.

Khan MS, Bryant R 3rd, Kim SH, et al. Contemporary outcomes of surgical repair of total anomalous pulmonary venous connection in patients with heterotaxy syndrome. Ann Thorac Surg. 2015;99:2134–9.

Kirshbom PM, Jaggers JJ, Ungerleider RM. Total anomalous pulmonary venous connection. In: Mavroudis C, Backer CL, editors. Pediatric cardiac surgery. 3rd ed. Philadelphia: Mosby, Inc; 2003.

Kobayashi D, Forbes TJ, Delius RE, et al. Amplatzer vascular plug for transcatheter closure of persistent unligated vertical vein after repair of infracardiac total anomalous pulmonary venous connection. Catheter Cardiovasc Interv. 2012;80:192–8.

Krabill KA, Lucas RV Jr. Abnormal pulmonary venous connections. In: Emmanouilides GC, Reimenschneider TA, Allen HD, et al., editors. Heart disease in infants, children and adolescents. Baltimore: Williams & Wilkins; 1995.

Kumar RN, Dharmapuram AK, Rao IM, et al. The fate of the unligated vertical vein after surgical correction of total anomalous pulmonary venous connection in early infancy. J Thorac Cardiovasc Surg. 2001;122:615–7.

Kyser JP, Bengur AR, Siwik ES. Preoperative palliation of newborn obstructed total anomalous pulmonary venous connection by endovascular stent placement. Catheter Cardiovasc Interv. 2006;67:473–6.

Lacour-Gayet F, Zoghbi J, Serraf AE, et al. Surgical management of progressive pulmonary venous obstruction after repair of total anomalous pulmonary venous connection. J Thorac Cardiovasc Surg. 1999;117:679–87.

Lim WK, Leong MC, Samion H. Stenting of vertical vein in an infant with obstructed supracardiac total anomalous pulmonary venous drainage. Ann Pediatr Cardiol. 2016;9:183–5.

Lo Rito M, Gazzaz T, Wilder T, et al. Repair type influences mode of pulmonary vein stenosis in total anomalous pulmonary venous drainage. Ann Thorac Surg. 2015;100:654–62.

Mathew R, Thilenius OG, Replogle RL, et al. Cardiac function in total anomalous pulmonary venous return before and after surgery. Circulation. 1977;55:361–70.

Moorman A, Webb S, Brown NA, et al. Development of the heart: (1) formation of the cardiac chambers and arterial trunks. Heart. 2003;89:806–14.

Murphy AM, Greeley WJ. Total anomalous pulmonary venous connection. In: Nichols DG, Cameron DE, Greeley WJ, et al., editors. Critical heart disease in infants and children. St Louis: Mosby, Inc; 1995.

Najm HK, Caldarone CA, Smallhorn J, et al. A sutureless technique for the relief of pulmonary vein stenosis with the use of in situ pericardium. J Thorac Cardiovasc Surg. 1998;115:468–70.

Nash D, Arrington CB, Kennedy BJ, et al. Shared segment analysis and next-generation sequencing implicates the retinoic acid signaling pathway in total anomalous pulmonary venous return (TAPVR). PLoS One. 2015;10:e0131514.

Neill CA. Development of the pulmonary veins; with reference to the embryology of anomalies of pulmonary venous return. Pediatrics. 1956;18:880–7.

Patel CR, Lane JR, Spector ML, et al. Totally anomalous pulmonary venous connection and complex congenital heart disease: prenatal echocardiographic diagnosis and prognosis. J Ultrasound Med. 2005;24:1191–8.

Peng Y, Ge Y, Zhang H, Liu J, Hong H, Lu Y. Positional relationship between the pulmonary venous confluence-vertical vein and atria in infracardiac total anomalous pulmonary venous connection. Pediatr Cardiol. 2016;37(2):372–7.

Rosenquist GC, Kelly JL, Chandra R, et al. Small left atrium and change in contour of the ventricular septum in total anomalous pulmonary venous connection: a morphometric analysis of 22 infant hearts. Am J Cardiol. 1985;55:777–82.

Seale AN, Uemura H, Webber SA, et al. Total anomalous pulmonary venous connection: morphology and outcome from an international population-based study. Circulation. 2010;122:2718–26.

Seale AN, Uemura H, Webber SA, et al. Total anomalous pulmonary venous connection: outcome of postoperative pulmonary venous obstruction. J Thorac Cardiovasc Surg. 2013;145:1255–62.

Smith B, Frye TR, Newton WA. Total anomalous pulmonary venous return: diagnostic criteria and a new classification. Am J Dis Child. 1961;101:41–51.

Stewart DL, Mendoza JC, Winston S, et al. Use of extracorporeal life support in total anomalous pulmonary venous drainage. J Perinatol. 1996;16:186–90.

Tucker BL, Lindesmith GG, Stiles QR, et al. The superior approach for correction of the supracardiac type of total anomalous pulmonary venous return. Ann Thorac Surg. 1976;22:374–7.

Valsangiacomo ER, Hornberger LK, Barrea C, et al. Partial and total anomalous pulmonary venous connection in the fetus: two-dimensional and Doppler echocardiographic findings. Ultrasound Obstet Gynecol. 2003a;22:257–63.

Valsangiacomo ER, Levasseur S, McCrindle BW, et al. Contrast-enhanced MR angiography of pulmonary venous abnormalities in children. Pediatr Radiol. 2003b;33:92–8.

van den Berg G, Moorman AF. Development of the pulmonary vein and the systemic venous sinus: an interactive 3D overview. PLoS One. 2011;6:e22055.

Vanderlaan RD, Caldarone CA. Total anomalous pulmonary venous connection. In: Mavroudis C, Backer CL, editors. Pediatric cardiac surgery. 5th ed. West Sussex: Wiley-Blackwell; 2023. p. 771–85.

Viola N, Caldarone CA. Total anomalous pulmonary venous connection. In: Mavroudis C, Backer CL, editors. Pediatric cardiac surgery. 4th ed. Oxford: Wiley-Blackwell; 2013. p. 659–73.

Yanagawa B, Alghamdi AA, Dragulescu A, et al. Primary sutureless repair for total anomalous pulmonary venous connection: midterm results in a single institution. J Thorac Cardiovasc Surg. 2011;141:1346–54.

Yun TJ, Coles JG, Konstantinov IE, et al. Conventional and sutureless techniques for management of the pulmonary veins: evolution of indications from postrepair pulmonary vein stenosis to primary pulmonary vein anomalies. J Thorac Cardiovasc Surg. 2005;129:167–74.

Zhang C, Ou Y, Zhuang J, et al. Comparison of sutureless and conventional techniques to repair total anomalous pulmonary venous connection. Semin Thorac Cardiovasc Surg. 2016;28(2):473–84.

Complications Associated with Repair of Cor Triatriatum

Constantine D. Mavroudis,
Constantine Mavroudis, and Amy Heincker

Abstract

The main complications to be avoided in repairing cor triatriatum are injury to the mitral valve and inadvertently exiting the atrial wall. Patients with long standing, undiagnosed cor triatriatum may have postoperative pulmonary hypertension requiring treatment.

Keywords

Congenital heart surgery · Cor triatriatum · Mitral valve · Outcomes

1 Introduction

Cor Triatriatum is a rare lesion where the left atrium is subdivided by a fibromuscular membrane into two separate chambers (Fig. 1). The pulmonary veins drain to a posterosuperior chamber, which then passes either around the membrane or through a fenestration to ultimately drain into the anteroinferior chamber that communicates with both the left atrial appendage and mitral valve. The origins of this membrane are thought to be related to an abnormal incorporation of the common pulmonary vein into the left atrium in-utero, similar to the proposed mechanism underlying the development of total anomalous pulmonary venous connection (Mavroudis et al. 2023). The extent to which this membrane causes inflow obstruction to the mitral valve determines the timing and severity of clinical presentation. In cases where there is no fenestration in the membrane, the pulmonary veins drain to an obligate interatrial communication and into the right atrium. While many patients present in early infancy, those with large fenestrations and low-pressure gradients can have a more indolent course and can present as adults. Typical presenting symptoms include those of pulmonary venous stenosis/obstruction: pulmonary hypertension, respiratory failure, low cardiac output, and failure to thrive. Echocardiogram is diagnostic. It is important to distinguish this lesion from supravalvar mitral ring (Slight et al. 2005). While these lesions can present similarly and demonstrate similar echocardiographic findings, the divided left atrium membrane arises, by definition, between the ostia of the pulmonary veins and the left atrial appendage. Any membrane that arises

C. D. Mavroudis
Pediatric Cardiothoracic Surgery, Children's Hospital of Philadelphia, Perelman School of Medicine, University of Pennsylvania, Philadelphia, PA, USA

C. Mavroudis (✉)
Chief of Pediatric Cardiothoracic Surgery (Retired), Peyton Manning Children's Hospital, Indianapolis, IN, USA

Professor Emeritus of Surgery, Johns Hopkins University School of Medicine, Baltimore, MD, USA

A. Heincker
Pediatric Cardiothoracic Surgery, Peyton Manning Children's Hospital, Indianapolis, IN, USA

C. L. Backer, C. Mavroudis (eds.), *Complications in Pediatric and Congenital Heart Surgery*,
https://doi.org/10.1007/978-3-032-02661-3_25

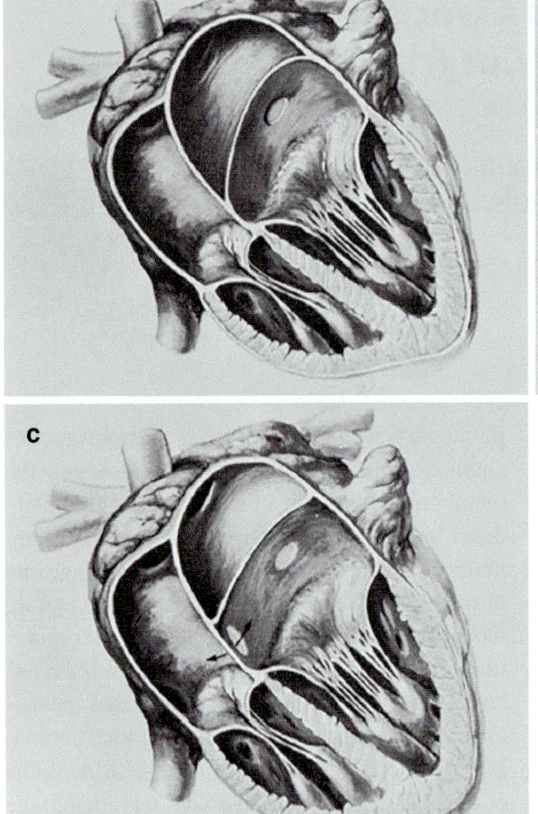

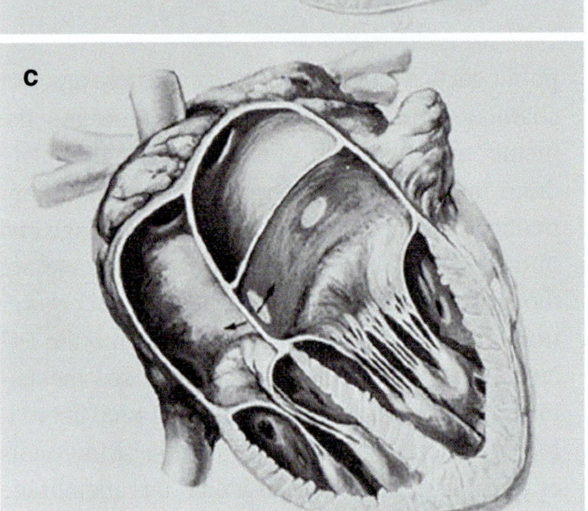

Fig. 1 (**a**) Cor triatriatum with intact atrial septum. (**b**) Cor triatriatum with atrial septal defect between the proximal left atrial chamber and the right atrium. (**c**) Cor triatriatum with atrial septal defect between distal chamber and the right atrium. *IVC* inferior vena cava, *LPV* left pulmonary vein, *RPV* right pulmonary vein. (Reproduced with permission from Arciniegas et al. 1981)

between the left atrial appendage and the annulus of the mitral valve is, therefore, considered a supravalvar ring, and is discussed separately in chapter "Complications Associated with Mitral Valve Surgery for Congenital Anomalies and Degenerative Diseases". The presence or absence of any additional pathology—especially interatrial communications and mitral regurgitation—should also be noted at the time of diagnosis (Saxena et al. 2014; Keeble et al. 2004).

The treatment for cor triatriatum is complete surgical excision of the membrane. The diagnosis is most often an indication for surgery, as many patients are infants who present with significant symptoms. The management of the rare, asymptomatic, adult patient is somewhat controversial. These patients should be watched closely for progression of stenosis and/or the development of atrial fibrillation, which can occur in untreated adult patients (Rudienė et al. 2019).

2 Complications Associated with Repair of Cor Triatriatum

Following establishment of aortobicaval cardiopulmonary bypass and cardioplegic arrest, the membrane can be approached through the left atrium, via the right atrium and a trans-septal exposure, or through a combination of both incisions. Proper visualization of the membrane is essential, as the orientation can be variable and the borders difficult to define. Figure 2 demonstrates a left atrial approach and subsequent surgical excision. Structures most at risk during surgical excision include the mitral valve and the external atrial wall. Because of the membrane's relative distance from the annulus of the mitral valve, the line of excision should be well away from periannular structures such as the circumflex coronary artery, although coronary injury is possible. Avoiding mitral valve injury is essential, as repair strategies are limited in scope and durability. Mitral valve injury can occur on initial incision into the membrane before the surgeon can appreciate the proximity of leaflets to the decompressed membrane. Figure 3 shows how a misplaced #11 blade can injure the anterior leaflet of the mitral valve. Such injuries tend to be small, and amenable to primary or patch leaflet repair using standard techniques as noted in Fig. 4. The larger the mitral injury the more necessity for patch augmentation. Because such injuries can be small, they may remain unnoticed. One should have a high degree of suspicion for such injuries. Following successful membrane excision, the mitral valve is routinely tested for regurgitation using bulb syringe saline insufflation. In addition the postoperative transesophageal echocardiogram should reveal injuries to the mitral valve causing regurgitation.

One method to avoid the potential for mitral valve injury is to incise the membrane at the fenestration while applying cranial traction. Employing a right-angle clamp within the orifice of the fenestration or a traction suture will help to open the membrane until the mitral valve can be completely visualized. Complete resolution of symptoms requires a thorough resection of all obstructing tissue. Because the border between the fibromuscular membrane and atrial wall can be difficult to discern, inadvertent atriotomy or creation of an atrial septal defect can occur. Such injuries are most problematic along the lateral and superior walls of the atrium, as these areas have no adjacent cardiac structures or pericardial reflections as noted in Fig. 5. These injuries, too, can be quite small and may only be discovered following cross-clamp removal and atrial filling. Posterior, bright red bleeding is near diagnostic for this complication. While some superior or anterior defects can be closed without the need to cross-clamp, it is typically necessary to re-arrest the heart to explore and repair the atrium primarily.

Additional postoperative complications may arise following repair of cor triatriatum. Atrioventricular block and atrial fibrillation may occur following resection of the fibrous membrane. Therefore, one should be mindful of the proximity to the conduction system; however, incomplete resection leads to persistent symptoms and should be avoided. A dila-

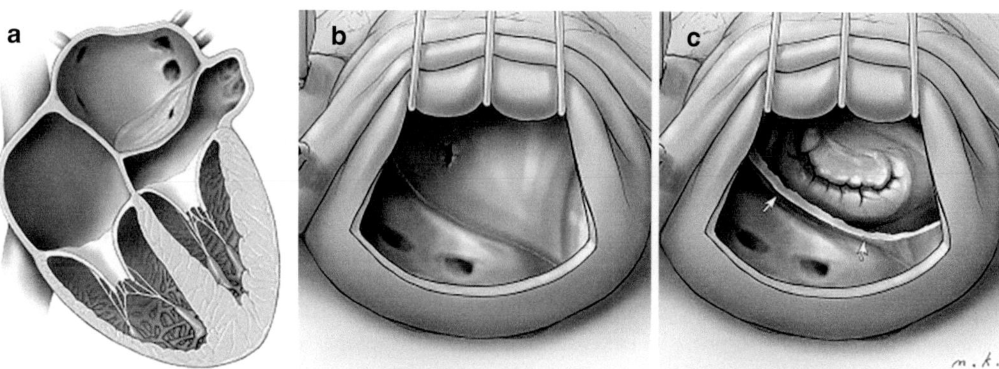

Fig. 2 Surgical approach to cor triatriatum. (**a**) Cor triatriatum with intact atrial septum and restrictive fenestration in the membrane. (**b**) Exposure and identification of the membrane via left atriotomy. Note small fenestration. (**c**) Complete resection of the membrane, allowing unobstructed mitral inflow (arrows mark line of excision). (Reprinted with permission Saxena et al. 2014)

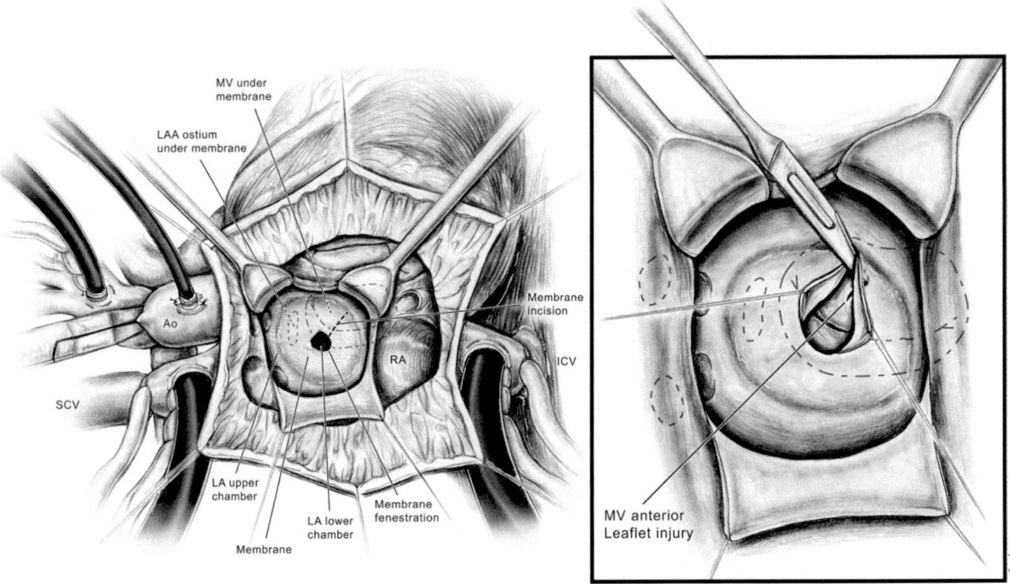

Fig. 3 Left panel shows transseptal left atrial exposure above the fenestrated membrane which is obstructing the entry to the mitral valve. The inset on the right panel shows how an unwanted injury to the anterior leaflet of the mitral valve can occur during membrane incision using an #11 blade. Careful and deliberate incisions can help to avoid this problem. The initial incision in the fenestration is best aimed posteriorly and laterally to the left. As the membrane is incised the exposure of the mitral valve becomes clearer. *Ao* aorta, *ICV* inferior caval vein, *LA* left atrium, *LAA* left atrial appendage, *MV* mitral valve, *RA* right atrium, *SCV* superior caval vein

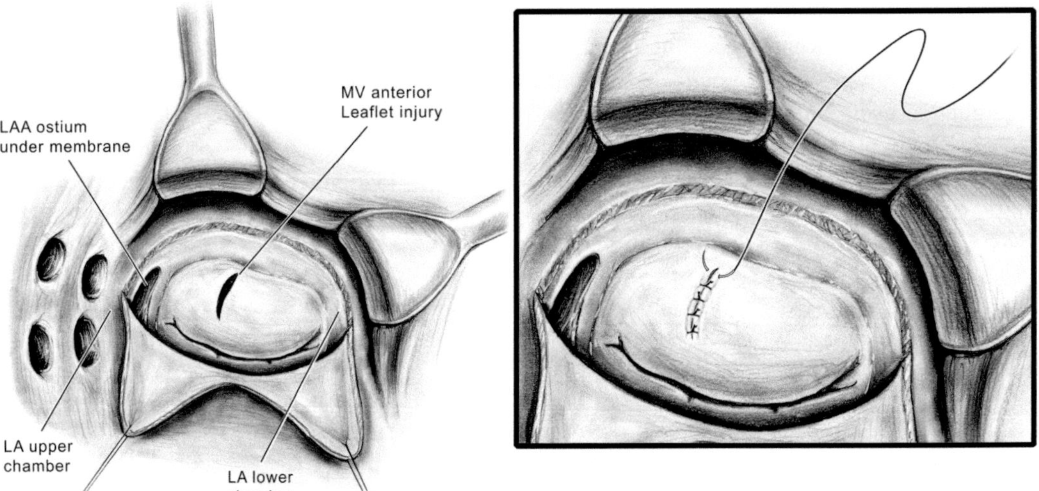

Fig. 4 Left panel shows the membrane partially resected and retracted thereby illustrating the incisional injury of the anterior leaflet of the mitral valve. In most cases, the incision is linear and can be repaired primarily as noted in the right panel inset. When the injury is uneven and large, the surgeon may elect a patch repair. *LA* left atrium, *LAA* left atrial appendage, *MV* mitral valve

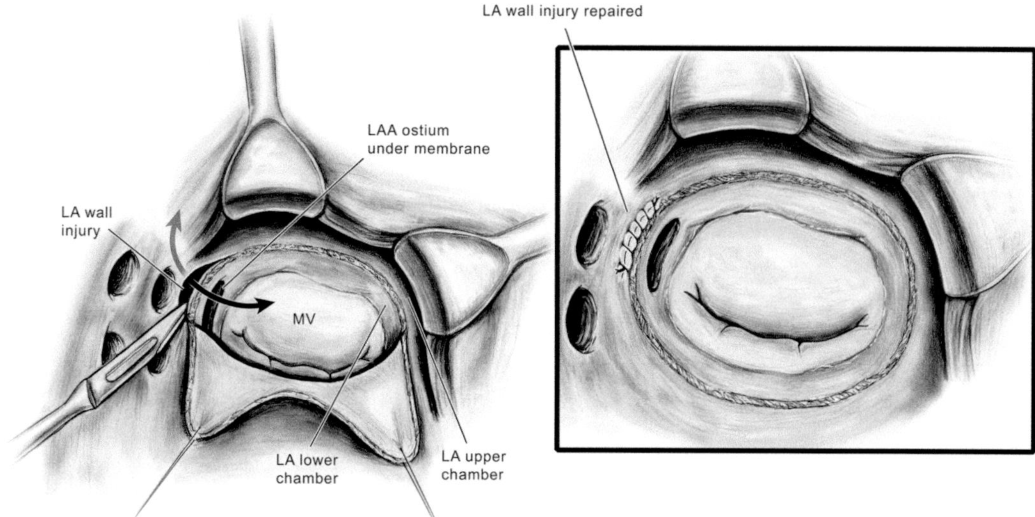

Fig. 5 The left panel illustrates an unwanted posterior left atriotomy caused by an unwanted incision during membrane resection. These injuries can be difficult to identify due to the anatomical proximity of the posterior pericardium. The actual injury may not look different from the correct membrane incisional pathway resection. Keen observation and anticipation will discover the injury and allow linear repair as shown in the right panel inset. *LA* left atrium, *LAA* left atrial appendage, *MV* mitral valve

tor can be used to assess the orifice size after resection to ensure that it is similar to, equal to, or greater than the mitral valve annulus. While complete resection of the membrane minimizes the risk of recurrence, restenosis is possible even with proper technique and may warrant reintervention. Pulmonary vasodilators may be necessary in the postoperative period in patients with preoperative pulmonary hypertension. All patients should be monitored closely for any echocardiographic or clinical evidence of pericardial effusion in the early postoperative period and for recurrent obstruction or valvar abnormalities.

In summary, cor triatriatum is a rare congenital anomaly that may be diagnosed at any age. Concomitant cardiac defects should be noted at the time of diagnosis and will help guide surgical approach and long-term prognosis (Saxena et al. 2014; Ozyuksel et al. 2015). Careful resection of the membranous obstruction leads to excellent outcomes, although the surgeon should be cognizant of the complications that may arise.

References

Arciniegas E, Farooki ZQ, Hakimi M, Perry BL, Green EW. Surgical treatment of cor triatriatum. Ann Thorac Surg. 1981;32:571–7.

Keeble W, Lundmark E, Dargie HJ. The paradoxical finding of mitral valve incompetence and cor triatriatum: a mechanism revealed? Heart. 2004;90(2):125.

Mavroudis CD, Anderson RH, Mavroudis C. Cor triatriatum, pulmonary vein stenosis and atresia of the common pulmonary vein. In: Mavroudis C, Backer CL, editors. Pediatric cardiac surgery. 5th ed. London: Wiley-Blackwell Inc; 2023.

Ozyuksel A, Yildirim O, Avsar M, Hayirlioglu M, Demiroluk S, Kucukosmanoglu O, Bilal MS. Surgical correction of cor triatriatum sinister in the paediatric population: mid-term results in 15 cases. Eur J Cardiothorac Surg. 2015;47(1):e25–8.

Rudienė V, Hjortshøj CMS, Glaveckaitė S, et al. Cor triatriatum sinistrum diagnosed in the adulthood: a systematic review. Heart. 2019;105:1197–202.

Saxena P, Burkhart HM, Schaff HV, Daly R, Joyce LD, Dearani JA. Surgical repair of cor triatriatum sinister: the Mayo Clinic 50-year experience. Ann Thorac Surg. 2014;97(5):1659–63.

Slight RD, Nzewi OC, Buell R, Mankad PS. Cor-triatriatum sinister presenting in the adult as mitral stenosis: an analysis of factors which may be relevant in late presentation. Heart Lung Circ. 2005;14(1):8–12.

Complications Associated with Repair of Congenital and Acquired Aortic Aneurysms

Constantine Mavroudis and Tomas D. Martin

Abstract

Congenital and acquired ascending aortic aneurysms in pediatric and young adults are generally encountered in those with Marfan, Lowes-Dietz, and Ehlers-Danlos syndromes as well as patients with sinus of Valsalva aneurysms who may require an aortic valve-sparing operation. Surgical management of these patients with aortic root and aortic wall pathology is dependent on aortic leaflet competence, annular size, and presence of dissection. This chapter will focus on whether a valve-sparing or valve-replacement strategy should be performed. In cases where aneurysms result in dissections into the transverse arch and descending aorta, a different and more extensive surgical strategy will be required to reestablish normal unobstructed flow into the brachiocephalic arteries and the descending aorta. Management schemes and complications relating thereto include myocardial preservation, cerebral protection, and establishing normal anatomic integrity. We will also discuss the importance of cardioplegic methods, "debranching" techniques, and operative hemostasis.

Keywords

Congenital heart surgery · Complications · Congenital aortic aneurysms · Florida sleeve operation · Bentall procedure · David operation · Debranching techniques · Branched endografts · Adult congenital heart surgery

1 Complications Associated with Pediatric, Congenital, and Acquired Aortic Aneurysms

The genetic origin for heart and vascular anatomic aberrations is diverse and includes inheritable as well as de novo mutations. Multiple inquires have shown that there are over 100 genes associated with congenital or progressive cardiovascular abnormalities (Jefferies et al. 2014; Van Laer et al. 2013). Of late, there has been intense interest and emphasis in children with hereditary connective tissue diseases in association with cardiovascular pathology (Svensson et al. 2013). Connective tissues are characterized as biologic tissues with an extracellular matrix (ECM) that supports and binds systemic structures and

C. Mavroudis (✉)
Chief of Pediatric Cardiothoracic Surgery (Retired), Peyton Manning Children's Hospital, Indianapolis, IN, USA

Professor Emeritus of Surgery, Johns Hopkins University School of Medicine, Baltimore, MD, USA

T. D. Martin
Division of Cardiovascular Surgery, University of Florida School of Medicine, Gainesville, FL, USA

C. L. Backer, C. Mavroudis (eds.), *Complications in Pediatric and Congenital Heart Surgery*,
https://doi.org/10.1007/978-3-032-02661-3_26

organs. The ECM is an organized multi-molecular structure that is essential for the normal functioning of organ systems (Wheeler et al. 2014). Genetic mutations that may affect vascular ECM structure generally give rise to arterial tortuosity, aneurysm formation, dissection and/or rupture. Moreover, a large number of connective tissue disorders can be associated with structural heart defects, which include but are not limited to patent ductus arteriosus (PDA), bicuspid aortic valve (BAV), coarctation of the aorta (CoA), and atrioventricular valve disease. Clinically, children with connective tissue disorders are at risk for aortic dissection, aneurysm, and aortic rupture which are the primary causes of morbidity and mortality (Milewicz et al. 2005; Everitt et al. 2009; Marfan 1896; Dietz et al. 1991). Mortality immediately after aortic catastrophic rupture in these individuals is very high, with up to 40% of pediatric patients dying immediately, and 1%–3% expiring every hour in the first 24 h following the initial event. Unfortunately, even if the child survives in time to reach the operating room, operative mortality has been reported to be as high as 25% (Milewicz et al. 2005). Diagnostic, therapeutic, and prophylactic interventions have been devised to alleviate the cardiovascular catastrophic outcomes involving these patients. Innovations that have provided improvements in genetic analysis have had a substantial impact on identification and management of children with connective tissue disorders. This has resulted in improved awareness of etiology and phenotypes and associated advanced management strategies resulting in enhanced long-term prognosis (Jefferies et al. 2014). The focus of this chapter revolves around complications associated with repair of congenital and acquired aortic aneurysms in the young. However, it is also important to consider the related connective tissue diseases that affect the pediatric patients and their associated cardiovascular manifestations. We will consider the most common forms of cardiovascular phenotype, namely proximal aortic pathology and mitral valve disease, to identify surgical indications and operative management.

In particular, congenital and acquired ascending aortic aneurysms in pediatric and young adult patients are generally encountered in those with Marfan (Judge and Dietz 2005; Faivre et al. 2008; Loeys et al. 2010; Silverman et al. 1995; van Karnebeek et al. 2001; Pyeritz and Wappel 1983; Morse et al. 1990; MacCarrick et al. 2014; Williams et al. 2007), Lowes-Dietz (van der Linde et al. 2013; Loeys et al. 2005, 2006; Patel et al. 2017; Parapia and Jackson 2008; Malfait et al. 2017), Ehlers-Danlos syndromes (Beighton et al. 1998; Royce and Steinmann 2002; Byers et al. 2017; Pepin et al. 2000), and Osteogenesis Imperfecta (Bonita et al. 2010) as well as patients with sinus of Valsalva aneurysms who may need an aortic valve-sparing operation. Surgical management of these patients with aortic root and aortic wall pathology is highly dependent on aortic leaflet competence, annular size, and presence of dissection. These considerations will determine whether a valve-sparing or valve-replacement strategy will be performed. In those cases when aneurysms result in dissections which extend into the transverse arch and descending aorta, a different and more extensive surgical strategy will be required to reestablish normal unobstructed flow into the brachiocephalic arteries and the descending aorta. Management schemes and complications relating thereto include myocardial preservation, cerebral protection, and establishing normal anatomic integrity. We will also discuss the importance of cardioplegic methods, "debranching" techniques, and operative hemostasis (Martin and Mavroudis 2020).

1.1 Aortic Valve Sparing Options

The surgical exposure and approach for an ascending aortic valve-sparing operation in patients with congenital aortopathy is median sternotomy, aortobicaval cardiopulmonary bypass, and left ventricular venting through the right superior pulmonary vein. The other important preoperative considerations are aortic valve competency, coronary artery anatomy, and mitral valve anomalies. There are many types of valve-sparing aortic aneurysm repairs (Vricella and Cameron 2017; Patel et al. 2011; Price et al.

2016). However, they share the idea that aortic wall resection or external aortic wall stabilization is paramount to a long-term outcome free of recurrent proximal aortic dilatation with all the complications thereto associated. In this section, we offer an operation that has come to be known as the "Florida Sleeve Operation" and is comprehensively described in the figures and legends noted in Figs. 1, 2, 3, 4, 5, 6, 7, 8, 9, 10, 11, 12, 13, 14, 15, 17 and 18 (Martin and Mavroudis 2020; Freeman et al. 2021).

The goals of this operation center around three principles that are paramount to a successful operation, namely (1) prevention of further aneurysmal dilatation and dissection (2) to remodel the aortic annulus in order to return it to normal or near normal size which will prevent further dilatation, and (3) to reconstruct the sinotubular junction and resuspend the aortic commissures to their proper functional orientation (Martin and Mavroudis 2020). While careful dissection and anatomic identification are intuitive for all parts of this operation, there are some potential complications that are emphasized herein which, if anticipated, can be avoided enroute to a complication free operation. For example, Fig. 4 reviews the topical coronary artery anatomy which will assist the surgeon for coronary artery fixation and protection during the external enveloping graft placement in association with the Florida Sleeve Operation. Preoperative identification of anomalous aortic origin of the coronary arteries will

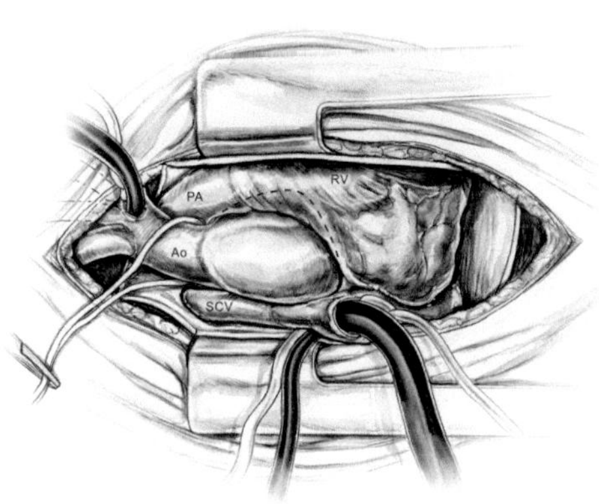

Fig. 1 Shows a large ascending aortic aneurysm weith high aortic cannulation, typically placed in the inferior transverse arch which will allow the surgeon to remove as much diseased aorta as possible without the necessity of circulatory arrest. Atrial or bicaval venous cannulation is determined by surgeon's preference. Comprehensive dissection of the aortic arch and proximal great vessels will allow greater facility in clamp placement and suture repair. *Ao* aorta, *PA* pulmonary artery, *RV* right ventricle, *SCV* superior caval vein. (With permission Martin and Mavroudis 2020)

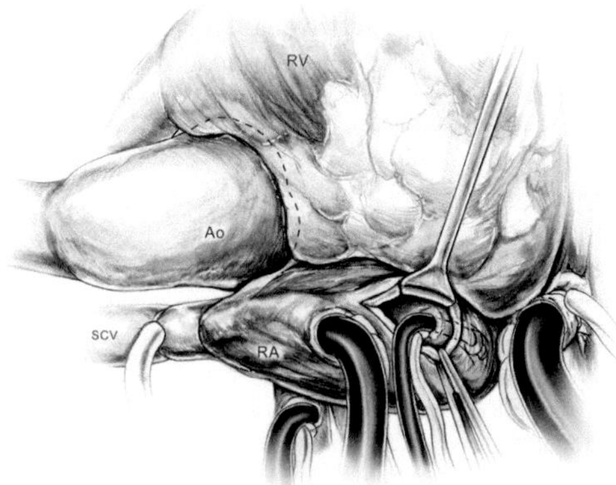

Fig. 2 Shows an open trans right atrial retrograde cardioplegic cannula which can be secured by the balloon only or by a purse-string suture which is shown as well. Successful institution of myocardial preservation techniques can be performed by antegrade or retrograde cardioplegia. We prefer retrograde cardioplegia in these circumstances which can be administered by a small right atrial incision and direct placement of the catheter. *Ao* aorta, *RA* right atrium, *RV* right ventricle, *SCV* superior caval vein. (With permission Martin and Mavroudis 2020)

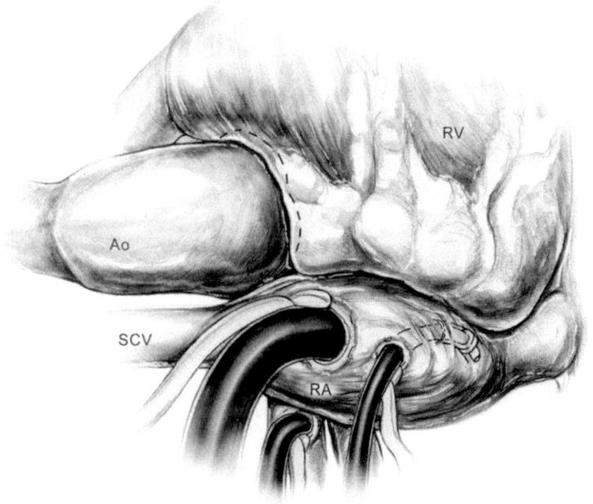

Fig. 3 Shows transatrial placement using palpation techniques to guide the catheter into the coronary sinus. *Ao* aorta, *RA* right atrium, *RV* right ventricle, *SCV* superior caval vein. (With permission Martin and Mavroudis 2020)

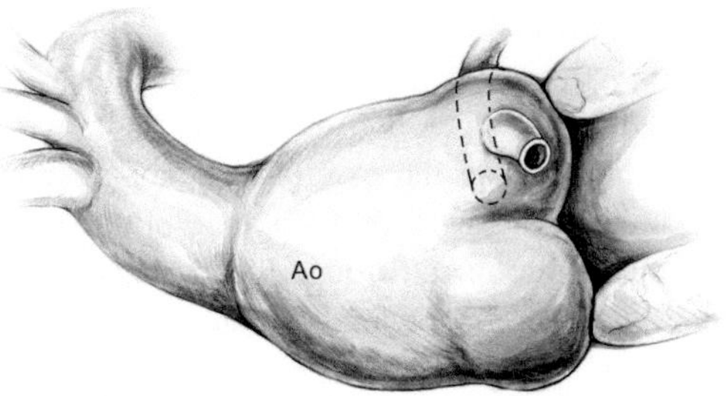

Fig. 4 Demonstrates a dilated aortic root and loss of the sinotubular junction with normal coronary artery anatomy. These anatomical features are important to note since there are three principles of this operation that will determine a successful short- and long-term outcome. The first is prevention of further aneurysmal dilatation and dissection; the second is to remodel the aortic annulus in order to return it to normal or near normal size which will prevent further dilatation; the third is to reconstruct the sinotubular junction and resuspend the aortic commissures to their proper functional orientation. The coronary artery depictions in the figure will assist the surgeon to plan for coronary artery reimplantation in the case of a David operation or coronary artery fixation and protection if a Florida Sleeve operation is elected. Anomalous aortic origin of the coronary arteries must be determined, preferably before the operation, to make technical adjustments. For instance, in the simple case, the origin of the coronary arteries may not be located centrally in the sinuses of Valsalva. Adjustments will be required for optimal location either for reimplantation or coronary fixation in the cases of the David operation or Florida Sleeve operation, respectively. Further to this theme, an anomalous circumflex coronary artery from the right coronary sinus will course posterior and close to the aortic root where subaortic sutures are generally placed for aortic graft fixation and annular reduction. Management of this anomaly will require mobilization and special consideration whether or not a David or Florida Sleeve operation is employed. Other coronary anomalies include intramural courses, high take-off origins, or unrecognized proximal stenoses. *Ao* aorta. (With permission Martin and Mavroudis 2020)

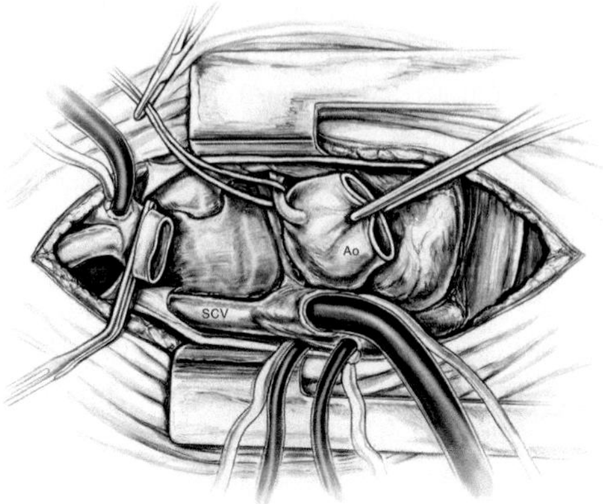

Fig. 5 After aortic cross-clamp application, retrograde cardioplegia, and left ventricular venting, the aorta is transected just proximal to the clamp with the aim of resecting all the diseased aorta distally and 1 cm above the sinotubular junction as shown in the figure. These guidelines will allow further aortic wall resection as necessary. Also shown is dissection and mobilization of the aortic root and left main coronary artery. During the left main dissection, care is taken to avoid injury to the left atrial wall which can be adherent to the aortic root and the course of the left main coronary artery. *Ao* aorta, *SCV* superior caval vein. (With permission Martin and Mavroudis 2020)

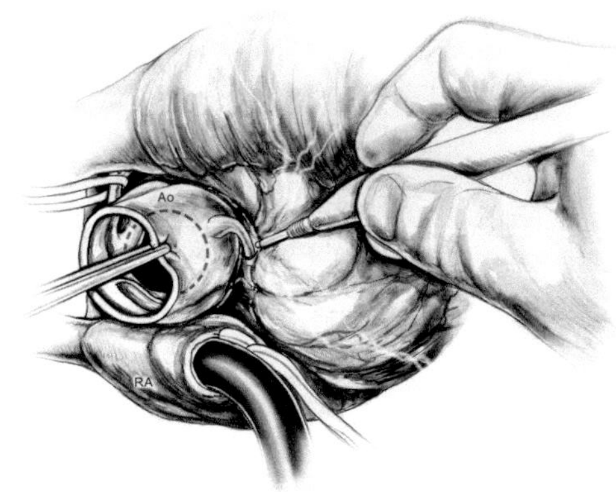

Fig. 6 Shows the use of low setting electrocautery to mobilize the course of the right coronary artery toward the epicardial surface of the myocardium. Care is also taken to avoid injury to the conal branch coronary artery which supplies the anterior right ventricular wall. Surgeons have noted that damage to the conal branch coronary artery is associated with an increased incidence of postoperative ventricular arrhythmias. Also shown in ghost profile are the leaflets of the aortic valve and the relationship to the coronary artery ostia. The surgeon can now perform either the David operation or the Florida Sleeve operation. *Ao* aorta, *RA* right atrium. (With permission Martin and Mavroudis 2020)

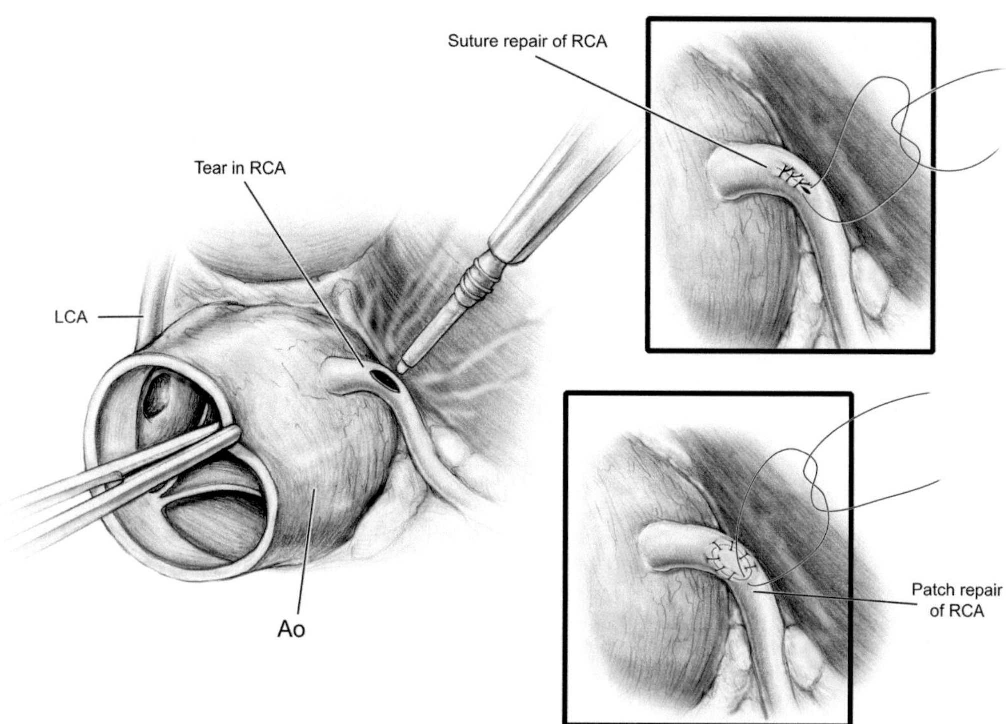

Fig. 7 The left panel shows an injury to the coronary artery during the dissection and the attempt to mobilize the proximal portion for the enveloping graft. The right upper inset shows interrupted suture technique. The right lower inset shows patch coronary artery arterioplasty. *Ao* aorta, *LCA* left coronary artery, *RCA* right coronary artery

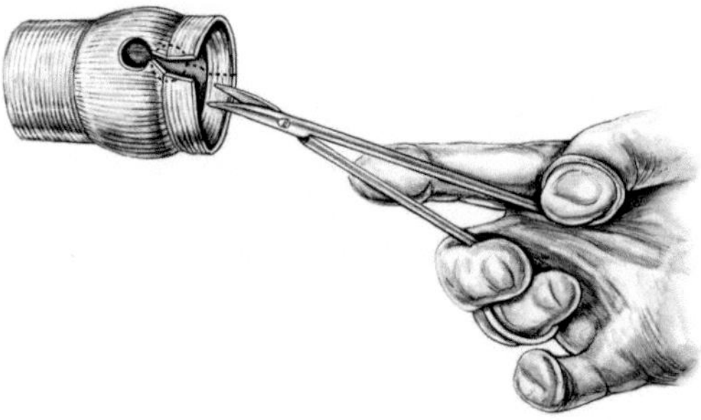

Fig. 8 Once the aortic root dissection and coronary artery mobilization are performed, a Vascutek® Gelweave Valsalva Dacron graft is prepared. The aim of the Florida Sleeve graft size is of some importance. The most common sizes are 32 and 34 mm. The selection is based on the maximum diameter of the aortic root at the sinuses of Valsalva. If the measurement is 4.5 cm or less, we recommend a 30-mm graft. If the measurement is between 4.5 and 6.0 cm, we recommend a 32-mm graft. And finally, for any measurement between 6.0 and 7.0 cm, we recommend a 34-mm graft. Any measurement above 7.0 cm should take into consideration aortic leaflet quality and anticipated function to proceed with a valve salvage operation. Sound judgment in these circumstances will help to determine and predict the long-term efficacy of this strategy. Figure 8 shows the Valsalva graft which is being contoured to provide appropriately placed "keyholes" for the exiting coronary arteries after the sleeve is placed completely around the aortic root. The height and diameter of the "keyholes" are a very important part of the operation. A "keyhole" that is too small will constrict the coronary; a keyhole that is too large leaves too much diseased aorta exposed to the dilatation effects of the native aortopathy. In our collective experience, the most common error is to make the "keyhole" too low or too far upstream. The consequence of this can lead to compression of the cephalad portion of the exiting coronary artery. In addition to the "keyhole" creation, we generally remove enough Dacron circumferentially to leave 3–4 mm connected to the Valsalva portion of the graft (not shown in the drawing). The Valsalva graft has three linear black markings to delineate the commissures which are 120° apart. In the case of unequal commissure distribution, the surgeon must adjust and mark the appropriate location. Occasionally, the surgeon will encounter a bicuspid valve which is competent and likely to perform well in the future. Adjustments will also have to be made under these circumstances which will not preclude a successful valve sparing repair. Once the "keyholes" are established, the graft is ready for implantation. (With permission Martin and Mavroudis 2020)

allow the surgeon to perform the most advantageous location for the graft "keyhole" placement (Fig. 8) which will ensure coronary artery flow and perfusion. The epicardial coronary artery dissection must be performed with the utmost care to avoid coronary injury and unwanted disruption of an early epicardial branch. Figures 5 and 6 illustrate the methods and results of coronary artery dissection which can be accomplished with careful scissor dissection and low-setting electrocautery. It is not always necessary to place a vessel loop around the proximal coronary artery; however, it can serve as a gentle retraction method to ensure proper enveloping graft placement which will prevent pericoronary artery dilation in the long term. If during the dissection the artery is injured as is noted in Fig. 7 (left panel), a careful and deliberate repair process is indicated. The right panel shows two methods of repair, namely, interrupted suture technique if the repair can be accomplished without resultant stenosis (right upper inset) or patch repair (right lower inset) if the injury is too large. Not shown is a PTFE interposition graft which may be performed if the injury is too extensive or too far posterior for a comfortable repair. Another option is coronary artery transection and end-to-end left internal thoracic artery-to-coronary artery anastomosis. Fortunately, these repair options are very rare; however, it is best to be advised and have options readily available for these unwanted circumstances.

The placement of the enveloping graft is shown in Figs. 8, 9 and 10. The optimal considerations for an accurate graft placement are proper size, absence of coronary artery obstruction, and proper resuspension of the aortic root. Figure 10 illustrates the ideal graft placement with encircling coronary artery graft placement and resuspension accuracy. Figure 11 left panel shows how the keyhole orifice in the graft placement can potentially obstruct the origin of the left main coronary artery

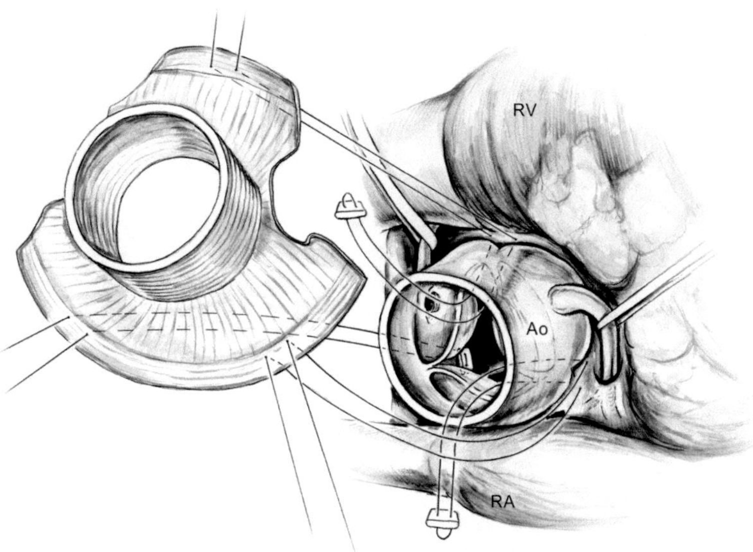

Fig. 9 Spatially demonstrates the placement of the subannular sutures at each commissure which will anchor the hovering graft into position. These pledgeted sutures are placed below the annulus from within the left ventricular outflow tract at the aortic-cardiac juncture and exit to the epicardial surface. They are then passed through the Dacron graft and the appropriate commissure marking. Occasionally, additional pledgeted sutures can be placed in the same manner in the noncoronary sinus if needed to reduce further the aortic annulus. In general, annular reduction is performed if the annulus is greater than 26 mm. *Ao* aorta, *RA* right atrium, *RV* right ventricle. (With permission Martin and Mavroudis 2020)

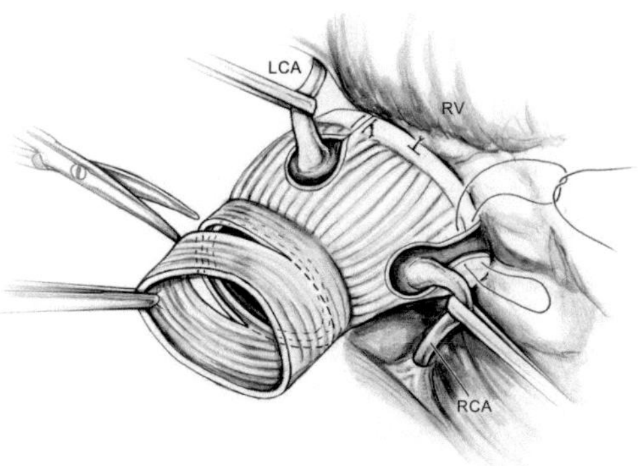

Fig. 10 Shows the graft being lowered over the entire aortic root and anchored to the aortic-cardiac juncture. Also noted are the coronary "keyholes" which are closed under the coronary arteries using monofilament suture. Care is taken to prevent inclusion of fibrous tissue in the suturing technique that might cause unwanted kinking or obstruction of the coronary artery orifice. If the superior lip of the graft appears to be obstructing the orifice, a vertical incision can be accomplished in order to prevent stenosis. The superior portion of the graft is then trimmed to align the orifice with the superior portion of the aortic root. The aortic root is pulled superiorly slightly to closely approximate the preferred level that will be fixed during the suture line that will attach the aorta to the encircling graft. *LCA* left coronary artery, *RCA* right coronary artery, *RV* right ventricle. (With permission Martin and Mavroudis 2020)

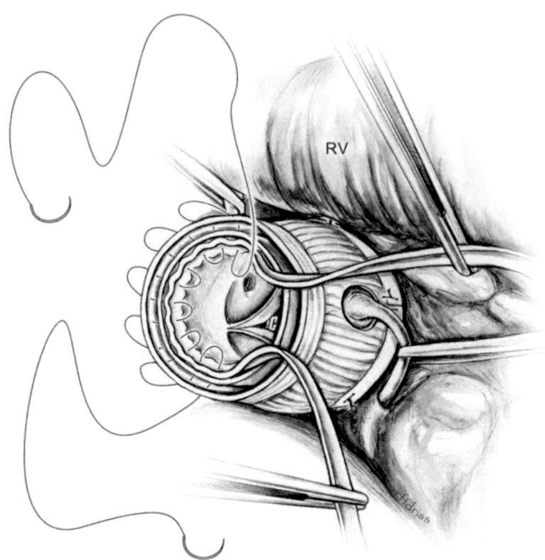

Fig. 12 Shows a strip of Teflon felt that is cut to size and used to bolster the anastomosis between the superior portion of the aortic root and neosinotubular junction and the investing graft. A running mattress monofilament suture line is being performed in the figure with the Teflon felt within the aorta. *RV* right ventricle. (With permission Martin and Mavroudis 2020)

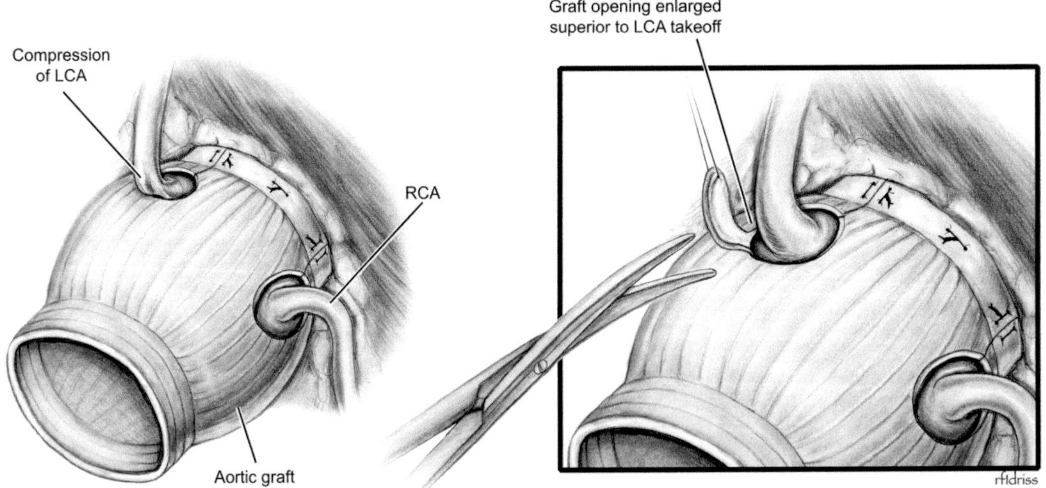

Fig. 11 Left panel shows the left main coronary artery being encumbered superiorly by the graft which was not cut high enough. The right panel inset shows the graft being enlarged by scissor dissection to allow unencumbered outflow of the coronary artery. *LCA* left coronary artery, *RCA* right coronary artery

which of course can happen for the right coronary artery as well. The right panel inset of Fig. 11 shows how judicious excision of the graft can enlarge the orifice to accommodate the size of the proximal coronary artery and still maintain the protective encircling function of the graft to prevent coronary artery dilatation in the long term.

The resuspension of the aortic root to the encircling graft is shown in Fig. 12. The running mattress suture technique with a strip of Teflon is illustrated to assure a leakproof anastomosis which will avoid disruption and leaking into the area between the graft and aortic root. This situation is shown in chapter "Complications Associated with Repair of Transposition of the Great Arteries and Associated Lesion", which highlights the results of a disrupted suture line which can cause internal leaking between the graft and the vessel resulting in obstruction and aortic valve regurgitation. Figure 13 highlights the proper method of securing the suture reconstruction of the neoaorta after resuspension of the aortic root to the encircling graft. The measured dilator is being used to prevent a "purse-string" effect. Figure 14 illustrates what can happen to the neoaortic reconstruction if the measured dilator is not used. Figure 15 shows how the proximal neoaorta, when properly constructed with a measured dilator to prevent the purse-string effect, aligns with the ascending aortic graft. Figures 16 and 17 illustrate the finishing maneuvers involving distal aortic anastomosis and separation from cardiopulmonary bypass. Not mentioned herein is the importance of conscientious cavitary air removal and effective hemostasis which are no doubt standard maneuvers for the experienced and cautious surgeon.

The short- and long-term excellent outcomes for the Florida Sleeve Operation have been reported (Price et al. 2016; Freeman et al. 2021; Hess Jr et al. 2009; Alhussaini et al. 2022; Uglov et al. 2021; Khvan et al. 2019; Kitaura et al. 2021; Aalaei-Andabili et al. 2017, 2019; Khvan et al. 2020). There is however a debate amongst experienced centers on whether the David operation (discussed in the following section) or the Florida Sleeve operation is superior. Holubec and associates from Frankfort, Germany (Holubec et al. 2022) have compared both operations in a large clinical series in which there were 285 patients who had the David operation and 57 patients who had the Florida Sleeve operation. They concluded that both the David operation and the Florida Sleeve operation resulted in similar early and longer-term outcomes with a trend to slightly better performance and survival in the David operation group. However, they also noted that the Florida Sleeve operation might be an alternative approach for patients with higher-risk profiles requiring valve-sparing aortic root replacement, which is essentially the main indication for application of the Florida Sleeve operation (Freeman et al. 2021; Hess Jr et al. 2009; Alhussaini et al. 2022; Uglov et al. 2021; Khvan et al. 2019; Kitaura et al. 2021; Aalaei-Andabili et al. 2017, 2019; Khvan et al. 2020). The differences between these two methods of valve-sparing ascending aorta and arch replacement is being debated in the literature (Holubec et al. 2022; Jahanyar et al. 2022; David et al. 2009) based on nonrandomized clinical series. At the moment, there appears to be indications for both operations. Time will tell which procedure will emerge as the preferred technique.

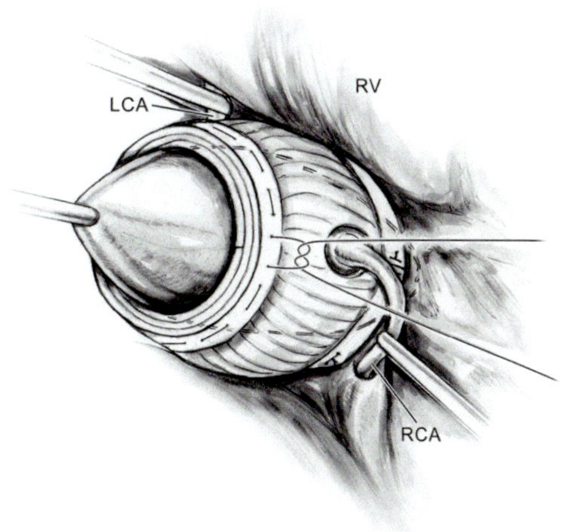

Fig. 13 Shows how a graded dilator can be placed within the distal reconstruction and the anastomosis is secured with the running suture. The dilator will prevent the "purse-string effect" that oftentimes accompanies such a repair. *LCA* left coronary artery, *RCA* right coronary artery, *RV* right ventricle. (With permission Martin and Mavroudis 2020)

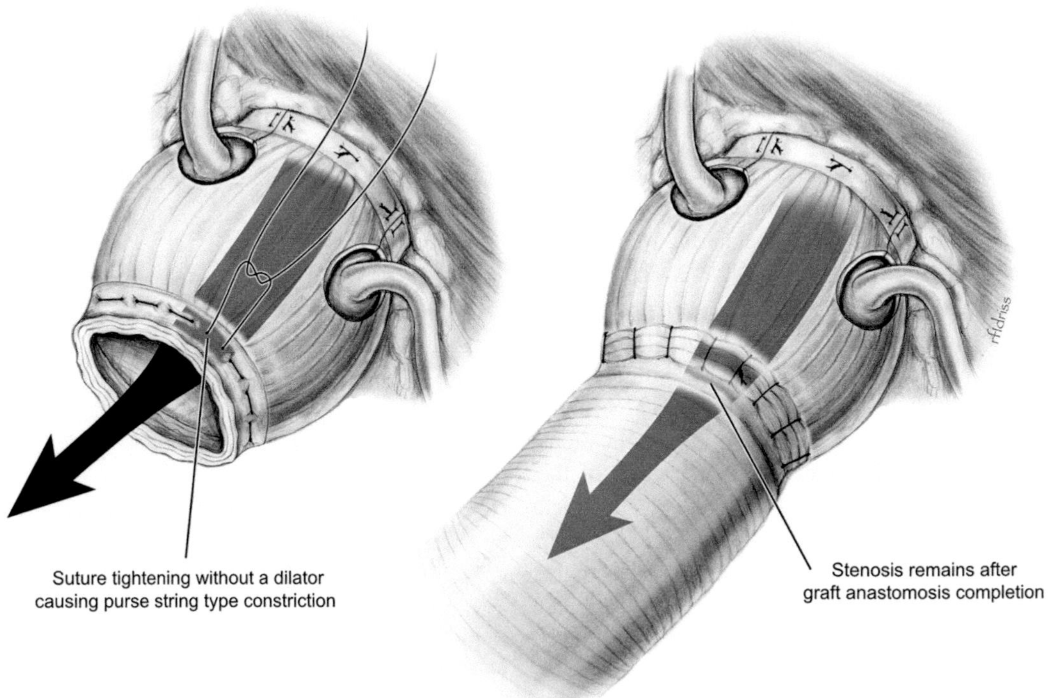

Fig. 14 A left panel shows the tying of the superior graft to aorta configuration without the dilator. The right panel shows the completed reconstruction significantly narrowed by the purse-string effect

1.2 David Valve Sparing Operation for Congenital Ascending Aortic Aneurysms

The David valve sparing operation for adult congenital ascending aortic aneurysms and aortic regurgitation due to annular dilatation is employed for the same indications as the Florida Sleeve operation (Freeman et al. 2021; Hess Jr et al. 2009; Alhussaini et al. 2022; Uglov et al. 2021; Khvan et al. 2019, 2020; Kitaura et al. 2021; Aalaei-Andabili et al. 2017, 2019; Holubec et al. 2022; Jahanyar et al. 2022). The choice between procedures is largely surgeon and institution dependent and is based on surgical experience/outcomes, individual preference, and facility with the potential complications. Multiple judgment-based decisions are involved including size of the graft, character of the aortic valve leaflets, and experience with valve leaflet repair should it be necessary. Much like the Florida Sleeve operation, the development of neoaortic regurgitation after root and arch repair is the most common cause of reoperation (Leontyev et al. 2012). The overwhelming benefit of this approach as with the Florida Sleeve operation is the sparring of the aortic valve which increases valve longevity, maintains excellent hemodynamics, and eliminates the problems of anticoagulation.

The operative exposure that will result in minimal potential complications is median sternotomy (although minimally invasive techniques have been advocated) (Cameron et al. 2009; Cameron and Vricella 2005), aortobicaval cardiopulmonary bypass, left ventricular vent, and antegrade/retrograde cardioplegia. Figures 18, 19, 20, 21 and 22 demonstrate the course of the operation with important procedural characteristics that are emphasized within the legends. It is important to confirm echocardiographic assessment of aortic valve regurgitation at close inspection of the aortic valve

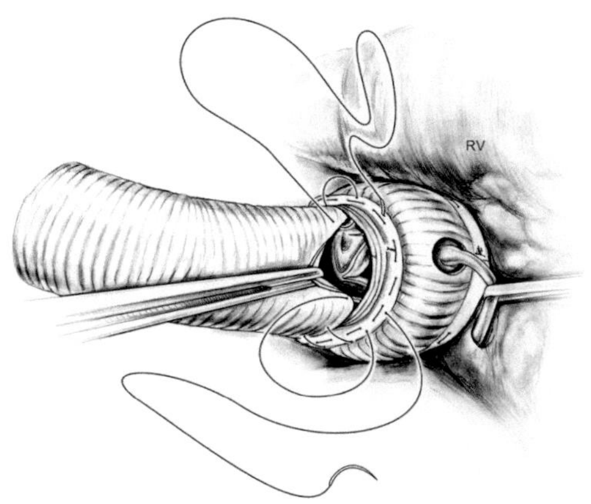

Fig. 15 Shows how the ascending aortic graft is anastomosed end-to-end to the reconstructed proximal aorta. *RV* right ventricle. (With permission Martin and Mavroudis 2020)

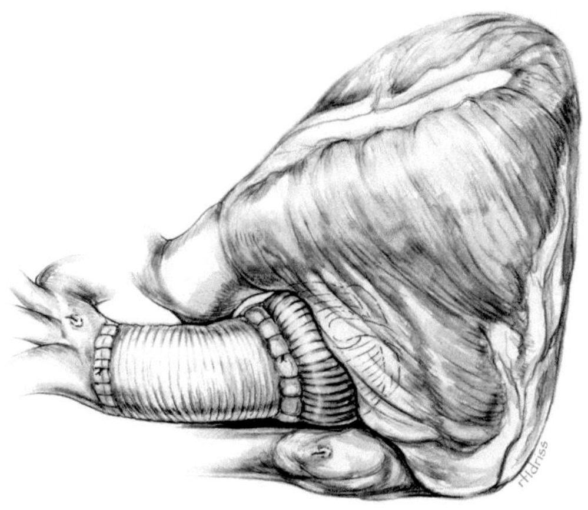

Fig. 17 Shows the completed repair after separation from cardiopulmonary bypass and decannulation. (With permission Martin and Mavroudis 2020)

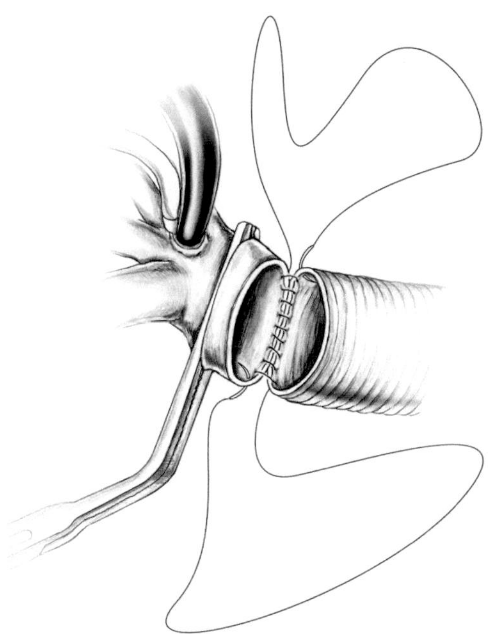

Fig. 16 The distal ascending aortic anastomosis as shown in the figure being performed with running suture technique. This will complete the repair after the necessary air evacuation techniques are completed. (With permission Martin and Mavroudis 2020)

after cardioplegic arrest and aortic transection (Fig. 18). In general, the preoperative assessment will determine whether valvuloplasty or whether aortic root replacement will be indicated. Aortic valve assessment has been discussed in chapter "Complications Associated with Repair of Transposition of the Great Arteries and Associated Lesion", and can be considered in evaluating aortic valve competency. Harvesting the coronary artery buttons and implanting the Dacron graft are shown in Fig. 19. The potential complications of this phase of the operation involve coronary artery button harvesting by button removal from the ascending aorta, epicardial dissection, and mobilization. This maneuver has been discussed in chapter "Complications Associated with Repair of Transposition of the Great Arteries and Associated Lesion", in association with coronary button harvesting in conjunction with the arterial switch operation. Excising the coronary artery button can result in inaccurate scissor dissection too close to the coronary orifice which complicates reimplantation. Figures 10, 11, 12, 13, 14, 15, 16, 17, 18 and 19 in chapter "Complications Associated with Repair of Transposition of the Great Arteries and Associated Lesion" show how these unwanted complications can be resolved without further problems.

The importance of a hemostatic stitch for attaching the graft to the scalloped proximal aortic root cannot be overstated. Figure 20 and the associated legend reviews the important steps to

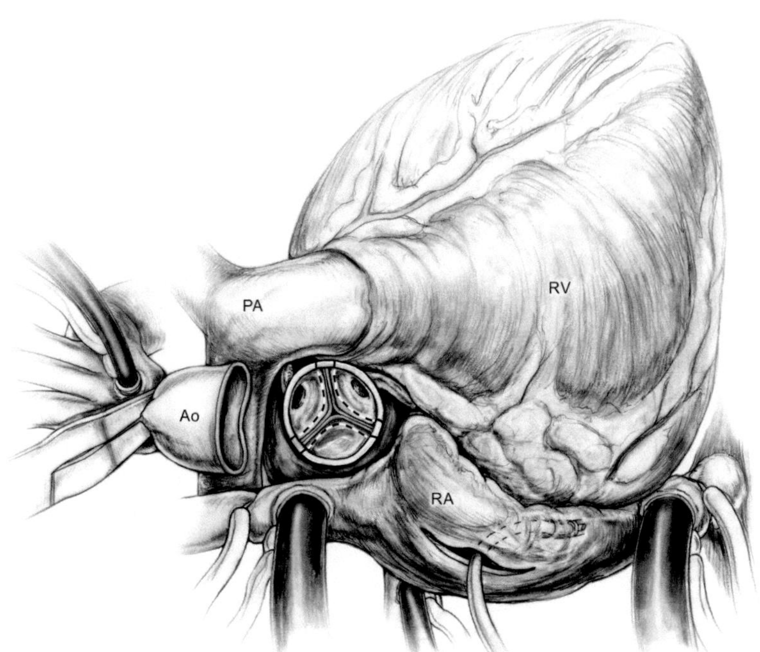

Fig. 18 Shows the operative aortic root exposure after aortobicaval cardiopulmonary bypass, left ventricular venting, antegrade/retrograde cardioplegia, ascending aortic aneurysmectomy, normal coronary artery anatomy. The aortic leaflets have not been involved in any dissection and the coronary artery orifices are normally situated and without proximal stenoses or dissections. *Ao* aorta, *PA* pulmonary artery, *RA* right atrium, *RV* right ventricle. (With permission Martin and Mavroudis 2020)

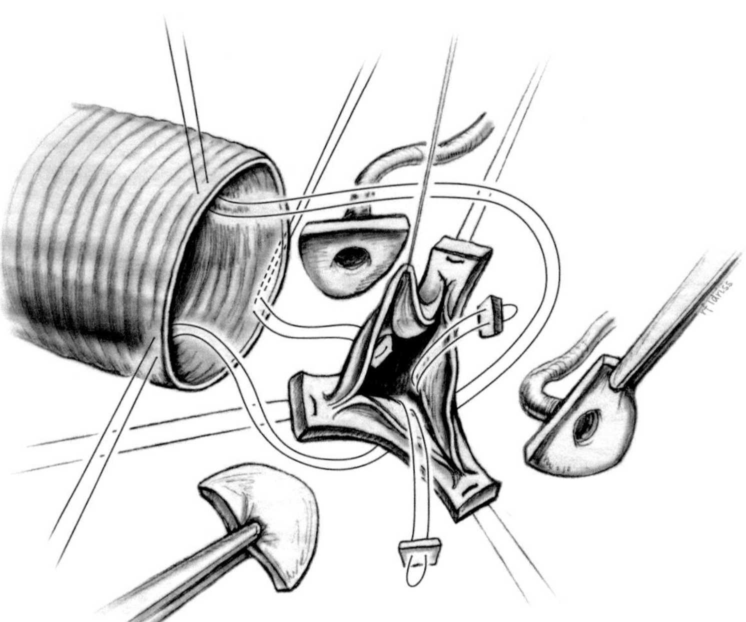

Fig. 19 Shows retraction sutures being placed at the commissures and the coronary artery buttons being harvested from their respective sinuses of Valsalva. The noncoronary cusp aortic wall is also resected to remove as much native aortic wall as is prudent since the remaining aortic wall must accept hemostatic sutures for the neoaortic reconstruction. An appropriately sized sinus of Valsalva graft is selected and pledgeted sutures are placed from within the aortic outflow tract at the nadir of each coronary cusp below the annulus to seat the graft. An additional pledgeted suture can be placed in the noncoronary cusp if an extensive annular reduction is required for aortic valve competency (not shown). (With permission Martin and Mavroudis 2020)

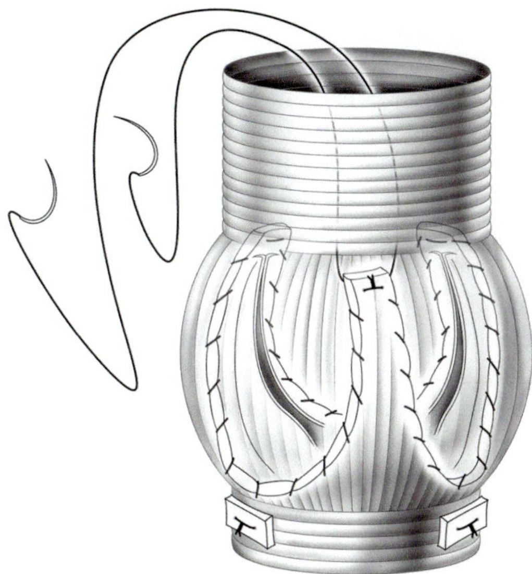

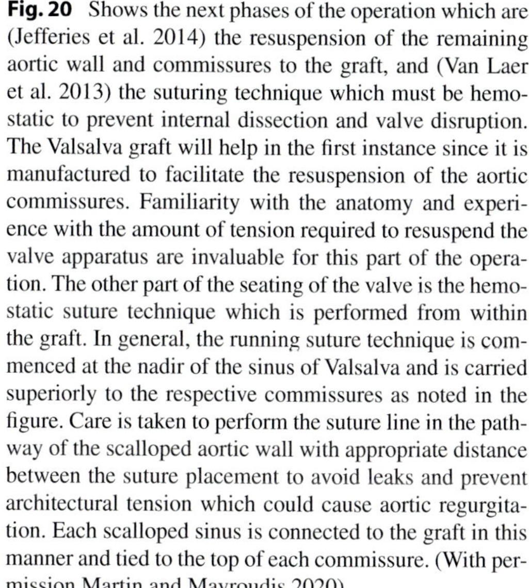

Fig. 20 Shows the next phases of the operation which are (Jefferies et al. 2014) the resuspension of the remaining aortic wall and commissures to the graft, and (Van Laer et al. 2013) the suturing technique which must be hemostatic to prevent internal dissection and valve disruption. The Valsalva graft will help in the first instance since it is manufactured to facilitate the resuspension of the aortic commissures. Familiarity with the anatomy and experience with the amount of tension required to resuspend the valve apparatus are invaluable for this part of the operation. The other part of the seating of the valve is the hemostatic suture technique which is performed from within the graft. In general, the running suture technique is commenced at the nadir of the sinus of Valsalva and is carried superiorly to the respective commissures as noted in the figure. Care is taken to perform the suture line in the pathway of the scalloped aortic wall with appropriate distance between the suture placement to avoid leaks and prevent architectural tension which could cause aortic regurgitation. Each scalloped sinus is connected to the graft in this manner and tied to the top of each commissure. (With permission Martin and Mavroudis 2020)

avoid suture disruption and proper aortic commissure resuspension. Careful attention to these two important steps will prevent internal disruption and root distortion leading to neoaortic regurgitation and potential coronary obstruction. Figure 67 (chapter "Complications Associated with Repair of Transposition of the Great Arteries and Associated Lesion", Transposition) demonstrates how a disrupted suture line can cause internal vascular mischief that is not always immediately discernable. Separation from cardiopulmonary bypass and transesophageal echo-

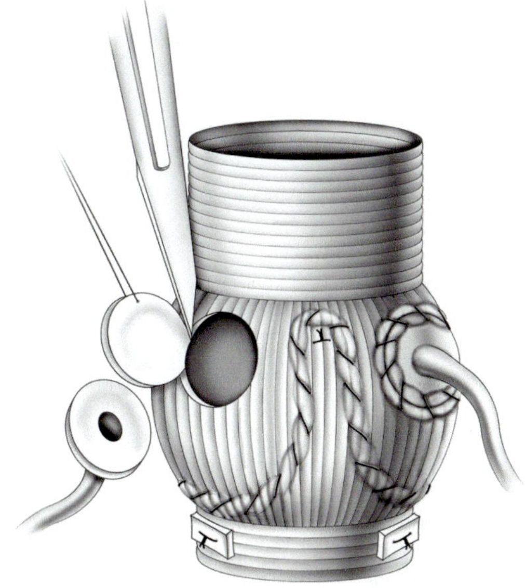

Fig. 21 Shows the remaining steps of the neoaortic reconstruction which are the implantation of the respective coronary artery buttons. Prior to the neoaortic reconstruction, the coronary buttons should have been carefully dissected to their attachments on the surface of the ventricular epicardium. In this manner, the coronaries can be anastomosed to the ascending portion of the Valsalva graft without tension and without concern of myocardial malperfusion postoperatively. Standard suturing techniques are employed while constant vigilance is afforded to assure that the aortic leaflets are not damaged during the graft orifice creation or suturing. (With permission Martin and Mavroudis 2020)

cardiography (TEE) interrogation generally identifies this problem which should trigger immediate return to cardiopulmonary bypass, aortic cross-clamping, cardioplegic arrest, and repair of the disrupted suture line.

Figure 21 reviews the coronary reimplantation technique for completion of the proximal neoaorta enroute to terminal aortic reconstruction as noted in Fig. 22. As noted, careful suturing technique will avoid unwanted aortic leaflet damage and ensure hemostasis. In addition, the coronary button should be aligned with the graft hole to avoid twisting and kinking. Oftentimes, a fine marker stitch can be placed to identify the superior portion of the coronary button which will instill confidence during the reimplantation maneuver. Proper de-airing maneuvers and aortic reanastomosis will complete the process. A liter-

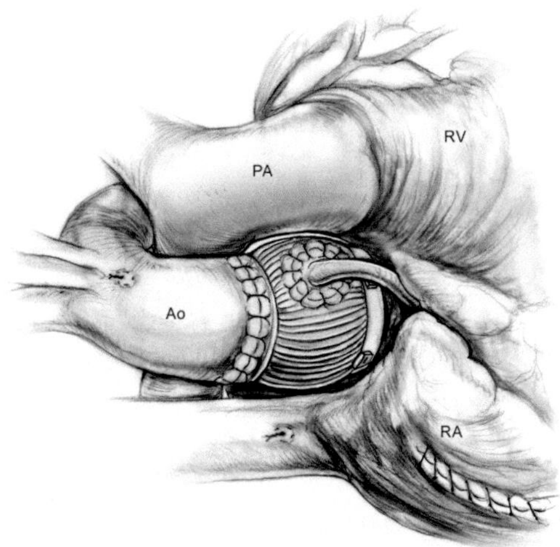

Fig. 22 Shows the completion of the operation by connection of the neoaorta with the ascending aorta, while performing all the de-airing maneuvers. Proper administration of myocardial protection strategies will insure prompt separation from cardiopulmonary bypass. Hemostasis is the staple of all operative and reoperative adult congenital heart operations. *Ao* aorta, *PA* pulmonary artery, *RA* right atrium, *RV* right ventricle. (With permission Martin and Mavroudis 2020)

ature review has confirmed the excellent short- and long-term outcomes of this operation (Pitts et al. 2022; Shrestha et al. 2022, 2023; Beckmann et al. 2021; Cardoso et al. 2021; David and Feindel 1992).

1.3 Bentall Procedure for Congenital Ascending Aortic Aneurysms and Aortic Regurgitation

The Bentall procedure was introduced in 1968 by Bentall and Debono in the United Kingdom which described a technique for complete replacement of the ascending aorta and aortic valve using a composite graft consisting of a prosthetic aortic graft sutured to a mechanical valve (Bentall and De Bono 1968). In that original operation, the coronary artery buttons were not implanted to the graft as they are in the current era. Rather, the aortic tissue surrounding the coronary arteries was sutured directly to openings in the aortic graft as a side-to-side anastomosis. The operation was completed by suturing the aneurysmal aortic wall around the graft to reduce the risk of bleeding. The ensuing clinical experience revealed anastomotic leaks arising at the coronary artery and distal aortic suture lines which resulted in false aneurysms that required reoperation (Kouchoukos et al. 1986). Christian Cabrol and associates in France introduced a modified operation for aortic root replacement that involved anastomosis of the ends of an 8-mm polyester tube graft to the aortic tissue surrounding the right and left coronary arteries with concurrent anastomosis of the midsegment of this graft to an opening in the composite graft (Cabrol et al. 1978). Consistent with the original Bentall procedure, the aneurysmal aortic wall was sutured over the aortic and coronary artery grafts to reduce blood loss. In an effort to avoid periaortic space thrombus, a fistula was created from the space surrounding the grafts to the right atrial appendage using a polyester tube graft. This modification however did not altogether prevent pseudoaneurysms leading to the further inquiries which triggered newer modifications.

The obvious solution to this problem is to anastomose the coronary arteries directly to the ascending aortic graft. However, significant impediments precluded this idea which included a large distance between the coronary arteries and the ascending graft, aortic dissection involving the coronary arteries, infection, extensive calcification of the aorta, and those undergoing reoperation with extensive scar tissue. Notable attempts to solve these problems involved interposition saphenous vein between the aortic graft and the coronary ostia (Blanco et al. 1976) suture occlusion of the coronary ostia and placement of saphenous vein bypass grafts from the aortic graft to the three major coronary arteries (Zubiate and Kay 1976), and use of short interposition grafts of polytetrafluoroethylene (PTFE) between the left coronary artery and the aortic graft (Piehler and Pluth 1982). All of these techniques proved useful, and they continue to be used on a selective basis.

Further improvements resulted in amending the idea of coronary management. Previously, grafts were used to bring the ascending aortic graft to the coronaries. Mobilization of the proximal portions of the coronary arteries by excision of a small cuff of surrounding aortic tissue, and direct attachment of these buttons of aortic tissue to openings in the composite graft was now used to bring the coronaries to the ascending aortic graft. New grafts and elimination of wrapping of the aortic wall around the grafts allowed direct coronary reimplantation into the ascending graft in much the same manner that is practiced for the arterial switch operation (chapter "Complications Associated with Repair of Transposition of the Great Arteries and Associated Lesion"). This idea was tested in a clinical study of 153 patients of whom 105 had the classic Bentall operation and 48 patients who had the coronary button transfer technique (Open Technique). Freedom from reoperation from whatever cause for the Bentall group was 67% at 8 years compared with 92% for the Open Technique group; the difference of which was highly significant (Kouchoukos et al. 1991). Furthermore, 9 patients in the Bentall operation group developed pseudoaneurysms of the aortic or coronary arterial suture lines, compared with the Open Technique which did not develop pseudoaneurysms. Subsequent studies confirmed these results leading to the wide acceptance of the current technique of direct coronary button implantation in association with aortic root replacement (Mookhoek et al. 2016; Maddalo et al. 2014; Victoria-Medina et al. 2022; Hosseinsabet et al. 2021)

In cases where an aortic valve has been damaged, a valve replacement strategy must be considered in association with the aneurysm repair. Indications include retrograde dissection, acute annular dilatation, leaflet foreshortening, prolapse, or endocarditis. As noted in the previous paragraphs, these situations generally require a Bentall procedure, which is based on prosthetic valve replacement, coronary artery reimplantation, and prosthetic ascending aortic arch replacement. Many surgeons select a prosthetic valve conduit for this reconstruction which necessitates lifelong anticoagulation. Alternatives exist (Chirichilli et al. 2020) and are being selected by an increasing number of patients due to improved bioprosthetic valves and the obvious freedom from anticoagulation strategies (Beliaev and Haydock 2020).

As with most binary decisions, there are advantages and disadvantages of the Bentall operation. In general, it is easier to perform than the Florida Sleeve and David operations due to fewer critical decisions involving commissure resuspension and neoaortic wall inclusion into the graft. In addition, coronary artery buttons do not have to be realigned with the sinuses of Valsalva when using a prosthetic valve, although they do have to be realigned if a stented bioprosthetic valve is employed.

Figures 23, 24 and 25 show the progression of the Bentall Procedure using a composite mechanical valve and ascending aortic graft. The principles for aortic valve replacement are in order. After aortobicaval cardiopulmonary bypass, moderate hypothermia, and left ventricular vent placement are accomplished, aortic cross clamp application is performed with a combination of antegrade and retrograde cardioplegia administration. Careful attention to the administration is imperative to avoid myocardial ischemia and postoperative dysfunction. Prompt cardiac arrest is anticipated and cardioplegia readministration is employed at appropriate time intervals which are largely dependent on the surgical team. Aortic transection slightly above the level of the commissures is performed with special care to identify the respective orifices of the coronary arteries. Frequently, the origin of the coronary arteries is not always in the center of the sinus of Valsalva. Important anomalies include intramural coronaries, high take off (above the commissures), and single coronary arteries. Deliberate aortic transection taking time to identify the coronary orifices will avoid potential complications. Coronary artery buttons are dissected and mobilized in preparation for transfer. Aortic leaflets are resected to avoid interference with the mechanical valve. Complications of composite aortic valve-ascending aortic graft placement include bleeding from the implantation sutures, the coronary button sites, and the distal aortic anastomosis. Coronary artery kinking, twisting, and malrotation can occur and have been discussed in association with repair of transposition of the great

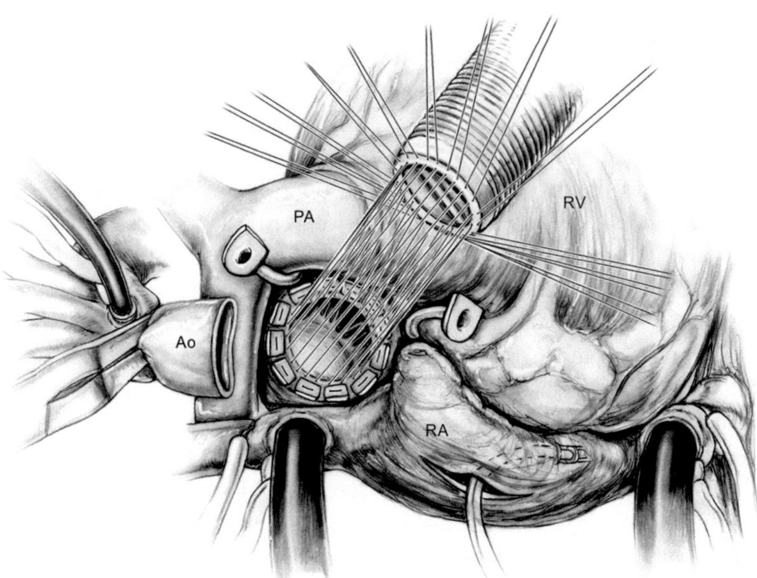

Fig. 23 Shows how pledgeted sutures are placed at 5–8 mm intervals with special care not to allow "gaps" which will cause postoperative bleeding. The sutures are placed in corresponding locations in the sewing ring of a composite valve-Dacron graft. After the sutures are tied and the valved conduit is seated, holes are made in the graft corresponding to the anticipated location for reimplantation of the coronary arteries. *Ao* aorta, *PA* pulmonary artery, *RA* right atrium, *RV* right ventricle. (With permission Martin and Mavroudis 2020)

Fig. 24 Demonstrates the reconstructed proximal neoaorta in preparation for reanastomosis to the ascending aorta. *Ao* aorta, *PA* pulmonary artery, *RA* right atrium, *RV* right ventricle. (With permission Martin and Mavroudis 2020)

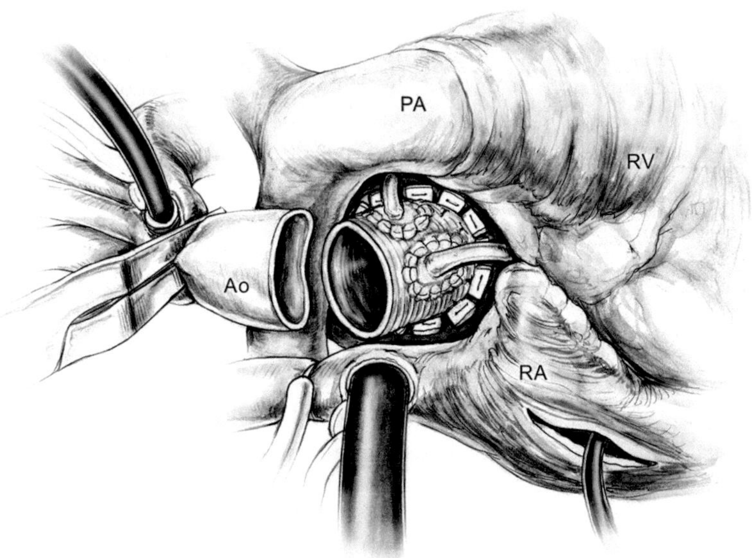

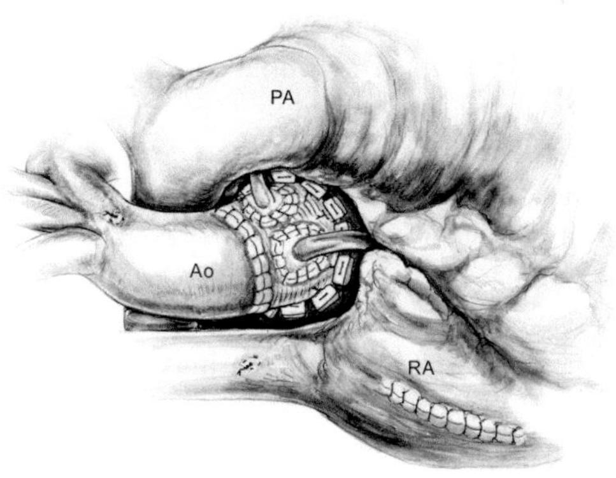

Fig. 25 Shows the completed repair. Unlike the Florida Sleeve and David operations which require an additional interposition between the proximal neoaorta and the distal aorta, the Bentall procedure does not require complex implantation and suspension of the proximal aorta and its commissures. Therefore, after the seating and coronary artery reimplantation, the graft can be measured to size and anastomosed to the ascending aorta or transverse arch as necessary. *Ao* aorta, *PA* pulmonary artery, *RA* right atrium. (With permission Martin and Mavroudis 2020)

arteries (chapter "Complications Associated with Repair of Transposition of the Great Arteries and Associated Lesion"). It is wise to place a tacking suture on the superior portion of the coronary button for proper alignment during the transfer. In addition, low setting electrocautery dissection should be judiciously used for mobilization to prevent unwanted coronary artery injury. In the event of considerable distance between the coronary orifice and the selected site on the graft, an interposition PTFE graft can be considered. This decision is made when the aortic implantation has been performed and the hole in the ascending graft has been made. Trying to readjust the resultant anatomic configuration will require considerably more cross clamp time making an interposition graft for the coronary artery more acceptable. Post repair TEE will confirm proper valve excursions and coaptation free of interference from errant sutures or unresected valve tissue. Any unwanted hemodynamic consequences should trigger a return to cardiopulmonary bypass, aortic cross clamping, and cardioplegic arrest to explore, identify, and repair any problems.

2 Debranching Techniques for Transverse Arch and Descending Aortic Dissections

As previously noted, aortic aneurysms or dissections in patients with congenital heart disease are generally seen in those individuals who have connective tissue disorders such as Marfan syndrome, Loeys-Dietz syndrome or Ehlers-Danlos syndrome. They can occur in childhood, adolescence, and young adults. Patients who exhibit significant symptoms and radiologic findings that threaten life, the cerebral circulation, aortic valve function, and coronary perfusion, should be considered for immediate repair (Srivastava and Bhan 2019). In particular dissecting aneurysms involving the transverse arch and descending aorta are the most vexing. Management schemes require careful perioperative planning, accurate surgical execution, and comprehensive postoperative management for optimal outcomes.

As noted, aortic arch repair is one of the most complex procedures with considerable rates of complications and mortality (Srivastava and Bhan 2019). In 1975, Randall B. Griepp introduced aortic arch repair using hypothermic circulatory arrest (Griepp et al. 1975). Since then, the introduction of antegrade and retrograde perfusion methods, improved surgical techniques, and innovative grafts, has helped to improve outcomes. However, mortality and complications rates remained high compared with other cardiac operations. Further developments concentrated on less invasive approaches resulting in endovascular aortic repair (TEVAR) with debranching of supra-aortic vessels as well as the frozen elephant trunk (Stepanenko et al. 2022; Papakonstantinou et al. 2018; Ramlawi and Reardon 2011; Smith et al. 2019; Chen et al. 2022; Chivasso et al. 2021; Redaelli et al. 2020; Çekmecelioğlu et al. 2020). At the present time, it is not clear whether the open procedure or the less invasive techniques are preferred. While many believe that the traditional open technique is the gold standard, others suggest that hybrid techniques such as the frozen elephant trunk and aortic arch vessel debranching are more appropriate procedures for high-risk patients whose comorbidities may contraindicate cardiopulmonary bypass and longer operative times required for traditional repair. No randomized trials have been performed to settle the equipoise that exists between the two approaches in normal or high-risk patients.

Aside from quoting the literature as to the ongoing developments to optimize therapy for patients with transverse arch pathologies, the chapter will not review all the extant issues that have been cited and offer any settled recommendations. Rather, this section of debranching techniques for aortic arch aneurysms will concentrate on the reparative procedure and the potential complications that should be avoided during the operation.

The initial consideration is to perform central and/or peripheral cannulation (femoral or axillary arteries) with a bifurcated arterial system that will allow regional perfusion during the debranching procedure. Oftentimes, some aortic root operation is performed as the initial part of the operation to repair the aortic arch pathology. This is generally performed during the cooling phase of cardiopulmonary bypass, using one of the aortic valve sparing operations (Florida Sleeve/David operation) or a Bentall operation in the event that the aortic valve cannot be preserved. The transverse arch reconstruction follows the proximal aortic root operation employing a series of regional perfusion maneuvers that are aimed at limiting the patient's exposure to deep hypothermia and circulatory arrest. Specialized grafts have been developed to facilitate arch reconstruction and are noted in the following description of the procedure.

3 Procedure

The patient is positioned in a comfortable supine position with groin access which will allow for central and/or peripheral cannulation. In general, both upper extremity and lower extremity arterial monitoring is established along with cerebrovascular monitoring. The arterial perfusion cannulation system is bifurcated in a "Y" configuration so that one arm of the "Y" will act as systemic perfusion and the other portion of the "Y" will function as regional cerebral perfusion.

Cardiac exposure is by median sternotomy and aorto-atrial or bicaval cardiopulmonary bypass which is commenced using one arm of the arterial "Y" perfusion system. Left ventricular venting through the right superior pulmonary vein is established with cooling to 18 °C. During the cooling stage of the operation, those patients with acquired aortic regurgitation will require immediate attention when ventricular fibrillation occurs. Timely aortic cross-clamping and retrograde cardioplegia will prevent left ventricular distention while initiating myocardial preservation for a valve sparing or valve replacement strategy, whichever is appropriate. The proximal aortic reconstruction can proceed in the usual fashion and with the proper myocardial preservation techniques as outlined in the previous parts of this chapter. Once the proximal part of the repair is concluded, preparations can be made for the debranching procedure.

When the core temperature reaches 18 °C, the patient is placed in a Trendelenburg position and circulatory arrest is induced. The Trendelenburg position is important to prevent complete cerebral vascular exsanguination which will help to avoid unwanted air embolism during the operation. The aortic cross-clamp is removed; the arterial cannula is removed; and the aorta is transected just upstream of the brachiocephalic artery. In some cases when the left brachiocephalic artery is involved in the dissection, the aorta can be transected downstream of the artery. This maneuver is more easily performed when the patient is young, and mobilization is easier. In this series of illustrations, the left subclavian artery is maintained connected to the descending aorta. In order to facilitate exposure and attention to the brachiocephalic arteries, the ascending portion of the transected aorta is retracted inferiorly to remove it from the field. The arch button is then created by sharp and electrocautery dissection with special care to perform hemostatic suturing of transected small arteries as needed. In most cases, the button will include the brachiocephalic artery together with the left common carotid artery. As discussed above, the left subclavian artery remains connected to the descending aorta. This is performed for two reasons: (1) mobilizing the left subclavian artery in adults can be hazardous and cause bleeding complications, as well as injury to the recurrent laryngeal nerve and (2) including the left subclavian artery in the arterial button will result in a more distal aortic anastomosis into the left thoracic cavity away from the surgeon thereby introducing more complexity to the procedure. Figure 26 illustrates the surgeon's view of the result of aneurysm resection and clarification of what will become necessary for the eventual aortic reconstruction.

A Vascutek® Gelweave™ Trifurcate arch graft is chosen for the arch reconstruction. In most cases for adults, a 14-mm graft is used with two 10 mm side arm branches. (Other sizes are available as well such as a 12 mm, 8 mm, 8 mm graft). Figure 27 shows how the graft is prepared by oversewing one of the side-arm grafts while using the other as the arterial cannulation site. The remaining step is to anastomose the beveled graft to the brachiocephalic vessels; the idea being that this reconstruction will result in regional perfusion to the cerebral vessels and brain thereby limiting the ischemic period. While it is easy to write that, "all the air maneuvers are then accomplished", it is more important to denotate what they actually are and how to prevent unwanted cerebral air embolism. Figure 27 shows the graft to brachiocephalic anastomosis in progress. The arterial catheter is shown to be filled, but there is a clamp upstream to the catheter to prevent air from tracking up the catheter. During the air removal maneuvers air must be purged from the arterial catheter, from the distal graft to brachiocephalic anastomosis, and from the proximal graft where the occlusive clamp is positioned. This is best per-

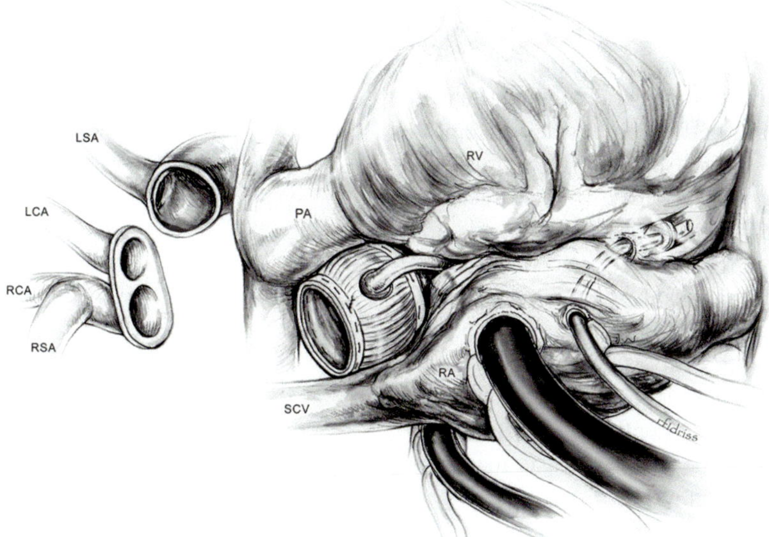

Fig. 26 Deep hypothermia, circulatory arrest, and retrograde cardioplegic arrest have been established. The figure shows isolation of the two brachiocephalic arteries in one island as a large aortic button. No clamps or snuggers are placed on the distal arteries. The descending aorta with the left subclavian connection is shown open without a clamp as well. The proximal Florida Sleeve operation has been completed in advance of the debranching procedure. *LCA* left coronary artery, *LSA* left subclavian artery, *PA* pulmonary artery, *RA* right atrium, *RCA* right coronary artery, *RSA* right subclavian artery, *RV* right ventricle, *SCV* superior caval vein. (With permission Martin and Mavroudis 2020)

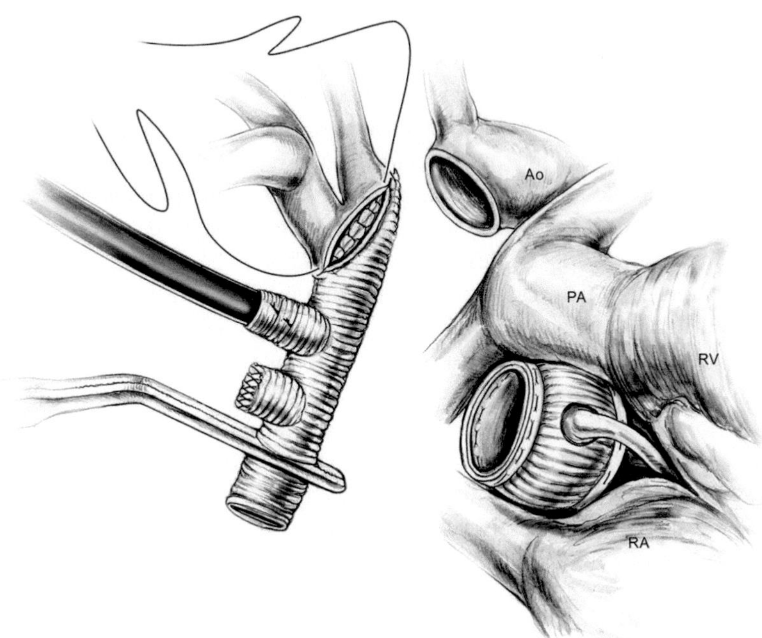

Fig. 27 The anastomosis of the brachiocephalic button to the beveled end of the 14 mm arm of the Vascutek graft is shown being performed during a short period of circulatory arrest. A 3/8″ plastic connector is attached to one of the branched 10 mm side arms which will serve as the arterial regional perfusion arm of the "Y" connection. *Ao* aorta, *PA* pulmonary artery, *RA* right atrium, *RV* right ventricle. (With permission Martin and Mavroudis 2020)

formed with vigorous arterial catheter purging to include exit from the proximal graft and the distal graft before the anastomosis is completed. A few concentrated moments to perform this important maneuver will help to prevent cerebral air embolism. Figure 28 illustrates the completed anastomotic reconstruction to establish regional cerebral perfusion. Besides air embolism, the surgeon will be wise to perform the anastomoses conscientiously to avoid bleeding by proper spacing of the suture technique and thorough inspection for bleeding points before the rest of the aortic reconstruction is continued. Figure 29 shows the established regional perfusion and the aortic reconstruction in progress. As noted in the figure legend, the other arterial cannula of the "Y" configuration has been placed into the aortic graft which is manufactured with a side arm to allow distal aortic perfusion. The principles of aortic suturing and air purging maneuvers are the same. Once the arterial catheter is placed and the distal aortic anastomosis is completed, full systemic perfusion can be established enroute to proximal aortic reconstruction which is partially shown in

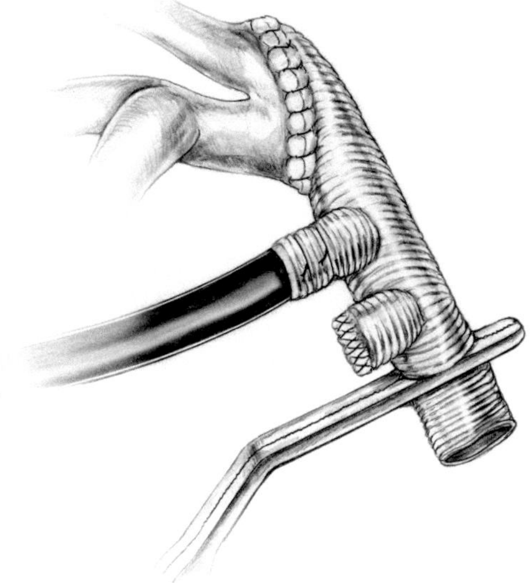

Fig. 28 Shows the completed brachiocephalic button to graft anastomosis and arterial line connection to the branched 10 mm graft. All the air maneuvers are performed as a vascular clamp is placed across the proximal 14 mm graft thereby establishing regional perfusion. This period of circulatory arrest should not exceed 10–15 min to perform the anastomosis, clear the air from the circuit, and establish regional flow at 10–15 cc/kg/min. (With permission Martin and Mavroudis 2020)

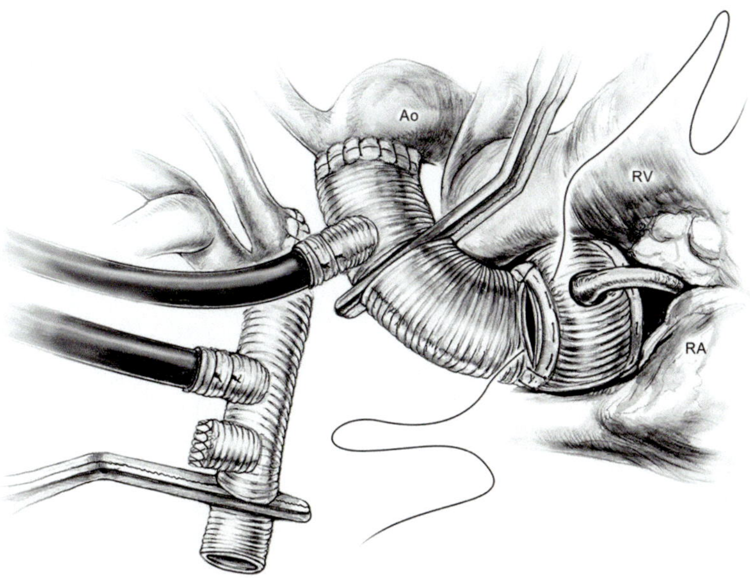

Fig. 29 A straight graft with a side arm is then chosen for the anastomosis between the proximal aortic root reconstruction and the descending aorta. The size of the graft ranges from 24 to 30 mm depending on the size of the patient and the caliber of the proximal aortic reconstruction. The side arm graft is connected to the other arm of the "Y" extension from the arterial line. After appropriate de-airing maneuvers, antegrade perfusion to the body is reestablished by clamping the graft as shown in Fig. 26. At this point, the patient can be rewarmed. *Ao* aorta, *RA* right atrium, *RV* right ventricle. (With permission Martin and Mavroudis 2020)

Fig. 30. The final stages of the operation require the important steps to attach the brachiocephalic graft to the ascending aortic graft. One might be tempted to remove the aortic cross clamp and establish coronary perfusion while using a side-biting clamp to perform the brachiocephalic to ascending graft anastomosis. The dangers of placing a side-biting clamp between the ascending aortic cannula and the proximal aortic anastomosis are too much to consider. First of all, the anastomosis will require a large hole in the ascending graft that will challenge placing a side-biting clamp. Furthermore, placing the clamp with enough room to complete the anastomosis will endanger the aortic cannula and the suture line of the graft to proximal neoaorta. In vernacular terms, it is not worth the effort. Better to leave the aortic cross-clamp in place, perform the open brachiocephalic graft to ascending graft anastomosis, and then release the cross-clamp after all the comprehensive air maneuvers have been performed. Suture line inspection for bleeding can then be performed. Figure 31 shows the completed neoaortic reconstruction which will allow rewarming and separation from cardiopulmonary bypass.

Oftentimes in these patients, aortic dissections or aneurysms can originate at the distal aortic anastomosis. These situations can be managed by endovascular graft techniques that will allow the endovascular graft to be attached to the existing transverse arch graft and engage the length of the aortic aneurysm. Clearly, this will result in entrapment of the left subclavian artery which can be managed by a localized graft between the left carotid and left subclavian arteries (Chadnick and Singh 2021). There have been recent ongoing clinical trials that have determined that branched endografts can be employed for distal dissections which will preserve subclavian artery perfusion by using a side arm projection into the orifice of the subclavian artery (Riesenman et al. 2007) (Fig. 32). Leaking endovascular grafts however have been described (Beeba 1996), which will require long term evaluation. Complications associated with descending thoracic aortic dissection will be considered in the next section.

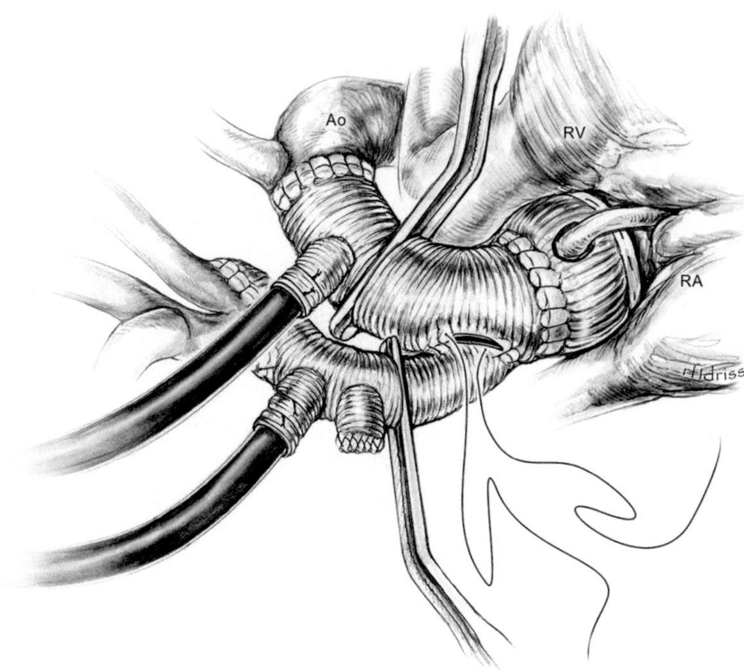

Fig. 30 The anastomosis between the aortic root reconstruction and the proximal straight graft is now performed. Once this is accomplished, the proximal portion of the 14 mm graft is anastomosed to the side of the ascending straight graft as shown in the figure. After appropriate de-airing maneuvers, all clamps are removed thereby reestablishing coronary perfusion. Hemostasis is optimized during the rewarming period. *Ao* aorta, *RA* right atrium, *RV* right ventricle. (With permission Martin and Mavroudis 2020)

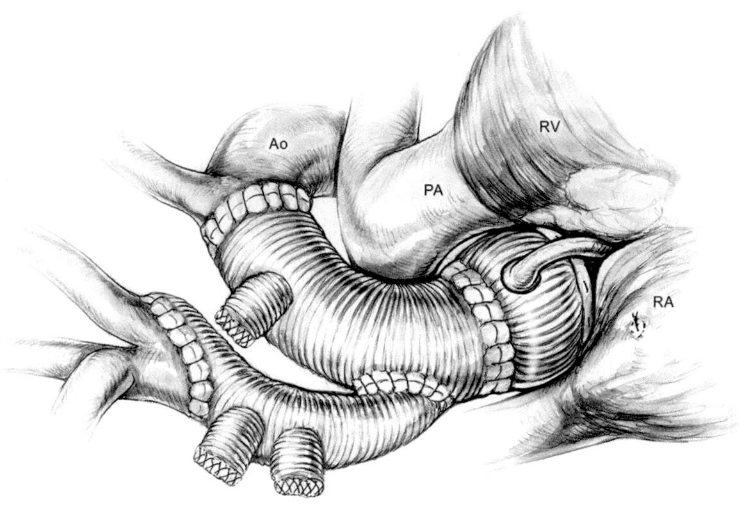

Fig. 31 Shows the completed repair after separation from cardiopulmonary bypass. *Ao* aorta, *PA* pulmonary artery, *RA* right atrium, *RV* right ventricle. (With permission Martin and Mavroudis 2020)

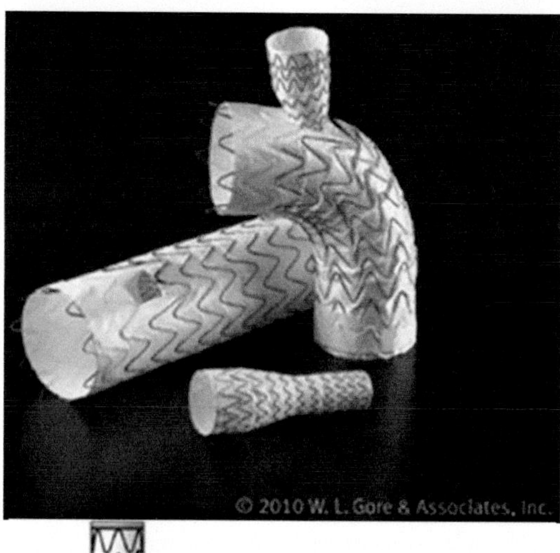

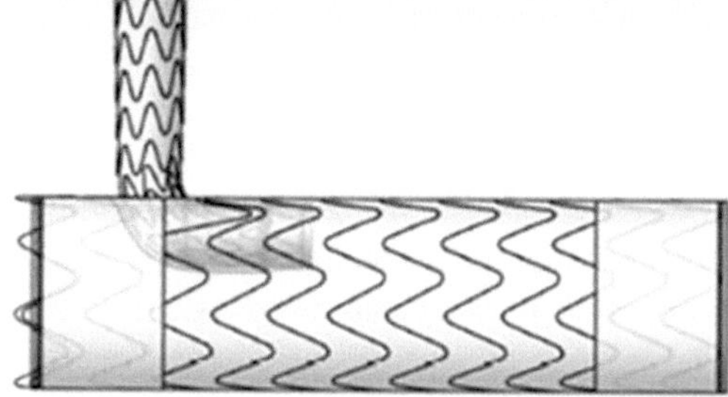

Fig. 32 As is so frequently the case, aortic dissections or aneurysms originating at the distal aortic anastomosis can occur in these patients. These conditions oftentimes can be managed by endovascular graft techniques that will join the existing transverse arch graft to the new descending endograft. This will result in obligatory left subclavian artery entrapment which can be managed by a localized graft between the left carotid and left subclavian arteries. Recent ongoing clinical trials however have shown that branched endografts can be used for distal dissections which will preserve subclavian artery perfusion using a side arm projection into the orifice of the subclavian artery. (With permission Martin and Mavroudis 2020)

4 Complications Associated with Repair of Descending Thoracic Aneurysm by Open and Transcatheter Techniques

4.1 Introduction and Anatomic Considerations

This chapter largely considers aneurysmal disease in young patients which is mostly caused by aortopathies and genetic tissue disorders. A review of complications associated with both open and transcatheter techniques by Zachary Chadnick and Kuldeep Singh which was published on April 28th, 2021 is extraordinarily comprehensive and is paraphrased extensively in this section involving descending thoracic aneurysms (Chadnick and Singh 2021).

Repair of descending aortic dissecting aneurysms is rather complex and is not associated with "one size fits all" solutions. For instance, the repair of a Type I ascending aortic dissection has a limited number of operative interventions which have been noted in this chapter. However, complications associated with open or endovascular repair of descending thoracic dissections and saccular aneurysms are highly dependent on the location, the extent of dissection especially to the aortic bifurcation, and presenting circumstances. This is not a "one size fits all" set of therapeutic interventions owing to the application of endovascular techniques, open techniques, and hybrid techniques which will be discussed.

Thoracic aneurysms are rarer than abdominal aneurysms in the adult population but tend to be more common in children and young adults due to the prevalence of dissection (Hiratzka et al. 2010). In general, endovascular repair of the thoracic aorta (TEVAR), when indicated and when possible, has fewer complications and associated morbidities than open repair. Multiple reports have registered mortality rates between 1.9% and 3.1% (Hiratzka et al. 2010; Schanzer et al. 2011; Howell et al. 2001; Orandi et al. 2009) with morbidity rates as low as 9% (Hess Jr et al. 2009). During the development of TEVAR, indications for open vs. endovascular are often unclear, especially in young patients leading experienced centers to take an individualized approach while considering many factors. This thoughtful approach led to hybrid techniques which feature a combination of open and endovascular methods (Hiratzka et al. 2010; Coady et al. 1999; Chung et al. 2010; Prinssen et al. 2004).

When considering the application of endovascular repair, anatomic landing zones should be considered. The thoracic aorta is divided into 4 landing zones (0–4) which defines the need for

Table 1 Thoracic aortic landing zones

Zone 0	Proximal to the origin of the brachiocephalic artery
Zone 1	Distal to the brachiocephalic but proximal to the left common carotid
Zone 2	Distal to the left common carotid but proximal to the left subclavian
Zone 3	Less than 2 cm from the left subclavian without coverage
Zone 4	More than 2 cm distal to the left subclavian but within the proximal half of the thoracic aorta

Reprinted with permission from Chadnick and Singh (2021)

aortic debranching and the problems of endovascular coverage as noted in Table 1.

There are a number of advantages of endovascular aneurysm repair, namely, (1) it avoids sternotomy and thoracotomy, (2) cardiopulmonary bypass and aortic cross-clamping are not necessary, and (3) postprocedural problems of respiratory dependency and operative pain are clearly improved. Authors have noted that endovascular repair is preferred for most descending aortic aneurysms except for patients with genetic connective tissue disorders which occur in younger age groups and are mostly caused by dissections (Milewicz et al. 2005; Pepin et al. 2000; Booher and Eagle 2011). In addition, TEVAR can result in conversion to open repair in conditions of endovascular leaks, the threat of spinal ischemia due to large spinal collateral arteries, and late rupture.

5 Complications Related to Endovascular Graft Placement

There are various graft devices available for thoracic aortic aneurysms each with their own advantages and disadvantages. Those grafts that are flexible are associated with favorable adaptability to aneurysm configuration. Others note that fully supported endografts are more resistant to kinking and thrombosis over time. In general, the more complex graft is, the more that it is associated with complications. In particular, an important risk of TEVAR is the entrapment of the left subclavian artery (Patterson et al. 2014). In many cases, subclavian artery entrapment is tolerated without sequelae or complications. In some cases, however, symptoms relating to subclavian artery coverage can include incapacitating arm pain, hand ischemia, and upper extremity exercise intolerance. Others may not tolerate coverage especially in those patients with a dominant left vertebral system, hypoplastic right vertebral artery, patent left internal thoracic artery after CABG, functioning left upper extremity dialysis AV-fistula or an incomplete Circle of Willis are at high risk of symptoms including stroke and paraplegia. Planned subclavian entrapment for aneurysm repair in these patients should be preceded by left carotid to subclavian bypass (Riesenman et al. 2007; Klocker et al. 2014; Maldonado et al. 2013).

When the dissection is extensive and endovascular procedures are contemplated, renal and visceral vessels must be considered. In cases where renal arteries or superior mesenteric artery are involved, a fenestrated or branched graft should be used if at all possible (Schanzer et al. 2011; Ricotta and Oderich 2008; Blankensteijn et al. 2005; Simonte et al. 2017). Alternatively, a hybrid procedure can be performed to restore adequate blood flow using

debranching, reimplantation, bypass techniques, and evaluation of the circulation for collateral flow (O'Callaghan et al. 2014; Leon et al. 2009).

6 Nongraft Related Complications

Placement of endovascular grafts are usually performed through the femoral vessels that require large bore sheaths with separate access for arteriography. Depending on patient age, complications associated with catheter placement can result in vessel disruption (especially the iliac artery). These complications can be mitigated by direct vascular exposure for sheath placement and creation of an iliac conduit. There is always a risk of delayed neurologic and vascular complications, as well as embolism during graft placement or from retrograde dissection (Coady et al. 1999; Klocker et al. 2014; Eggebrecht et al. 2009). It is for these aforementioned reasons that patients are monitored in an intensive care unit before discharge from the hospital (Najibi et al. 2002; Cheung 2010; Acher and Wynn 2009).

7 Ischemic and Neurologic Complications

As in the repair of coarctation of the aorta, devastating complications of descending thoracic aortic aneurysm repair are paresis and paraplegia. These consequences relate to the extent of aortic involvement and can occur along any aortic segment. The estimated incidence is between 8% and 30%. Spinal cord ischemia is less for endovascular repair registering at a rate of 3%–11% according to literature reports (Patterson et al. 2014; Acher and Wynn 2009; Connolly 1998; Czerny et al. 2012; Buth et al. 2007). In general, spinal cord ischemia and symptoms relating thereto occur at a mean onset time of 10.6 hours after repair (Maldonado et al. 2013).

To consider the origin of cord ischemia in anatomic terms and situational perspective, it is important to review the major blood supply to the spinal cord. As Chadnick and Singh (Chadnick and Singh 2021) note,

> There are three major blood supplies to the spinal cord, the vertebral arteries in the neck, the anterior spinal artery and the two posterior spinal arteries that anastomose distally at the conus medularis. The anterior spinal artery supplies the anterior two-thirds. The thoracic spinal cord is especially dependent on radicular contributions to the anterior spinal artery, namely the Artery of Adamkiewicz between T9-T12. There are reserves with collateral circulation however as more of the arterial system is disturbed the higher the likelihood of injury. If able to limit the disruption to 8 or fewer segments, then the risk of paresis and paraplegia are low. Crawford Type II aneurysms have the highest risk. (Chadnick and Singh 2021)

Spinal cord safety measures during repair of descending thoracic aortic aneurysms have been implemented in both open and endovascular repairs to moderate risks. The extent of coverage with either endovascular or open techniques is the highest associated risk factor for paralysis (Greenberg et al. 2008; Zoli et al. 2010). In addition, hypotension, procedural duration, need for reimplantation and renal insufficiency are all associated risk factors (Acher and Wynn 2009; Czerny et al. 2012; Zoli et al. 2010). Risk of paraplegia can be mitigated with cerebrospinal fluid drainage using a lumbar drain (Zoli et al. 2010). Perioperative monitoring using spinal perfusion pressure is also recommended with an intrathecal pressure recommended to be ≤10 mmHg (Takayama and Borger 2015; Di Luozzo 2013). Of note, reimplantation of lower intercostal arteries (T8–T12) is associated with decreased risk of neurologic deficits. Ischemic complications associated with TEVAR can also occur in the extremities, visceral organs, and cerebrovascular system due to emboli to the brain (Svensson et al. 2008).

Fortunately, complications can be delayed, and patients should be monitored for occurrence. CT scan imaging is employed for surveillance and is generally performed at 1-, 6-, and 12-months postoperatively and annually thereafter. Reintervention is not uncommon, and evidence of endovascular leaks will oftentimes require prompt attention (Hiratzka et al. 2010; Prinssen et al. 2004; Svensson et al. 2008; Nordon et al. 2010). Late clinical outcomes are related to the natural history of the disease process and graft choice. Late endovascular leaks are associated with device migration (1%–3% over a 1-year period associated with oversized grafts), collapse, or infolding (occurring in younger patients with proximal angulation) (Bavaria et al. 2007; Ultee et al. 2016). Symptoms can occur and are caused by aortic occlusion and require timely attention and intervention. Another problem which has been reported (Matsumura et al. 2008; Makaroun et al. 2008; Scali et al. 2014; Szeto et al. 2013) relates to endovascular device separation, which fortunately, can be managed by secondary intervention using endovascular techniques (Perek et al. 2014; Shukla et al. 2011). In general, secondary endovascular intervention due to the accumulated experience ranges from 3.6% to 24%. As noted, important complications include an overall mortality of 4% due to aneurysmal rupture, stent erosion into the esophagus, bleeding and arterial injury (Dake et al. 1998). Late endovascular complications occur in 38% of patients and are due to malposition, endovascular leaks, dissection, distal embolization, gut ischemia, and infection. Furthermore, aortobronchial and aortopulmonary fistulas can occur due to contained endovascular leaks which can lead to lethal hemoptysis.

8 Complications Relating to Open Descending Aortic Aneurysm Repair

There is no doubt that the successful introduction of endovascular techniques has had a positive influence on the treatment of descending thoracic aortic aneurysms as noted in the previous section. However, there are still many remaining indications for open techniques which have also been noted. Certainly, surgery is the standard of care for ascending aneurysms >5.5 cm, >4.5 cm with associated genetic anomalies (>4.2 cm with patients with Loeys-Dietz Syndrome), and rapid expansion. Patient selection, especially for patients with descending thoracic aortic aneurysms, is an important factor, since many of the required operations involve cardiopulmonary bypass, hypothermic circulatory arrest, and complications thereto pertaining (Hiratzka et al. 2010; Cheung 2010). As noted, and as inferred, patients who are not candidates and do not meet anatomic criteria for endograft placement, will require open techniques.

As a matter of review, perioperative bleeding complications occur in 10% of patients who require emergent repair and 3% for those who had elective repair. Management of bleeding complications often results in shock, dilutional coagulopathy, and transfusion related complications. Moreover, bleeding complications can also occur in a delayed fashion which can result in hemothorax, drainage, and likely reintervention. The best prevention for such bleeding complications is conscientious surgical hemostasis, correction of inherent and acquired coagulation disorders, and use of local hemostatic agents (Hiratzka et al. 2010; Shapira et al. 1999; Achneck et al. 2007). Besides ischemic renal, visceral organ, and neurological injuries which have been discussed, other complications can occur as well. Excessive traction during the operation can result in peripheral nerve injuries which fortunately generally resolve with observation (Faure et al. 2015; Rayt et al. 2008). The recurrent laryngeal nerve is also at risk when the aneurysm takes origin at the level of the distal aortic arch which results in hoarseness and vocal cord paralysis. In addition, the phrenic nerve is at risk for injury and respiratory distress, especially in those cases where the dissection causes obliteration of para-aortic structures (Svensson et al. 2013). Furthermore, anastomotic pseudoaneurysm formation can occur especially in the presence of graft infection (Coscas et al. 2010).

As discussed, the types of operations that are used for the repair of descending thoracic aortic aneurysms are highly dependent on the extent, location, and associated risk factors. We will review the series of operations in a 13-year-old girl with Loeys-Dietz Syndrome who underwent valve-sparing ascending aortic arch replacement with brachiocephalic artery debranching (Florida Sleeve Operation), thoracoabdominal descending thoracic aortic replacement from the subclavian artery to the aortic bifurcation, and eventual thoracic exploration and lobectomy for hemoptysis due to graft-bronchial fistula. Between the ascending aortic arch repair and descending dissection repair, she underwent extensive spine repair for severe scoliosis.

Because of enlargement of the ascending aorta, she underwent the valve-sparing Florida Sleeve operation with debranching of the brachiocephalic vessels as noted in Figs. 1, 2, 3, 4, 5, 6, 7, 8, 9, 10, 11, 12, 13, 14, 15, 16, 17, 26, 27, 28, 29, 30 and 31 without complications. Because the operation was performed with regional perfusion and a minimum of circulatory arrest, comprehensive antegrade and retrograde cardioplegia, and conscientious hemostasis, the patient did well. The aortic valve function was maintained, the coronary arteries were appropriately enforced to prevent recurrent aneurysms, and heart function was preserved. After 8 weeks, she underwent successful spine surgery. Two months later, she presented with back pain and underwent CT scan which showed descending thoracic aortic dissection originating from the left subclavian artery which was not debranched at the original mediastinal corrective operation. After a period of medical blood pressure management, the aortic dissection extended making an emergency operation necessary.

The preoperative CT scan is shown in Fig. 33 which identifies the extent of the dissection and allowed the opportunity for careful planning of the open repair. The important preoperative anatomic and procedural considerations include peripheral cannulation techniques for cardiopulmonary bypass, downstream aortic clamping sequence, management of thoracic intercostal arteries for spinal cord preservation, and visceral arterial reimplantation. Further important considerations include careful spacing for the suture technique to avoid bleeding; constant assessment of perfusion techniques that limit circulatory arrest time, ensuring intercostal artery reimplantation for spinal perfusion, and avoidance of air embolism. Oftentimes, these preservation techniques require time to perform which can lead the impatient surgeon to cut corners and omit precautionary procedures to limit circulatory arrest time, cross-clamp time, and time on cardiopulmonary bypass. Prudence will determine how the surgeon will proceed in light of these considered tensions.

The operation begins with the proper positioning and preparation techniques. To begin with, a cerebrospinal fluid (CSF) drainage catheter is inserted which is associated with improved neurologic outcomes (Coselli et al. 2002). However, complications can occur with this management scheme and include headache (2.1%–3.0%), intracranial hemorrhage (0.3%–1.5%), CSF leak (0.9%–1.1%), epidural hematoma (0.4%–0.8%), and neurologic deficit (0.1%–0.6%) (Rong et al. 2018). These potential complications are noted not to avoid this management scheme, but rather to alert the operative team that complications can occur and will require diagnostic inquiries and supportive care. Perioperative CSF drainage in association with thoracoabdominal repair techniques is an important part of thoracoabdominal aneurysm management and should be considered. A transesophageal echocardiogram probe is placed and the patient is positioned for a modified right lateral decubitus position with the shoulders rotated to a 60° from horizontal and the hips rotated to a 30° from horizontal. This allows groin access for cannulation (Ouzounian et al. 2018). The left arm of the patient is suspended on an elevated arm board in a standard manner for a left thoracotomy incision. The patient is then

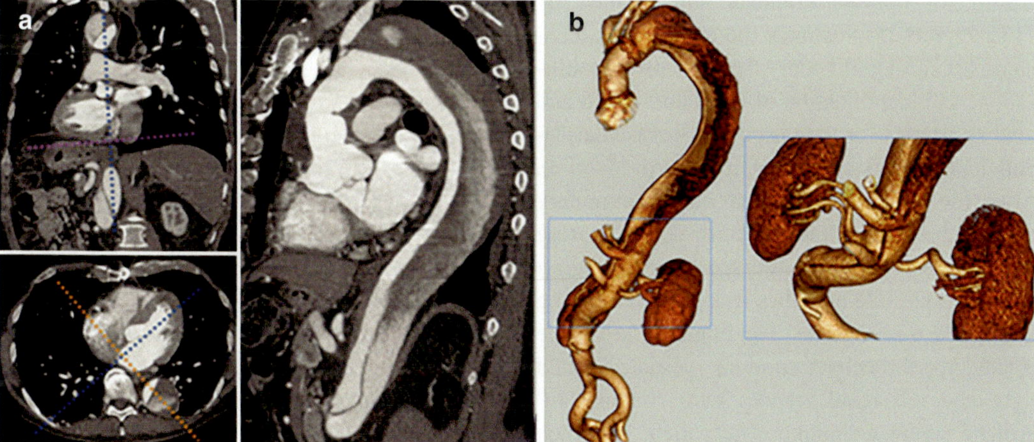

Fig. 33 Shows the CT scan which identifies the extent of descending thoracic aortic aneurysm 6 months after ascending aortic aneurysm repair with brachiocephalic debranching techniques. The scan shows the enlarged aneurysm. (With permission Diletta et al. 2022)

prepped and draped in the usual sterile fashion. A standard thoracoabdominal incision is performed and carried down sharply through the skin followed by electrocautery through the subcutaneous tissues, through all the muscles of the chest wall, into the paramedian space, and through the bed of the rectus muscle. The retroperitoneum is identified through the posterior rectus sheath and a standard retroperitoneal approach is undertaken. All viscera are mobilized off the diaphragm and the exposure is extended to the iliac vessels. The chest is entered above the 7th rib and the costochondral margin is divided. The diaphragm is divided in a circumferential radial fashion utilizing the GIA staplers (Ziganshin 2013). The chest is opened widely and retraction is performed with an Omni retractor. The thoracoabdominal dissecting aortic aneurysm can be identified and assessed as noted in Fig. 34. The ureter, not shown, is identified and preserved.

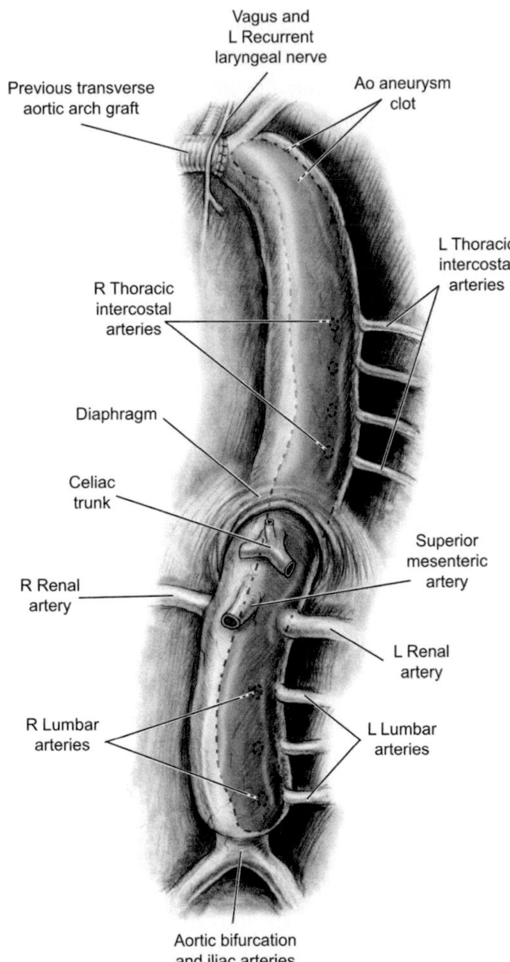

Fig. 34 Illustrates the thoracoabdominal exposure for extensive repair of the dissected descending thoracic and abdominal aorta. *Ao* aorta

Heparin is administrated. In this specific case, the operative report will be paraphrased to emphasize the particulars of the operation such as cannula size, type of grafts, and sequence of the operation. The patient had small vessels for peripheral cannulation necessitating common left iliac artery cannulation with a #15 Bio-Medicus arterial cannula and the iliac vein was cannulated with at #21 Bio-Medicus catheter. The venous catheter was advanced superiorly into the right atrium for optimal drainage and verified by TEE. Figure 35 illustrates the cannulation technique for cardiopulmonary bypass, aortic mobilization, and identification of large intercostal and lumbar arteries for the purpose of revascularization and preservation of spinal cord function. After the commencement of cardiopulmonary bypass, the patient was cooled to 20 °C. During the time of cooling, a thoracoabdominal graft with multiple side branches was created utilizing 8 mm and 6 mm grafts. The branch grafts were created for the celiac; superior mesenteric; and right and left renal arteries with running 4-0 Prolene suture technique. The patient was then placed in the Trendelenburg position and the mid-descending thoracic aorta was cross-clamped. Perfusion remained to the lower body. The descending thoracic was opened longitudinally towards the distal aortic arch. The distal aortic arch was resected with exposure to normal tissue past the original fenestration that caused the dissection. A 22 mm Dacron graft was chosen with a side arm graft to be used for regional perfusion. The graft was anastomosed to the underneath side of the aortic arch and into the orifice of the left subclavian artery. Once this was accomplished, the side arm was connected to a "Y" cannula from the arterial line and, after appropriately

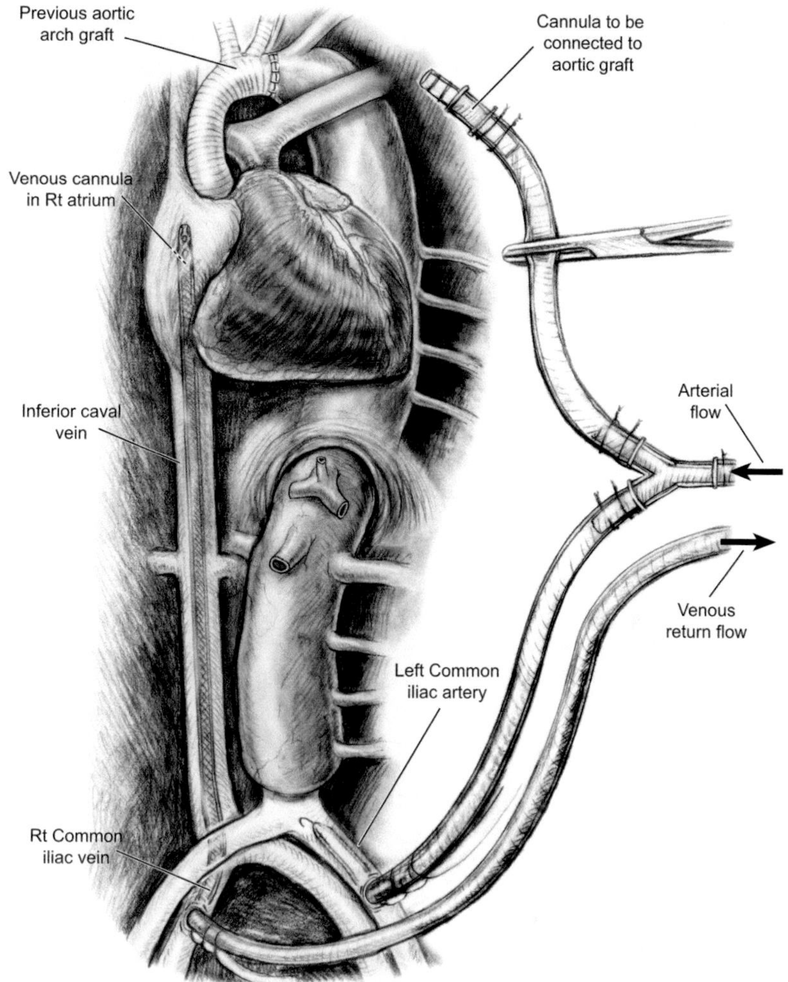

Fig. 35 Illustrates the cannulation technique for cardiopulmonary bypass and the mobilization maneuvers to safely expose the descending thoracic and abdominal aorta. *Rt* right

de-airing the arch and the graft, the graft was clamped and antegrade perfusion was reestablished through the "Y" graft as noted in Fig. 36. The iliac artery cannula "Y" was then clamped and the descending clamp was removed. The remainder of the aorta was opened from the diaphragm distally to the iliac arteries. The false lumen ended at the iliac arteries. All of the dissected septum was resected and each individual visceral vessel was identified as shown in Fig. 37. The 16 mm multi-branch graft was then cut to the appropriate length and anastomosed end-to-end to the distal aorta upstream to the level of the iliac origins utilizing a running 4-0 Prolene suture. This was then clamped and reperfusion to the lower body was reestablished. Each side branch was then anastomosed to the visceral vessel starting with the right renal artery, the superior mesenteric artery second, and the celiac artery third with end-to-end anastomoses sewing the end of the graft directly into the ostia of each of the visceral vessels using 3-0 Prolene suture. The left renal artery was buttoned down over the sidewall of the aorta and this was anastomosed end-to-end to the left renal Dacron graft utilizing running 4-0 Prolene suture. Each vessel was perfused as the

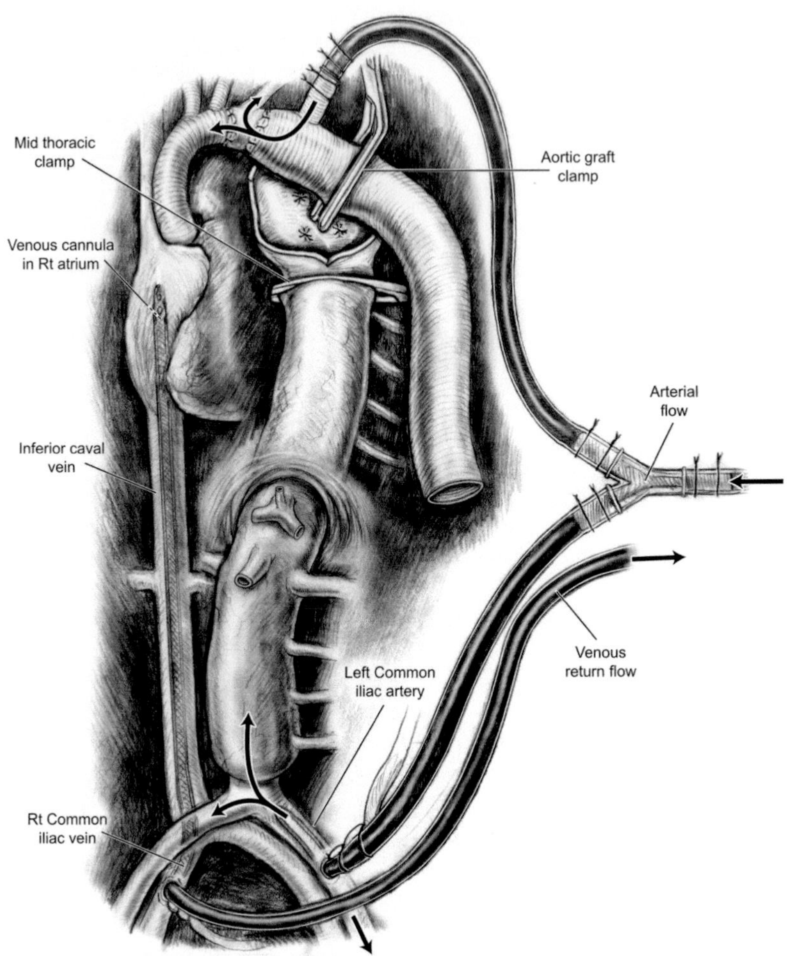

Fig. 36 Shows the regional perfusion to the brachiocephalic vessels after a brief period of deep hypothermic circulatory arrest and proximal anastomosis of the thoracic graft to the transverse arch. The regional perfusion is through a side branch of the graft as noted in the upper part of the figure. *Rt* right

anastomosis was completed by adjusting the cross-clamp. The 22 mm and 16 mm grafts were then cut to the appropriate length and anastomosed together. This was performed with running 3-0 Prolene (Fig. 38). A 10 mm Dacron graft which was anastomosed on the ventral portion of the proximal portion of the 22 mm graft was modified with a large slit on the back side of the graft and the left T-7 through T-11 intercostal arteries were anastomosed to the side of the Dacron graft with a running 3-0 Prolene suture. Once the visceral component was completed, we noted that there were large lumbar vessels. We then cut another slit in the 10 mm Dacron graft and anastomosed this to the sidewall of the aorta incorporating T-12 through L-4. The distal end of the 10 mm graft was then anastomosed end-to-side to the infrarenal 16 mm graft with a running 3-0 Prolene suture (Fig. 39). This was performed since there was too much distance between the right and left intercostals or lumbar vessels and this created too much of a possibility for a patch aneurysm. The origins of the right intercostal and lumbar arteries were therefore ligated. The patient was rewarmed to 36° and spontaneously returned to normal sinus rhythm. When full perfusion is engaged, bleeding points need to be assessed and controlled. In particular, the long suture line for the 10 mm graft supplying the intercostal and lumbar arteries tend to leak owing to the long running suture technique and the uneven aortic wall where the dissection occurred.

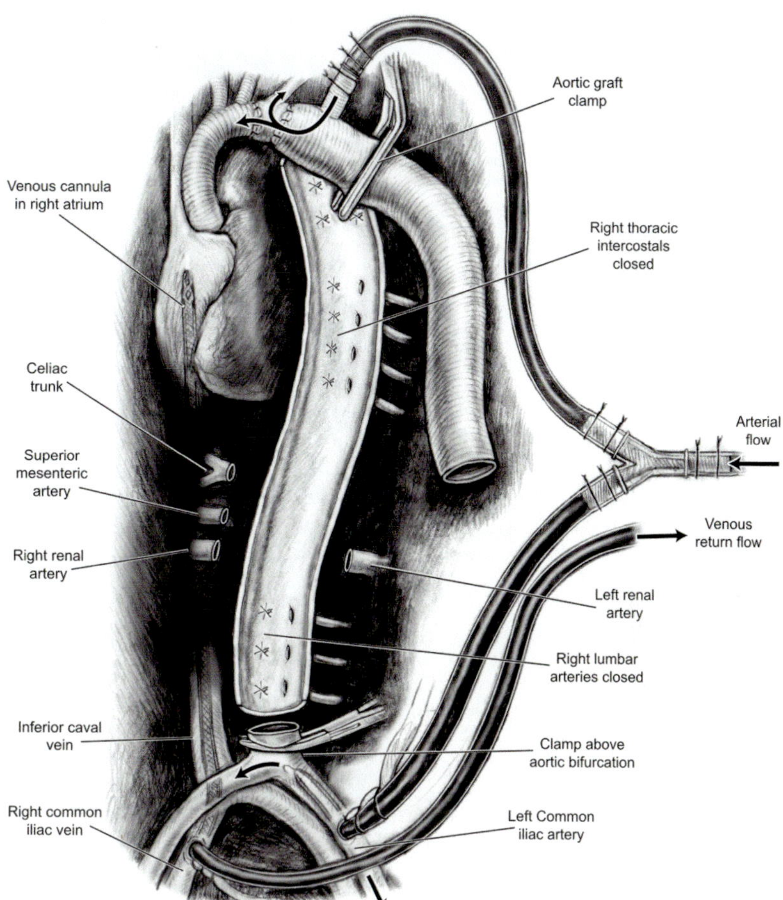

Fig. 37 Illustrates the completed proximal aortic anastomosis with perfusion through a side graft enabling regional perfusion to the brachiocephalic vessels and the lower extremities using bi-arterial cannulation. All the visceral vessels are exposed before the anastomoses. In addition, the right thoracic intercostal arteries and the right lumbar arteries are oversewn in anticipation of graft reperfusion to the intercostal and lumbar arteries

Under these circumstances, a nerve hook can be used to increase the tension of the suture line by gentle traction and tying the loop generated by traction to another well-placed suture as noted in Fig. 40. Other bleeding points need to be managed judiciously and conscientiously to limit the amount of bleeding that will eventually be managed by administration of clotting factors. The patient was ultimately weaned from cardiopulmonary bypass without difficulty. All cannulas were removed. Systemic heparinization was reversed with protamine. The cannulation sites were secure and there was adequate hemostasis. The chest was drained with two #24 Argyle chest tubes. The diaphragm was closed with running #2 Prolene suture, the abdomen was closed with running #1 looped PDS suture and the chest was closed with figure of 8 #2 Vicryl pericostal sutures.

The patient had an uncomplicated postoperative course without complications and was discharged on the 7th postoperative day.

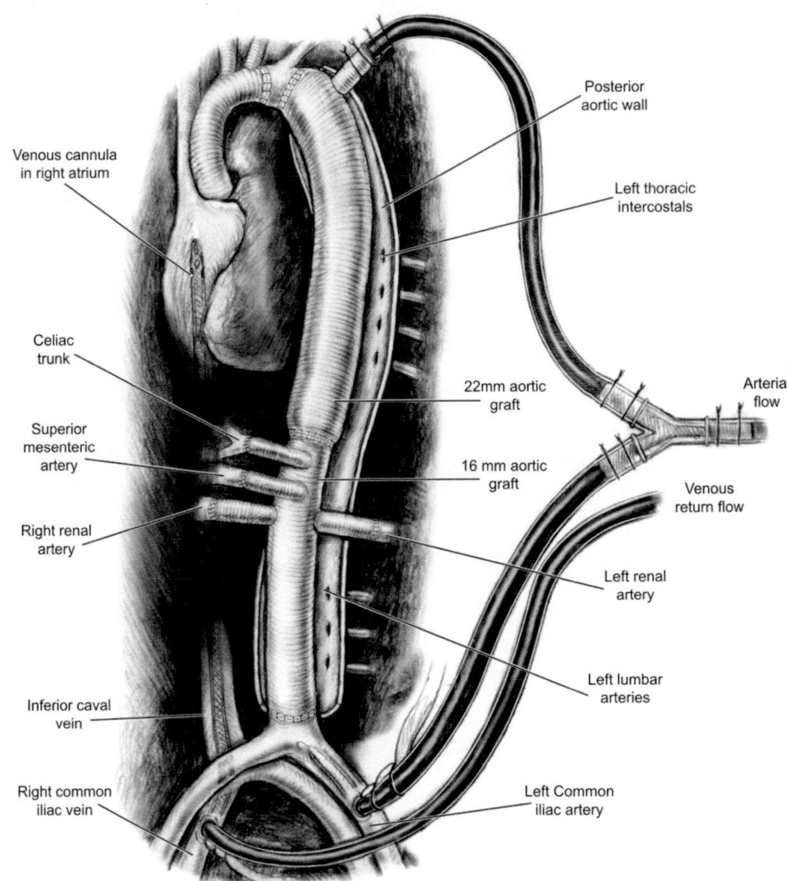

Fig. 38 Shows the operation mostly completed with the exception of the graft to the intercostals and the lumbar vessels. The abdominal graft was pre-arranged with the appropriately sized grafts to the celiac trunk, the superior mesenteric artery, and both renal arteries. The next phase of the operation is to connect the left intercostal and left lumbar arteries to an additional graft taking origin from the thoracic aortic graft

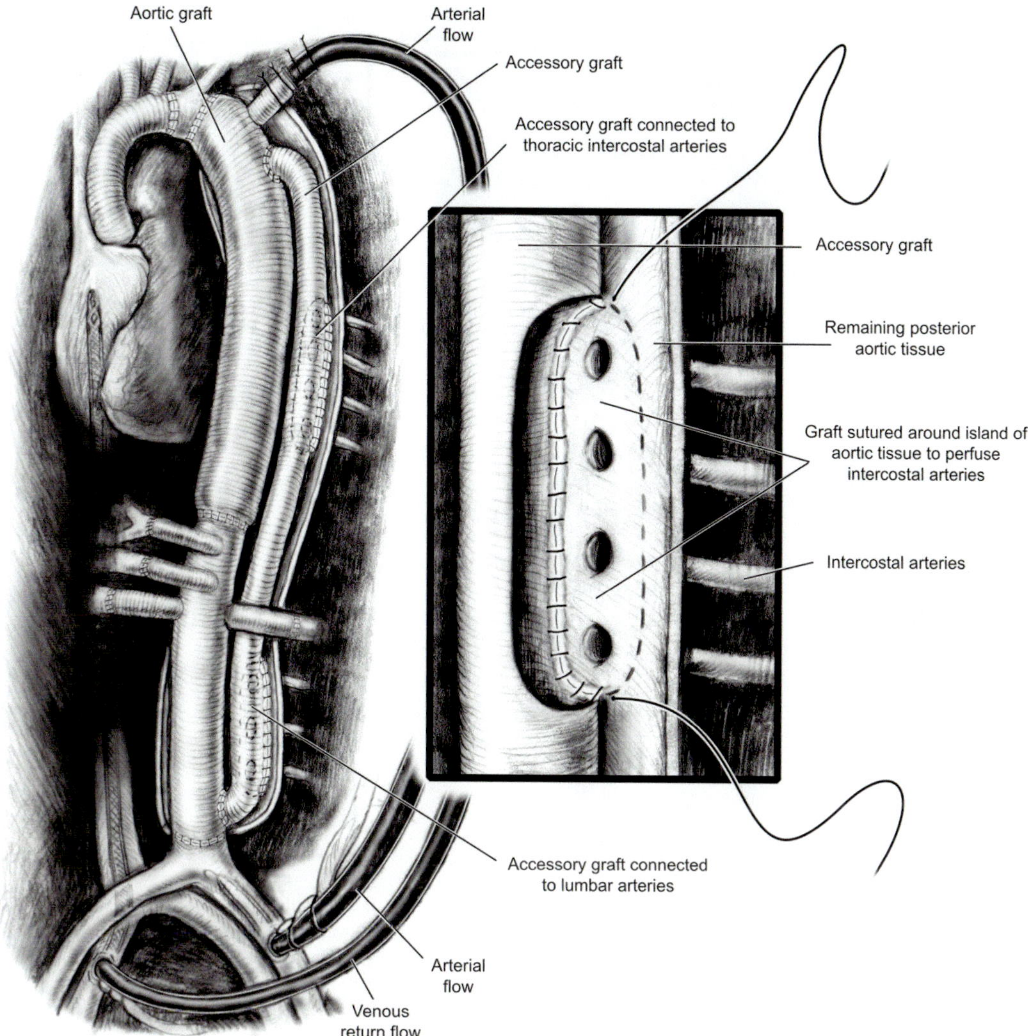

Fig. 39 Shows the entire operation completed including the graft to the intercostals and the lumbar arteries. The inset demonstrates the anastomotic technique that is used to sew the island of intercostal vessels to the graft

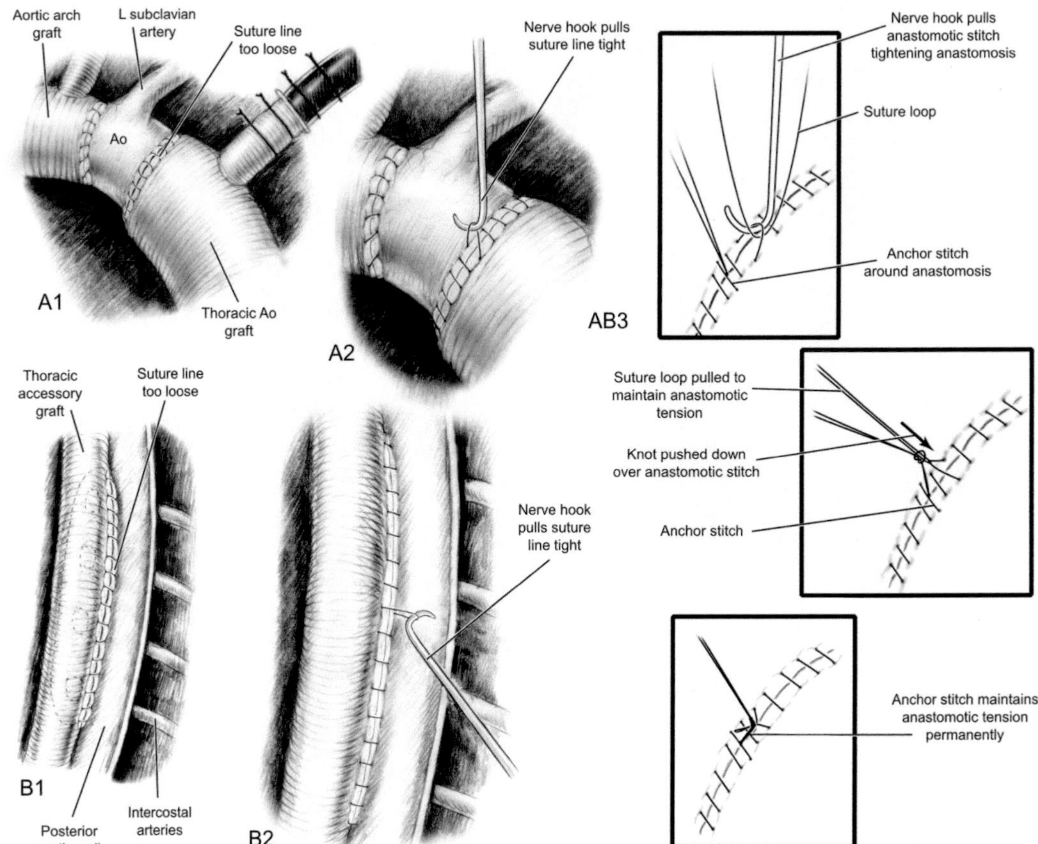

Fig. 40 Final reconstruction showing the tenting up of the suture to stop the bleeding and tying the loop to another suture. Figures A1 and B1show the loose suture line which can cause unwanted bleeding. Figures A2 and B2 demonstrate how the nerve hook can lasso the loose suture line and apply tension to stop the bleeding. Figure AB3 shows how another nearby suture can be placed through the anastomotic suture line while tying this suture to the lassoed anastomotic suture. This will result in anchoring and tightening of the loose suture line to stop the bleeding. *Ao* aorta

9 Postoperative Hemoptysis After Open Repair of Thoracoabdominal Aneurysm

The patient, relating to the previous description of open thoracoabdominal dissecting aneurysm repair developed postoperative recurrent hemoptysis which was thought to be due to left upper lobe injury secondary to the previous 8 mm side-arm graft from the 22 mm Dacron graft that was used for arterial perfusion during the aneurysm repair. Hemoptysis progressed and the patient required operative intervention. The MRI is shown in Fig. 41. The patient underwent a left thoracotomy where an injury site to the left upper lobe was identified from the 8 mm side-arm graft that was used for regional perfusion at the original thoracoabdominal aneurysm repair. The side-arm graft was rigid owing to two previously placed titanium clips which caused the lung injury. The clips were removed and the side-arm graft was tacked down to the larger Dacron graft keeping it relatively flat. Then a piece of Gore-Tex patch material was sutured over the exposed Daron in order to protect the lung. The injury site to the lung measured 8 mm and this was oversewn with a pledgeted 3-0 Prolene suture. After

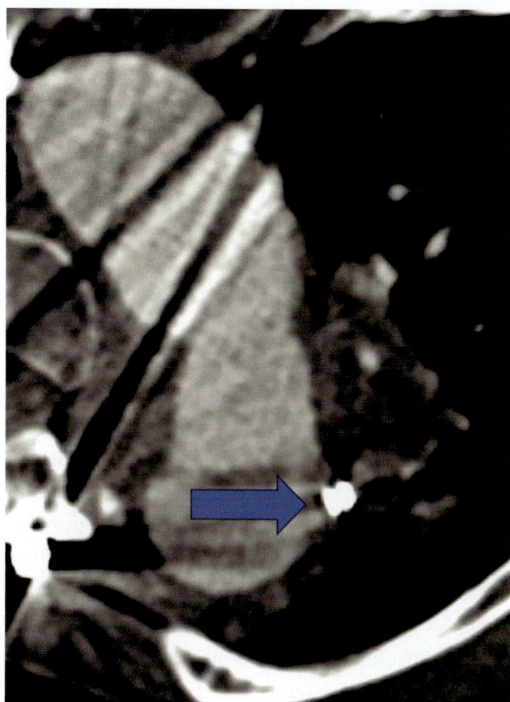

Fig. 41 Shows the magnetic resonance imaging of the left chest diagnosing the lung injury. The blue arrow shows the clip eroding into the lung

drainage tubes were placed the chest was closed uneventfully. The patient had an uncomplicated postoperative course.

This complication was unanticipated; however, any rigid tube or metal projection that can potentially extend into the lung should be suspected of such a complication. Other causes of postoperative hemoptysis brought about by an aortobronchial fistula have been linked to infection and false aneurysms. Oftentimes, the causative agent has been noted to be inflammatory lung disease. These possibilities require extensive diagnostic inquiry to plan an accurate therapeutic course (Ishikawa et al. 2020).

Most clinical reports concerning clinical outcomes of thoracoabdominal aortic aneurysm repair involve older patients (Coselli et al. 2016; Rosenblum and Chen 2019) and have only partial relevance to younger patients with connective tissue disorders. However, Glebova, Cameron, and Black (Glebova et al. 2018) have offered a comprehensive review of 28 studies which reviewed the treatment of thoracoabdominal aortic disease in patients with connective tissue disorders. The authors reviewed the clinical results for both open procedures and endovascular aortic repair. Of the eight studies that specifically reported the outcomes of open repair of thoracoabdominal aortic disease in patients with connective tissue disorders, the perioperative mortality ranged between 0% and 11.5% with an overall survival of 53%–96%. Perioperative morbidity ranged from 0% to 65% for paraplegia, 0–13% for permanent renal failure, and 0–11% for reexploration for bleeding. The authors identified 12 studies that reported the outcomes of endovascular treatment of thoracoabdominal aortic disease in patients with connective tissue disease. The technical success rate of endovascular treatment varied from 38% to 100%. Perioperative mortality ranged from 0% to 14%, with overall survival between 67% and 100%. Perioperative morbidity varied from 0% to 33% for paraplegia, 0–6.7% for permanent renal failure, and 0–14% for reexploration for bleeding. Type I Endo leaks occurred in 8%–30% and new dissections were noted in 17% of patients. The authors concluded with the following,

> Patients with connective tissue disorders (CTDs) are living longer and require durable aortic reconstruction. There is currently a lack of high quality evidence to support any particular approach to aortic repair in patients with CTD and a dearth of comparative data between open repair and endovascular repair. There are distinct differences in the published lengths of follow-up between the two repair approaches as well as in the prevalence of their use in an acute vs elective setting. Published reports on endovascular techniques describe largely limited extent aortic repairs in contrast to full aortic repairs for open surgical techniques. Endovascular repair is associated with less significant immediate physiologic demand on the cardiovascular system and decreased perioperative morbidity, whereas open repair affords greater durability with fewer reinterventions.
>
> Currently, repair of thoracoabdominal aneurysms in patients with CTDs can be performed safely with branched grafts, allowing low morbidity and mortality and excellent branch patency. Branched grafts should be used preferentially over traditional open repair with a Carrell patch to reduce the risk of patch aneurysms and the need for reoperation. Endovascular approaches for CTD patients should

be used with caution for specific anatomic circumstances in which surgical graft is available for fixation because of frequent endograft-related complications with native aortic tissue. (Glebova et al. 2018)

10 Complications Associated with Repair of Sinus of Valsalva Aneurysm

10.1 Anatomy, Associated Lesions, Classification

Sinus of Valsalva Aneurysm (SVA) is a rare intracardiac anomaly that is found in patients ranging from the teenage years to 50 years of age and beyond. Anatomic characterization of this entity is defined by dilatation of the aortic root, which is bounded by the aortic cusp, the aortic valve annulus, and the sinotubular ridge. Congenital SVA aneurysms generally have a thin-walled extension of the aortic wall that arises from the base of a single aortic sinus. In rare cases of SVA a small fistulous tract between an aortic sinus and an adjacent cardiac chamber can develop. The fistula typically arises from the right sinus of Valsalva or the noncoronary sinus of Valsalva and penetrates to the adjacent low-pressure chambers, which by anatomic proximity are the right atrium or right ventricle. This results in cardiac distention and heart failure owing to the resultant large left to right shunts, and para-aortic regurgitation. In unusual cases, free rupture into the pericardial cavity can occur and cause catastrophic outcomes (Serban et al. 2019; Galeczka et al. 2019; Wierda et al. 2018; Hajizeinali and Hosseinsabet 2019; Wingo et al. 2019; Ohno et al. 2019; Urbanski et al. 2020; Seo and Park 2019; Stöger et al. 2019; Diwakar et al. 2019; Chen et al. 2019; Stróżyk et al. 2018; Sarkar et al. 2019; Chan et al. 2020; Weinrich et al. 2015).

The incidence of SVA varies amongst geographic and cultural divides. Frequency has been reported to be 0.26% in Western patients (van Son et al. 1994), 1.37% to 1.5% in patients from India (Pannu et al. 1995; Verghese et al. 1986), and 2.0%–3.57% in patients from Japan (Taguchi et al. 1969; Tanabe et al. 1979). Interestingly, associated cardiac lesions are common in patients with SVA. For example, ventricular septal defect (VSD) occurs in approximately 40%–60% of Asian patients with SVA and in 35%–40% in Western populations with SVA. Furthermore, aortic regurgitation occurs according to two manifestations, namely, (1) from the fistulous tract into the low-pressure chamber and (2) due to bicuspid aortic valves with incomplete commissures. Other associated lesions include pulmonary stenosis, atrial septal defect, patent ductus arteriosus, and coarctation of the aorta (Serban et al. 2019; Weinrich et al. 2015). Some authors have noted the unusual circumstances that the incidence of SVA aneurysms in the Asian population is 5 times greater than in Western populations (Chu et al. 1990). In addition, other important differences are a higher incidence of right SVAs, more common penetration into the right ventricle, and a higher association with ventricular septal defects (Serban et al. 2019; Galeczka et al. 2019; Wierda et al. 2018; Hajizeinali and Hosseinsabet 2019; Wingo et al. 2019; Ohno et al. 2019; Urbanski et al. 2020; Seo and Park 2019; Stöger et al. 2019; Diwakar et al. 2019; Chen et al. 2019; Stróżyk et al. 2018; Sarkar et al. 2019; Chan et al. 2020; Weinrich et al. 2015). The speculative reason for these variations is unclear and may be due to the higher incidence of supracristal (subarterial) ventricular septal defects that are found in the Asian population. The natural history of this disease is unclear due to the many etiological factors that defy a settled scientific explanation.

The pathologic phase of an unruptured SVA begins with an enlargement stage during which time the patient is generally asymptomatic and can be diagnosed by incidental routine echocardiography, even in patients older than 60 years (Wingo et al. 2019). SVAs, like many aneurysmal dilatations, can rupture and cause catastrophic consequences. These situations, however present in younger patients, namely from puberty to 30 years of age. The median age of repair is in the third or fourth decades of life (Chu et al. 1990; Nowicki et al. 1977).

Classification of SVA is multifactorial and includes sinus of origin, chamber of penetration, and acuity (ruptured versus nonruptured)

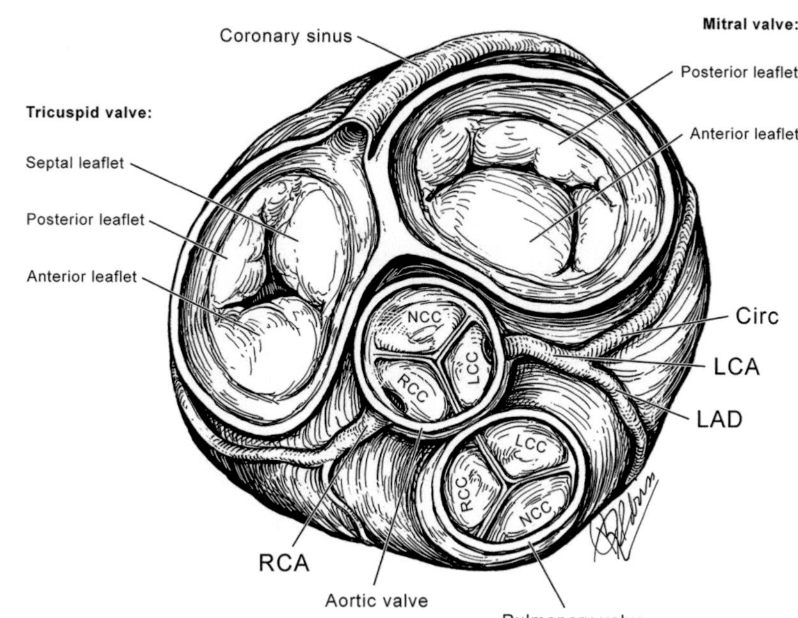

Fig. 42 Demonstrates a coronal section through the base of the heart which shows the inter-relational cardiac structures, which include the close anatomic proximity between the right and noncoronary sinuses with the right atrium and right ventricle, the most commonly penetrated sites. *LAD* left anterior descending artery, *LCA* left coronary artery, *LCC* left coronary cusp, *NCC* noncoronary cusp, *RCA* right coronary artery, *RCC* right coronary cusp. (With permission Martin and Mavroudis 2020)

(Sakakibara and Konno 1968). Other etiologic factors that weigh into the classification scheme relate to atherosclerosis, congenital lesions, connective tissue defects (Marfan Disease), inflammatory conditions, infectious causes, and trauma (Ring 2000). A comprehensive understanding of the anatomic interrelationships between the aortic sinuses and the adjoining cardiac chambers is shown in Fig. 42 and forms the basis and intuitive insight into the extant pathological anatomy, pathophysiology, and options for surgical treatment of SVAs.

11 Evaluation

The diagnostic test best suited for quantifying size and morphology of sinus of Valsalva aneurysm is cardiac computed tomography. Concurrently, transesophageal echocardiography can evaluate flow and hemodynamic impact if SVA rupture is being considered. In addition, cardiac MRI will determine the anatomy and hemodynamic significance. The gold standard for diagnosis is considered to be Cine Cardiac MRI, although it is not required if other imaging techniques adequately provide the diagnostic anatomic and physiologic details. Assessment of coronary artery anatomy can be determined by cardiac computed tomography for low-risk patients or coronary angiography in the event that coronary artery bypass might be anticipated (Wierda et al. 2018; Taguchi et al. 1969).

12 Surgical Repair of Sinus of Valsalva Aneurysms

12.1 General Principles and Surgical Repair

Operative exposure for repair of SVA is attained through a median sternotomy. Cannulation and execution of cardiopulmonary bypass takes into consideration that a transaortic, transcavitary (in the case of fistulous formation) approach will be necessary with appropriate cardioplegic administration. Aortobicaval cardiopulmonary bypass, left ventricular venting, and a combination of antegrade/retrograde cardioplegia is therefore established as shown and described in Fig. 43. Transesophageal echocardiography is essential to further assess preoperative and perioperative findings that can help to guide the operation and evaluate the intraoperative results after separation from cardiopulmonary bypass. Taking a

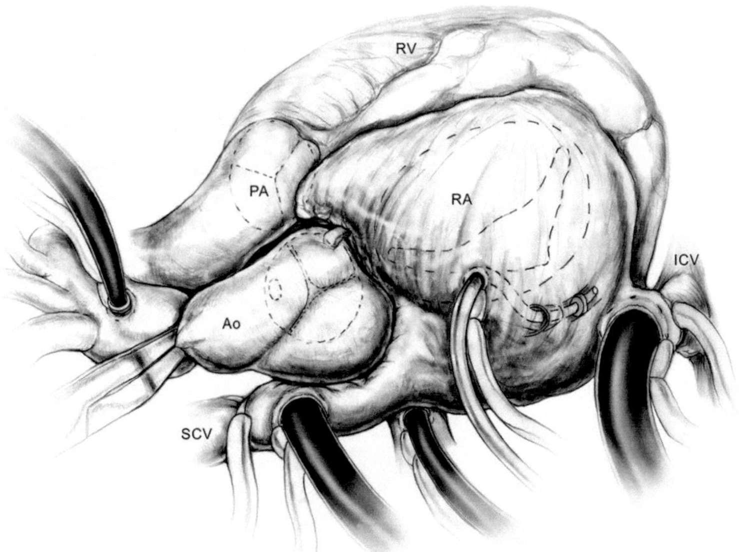

Fig. 43 The unruptured sinus of Valsalva aneurysm (SVA) tends to be confined to the noncoronary sinus which presents with a large dilatation as noted in the figure. This large aneurysm is thin-walled and subject to fistulous formation or free rupture. Once aortic cross-clamping with cardioplegic arrest is established, the involved wall can be resected and replaced with a PTFE or Dacron patch which will effectively restore the strength and size of the aortic wall towards a more normal *contour*. *Ao* aorta, *ICV* inferior caval vein, *PA* pulmonary artery, *RA* right atrium, *RV* right ventricle, *SCV* superior caval vein. (With permission Martin and Mavroudis 2020)

moment to perform epicardial inspection and gentle palpation can reveal the presence and location of turbulence which will help with intracardiac location in the event that a penetrating (ruptured) aneurysm is suspected.

As mentioned, SVAs can be categorized by those presenting as unruptured vs. ruptured. The repair of the unruptured SVA is noted in Figs. 43 and 44 that highlights the resection of the thin-walled aneurysm and replacement with a PTFE graft to remove the aneurysmal bulge and restore the proper aortic contour. In general, aneurysm can occur in the noncoronary cusp or the right coronary cusp. These locations have unwanted deleterious exposure for harm to the aortic valve leaflets, commissures, and coronary arteries during repair. These anatomic structures require careful attention to the PTFE placement, and demand avoidance of disruptive instrumentation. Nevertheless, the presence of antecedent aortic valve regurgitation and a bicuspid valve may result in a Bentall operation as reported by Wingo and associates (2019).

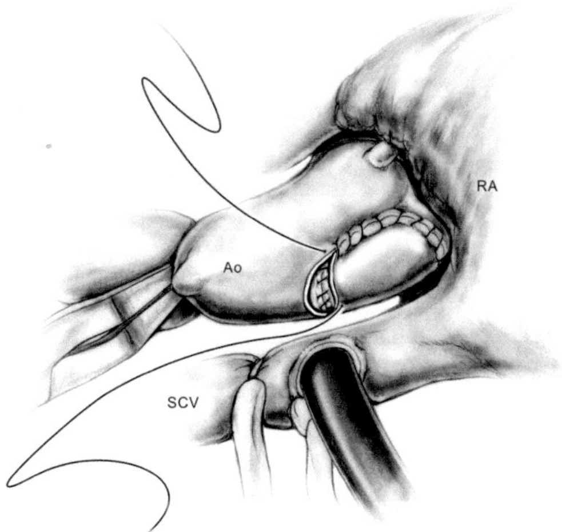

Fig. 44 Clearly, repair of this type of sinus of Valsalva aneurysm (SVA) is easier to perform than the ruptured type since there is no associated cavitary penetration or aortic valve involvement. The figure shows the normal contour of the ascending aorta being restored with a graft. *Ao* aorta, *RA* right atrium, *SCV* superior caval vein. (With permission Martin and Mavroudis 2020)

In those cases where the patient presents with ruptured SVA, the situation is more complicated. As a matter of review, a ruptured SVA can result in a confined rupture into a neighboring cardiac chamber (mostly the right atrium and right ventricle) without escape into the pericardial cavity. Left SVA rupture causing communication to the left atrium or left ventricular outflow tract (Stöger et al. 2019; Diwakar et al. 2019; Chen et al. 2019), is rare but can still cause significant findings and symptoms. In addition, the enlarged aneurysm can cause superior caval vein obstruction and arrhythmias. When free rupture into the pericardial cavity occurs, pericardial tamponade results in raising the acuity which requires immediate operation. Interestingly, case reports (Iida et al. 2006; Uesugi et al. 2017), have described successful outcomes under these circumstances.

Figures 45, 46, 47, 48, 49, 50, 51 and 52 show the procedural characteristics and techniques that are used to repair ruptured SVA into an adjacent cavity. In particular, Fig. 45 demonstrates trans-aortic, trans-right atrial exposure of a fistulous tract taking origin from the right coronary cusp, adjacent to the right coronary artery orifice and penetrating to the right ventricle behind the anterior leaflet of the tricuspid valve. The legend outlines the procedural steps to avoid complications. Clearly, the adjacent structures and orifices such as the right coronary artery orifice, the aortic valve leaflets, and the conduction system are at risk for injury and will require careful attention to

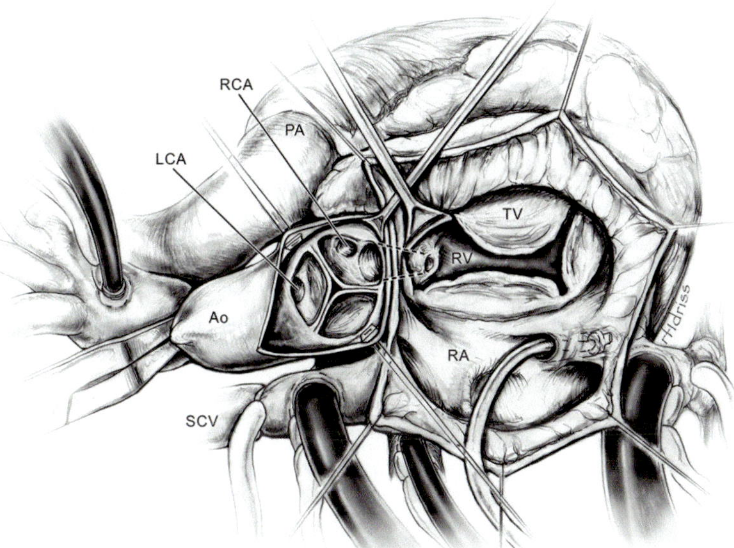

Fig. 45 Repair of sinus of Valsalva aneurysms (SVAs) with cavitary rupture and aortic valve involvement is another matter and must be approached with caution. At the beginning of CPB, special care is taken to avoid ventricular fibrillation and ventricular dilatation due to native aortic valve regurgitation and fistula flow to the affected chamber. The left ventricular vent will help to decompress the chamber, but the best way to deal with this situation is to apply the aortic cross-clamp with a combination of antegrade and retrograde administration of cardioplegia. The aorta can then be transversely incised upstream to the affected SVA for suitable exposure and exploration of the fistulous track. This will allow proper inspection of the aortic valve leaflets and the fistulous tract connecting to the affected chamber. Most often, the fistula tract takes origin at the aortic annulus in close proximity to the aortic leaflets or above the aortic annulus and may track near the right coronary artery orifice. In general, the aortic leaflets are not directly involved by the rupture. The leaflets however can be distorted by the fistulous tract which can cause important regurgitation. *Ao* aorta, *LCA* left coronary artery, *PA* pulmonary artery, *RA* right atrium, *RCA* right coronary artery, *RV* right ventricle, *SCV* superior caval vein, *TV* tricuspid valve. (With permission Martin and Mavroudis 2020)

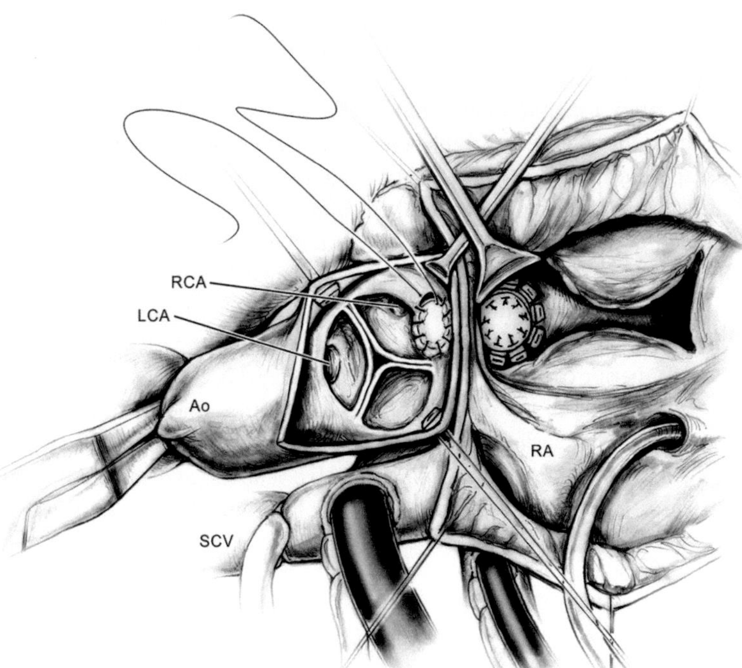

Fig. 46 Transaortic exposure in this fashion allows the surgeon to close the origin of the fistulous tract using a pericardial patch or PTFE material as shown in the figure. At this point, the surgeon can assess the valve leaflets for repair or replacement. Assuming that the aortic valve retains competency with this patch, many surgeons will accept this well-placed patch as the definitive operation and not explore the fistulous tract chamber of destination. Other surgeons, however, reason that the chamber of destination should be explored and closed to ensure obliteration of the ruptured tract. This is especially important since oftentimes, the fistulous tract is very close to a perimembranous ventricular septal defect (VSD). The figure also shows the trans-tricuspid valve closure of the fistulous tract in proximity to an associated VSD. *Ao* aorta, *LCA* left coronary artery, *RA* right atrium, *RCA* right coronary artery, *SCV* superior caval vein. (With permission Martin and Mavroudis 2020)

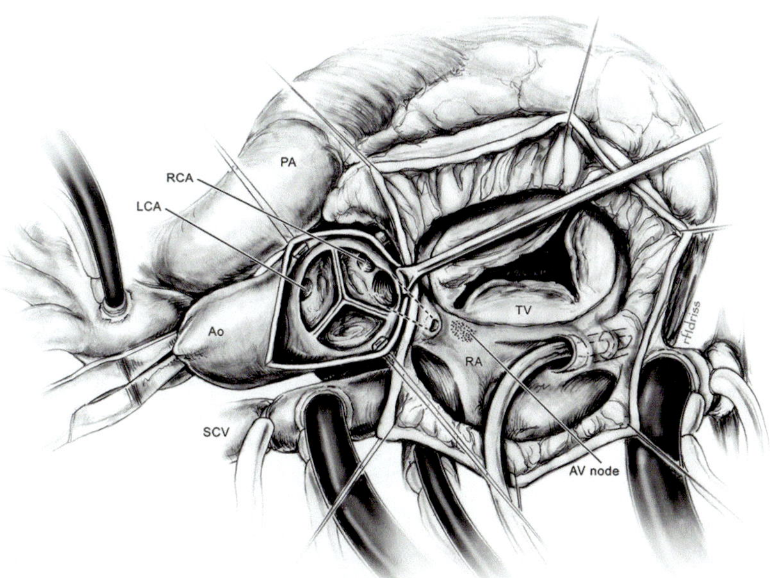

Fig. 47 Other cavitary fistulous tract penetrations include: the right atrium, the high subpulmonic right ventricular outflow tract, and the mid-right ventricular location. Cavitary penetrations other than these are extremely rare. Fistulas that perforate the right atrium are mostly located near the area of the tricuspid valve septal and anterior leaflets as noted in the figure. The "wind-sock" protrusion is located and resected. *Ao* aorta, *AV* atrioventricular, *LCA* left coronary artery, *PA* pulmonary artery, *RA* right atrium, *RCA* right coronary artery, *SCV* superior caval vein, *TV* tricuspid valve. (With permission Martin and Mavroudis 2020)

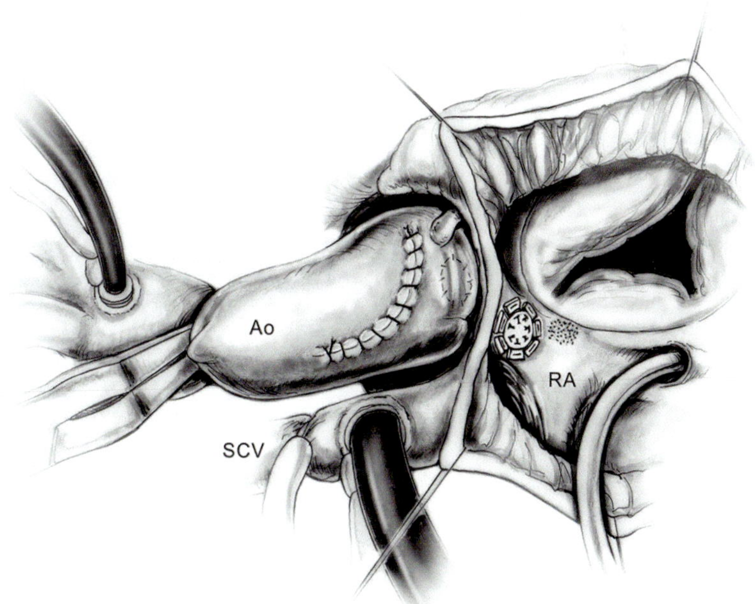

Fig. 48 Shows how the remaining hole is closed using a pericardial or PTFE patch and interrupted pledgeted suture technique with special care to avoid the conduction system as noted in the figure. *Ao* aorta, *RA* right atrium, *SCV* superior caval vein. (With permission Martin and Mavroudis 2020)

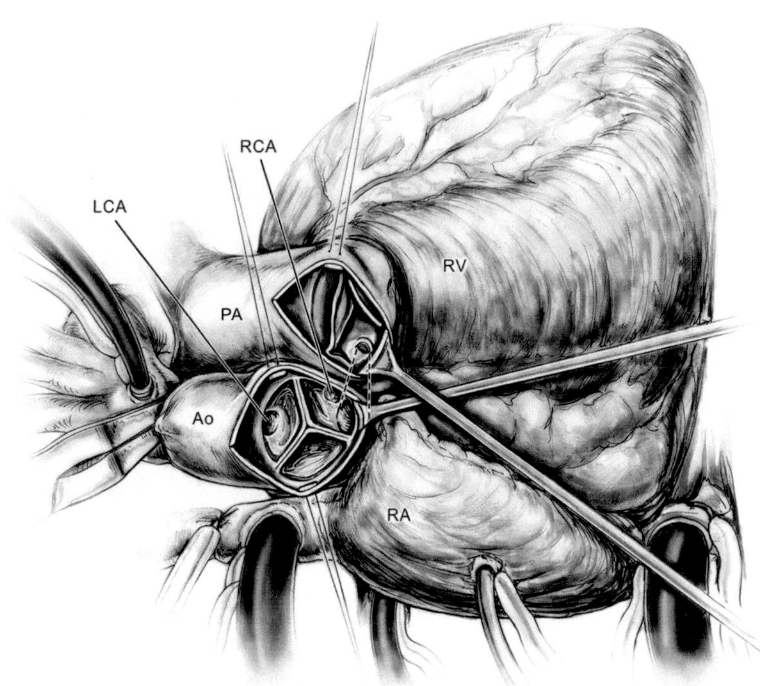

Fig. 49 For those fistulas that perforate the subpulmonic area of the right ventricle as shown in the figure, a transpulmonary artery approach is used to expose the fistulous tract and an associated juxta-arterial ventricular septal defect (VSD) if present. After "wind-sock" resection, the fistulous tract can be closed in association with the VSD if present. *Ao* aorta, *LCA* left coronary artery, *PA* pulmonary artery, *RA* right atrium, *RCA* right coronary artery, *RV* right ventricle. (With permission Martin and Mavroudis 2020)

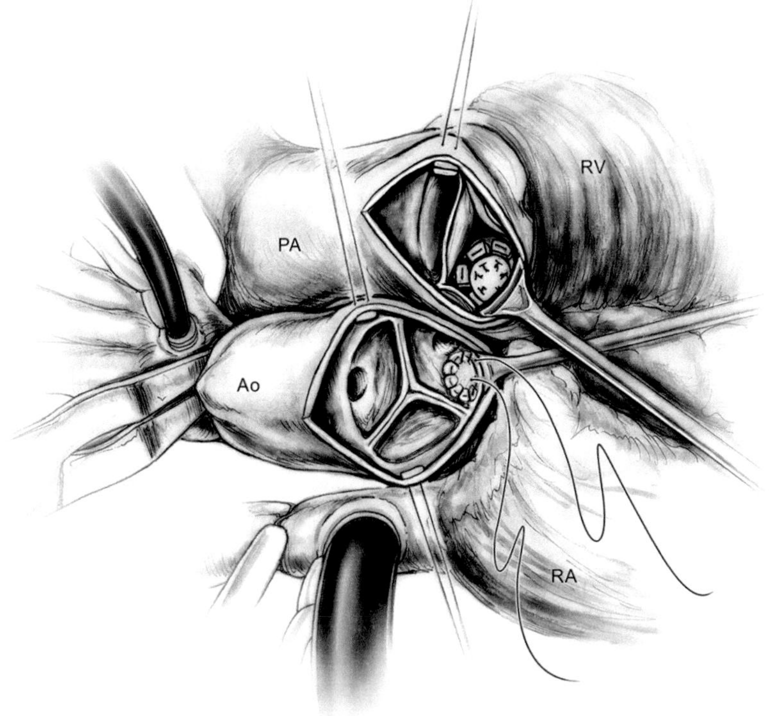

Fig. 50 Shows the completed patch repair using interrupted pledgeted suture technique in the subpulmonic area. In addition, the proximal fistulous tract is shown being closed with a PTFE patch using running suture technique. *Ao* aorta, *PA* pulmonary artery, *RA* right atrium, *RV* right ventricle. (With permission Martin and Mavroudis 2020)

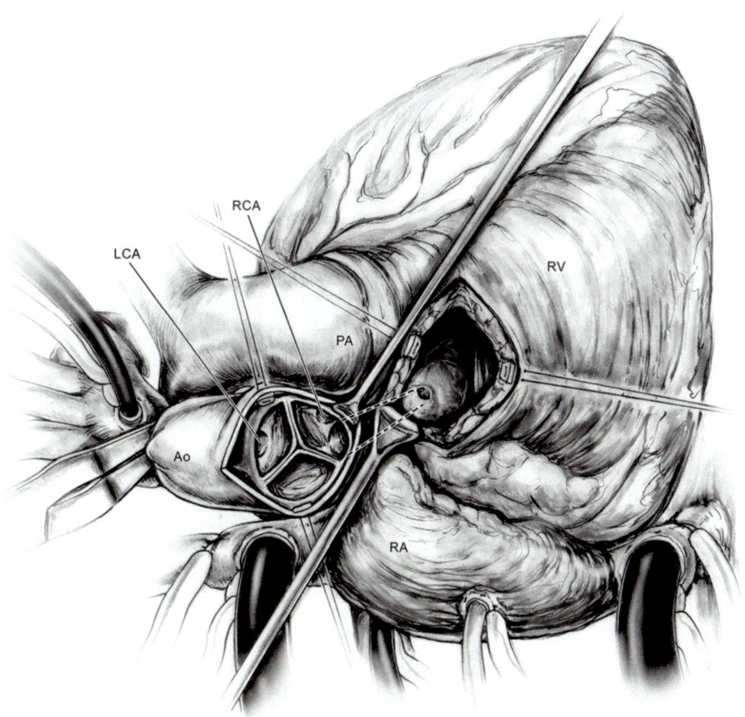

Fig. 51 A fistulous tract that penetrates into the mid-right ventricular area as shown in the figure may require a localized ventriculotomy to expose the fistula and an associated perimembranous ventricular septal defect if present. *Ao* aorta, *LCA* left coronary artery, *PA* pulmonary artery, *RA* right atrium, *RCA* right coronary artery, *RV* right ventricle. (With permission Martin and Mavroudis 2020)

prevent unwanted indiscriminate manipulation. Figure 46 demonstrates the repair of the aforementioned ruptured SAV as noted in Fig. 45. In this case the ruptured tract is closed at the origin which is adjacent to the right coronary artery orifice and the right ventricle communication. It is prudent to explore the right ventricle through the tricuspid valve in order to simultaneously close the distal fistula and the VSD, assuming that it is present, with one patch as noted in the drawing. The complications associated with this operation are the possibility of (1) causing right coronary artery orifice stenosis or disruption, (2) causing heart block due to unwanted suture placement through either the aorta or the right ventricle, residual VSD. These complications can be avoided with the proper knowledge of anatomy, careful suturing technique, and vigilance to avoid retraction injury. Figure 47 shows another form of a ruptured SVA with a fistulous tract from the right coronary sinus adjacent to the right coronary artery orifice to the right atrium near the tricuspid annulus with proximity to the atrioventricular node. The figure legend makes reference to the location and the "wind-sock" protrusion which forms as a result of the penetrating pathologic characteristics during the process of rupture. The wind-sock is resected to expose the atrial orifice of the channel that will allow proper suture placement. Figure 48 demonstrates the repaired lesion using the principles of the two-patch technique of aortic patch placement and right atrial patch placement. The potential complications are the same as described for the aortic to right ventricle fistula repair. Notice in the figure the right atrial patch repair is close but not adjacent to the atrioventricular node. Practical wisdom should guide the surgeon to either close the right atrial side of the fistula or to leave it in place without a patch owing to the proximity of the conduction system. As long as the aortic fistulous closure is secure, the right atrial patch may not be necessary. Another location of a ruptured SVA is the fistulous tract that connects the right coronary sinus of Valsalva to the subpulmonic area in the right ventricular outflow tract. The exposure for this type of fistula is different from the other descriptions since this area of fistulous tract is often

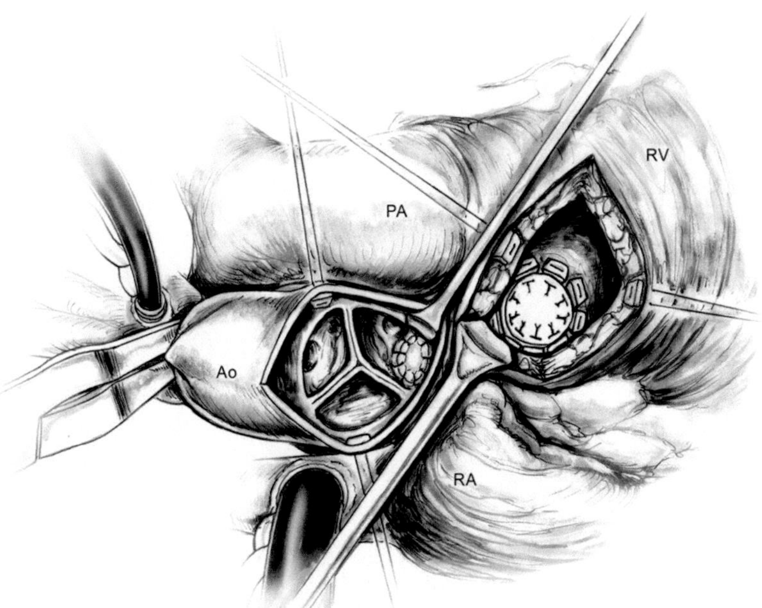

Fig. 52 Shows closure of the fistulous tract using a patch and interrupted pledgeted suture technique as well as transaortic closure of the proximal fistula at the aortic annulus using running suture technique. The ventricular septal defect (VSD), if present, can be closed simultaneously. Practical wisdom will guide the surgeon's approach in the event of the need to repair associated lesions. Most surgeons will first explore the aorta and place a patch at the fistulous origin using PTFE or autologous pericardium. The affected chamber can then be explored to resect the wind-sock protrusion and place another patch to close the fistulous tract at the affected chamber. In general, transaortic patch closure of the fistulous tract will suffice. However, exploration of the affected chamber will allow further inspection for closure of an associated atrial septal defect or VSD as well as patch closure of the entry site of the fistula. Separation from cardiopulmonary bypass is accomplished and the integrity of the repair is confirmed by transesophageal echocardiography. *Ao* aorta, *PA* pulmonary artery, *RA* right atrium, *RV* right ventricle. (With permission Martin and Mavroudis 2020)

associated with a conal or subarterial VSD. Figure 49 and the accompanying legend describe the anatomic landmarks of such a ruptured SVA. Notice that the exposure is transaortic and transpulmonary much like the exposure for repair of conal or subarterial VSD. In general, the orifice of the fistula is very close to the origin of the right coronary artery. Figure 50 illustrates the combined cavitary approach with PTFE patches placed in the right sinus of Valsalva and the subpulmonic area of the right ventricular outflow tract, respectively. The potential complications involving this repair are mostly procedure oriented and involve coronary orifice stenosis due to patch proximity and pulmonary valve disruption due to overzealous retraction. The surgeon is responsible for retractors and those who hold them. If exposure proves to be daunting for accurate repair, a small vertical subpulmonic ventriculotomy can be performed to enhance exposure and allow proper suture placement. The ventriculotomy can then be closed primarily or with PTFE patch augmentation. We prefer PTFE patch augmentation under these circumstances.

Another exposure problem is defined by a fistulous tract that takes origin from the right coronary sinus of Valsalva with penetration to the mid-right ventricle. Bicameral exposure can be accomplished by aortotomy and either right atrium or right ventricle. Figure 51 shows the distal exposure of the penetrating fistulous tract through a right ventriculotomy. This allows extended exposure for wind-sock excision, fistulous track identification, and evaluation of the

VSD anatomy which is oftentimes present. Figure 52 and the accompanying figure legend demonstrate the repaired lesion using two PTFE patches. The ventricular patch is large enough to close both the distal fistulous patch and the VSD using interrupted suture technique. The potential complications are similar to those described for the previous types of SVA repairs.

To be complete, percutaneous transcatheter closure of a ruptured right SVA has been reported (Galeczka et al. 2019; Hajizeinali and Hosseinsabet 2019) however follow-up has been limited. Concerns of endocarditis and hemolysis have been reported (Arora et al. 2004) and remain unresolved. More importantly, device closure is not appropriate for patients with significant aortic insufficiency or ventricular septal defect. Consequently, surgery remains the standard therapy (Wang et al. 2007).

References

Aalaei-Andabili SH, Martin T, Hess P, Klodell C, Karimi A, Arnaoutakis G, Lee T, Beaver T. Florida sleeve procedure is durable and improves aortic valve function in Marfan syndrome patients. Ann Thorac Surg. 2017;104(3):834–9.

Aalaei-Andabili SH, Martin TD, Hess PJ, Karimi A, Bavry AA, Arnaoutakis GJ, Beaver TM. The Florida Sleeve procedure is durable and improves aortic valve function. Aorta (Stamford). 2019;7(2):49–55.

Acher CW, Wynn M. A modern theory of paraplegia in the treatment of aneurysms of the thoracoabdominal aorta: an analysis of technique specific observed/expected ratios for paralysis. J Vasc Surg. 2009;49(5):1117–24.

Achneck HE, Rizzo JA, Tranquilli M, Elefteriades JA. Safety of thoracic aortic surgery in the present era. Ann Thorac Surg. 2007;84(4):1180–5.

Alhussaini M, Jeng EI, Martin TD, Fillion A, Beaver TM, Arnaoutakis GJ. Florida sleeve is a safe and effective technique for valve salvage in acute stanford type A aortic dissection. J Card Surg. 2022;37(1):39–46.

Arora R, Trehan V, Rangasetty UM, Mukhopadhyay S, Thakur AK, Kalra GS. Transcatheter closure of ruptured sinus of Valsalva aneurysm. J Interv Cardiol. 2004;17(1):53–8.

Bavaria JE, Appoo JJ, Makaroun MS, Verter J, Yu Z-F, Mitchell RS, et al. Endovascular stent grafting versus open surgical repair of descending thoracic aortic aneurysms in low-risk patients: a multicenter comparative trial. J Thorac Cardiovasc Surg. 2007;133(2):369–77.

Beckmann E, Martens A, Krüger H, Korte W, Kaufeld T, Stettinger A, Haverich A, Shrestha ML. Aortic valve-sparing root replacement with Tirone E. David's reimplantation technique: single-centre 25-year experience. Eur J Cardiothorac Surg. 2021;60(3):642–8.

Beeba HG. Leaks after endovascular therapy for aneurysm: detection and classification. J Endovasc Surg. 1996;3:445–8.

Beighton P, De Paepe A, Steinmann B, Tsipouras P, Wenstrup RJ. Ehlers-Danlos syndromes: revised nosology, Villefranche, 1997. Ehlers-Danlos National Foundation (USA) and Ehlers-Danlos Support Group (UK). Am J Med Genet. 1998;77(1):31–7.

Beliaev AM, Haydock DA. How to replace a bioprosthetic aortic valve within the Bentall graft. J Card Surg. 2020;35(3):656–8.

Bentall H, De Bono A. A technique for complete replacement of the ascending aorta. Thorax. 1968;23(4):338–9.

Blanco G, Adam A, Carlo V. A controlled surgical approach to annulo aortic ectasia. Ann Surg. 1976;183:174–8.

Blankensteijn JD, de Jong SECA, Prinssen M, van der Ham AC, Buth J, van Sterkenburg SMM, et al. Two-year outcomes after conventional or endovascular repair of abdominal aortic aneurysms. N Engl J Med. 2005;352(23):2398–405.

Bonita RE, Cohen IS, Berko BA. Valvular heart disease in osteogenesis imperfecta: presentation of a case and review of the literature. Echocardiography. 2010;27(1):69–73.

Booher AM, Eagle KA. Diagnosis and management issues in thoracic aortic aneurysm. Am Heart J. 2011;162(1):38–46.e1.

Buth J, Harris PL, Hobo R, van Eps R, Cuypers P, Duijm L, et al. Neurologic complications associated with endovascular repair of thoracic aortic pathology: incidence and risk factors. A study from the European Collaborators on Stent/Graft Techniques for Aortic Aneurysm Repair (EUROSTAR) registry. J Vasc Surg. 2007;46(6):1103–10; discussion 1110–1111.

Byers PH, Belmont J, Black J, et al. Diagnosis, natural history, and management in vascular Ehlers-Danlos syndrome. Am J Med Genet Part C Semin Med Genet. 2017;175(1):40–7.

Cabrol C, Gandjbakhch I, Cham B. Aneurysms of the ascending aorta; total replacement with reimplantation of the coronary arteries. (Author's transl). Nouv Press Med. 1978;7:363–5.

Cameron D, Vricella L. Valve-sparing aortic root replacement with the Valsalva graft. Oper Tech Thorac Cardiovasc Surg. 2005;10(4):259–71.

Cameron DE, Alejo DE, Patel ND, et al. Aortic root replacement in 372 Marfan patients: evolution of operative repair over 30 years. Ann Thorac Surg. 2009;87(5):1344–50.

Cardoso LF, Dias RR, Dinato FJ, Duncan JA, Fernandes F, Ramires FJA, Mady C, Jatene FB. Impact of aortic valve function and the need for aortic valve repair on long-term outcomes of valve-sparing aortic root replacement: 13-year experience of David operation. Heart Lung Circ. 2021;30(6):902–8.

Çekmecelioğlu D, Köksoy C, Coselli J. The frozen elephant trunk technique in acute DeBakey type I aortic dissection. Turk Gogus Kalp Damar Cerrahisi Derg. 2020;28(3):411–8.

Chadnick Z, Singh K. Complications associated with aortic aneurysm repair. In: Terezinha G, editor. Aortic aneurysm Intech Open. Clinical findings, diagnostic, treatment and special situations. Google Books; 2021.

Chan N, Charalambous M, Fuschetto DP, Fuschetto O, Makaryus JN. Severe compression of the left circumflex coronary artery by a large sinus of Valsalva aneurysm. J Cardiovasc Comput Tomogr. 2020;14(5):e26–8.

Chen J, Liang HN, Wu L, Dong SH, Li JH. Right sinus of Valsalva aneurysm spontaneously dissecting into the interventricular septum in a rare case of Behcet's disease. Eur Heart J Cardiovasc Imaging. 2019;20(5):601.

Chen JF, Tan KT, Lindsay TF, Ouzounian M, Chung JC. Surgery for complications after thoracic endovascular aortic repair with arch vessel debranching: role of imaging in preoperative planning. J Card Surg. 2022;37(12):4144–9.

Cheung AT. An evolving role of anesthesiologists in the management of thoracic aortic diseases. Anesth Analg. 2010;111(2):259–60.

Chirichilli I, Irace FG, D'Aleo S, Folino G, Weltert LP, Scaffa R, Nardella S, De Paulis R. Long-term follow-up of Bentall procedure using the Perimount bioprosthesis and the Valsalva graft. Interact Cardiovasc Thorac Surg. 2020;30(5):679–84.

Chivasso P, Mastrogiovanni G, Miele M, et al. Frozen elephant trunk technique in acute type A aortic dissection: is it for all? Medicina (Kaunas). 2021;57(9):894.

Chu SH, Hung CR, How SS, Chang H, Wang SS, Tsai CH, et al. Ruptured aneurysms of the sinus of Valsalva in oriental patients. J Thorac Cardiovasc Surg. 1990;99(2):288–98.

Chung J, Corriere MA, Veeraswamy RK, Kasirajan K, Milner R, Dodson TF, et al. Risk factors for late mortality after endovascular repair of the thoracic aorta. J Vasc Surg. 2010;52(3):549–54; discussion 555.

Coady MA, Rizzo JA, Hammond GL, Kopf GS, Elefteriades JA. Surgical intervention criteria for thoracic aortic aneurysms: a study of growth rates and complications. Ann Thorac Surg. 1999;67(6):1922–6; discussion 1953–1958.

Connolly JE. Hume memorial lecture. Prevention of spinal cord complications in aortic surgery. Am J Surg. 1998;176(2):92–101.

Coscas R, Greenberg RK, Mastracci TM, Eagleton M, Kang WC, Morales C, et al. Associated factors, timing, and technical aspects of late failure following open surgical aneurysm repairs. J Vasc Surg. 2010;52(2):272–81.

Coselli JS, LeMaire SA, Koksoy C, Schmittling ZC, Curling PE. Cerebrospinal fluid drainage reduces paraplegia after thoracoabdominal aortic aneurysm repair: results of a randomized clinical trial. J Vasc Surg. 2002;35(4):631–9.

Coselli JS, LeMaire SA, Preventza O, et al. Outcomes of 3309 thoracoabdominal aortic aneurysm repairs. J Thorac Cardiovasc Surg. 2016;151(5):1323–37.

Czerny M, Eggebrecht H, Sodeck G, Verzini F, Cao P, Maritati G, et al. Mechanisms of symptomatic spinal cord ischemia after TEVAR: insights from the European Registry of Endovascular Aortic Repair Complications (EuREC). J Endovasc Ther. 2012;19(1):37–43.

Dake MD, Miller DC, Mitchell RS, Semba CP, Moore KA, Sakai T. The "first generation" of endovascular stent-grafts for patients with aneurysms of the descending thoracic aorta. J Thorac Cardiovasc Surg. 1998;116(5):689–703; discussion 703–704.

David TE, Feindel CM. An aortic valve-sparing operation for patients with aortic incompetence and aneurysm of the ascending aorta. J Thorac Cardiovasc Surg. 1992;103(4):617–22.

David TE, Armstrong S, Maganti M, Colman J, Bradley TJ. Long-term results of aortic valve–sparing operations in patients with Marfan syndrome. J Thorac Cardiovasc Surg. 2009;138(4):859–64.

Di Luozzo G. Visceral and spinal cord protection during thoracoabdominal aortic aneurysm repair: clinical and laboratory update. J Thorac Cardiovasc Surg. 2013;145(3 Suppl):S135–8.

Dietz HC, Cutting CR, Pyeritz RE, et al. Marfan syndrome caused by a recurrent de novo missense mutation in the fibrillin gene. Nature. 1991;352(6333):337–9.

Diletta L, Enrico R, Germano M. Thoracoabdominal aortic aneurysm in connective tissue disorder patients. Indian J Thorac Cardiovasc Surg. 2022;38(Suppl 1):146–56.

Diwakar A, Patnaik SS, Hiremath CS, Chalam KS, Dash P. Rupture of sinus of Valsalva—a 15 years single institutional retrospective review: preoperative heart failure has an impact on post operative outcome? Ann Card Anaesth. 2019;22(1):24–9.

Eggebrecht H, Thompson M, Rousseau H, Czerny M, Lönn L, Mehta RH, et al. Retrograde ascending aortic dissection during or after thoracic aortic stent graft placement: insight from the European registry on endovascular aortic repair complications. Circulation. 2009;120(11 Suppl):S276–81.

Everitt MD, Pinto N, Hawkins JA, Mitchell MB, Kouretas PC, Yetman AT. Cardiovascular surgery in children with Marfan syndrome or Loeys-Dietz syndrome. J Thorac Cardiovasc Surg. 2009;137(6):1327–33.

Faivre L, Collod-Beroud G, Child A, et al. Contribution of molecular analyses in diagnosing Marfan syndrome and type I fibrillinopathies: an international study of 1009 probands. J Med Genet. 2008;45(6):384–90.

Faure EM, Becquemin J-P, Cochennec F, ENGAGE collaborators. Predictive factors for limb occlusions after endovascular aneurysm repair. J Vasc Surg. 2015;61(5):1138–1145.e2.

Freeman KA, Arnaoutakis GJ, Jeng EI, Martin TD, Beaver TM. Florida Sleeve operative techniques. Op Tech Thorac Cardiovasc Surg. 2021;26:306–21.

Galeczka M, Glowacki J, Yashchuk N, et al. Medium- and long-term follow-up of transcatheter closure of ruptured sinus of Valsalva aneurysm in Central Europe population. J Cardiol. 2019;74(4):381–7.

Glebova NO, Cameron DE, Black JH 3rd. Treatment of thoracoabdominal aortic disease in patients with connective tissue disorders. J Vasc Surg. 2018;68(4):1257–67.

Greenberg RK, Lu Q, Roselli EE, Svensson LG, Moon MC, Hernandez AV, et al. Contemporary analysis of descending thoracic and thoracoabdominal aneurysm repair: a comparison of endovascular and open techniques. Circulation. 2008;118(8):808–17.

Griepp RB, Stinson EB, Hollingsworth JF, Buehler D. Prosthetic replacement of the aortic arch. J Thorac Cardiovasc Surg. 1975;70(6):1051–63.

Hajizeinali A, Hosseinsabet A. Percutaneous device closure of a ruptured aortic sinus of Valsalva aneurysm in a patient with a mechanical bileaflet aortic valve. Turk Kardiyol Dern Ars. 2019;47(3):243.

Hess PJ Jr, Harman PK, Klodell CT, Beaver TM, Bologna MT, Mikhail P, Tribble CG, Martin TD. Early outcomes using the Florida sleeve repair for correction of aortic insufficiency due to root aneurysms. Ann Thorac Surg. 2009;87(4):1161–9.

Hiratzka LF, Bakris GL, Beckman JA, Bersin RM, Carr VF, Casey DE, et al. ACCF/AHA/AATS/ACR/ASA/SCA/SCAI/SIR/STS/SVM guidelines for the diagnosis and management of patients with Thoracic Aortic Disease: a report of the American College of Cardiology Foundation/American Heart Association Task Force on Practice Guidelines, American Association for Thoracic Surgery, American College of Radiology, American Stroke Association, Society of Cardiovascular Anesthesiologists, Society for Cardiovascular Angiography and Interventions, Society of Interventional Radiology, Society of Thoracic Surgeons, and Society for Vascular Medicine. Circulation. 2010;121(13):e266–369.

Holubec T, Rashid H, Hecker F, et al. Early- and longer-term outcomes of David versus Florida sleeve procedure: propensity-matched comparison. Eur J Cardiothorac Surg. 2022;62(3):ezac104.

Hosseinsabet A, Bagheri J, Shirani S. A mediastinal hematoma after the Bentall operation detected by transthoracic echocardiography. J Cardiovasc Echogr. 2021;31(2):96–7.

Howell M, Villareal R, Krajcer Z. Percutaneous access and closure of femoral artery access sites associated with endoluminal repair of abdominal aortic aneurysms. J Endovasc Ther. 2001;8(1):68–74.

Iida Y, Sugimoto T, Katsu M, Shimada K, Yamamoto K, Yoshii S, Kasuya S. Extracardiac rupture of aneurysm of the noncoronary sinus of Valsalva: report of a case. Kyobu Geka. 2006;59(7):580–4. Japanese. PMID: 16856535.

Ishikawa N, Hirofuji A, Wakabayashi N, Nakanishi S, Kamiya H. The cause of massive hemoptysis after thoracic endovascular aortic repair may not always be an aortobronchial fistula: report of a case. Clin Med Insights Case Rep. 2020;13:1179547620939078. https://doi.org/10.1177/1179547620939078.

Jahanyar J, El Khoury G, de Kerchove L. Is extension of Florida Sleeve indications taking us in the right direction? Eur J Cardiothorac Surg. 2022;62(3):ezac247.

Jefferies JL, Martinez HR, Towbin JA. Genetics of congenital and acquired cardiovascular disease. In: Pediatric and congenital cardiology, cardiac surgery and intensive care. London: Springer London; 2014. p. 3–16.

Judge DP, Dietz HC. Marfan's syndrome. Lancet. 2005;366(9501):1965–76.

Khvan DS, Sirota DA, Liashenko MM, Al'sov SA, Cherniavskiĭ AM. Operatsiia po metodike Florida Sleeve u patsienta s vyrazhennym kal'tsinozom kornia aorty [Florida sleeve operation in a patient with pronounced aortic root calcification]. Angiol Sosud Khir. 2019;25(2):171–4. Russian.

Khvan DS, Sirota DA, Zhul'kov MO, Liashenko MM, Cherniavskiĭ AM. Remote results of Florida Sleeve technique in patients with ascending aortic aneurysms and aortic insufficiency. Angiol Sosud Khir. 2020;26(4):108–18. English, Russian.

Kitaura J, Mukai S, Morimoto H, Futagami D, Furuta A. Florida Sleeve technique concomitant with total aortic arch replacement. Kyobu Geka. 2021;74(13):1063–6. Japanese.

Klocker J, Koell A, Erlmeier M, Goebel G, Jaschke W, Fraedrich G. Ischemia and functional status of the left arm and quality of life after left subclavian artery coverage during stent grafting of thoracic aortic diseases. J Vasc Surg. 2014;60(1):64–9.

Kouchoukos NT, Marshall WG Jr, Wedige-Stecher TA. Eleven-year experience with composite graft replacement of the ascending aorta and aortic valve. J Thorac Cardiovasc Surg. 1986;92:691–705.

Kouchoukos NT, Wareing TH, Murphy SF, et al. Sixteen-year experience with aortic root replacement. Results of 172 operations. Ann Surg. 1991;214:308–18.

Leon LR, Mills JL, Jordan W, Morasch MM, Kovacs M, Becker GJ, et al. The risks of celiac artery coverage during endoluminal repair of thoracic and thoracoabdominal aortic aneurysms. Vasc Endovasc Surg. 2009;43(1):51–60.

Leontyev S, Trommer C, Subramanian S, et al. The outcome after aortic valve-sparing (David) operation in 179 patients: a single-centre experience. Eur J Cardiothorac Surg. 2012;42(2):261–7.

Loeys BL, Chen J, Neptune ER, et al. A syndrome of altered cardiovascular, craniofacial, neurocognitive and skeletal development caused by mutations in TGFBR1 or TGFBR2. Nat Genet. 2005;37(3):275–81.

Loeys BL, Schwarze U, Holm T, et al. Aneurysm syndromes caused by mutations in the TGF-β receptor. N Engl J Med. 2006;355(8):788–98.

Loeys BL, Dietz HC, Braverman AC, et al. The revised Ghent nosology for the Marfan syndrome. J Med Genet. 2010;47(7):476–85.

MacCarrick G, Black JH, Bowdin S, et al. Loeys–Dietz syndrome: a primer for diagnosis and management. Genet Med. 2014;16(8):576–87.

Maddalo S, Beller J, DeAnda A. A Bentall is not a Bentall is not a Bentall: the evolution of aortic root surgery. Aorta (Stamford). 2014;2(5):169–78.

Makaroun MS, Dillavou ED, Wheatley GH, Cambria RP, Gore TAG Investigators. Five-year results of endovascular treatment with the Gore TAG device compared with open repair of thoracic aortic aneurysms. J Vasc Surg. 2008;47(5):912–8.

Maldonado TS, Dexter D, Rockman CB, Veith FJ, Garg K, Arko F, et al. Left subclavian artery coverage during thoracic endovascular aortic aneurysm repair does not mandate revascularization. J Vasc Surg. 2013;57(1):116–24.

Malfait F, Francomano C, Byers P, et al. The 2017 international classification of the Ehlers-Danlos syndromes. Am J Med Genet Part C Semin Med Genet. 2017;175(1):8–26.

Marfan A. "Un cas de déformation congénitale des quartre membres, plus prononcée aux extrémitiés, caractérisée par l'allongement des os avec un certain degré d'amincissement" [A case of congenital deformation of the four limbs, more pronounced at the extrem]. Bull Mem la Société medicale des hôspitaux Paris; 1896.

Martin T, Mavroudis C. Congenital aortic aneurysms. In: Mavroudis C, Dearani J, editors. Atlas of adult congenital heart surgery. Cham: Springer; 2020. p. 359–82.

Matsumura JS, Cambria RP, Dake MD, Moore RD, Svensson LG, Snyder S, et al. International controlled clinical trial of thoracic endovascular aneurysm repair with the Zenith TX2 endovascular graft: 1-year results. J Vasc Surg. 2008;47(2):247–57.

Milewicz DM, Dietz HC, Miller DC. Treatment of aortic disease in patients with Marfan syndrome. Circulation. 2005;111(11):e150–7.

Mookhoek A, Korteland NM, Arabkhani B, et al. Bentall procedure: a systematic review and meta-analysis. Ann Thorac Surg. 2016;101(5):1684–9.

Morse RP, Rockenmacher S, Pyeritz RE, et al. Diagnosis and management of infantile Marfan syndrome. Pediatrics. 1990;86(6):888–95.

Najibi S, Terramani TT, Weiss VJ, Mac Donald MJ, Lin PH, Redd DC, et al. Endoluminal versus open treatment of descending thoracic aortic aneurysms. J Vasc Surg. 2002;36(4):732–7.

Nordon IM, Karthikesalingam A, Hinchliffe RJ, Holt PJ, Loftus IM, Thompson MM. Secondary interventions following endovascular aneurysm repair (EVAR) and the enduring value of graft surveillance. Eur J Vasc Endovasc Surg. 2010;39(5):547–54.

Nowicki ER, Aberdeen E, Friedman S, Rashkind WJ. Congenital left aortic sinus-left ventricle fistula and review of aortocardiac fistulas. Ann Thorac Surg. 1977;23(4):378–88.

O'Callaghan A, Mastracci TM, Greenberg RK, Eagleton MJ, Bena J, Kuramochi Y. Outcomes for supra-aortic branch vessel stenting in the treatment of thoracic aortic disease. J Vasc Surg. 2014;60(4):914–20.

Ohno N, Watanabe K, Maeda T, et al. A rare case of unruptured extracardiac multiple sinus of Valsalva aneurysms originating from the orifices with partial aortic wall defects. Surg Case Rep. 2019;5(1):47.

Orandi BJ, Dimick JB, Deeb GM, Patel HJ, Upchurch GR. A population-based analysis of endovascular versus open thoracic aortic aneurysm repair. J Vasc Surg. 2009;49(5):1112–6.

Ouzounian M, LeMair SA, Welson S, Coselli JS. Open repair of thoracoabdominal aoritc aneurysm: step-by-step. Oper Tech Thorac Cardiovasc Surg. 2018;23:2–20.

Pannu HS, Shivaprakash K, Bazaz S, Bedi HS, Dhaliwal RS, Singh H, et al. Geographical variations in the presentation of ruptured aneurysms of sinuses of Valsalva: evaluation of surgical repair. J Card Surg. 1995;10(4 Pt 1):316–24.

Papakonstantinou NA, Antonopoulos CN, Baikoussis NG, Kakisis I, Geroulakos G. Aortic arch reconstruction: are hybrid debranching procedures a good choice? Heart Lung Circ. 2018;27(11):1335–49.

Parapia LA, Jackson C. Ehlers-Danlos syndrome—a historical review. Br J Haematol. 2008;141(1):32–5.

Patel ND, Arnaoutakis GJ, George TJ, et al. Valve-sparing aortic root replacement in children: intermediate-term results. Interact Cardiovasc Thorac Surg. 2011;12(3):415–9.

Patel ND, Alejo D, Crawford T, et al. Aortic root replacement for children with Loeys-Dietz syndrome. Ann Thorac Surg. 2017;103(5):1513–8.

Patterson BO, Holt PJ, Nienaber C, Fairman RM, Heijmen RH, Thompson MM. Management of the left subclavian artery and neurologic complications after thoracic endovascular aortic repair. J Vasc Surg. 2014;60(6):1491–1497.e1.

Pepin M, Schwarze U, Superti-Furga A, Byers PH. Clinical and genetic features of ehlers–danlos syndrome type IV, the vascular type. N Engl J Med. 2000;342(10):673–80.

Perek B, Juszkat R, Kulesza J, Jemielity M. Stent grafts separation 6 years after endovascular repair of a thoracic aortic aneurysm. J Vasc Interv Radiol. 2014;25(10):1650–2.

Piehler JM, Pluth JR. Replacement of the ascending aorta and aortic valve with a composite graft in patients with displaced coronary ostia. Ann Thorac Surg. 1982;33:406–9.

Pitts L, Van Praet KM, Montagner M, Kofler M, Falk V, Kempfert J. David procedure as valve-sparing root replacement. Surg Technol Int. 2022;41:sti41/1593.

Price J, Magruder JT, Young A, et al. Long-term outcomes of aortic root operations for Marfan syndrome: a comparison of Bentall versus aortic valve-sparing procedures. J Thorac Cardiovasc Surg. 2016;151(2):330–8.

Prinssen M, Verhoeven ELG, Buth J, Cuypers PWM, van Sambeek MRHM, Balm R, et al. A randomized trial comparing conventional and endovascular

repair of abdominal aortic aneurysms. N Engl J Med. 2004;351(16):1607–18.
Pyeritz RE, Wappel MA. Mitral valve dysfunction in the Marfan syndrome. Clinical and echocardiographic study of prevalence and natural history. Am J Med. 1983;74(5):797–807.
Ramlawi B, Reardon MJ. Aortic arch debranching: advanced and hybrid techniques. Methodist Debakey Cardiovasc J. 2011;7(3):43–7.
Rayt HS, Bown MJ, Lambert KV, Fishwick NG, McCarthy MJ, London NJM, et al. Buttock claudication and erectile dysfunction after internal iliac artery embolization in patients prior to endovascular aortic aneurysm repair. Cardiovasc Intervent Radiol. 2008;31(4):728–34.
Redaelli P, Belluschi I, Bertoglio L, Verzini A, Chiesa R, Castiglioni A. Frozen elephant trunk: debranch first technique. Ann Cardiothorac Surg. 2020;9(3):257–8.
Ricotta JJ, Oderich GS. Fenestrated and branched stent grafts. Perspect Vasc Surg Endovasc Ther. 2008;20(2):174–87; discussion 188–189.
Riesenman PJ, Farber MA, Mendes RR, Marston WA, Fulton JJ, Keagy BA. Coverage of the left subclavian artery during thoracic endovascular aortic repair. J Vasc Surg. 2007;45(1):90–4; discussion 94–95.
Ring WS. Congenital heart surgery nomenclature and database project: aortic aneurysm, sinus of Valsalva aneurysm, and aortic dissection. Ann Thorac Surg. 2000;69(4 Suppl):S147–63.
Rong LQ, Kamel MK, Rahouma M, et al. Cerebrospinal-fluid drain-related complications in patients undergoing open and endovascular repairs of thoracic and thoraco-abdominal aortic pathologies: a systematic review and meta-analysis. Br J Anaesth. 2018;120(5):904–13.
Rosenblum JM, Chen EP. Thoracoabdominal aortic aneurysm repair: open, endovascular, or hybrid? Gen Thorac Cardiovasc Surg. 2019;67:175–9.
Royce PM, Steinmann B, editors. Connective tissue and its heritable disorders. Hoboken: Wiley; 2002.
Sakakibara S, Konno S. Congenital aneurysm of the sinus of Valsalva associated with ventricular septal defect: anatomical aspects. Am Heart J. 1968;75:595–603.
Sarkar M, Wehman B, Mukherjee R, Taylor BS. Left sinus of Valsalva aneurysm presenting as myocardial ischemia. J Thorac Cardiovasc Surg. 2019;157(3):e167–8.
Scali ST, Beck AW, Butler K, Feezor RJ, Martin TD, Hess PJ, et al. Pathology-specific secondary aortic interventions after thoracic endovascular aortic repair. J Vasc Surg. 2014;59(3):599–607.
Schanzer A, Greenberg RK, Hevelone N, Robinson WP, Eslami MH, Goldberg RJ, et al. Predictors of abdominal aortic aneurysm sac enlargement after endovascular repair. Circulation. 2011;123(24):2848–55.
Seo KW, Park JS. Sinus of Valsalva aneurysm and multiple aortic aneurysms provoked by viral myocarditis. Korean Circ J. 2019;49(2):194–6.
Serban AM, Bătrâna N, Cocoi M, et al. The role of echocardiography in the diagnosis and management of a giant unruptured sinus of Valsalva aneurysm. Med Ultrason. 2019;21(2):194–6.
Shapira OM, Aldea GS, Cutter SM, Fitzgerald CA, Lazar HL, Shemin RJ. Improved clinical outcomes after operation of the proximal aorta: a 10-year experience. Ann Thorac Surg. 1999;67(4):1030–7.
Shrestha M, Kaufeld T, Shrestha P, et al. Valve-sparing David procedure via minimally invasive access does not compromise outcome. Front Cardiovasc Med. 2022;14(9):966126. https://doi.org/10.3389/fcvm.2022.966126. PMID: 36312253.
Shrestha M, Boethig D, Krüger H. Valve-sparing aortic root replacement using a straight tube graft (David I procedure). J Thorac Cardiovasc Surg. 2023;66(5):1387–97.
Shukla AJ, Jeyabalan G, Cho J-S. Late collapse of a thoracic endoprosthesis. J Vasc Surg. 2011;53(3):798–801.
Silverman DI, Burton KJ, Gray J, et al. Life expectancy in the Marfan syndrome. Am J Cardiol. 1995;75(2):157–60.
Simonte G, Parlani G, Farchioni L, Isernia G, Cieri E, Lenti M, et al. Lesson learned with the use of iliac branch devices: single centre 10 year experience in 157 consecutive procedures. Eur J Vasc Endovasc Surg. 2017;54(1):95–103.
Smith T, van der Weijde E, Heijmen RH. Surgical debranching for endovascular arch penetrating ulcer management. Ann Cardiothorac Surg. 2019;8(4):512–5.
Srivastava S, Bhan A. Aortic arch aneurysms and dissection-open repair is the gold standard. Indian J Thorac Cardiovasc Surg. 2019;35(Suppl 2):136–55.
Stepanenko AB, Charchyan ER, Gens AP, Fedulova SV, Timofeeva IE, Belov YV. Aortic arch debranching in hybrid thoracic aortic replacement. Khirurgiia (Mosk). 2022;6:32–9. English, Russian.
Stöger G, Borger MA, Misfeld M. A giant aneurysm of the left sinus of Valsalva. Eur J Cardiothorac Surg. 2019;56(3):627.
Stróżyk A, Kołaczkowska M, Fijałkowska J, Siondalski P, Fijałkowski M. Sinus of Valsalva rupture in a patient with a mechanical aortic prosthesis: aneurysm dissecting into the interventricular septum. Kardiol Pol. 2018;76(12):1742.
Svensson LG, Kouchoukos NT, Miller DC, Bavaria JE, Coselli JS, Curi MA, et al. Expert consensus document on the treatment of descending thoracic aortic disease using endovascular stent-grafts. Ann Thorac Surg. 2008;85(1 Suppl):S1–S41.
Svensson LG, Blackstone EH, Alsalihi M, et al. Midterm results of David reimplantation in patients with connective tissue disorder. Ann Thorac Surg. 2013;95(2):555–62.
Szeto WY, Desai ND, Moeller P, Moser GW, Woo EY, Fairman RM, et al. Reintervention for endograft failures after thoracic endovascular aortic repair. J Thorac Cardiovasc Surg. 2013;145(3 Suppl):S165–70.
Taguchi K, Sasaki N, Matsuura Y, Uemura R. Surgical correction of aneurysm of the sinus of Valsalva. A report of forty-five consecutive patients including

eight with total replacement of the aortic valve. Am J Cardiol. 1969;23(2):180–91.

Takayama H, Borger MA. Preventing spinal cord injury during thoracic aortic surgery: simpler than we thought? J Thorac Cardiovasc Surg. 2015;149(1):366–8.

Tanabe T, Yokota A, Sugie S. Surgical treatment of aneurysms of the sinus of Valsalva. Ann Thorac Surg. 1979;27(2):133–6.

Uesugi S, Kawahito K, Sato H, Sugaya A, Misawa Y. Rupture of an aneurysm of the right sinus of Valsalva into the pericardium; Report of a case. Kyobu Geka. 2017;70(5):385–8. Japanese. PMID: 28496087.

Uglov KA, Sorokina AA, Konoval'chuk EV, Voronova OV, Sidorov RV, Uglov AI. Operatsiia pri ostrom rassloenii aorty I tipa po DeBeĭki po metodike Florida Sleeve [Operation in DeBakey type I acute aortic dissection according to the Florida Sleeve technique]. Angiol Sosud Khir. 2021;27(4):118–24. Russian.

Ultee KHJ, Soden PA, Zettervall SL, Darling J, Verhagen HJM, Schermerhorn ML. Conversion from endovascular to open abdominal aortic aneurysm repair. J Vasc Surg. 2016;64(1):76–82.

Urbanski PP, Hirao S, Irimie V. Root repair in patient with huge sinus Valsalva aneurysm and severe aortic regurgitation. Gen Thorac Cardiovasc Surg. 2020 May;68(5):530–3.

van der Linde D, Bekkers JA, Mattace-Raso FUS, et al. Progression rate and early surgical experience in the new aggressive aneurysms-osteoarthritis syndrome. Ann Thorac Surg. 2013;95(2):563–9.

van Karnebeek CD, Naeff MS, Mulder BJ, Hennekam RC, Offringa M. Natural history of cardiovascular manifestations in Marfan syndrome. Arch Dis Child. 2001;84(2):129–37.

Van Laer L, Proost D, Loeys BL. Educational paper. Connective tissue disorders with vascular involvement: from gene to therapy. Eur J Pediatr. 2013;172(8):997–1005. https://doi.org/10.1007/s00431-012-1773-x.

van Son JA, Danielson GK, Schaff HV, Orszulak TA, Edwards WD, Seward JB. Long-term outcome of surgical repair of ruptured sinus of Valsalva aneurysm. Circulation. 1994;90(5 Pt 2):II20–9.

Verghese M, Jairaj PS, Babuthaman C, Sukumar IP, John S. Surgical treatment of ruptured aneurysms of the sinus of Valsalva. Ann Thorac Surg. 1986;41(3):284–6.

Victoria-Medina WL, Quispe-Vizcarra C, Rojas-Huillca M, Moreno-Loaiza M, Cubas WS. Bentall surgery and total arch repair with debranching of supra-aortic vessels: a case report. Egypt Heart J. 2022;74(1):12.

Vricella LA, Cameron DE. Valve-sparing aortic root replacement in pediatric patients: lessons learned over two decades. Semin Thorac Cardiovasc Surg Pediatr Card Surg Annu. 2017;20:56–62.

Wang ZJ, Zou CW, Li DC, Li HX, Wang AB, Yuan GD, et al. Surgical repair of sinus of Valsalva aneurysm in Asian patients. Ann Thorac Surg. 2007;84:156–60.

Weinrich M, Yu PJ, Trost B. Sinus of Valsalva aneurysms: review of the literature and an update on management. Clin Cardiol. 2015;38(3):185–9.

Wheeler JB, Ikonomidis JS, Jones JA. Connective tissue disorders and cardiovascular complications: the indomitable role of transforming growth factor-beta signaling. Adv Exp Med Biol. 2014;802:107–27.

Wierda E, Koolbergen DR, de Mol BAJM, Bouma BJ. Rupture of a giant aneurysm of the sinus of Valsalva leading to acute heart failure: a case report demonstrating the excellence of echocardiography. Eur Heart J Case Rep. 2018;2(3):yty090. https://doi.org/10.1093/ehjcr/yty090. PMID: 31020167; PMCID: PMC6177027.

Williams JA, Loeys BL, Nwakanma LU, et al. Early surgical experience with Loeys-Dietz: a new syndrome of aggressive thoracic aortic aneurysm disease. Ann Thorac Surg. 2007;83(2):S757–63.

Wingo M, de Angelis P, Worku BM, et al. Sinus of Valsalva aneurysm repairs: operative technique and lessons learned. J Card Surg. 2019;34(6):400–3.

Ziganshin BA. How do you manage the diaphragm during open thoracoabdominal interventions on the aorta? Aorta (Stamford). 2013;1(1):67–8. https://doi.org/10.12945/j.aorta.2013.13.021. PMID: 26798676; PMCID: PMC4682702.

Zoli S, Roder F, Etz CD, Brenner RM, Bodian CA, Lin H-M, et al. Predicting the risk of paraplegia after thoracic and thoracoabdominal aneurysm repair. Ann Thorac Surg. 2010;90(4):1237–44; discussion 1245.

Zubiate P, Kay JH. Surgical treatment of aneurysm of the ascending aorta with aortic insufficiency and marked displacement of the coronary ostia. J Thorac Cardiovasc Surg. 1976;71:415–21.

Complications Associated with Repair of Congenital and Acquired Coronary Artery Anomalies

Constantine Mavroudis, Carlos M. Mery, and Constantine D. Mavroudis

Abstract

Congenital coronary artery malformations can take several forms: (1) anomalous left or right coronary artery arising from the pulmonary artery, (2) anomalous aortic origin of the coronary arteries, (3) single coronary artery with or without anomalous course between the aorta and pulmonary artery, congenital atresia or stenosis of the left main coronary artery, (4) coronary artery fistulas, and (5) coronary artery bridging. Acquired coronary lesions include: (1) coronary artery aneurysms and stenoses associated with Kawasaki Disease, (2) iatrogenic injuries caused by transcutaneous invasive procedures or surgical complications, and (3) rare instances of sharp or blunt trauma. This chapter will highlight the necessary extant reparative procedures to repair congenital and acquired coronary artery lesions and show how complications can occur. New illustrations will show actual drawings of surgical complications that will require successful resolution.

Keywords

Anomalous aortic origin · Coronary artery · Congenital heart surgery · Coronary artery fistula · Coronary artery bridging · Kawasaki disease · Complications

C. Mavroudis (✉)
Chief of Pediatric Cardiothoracic Surgery (Retired), Peyton Manning Children's Hospital, Indianapolis, IN, USA

Professor Emeritus of Surgery, Johns Hopkins University School of Medicine, Baltimore, MD, USA

C. M. Mery
Dell Medical School, The University of Texas at Austin, Austin, TX, USA

Dell Children's Medical Center, Austin, TX, USA

C. D. Mavroudis
Pediatric Cardiothoracic Surgery, Children's Hospital of Philadelphia, Perelman School of Medicine, University of Pennsylvania, Philadelphia, PA, USA

C. L. Backer, C. Mavroudis (eds.), *Complications in Pediatric and Congenital Heart Surgery*, https://doi.org/10.1007/978-3-032-02661-3_27

1 Introduction

Anomalies of the coronary arteries can be described as congenital or acquired and are characterized as abnormalities of the normal anatomy of two patent and separately arising right and left arterial blood vessels. The coronary arteries represent the first branches of the ascending aorta, arise from their respective sinuses of Valsalva, and gradually branch distally to supply the myocardium. The anatomical substrates are characterized by a lack of origin, abnormal origin, anomalous course, lack of patency, abnormal connections, and/or abnormal drainage of the coronary vessels. Interruptions or lack of flow can cause significant morbidity and mortality due to ischemia, infarction, and fistulous connections, which can lead to cardiac failure (Ogden 1970; Dodge-Khatami et al. 2000; Friedman et al. 2007; Post et al. 1995; Le Roy et al. 2019; Mavroudis 2015).

The array of congenital coronary artery malformations includes: (1) anomalous left or right coronary artery (RCA) arising from the pulmonary artery (Mavroudis 2015; Brooks 1885; Dodge-Khatami et al. 2002; Walker et al. 2016; Bland et al. 1933; Edwards 1964; Fudulu et al. 2015; Bunton et al. 1987; Levitas et al. 2016; Sauer et al. 1992; Mavroudis et al. 1988, 1996, 2003; Backer et al. 1992, 2000; Vouhé et al. 1987, 1992; Potts et al. 1955; Mustard 1962; Sabiston Jr et al. 1960; Cooley et al. 1966; Meyer et al. 1968; Fortune et al. 1987; Neches et al. 1974; Takeuchi et al. 1979; Arciniegas et al. 1980; Turley et al. 1995; Alexi-Meskhishvili et al. 1995; Moodie et al. 1983; Kitamura et al. 1992; Mavroudis and Dearani 2020; Lambert et al. 1996; Schwartz et al. 1997; Singh et al. 1998; Stern et al. 1993; Carvalho et al. 1991; Laks et al. 1995; Paridon et al. 1990; Rein et al. 1987; Mongé et al. 2015; Huddleston et al. 2001; Isomatsu et al. 2001; Naimo et al. 2016; Bravo-Valenzuela and Silva 2015; Cochrane et al. 1999; del Nido et al. 1999; Karl et al. 1991; Zhang et al. 2020; Stephens and Dearani 2020; Agrawal et al. 2019; Ben Ali et al. 2009; Secinaro et al. 2011), (2) anomalous aortic origin of the coronary arteries (Williams et al. 2006; Chernogrivov et al. 2015; Taylor et al. 1992; Cohen et al. 1989; Angelini and Flamm 2007; Brothers et al. 2007, 2010, 2015, 2017; Davis et al. 2001; Eckart et al. 2004; Erez et al. 2006; Fedoruk et al. 2007; Jaggers and Lodge 2005; Jokl et al. 1962; Liberthson et al. 1979a; Angelini et al. 2018; Mustafa et al. 1981; Roberts et al. 1982; Kimbiris 1985; Ueyama et al. 1997; Barth 3rd and Roberts 1986; Moodie et al. 1980; Turner et al. 2011; Mavroudis et al. 2015; Lorber et al. 2015; Benge et al. 1980; Bett et al. 1985; Bloomfield et al. 1983; Jacobs 2017; Jegatheeswaran et al. 2019, 2020; Mavroudis and Backer 2010; Meza et al. 2017; Elias et al. 2017; Wilder and Williams 2016; Poynter et al. 2014a, b) (3) single coronary artery with or without anomalous course between the aorta and pulmonary artery (Brothers et al. 2009; Mumtaz et al. 2011; Sharbaugh and White 1974; Akcay et al. 2008; Desmet et al. 1992; Lipton et al. 1979; Yamanaka and Hobbs 1990; Smith 1950; Aldana-Sepulveda et al. 2013; Corbett et al. 2009), (4) congenital atresia/stenosis of the left main coronary artery (Unzué et al. 2015; Lurie 1977; Ghosh et al. 1993; Tanawuttiwat et al. 2013; D'Souza et al. 2016; Musiani et al. 1997; Byrum et al. 1980; Koh et al. 1989; Rosenkranz et al. 1992; Dymond et al. 1980; Gay et al. 1989; Kaczorowski et al. 2012), (5) coronary artery fistulas (Fernandes et al. 1992; Olearchyk et al. 1997; Krause 1865; Urrutia-S et al. 1983; Mavroudis et al. 1997; Harris et al. 1996; Lowe et al. 1981; Schumacher et al. 1997; Kamiya et al. 2002; Tkebuchava et al. 1996; Sakakibara et al. 1966; Dodd et al. 2008; Bauer et al. 1996; Liberthson et al. 1979b; Biörck and Crafoord 1947; Cooley and Ellis Jr. 1962; Reidy et al. 1983; Alkhulaifi et al. 1995; Fetter et al. 1994; Bogers et al. 1987; Crainicianu 1922), and

(6) coronary artery bridging (Angelini et al. 1983; Bourassa et al. 2003; den Dulk et al. 1983; Mookadam et al. 2009; Pey et al. 1985; Schwarz et al. 1996; Kardasz and De Caterina 2007; Y-Hassan 2014; Brolin et al. 2015; Geiringer 1951; Kramer et al. 1982; Ferreira Jr et al. 1991; Betriu et al. 1980; Hill et al. 1981; Hillman et al. 1999; Feld et al. 1991; Vasan et al. 1989; Von Poláček and Zechmeister 1968; Hakeem et al. 2010; Huang et al. 2007; Lee and Chen 2015; Binet et al. 1975; Haager et al. 2000). The range of acquired coronary lesions includes: (1) coronary artery aneurysms (Munkner et al. 1958; Aintablian et al. 1978; Anabtawi and de Leon 1974; Befeler et al. 1977; Falsetti and Carrol 1976; Hartnell et al. 1985; Kosar and Chandraratna 1997; Swaye et al. 1983; Markis et al. 1976; Rab et al. 1991; Cohen and O'Gara 2008; Ayusawa et al. 2008; Tunick et al. 1989; Boyer et al. 2014; Heuser 2015) and stenoses associated with Kawasaki Disease (Kato et al. 1975; Akagi et al. 1992; Beiser et al. 1998; Burns et al. 1996; Gersony 1998; Suzuki et al. 1986; Checchia et al. 1997; Dajani et al. 1993; Dajani et al. 1994; Harada et al. 1993; Kato et al. 1982; Nakamura et al. 1998; Newburger et al. 2004; Pahl 1997; Satou et al. 2007; Suzuki et al. 1990; Newburger et al. 2016; Kitamura et al. 1990; Ino et al. 1996; Mavroudis et al. 2023), (2) iatrogenic injuries caused by transcutaneous invasive procedures or surgical complications, and (3) the rare instances of sharp or blunt trauma.

Congenital and acquired congenital coronary artery anomalies come to the attention of diagnosticians and theoreticians based on coronary under-perfusion and related symptoms. Reparative operative techniques are focused on the particular lesion that will resolve the problem (Mavroudis 2015; Mavroudis and Dearani 2020). This chapter will highlight the necessary extant reparative procedures to repair congenital and acquired coronary artery lesions and show how complications can occur. Previous drawings from our atlases (Mavroudis 2015; Mavroudis and Dearani 2020) are repeated herein to establish the operation while new illustrations will show actual drawings of complications that will require successful resolution.

2 Anomalous Left Coronary Artery from the Pulmonary Artery (ALCAPA)

Anomalous left coronary artery originating from the pulmonary artery (ALCAPA) is the most common cause of myocardial ischemia and infarction in infants and children. These conditions can cause mitral insufficiency, congestive heart failure, and death in early infancy if not treated (Dodge-Khatami et al. 2002; Walker et al. 2016). The physiologic consequence of this pathoanatomy is characterized by desaturated blood perfusion to the myocardium from the left main coronary artery which arises from the pulmonary artery. Early survival is conditional on the size of intercoronary collaterals which arise from the right coronary artery. They then connect through open channels to the left coronary system which allows perfusion of the myocardium. While some collateral vessels are adequate to perfuse the myocardium over the long term; most are not. In general, patients with ALCAPA should be repaired at diagnosis assuming that the very rare condition of left main coronary artery atresia has been ruled out.

In the greater majority of cases, ALCAPAs take their origin from the posterior pulmonary artery sinus. This anatomic configuration allows direct implantation into the ascending aorta in most of these of cases (Fig. 1). In cases where the ALCAPA arises from other sinuses, lengthening procedures may become necessary (Turley et al. 1995; Laks et al. 1995). These maneuvers involve fashioning an extension of the coronary artery by incorporating pulmonary artery tissue.

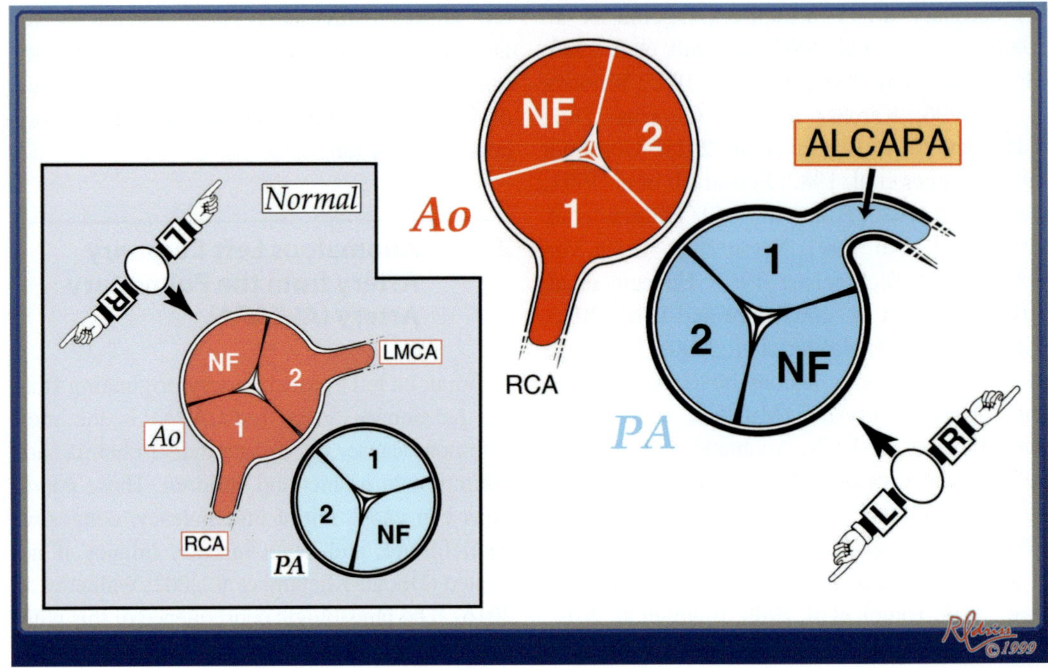

Fig. 1 Shows a diagrammatic scheme for identifying and naming the ALCAPA in relationship to the pulmonary artery and the ascending aorta. The reader is asked to assume that a surgeon is standing in the non-facing sinus looking toward the opposite great vessel (aorta to the pulmonary artery and vice versa). The sinus to the right of the surgeon is by convention sinus 1 and correspondingly, the other sinus to the left of the surgeon is sinus 2. *ALCAPA* anomalous left coronary artery from the pulmonary artery, *Ao* aorta, *LMCA* left main coronary artery, *NF* non-facing, *PA* pulmonary artery, *RCA* right coronary artery. (With permission Mavroudis 2015)

The operation to repair ALCAPA by coronary reimplantation to the ascending aorta is started through a median sternotomy and aortobicaval cannulation techniques as noted in Figs. 2, 3, 4, 5 and 6. The particulars of pulmonary artery control, proper cardioplegic administration, coronary artery transfer without tension, and pulmonary artery reconstruction are carefully reviewed within the legends. There are however complications that can occur, which of course, is the focus

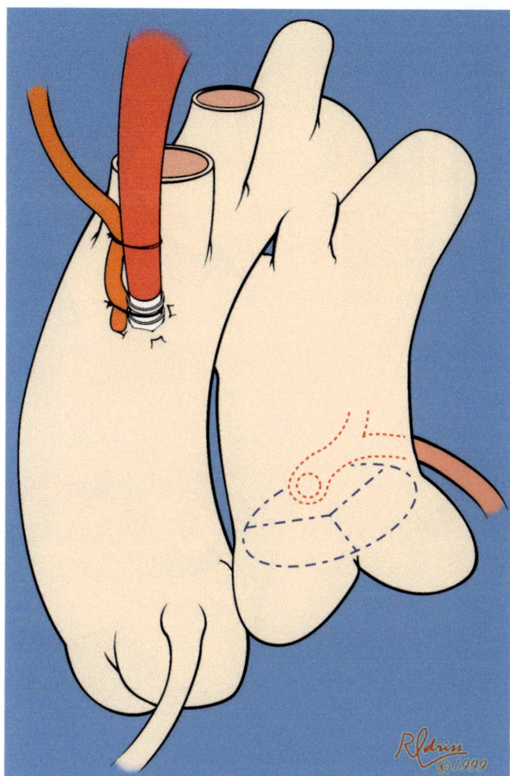

Fig. 2 This is a diagrammatic representation of aortic cannulation and the ghost representation (dotted lines) of the left main coronary artery arising from the posterior pulmonary artery sinus. (With permission Mavroudis 2015)

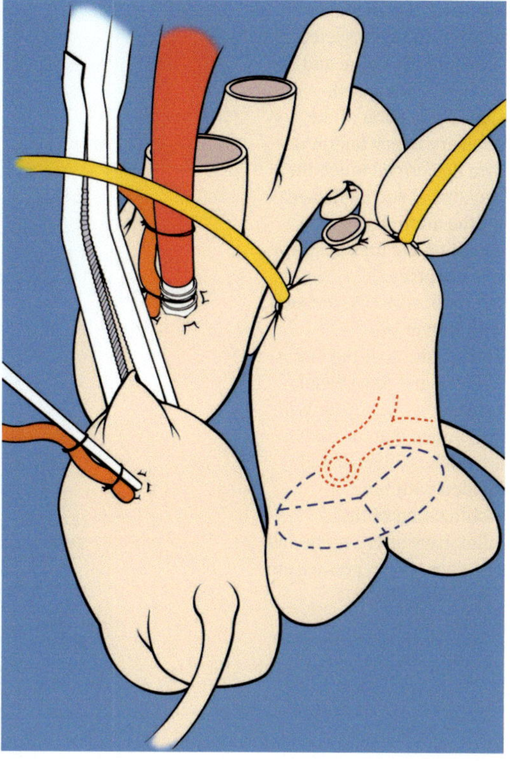

Fig. 3 Prior to the commencement of cardiopulmonary bypass (CPB), the right and left main pulmonary arteries are controlled with snuggers in anticipation of engagement shortly after the initiation of CPB. The cardioplegic catheter is placed in the ascending aorta, also before the commencement of CPB. The cardioplegia issue must be resolved with the perfusion team since blood cardioplegia is prepared shortly after the commencement of CPB. The idea in this case is to start antegrade cardioplegia immediately after the start of CPB to prevent coronary run off and ischemia. This may require crystalline cardioplegia or special measures to establish blood cardioplegia. So, the following steps are taken in short order to infuse antegrade cardioplegia before any period of ischemia is experienced by the patient. CPB is commenced with cooling to 32° or 28 °C. Proper venous drainage is established; the aorta is immediately cross-clamped and antegrade cardioplegia is started as shown in the figure; the right and left pulmonary arteries are completely snugged thereby preventing cardioplegia run-off through the intercoronary collaterals from the right coronary artery. A vent is then placed in the right superior pulmonary vein into the left ventricle. The administration of cardioplegia is completed with epicardial iced saline. (With permission Mavroudis 2015)

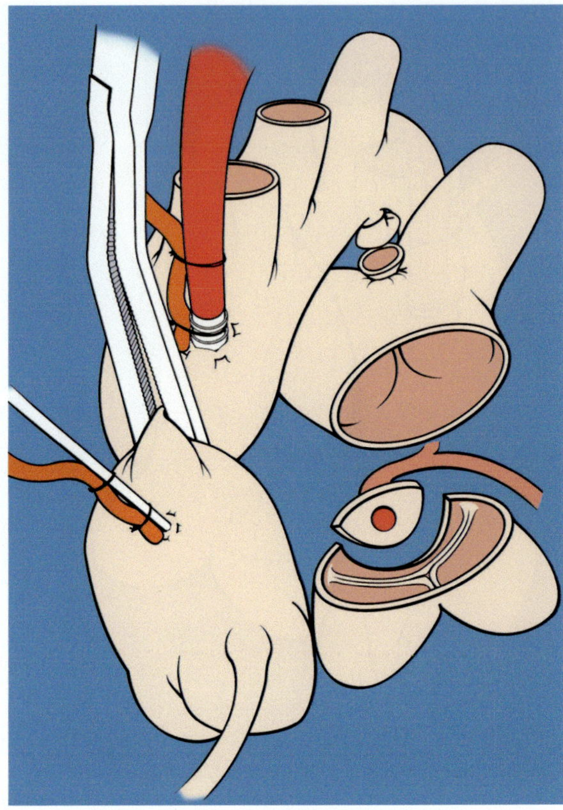

Fig. 4 The pulmonary artery is then transected as shown in the figure and the ALCAPA is located. Careful excision of the coronary artery button is then performed much the way that is accomplished for the arterial switch operation for transposition (see chapter "Complications Associated with Repair of Transposition of the Great Arteries and Associated Lesions"). The reader will also notice that the ductus arteriosus is ligated and divided with full mobilization of the pulmonary artery trunk and branches. (With permission Mavroudis 2015)

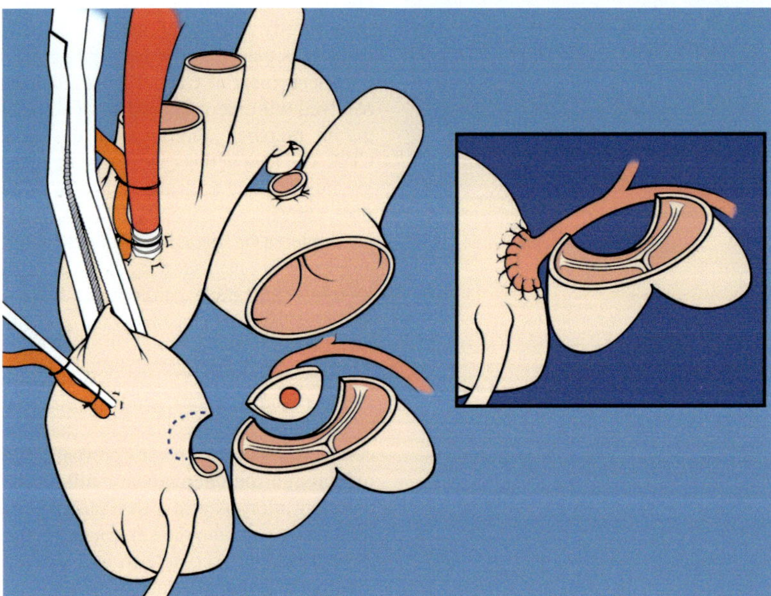

Fig. 5 Shows the excised portion of the ascending aorta in preparation for the end-to-side anastomosis between the coronary artery button and the side of the ascending aorta. Great care is taken to perform the ascending aortic wall excision to avoid any injury to the aortic valve commissures and leaflets. This requires proper aortic retraction and segmental cuts while locating and respecting the structures as the excision progresses. The anastomosis can be performed with running suture technique using fine suture material. (With permission Mavroudis 2015)

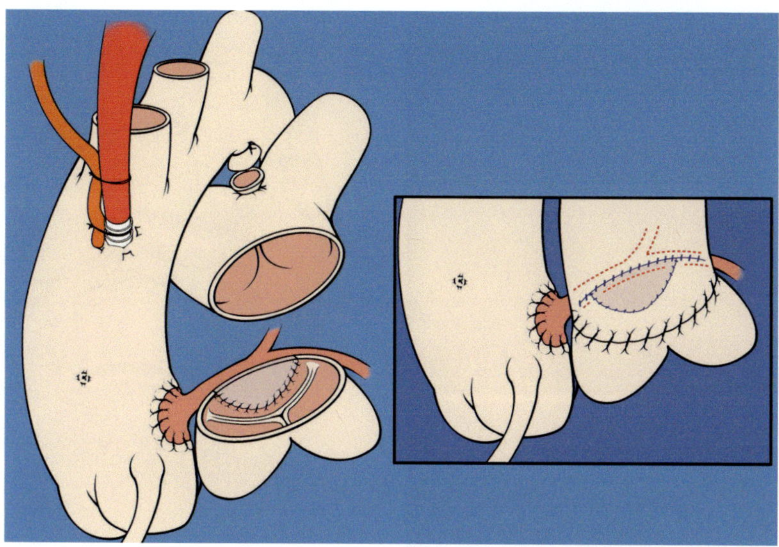

Fig. 6 Shows removal of the aortic cross-clamp and myocardial reperfusion after successful ALCAPA transfer to the ascending aorta. Special care is now taken to avoid pulmonary artery compression of the course of the left main coronary artery. This is performed by a generous piece of pericardium which can be used to augment the dissected sinus of Valsalva from where originated the ALCAPA. The diagrammatic figure shows a tapered patch which is flush with the proximal pulmonary artery. In practice, we fashion a much larger patch with a superior extension to lengthen the posterior portion of the pulmonary trunk. This maneuver minimizes the chances of coronary compression. The majority of patients do well with this operation despite significant myocardial depression and mitral regurgitation. The function and regurgitation improve over time leading to excellent function, minimal mitral regurgitation and near normal clinical functional status. Occasionally, ECMO will be needed for a few days to unload the left ventricle in anticipation of recovery and ECMO cessation. *ALCAPA* anomalous left coronary artery from the pulmonary artery, *ECMO* extracorporeal membrane oxygenation. (With permission Mavroudis 2015)

of this textbook. Figures 7 and 8 show the complications of coronary button tension and coronary button malrotation, respectively. Either complication can occur independently or in combination with resultant poor myocardial perfusion. This complication does not necessarily present in the immediate postoperative period since ventricular function was dependent on right coronary artery collaterals preoperatively and will persist postoperatively. Moreover, myocardial improvement may take more time than is expected intraoperatively. Oftentimes, the flow can be assessed by echocardiographic methods. Probably more important is the epicardial assessment of the surgeon who can evaluate malrotation and tension causing coronary obstruction by visual clues. When this situation is not repaired at the initial operation, persistent myocardial dysfunction in the postoperative period should lead the clinical team towards diagnostic evaluation to determine coronary artery flow and possible obstruction. Consideration should be made to

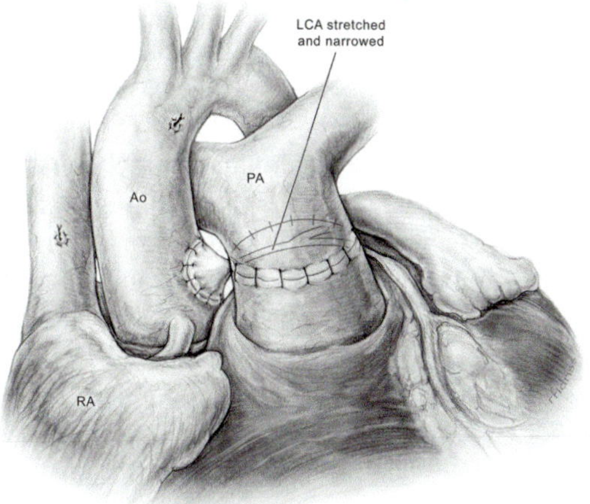

Fig. 7 Shows malrotation and stretching of the coronary artery button that can be discovered in the operating room after separation from cardiopulmonary bypass or in the immediate postoperative period. When preoperative ventricular dysfunction does not improve after the operation, diagnostic methods should be implemented to determine the anastomotic anatomy and determine if there is a perfusion problem. *Ao* aorta, *LCA* left coronary artery, *PA* pulmonary artery, *RA* right atrium

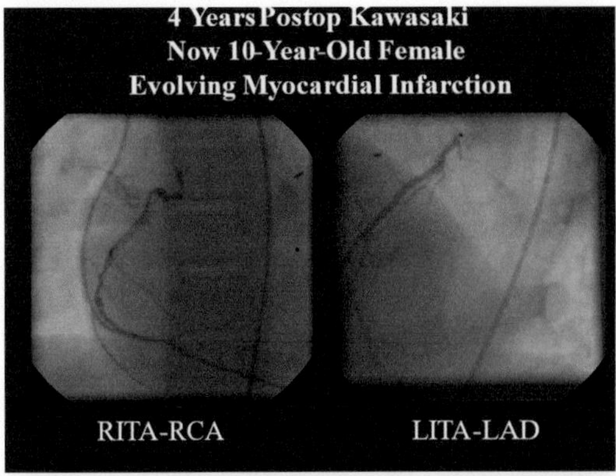

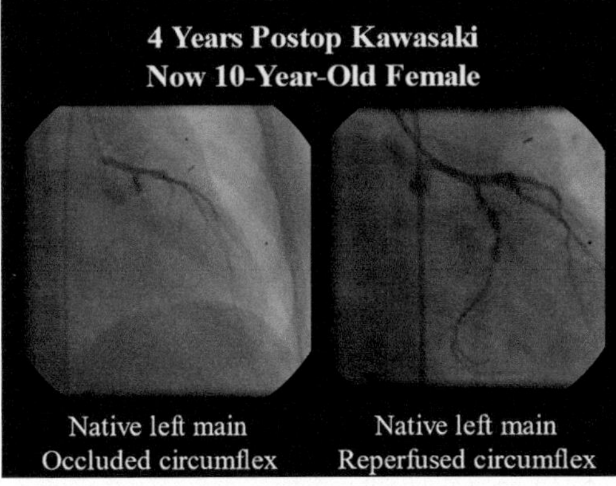

Fig. 8 Shows an unwanted 180-degree coronary button malrotation which can cause coronary artery stenosis and poor myocardial perfusion. The best course of action is to repair the malrotation by reanastomosis or patch angioplasty or both as noted in Fig. 9. *Ao* aorta, *CA* coronary artery, *LCA* left coronary artery, *PA* pulmonary artery, *RAA* right aortic arch

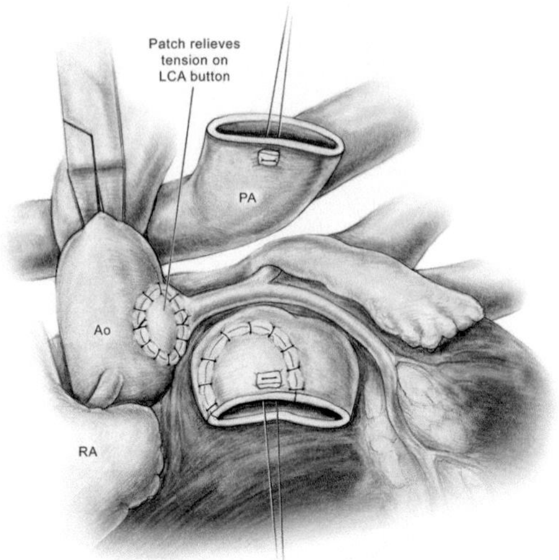

Fig. 9 Shows repair of the rotated and stretched coronary artery button by anastomotic takedown and patch arterioplasty. Aortic cross-clamping with cardioplegic arrest is necessary to perform an accurate and tension free reconstruction. *Ao* aorta, *LCA* left coronary artery, *PA* pulmonary artery, *RA* right arch

repair the stenosis by malrotation correction and patch arterioplasty which is shown in Fig. 9.

In rare cases, ALCAPA takes origin from the right pulmonary artery and will require special surgical consideration which includes ascending aortic implantation (Agrawal et al. 2019) and in some cases, unroofing of an intramural coronary artery (Agrawal et al. 2019). These unusual cases require conscientious preoperative evaluation and identification that will require a complex solution. Repair of ALCAPA origin from the right pulmonary artery is shown in Figs. 10, 11, 12, 13, 14 and 15. The administration of cardioplegia, special attention to avoid coronary button malrotation, and assessment of resultant perfusion have been discussed herein and apply.

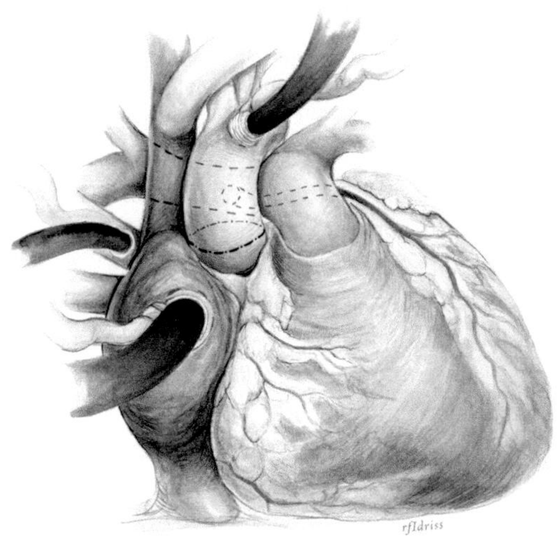

Fig. 10 Shows the ghost origin (dotted lines) of the ALCAPA originating from the right pulmonary artery. The techniques of CPB and cardioplegia administration are the same as previously discussed for this anomaly. *ALCAPA* anomalous left coronary artery from the pulmonary artery, *CPB* cardiopulmonary bypass. (With permission Mavroudis 2015)

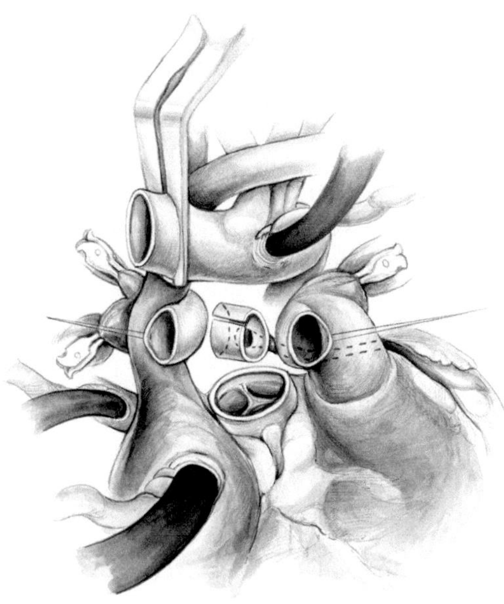

Fig. 11 Shows the resultant anatomy after aortic transection, pulmonary artery mobilization, and segmental resection of the right pulmonary artery together with the ALCAPA origin. *ALCAPA* anomalous left coronary artery from the pulmonary artery. (With permission Mavroudis 2015)

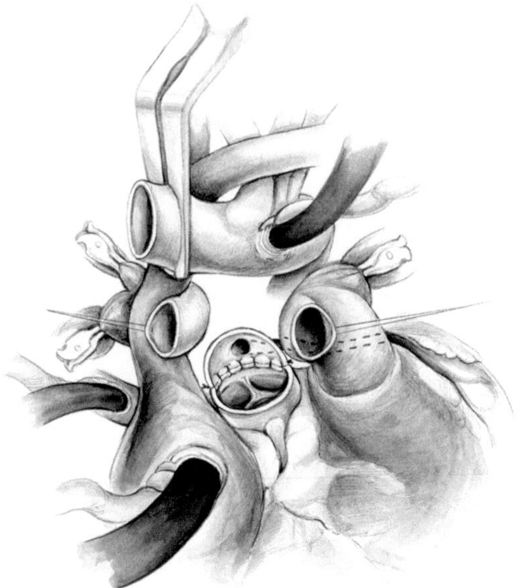

Fig. 12 Shows the reconstruction in progress. The coronary artery is rotated clockwise 90° and sutured to the ascending aorta as noted. This configuration will allow an end-to-end anastomosis with the ascending aorta after the pulmonary artery is reconstructed. (With permission Mavroudis 2015)

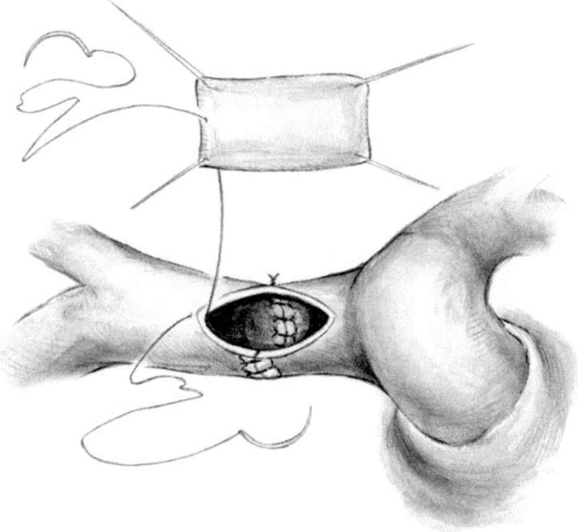

Fig. 13 Depicts the right pulmonary artery reconstruction by a combined end-to-end anastomosis using interrupted suture technique and the initiation of pericardial augmentation using running suture technique. (With permission Mavroudis 2015)

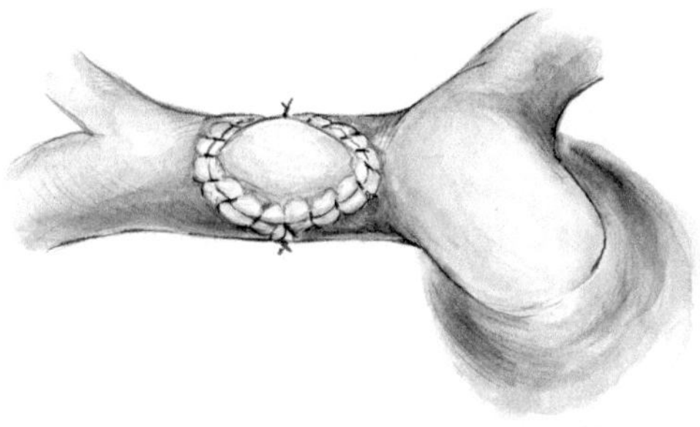

Fig. 14 Shows the reconstructed right pulmonary artery with anterior pericardial patch arterioplasty. (With permission Mavroudis 2015)

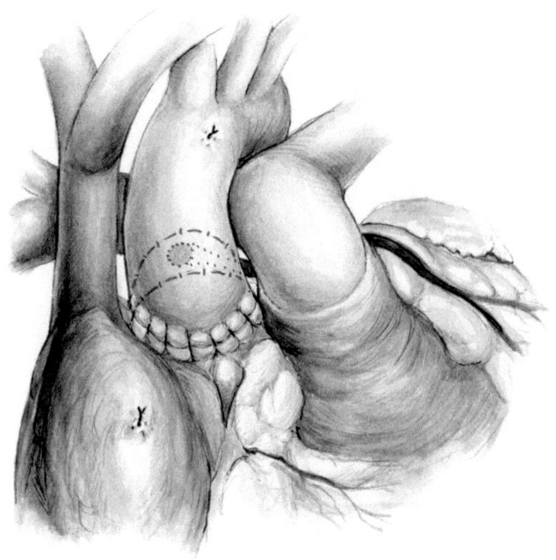

Fig. 15 Once the right pulmonary artery reconstruction is completed, the surgeon can perform the aortic reanastomosis, remove the cross-clamp, rewarm, and separate from cardiopulmonary bypass. The end result after decannulation is shown in the figure. (With permission Mavroudis and Dearani 2020)

3 Anomalous Coronary Artery Arising from the Pulmonary Artery in the Adult

The greater majority of cases with anomalous coronary artery arising from the pulmonary artery occur in newborns and infants as noted previously in this chapter. There are some patients however who present later in life owing to rich collateral vessels from the right coronary artery that provide adequate myocardial perfusion to the left coronary artery circulation (Mavroudis 2015; Mavroudis et al. 2003; Alexi-Meskhishvili et al. 1995; Mavroudis and Dearani 2020). Previous categorization of ALCAPA recognized two types; namely, the infantile form and the adult form (Dodge-Khatami et al. 2000, 2002; Backer et al. 1992; Alexi-Meskhishvili et al. 1995). This classification is neither anatomic nor physiologic since those individuals with collaterals matured to older ages while those without collaterals presented earlier with heart failure and ischemic mitral regurgitation. In the present era, early detection with diagnostic echocardiography allows virtually all patients with ALCAPA to be diagnosed and treated in early infancy. As a result, the old categorization has been relegated to historical interest only.

As noted, adults with ALCAPA are generally well balanced and without symptoms due to the extensive collateral circulation from the enlarged right coronary artery. It would seem therefore that no further therapeutic intervention would be necessary. However, reports of sudden death in this group of patients have resulted in indications for surgery to establish a two coronary system in all patients with ALCAPA regardless of age or symptoms (Schwartz et al. 1997; Singh et al. 1998; Stern et al. 1993; Carvalho et al. 1991; Laks et al. 1995; Paridon et al. 1990; Rein et al. 1987)

The principles for repair of ALCAPA in adults is largely the same as is described herein for neonates and infants with some notable exceptions (Mavroudis and Dearani 2020). The operative procedure and particulars of each stage are shown in Figs. 16, 17, 18, 19, 20 and 21. The most com-

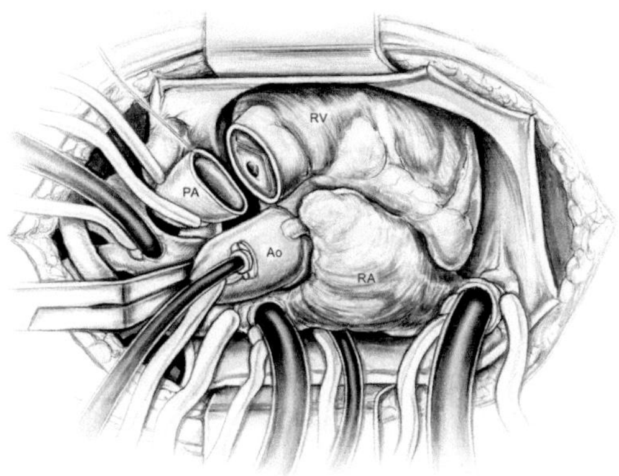

Fig. 16 In adults, the operation to repair anomalous left coronary artery from the pulmonary artery (ALCAPA) by coronary reimplantation to the ascending aorta is started through a median sternotomy. Cardiopulmonary bypass techniques and aortic cross-clamping require important considerations to avoid unsuspected myocardial ischemia. Before cardiopulmonary bypass (CPB) is performed, the right and left main pulmonary arteries are controlled with snuggers in anticipation of engagement shortly after the initiation of CPB. The cardioplegic catheter is placed in the ascending aorta, also before the commencement of CPB. The cardioplegia administration must be coordinated with the perfusion team since blood cardioplegia is prepared shortly after the commencement of CPB. The intent, however, in ALCAPA repair is to commence antegrade cardioplegia immediately after the start of CPB to prevent coronary run off and ischemia. The surgeon may elect to use crystalline cardioplegia or employ other special measures to establish blood cardioplegia. The following stages are used in short order to administer antegrade cardioplegia before any period of ischemia can occur. CPB is initiated with cooling to 32 °C with proper venous drainage; the aorta is immediately cross-clamped and antegrade cardioplegia is started; the right and left pulmonary arteries are completely snugged thereby preventing cardioplegia runoff through the intercoronary collaterals from the right coronary artery. A vent is then placed in the right superior pulmonary vein into the left ventricle. The administration of cardioplegia is completed with epicardial iced saline. If there are any problems with cardiac arrest, the team can infuse retrograde cardioplegia which should be available. The pulmonary artery is then transected as seen in the figure and the ALCAPA is noted. *Ao* aorta, *PA* pulmonary artery, *RA* right atrium, *RV* right ventricle. (With permission Mavroudis and Dearani 2020)

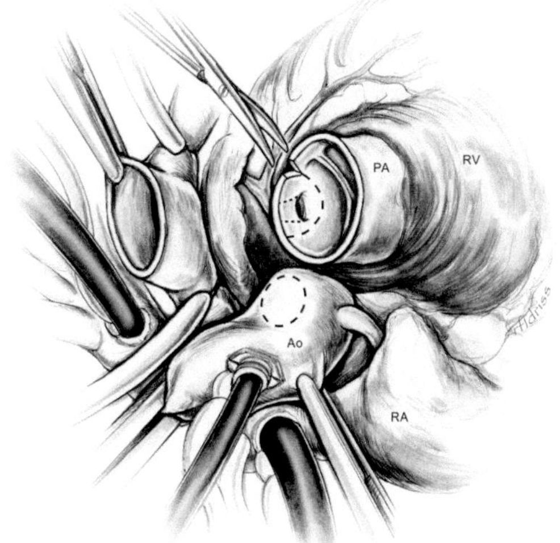

Fig. 17 Careful excision of the coronary artery button is performed making sure to avoid any injury to the pulmonary valve leaflets as noted in the figure. The dotted line in the ascending aorta identifies the location of the aortotomy for the eventual reimplantation. *Ao* aorta, *PA* pulmonary artery, *RA* right atrium, *RV* right ventricle. (With permission Mavroudis and Dearani 2020)

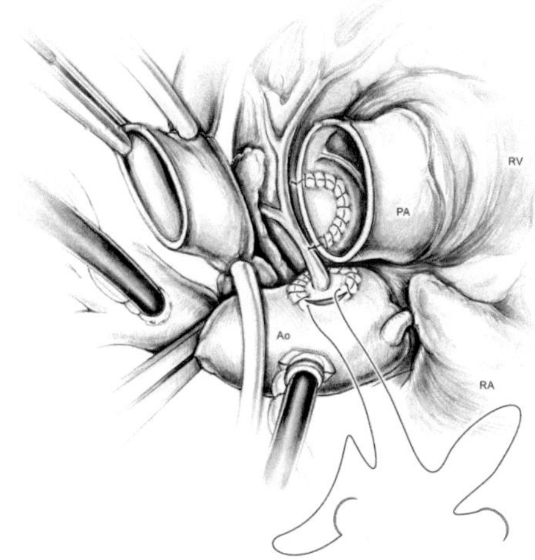

Fig. 18 Shows the coronary to ascending aortic anastomosis being performed. Also noted is the pericardial patch in the pulmonary artery moiety that was the result of the coronary artery mobilization. Once the coronary artery implantation is completed, the air maneuvers can be instituted and followed by cross-clamp removal. *Ao* aorta, *PA* pulmonary artery, *RA* right atrium, *RV* right ventricle. (With permission Mavroudis and Dearani 2020)

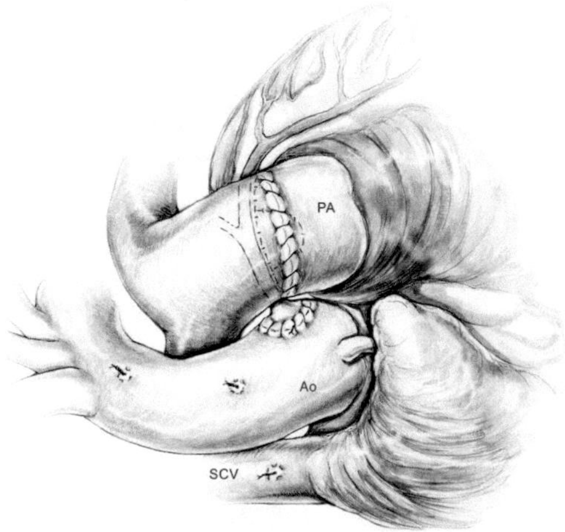

Fig. 19 The end-to-end pulmonary artery reconstruction is completed and followed by separation from cardiopulmonary bypass. Oftentimes, the surgeon will find extensive venous and arterial collateral vessels surrounding the anomalous coronary artery. In addition, mobilization may prove to be too hazardous for safe primary reimplantation. Under these circumstances, careful and individual ligation of the collaterals will be required. Coagulating these vessels rarely stops the bleeding. When the distance is too long for primary reimplantation, a PTFE interposition graft is used for a safe and untethered anastomosis as shown in Fig. 20. *Ao* aorta, *PA* pulmonary artery, *SCV* superior caval vein. (With permission Mavroudis and Dearani 2020)

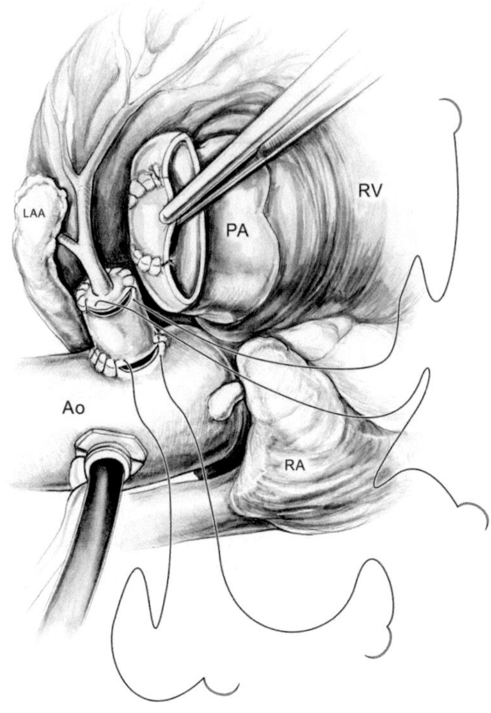

Fig. 20 Shows the PTFE interposition graft being anastomosed to both the coronary artery and the ascending aorta. Sound judgment will determine the caliber and length of the graft. A 4–8 mm graft can be used under these circumstances. *Ao* aorta, *LAA* left atrial appendage, *PA* pulmonary artery, *RA* right atrium, *RV* right ventricle. (With permission Mavroudis and Dearani 2020)

mon problem involving this procedure in adults is evaluating the length of the coronary artery button for translocation. A short coronary artery button when implanted into the ascending aorta will cause anastomotic tension and possible poor perfusion as noted in Fig. 7. As noted in Figs. 9, 20 and 21, coronary patch arterioplasty or an interposition graft will solve this problem and ensure myocardial perfusion.

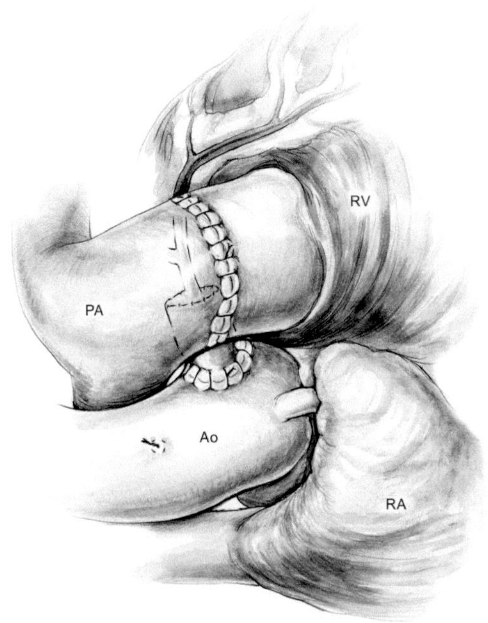

Fig. 21 Depicts the completed graft after the separation from cardiopulmonary bypass. Unlike neonates and infants undergoing this operation, adults with ALCAPA have normal or near-normal ventricular function owing to the rich collaterals. Usually, prompt separation from cardiopulmonary bypass can be anticipated with only very rare cases requiring extracorporeal membrane oxygenation. *ALCAPA* anomalous left coronary artery from the pulmonary artery, *Ao* aorta, *PA* pulmonary artery, *RA* right atrium, *RV* right ventricle. (With permission Mavroudis and Dearani 2020)

4 Anomalous Right Coronary Artery from the Pulmonary Artery (ARCAPA)

The most common variant of pulmonary artery origin of the coronary artery involves the left main coronary artery, described as Type 1 by some authors (Williams et al. 2006; Chernogrivov et al. 2015). Type 2, or anomalous RCA from the pulmonary artery (ARCAPA), is a very rare congenital anomaly, first described by Brooks (Brooks 1885). The potential complications involving the management of the patient with an anomalous origin of the right coronary artery from the pulmonary artery are medical and surgical. Williams and colleagues analyzed 70 cases of ARCAPA in a metanalysis: 40 were children less than 18 years, and 11 were infants (Williams et al. 2006). More recently, Chernogrivov and colleagues performed a meta-nalysis of ARCAPA involving 200 cases concentrating on surgical indications and techniques (Chernogrivov et al. 2015). The majority of patients were asymptomatic while others had presenting findings of angina, congestive heart failure, cyanosis, palpitations, myocardial infarction, and sudden death (Williams et al. 2006; Chernogrivov et al. 2015; Taylor et al. 1992). The reports noted that electrocardiogram (ECG) findings are nonspecific, but echocardiography with Doppler flow color mapping, computed tomography (CT), or magnetic resonance imaging (MRI) is diagnostic (Secinaro et al. 2011). ARCAPA was initially thought to be a benign lesion, but the potential for sudden death as an initial and terminal event has been determined and realized in patients. In keeping with the excellent outcomes achieved with surgical interventions for ALCAPA, coronary reimplantation of ARCAPA is indicated on diagnosis (Williams et al. 2006; Chernogrivov et al. 2015). Diagrammatic representation of the repair sequence is shown in Figs. 22, 23 and 24.

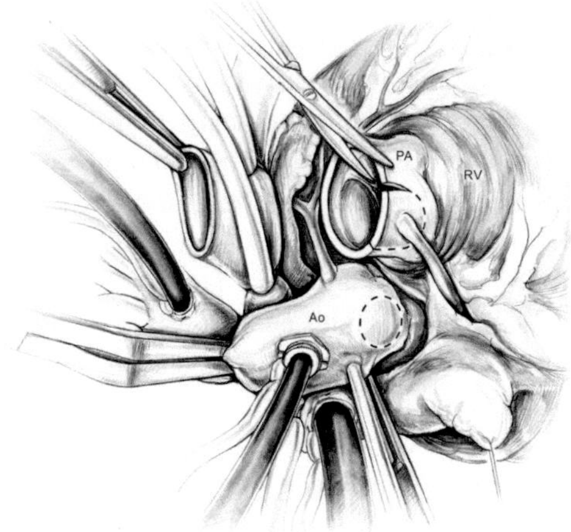

Fig. 22 Shows the anomalous right coronary artery arising from the pulmonary artery. In the adult this is quite rare; however the same principles and techniques apply. In this case, the rich collaterals arise from the left coronary artery and perfuse the right coronary artery distribution. All the protective techniques of cardiopulmonary bypass and myocardial preservations as noted should be employed. The figure shows aortobicaval cardiopulmonary bypass, right and left pulmonary artery snuggers, aortic cross-clamping, antegrade cardioplegia, coronary artery button harvesting, and the location (dotted lines) where the right coronary artery button is to be implanted. *Ao* aorta, *PA* pulmonary artery, *RV* right ventricle. (With permission Mavroudis and Dearani 2020)

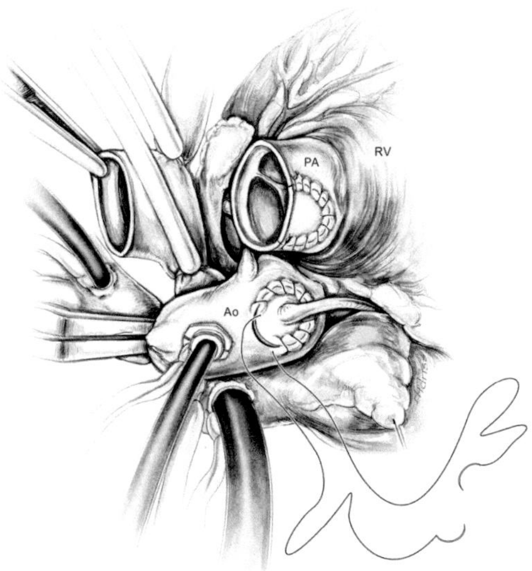

Fig. 23 Demonstrates the right coronary button being anastomosed to the ascending aorta and the completed pulmonary artery pericardial patch to augment the proximal pulmonary artery trunk. *Ao* aorta, *PA* pulmonary artery, *RV* right ventricle. (With permission Mavroudis and Dearani 2020)

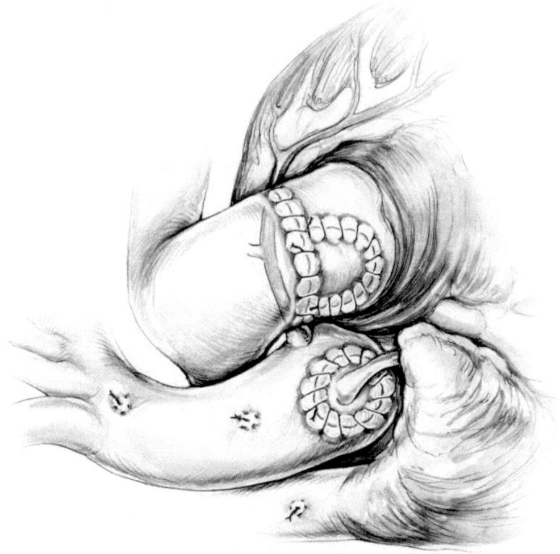

Fig. 24 Shows the completed repair of anomalous pulmonary artery origin of the right coronary artery after separation from cardiopulmonary bypass. (With permission Mavroudis and Dearani 2020)

5 Anomalous Aortic Origin of the Coronary Arteries (AAOCA)

Anomalous aortic origins of the coronary arteries (AAOCA) are found in approximately one-third of all congenital coronary artery anomalies (Taylor et al. 1992; Cohen et al. 1989). All three coronary artery branches can be involved, and essentially every combination of coronary anatomy and origin has been reported. In general, anomalous aortic origins of the coronary arteries are presumed to be benign, except anomalous origin of the left main coronary artery (LMCA) from the right aortic sinus of Valsalva (RASV) and anomalous origin of the RCA from the left aortic sinus of Valsalva (LASV), which are linked to cardiac symptoms and sudden death (Friedman et al. 2007; Taylor et al. 1992; Cohen et al. 1989; Angelini and Flamm 2007; Brothers et al. 2007; Davis et al. 2001; Eckart et al. 2004; Erez et al. 2006; Fedoruk et al. 2007; Jaggers and Lodge 2005; Jokl et al. 1962; Liberthson et al. 1979a; Angelini et al. 2018; Mustafa et al. 1981; Roberts et al. 1982). The troubling problem in these patients is that, in some individuals, the first symptom is sudden death. This has resulted in clinical advocacy in many centers, but not all, for prophylactic coronary artery unroofing in all cases of "left from right" and in selected cases of "right from left" AAOCA (Mavroudis and Dearani 2020).

The potential for mortality of theses seemingly minor coronary abnormalities was first reported by Jokl and associates in 1962 (Jokl et al. 1962). Later in 1992, Taylor and colleagues proposed a classification of anomalous aortic origins (Taylor et al. 1992; Kimbiris 1985; Ueyama et al. 1997; Barth 3rd and Roberts 1986). The accepted, inclusive, and preferred nomenclature system including all possible variations of AAOCA was described in the Congenital Heart Surgery Nomenclature and Database Project and is used up to the time of this publication (Dodge-Khatami et al. 2000).

The diagnostic inquiry for AAOCA usually starts with chest roentgenography and ECG which are generally noncontributory. A stress ECG may suggest ischemia, however, in many cases of AAOCA, the potential clinical ischemic episode is unpredictable (Mustafa et al. 1981; Moodie et al. 1980). Cardiac catheterization was the accepted diagnostic method (Taylor et al. 1992; Cohen et al. 1989; Liberthson et al. 1979a; Mustafa et al. 1981; Ueyama et al. 1997; Moodie et al. 1980; Turner et al. 2011) in the recent past, however, current transthoracic echocardiography using contrast-enhanced, color-guided, pulse-wave Doppler flow interrogation is increasingly relied upon as a noninvasive imaging modality (Taylor et al. 1992; Moodie et al. 1980; Mavroudis et al. 2015). For complete anatomic diagnosis, CT angiography and MRI have become the diagnostic procedures of choice (Angelini and Flamm 2007; Lorber et al. 2015).

These aforementioned diagnostic criteria have resulted in a large number of patients who have been identified and have come to the attention of clinicians leading to the question, "What needs to be done?" Some retrospective observational studies have shown the threat of unfortunate outcomes in this set of patients; however, no prospective and consistent agreement has emerged with the exception that surgery should be offered for left from right AAOCA even if asymptomatic. Moreover, there is no comprehensive study to evaluate the operations that are performed for this entity. The dilemma is that in most cases, the operation is being performed for potential complications in asymptomatic patients. The operation therefore should be performed with the minimum of operative complications. This section of this chapter explores the methods of AAOCA repair and how to avoid complications and treat them if and when they occur.

5.1 Right Coronary Artery from Left Aortic Sinus of Valsalva

Anomalous RCA arising from the left aortic sinus of Valsalva is estimated to be found in 6%–27% of all congenital coronary anomalies (Davis et al. 2001) and in 0.33% of the general population of adolescents (Angelini et al. 2018). Symptoms and clinical findings include myocardial ischemia leading to infarction, syncope, and atrioventricular block. The causative pathoanatomic condition may be characterized by a slit-like and stenotic orifice within the left coronary sinus as well as an associated intramural course within the wall of the aorta of varying distances enroute to the right coronary sinus where it exits to the epicardial surface (Mavroudis and Dearani 2020). Ischemic symptoms which can lead to sudden death occur due to intermittent closure/stenosis of the anomalous ostium or intramural segment within the aortic wall during exercise or hypertensive crises. While not common, pulmonary stenosis with post-stenotic dilatation can also cause pressure on the anomalous coronary artery. Left ventricular dysfunction during exertion can also occur owing to aortic root dilatation with relation to the pulmonary artery or the intercoronary pillar thereby contributing to coronary compression (Mavroudis et al. 2023).

The anatomic pathway of the anomalous RCA in most cases crosses above or downstream of the commissure between the left and right coronary sinuses. Generally, the intramural coronary pathway traverses 1–2 mm downstream of the commissure and thus represents no anatomic risk to aortic leaflet function during the unroofing proce-

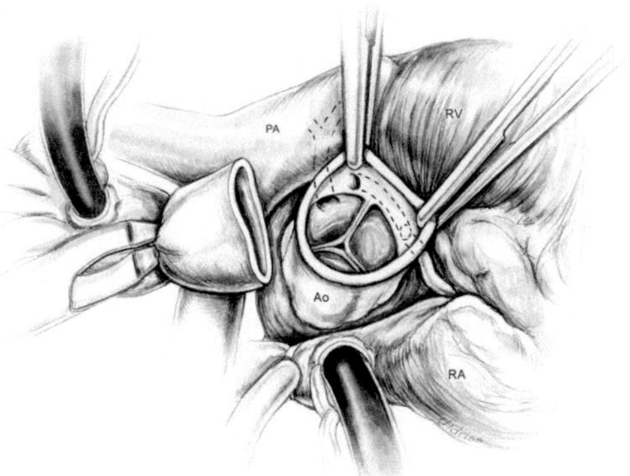

Fig. 25 Shows the operative techniques for repair of AAOCA which are straightforward and involve aortobicaval CPB, left ventricular venting, antegrade/retrograde cardioplegia, and aortic transection or near transection. In the case of aortic transection, corresponding marking sutures (not shown in the drawing) are placed at the respective ascending and proximal aorta sites to facilitate accurate reanastomosis. The anomalous right coronary orifice and the left coronary orifice are measured by graduated dilators and recorded. A dilator is then advanced into the tunnel to confirm the intramural course to the right coronary cusp. The length of the intramural tunnel is also measured by a ruler. The figure shows the intramural course of the anomalous right coronary artery as depicted by the dashed lines. *Ao* aorta, *PA* pulmonary artery, *RA* right atrium, *RV* right ventricle. (With permission Mavroudis and Dearani 2020)

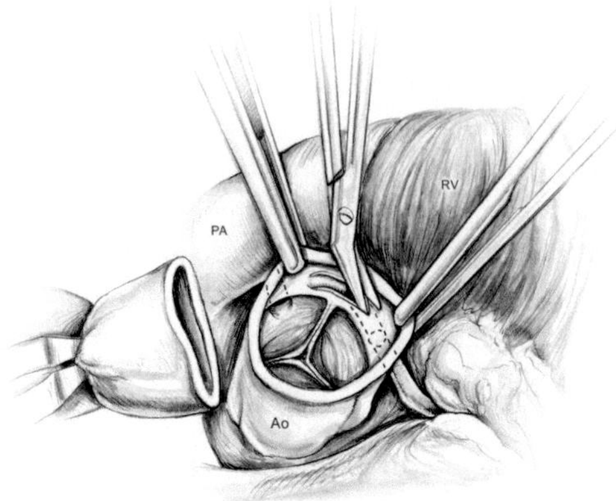

Fig. 26 The unroofing procedure is shown in the figure which demonstrates the unroofed segment as it courses from the left coronary cusp to the right coronary cusp where upon it exits onto the epicardial surface. The incision into the slit-like orifice commences with a scalpel or scissors (noted in the drawing) and progresses downstream superior to the aortic commissure and subsequently to the coronary artery exit site. *Ao* aorta, *PA* pulmonary artery, *RV* right ventricle. (With permission Mavroudis and Dearani 2020)

dure. In unusual cases, the intramural course will traverse from one sinus of Valsalva to the other below or upstream to the commissure. Surgical management of this anatomic entity requires more challenging techniques that will spare the aortic valve leaflets. These techniques are well described and shown in Figs. 25, 26, 27, 28, 29 and 30. The principles of the unroofing procedure can be paraphrased by the carpenter's adage, namely, "measure ten times; cut once". This is sound advice. The unroofing technique is designed to extend into the exiting portion of the anomalous coronary artery to achieve an unobstructed pathway. This maneuver requires careful consideration to unroof the pathway adequately enough to create a neo-orifice without extending the incision too far into the aorta/coronary junction and therefore into the epicardial surface of the heart. The unroofing incision into the neo-ostium needs to be performed using a gradual process and ceased when the orifice is identified short of transmural incision towards the epicardial surface. This process will allow gradual inspection to allow an appropriately sized dilator to pass into the coronary artery without difficulty

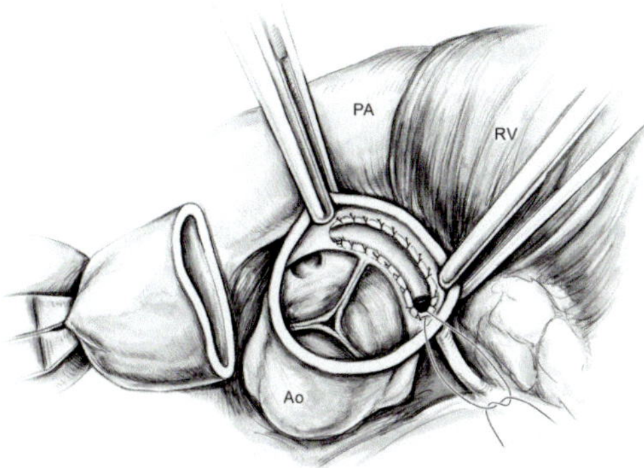

Fig. 27 Once the intramural segment is safely and effectively unroofed, the distance is measured and recorded. Occasionally, the common wall (tunica media) is very thick; and leaving it simply unroofed could threaten the neo-orifice by obstruction. The sides of the tunica media could just flap back and recreate the original stenosis. It is therefore wise and prudent to consider resection of a large portion of the common wall using endarterectomy techniques. The unroofed segment may result in an intimal gap between the coronary artery wall and the aortic wall. This necessitates "tacking sutures" which are placed to reapproximate the intimal edges to avoid dissection and bleeding after separation from CPB. The figure shows the interrupted tacking sutures placed at the neo-orifice of the right coronary artery in the right coronary cusp. The rest of the unroofed segment will also require tacking sutures to complete this part of the operation as noted. Some surgeons prefer a running suture technique for this part of the operation. Most prefer fine monofilament interrupted suture technique. *Ao* aorta, *PA* pulmonary artery, *RV* right ventricle. (With permission Mavroudis and Dearani 2020)

and without unwanted disruption. Placement of a transmural fine suture from outside the aorta where the coronary leaves the aorta is helpful in demonstrating the course and length of the intramural segment. In the case of an unintended disruption to and through the epicardial arterial surface, the intimal edges must be reattached using interrupted monofilament suture before the

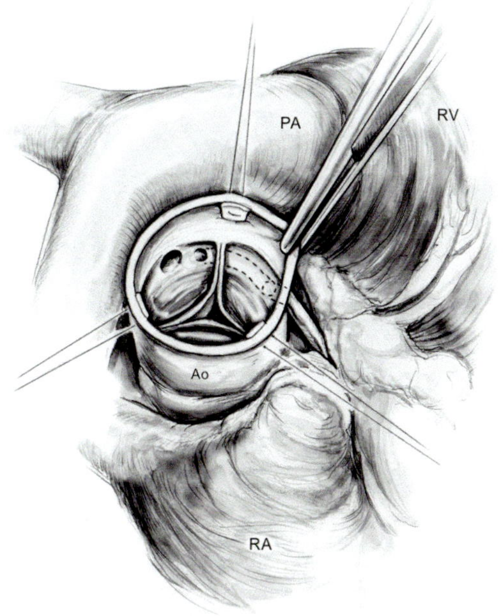

Fig. 28 In very rare circumstances, the right from left anomalous aortic origin of the coronary artery courses from the left coronary cusp to the right coronary cusp upstream or below the commissure. Repair of this configuration is more challenging since the aortic commissure and associated leaflets are subject to injury during the unroofing procedure. More thoughtful reparative techniques are required. The figure demonstrates the aortic root exposure after all of the preparatory maneuvers have been employed such as cardiopulmonary bypass, cardioplegia, and the like. *Ao* aorta, *PA* pulmonary artery, *RA* right atrium, *RV* right ventricle. (With permission Mavroudis and Dearani 2020)

operation continues. Failure to perform this reparative stage of the procedure will likely result in dissection, bleeding, and coronary occlusion at the time of separation from cardiopulmonary bypass (CPB). Timely identification of the problem and resumption of CPB, aortic cross-

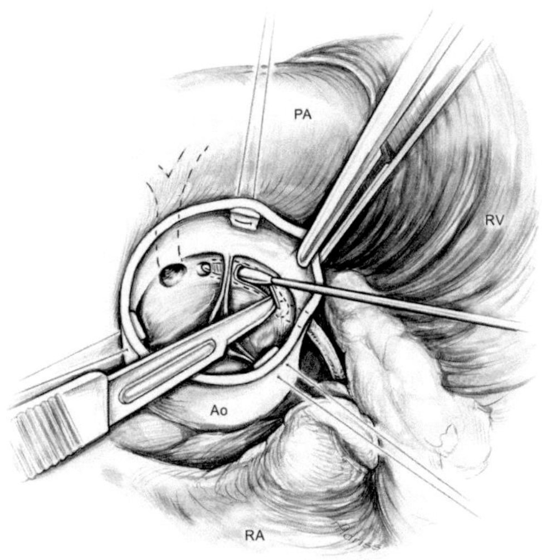

Fig. 29 Shows how a calipered probe measures the orifice diameter and when advanced past the commissure, an incision can be made in the tunica media (shared wall between the coronary artery and the aorta) which can expose the course of the intramural coronary artery. The figure also demonstrates incision and unroofing of the proximal tunnel within the left coronary sinus and complete unroofing within the right coronary sinus. A probe is placed into the unroofed coronary artery to demonstrate the arterial course. Careful incisions will avoid injury to the aortic valve leaflets and prevent any transmural incisions to the epicardial surface of the heart. The same recommendations are advocated for this part of the procedure as noted previously. *Ao* aorta, *PA* pulmonary artery, *RA* right atrium, *RV* right ventricle. (With permission Mavroudis and Dearani 2020)

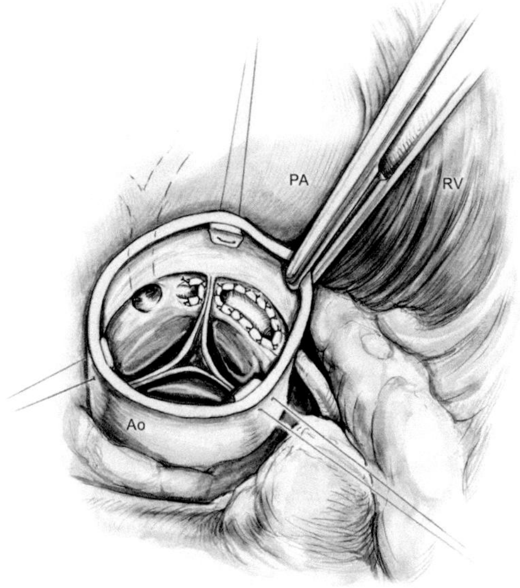

Fig. 30 Shows the completed unroofing procedure which features tacking sutures to approximate the respective intimal flaps of the coronary artery and the aorta. As previously noted, these interrupted sutures along the entire length of unroofing will prevent dissection, hemorrhage, and coronary artery occlusion. Once the operation is completed, the aorta can be reapproximated. After separation from cardiopulmonary bypass (CPB), any unanticipated bleeding or echocardiographic evidence of ventricular dysfunction should result in reinstitution of CPB and exploration of the repair to rule out dissection, anastomotic disruption, and coronary artery occlusion. Excellent results can be anticipated with this operation. Rarely, the intramural orifice can be camouflaged behind the commissure between the right and left coronary cusps. This challenging anatomic variant will be discussed in a subsequent section (Figs. 56, 57, 58, 59, 60, 61 and 62). *Ao* aorta, *PA* pulmonary artery, *RV* right ventricle. (With permission Mavroudis and Dearani 2020)

clamping, and effective repair of the coronary/aortic tear with a biological patch will be required to rectify the situation. This reparative process is reviewed and illustrated in Figs. 54, 55, 56, 57, 58, 59, 60 and 61, which is discussed in a subsequent section of this chapter.

It is important for the unroofing procedure to virtually move the ostium of the anomalous coronary artery beyond the level of the intercoronary commissure or intercoronary pillar (a variable thickening of the aortic wall that travels cranially or downstream from the intercoronary commissure up to the sinotubular junction). Failure to do so, as it occurs with shorter intramural segments, may risk persistent compression of the coronary artery by that pillar (Mery et al. 2018; Agrawal et al. 2017). Figure 31a shows the partial unroofing of an anomalous "right from left" intramural coronary artery that is encumbered by the thickened aortic wall that arises from the commissure and is continuous downstream onto the aortic wall. Two issues arise. First, the orifice of the right coronary artery arises very close to the commissure making an adequate unroofing maneuver unattractive since the thickened course of the intramural segment may still be obstructive. Second, the course of the unroofing procedure may cause unwanted aortic insufficiency if the surgeon is too aggressive in resecting the tunica. Figure 31b shows the first stages of neo-orifice creation by punch technique. Figure 32a illustrates the continuation of the coronary reimplantation procedure (Bonilla–Ramirez et al. 2021). In this technique, the coronary artery is transected as it arises from the aorta, the proximal stump is sutured closed, and the coronary is reimplanted with a direct end-to-side anastomosis to the correct sinus as shown in Fig. 32b. If the surgeon thinks that this procedure may be a possibility based on preoperative imaging, it is useful to place a marking stitch on the external surface of the aorta at the possible site of reimplantation prior to cross-clamping to determine, with the aorta and the coronary artery distended, the ideal location for reimplantation. The perforation on the aorta is performed with an aortic punch the size or slightly smaller than the coronary artery to avoid "flattening" of the coronary artery. It is important to keep an adequate orientation of the coronary artery through the process of reimplantation. Placing a fine stay suture on the adventitia of the vessel prior to transection is helpful for this purpose. If the intramural segment is very short or nonexistent and there is a reasonable segment of the coronary artery wrapping around and touching the aorta, one can create a long oblique

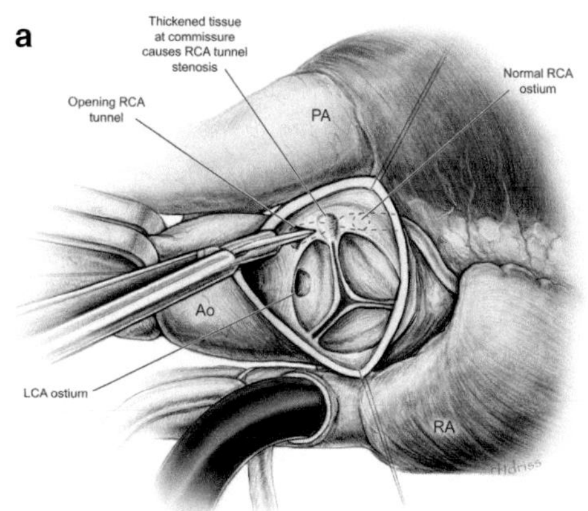

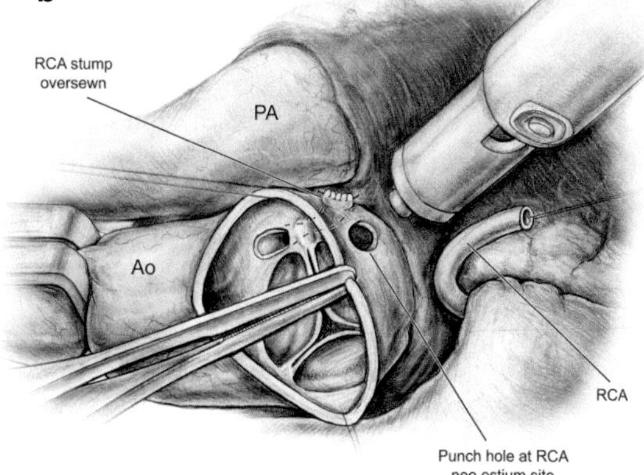

Fig. 31 (**a**) Shows the partially unroofed right from left intramural coronary artery with an endovascular thickening at the commissure extending downstream that could obstruct the coronary artery orifice. (**b**) Shows the aortic epicardial surface with the proximal artery transected at the origin, ligated, and a punch hole being made in the correct sinus. This neo-orifice is generally made nearer to the aortic commissure owing to the anatomic configuration and course of the epicardial coronary artery. *Ao* aorta, *LCA* left coronary artery, *PA* pulmonary artery, *RA* right atrium, *RCA* right coronary artery

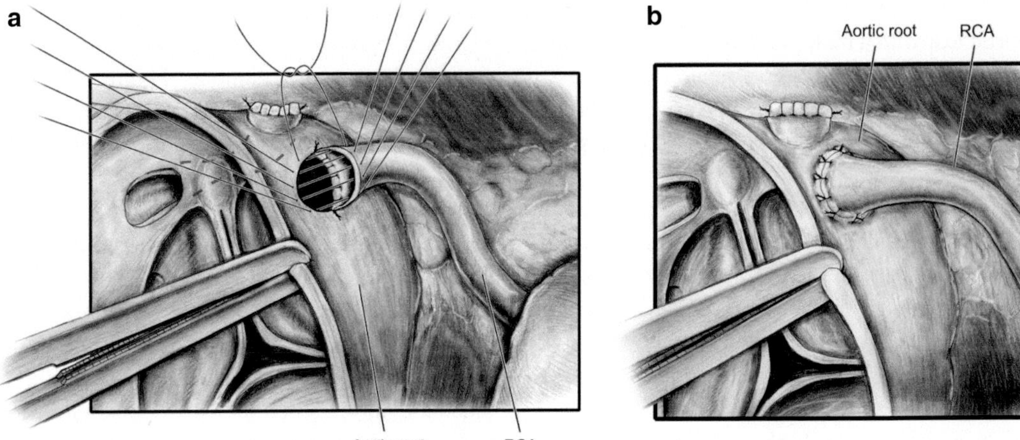

Fig. 32 (**a**) Shows the suturing of the coronary artery into the correct sinus in action with running suture technique for the posterior segment of the anastomosis and interrupted sutures in the anterior portion of the anastomosis. (**b**) Shows the completed anastomosis without any kinks. Any abnormality of this coronary artery reimplantation should signal recommencement of cardiopulmonary bypass, aortic cross-clamping, and cardioplegic arrest to repair the anastomosis by patch arterioplasty or coronary bypass if necessary. *RCA* right coronary artery

anastomosis between the coronary artery and the aorta rather than a round anastomosis. This allows for a wider opening. The major potential complications of this technique involve torsion of the anastomosis, which can be more apparent once the aortic root is distended, and bleeding. These complications require immediate revision with replacement of the cross-clamp. The optimal management of these complications may require placement of a small patch into the proximal coronary artery as noted in Figs. 55, 56, 57 and 58 or placement of a coronary artery bypass graft. This technique of coronary reimplantation can also be used in cases where the intramural segment travels below (upstream to) the aortic valve but the intramural segment is not long enough to allow a partial unroofing of the vessel on the correct sinus as described in Figs. 28, 29 and 30.

5.2 Left Coronary Artery from Right Aortic Sinus of Valsalva

Left Coronary Artery Arising from the Right Aortic Sinus of Valsalva (AAOCA; Left from Right) is the most life-threatening anomaly of congenital aortic coronary origin and is correlated with the highest incidence of symptoms and sudden death (Friedman et al. 2007; Taylor et al. 1992; Cohen et al. 1989; Angelini and Flamm 2007; Brothers et al. 2007; Davis et al. 2001; Eckart et al. 2004; Erez et al. 2006; Fedoruk et al. 2007; Jaggers and Lodge 2005; Jokl et al. 1962; Liberthson et al. 1979a; Angelini et al. 2018; Mustafa et al. 1981; Roberts et al. 1982; Turner et al. 2011; Lorber et al. 2015). The incidence of sudden death in untreated patients can be as high as 57%, and up to 66% are related to exercise (Taylor et al. 1992; Mustafa et al. 1981; Moodie et al. 1980). In a subgroup of patients, the risk of sudden death is reported to be as high as 82% if the LMCA courses between the great vessels (Taylor et al. 1992; Moodie et al. 1980; Turner et al. 2011).

The nomenclature system for "left from the right" AAOCA has been proposed. It is characterized by the course of the left main coronary artery in relation to the great vessels and is noted by: (1) anterior to the pulmonary artery; (2) posterior to the aorta; (3) between the great vessels; and (4) trans-septal course through the conal septum (beneath the right ventricular infundibulum) (Moodie et al. 1980). Furthermore, the myocardial distribution of the branch coronary arteries is also affected. In the case that the LMCA courses between the great vessels, it provides one or two branches to the proximal ventricular septum. On the other hand, when the anomalous LMCA is posterior to the aorta, there are no septal branches from the left coronary system, rising rather from the RCA (Ueyama et al. 1997). As described earlier, the principle pathoanatomic characteristic of an anomalous coronary artery is an intramural course that is almost always stenotic, both at its orifice and over the intramural course. Complicating the matter further is that the intramural course can be above the commissure, between the left and right coronary cusps, or below the commissure. In particular, the recognized causes of myocardial ischemia and sudden death are multifactorial and include an acute angular origin of the anomalous vessel causing a slit-like orifice (Taylor et al. 1992; Cohen et al. 1989; Mustafa et al. 1981; Ueyama et al. 1997; Moodie et al. 1980; Turner et al. 2011; Lorber et al. 2015), compression of the coronary artery by aortic root distension at the onset of diastole (Taylor et al. 1992; Moodie et al. 1980), exercise-induced expansion of both the aortic root and the pulmonary trunk causing compression of the LMCA (Mustafa et al. 1981), effort-related stretching of the intramural LMCA segment adherent to the aorta along its first 1.5 cm of length (Mustafa et al. 1981; Moodie et al. 1980), and compression of the LMCA by the intercoronary commissure, predominantly during diastole when the aortic valve is closed (Mustafa et al. 1981), with resultant spasm, torsion, or kinking (Taylor et al. 1992; Ueyama et al. 1997).

In adults, the prevalence of atherosclerosis is higher in those patients with aberrant LMCA than in age-matched controls (Liberthson et al. 1979a; Ueyama et al. 1997) making the risk of complications all the more frequent. Symptoms are common and can be experienced in as many as 54% of patients (Taylor et al. 1992; Eckart et al. 2004; Liberthson et al. 1979a). Predictably, symptoms include angina during exercise, congestive heart failure, syncope, palpitations, gastrointestinal symptoms (Benge et al. 1980), myocardial infarction, and sudden death (Taylor et al. 1992; Cohen et al. 1989). Angina and syncope are more common in younger patients, in contrast to older patients (greater than 30 years of age) who experience angina and myocardial infarction (Cohen et al. 1989). Furthermore, younger patients are more prone to sudden death, which may occur as a presenting symptom (Taylor et al. 1992; Cohen et al. 1989). Probably the most revealing postmortem study in young patients involved 6.3 million US military recruits (ages 17–35 years) undergoing basic military training between 1977 and 2001 (Eckart et al. 2004) There were 64 sudden cardiac deaths and among these, the majority (61%) were related to coronary artery pathology, of which 54% had anomalous aortic coronary origins.

In summary, anomalous left main coronary artery origin with an intramural course from the right aortic sinus of Valsalva is associated with the highest incidence of cardiac ischemic symptoms and sudden death. The anatomic configurations that result in ischemic complications in "Left from Right" AAOCA are similar to those that occur in patients with "Right from Left" AAOCA.

The operative management of "Left from Right" intramural AAOCA is reviewed in Figs. 33, 34, 35, 36, 37, 38, 39, 40, 41 and 42 When the intramural segment of the coronary artery traverses below the intercoronary commissure (Fig. 39), the surgeon can use a technique of partial unroofing to the correct sinus (Figs. 40 and 41) or if the intramural segment is not long enough, transection of the coronary artery as it arises from the sinus with reimplantation into the correct sinus can be performed. This scenario does not allow harvesting of the coronary artery as a button as described for extramural coronary arteries (Figs. 68, 69 and 70) due to the relationship between the anomalous coronary artery and the aortic valve.

Included in this review is the complication of unwanted injury to the aortic commissure during the unroofing procedure as noted in Fig. 42. The repair technique involves suture resuspension of the damaged commissure to the aortic wall by suture approximation of the commissure to the original site using transaortic sutures with pledgets on the epicardial surface to prevent tearing

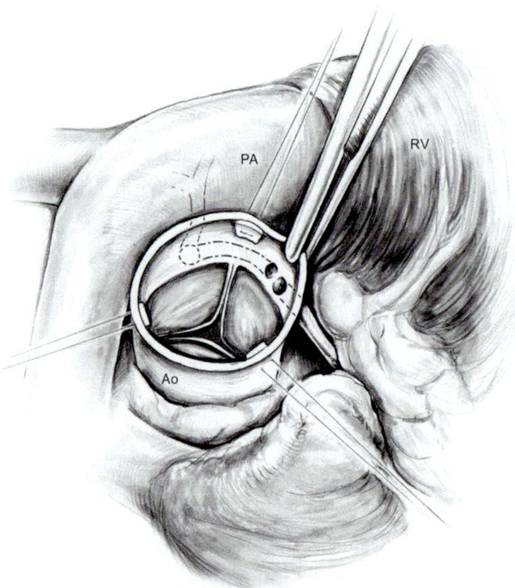

Fig. 33 The operative approach and exposure is the same as previously described. The anatomic specifics for "left from right" AAOCA are demonstrated in the figure. In particular, the anomalous left coronary orifice is stenotic with a slit-like opening; the course slightly above the commissure is depicted by the dashed lines and ghost-like appearance. *Ao* aorta, *PA* pulmonary artery, *RV* right ventricle. (With permission Mavroudis and Dearani 2020)

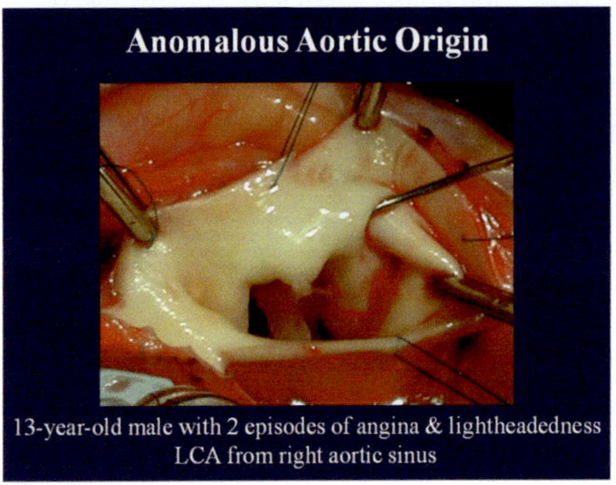

Fig. 34 Photograph showing anomalous left main coronary artery from the right coronary sinus. The coronary probe instrument is entering the orifice of the left main coronary artery from the right coronary sinus of Valsalva. *LCA* left coronary artery

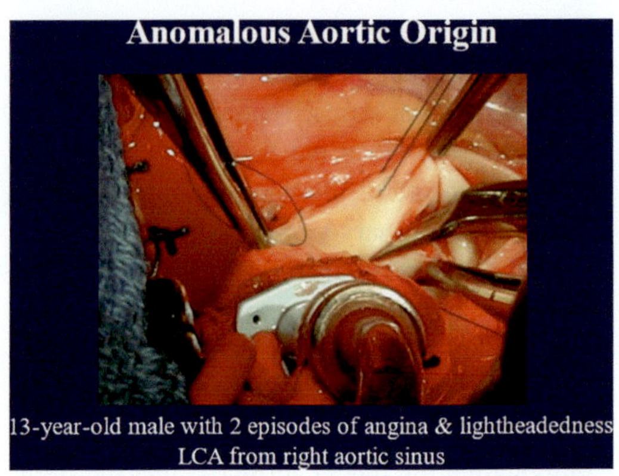

Fig. 35 Photograph showing scissor incision along the course of the anomalous left main coronary artery from the right coronary sinus. *LCA* left coronary artery

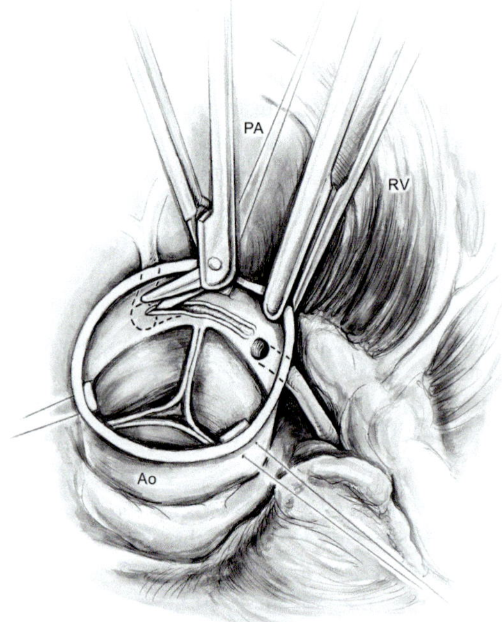

Fig. 36 Depicts the unroofing procedure using sharp scissors incision. Similar safeguards are undertaken as previously described to avoid an unwanted transaortic/transcoronary incision to the epicardial surface of the heart. A transmural incision at this point in the operation will require proper identification of the problem and careful repair as will be discussed in Figs. 49, 50, 51, 52, 53, 54 and 55. *Ao* aorta, *PA* pulmonary artery, *RV* right ventricle. (With permission Mavroudis and Dearani 2020)

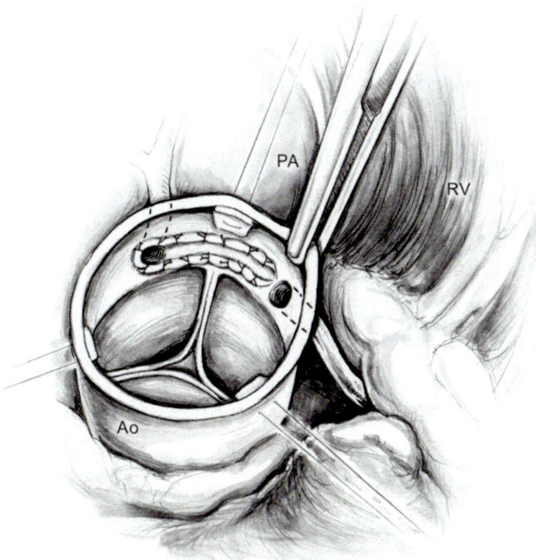

Fig. 37 Demonstrates the unroofing procedure with tacking sutures at the left main coronary artery neo-orifice. The rest of the tacking sutures are placed to complete the procedure. *Ao* aorta, *PA* pulmonary artery, *RV* right ventricle. (With permission Mavroudis and Dearani 2020)

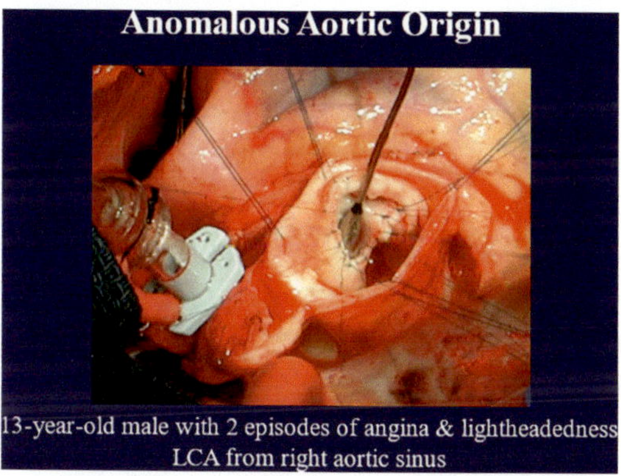

Fig. 38 Photograph showing completed tacking sutures along the length of the unroofed course of the left intramural coronary artery which originated from the right coronary sinus. The coronary probe instrument shows the widely patent left main coronary artery orifice in the appropriate sinus. *LCA* left coronary artery

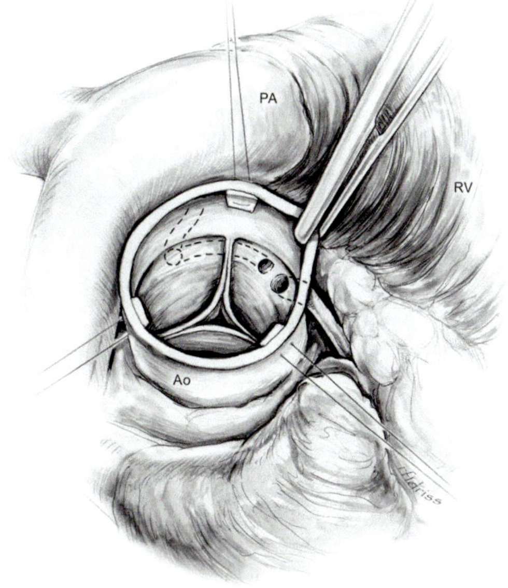

Fig. 39 In the case that the left main coronary artery arises from the right coronary sinus and traverses below the commissure to the left coronary sinus, the same techniques are employed as have been described in the "right from left" anatomic details. The figure shows the "left from right" AAOCA anomalous anatomy coursing below the commissure. *Ao* aorta, *PA* pulmonary artery, *RV* right ventricle. (With permission Mavroudis and Dearani 2020)

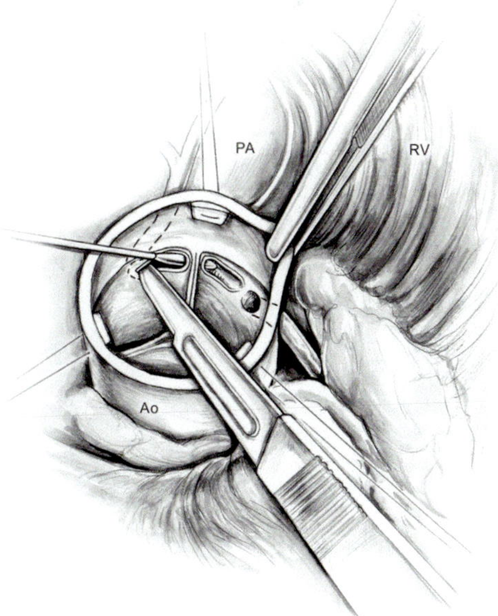

Fig. 40 Shows how the incisions of the tunica media and unroofing procedure are performed in both sinuses of Valsalva. *Ao* aorta, *PA* pulmonary artery, *RV* right ventricle. (With permission Mavroudis and Dearani 2020)

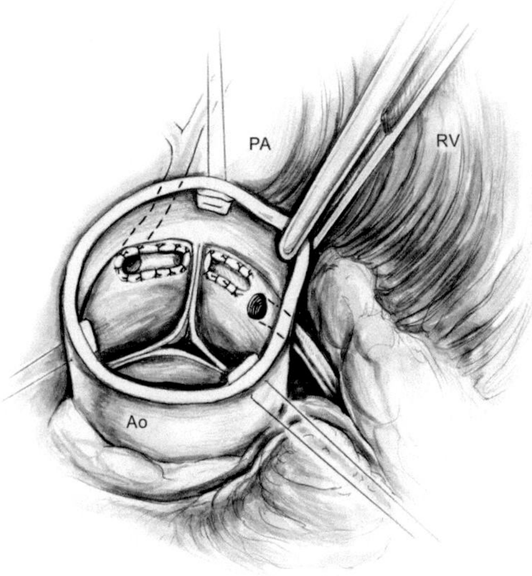

Fig. 41 Shows how tacking sutures are placed which ensure integrity of the intimal surfaces. The rest of the tacking sutures are required along the entire unroofed segment to prevent dissection and bleeding. *Ao* aorta, *PA* pulmonary artery, *RV* right ventricle. (With permission Mavroudis and Dearani 2020)

and disruption of the repair. If the injury is not recognized during the procedure, intraoperative post-procedural TEE can identify new onset of aortic regurgitation. Consideration should be given to aortic root reexploration and repair of the aortic leaflet injury by commissure resuspension. Rarely, an aortic valve replacement might be indicated.

A very rare type of AAOCA "left from right" is demonstrated in the coronary artery angiogram in Fig. 43 which shows the retroaortic course of the left main coronary artery arising from the right coronary sinus. The patient is a 19-year-old presenting with exertional angina.

The anatomic details of this anomaly are noted in Fig. 44 which shows acute angulation of the left main coronary artery at its origin from the right coronary sinus with a long retroaortic course to the bifurcation. Ischemic symptoms and complications are thought to be intermittent compression of the long segment enroute to the bifurcation

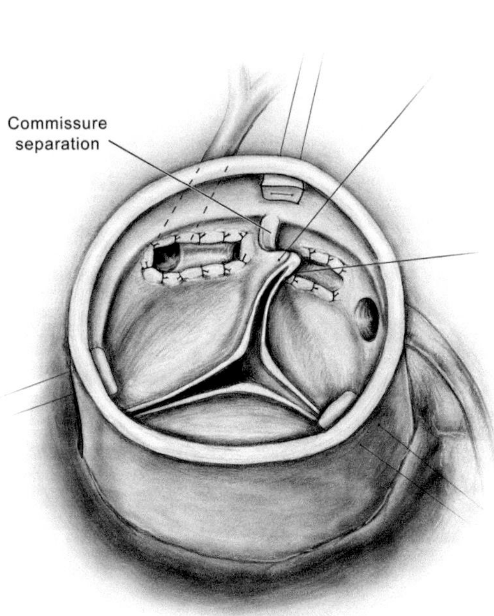

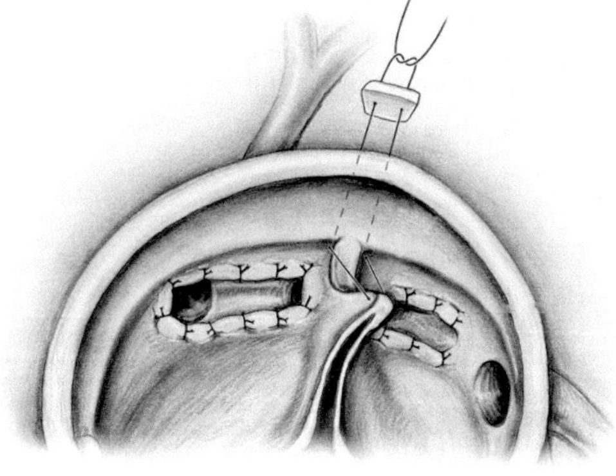

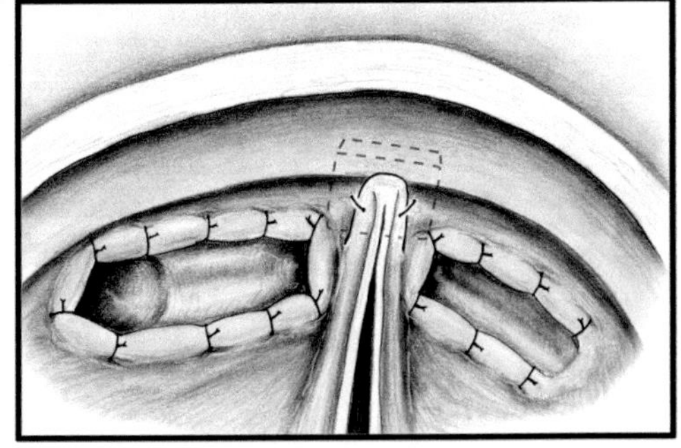

Fig. 42 Left panel shows how an unwanted injury can occur at the aortic commissure during the unroofing procedure. The right panel shows the injured commissure being resuspended to avoid aortic regurgitation. The inset demonstrates the repaired dislodged commissure using suture technique using a pledget on the epicardial surface of the aorta. The pledget offers tensile strength to avoid sutures ripping through the wall of the aorta

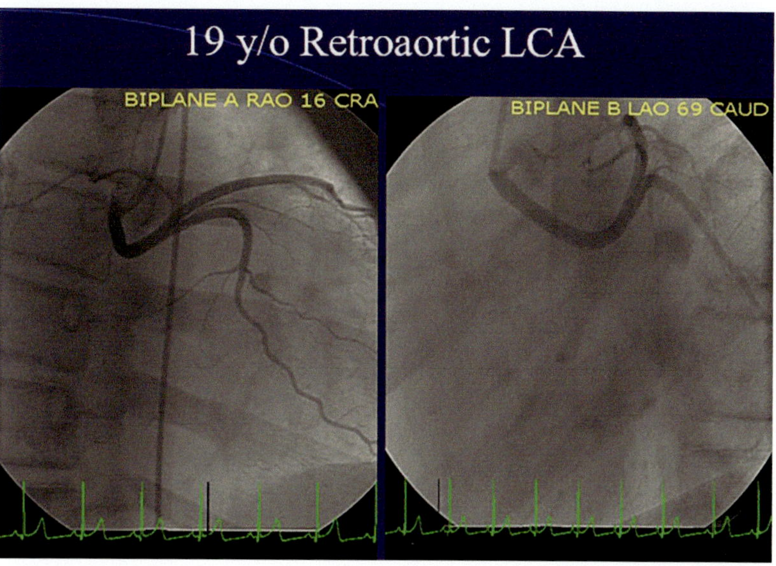

Fig. 43 Shows an angiogram of a retroaortic course of the left main coronary artery arising from the right coronary sinus in a symptomatic 19-year-old patient (angiogram). *LCA* left coronary artery

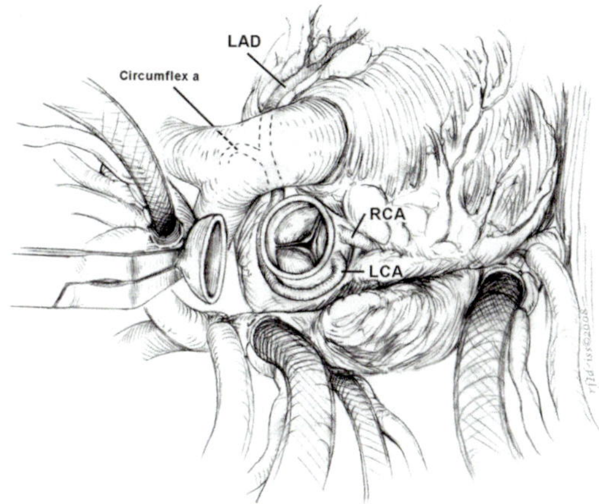

Fig. 44 Another very rare AAOCA "left from right" is demonstrated in the figure. The anatomic details of this anomaly are acute angulation of the left main coronary artery as it emerges from the right coronary sinus with a long course to the bifurcation. Ischemic complications are thought to be induced by the long segment enroute to the left anterior and circumflex coronary arteries. In this anatomic variation, there is no intramural segment. However, the course of the left main coronary starts at the right coronary sinus of Valsalva and makes a rightward turn around the ascending aorta with posterior and transverse extensions to the bifurcation. *Circumflex a* circumflex aorta, *LAD* left anterior descending, *LCA* left coronary artery, *RCA* right coronary artery. (With permission Mavroudis and Dearani 2020)

of the left anterior and circumflex coronary arteries. This anatomic variation is not associated with an intramural segment. However, the course of the left main coronary takes its origin at the right coronary sinus of Valsalva and makes an acute rightward turn around the ascending aorta with posterior and transverse extensions to the bifurcation which subjects the artery to origin stenosis and compression during systole and diastole (Khan et al. 2020)

Figure 45 (left panel) shows the start of a side-to-side anastomosis of the anomalous left coronary artery to the left coronary sinus of Valsalva. The right panel shows the completion repair. The potential complications of this procedure are intuitive and include injury to the left coronary aortic leaflet while creating an orifice for the anastomosis, avoiding unwanted kinking of the coronary artery during the side-to-side anastomosis, and bleeding. In general, accurate estimation of anastomotic location and careful suture technique will result in an excellent outcome.

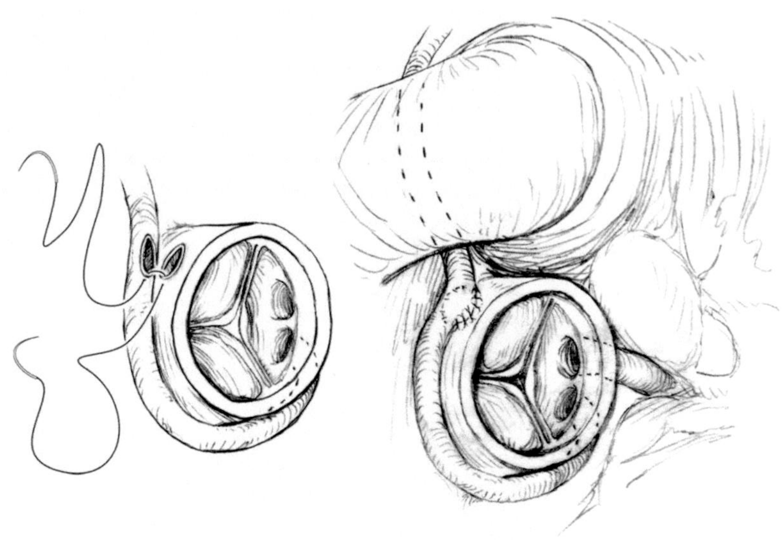

Fig. 45 Left panel indicates the preparatory stages that will facilitate the side-to-side anastomosis between the coronary artery and the aortic wall in the left sinus of Valsalva. The right panel demonstrates the completed side-to-side anastomosis with continuation of the left main to the bifurcation. (With permission Mavroudis and Dearani 2020)

5.3 Unroofing of Anomalous Origin of the Left Main Coronary Artery with Intrainfundibular (Transseptal or Intraconal) Course of the Left Anterior Descending Coronary Artery

The rare condition of a left anterior descending (LAD) coronary artery coursing through the infundibular septum has been associated with angina, especially in older patients. Literature reports have noted that although rare, this condition is being recognized to a greater degree owing to improved imaging techniques (Marey and Said 2021; Mainwaring and Hanley 2019). Anginal symptoms in patients with this anatomic entity present a clinical dilemma since there are no settled treatment plans which can include clinical observation or surgical intervention. Even surgical intervention is not agreed upon which includes coronary bypass as well as coronary unroofing. It is generally assumed that coronary stenosis in these patients is intermittent. Coronary bypass can be performed but it will establish a competitive hemodynamic flow situation during times of absence of dynamic stenosis. Coronary bypass in these circumstances can result in bypass occlusion. Some authors (Marey and Said 2021; Mainwaring and Hanley 2019) have advocated coronary artery unroofing as noted in Figs. 46, 47, 48 and 49. While it is possible to perform a significant portion of the unroofing procedure without pulmonary artery transection, anatomic exposure is improved with transection and will enhance a controlled and accurate unroofing operation. Even so, complications can occur, especially if the dissection and unroofing of the coronary artery causes arterial injury as noted in Fig. 48a. The illustration shows how an unwanted incision into the anterior portion of the coronary artery can result from deep dissection. Interrupted suture technique may seem to be indicated but in general this will cause localized stenosis. Better to use a pericardial patch to repair the injury which will result in an unobstructed pathway as noted in the inset of Fig. 48b. Care must be taken to perform a hemostatic anastomo-

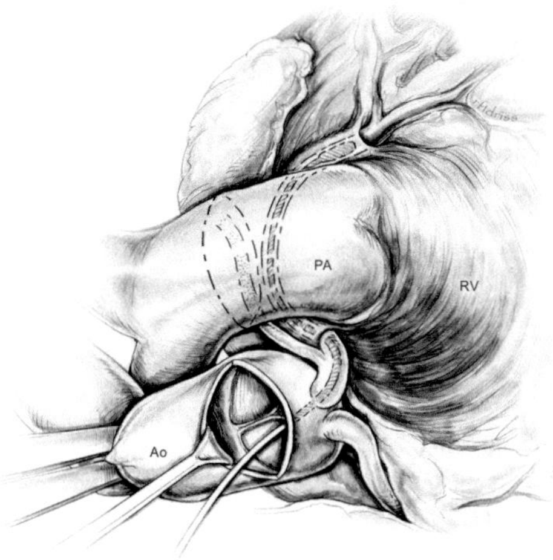

Fig. 46 Shows transaortic exposure of an anomalous left main coronary artery arising from the right coronary sinus after aortic cross-clamping and cardioplegic arrest. A coronary dilator is shown within the course of the left anterior descending coronary artery that traverses within the infundibulum along the arterial pathway. This course with intermittent coronary compression is thought to be the cause of angina and ischemic episodes that occur in patients with this anomaly. *Ao* aorta, *PA* pulmonary artery, *RV* right ventricle. (With permission Mavroudis and Dearani 2020)

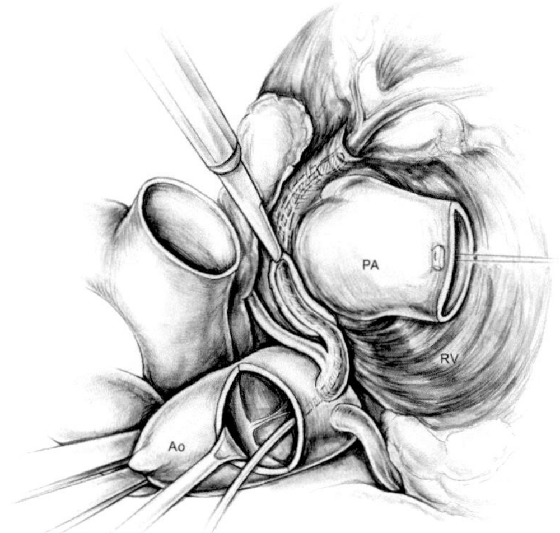

Fig. 47 While it is possible to partially unroof the proximal coronary artery without pulmonary artery transection, a greater degree of exposure will allow a more comprehensive unroofing operation with pulmonary artery transection as noted in the figure. The course of the intra-infundibular coronary artery has been shown to be relatively constant in previous anatomic studies; however, the surgeon should use prudence to avoid an unwanted posterior right ventricular entry below the pulmonary outflow tract. Other authors have used the anterior approach by detaching the pulmonary artery and coronary unroofing through the inside of the right ventricle. *Ao* aorta, *PA* pulmonary artery, *RV* right ventricle. (With permission Mavroudis and Dearani 2020)

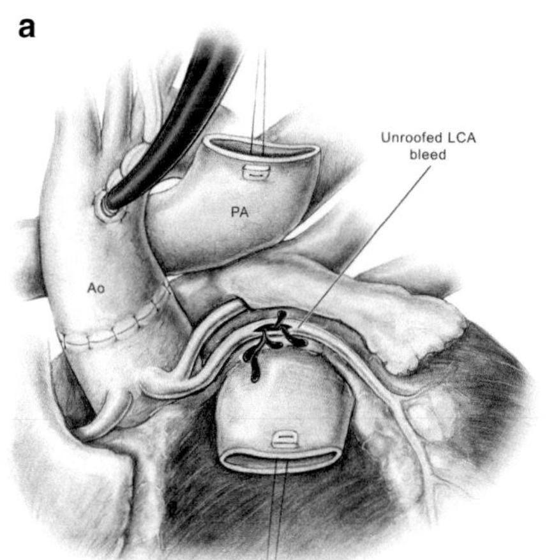

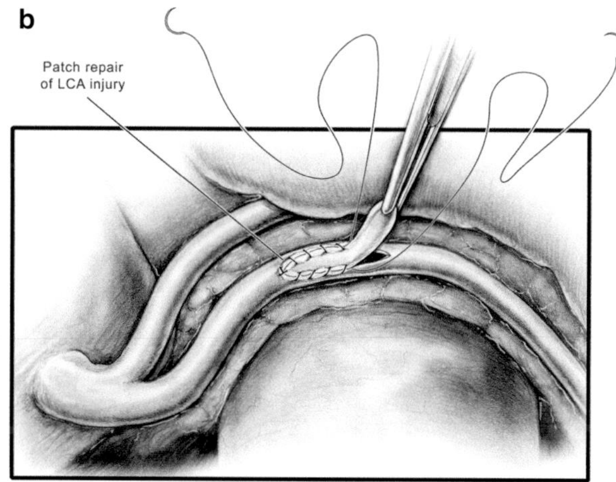

Fig. 48 (**a**) Shows coronary artery injury with bleeding after release of the cross-clamp. The injury was caused by an overzealous unroofing maneuver which can result in a partial incision which may not become manifest until cross-clamp removal and systemic pressure. (**b**) Shows the pericardial patch arterioplasty of the injured coronary artery during a renewed period of aortic cross-clamping and cardioplegic arrest. *Ao* aorta, *LCA* left coronary artery, *PA* pulmonary artery

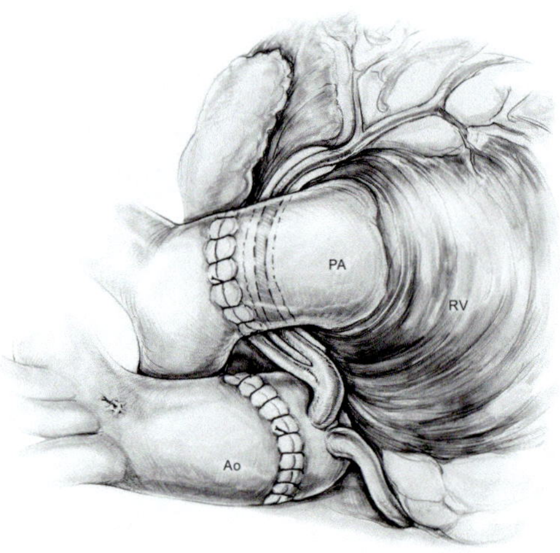

Fig. 49 Demonstrates the extensive unroofing of the anomalous left anterior coronary artery after successful unroofing and reapproximation of the pulmonary artery trunk. *Ao* aorta, *PA* pulmonary artery, *RV* right ventricle. (With permission Mavroudis and Dearani 2020)

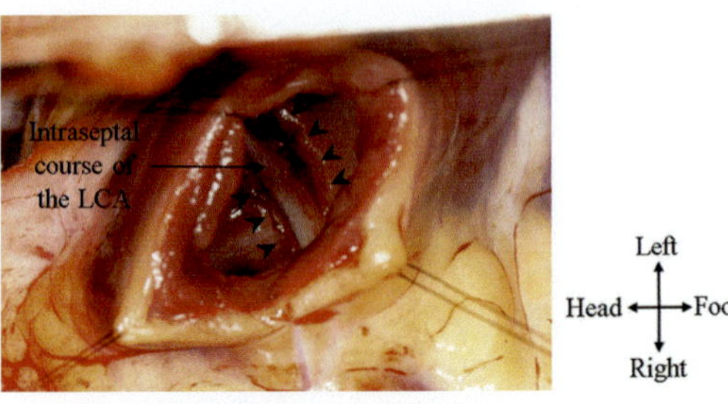

Fig. 50 Shows an operative photograph of a patient with anomalous intramyocardial trans-septal course of the left main coronary artery. The exposure is by a transverse right ventriculotomy. The completed unroofing procedure is shown with clear identification of the left main coronary artery which has been freed from the surrounding conal muscle. *LCA* left coronary artery. (With permission Doan et al. 2020)

sis since the repaired artery will be camouflaged under the main pulmonary artery after the reanastomosis is completed as shown in Fig. 49. Another potential complication could result from entry into the right ventricular outflow tract while unroofing the coronary as the wall of the outflow tract can be quite thin at this level. The best approach for this complication would be to open the outflow tract anteriorly and repair the area of injury with a small pericardial patch, analogous to the technique illustrated in Fig. 50. Another procedure to accomplish transconal unroofing is shown in Fig. 50 which depicts an operative photograph of a patient with a transseptal anomalous left coronary artery from the right sinus. The exposure is through a transverse right ventriculotomy inferior to the pulmonary valve annulus. The unroofing procedure is performed using a sharp blade which is clearly shown in the photograph (Doan et al. 2020). Najm and associates (Najm and Ahmad 2019; Najm et al. 2021, 2023) have presented their modified reconstruction of the transconal unroofing procedure which is shown in Figs. 51 and 52a–c. The repair involves

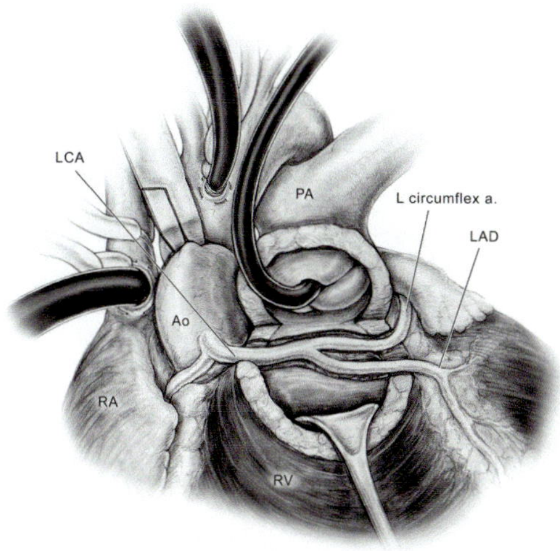

Fig. 51 Shows the modified method of intramural septal unroofing of the anomalous left main coronary artery. The exposure is through a transverse right ventriculotomy inferior to the pulmonary valve annulus. The course of the unroofed left main coronary artery and the early takeoff of the left anterior descending coronary artery are clearly shown. The catheter through the pulmonary valve keeps the valve competent to ensure an anatomical configuration that will avoid valvar injury during the unroofing procedure. *Ao* aorta, *LAD* left anterior descending, *LCA* left coronary artery, *L* circumflex a, left circumflex aorta, *PA* pulmonary artery, *RA* right atrium, *RV* right ventricle

anterior subpulmonic right ventricular exposure to identify the intramural septal course of the left main coronary artery and in some cases an early take-off of the left anterior descending coronary artery as shown in Fig. 51. The essence of the procedure requires extensive coronary unroofing and autologous pericardial reconstruction to reconnect the right ventricle to the pulmonary artery while keeping the course of the left main coronary artery posterior to the reconstructed right ventricular-to-pulmonary artery continuity. Essentially, the left main coronary artery is excluded from the enveloping muscle and outside of the right ventricular-to-pulmonary artery circulation as shown in Fig. 52a–c. Najm and associates (Najm and Ahmad 2019; Najm et al. 2021, 2023) have reported excellent results with this technique as documented in pre- and postoperative imaging. While their group reported no important complications, potential problems involving anastomotic bleeding from the pericardial reconstruction site, false aneurysm involving the right ventricular outflow tract, and possible acquired subpulmonic stenosis should be monitored to assure proper long-term success.

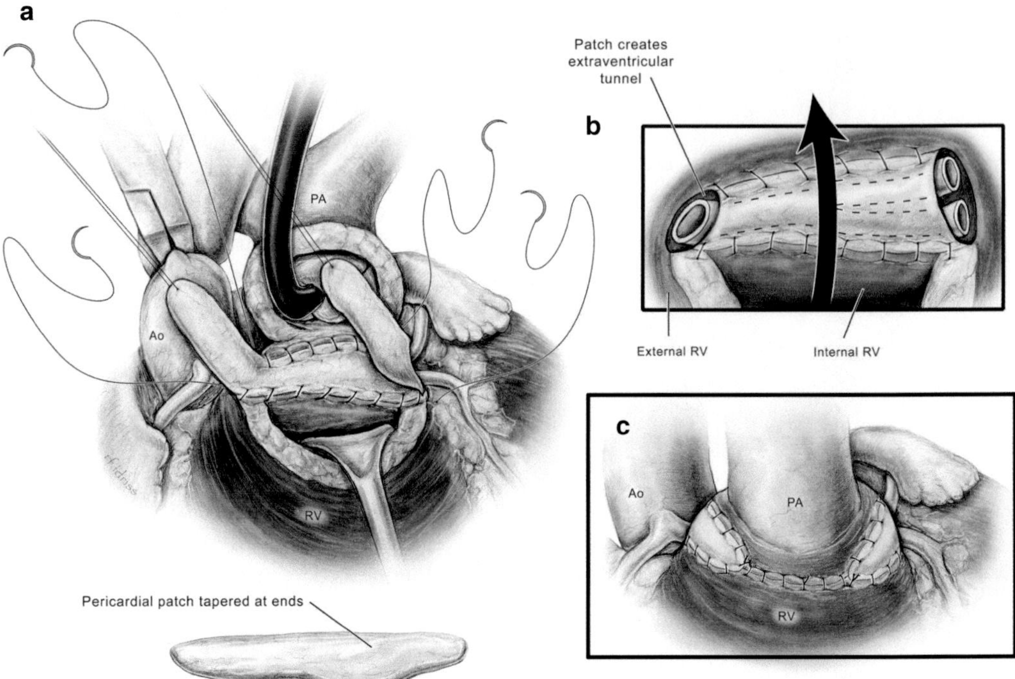

Fig. 52 (**a–c**) (**a**) demonstrates how the autologous pericardium is cut to size and sutured in place to reconstruct the continuity between the pulmonary annulus and the right ventricle while excluding the unroofed anomalous coronary artery from the circulation. In essence, the unroofed coronary has been freed from the enveloping muscle and courses to the epicardial surface external to the right ventricular to pulmonary artery circulation. The (**b**) inset shows how the patch creates an extraventricular tunnel which basically frees the course of the coronary artery from the pressure conditions of the right ventricle. The inset (**c**) shows the completed reconstruction which highlights the tapered pericardial patches which allow native pulmonary artery to right ventricular anastomosis for continued growth potential. The possible complications, although not experienced by authors are bleeding at the anastomotic sites, development of false aneurysms in the long term, and subpulmonic stenosis. *Ao* aorta, *PA* pulmonary artery, *RV* right ventricle

5.4 Right Coronary Artery from the Left Coronary Sinus Complicated by Unwanted Transaortic, Transcoronary Incision

Although there are no long-term clinical results of transaortic unroofing of an intramural coronary artery, the procedure has been shown to be safe and effective in the short term (Poynter et al. 2014a; Sharma et al. 2014; Romp et al. 2003; Padalino et al. 2019). Infrequently, however, the unroofing procedure may result in an unwanted transmural incision through the intimal layers of the aorta and coronary artery resulting in disruption at the site of coronary artery to aorta connection. This situation, if not effectively repaired, can have significant and serious consequences that can lead to uncontrolled bleeding and myocardial infarction both of which can result in extracorporeal membrane oxygenation and death. Figures 53, 54, 55, 56, 58, 59 and 60 show the stages of unroofing an anomalous intramural right coronary artery taking its origin from the left coronary sinus. The progression of the operation is standard until the unroofing incision is carried too far into the connection between the aorta and the coronary artery as shown in Fig. 54. The attempts at repair are shown in Figs. 55 and 56 which are oftentimes sufficient for resolution of the problem. However, when the attempted repair is completed and the cross-clamp is removed, bleeding at the site of injury can occur as shown in Fig. 57. Attempts at suture repair without a cross-clamp will generally result in further bleeding and anastomotic disruption. Figures 58, 59 and 60 show how the problem can be resolved with careful planning and use of a pulmonary artery patch arterioplasty (Mavroudis 2015).

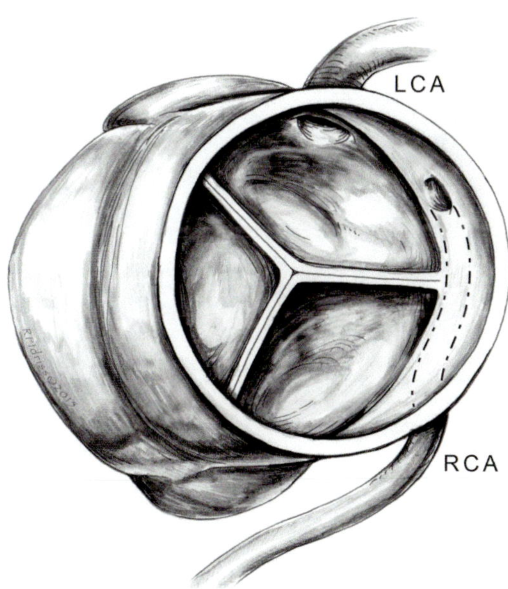

Fig. 53 Demonstrates the usual and expected intramural course of an anomalous right coronary artery with a slit-like opening arising from the left coronary cusp. *LCA* left coronary artery, *RCA* right coronary artery. (With permission Mavroudis and Dearani 2020)

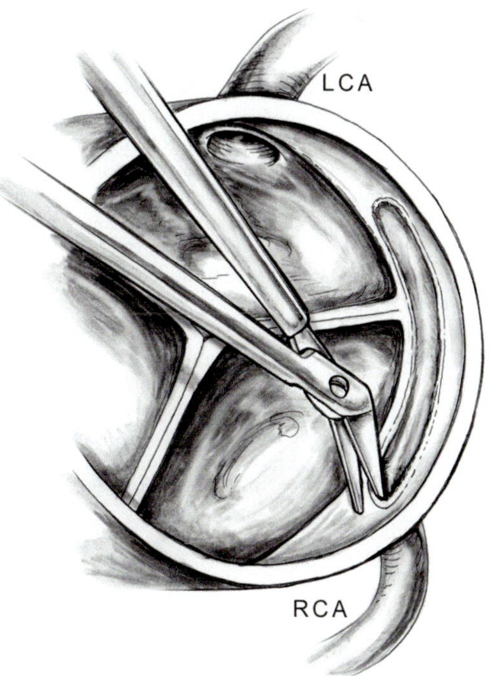

Fig. 54 Shows the unroofing procedure, which in this case is performed with a scissors. This part of the procedure can also be performed sharply with a scalpel. Infrequently, the incision can be taken too far, even for 1 mm. This can result in intimal coronary-aortic disruption which may become transmural or practically transmural, the disruption being bridged by a thin piece of epicardial tissue with no vascular integrity. *LCA* left coronary artery, *RCA* right coronary artery. (With permission Mavroudis and Dearani 2020)

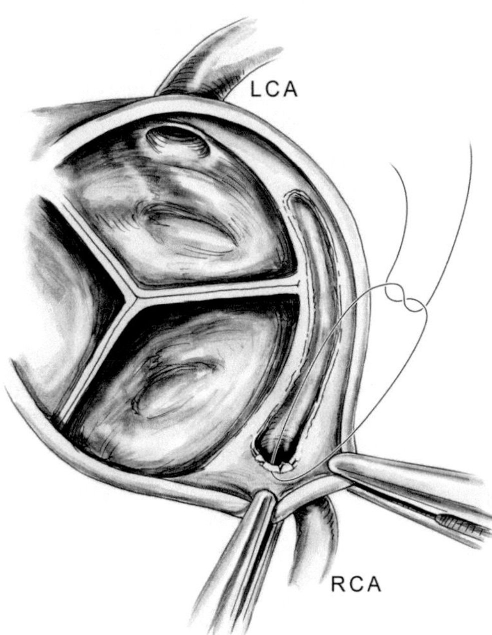

Fig. 55 Shows transaortic intimal repair of the coronary-aortic disruption with multiple fine sutures which, for the most part, effectively manage this potentially dangerous problem. After cross-clamp removal, the completed repair can be visually assessed and if the integrity of the repair is questionable or unacceptable, further measures must be undertaken. What is meant by "questionable" or "unacceptable" is challenging and requires a high level of intuitive observation. One relatively easy assessment is the visualization of blood swirling under the epicardial surface of the repair. Other assessments can be obvious which include epicardial kinking, stenosis, or suspected intimal integrity. Reexploration of the anastomosis should not be delayed. *LCA* left coronary artery, *RCA* right coronary artery. (With permission Mavroudis and Dearani 2020)

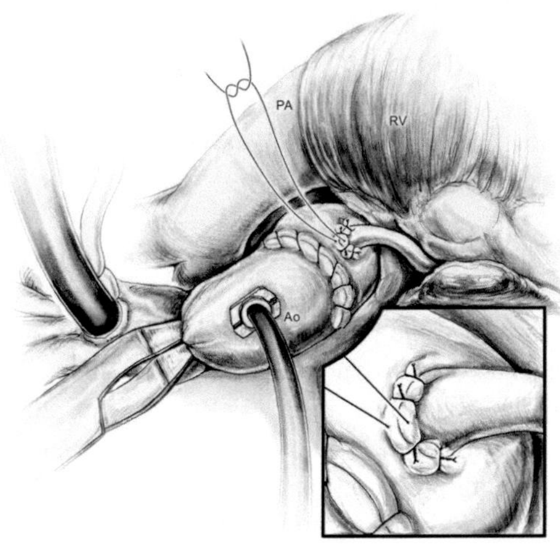

Fig. 56 Shows attempted repair of the disrupted suture line with multiple external fine sutures on the epicardial aortic-coronary junctional surface. This should be performed during a period of cross-clamp and cardioplegic arrest. The inset drawing highlights the suture placement. While this repair action may seemingly settle the problem, internal and external sutures can disrupt the integrity of the anastomotic suture line further and result in more bleeding after the cross-clamp has been removed as shown in Fig. 52a–c. *Ao* aorta, *PA* pulmonary artery, *RV* right ventricle. (With permission Mavroudis and Dearani 2020)

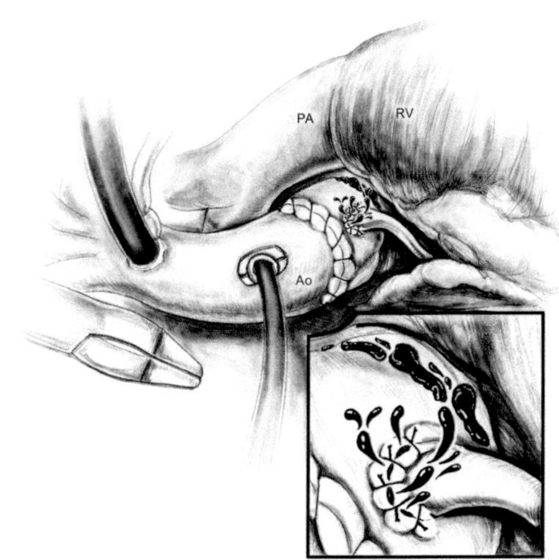

Fig. 57 Emphasizes the continued bleeding problem after the cross-clamp has been removed. The inset demonstrated localized hemorrhage between the sutures due to intimal disruption. Further suturing will not resolve the problem. Another period of cross-clamp application and cardioplegic arrest with exploration and removal of all reparative sutures is recommended. *Ao* aorta, *PA* pulmonary artery, *RV* right ventricle. (With permission Mavroudis and Dearani 2020)

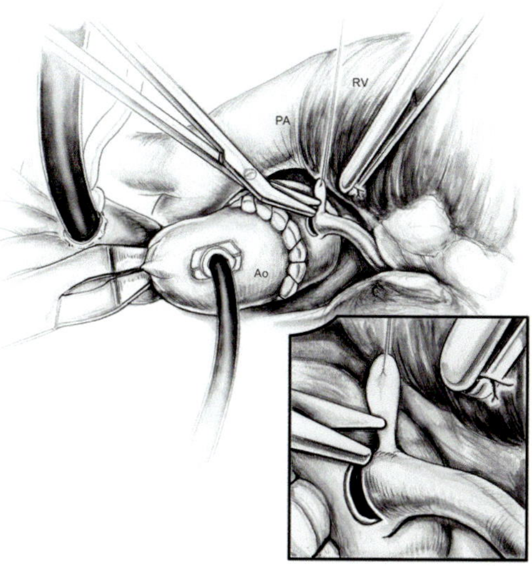

Fig. 58 Careful debridement of the suture line to remove the sutures and the uneven edges is shown in this figure. Necessarily, this results in a large defect which cannot be bridged by direct anastomosis. Some kind of patch material will be required to augment the anastomotic suture line. PTFE, autologous pericardium, and other biologic material have been advocated. The editors have used an autologous piece of pulmonary artery trunk which we feel is optimal patch material for this purpose. *Ao* aorta, *PA* pulmonary artery, *RV* right ventricle. (With permission Mavroudis and Dearani 2020)

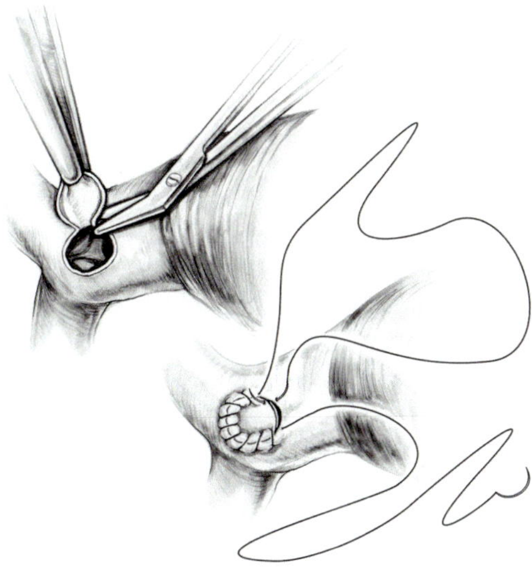

Fig. 59 Demonstrates the pulmonary artery wall harvest which can be replaced using autologous pericardium as noted in the figure. (With permission Mavroudis and Dearani 2020)

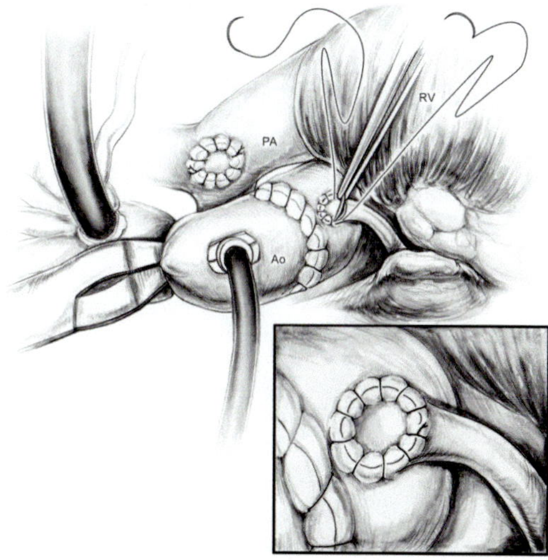

Fig. 60 The pulmonary artery patch can now be employed for the coronary artery aortic wall patch repair as noted in the figure. The repair can be accomplished without suture line tension and with excellent flow characteristics. The inset shows the completed repair without bleeding. *Ao* aorta, *PA* pulmonary artery, *RV* right ventricle. (With permission Mavroudis and Dearani 2020)

5.5 The Camouflaged Coronary Intramural Orifice by the Aortic Commissure

In rare cases, the orifice of an intramural coronary artery may arise at the commissure between the right and left coronary cusps (Muriago et al. 1997). The unsuspecting surgeon may not immediately discover the orifice since the slit-like opening is small and is camouflaged behind the leaflet. This situation, when not immediately discovered, can be quite disturbing since at first glance, the preoperative diagnosis and purported reason for performing the operation are now in question. Attempts to locate the intramural coronary artery generally leads to the area behind the commissure which confirms the precise diagnosis which will lead to the appropriate operation. This diagnostic problem is illustrated in Fig. 61. The dotted/dashed lines reveal the intramural course of the anomalous right coronary artery which takes its origin from the camouflaged slit-like orifice behind the aortic commissure. Since

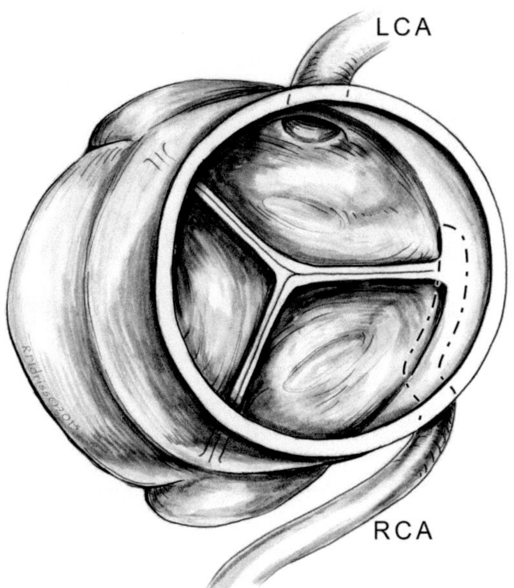

Fig. 61 In rare cases, the orifice of an intramural coronary artery may arise at the commissure between the right and left coronary cusps which can obstruct the surgeon's view of the slit-like orifice. Efforts to find the intramural coronary artery usually lead to the area behind the commissure which confirms the correct diagnosis and subsequent appropriate operation. This diagnostic dilemma is noted in the figure. The dotted/dashed lines demonstrate the intramural course of the anomalous right coronary artery arising from the left coronary sinus with the slit-like orifice camouflaged by the aortic commissure. *LCA* left coronary artery, *RCA* right coronary artery. (With permission Mavroudis and Dearani 2020)

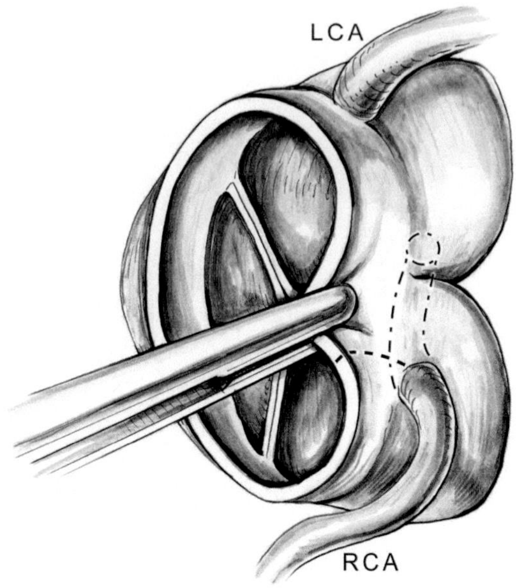

Fig. 62 Further inspection of the epicardial surface results in identification of the right coronary artery which appears to arise from the right coronary cusp as shown in the figure. In fact, as the dotted/dashed line suggests, the epicardial right coronary artery is the continuation of the intramural portion, the origin of which is camouflaged behind the commissure. It is important to identify whether the intramural segment is above the commissure or traverses below the commissure. If above the commissure, a simple unroofing procedure can be accomplished without injury to the aortic valve integrity. If below the commissure, more creative options will be required. *LCA* left coronary artery, *RCA* right coronary artery. (With permission Mavroudis and Dearani 2020)

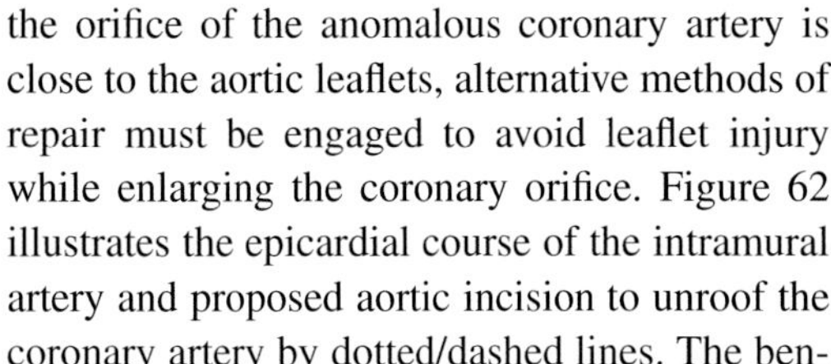

the orifice of the anomalous coronary artery is close to the aortic leaflets, alternative methods of repair must be engaged to avoid leaflet injury while enlarging the coronary orifice. Figure 62 illustrates the epicardial course of the intramural artery and proposed aortic incision to unroof the coronary artery by dotted/dashed lines. The benefit of aortic transection for operative exposure allows for creative maneuvers that require exact incisions and precise coronary artery reconstruction. Figure 63 illustrates the aortic coronal incision which is carried into the body of the right coronary artery thereby enlarging the orifice widely. The probe confirms the slit-like orifice of

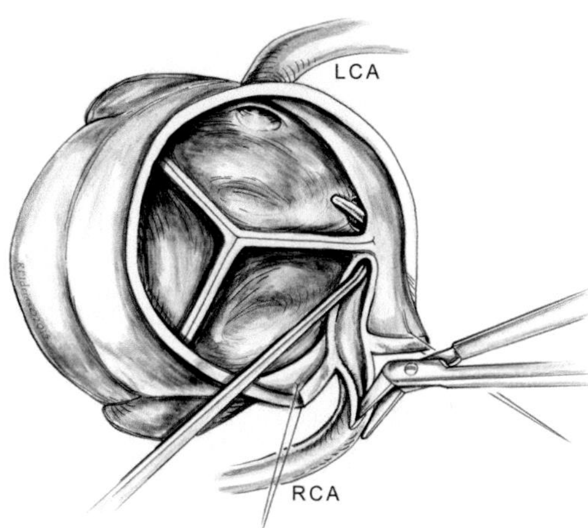

Fig. 63 One option to repair this anatomic dilemma is to apply accepted surgical solutions for coronary artery orifice atresia. The dotted line in Fig. 57 from the transected aorta to the epicardial surface of the right coronary artery demonstrates the proposed incision which will unite the aorta and the coronary artery enroute to repair. For reference, the other dotted/dashed lines demonstrate the intramural coronary course. The incision is performed as demonstrated in the figure onto the surface of the right coronary artery. This maneuver can now help to identify the intramural course of the right coronary artery and by a probe demonstrate the camouflaged origin behind the affected commissure. *LCA* left coronary artery, *RCA* right coronary artery. (With permission Mavroudis and Dearani 2020)

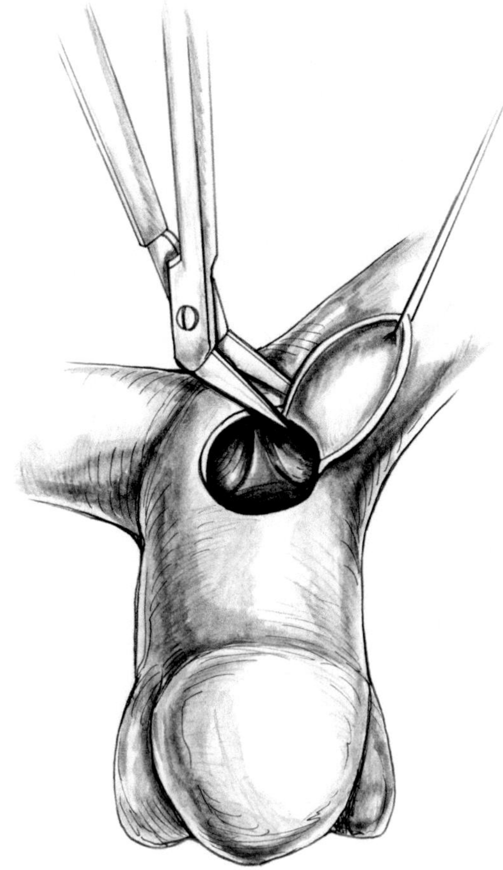

Fig. 64 The coronary neo-orifice can now be reconstructed using a biologic patch. The figure shows the harvest of a piece of autologous pulmonary trunk for repair. (With permission Mavroudis and Dearani 2020)

the intramural coronary artery origin behind the aortic commissure. It is important to select a suitable biologic patch to perform the coronary artery arterioplasty. Autologous pericardium, internal thoracic artery (Anagnostopoulos et al. 2004), or a piece of harvested pulmonary artery wall as noted in Fig. 64 can be used for coronary artery arterioplasty. The pulmonary artery patch or the internal thoracic artery are preferred since these are viable grafts with excellent sewing characteristics. The material that the surgeon prefers is the more important consideration, however. Figure 65 shows the tacking sutures of the intramural unroofing to prevent aortic wall dissection and the biologic patch being used to form the coronary artery arterioplasty. Care is taken to use

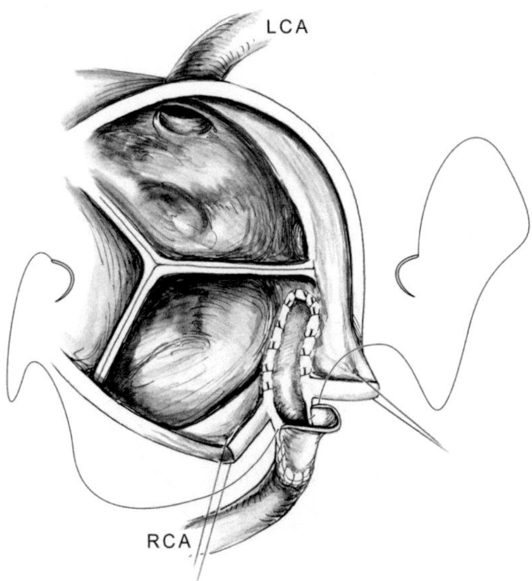

Fig. 65 This pulmonary artery patch is then used to augment the orifice of the right coronary artery with anastomotic extension to the aortic wall as shown in the figure. Tacking sutures are placed within the aorta at the unroofing site. *LCA* left coronary artery, *RCA* right coronary artery. (With permission Mavroudis and Dearani 2020)

fine 7-0 monofilament suture for the arterioplasty. Figure 66 illustrates the completed arterioplasty before the aortic reanastomosis as shown in Fig. 67. Complications concerning this procedure have been previously noted and include anastomotic bleeding, aortic leaflet injury, and twisting of the aortic reconstruction. If the hidden orifice is discovered preoperatively, the operating team may consider coronary artery reimplantation as discussed in Figs. 31 and 32. While coronary

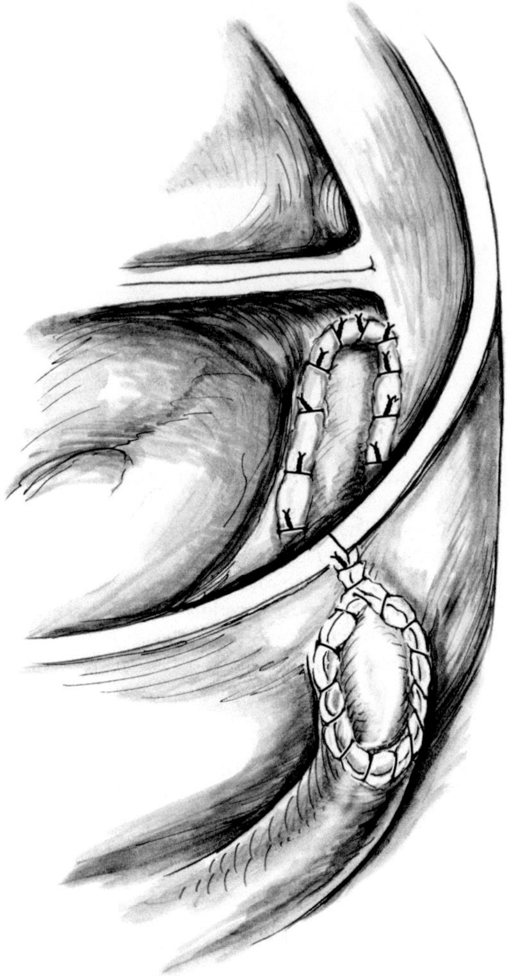

Fig. 66 The right coronary artery neo-orifice is augmented, and, in this manner, the neo-coronary orifice is formed as shown in the figure. (With permission Mavroudis and Dearani 2020)

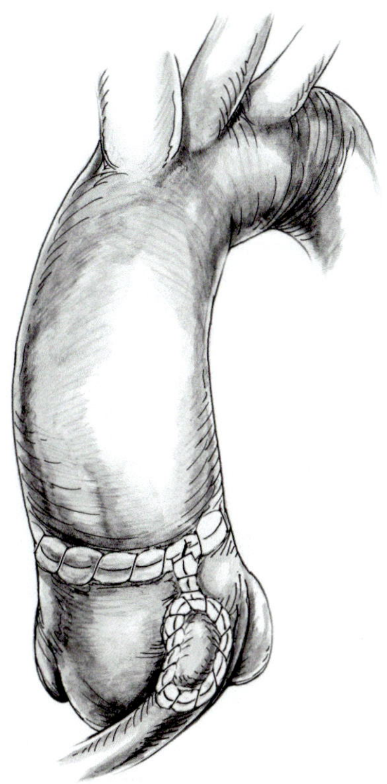

Fig. 67 Shows the completed reconstruction after separation from cardiopulmonary bypass. It is not altogether apparent whether this coronary aortic reconstruction is the preferred resolution for this kind of anatomic problem. On the positive side, the affected commissure is not manipulated and consequently the possibility of resultant aortic regurgitation is unlikely. In addition, the neocoronary orifice is large and is not at risk for a stenotic internal orifice by a side-to-side anastomosis. Conversely, the possibility of epicardial bleeding using the autologous pulmonary patch and coronary distortion are always potential complications. Whatever operative choice is applied, postoperative myocardial function as evaluated by transesophageal echocardiography, electrocardiography, and timely cardiac catheterization are all important diagnostic tools to verify adequate coronary flow to avoid perioperative complications. (With permission Mavroudis and Dearani 2020)

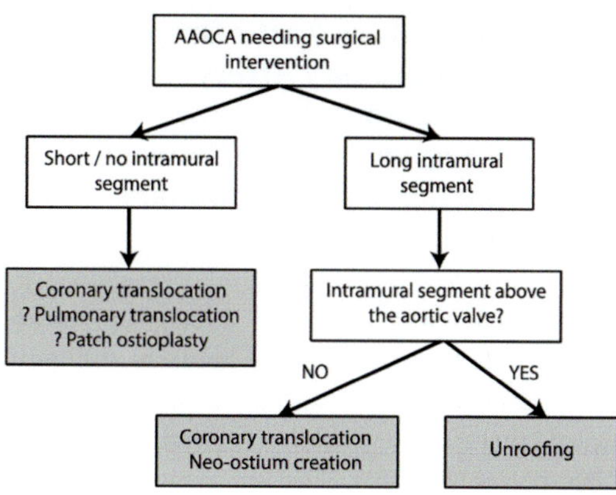

Fig. 68 Proposed algorithm to select optimal surgical intervention for patients with anomalous aortic origin of the coronary artery (AAOCA) requiring intervention. (With permission Mery et al. 2018)

reimplantation is the better option, the surgeon is wise to know both techniques in the event that circumstances require more creative techniques to resolve the problem.

Mery, De Leon, and associates (2018) have offered an algorithm (Fig. 68) for management of anomalous aortic origin of the coronary arteries which is quite helpful in applying operative schemes.

5.6 Anomalous Aortic Origin of a Coronary Artery with a Nonintramural Malignant Course Between the Aorta and Pulmonary Artery

Anomalous aortic origin of a coronary artery with a nonintramural course between the aorta and pulmonary artery can be a difficult diagnostic and therapeutic problem (Hatoum et al. 2022; Gharibeh et al. 2021).

Recent advances have allowed clinicians to distinguish between an intramural and extramural course of a coronary artery which traverses between the great vessels (Albuquerque et al. 2021). When an extramural course is found, coronary reimplantation is the procedure of choice to correct the constrictive actions of the great arteries and the angulation of the coronary origin. This can be achieved by forming a neo-orifice to a favorable site on the ascending aorta within the proper sinus of Valsalva. Figure 69 shows how the anomalous right coronary artery is being harvested from the left coronary sinus of Valsalva with the target area for anastomosis higher in the right coronary sinus of Valsalva. Care is taken to perform a hemostatic anastomosis at both the harvested area in the left sinus of Valsalva as well as the anastomotic site in the right sinus of Valsalva. Failure to perform an adequate epicardial mobilization of the right coronary artery may result in kinking and decreased flow as noted in Fig. 70. This situation can generally be identified by visual inspection which should promote reparative procedures to straighten the artery towards a gentler curve to enhance coronary flow. This maneuver can be performed using low set-

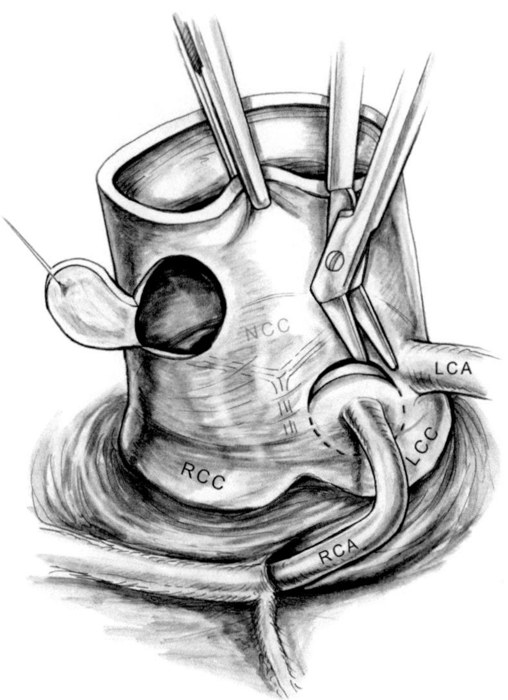

Fig. 69 Demonstrates a characteristic course of an extramural anomalous right coronary artery arising from the left coronary sinus. The figure shows important anatomic features that includes the internal aortic cusps (demonstrated in ghost techniques), the anomalous right coronary artery with a camouflaged intramyocardial course, and the proposed target site of reimplantation on the ascending aorta more superior in the right coronary cusp away from the potential constriction effects between the aorta and pulmonary artery. It is advisable to carefully dissect and mobilize the anomalous coronary artery to the epicardial surface. In this drawing, an extensive dissection and mobilization of the coronary artery is intentionally not demonstrated to highlight the potential unfavorable reconstruction and distortion that can occur when the coronary artery button is transferred to the intended site of implantation. *LCA* left coronary artery, *LCC* left coronary cusp, *NCC* noncoronary cusp, *RCA* right coronary artery, *RCC* right coronary cusp. (With permission Mavroudis and Dearani 2020)

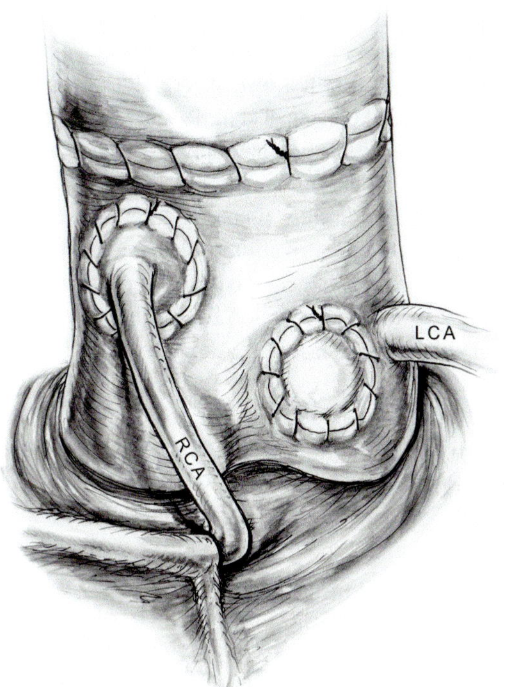

Fig. 70 Shows the resultant coronary artery kinking that can occur after coronary artery button transfer. This suboptimal epicardial coronary dissection and mobilization can result in unfavorable flow characteristics. *LCA* left coronary artery, *RCA* right coronary artery. (With permission Mavroudis and Dearani 2020)

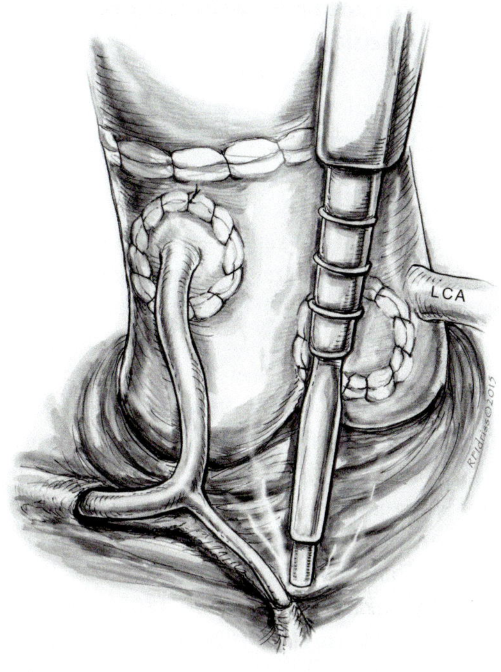

Fig. 71 Shows how more comprehensive epicardial electrocautery dissection and mobilization can free the coronary artery to improve flow. The operative principles for coronary reimplantation under these circumstances require significant coronary artery mobilization, proper location of the neo-orifice, and careful assessment of ventricular function and coronary flow. All surgeons who perform these operations should be cognizant of these aforementioned techniques and apply them as indicated. *LCA* left coronary artery. (With permission Mavroudis and Dearani 2020)

ting electrocautery with special attention not to cause injury to the coronary artery as noted in Fig. 71. If there is any doubt, it is advisable to finish the operation and commit to coronary angiography with return to the operating room if repair proves to be necessary.

6 Coronary Arteriovenous Fistulas

Coronary arteriovenous fistulas (CAVF), sometimes called Coronary Cameral Fistulas represent an anomaly of coronary origin and cavitary cardiac termination. This entity was first described by Krause in 1865 (Krause 1865). The incidence is 1%–2% of the general population while angiographic series show an incidence of 0.2%–0.85% (Fernandes et al. 1992; Olearchyk et al. 1997; Krause 1865; Urrutia-S et al. 1983; Mavroudis et al. 1997; Harris et al. 1996; Lowe et al. 1981). Coronary cameral fistulas are common and represent approximately 50% of all congenital coronary artery anomalies (Schumacher et al. 1997), some of which are hemodynamically significant coronary anomalies (Fernandes et al. 1992; Olearchyk et al. 1997; Krause 1865; Urrutia-S et al. 1983; Harris et al. 1996; Lowe et al. 1981; Schumacher et al. 1997).

About two-thirds of fistulas are congenital; however, acquired lesions are steadily increasing in number owing to trauma, catheterization procedures, and Takayasu arteritis (Kamiya et al. 2002). Most CAVFs occur in isolation (55%–80%) (Fernandes et al. 1992; Olearchyk et al. 1997; Krause 1865; Urrutia-S et al. 1983; Schumacher et al. 1997; Tkebuchava et al. 1996) or in association with other congenital heart anomalies which include tetralogy of Fallot, atrial septal defect, patent arterial duct, ventricular septal defect, and other coronary artery lesions (Urrutia-S et al. 1983; Kamiya et al. 2002).

Fistulas can be single, ranging from 74% to 90% of cases (Urrutia-S et al. 1983; Mavroudis et al. 1997; Harris et al. 1996; Kamiya et al. 2002; Sakakibara et al. 1966; Bauer et al. 1996), multiple, occurring in 10.7%–16% of cases (Fernandes et al. 1992; Olearchyk et al. 1997; Tkebuchava et al. 1996), or taking origin from both coronaries in 4%–18% (Fernandes et al. 1992; Olearchyk et al. 1997; Krause 1865; Urrutia-S et al. 1983; Tkebuchava et al. 1996). The RCA and LAD are the most common sites of vascular origin (Kamiya et al. 2002). The most common sites of termination are the pulmonary artery and right ventricle (Kamiya et al. 2002). Drainage into the right side of the heart is more prevalent (92%) due to the lower pressures (Olearchyk et al. 1997; Harris et al. 1996; Lowe et al. 1981; Kamiya et al. 2002; Tkebuchava et al. 1996). While proximal coronary artery dilatation is the norm, the extent of dilatation is not proportional to the amount of shunting (Olearchyk et al. 1997). Anatomic characterization is determined by the vessel of origin and chamber of termination. One angiographic classification has been reported by Sakakibara and associates in 1966 (Sakakibara et al. 1966).

Diagnosis can often be inferred clinically with the finding of a nonspecific continuous machinery type murmur heard best at the second and third right or left parasternal border. ECG changes are present in about two-thirds of patients and include ischemia, chamber overload, infarction, and arrhythmias (Fernandes et al. 1992). Cardiomegaly on chest radiograph is often present owing to intracardiac shunting (Fernandes et al. 1992). Color flow Doppler echocardiography is a very effective diagnostic modality and can define the exact anatomy in CAVF. Most surgeons however concur that preoperative cardiac catheterization is needed to define multiple fistulas, assess hemodynamics, determine the degree of left-to-right shunting (Olearchyk et al. 1997) as shown in Fig. 72, and to evaluate the feasibility of transcatheter device closure of solitary distal fistulous lesions (Mavroudis et al. 1997; Schumacher et al. 1997; Kamiya et al. 2002). Recent advances have shown that MR angiography and 64-slice CT is an excellent diagnostic tool for precise anatomic delineation of coronary fistula origins and sites of termination, which can help to define therapeutic strategy (Mavroudis et al. 1997; Dodd et al. 2008).

Coronary fistulas rarely close spontaneously (Urrutia-S et al. 1983; Mavroudis et al. 1997). The natural history of patients with CAVF is associated with a shorter life span (Harris et al. 1996). Symptoms and complications in untreated patients generally occur during their second or third decades of life (Fernandes et al. 1992; Harris et al. 1996; Lowe et al. 1981; Schumacher et al. 1997; Tkebuchava et al. 1996), which include myocardial infarction (3%–11%), subacute bacterial

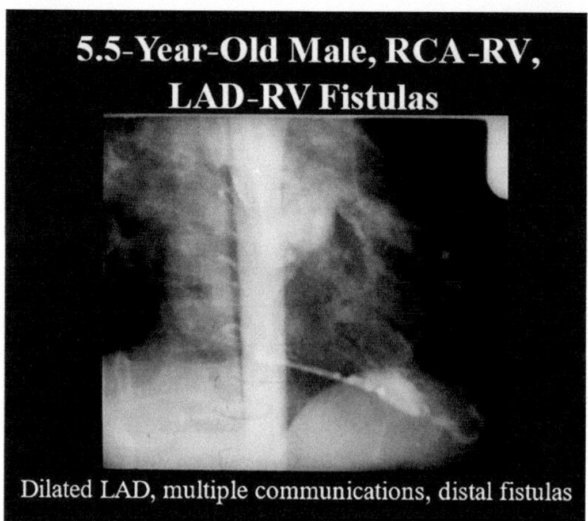

Fig. 72 Shows the coronary angiogram of a 5.5-year-old boy who had two demonstrated coronary fistulas that drained to the right ventricle. The right coronary artery is shown with termination into the right ventricle. The left anterior descending artery shows proximal dilatation and termination in the same area of the right ventricle. *LAD* left anterior descending, *RCA* right coronary artery, *RV* right ventricle

endocarditis (5%–20%), aneurysm formation (19%–26%), rupture with tamponade, and death (7%–14%) (Fernandes et al. 1992; Sakakibara et al. 1966; Liberthson et al. 1979b).

7 Historical Accounts, Operative Procedures, and Management of Operative Complications

The first surgical correction of CAVF by epicardial ligation, was reported by Biörck and Crafoord in 1947 (Biörck and Crafoord 1947) which was serendipitously found during an operation to close a patent arterial duct. The first tangential arteriorrhaphy was reported by Cooley and Ellis in 1962 (Cooley and Ellis Jr. 1962), and the first successful embolization using transcatheter techniques was performed in 1983 by Reidy (Reidy et al. 1983). Therapeutic interventions such as surgical or transcatheter device closure must be performed without compromising normal coronary flow which is oftentimes very close to the fistulous tract (Fernandes et al. 1992; Olearchyk et al. 1997; Krause 1865; Urrutia-S et al. 1983; Mavroudis et al. 1997; Harris et al. 1996; Lowe et al. 1981; Schumacher et al. 1997). Therapeutic intervention is indicated in patients with symptoms and can be controversial in patients without symptoms although many surgical reports advocate for early prophylactic closure, due to near-zero morbidity and mortality in cases of isolated fistulas (Urrutia-S et al. 1983; Mavroudis et al. 1997; Lowe et al. 1981; Dodd et al. 2008; Alkhulaifi et al. 1995). The reported techniques depend on the anatomic circumstances and include distal ligation, proximal and distal ligation, tangential arteriorrhaphy with or without bypass, and intracardiac closure with CPB (Mavroudis et al. 2023). Figure 73 shows the preferred method for epicardial fistula location and ligation without the use of cardiopulmonary bypass. The intraoperative management using this technique is described in the figure which includes the dissection, temporary trial occlusion, and observation for the development of ischemic findings before actual ligation. Complications associated with epicardial ligation include unwanted ligation or injury to parallel coronary arteries arising close to the fistula which can result in myocardial infarction. This is the reason why the fistula should be temporarily compressed with a tourniquet to observe the results of the intervention. Other potential complications include bleeding which may require emergency cardiopulmonary bypass, cardioplegic arrest, and exploration of the bleeding site. There are occasions when elective cardiopulmonary bypass with intracavitary fistula ligation and possible distal coronary bypass may be required (Lowe et al. 1981; Schumacher et al. 1997; Bogers et al. 1987). Figure 74 reviews the comprehensive operative techniques of intracardiac fistula ligation to ensure the proper steps of the operation which will lead to complete occlusion. Figure 75 shows the preoperative and postoperative results of an unwanted injury to the posterior aspect of the anomalous left anterior descending coronary artery during transatrial resection of the right ventricular outflow tract during repair of tetralogy of Fallot in a 6.4-year-old male. During the repair, the injury to the artery was not recognized which created a fistulous tract from the

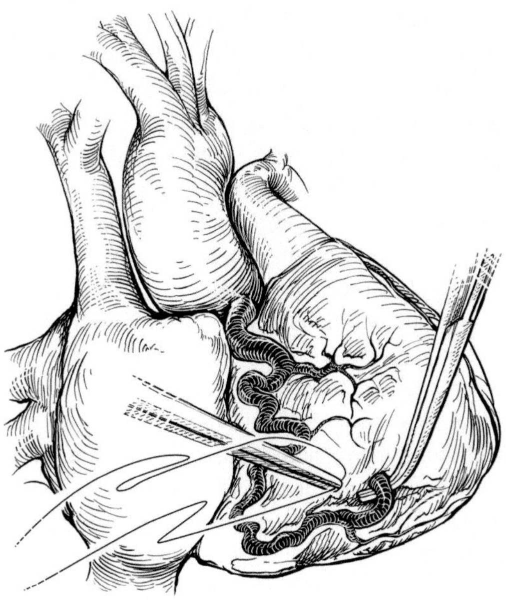

Fig. 73 The preferred procedure is to perform epicardial fistula location and ligation without the use of cardiopulmonary bypass (CPB) and systemic heparin. Patients are approached through a median sternotomy with CPB standby. Transesophageal echocardiography (TEE) is very helpful in these situations since the fistula can readily be identified and monitored. The coronary artery in question is usually very large and can easily be tracked to the entry point as shown in the figure. The electrocautery dissector should be adjusted to low power for the epicardial dissection enroute to identifying the entry point of the fistula into the chamber in question. Once the most distal entry point is identified, a clamp is placed around the vessel and a vessel loop is used to control the flow with a snugger. No effort to ligate the vessel is made at this point. Using TEE and surface electrocardiogram (EKG) monitoring the fistula is snugged. If the flow is interrupted by TEE, if no EKG evidence of ischemia is noted, and if no ventricular dysfunction occurs, then the fistula can be ligated thereby completing the operation. (With permission Mavroudis and Dearani 2020)

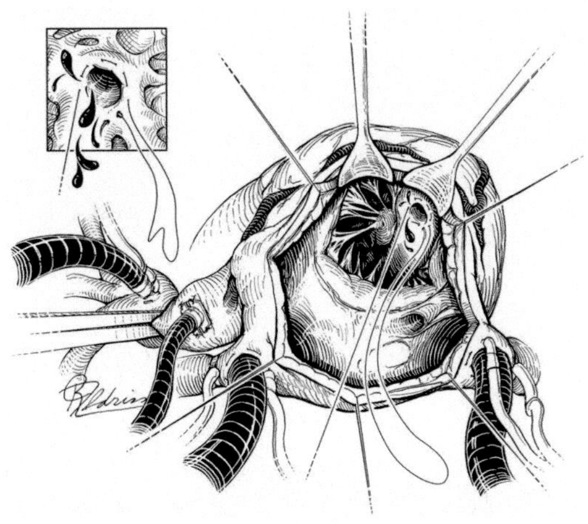

Fig. 74 For those patients, whose fistulas are poorly defined at the epicardial surface and are at risk for collateral coronary artery injury, the surgeon may elect to perform endocardial ligation. The perioperative monitoring procedures are different from epicardial ligation, however. TEE can be used to identify the fistula, but its role will be relegated to postoperative verification. The patient is prepared for aortobicaval cardiopulmonary bypass (CPB) and antegrade cardioplegia. CPB is commenced with a left ventricular vent and mild hypothermia. The aortic cross-clamp is applied and cardioplegia is administered. If the coronary runoff is too great temporary finger occlusion of the fistula might help. Otherwise, a retrograde catheter may be required to complete the cardioplegia administration. In the case of a right coronary artery fistula to the right ventricle, as noted in the figure, a transatrial exposure is established with fistula visualization through the tricuspid valve. Usually there is a white fibrous hue to the entry point which we refer to as the area of "hemodynamic changes." The experienced cardiac surgeon will see these intracardiac hemodynamic changes in areas of turbulence such as right and left ventricular outflow tract obstructions and the result of jet lesions from ventricular septal defects. A purse string suture is placed around the fistula orifice and the suture is controlled with a snugger. At this point, antegrade cardioplegia is administered and the flow into the fistula is noted. During the cardioplegia administration, the snugger is engaged and flow is assessed to determine complete closure. Once the surgeon is satisfied that complete closure has been achieved, the fistula is closed. Epicardial inspection is performed to rule out unwanted collateral damage to the normal epicardial coronaries. A final small dose of antegrade cardioplegia will confirm the integrity of the ligation. The atrium is then closed, the air maneuvers are performed, and the cross-clamp is removed. This is followed by separation from CPB and transesophageal echocardiogram assessment. (With permission Mavroudis and Dearani 2020)

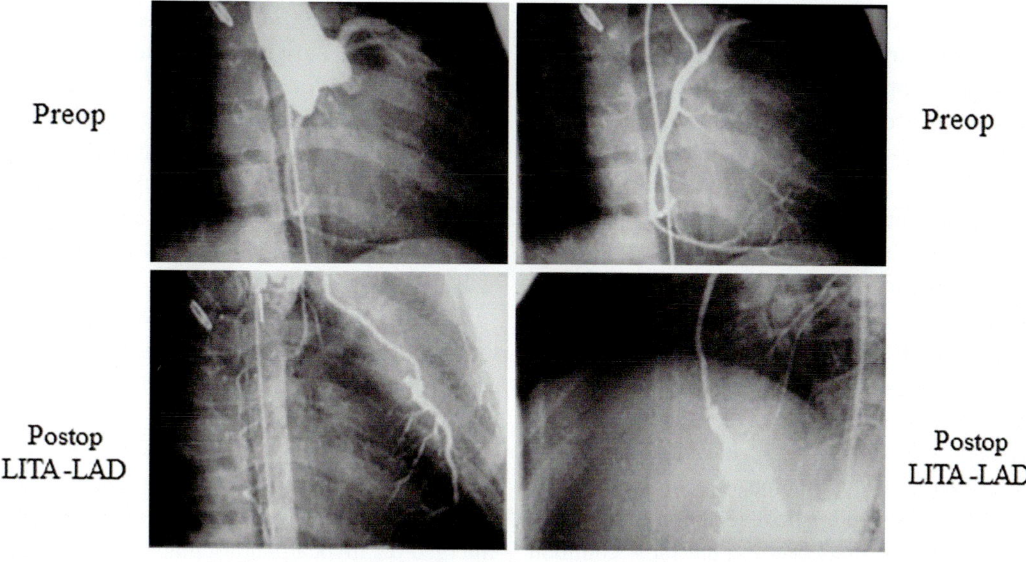

Fig. 75 Shows the preoperative and postoperative coronary angiograms of an unwanted injury to the posterior aspect of the anomalous left anterior descending coronary artery during transatrial resection of the right ventricular outflow tract during repair of tetralogy of Fallot in a 6.4-year-old male. The postoperative angiogram shown in the lower panels shows the result of transatrial fistula ligation and an internal thoracic coronary bypass graft to the left anterior descending coronary artery. This is an example of an acquired coronary to cameral fistula which requires a careful assessment and comprehensive solution. *LAD* left anterior descending, *LITA* Left Internal Thoracic Artery

artery to the right ventricle. The patient had a difficult postoperative course with ventricular arrhythmias and eventually was discharged with premature ventricular contractions. At reoperation, the fistula was ligated from within the right ventricle which was accompanied by an internal thoracic coronary bypass graft to the left anterior descending coronary artery which is shown in the postoperative angiogram. The patient recovered without persistence of the premature ventricular contractions. This is an example of an acquired coronary to cameral fistula which requires a careful assessment and comprehensive solution.

In the majority of cases, cardiopulmonary bypass is not necessary assuming that epicardial ligation or tangential arteriorrhaphy (Fernandes et al. 1992; Olearchyk et al. 1997; Schumacher et al. 1997; Tkebuchava et al. 1996; Cooley and Ellis Jr. 1962) can be performed safely. Nevertheless, cardiopulmonary bypass capabilities should be immediately available. As noted, cardiopulmonary bypass is required if associated intracardiac lesions are to be addressed concurrently. Recent innovation techniques have allowed for transcatheter device or coil occlusion methods as a safe alternative to surgery, assuming that the anatomy is judged to be favorable. Mortality approaches zero and complications are rare (Urrutia-S et al. 1983; Mavroudis et al. 1997). However, it should be noted that no randomized studies have compared surgery with interventional techniques. In addition, no guidelines have been developed for a treatment algorithm depending on shunt size or anatomy. Therapeutic strategies in the current era are institution dependent.

As we have shown, operative or interventional mortality for isolated CAVF closure has been shown to be low. There are still controversial issues regarding treatment for asymptomatic patients even though the natural history of these patients is not equivalent to that of the general population. In general, most surgeons promote operative or transcatheter intervention before the onset of symptoms to avoid the increased incidence in operative complications and death, which tend to be more common in patients older than 20–30 years of age (Urrutia-S et al. 1983; Mavroudis et al. 1997; Harris et al. 1996; Tkebuchava et al. 1996; Cooley and Ellis Jr. 1962; Reidy et al. 1983).

Reported results show that all surgically closed CAVFs remained closed, and late death is rare (Kaczorowski et al. 2012). For those patients with preoperative symptoms, improvement of functional class has been achieved (Tkebuchava et al. 1996). Owing to improvement in transcatheter techniques and patient selection, transcatheter embolization has become the most common initial procedure of choice for these patients. Surgical intervention is therefore reserved for patients who fail or who are not amenable for transcatheter occlusion (Mavroudis et al. 1997; Harris et al. 1996; Reidy et al. 1983; Alkhulaifi et al. 1995).

8 Intramyocardial Course of Coronary Arteries (Bridging)

Intramural (intramyocardial) segments of epicardial coronary arteries, also referred to as bridging, were first described by Crainicianu in 1622 (Crainicianu 1922). The incidence of intramyocardial bridging in the general population has been estimated to be between 5.4% and 85.7% (Crainicianu 1922; Angelini et al. 1983; Bourassa et al. 2003; den Dulk et al. 1983; Mookadam et al. 2009; Pey et al. 1985; Schwarz et al. 1996; Kardasz and De Caterina 2007), which offers pause in determining the clinical importance of this entity. Nevertheless, there are some patients in whom coronary bridging may play an important role in explaining angina and heralding other associated lesions. Bridging is most commonly seen in the mid-segment of the LAD, however other locations include LAD diagonal branches, the posterior descending artery of the RCA, and marginal arteries of the circumflex coronary (Bourassa et al. 2003). Symptoms can occur in children but are most commonly seen in patients in their third or fourth decade of life (Schwarz et al. 1996). Coronary bridging can be seen in association with hypertrophic cardiomyopathy, ischemic cardiomyopathy, idiopathic cardiomyopathy, mitral valve prolapse, and muscular subaortic stenosis (Angelini et al. 1983; den Dulk et al. 1983; Pey et al. 1985).

There have been many studies to consider anatomic variations, denotative nomenclature, and associated syndromes (Kardasz and De Caterina 2007; Y-Hassan 2014; Brolin et al. 2015; Geiringer 1951; Kramer et al. 1982; Ferreira Jr et al. 1991) which are out of the scope of this chapter. However, anatomic considerations emerged for myocardial bridging that may cause symptoms due to the constricting actions of the surrounding myocardial fibers (Y-Hassan 2014; Brolin et al. 2015; Geiringer 1951; Kramer et al. 1982; Ferreira Jr et al. 1991; Betriu et al. 1980; Hill et al. 1981; Hillman et al. 1999; Feld et al. 1991; Vasan et al. 1989; Von Poláček and Zechmeister 1968; Hakeem et al. 2010; Huang et al. 2007; Lee and Chen 2015). The mechanisms of action that cause ischemia in coronary bridging are not universal in agreement since not all patients with myocardial bridging have demonstrable symptoms and ischemia either by exercise or cardiac pacing (Angelini et al. 1983; Bourassa et al. 2003). It follows then that indications for surgery are controversial. Nevertheless, angiographic evidence of systolic narrowing of coronary arteries caused by bridging has been associated with symptomatic ischemia and should not be overlooked (Mookadam et al. 2009; Schwarz et al. 1996; Kardasz and De Caterina 2007; Y-Hassan 2014; Betriu et al. 1980; Feld et al. 1991; Vasan et al. 1989; Von Poláček and Zechmeister 1968; Hakeem et al. 2010; Huang et al. 2007; Lee and Chen 2015; Binet et al. 1975; Haager et al. 2000), especially since systolic coronary flow represents 5%–30% of total coronary flow. In those patients with coronary bridging, it is estimated that one-half of the flow in septal vessels is impaired during diastole (Binet et al. 1975). Further to the proposed mechanisms is that turbulent flow can occur through the bridge which can enhance intimal trauma and possible platelet aggregation (Pey et al. 1985; Geiringer 1951; Haager et al. 2000). This may result in impaired local oxygen delivery, leading to ischemia, conduction abnormalities, tachyarrhythmias, or syncope (Pey et al. 1985; Schwarz et al. 1996; Geiringer 1951; Hakeem et al. 2010; Lee and Chen 2015).

In the present era, angiography and intravascular ultrasound (IVUS) are considered to be the optimal diagnostic tools to measure bridging (Bourassa et al. 2003). For all the reasons noted in the literature concerning these measurements (Bourassa et al. 2003; Pey et al. 1985; Schwarz et al. 1996; Kardasz and De Caterina 2007), it is important to measure diastolic fractional flow reserve by angiography under dobutamine provocation, to document the physiologic assessment of myocardial bridges (Hakeem et al. 2010), which will help to determine therapeutic options.

In general, initial treatment for symptomatic or asymptomatic patients with bridging is medical (Bourassa et al. 2003; Lee and Chen 2015), which involves beta blockers and calcium channel blockers. The mechanism of action of these medications is through their negative chronotropic and inotropic effects, which reduce tachycardia, prolong diastole, and reduce circumferential myocardial muscle compression (Bourassa et al. 2003; Schwarz et al. 1996; Betriu et al. 1980; Vasan et al. 1989), and calcium channel blockers have also been used with success (Bourassa et al. 2003). Nitrites, however, have been shown to be contraindicated because of the association with worsening angina (Schwarz et al. 1996; Lee and Chen 2015). Some have advanced pacemaker implantation for syncope and conduction disturbances (Bourassa et al. 2003). However, when symptoms persist, most practitioners advocate surgical therapy to unroof the course of the bridged coronary artery. Binet, in 1975 first reported surgical myotomy to unroof the investing myocardial bridge in the involved coronary artery (Binet et al. 1975). Various other therapeutic interventions have been reported and include distal coronary artery bypass and interventional percutaneous stenting of bridged vessels although the mid-term results are still unknown (Haager et al. 2000). In general, however, the literature supports surgical myotomy and bypass grafting, with or without cardiopulmonary bypass which have shown satisfactory results at follow-up evaluation as determined by disappearance of symptoms and normalization of electrocardiogram and angiographic findings (Pey et al. 1985; Schwarz et al. 1996; Ferreira Jr et al. 1991; Betriu et al. 1980; Hillman et al. 1999; Huang et al. 2007; Binet et al. 1975). Figure 76 shows the difference in coronary filling

15-Year-Old Male, Preop Middle Diastole

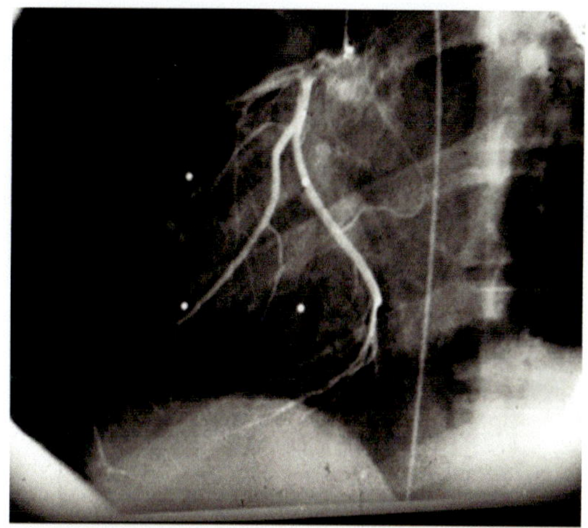

15-Year-Old Male, Preop Early Systole

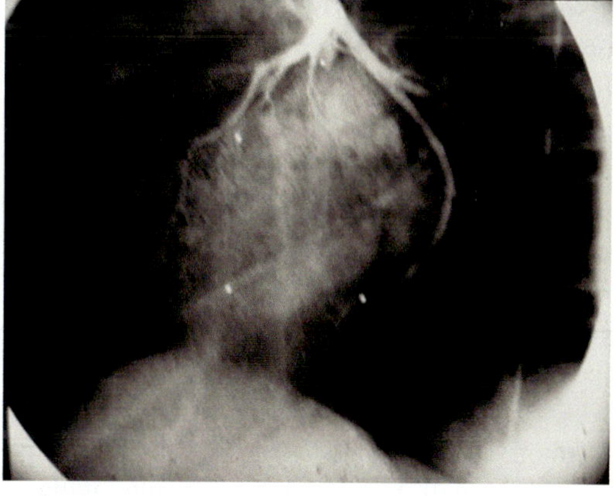

Fig. 76 Shows a coronary angiogram in a symptomatic 15-year-old male in mid-diastole in the upper portion indicating excellent coronary filling. During systole (lower portion), however, the filling of the coronary arteries is obliterated due to myocardial compression of the bridging intramural coronary artery

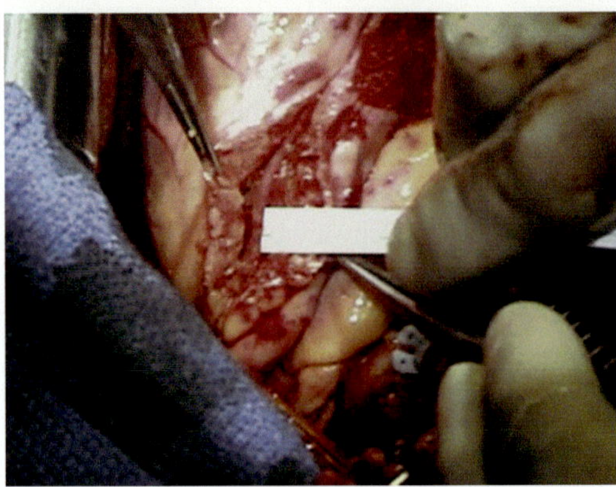

Fig. 77 This is an intraoperative photograph after extensive epicardial unroofing of the length of the left anterior descending coronary artery to the depth of 2.5 cm (the ruler measurement indicators are faded and not clearly seen). The epicardial dissection should be performed carefully to avoid unwanted entry through the anterior portion of the coronary artery

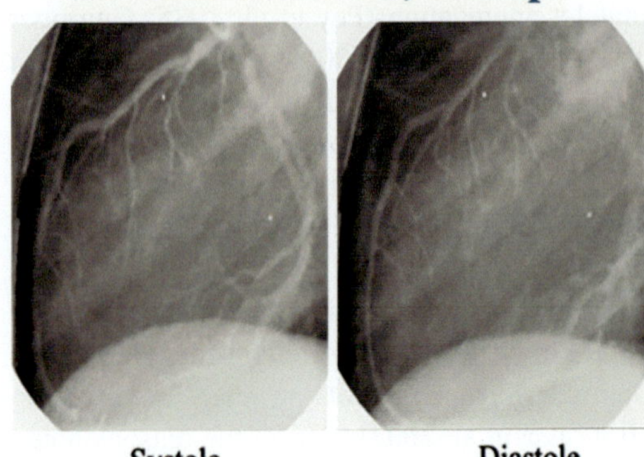

Fig. 78 Shows the postoperative angiogram after extensive unroofing of the entire length of the left anterior descending coronary artery during systole (left frame) and diastole (right frame). Notice that there is no difference in coronary artery filling between systole and diastole indicating that the myocardial bridging was resolved during the operation thereby eliminating the constricting effects of the surrounding muscular tissue. The patient's symptoms resolved

during diastole and systole in a symptomatic 15-year-old. Normal coronary filling is noted in diastole, but coronary filling is obliterated in systole. Figure 77 shows an intraoperative photograph of an extensive unroofing procedure of the left anterior descending artery without unwanted complications. Figure 78 demonstrates the angiographic results of clear coronary filling in both systole and diastole. This patient had resolution of symptoms. Complications associated with this operation stem from the possible injury to the anterior portion of the involved coronary artery during the unroofing procedure. The process is similar to coronary identification and superficial dissection in preparation for coronary artery bypass. Unroofing of the course of an embedded coronary, however, is not always obvious due to the deep intramural course of the coronary artery which can be deep in one location and superficial in another. Deliberate unroofing by epicardial dissection will yield the best results without unwanted entry into the artery. Should entry occur however, patch arterioplasty using a portion of the internal thoracic artery can be performed with acceptable results.

In the modern era, there is no consensus and no randomized studies to guide treatment for patients with coronary artery bridging regardless of symptomatic status. For patients with demonstrated angiographic findings and significant ischemic symptoms, coronary artery unroofing should be seriously considered.

9 Coronary Bypass for Acquired and Congenital Heart Disease After Surgical Coronary Manipulation in Infants, Children, and Young Adults

Coronary artery bypass in infants, children, and young adults with congenital coronary artery malformations is employed to treat the ischemic effects of coronary insufficiency for whatever cause and condition (Mavroudis and Dearani 2020). The focus of this section is on the indications for coronary bypass and the complications that can occur. Some clinical examples that require coronary bypass include obstructive aneurysms for Kawasaki Disease, obstructions to coronary flow due to remote operations requiring coronary button manipulations as seen after the arterial switch operation or Ross operation, and remote coronary artery injury as found in transatrial repair of tetralogy of Fallot (coronary to right ventricular fistula), to name but a few (Mavroudis 2015; Dodge-Khatami et al. 2002; Mavroudis et al. 2003; Mavroudis and Dearani 2020). Coronary bypass therefore is an important therapeutic intervention to treat ischemic clinical conditions that threaten life and should be mastered and practiced by pediatric and adult congenital heart surgeons for the unlikely necessity that will require myocardial revascularization. In the present era, pediatric and adult congenital heart surgeons may need to perform coronary bypass in emergent conditions such as for circumstance involving: (1) acute Type I aortopathy dissections with extension to the coronary arteries, (2) iatrogenic injury during a complex dissection/operation, and (3) iatrogenic injuries due to complications in the catheterization laboratory from unwanted coronary dissection due to catheter manipulation, coronary disruption due to over dilatation of the aortic root, and coronary compression due to device placement (Mavroudis 2015; Mavroudis and Dearani 2020).

9.1 Technique of Internal Thoracic to Coronary Bypass

Coronary bypass in infants, children, and adults with congenital heart disease requires demonstrable patency of both internal thoracic artery (ITA) branches whenever possible by preoperative cardiac catheterization or other diagnostic measures such as CT angiography.

Intraoperative preparation of the ITA requires careful dissection to avoid arterial electrocautery burns and traction injury to the intima. The dissection should proceed towards the origin of the ITA from the subclavian artery by isolating the graft from the underside of the sternum and to avoid injury to the phrenic nerve. Some surgeons prefer to transect the distal graft during the dissection; others prefer to transect the distal graft after cardiopulmonary bypass is instituted and just before the anastomosis is being prepared. The ITA to coronary artery anastomosis demands deliberate and time-consuming steps, especially in infants and children. The denotative steps of the operation are quoted from the *Atlas of Adult Congenital Heart Surgery* (Mavroudis and Dearani 2020),

> CPB is commenced with moderate cooling. The ITA is transected at the distal end and the tip of the vessel is skeletonized. Traction sutures are placed at the pedicle which will insure proper orientation and gentle retraction. An incision is made posteriorly to form angled opening for the end to side anastomosis. The flow is controlled by a small self-occluding clamp. A vent is placed into the right superior pulmonary vein to the left ventricle. Antegrade cardioplegia is administered and quiet, bloodless conditions are established. The heart is positioned to identify the target vessel and prepare for entry. Antegrade cardioplegia is given to distend the coronary vessel while a sharp blade is used for the coronary incision. The arteriotomy is then enlarged as indicated depending on the size of the ITA. The anastomosis may take some time to perform owing to size and friability of the native and ITA vessels. The time that it takes to perform a perfect anastomosis is clearly more important than the cross-clamp time that it required to complete the process. (Mavroudis and Dearani 2020)

Complications associated with coronary bypass involve anastomotic tension, bleeding, unwanted posterior coronary artery disruption during the arterial entry, and failure to ligate all branches of the graft which may result in flow runoff and under-perfusion of the intended coronary artery. Careful planning and execution of the operation will avoid these complications.

9.2 Technique of Proximal Coronary Interposition Grafts

Multiple redo sternotomies for patients with congenital heart disease who require reparative procedures such as conduit replacement, aortic root procedures, repair of residual defects, and obstructive lesions, to name but a few, are at risk for coronary artery injury during redo sternotomy and mediastinal dissection. Aside from the bleeding that occurs, myocardial under- perfusion can cause acute cardiac failure that will require immediate CPB at a time when the conditions are most unfavorable. When one considers 3rd or 4th time redo operations, cardiac injuries are inevitable. Proper planning for emergency CPB, and repair techniques for unwanted injuries are essential. In the course of cardiac dissection in the presence of dense adhesions, coronary injury is most likely to involve the proximal coronary artery near its origin from the ascending aorta especially during proximal aortic root dissection to replace an aortic valve or to perform one of the aortic root operations (valve sparing or root replacement). During exploratory dissection in the aforementioned area, the superior-anterior portion of the coronary artery origin can be entered resulting in a jagged laceration and intimal disruption. After emergency CPB, aortic cross-clamping, and cardioplegic arrest, the choice of coronary repair must be considered which involves patch arterioplasty or interposition graft. The chance of patch arterioplasty is hampered by the likely uneven and jagged injury to the coronary. The injury is best repaired by completion transection, freshening the two resultant arterial ends and performing an interposition graft using an autonomous saphenous vein harvested from the thigh or a PTFE ribbed graft (Mavroudis and Dearani 2020). Proximal grafts in coronary arteries have better flow characteristics and are likely to maintain long-term patency. Figures 20 and 21 show how a similar situation during the repair of anomalous left coronary artery from the pulmonary artery (ALCAPA) can be repaired with a PTFE interposition graft. When recognized to be a better solution to patch arterioplasty, an interposition graft for proximal coronary artery problems is quicker to perform, saves important cross-clamp time, and generally will result in an acceptable coronary artery reconstruction.

10 Coronary Aneurysms

The historical accounts of coronary aneurysms are well documented and include etiology (Munkner et al. 1958), diagnosis (Munkner et al. 1958), incidence (Aintablian et al. 1978; Anabtawi and de Leon 1974; Befeler et al. 1977; Falsetti and Carrol 1976), anatomic characteristics (Aintablian et al. 1978; Anabtawi and de Leon 1974; Befeler et al. 1977; Falsetti and Carrol 1976; Hartnell et al. 1985; Kosar and Chandraratna 1997; Swaye et al. 1983; Markis et al. 1976; Rab et al. 1991; Cohen and O'Gara 2008), angiographic classification (Haager et al. 2000). and histological findings (Lee and Chen 2015; Binet et al. 1975; Haager et al. 2000; Munkner et al. 1958; Aintablian et al. 1978; Anabtawi and de Leon 1974; Befeler et al. 1977; Falsetti and Carrol 1976; Hartnell et al. 1985; Kosar and Chandraratna 1997; Swaye et al. 1983; Markis et al. 1976; Rab et al. 1991; Cohen and O'Gara 2008). Acquired coronary aneurysms in the pediatric population are due to Kawasaki disease, trauma, polyarteritis nodosa, Takayasu's disease, bacterial infection, septic embolism, dissection, and iatrogenic insults after angioplasty or stent placement (Hartnell et al. 1985; Kosar and Chandraratna 1997; Swaye et al. 1983; Markis et al. 1976; Rab et al. 1991). Congenital aneurysms account for 20%–30% of coronary aneurysms (Rab et al. 1991), and are associated with Ehlers–Danlos syndrome, Marfan disease, cyanotic congenital heart disease, and supravalvar aortic stenosis (Munkner et al. 1958; Befeler et al. 1977). Kawasaki disease accounts for the majority of coronary aneurysms found in children (Hartnell et al. 1985; Kosar and Chandraratna 1997; Markis et al. 1976; Ayusawa et al. 2008).

Symptoms and risk factors include angina, congestive heart failure, and myocardial infarction (Aintablian et al. 1978; Rab et al. 1991). Diagnosis can be made by echocardiography (Hartnell et al. 1985; Kosar and Chandraratna 1997; Markis et al. 1976; Rab et al. 1991; Ayusawa et al. 2008; Tunick et al. 1989), angiography, MRI, and CT scanning. Localized changes in flow and thrombosis in an aneurysm with subsequent embolization to the distal coronary artery may cause ischemia and left ventricular dysfunction (Munkner et al. 1958; Aintablian et al. 1978; Rab et al. 1991). In adult patients with or without congenital heart disease, aneurysms are more frequently associated with three-vessel coronary artery disease (42.3%). Myocardial infarction is observed more frequently in patients with aneurysms, but this finding may be due to a higher prevalence of three-vessel coronary artery disease.

Medical therapy has not been effective for improving functional class of patients with aneurysms (Munkner et al. 1958; Befeler et al. 1977; Hartnell et al. 1985; Rab et al. 1991). In patients with symptoms, prognosis is poorer and death from myocardial infarction more probable without surgery (Swaye et al. 1983). Surgery is recommended for patients with coronary aneurysms with or without associated atherosclerosis for ischemic conditions (Munkner et al. 1958; Aintablian et al. 1978; Befeler et al. 1977; Falsetti and Carrol 1976; Hartnell et al. 1985; Swaye et al. 1983). For those individuals with isolated coronary aneurysms, it is unclear if prophylactic surgery is indicated. Symptomatic patients, however, will benefit from bypass surgery which is associated with a reported low 5-year mortality and incidence of postoperative myocardial infarction similar to coronary bypass for atherosclerosis (Kosar and Chandraratna 1997). Repair techniques for saccular aneurysms are more complicated than just coronary bypass and include lateral aneurysmorrhaphy, thrombectomy, and endarterectomy. Recently however, improved techniques with covered intracoronary stents with drug-eluting therapy have been reported. However, the mid- to long-term results are yet to be assessed (Boyer et al. 2014). Surgical consideration for complicated aneurysms, namely those which are thrombosed, occluded, or ruptured require specialized care to resolve the specific conditions. As a result, there is no consensus to recommend the advantage of thrombectomy, endarterectomy, ligation, or aneurysmorrhaphy in addition to bypass of a stenotic aneurysm. Alternatively, catheter-based techniques using drug-eluting stents are increasingly being applied and are under continued evaluation (Heuser 2015).

11 Coronary Aneurysms in Association with Kawasaki Disease

Coronary artery involvement in Kawasaki Disease was first reported by Kato in 1975 (Kato et al. 1975). The incidence, clinical findings (Kato et al. 1975, 1982; Akagi et al. 1992; Beiser et al. 1998; Burns et al. 1996; Gersony 1998; Suzuki et al. 1986; Checchia et al. 1997; Dajani et al. 1993, 1994; Harada et al. 1993; Nakamura et al. 1998; Newburger et al. 2004; Pahl 1997; Satou et al. 2007; Suzuki et al. 1990; Newburger et al. 2016; Kitamura et al. 1990; Ino et al. 1996), and pathologic characteristics (Kato et al. 1975; Beiser et al. 1998) have been further defined and categorized.

Diagnosis is established by echocardiography and coronary angiography (Newburger et al. 2004). In addition, left ventricular function, mitral valve insufficiency, and pericardial effusion may be assessed. The American Heart Association has classified aneurysms as small (<5 mm internal diameter), medium (5–8 mm), or giant (>8 mm internal diameter). The most common anatomic sites for coronary artery involvement are the proximal LAD and the proximal RCA, followed by the LMCA (Newburger et al. 2004). The LMCA is usually spared except for the rare situation that involves the common orifice of both LAD and circumflex artery (Newburger et al. 2004). In addition to coronary artery aneurysms systemic aneurysms may occur (Dajani et al. 1994; Newburger et al. 2004; Satou et al. 2007) and involve the subclavian artery, the internal mammary artery, the iliofemoral arteries, the abdominal aorta, and the renal arteries (Pahl 1997). Males are more likely to develop aneurysms than females, and infants younger than 6 months, as well as those older than 8 years, are associated with the highest risk (Newburger et al. 2016).

While this chapter on coronary problems has centered on surgical complications, it is also important to understand some of the anatomic and clinical findings at follow-up (Kato et al. 1982) which will guide possible surgical intervention and highlight the possible complications that may occur during therapeutic measures. Four angiographic groups have been identified by Kato and associates (1982): Group I represents 50% of Kawasaki patients, who have regression of aneurysm, no symptoms, no ECG changes, and a negative thallium test result. Group II Kawasaki patients (24%) have an unobstructed aneurysm. Group III patients (17%) have an obstructed aneurysm. Group IV patients (9%) have a non-stenotic irregular arterial wall. Risk stratification as measured by z-scores (<2 to >10 or absolute dimensions >8 mm), corresponding to risk levels 1–5 (normal coronary arteries, transient dilatation, small aneurysm, medium aneurysm, large or giant aneurysm), and suggest management strategies for treatment and follow-up (Newburger et al. 2016; Kitamura et al. 1990; Ino et al. 1996).

The natural history of untreated coronary aneurysms is varied. Aneurysms can progress and cause thrombosis of the lumen and stenosis, or more rarely expand and rupture (Newburger et al. 2004). Occlusion of the coronary arteries can occur, most commonly of the RCA (61.5%), followed by LAD, and the circumflex coronary artery involvement (Burns et al. 1996; Pahl 1997). Giant aneurysms (>8 mm) are rare (1% of patients), but they may develop into life-threatening coronary lesions (Beiser et al. 1998; Newburger et al. 2004; Pahl 1997) and generally do not regress (Akagi et al. 1992; Checchia et al. 1997; Dajani et al. 1993; Pahl 1997). These giant aneurysms can progress to occlusion, myocardial infarction, and sudden death (Akagi et al. 1992; Checchia et al. 1997; Dajani et al. 1994). On the other hand, about 50% of smaller aneurysms regress within 1 year (Kato et al. 1975, 1982; Beiser et al. 1998; Nakamura et al. 1998). The actuarial persistence of all aneurysms combined is 72% at 1 year and 41% at 5 years (Akagi et al. 1992; Dajani et al. 1993, 1994).

In the present era, the greater majority of children who are treated with intravenous gammaglobulins and aspirin in the acute phase of illness never develop aneurysms (Kato et al. 1975; Beiser et al. 1998; Dajani et al. 1994; Newburger et al. 2004; Pahl 1997; Newburger et al. 2016). Furthermore, therapeutic advances have emerged which are undergoing evaluation and include plasma exchange, cyclophosphamide, and an interleukine-1 receptor antagonist anakinra (Newburger et al. 2004, 2016). Aneurysm regression has been associated with smaller initial size, age at onset of Kawasaki disease less than 1-year, female sex, fusiform rather than saccular anatomic configuration, and distal segment aneurysms (Akagi et al. 1992; Newburger et al. 2004).

Myocardial infarction occurs in 1.5% of all patients with Kawasaki disease and 11.3% of those with documented coronary disease. Those patients with giant aneurysms (Akagi et al. 1992) are at the highest risk for infarction within the first year after presentation (Satou et al. 2007). Mortality from myocardial infarction under these circumstances remains high and can reach 25% (Dajani et al. 1993; Kato et al. 1982).

12 Surgical Management in Patients with Kawasaki Coronary Disease

Surgical therapy involving excision or plication of coronary aneurysms has been attempted with poor results and has been abandoned. Coronary bypass has been established for ischemic complications of Kawasaki Disease despite the absence of clinical trials. Indications include severe proximal stenosis (>75%), left main stenosis, proximal LAD stenosis, ischemia after percutaneous coronary angioplasty, and proximal aneurysms (Akagi et al. 1992; Checchia et al. 1997; Newburger et al. 2004; Pahl 1997). Coronary bypass indications have evolved because of the unacceptable rate of myocardial infarction or sudden death without surgery (Akagi et al. 1992). Saphenous vein bypass has been largely abandoned since the internal thoracic artery to coronary artery bypass has far better long-term patency and growth potential (86%–100% at 1 year) (Harada et al. 1993; Suzuki et al. 1990;

Kitamura et al. 1990). Furthermore, bilateral internal thoracic artery bypass grafts have been performed and advocated by Kitamura and associates with excellent results including absence of sternal infections and adverse effects of chest wall development in children (Kitamura et al. 1990). Percutaneous transluminal coronary angioplasty has been used in patients with Kawasaki disease for indications similar to atherosclerotic coronary artery disease; for example, lesions with localized proximal stenosis (Ino et al. 1996). However, no randomized trials exist comparing bypass surgery with percutaneous coronary interventions in Kawasaki disease (Newburger et al. 2016). There are, however, many complicating factors which favor coronary bypass such as propensity of aneurysms to cause distal clot embolization and long-term antiplatelet therapy.

The presence of aneurysms, no matter how small, are a cause of clinical dilemmas. For instance, patent and non-stenotic aneurysms present a particular problem, since localized flow patterns and stasis may be responsible for acute coronary events. In other words, coronary bypass distal to an obstructed coronary aneurysm does not protect against postoperative thrombosis, embolization, and resultant myocardial infarction and possible death. Therefore, the current recommendation is to perform bypass grafts for only stenotic vessels (Newburger et al. 2004; Suzuki et al. 1990). Percutaneous transluminal coronary angioplasty is generally not indicated in the treatment of children younger than 10 years, in those whose coronary arteries reveal calcification on fluoroscopy, or when multiple stenosis or long-segment stenosis is present (Newburger et al. 2016).

Transplantation has been performed for end-stage ischemic cardiomyopathy, much like the indications for other conditions with poor ventricular function, no matter the cause. Indications for cardiac transplantation in this group of patients however have been developed. They include left ventricular dysfunction from myocardial infarction, ventricular arrhythmias and cardiac arrest, as well as multivessel or inoperable coronary artery disease (Checchia et al. 1997). The fear of recurrent Kawasaki coronary artery disease in the transplanted heart has been assessed and dispelled without evidence of recurrent disease over 1–6 years of follow-up (Checchia et al. 1997).

13 Coronary Bypass for Kawasaki Disease, Operations That Require Coronary Button Translocation (Arterial Switch and Ross Operation), Left Coronary Artery Atresia, and Iatrogenesis

As noted previously, coronary artery bypass in infants, children, and young adults is a therapeutic measure to treat localized coronary ischemia for whatever cause that can threaten life (Mavroudis 2015; Mavroudis and Dearani 2020). The more common indication is for patients with Kawasaki disease who develop giant aneurysms and hemodynamically stenotic vessels as discussed. Coronary bypass can also be lifesaving for infants presenting with left main coronary artery atresia as well as for patients who have experienced unwanted iatrogenic coronary injuries. These injuries can be due to catheter procedures, acute intraoperative surgical mishaps, or remote coronary artery manipulations as can be seen in patients who present status post arterial switch, Ross operation, and other operations that require coronary button translocation (Mavroudis 2015; Mavroudis and Dearani 2020).

Coronary bypass for the complications of Kawasaki disease can be performed in very young patients Fig. 79 who have experienced significant ischemic complications. Figure 80 illustrates a left internal thoracic artery to left anterior

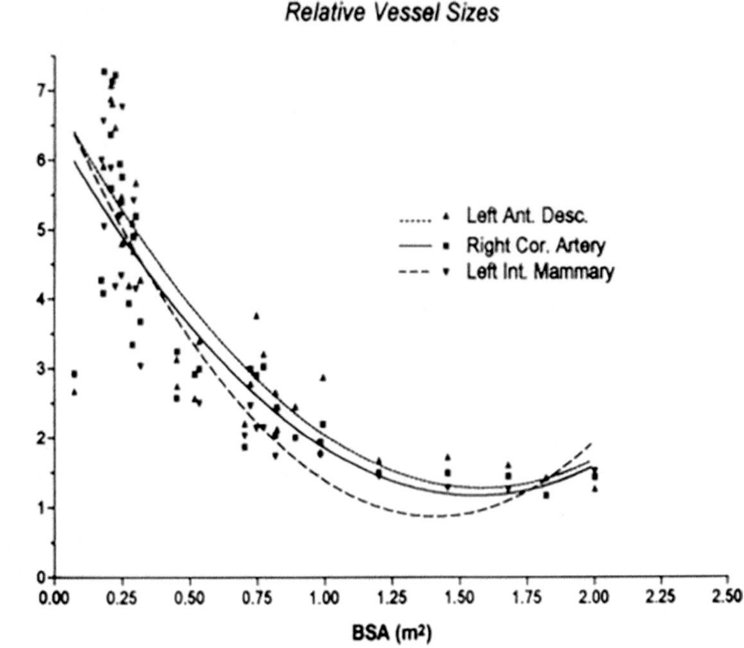

Fig. 79 Shows a graph that correlates vessel diameter mm/BSA and BSA based on angiographic measurements in normal patients from early infancy to adulthood. The data shows that coronary artery (left and right) and left internal mammary artery measurements larger in infancy and childhood based on their mass than in adults. The implication is that coronary bypass in infants and children can be performed since the arteries are larger than what one would expect based on body mass

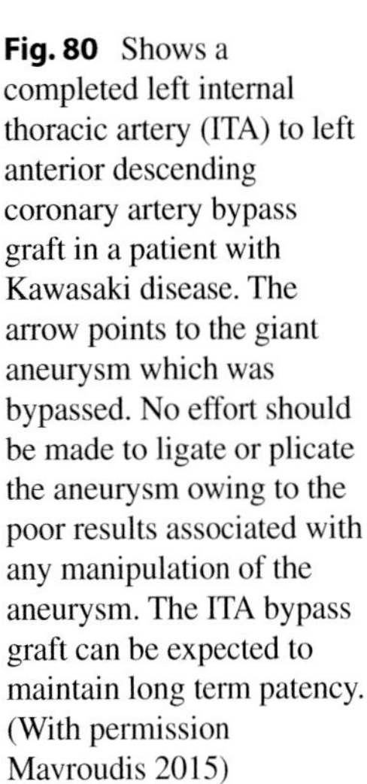

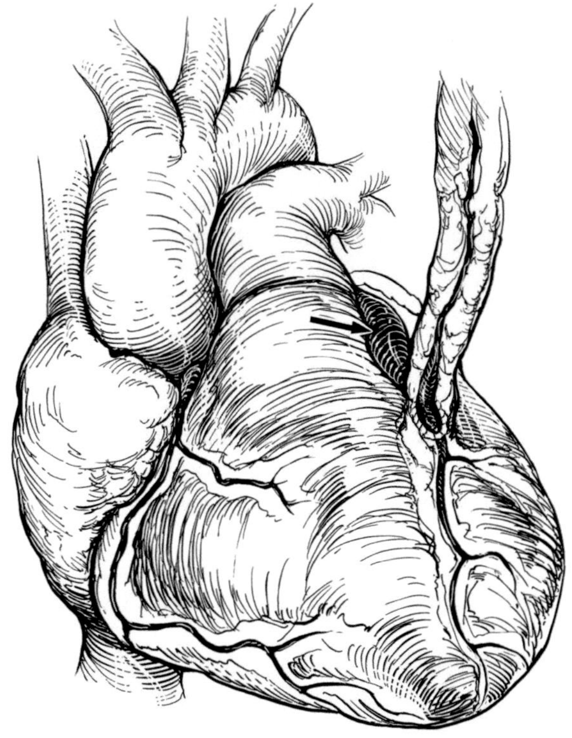

Fig. 80 Shows a completed left internal thoracic artery (ITA) to left anterior descending coronary artery bypass graft in a patient with Kawasaki disease. The arrow points to the giant aneurysm which was bypassed. No effort should be made to ligate or plicate the aneurysm owing to the poor results associated with any manipulation of the aneurysm. The ITA bypass graft can be expected to maintain long term patency. (With permission Mavroudis 2015)

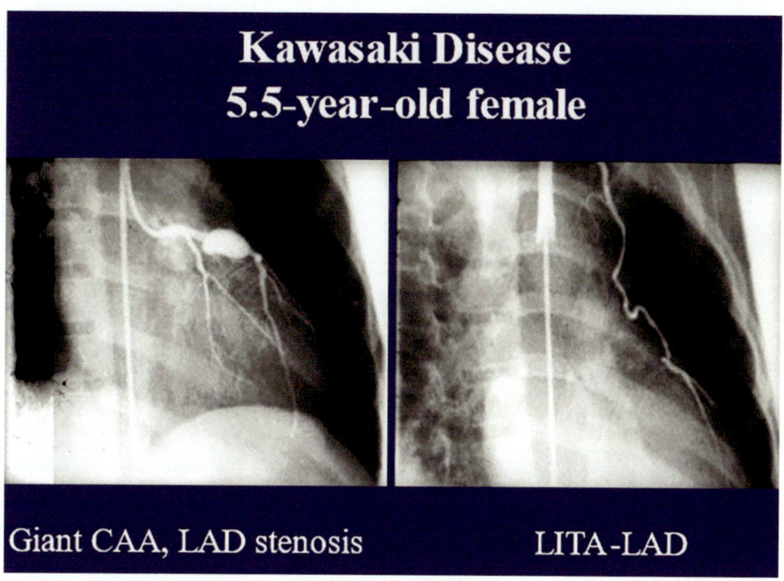

Fig. 81 Left frame shows a coronary arteriogram in a 5.5-year-old female with a giant left anterior descending coronary artery aneurysm due to Kawasaki Disease. The aneurysm is also associated with critical stenosis. The right frame shows a postoperative patent left internal thoracic artery to left anterior descending coronary artery bypass. *CAA* coronary anterior aneurysm, *LAD* left anterior descending, *LITA* left internal thoracic artery

descending coronary artery bypass in a patient with Kawasaki disease and associated proximal coronary aneurysm. Figures 81, 82, 83, 84, 85, 86, 87 and 88 demonstrate a series of pre- and postoperative angiograms showing patients with Kawasaki disease who had coronary bypass at different ages, for a variety of indications, often with bilateral ITA to coronary bypass, and universal midterm follow-up. All patients in this series of patients had confirmation of patency.

Coronary bypass is also indicated for patients who experienced complications of coronary button transfer during the arterial switch or Ross operations resulting in severe stenosis or occlu-

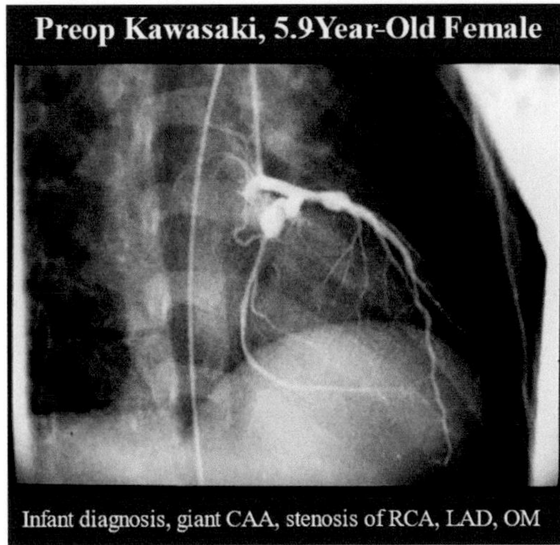

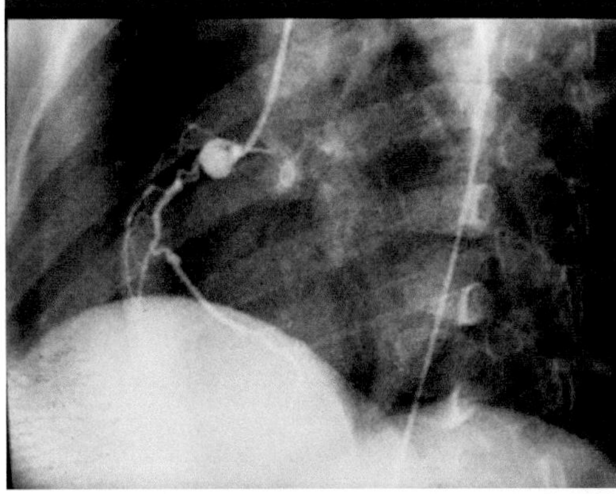

Fig. 82 Shows a preoperative coronary angiogram showing aneurysms of the LAD, Circumflex (upper frame) and RCA. The operative plan was to perform bilateral ITA grafts to the LAD and RCA and not bypass the circumflex artery. This plan would unfold in the next series of arteriograms. *CAA* coronary artery aneurysm, *LAD* left anterior descending, *OM* obtuse marginal, *RCA* right coronary artery

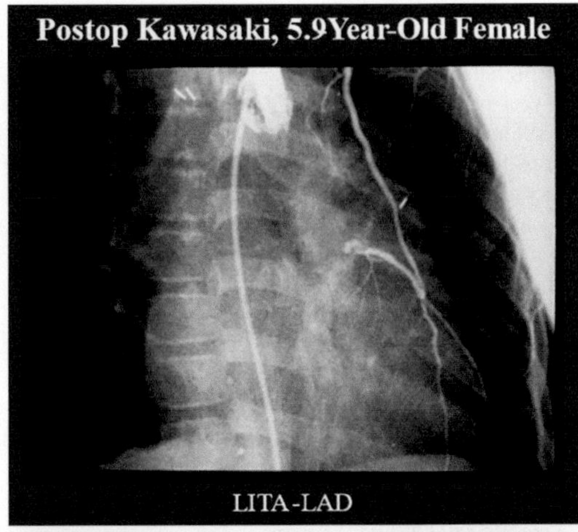

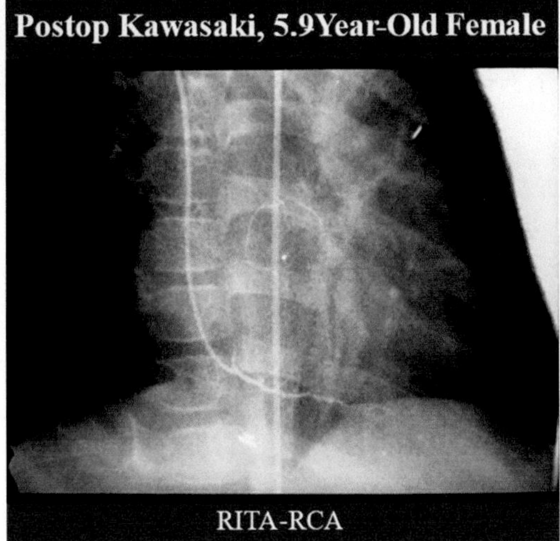

Fig. 83 Shows completed left LITA-LAD (upper frame) and RITA-RCA (lower frame) bypass grafts in a patient with Kawasaki disease. Both grafts are patent with excellent distal run off. *LAD* left anterior descending, *LITA* left internal thoracic artery, *RCA* right coronary artery, *RITA* right internal thoracic artery

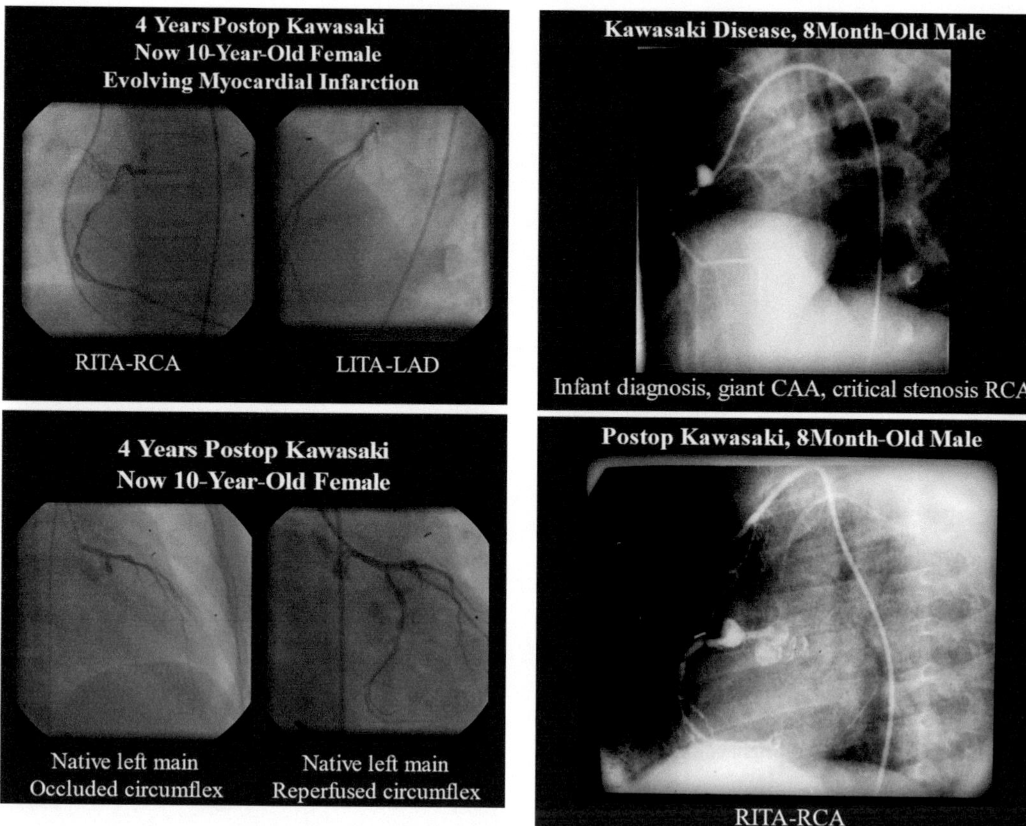

Fig. 84 Shows coronary angiograms of a patient 4 years postoperatively which was performed for clinical evidence of an evolving myocardial infarction. Both bypass grafts are shown in the upper frame to be widely patent with excellent flow patterns. The lower frame, however, shows occlusion of the circumflex coronary (left) which was not bypassed during the first operation. The patient responded to medical therapy. *LAD* left anterior descending, *LITA* left internal thoracic artery, *RCA* right coronary artery, *RITA* right internal thoracic artery

Fig. 85 Shows coronary arteriograms in an 8-month-old infant with a giant RCA aneurysm with critical stenosis (upper frame). A RITA-RCA bypass graft was performed with demonstrated patency (lower frame) The bypass graft was performed distal to the significant stenosis. *CAA* coronary artery aneurysm, *RCA* right coronary artery, *RITA* right internal thoracic artery

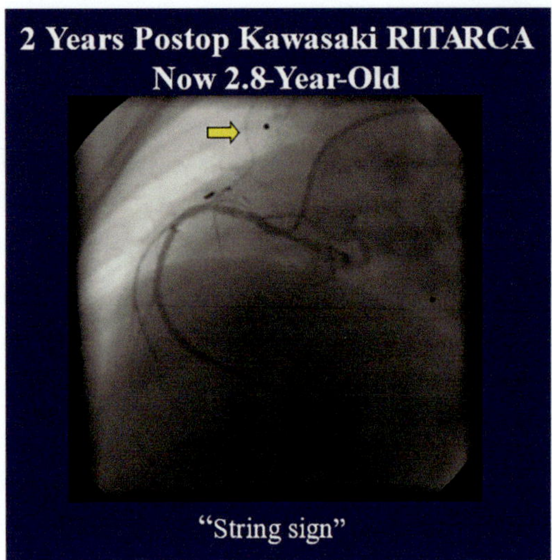

Fig. 86 Shows a 2-year follow-up coronary arteriogram. The RCA has been remodeled and displays no evidence of a prior aneurysm or stenosis. As expected, the improved circulation through the native coronary artery resulted in an RTA "string sign" which was associated with patency regression due to competitive flow which favored the RCA. This shows clear evidence that Kawasaki aneurysms can be remodeled. *RCA* right coronary artery, *RITA* right internal thoracic artery

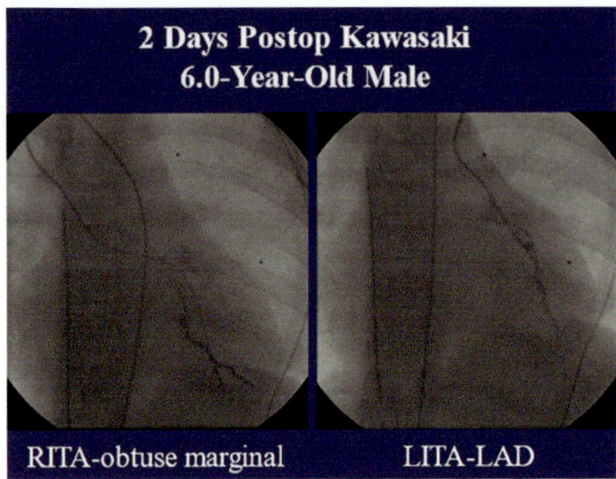

Fig. 87 Shows widely patent postoperative coronary bypass angiograms that were performed for severely stenotic LAD and obtuse marginal (OM) coronary arteries in a 6-year-old male. The angiograms are displayed to show that the OM coronary artery can be bypassed with the RITA despite the technical challenges associated with completion of this graft. *RITA* right internal thoracic artery, *LAD* left anterior descending, *LITA* left internal thoracic artery

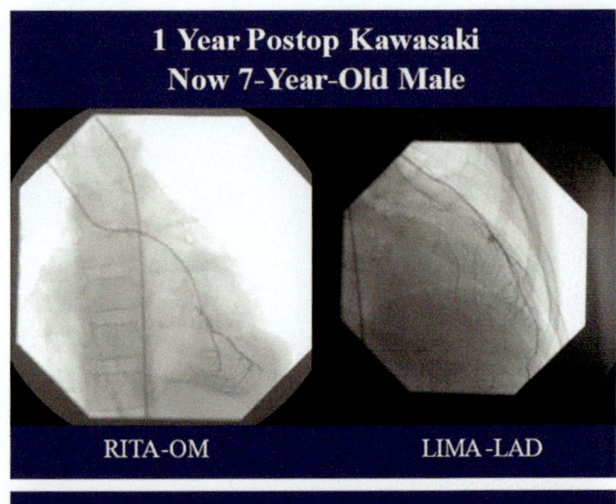

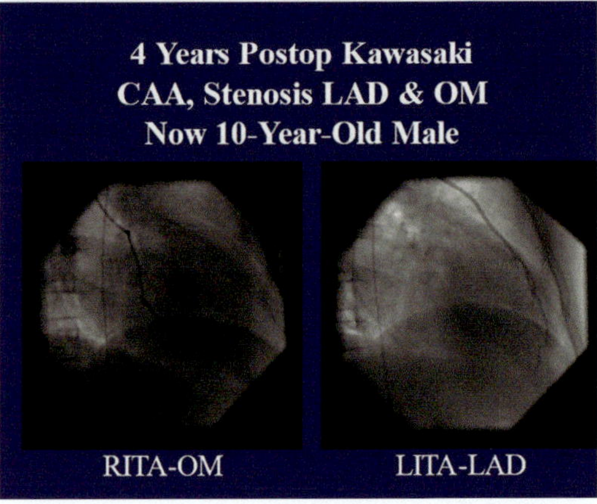

Fig. 88 Shows routine follow-up of 1 year and 4-year postoperative coronary angiograms. Both bypass grafts are widely patent with excellent distal flow patterns. *LAD* left anterior descending, *OM* obtuse marginal, *RITA* right internal thoracic artery

sion (Mavroudis 2015; Mavroudis and Dearani 2020). Figures 89, 90, 91, 92, 93, 94 and 95 show the various coronary artery problems that can occur during and after coronary artery button transfer for the arterial switch operation. Coronary problems not requiring coronary bypass associated with the arterial switch operation include intraoperative twisted button transfer, neopulmonary artery compression of the proximal coronaries, and management of the single coronary artery have been discussed in the transposition chapter in Figs. 11, 15, 24, 33, 75 and 94. Patients who are likely to require coro-

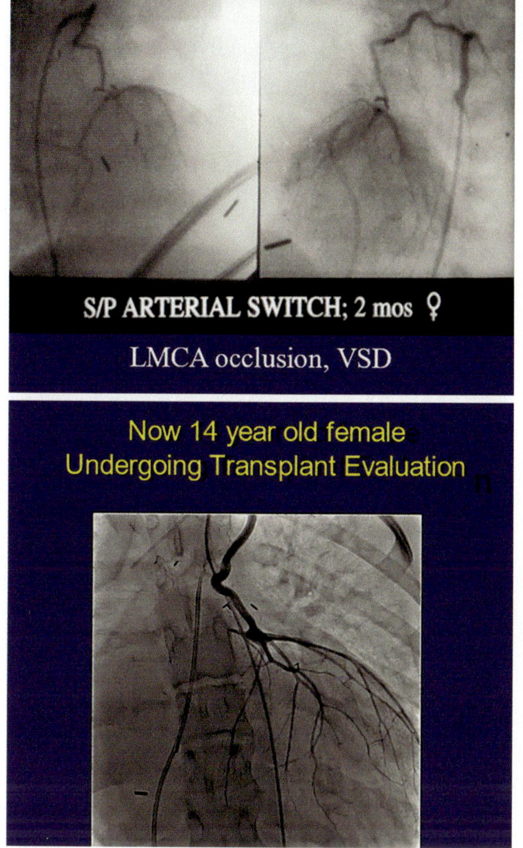

Fig. 89 Shows an angiogram of a completed LITA LAD that was performed in a patient who had been referred for a complicated arterial switch-VSD operation. The patient had severe ventricular dysfunction and an occluded left main coronary artery. The LITA-LAD graft was accomplished with demonstrated postoperative patency and mildly improved ventricular function (upper frame). Fourteen years after the arterial switch and subsequent LITA-LAD bypass graft, the patient underwent cardiac catheterization for cardiac transplant evaluation which showed poor ventricular dysfunction despite a patent LITA-LAD graft (lower frame) which had grown considerably during the follow up period. *LMCA* left main coronary artery, *VSD* ventricular septal defect

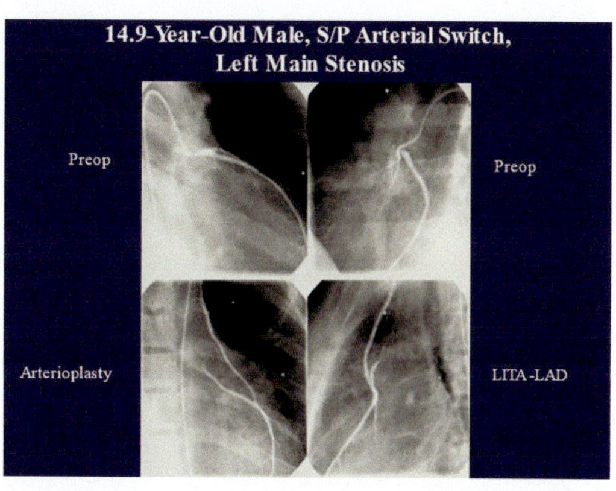

Fig. 90 Shows pre- and postoperative coronary angiograms of a symptomatic 14.9-year-old male. The preoperative angiograms show severe left main coronary artery stenosis. The operation that was performed was a left main coronary artery arterioplasty and concomitant LITA-LAD bypass graft in a "belt and suspenders" approach to vascular revascularization. The idea was that the proximal coronary arterioplasty might not be optimal and if not, the LITA-LAD bypass graft would provide the necessary perfusion. *LAD* left anterior descending, *LITA* left internal thoracic artery

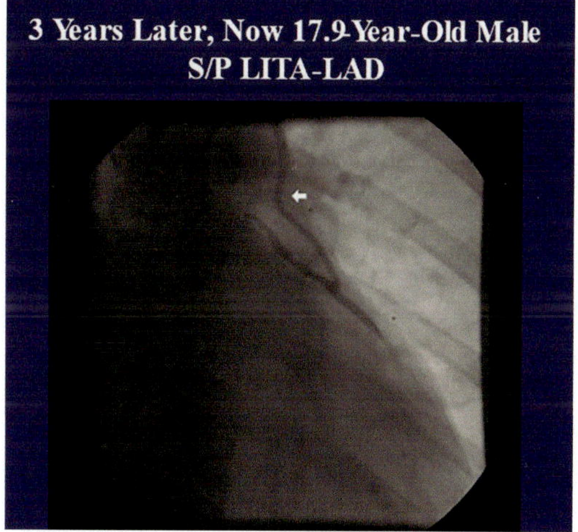

Fig. 91 Shows a routine 3-year postoperative coronary angiogram. As predicted the proximal left main coronary arterioplasty was insufficient and still stenotic despite the arterioplasty. The LITA-LAD bypass graft however remained patent with excellent run-off characteristics. The proximal arterioplasty in combination with coronary artery bypass is controversial and has not been resolved, leading the clinician to use best judgment indications during the planning and the course of the operation. *LAD* left anterior descending, *LITA* left internal thoracic artery

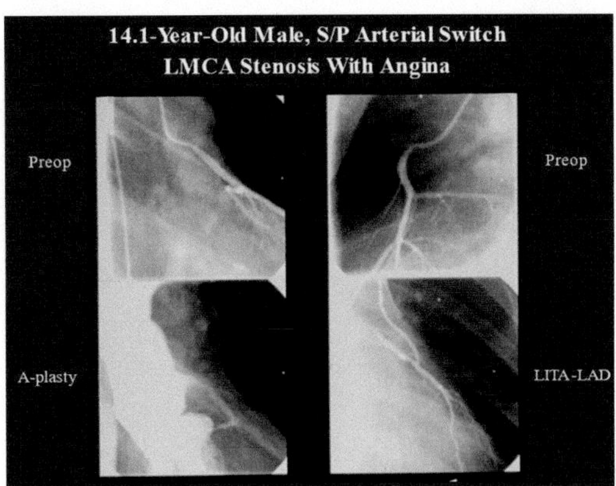

Fig. 92 Shows a similar dilemma of left main coronary artery stenosis in a symptomatic 14.1-year-old male S/P arterial switch. The left main stenosis is shown to be at the orifice which appears to be amenable to a proximal arterioplasty. The reparative operation was a "belt and suspenders" approach with proximal coronary arterioplasty and LITA-LAD bypass graft. The postoperative patency of the proximal coronary arterioplasty and the LITA-LAD bypass graft is shown with excellent patency characteristics. *LAD* left anterior descending, *LITA* left internal thoracic artery, *LMCA* left main coronary artery

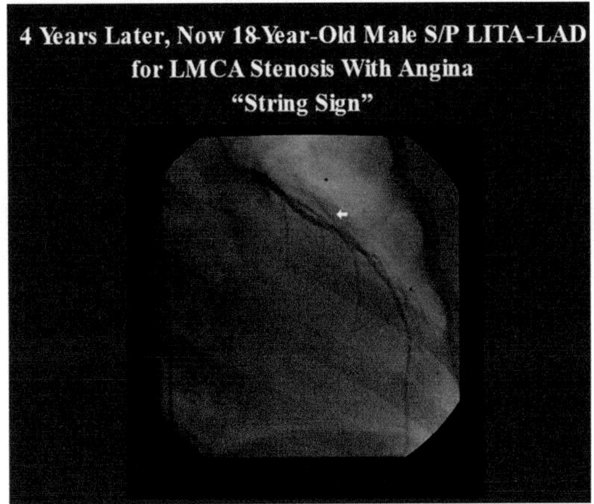

Fig. 93 Shows a routine 4-year follow-up coronary arteriogram. A widely patent proximal left main coronary arterioplasty is illustrated with an associated "string-sign" LITA-LAD graft which underwent anatomic regression during the interim due to competitive flow. This series of coronary artery reconstructive procedures shows how unpredictable proximal coronary artery arterioplasty versus coronary bypass surgery can be. Practical wisdom and anatomic analysis will guide the surgeon as to what operation to perform. In the case of extensive proximal coronary stenosis, it would seem prudent to perform only a coronary bypass. In the event of reparable proximal stenosis by arterioplasty, one could consider the "belt and suspender" technique. *LAD* left anterior descending, *LITA* left internal thoracic artery, *LMCA* left main coronary artery

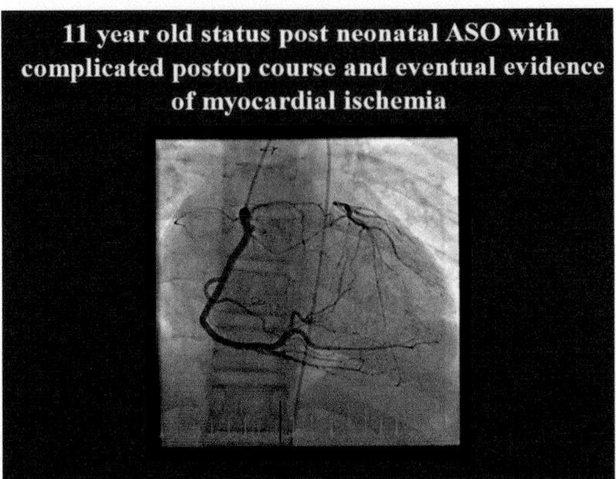

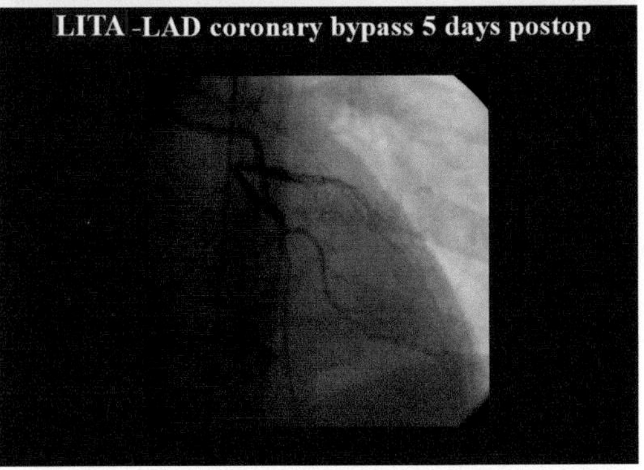

Fig. 94 Shows a pre- and postoperative angiogram of an 11-year-old patient who had remote neonatal arterial switch with a complicated postoperative course. He developed severe angina and was found to have long segment left main occlusion with significant collaterals from the right coronary artery to the left anterior descending artery (upper panel). At operation, no effort was made to perform a proximal left main arterioplasty. The LITA-LAD graft was performed without incident and the postoperative angiogram is shown (lower panel). *ASO* arterial switch operation, *LAD* left anterior descending, *LITA* left internal thoracic artery

nary bypass involve those who have survived coronary occlusion or severe stenosis at the original operation as shown in Figs. 89, 90, 91, 92, 93, 94 and 95. Patient selection for coronary bypass under these circumstances involves the accepted maxim that, when possible, a two coronary artery should be maintained and established. Perhaps, the most common dilemma that arises is whether to perform proximal arterioplasty, distal ITA-coronary artery bypass, or both (Mavroudis 2015; Mavroudis and Dearani 2020). The included angiograms show that a certain amount of uncertainty and anxiety attends this dilemma. Our

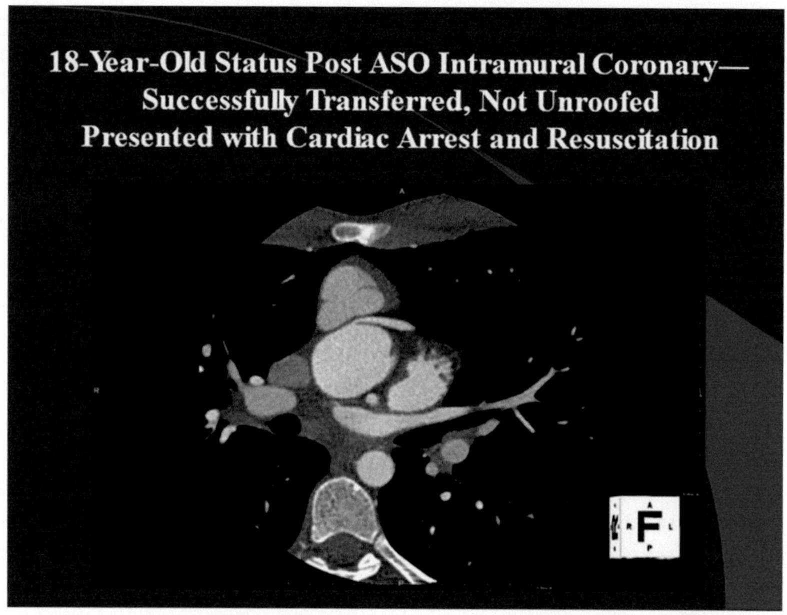

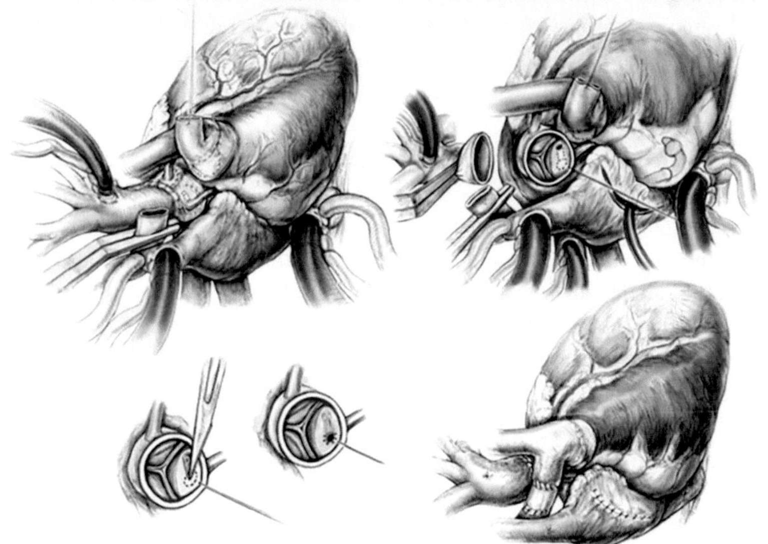

Fig. 95 Shows a CT coronary angiogram of a patient who had remote infant ASO in whom an intramural left main coronary button was successfully transferred but not unroofed (upper panel). He presented 18 years postop with cardiac arrest, resuscitation, ECMO and eventual recovery albeit with a below the knee amputation from the femoral-femoral ECMO. He underwent coronary unroofing as shown in the lower panel without complications

experience has shown that performing proximal arterioplasty and coronary bypass has resulted in proximal repair failure with coronary artery patency in one patient and successful proximal arterioplasty with eventual "string sign" of the bypass graft in the other, indicating that the bypass graft regressed owing to competitive flow from the proximal arterioplasty. In other patients, the proximal stenosis was so extensive that contemplating proximal arterioplasty would have been folly. In these patients, coronary bypass only was performed with excellent results. We have concluded, without clear-cut evidence, that practical wisdom and excellent clinical judgment should guide the surgeon as to what course to take in these very challenging cases.

Complications associated with ITA-coronary bypass involve the ITA harvest and the distal anastomosis. Those surgeons with extensive experience with harvesting the ITA will understand that careful use of electrocautery, especially in very young children, will avoid thermal injury and yield the best results. Injury to the harvested ITA will require special attention which can be resolved with a suture or two for a small injury to resection and end-to-end anastomosis. In addition, the ITA must be harvested up to the origin from the subclavian artery to prevent competitive flow if a major branch is not divided. The ITA to coronary artery anastomosis in an infant and young child has many pitfalls that must be respected. First of all, coronary entry using a Beaver blade requires utmost attention since an unwanted deep cut can injure the posterior portion of the coronary artery, cause dissection, and thrombosis. Better to administer cardioplegia during the entry and use caution. Each surgeon has his/her own way to perform coronary bypass anastomosis which involves various practices of the starting point, inside-out suturing, and interrupted versus running technique. We have used interrupted 8-0 monofilament suture technique for young infants and running suture technique (8-0 monofilament suture) for older children based on the operative findings. Recently, Iwata and colleagues (2021) have performed infant coronary artery bypass grafting completely under surgical microscope. There truly is no reason not to apply this technology for these challenging anastomoses. Like most new technologies, there will be a learning curve and an administrative acceptance to support these important improvements.

Rarely, during the arterial switch operation, an intramural coronary artery will be encountered as noted in Fig. 95. The artery was successfully transferred at the original operation, but the intramural segment was not unroofed. As noted in the figure legend, the patient presented with a myocardial infarction, cardiogenic shock, and required ECMO. The patient underwent unroofing without complication as shown in the figure. However, one may consider if this complication might not have occurred if the intramural artery was indeed unroofed at the original operation. On the other side of this dilemma is the ever-present danger of a potential technical mishap of the unroofing procedure at the original operation. Unfortunately, we will never know since there are very few patients with transposition that present with this very rare coronary artery anomaly. It is left to the prudent surgeon to decide whether to perform the unroofing procedure at the initial operation for arterial switch. From our point of view, the unroofing procedure is worth the effort.

Patients undergoing the Ross operation require pulmonary artery autograft translocation and coronary button reimplantation in much the same manner as for the arterial switch operation which is discussed in the previous paragraph. The key to making sure that autograft coronary reimplantation is successful is the proper alignment of the autograft into the aortic annulus. An unwanted rotation can cause poor alignment of the coronary artery buttons into the proper sinus of Valsalva. Even so, there are situations in which the autograft is aligned perfectly for the left main coronary artery button attachment but not perfectly aligned for the right coronary artery button attachment. Further dissection of the right coronary artery button in this situation may afford a tension-free anastomosis to the neoaorta. However, the surgeon should not hesitate to perform a coronary PTFE interposition graft which can rectify a very difficult situation. Sometimes coronary artery implantation can result in severe proximal stenosis as noted in Fig. 96. While a proximal coronary artery arterioplasty might be considered, one has to take into account the autograft thin-walled characteristics and proximity to the neoaortic valve leaflets which might result in unwanted injury to one or both structures. Better to perform an ITA-coronary artery bypass as noted in the lower frame of Fig. 96.

Left main coronary artery atresia is extraordinarily rare and can be confused with ALCAPA since there is no demonstrable flow from the aorta. Echocardiography can show retrograde flow into the pulmonary artery from the ALCAPA which can rule out left main coronary artery atresia; however, in the absence of retrograde flow, this diagnosis may be difficult. When in doubt CT angiography or cardiac catheterization may differentiate between the two diagnoses. Figure 97 shows the results of pre- and postoperative arteriograms in a patient who was diagnosed with atresia of the left main coronary artery. In particular, the preoperative frames show right coronary flow from the aorta with collateral flow to the LAD and no left main antegrade flow. The pulmonary artery preoperative frame shows no coronary flow indicating that the diagnosis is more likely to be left main coronary artery atresia. At operation, there was left main coronary artery obstruction (atresia) very close to the distal left main coronary artery which was amenable to proximal coronary artery patch arterioplasty which was performed. In addition, a left internal thoracic artery-left anterior descending (LITA-LAD) bypass graft was also performed in a "belt and suspenders" solution as has been described in previous paragraphs along with the advantages and disadvantages of such an operative approach. The postoperative angiograms are noted in the lower frames which show patency of both the proximal patch arterioplasty and the LITA-LAD bypass graft. The potential complications of these operations are mostly technical and involve postoperative bleeding, thrombosis, and unwanted stenosis as a result of inaccurate suturing. On occasion, left main coronary atresia may be encountered serendipitously in adults as noted in Fig. 98 which highlights pre- and postoperative coronary arteriograms in a 28-year-old male

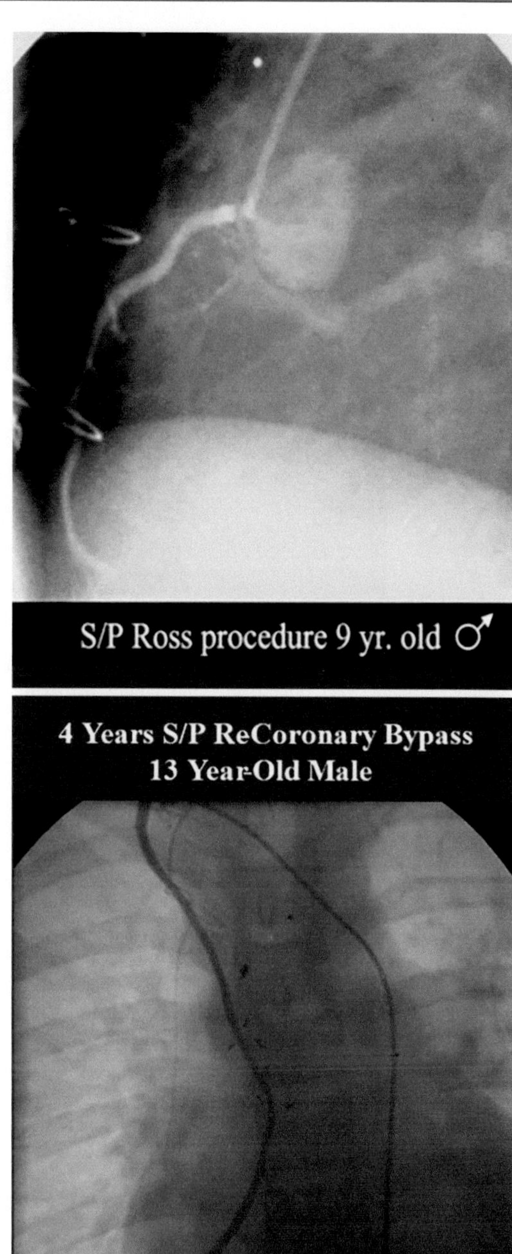

Fig. 96 Other forms of coronary button translocation can also be associated with proximal stenoses as noted in this symptomatic 9-year-old patient who had a remote Ross operation and severe right coronary artery orifice stenosis (upper panel). It was determined that he should undergo a RITA-RCA bypass operation without consideration for a proximal arterioplasty owing to the unfavorable characteristics of the proximal neoaorta (pulmonary autograft). The routine 4-year follow-up coronary angiogram is shown with a widely patent bypass graft (lower panel). *RCA* right coronary artery, *RITA* right internal thoracic artery

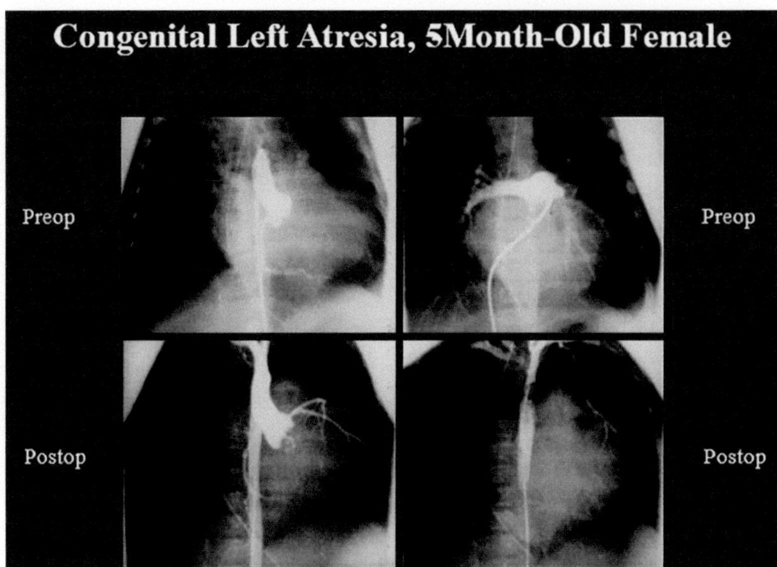

Fig. 97 Shows preoperative and postoperative cardiac catheterization in a 5-month-old female with left main coronary atresia with operative management involving proximal left main patch arterioplasty and concomitant left internal thoracic artery-left anterior descending artery (LITA-LAD) bypass graft. The operative procedure was performed as a "belt and suspenders" type of solution to make sure that flow to the coronary artery would be assured. The postoperative angiograms show a widely patent proximal patch arterioplasty and a patent LITA-LAD graft. *LAD* left anterior descending, *LITA* left internal thoracic artery

who underwent reoperation to replace an aortic homograft and apply a Bentall aortic root replacement. Preoperatively, a large RCA was noted with collateral flow to the left-sided coronary arteries. At operation, left main coronary artery atresia was found which was not due to the previous operation. The Bentall operation was performed with LITA-LAD bypass graft with postoperative arteriogram shown in the lower frame of the figure. It is not entirely clear that this left main atresia was congenital in nature since there was a prior operation in the vicinity. However, the area from where the presumed coronary orifice was to originate was smooth and without evidence of prior vascular injury. And as the adage goes, "that's my story and I am sticking with it." On a more serious side, whatever the cause of the left main atresia whether it be congenital or acquired, the treatment is the same. The potential complication of coronary revascularization in this type of case is to avoid proximal coronary arterioplasty if the atretic segment is too long and not amenable to proximal arterioplasty. The coronary bypass solution is therefore the better option.

Unwanted coronary artery injuries can occur during surgical mishaps or by cardiac catheterization injury. Figure 99 shows a patent postoperative right internal thoracic artery-right coronary artery (RITA-RCA) bypass graft which was necessarily and emergently performed during an operation to replace the mitral valve in an 18-year-old female with Marfan syndrome. An unwanted maneuver during the course of the operation resulted in avulsion of the RCA necessitating immediate cardiopulmonary bypass, aortic cross-clamping, retrograde cardioplegia, mitral valve replacement, and RITA-RCA bypass. Despite the elongated cross- clamp time, the patient made an uneventful recovery. As noted in the angiogram, the bypass graft is widely patent with excellent flow characteristics. The complication described herein was clearly undesirable like most complications. The important issue, however, after the event is to pro-

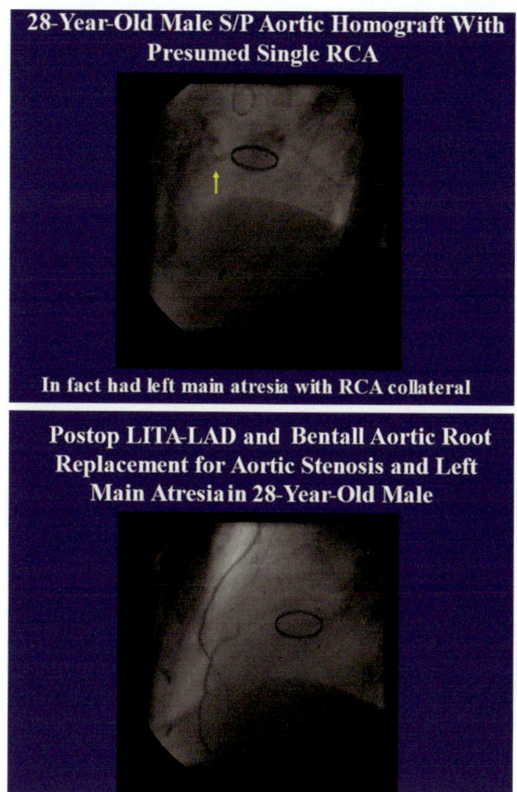

Fig. 98 Shows left main atresia which was discovered at exploration of the aortic root during reoperation to replace an aortic homograft using a Bentall operation. Arteriography (upper frame) shows a large RCA with collateral flow to the LAD. At reoperation, the Bentall procedure was performed without incident and the LITA-LAD graft (lower frame) revascularized flow to the left side of the heart. *LAD* left anterior descending, *LITA* left internal thoracic artery, *RCA* right coronary artery

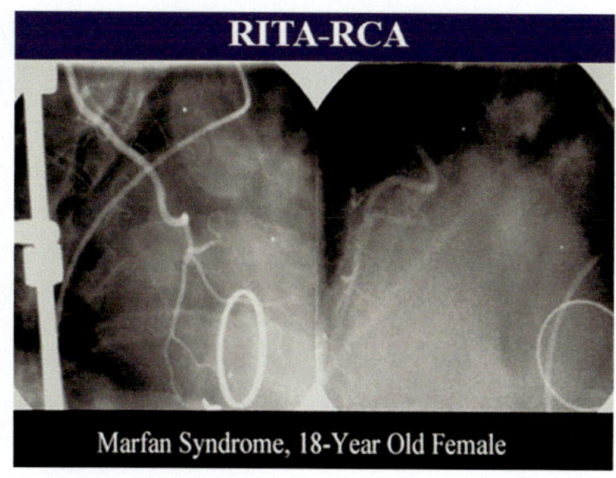

Fig. 99 Shows a postoperative RITA-RCA bypass graft which was required during an operation to replace the mitral valve in an 18-year-old female with Marfan syndrome. During the course of the operation the right coronary artery was disrupted by an unwanted maneuver that resulted in avulsion of the RCA. The situation was immediately recognized which was attended by immediate cross-clamp, retrograde cardioplegia, mitral valve replacement, and RITA-RCA bypass. As noted in the angiogram, the bypass graft is widely patent with excellent flow characteristics. *RCA* right coronary artery, *RITA* right internal thoracic artery

ceed with the necessary procedures to rectify the dilemma which was done in this case. This particular case was not a redo operation. In those patients who are undergoing resternotomy, it is wise to ascertain ITA patency in the event that coronary artery bypass for an injured coronary artery can be performed.

Coronary artery catheterization can result in coronary artery dissection, especially if the coronary artery wall structure is weakened due to antirejection medications as has been inferred by Sbitli and associates who documented spontaneous coronary artery dissection in a transplanted heart (Sbitli et al. 2022). Figure 100 shows a routine postoperative coronary arteriogram in a 7-year-old female 4 years after cardiac transplantation who is undergoing screening for transplant coronary artery disease. During the course of the coronary artery contrast injection into the left main coronary artery a dissection occurred as noted in the figure (upper panel). The patient was hemodynamically stable, but the dissection was deemed to be dangerous especially if it dissected further into the vessel. It was deemed prudent to perform coronary bypass which was accomplished without incident. The postoperative arteriogram is shown in the lower panel of the figure highlighting a widely patent LITA-LAD bypass graft with retrograde flow into the proximal LAD and thence into the left main coronary artery. The dissection appears to have been resolved, likely due to the retrograde flow from the bypass graft thereby establishing favorable union of the dissected layers of the artery. Fortunately, this complication is rare owing to increased awareness and improved techniques as well as new methods of detecting coronary vasculopathy such as intravascular ultrasound and coronary flow reserve (Hussain et al. 2012).

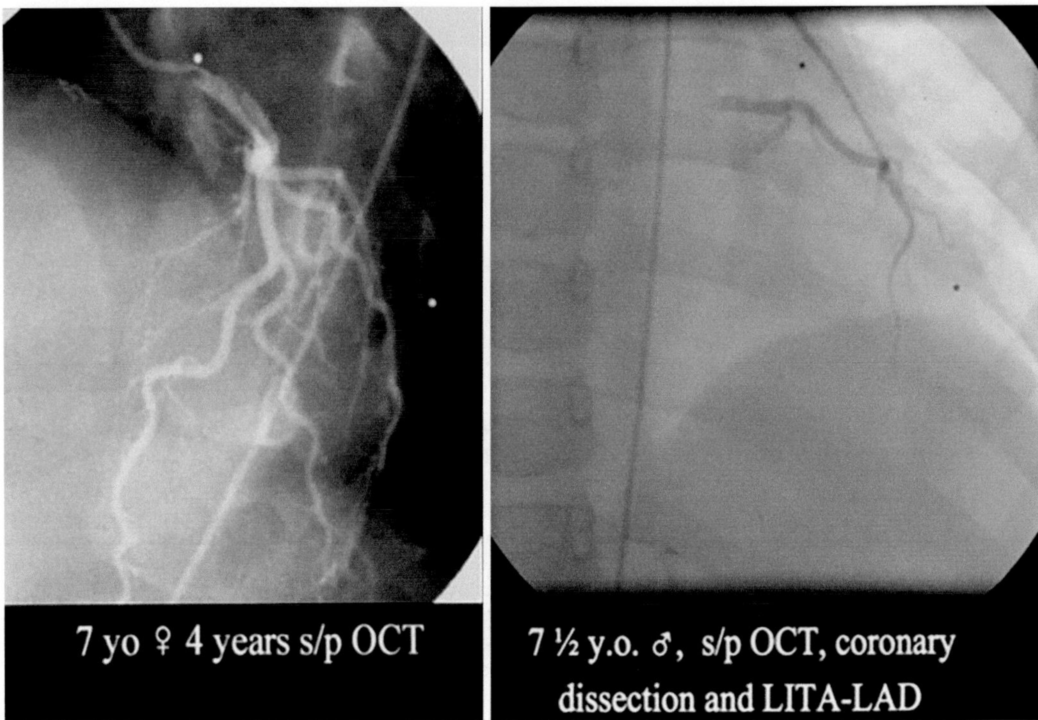

Fig. 100 Unwanted coronary mishaps can also occur in the cath lab. Shown here is a routine follow-up cardiac catheterization to evaluate hemodynamics and coronary artery anatomy that was performed in a 7-year-old female 4 years S/P cardiac transplant. The left panel shows a long segment left main coronary artery dissection to the bifurcation. While the patient was hemodynamically stable, a LITA-LAD coronary bypass was performed (right panel). *LAD* left anterior descending, *LITA* left internal thoracic artery

References

Agrawal H, Sexson-Tejtel SK, Qureshi AM, et al. Aborted sudden cardiac death after unroofing of anomalous left coronary artery. Ann Thorac Surg. 2017;104(3):e265–7.

Agrawal V, Vaidhya N, Patel M, Mishra A, Patel D. Intramural aortic course should always be considered for anomalous origin of the left coronary artery from the right pulmonary artery. World J Pediatr Congenit Heart Surg. 2019;10(4):508–12.

Aintablian A, Hamby RI, Hoffman I, Kramer RJ. Coronary ectasia: incidence and results of coronary bypass surgery. Am Heart J. 1978;96:309–15.

Akagi T, Rose V, Benson LN, Newman A, Freedom RM. Outcome of coronary artery aneurysms after Kawasaki disease. J Pediatr. 1992;121(5 Pt 1):689–94.

Akcay A, Tuncer C, Batyraliev T, et al. Isolated single coronary artery: a series of 10 cases. Circ J. 2008;72:1254–8.

Albuquerque F, de Araújo Gonçalves P, Marques H, et al. (2021) Anomalous origin of the right coronary artery with interarterial course: a mid-term follow-up of 28 cases. Sci Rep. 2021;11:18666. https://doi.org/10.1038/s41598-021-97917-w.

Aldana-Sepulveda N, Restrepo CS, Kimura-Hayama E. Single coronary artery: spectrum of imaging findings with multidetector CT. J Cardiovasc Comput Tomogr. 2013;7:391–9.

Alexi-Meskhishvili V, Berger F, Weng Y, Lange PE, Hetzer R. Anomalous origin of the left coronary artery from the pulmonary artery in adults. J Card Surg. 1995;10(4 Pt 1):309–15.

Alkhulaifi AM, Horner SM, Pugsley WB, Swanton RH. Coronary artery fistulas presenting with bacterial endocarditis. Ann Thorac Surg. 1995;60:202–4.

Anabtawi IN, de Leon JA. Arteriosclerotic aneurysms of the coronary arteries. J Thorac Cardiovasc Surg. 1974;68:226–8.

Anagnostopoulos PV, Pigula FA, Myers JL, Beerman LB, Siewers RD, Gandhi SK. Autologous patch angioplasty of the left main coronary artery in a pediatric patient: 7-year follow-up. Ann Thorac Surg. 2004;77(4):1457–9.

Angelini P, Flamm SD. Newer concepts for imaging anomalous aortic origin of the coronary arteries in adults. Catheter Cardiovasc Interv. 2007;69:942–54.

Angelini P, Trivellato M, Donis J, Leachman RD. Myocardial bridges: a review. Prog Cardiovasc Dis. 1983;26:75–88.

Angelini P, Cheong BY, Lenge De Rosen VV, et al. Magnetic resonance imaging–based screening study in a general population of adolescents. J Am Coll Cardiol. 2018;71(5):579–80.

Arciniegas E, Farooki ZQ, Hakimi M, Green EW. Management of anomalous left coronary artery from the pulmonary artery. Circulation. 1980;62(2 Pt 2):I180–9.

Ayusawa M, Sato Y, Kanamaru H, et al. Multidetector–row computed tomographic depiction of congenital coronary artery aneurysms and ectasia. Int J Cardiol. 2008;127(3):e172–4.

Backer CL, Stout MJ, Zales VR, et al. Anomalous origin of the left coronary artery. A twenty-year review of surgical management. J Thorac Cardiovasc Surg. 1992;103:1049–58.

Backer CL, Hillman N, Dodge-Khatami A, Mavroudis C. Anomalous origin of the left coronary artery from the pulmonary artery: successful surgical strategy without assist devices. Semin Thorac Cardiovasc Surg Pediatr Card Surg Annu. 2000;3:165–72.

Barth CW 3rd, Roberts WC. Left main coronary artery originating from the right sinus of Valsalva and coursing between the aorta and pulmonary trunk. J Am Coll Cardiol. 1986;7:366–73.

Bauer HH, Allmendinger PD, Flaherty J, et al. Congenital coronary arteriovenous fistula: spontaneous rupture and cardiac tamponade. Ann Thorac Surg. 1996;62:1521–3.

Befeler B, Aranda MJ, Embi A, et al. Coronary artery aneurysms: study of the etiology, clinical course and effect on left ventricular function and prognosis. Am J Med. 1977;62:597–607.

Beiser AS, Takahashi M, Baker AL, Sundel RP, Newburger JW. A predictive instrument for coronary artery aneurysms in Kawasaki disease. US Multicenter Kawasaki Disease Study Group. Am J Cardiol. 1998;81:1116–20.

Ben Ali W, Metton O, Roubertie F, et al. Anomalous origin of the left coronary artery from the pulmonary artery: late results with special attention to the mitral valve. Eur J Cardiothorac Surg. 2009;36:244–9.

Benge W, Martins JB, Funk DC. Morbidity associated with anomalous origin of the right coronary artery from the left sinus of Valsalva. Am Heart J. 1980;99:96–100.

Betriu A, Tubau J, Sanz G, Magriña J, Navarro-Lopez F. Relief of angina by periarterial muscle resection of myocardial bridges. Am Heart J. 1980;100:223–6.

Bett JH, O'Brien MF, Murray PJ. Surgery for anomalous origin of the right coronary artery. Br Heart J. 1985;53:459–61.

Binet JP, Planche C, Leriche H, et al. Myocardial bridge compressing the anterior inter-ventricular artery. Apropos of a successfully operated case. Arch Mal Coeur Vaiss. 1975;68:85–90.

Biörck G, Crafoord C. Arteriovenous aneurysm on the pulmonary artery simulating patent ductus arteriosus Botalli. Thorax. 1947;2:65–74.

Bland EF, White PD, Garland J. Congenital anomalies of the coronary arteries: report of an unusual case associated with cardiac hypertrophy. Am Heart J. 1933;8:787–801.

Bloomfield P, Erhlich C, Folland ED, et al. Anomalous right coronary artery: a surgically correctable cause of angina pectoris. Am J Cardiol. 1983;51:1235–7.

Bogers AJ, Quaegebeur JM, Huysmans HA. Early and late results of surgical treatment of congenital coronary artery fistula. Thorax. 1987;42:369–73.

Bonilla-Ramirez C, Molossi S, Sachdeva S, et al. Outcomes in anomalous aortic origin of a coronary artery after surgical reimplantation. J Thorac Cardiovasc Surg. 2021;162(4):1191–9.

Bourassa MG, Butnaru A, Lesperance J, Tardif JC. Symptomatic myocardial bridges: overview of ischemic mechanisms and current diagnostic and treatment strategies. J Am Coll Cardiol. 2003;41:351–9.

Boyer N, Gupta R, Schevchuck A, et al. Coronary artery aneurysms in acute coronary syndrome: case series, review and proposed management strategy. J Invasive Cardiol. 2014;26:283–90.

Bravo-Valenzuela NJ, Silva GR. Aneurysm of the left coronary artery in postoperative Bland–White–Garland syndrome. Case Rep Cardiol. 2015;2015:568014. https://doi.org/10.1155/2015/568014.

Brolin EB, Brismar TB, Collste O, et al. Prevalence of myocardial bridging in patients with myocardial infarction and nonobstructed coronary arteries. Am J Cardiol. 2015;116:1833–9.

Brooks HS. Two cases of an abnormal coronary artery of the heart arising from the pulmonary artery: with some remarks upon the effect of this anomaly in producing cirsoid dilatation of the vessels. J Anat Physiol. 1885;20(Pt 1):26–9.

Brothers JA, McBride MG, Seliem MA, et al. Evaluation of myocardial ischemia after surgical repair of anomalous aortic origin of a coronary artery in a series of pediatric patients. J Am Coll Cardiol. 2007;50:2078–82.

Brothers J, Gaynor JW, Paridon S, Lorber R, Jacobs M. Anomalous aortic origin of a coronary artery with an interarterial course: understanding current management strategies in children and young adults. Pediatr Cardiol. 2009;30:911–21.

Brothers JA, Gaynor JW, Jacobs JP, et al. Anomalous Coronary Artery Working Group. The Registry of Anomalous Aortic Origin of the Coronary Artery of the Congenital Heart Surgeons' Society. Cardiol Young. 2010;20(suppl 3):50–8.

Brothers JA, Gaynor JW, Jacobs JP, Poynter JA, Jacobs ML. The Congenital Heart Surgeons' Society Registry of Anomalous Aortic Origin of a Coronary Artery: an update. Cardiol Young. 2015;25:1567–71.

Brothers JA, Frommelt MA, Jaquiss RDB, et al. Expert consensus guidelines: anomalous aortic origin of a coronary artery. J Thorac Cardiovasc Surg. 2017;153:1440–57.

Bunton R, Jonas RA, Lang P, Rein AJ, Castaneda AR. Anomalous origin of left coronary artery from pulmonary artery. Ligation versus establishment of a two coronary artery system. J Thorac Cardiovasc Surg. 1987;93:103–8.

Burns JC, Shike H, Gordon JB, et al. Sequelae of Kawasaki disease in adolescents and young adults. J Am Coll Cardiol. 1996;28:253–7.

Byrum CJ, Blackman MS, Schneider B, Sondheimer HM, Kavey RE. Congenital atresia of the left coronary ostium and hypoplasia of the left main coronary artery. Am Heart J. 1980;99:354–8.

Carvalho JS, Redington AN, Oldershaw PJ, et al. Analysis of left ventricular wall movement before and after reimplantation of anomalous left coronary artery in infancy. Br Heart J. 1991;65:218–22.

Checchia PA, Pahl E, Shaddy RE, Shulman ST. Cardiac transplantation for Kawasaki disease. Pediatrics. 1997;100:695–9.

Chernogrivov AE, Gornostaev AA, Chernogrivov IE, et al. Anomalous origin of the right coronary artery from the pulmonary artery: surgical re-implantation into the aorta. Multimed Man Cardiothorac Surg. 2015;2015:mmv024. https://doi.org/10.1093/mmcts/mmv024. PMID: 26358324.

Cochrane AD, Coleman DM, Davis AM, et al. Excellent long-term functional outcome after an operation for anomalous left coronary artery from the pulmonary artery. J Thorac Cardiovasc Surg. 1999;117:332–42.

Cohen P, O'Gara PT. Coronary artery aneurysms: a review of the natural history, pathophysiology, and management. Cardiol Rev. 2008;16:301–4.

Cohen AJ, Grishkin BA, Helsel RA, Head HD. Surgical therapy in the management of coronary anomalies: emphasis on utility of internal mammary artery grafts. Ann Thorac Surg. 1989;47:630–7.

Cooley DA, Ellis PR Jr. Surgical considerations of coronary arterial fistula. Am J Cardiol. 1962;10:467–74.

Cooley DA, Hallman GL, Bloodwell RD. Definitive surgical treatment of anomalous origin of left coronary artery from pulmonary artery: indications and results. J Thorac Cardiovasc Surg. 1966;52:798–808.

Corbett M, Powers J, King S, Quinn M, Harris D. Images in cardiology. Single coronary artery. J Am Coll Cardiol. 2009;53:455.

Crainicianu A. Antomische Studien über die Coronararterien und experimentelle Untersuchungen über ihre Durchgangigkeit. Virchows Arch Path Anat. 1922;238:1–75.

Dajani AS, Taubert KA, Gerber MA, et al. Diagnosis and therapy of Kawasaki disease in children. Circulation. 1993;87:1776–80.

Dajani AS, Taubert KA, Takahashi M, et al. Guidelines for long-term management of patients with Kawasaki disease. Report from the Committee on Rheumatic Fever, Endocarditis, and Kawasaki Disease, Council on Cardiovascular Disease in the Young, American Heart Association. Circulation. 1994;89:916–22.

Davis JA, Cecchin F, Jones TK, Portman MA. Major coronary artery anomalies in a pediatric population: incidence and clinical importance. J Am Coll Cardiol. 2001;37:593–7.

del Nido PJ, Duncan BW, Mayer JE Jr, et al. Left ventricular assist device improves survival in children with left ventricular dysfunction after repair of anomalous origin of the left coronary artery from the pulmonary artery. Ann Thorac Surg. 1999;67:169–72.

den Dulk K, Brugada P, Braat S, Heddle B, Wellens HJ. Myocardial bridging as a cause of paroxysmal atrioventricular block. J Am Coll Cardiol. 1983;1:965–9.

Desmet W, Vanhaecke J, Vrolix M, et al. Isolated single coronary artery: a review of 50,000 consecutive coronary angiographies. Eur Heart J. 1992;13:1637–40.

Doan TT, Molossi S, Qureshi AM, McKenzie ED. Intraseptal anomalous coronary artery with myocardial infarction: novel surgical approach. Ann Thorac Surg. 2020;110(4):e271–4.

Dodd JD, Ferencik M, Liberthson RR, et al. Evaluation of efficacy of 64-slice multidetector computed tomography in patients with congenital coronary fistulas. J Comput Assist Tomogr. 2008;32:265–70.

Dodge-Khatami A, Mavroudis C, Backer CL. Congenital Heart Surgery Nomenclature and Database Project: anomalies of the coronary arteries. Ann Thorac Surg. 2000;69(4 suppl):S270–97.

Dodge-Khatami A, Mavroudis C, Backer CL. Anomalous origin of the left coronary artery from the pulmonary artery: collective review of surgical therapy. Ann Thorac Surg. 2002;74:946–55.

D'Souza TF, Samuel BP, Vettukattil JJ, Haw MP. Surgical treatment of neonate with congenital left main coronary artery atresia. Ann Thorac Surg. 2016;101:352–5.

Dymond D, Camm J, Stone D, et al. Dual isotope stress testing in congenital atresia of left coronary ostium. Applications before and after surgical treatment. Br Heart J. 1980;43:270–5.

Eckart RE, Scoville SL, Campbell CL, et al. Sudden death in young adults: a 25-year review of autopsies in military recruits. Ann Intern Med. 2004;141:829–34.

Edwards JE. The direction of blood flow in coronary arteries arising from the pulmonary trunk. Circulation. 1964;29:163–6.

Elias MD, Meza J, McCrindle BW, et al. Effects of exercise restriction on patients with anomalous aortic origin of a coronary artery. World J Pediatr Congenit Heart Surg. 2017;8:18–24.

Erez E, Tam VK, Doublin NA, Stakes J. Anomalous coronary artery with aortic origin and course between the great arteries: improved diagnosis, anatomic findings, and surgical treatment. Ann Thorac Surg. 2006;82:973–7.

Falsetti HL, Carrol RJ. Coronary artery aneurysm. A review of the literature with a report of 11 new cases. Chest. 1976;69:630–6.

Fedoruk LM, Kern JA, Peeler BB, Kron IL. Anomalous origin of the right coronary artery: right internal thoracic artery to right coronary artery bypass is not the answer. J Thorac Cardiovasc Surg. 2007;133:456–60.

Feld H, Guadanino V, Hollander G, et al. Exercise-induced ventricular tachycardia in association with a myocardial bridge. Chest. 1991;99:1295–6.

Fernandes ED, Kadivar H, Hallman GL, et al. Congenital malformations of the coronary arteries: the Texas Heart Institute experience. Ann Thorac Surg. 1992;54:732–40.

Ferreira AG Jr, Trotter SE, König B Jr, et al. Myocardial bridges: morphological and functional aspects. Br Heart J. 1991;66:364–7.

Fetter JE, Backer CL, Muster AJ, Weigel TJ, Mavroudis C. Successful repair of congenital left ventricle-to-coronary sinus fistulas. Ann Thorac Surg. 1994;57:757–8.

Fortune RL, Baron PJ, Fitzgerald JW. Atresia of the left main coronary artery: repair with left internal mammary artery bypass. J Thorac Cardiovasc Surg. 1987;94:150–1.

Friedman AH, Fogel MA, Stephens P Jr, et al. Identification, imaging, functional assessment and management of congenital coronary arterial abnormalities in children. Cardiol Young. 2007;17(suppl 2):56–67.

Fudulu DP, Tulloh RM, Wolf AR, Parry AJ, Stoica SC. Anomalous left coronary from the pulmonary artery presenting as ventricular fibrillation after persistent ductus arteriosus ligation. Ann Thorac Surg. 2015;100(1):e9–e10. https://doi.org/10.1016/j.athoracsur.2015.04.015. PMID: 26140805.

Gay F, Vouhé P, Lecompte Y, et al. Atresia of the left coronary ostium. Repair in a 2-month-old infant. Arch Mal Coeur Vaiss. 1989;82:807–10.

Geiringer E. The mural coronary. Am Heart J. 1951;41:359–68.

Gersony WM. Predicting coronary aneurysms in Kawasaki disease. Am J Cardiol. 1998;81:1162–4.

Gharibeh L, Rahmouni K, Hong SJ, Crean AM, Grau JB. Surgical techniques for the treatment of anomalous origin of right coronary artery from the left sinus: a comparative review. J Am Heart Assoc. 2021;10(22):e022377. https://doi.org/10.1161/JAHA.121.022377. Epub 2021 Nov 2. PMID: 34726074; PMCID: PMC8751967.

Ghosh PK, Friedman M, Vidne BA. Isolated congenital atresia of the left main coronary artery and atherosclerosis. Ann Thorac Surg. 1993;55:1564–5.

Haager PK, Schwarz ER, vom Dahl J, et al. Long term angiographic and clinical follow up in patients with stent implantation for symptomatic myocardial bridging. Heart. 2000;84:403–8.

Hakeem A, Cilingiroglu M, Leesar MA. Hemodynamic and intravascular ultrasound assessment of myocardial bridging: fractional flow reserve paradox with dobutamine versus adenosine. Catheter Cardiovasc Interv. 2010;75:229–36.

Harada K, Yamaguchi H, Kato H. Indication for intravenous gamma globulin treatment for Kawasaki disease. In: Takahashi M, Taubert K, editors. Proceedings of the fourth international symposium on Kawasaki disease. Dallas: American Heart Association; 1993. p. 459–62.

Harris WO, Andrews JC, Nichols DA, Holmes DR Jr. Percutaneous transcatheter embolization of coronary arteriovenous fistulas. Mayo Clin Proc. 1996;71:37–42.

Hartnell GG, Parnell BM, Pridie RB. Coronary artery ectasia. Its prevalence and clinical significance in 4993 patients. Br Heart J. 1985;54:392–5.

Hatoum H, Krishnamurthy R, Parthasarathy J, et al. Flow dynamics in anomalous aortic origin of a coronary artery in children: importance of the intramural segment. Semin Thorac Cardiovasc Surg. 2022;34(1):226–35.

Heuser RR. Treatment for coronary aneurysms: twenty years of experience with covered stents. J Invasive Cardiol. 2015;27(2):E36.

Hill RC, Chitwood WR Jr, Bashore TM, et al. Coronary flow and regional function before and after supraarterial myotomy for myocardial bridging. Ann Thorac Surg. 1981;31:176–81.

Hillman ND, Mavroudis C, Backer CL, Duffy CE. Supraarterial decompression myotomy for myocardial bridging in a child. Ann Thorac Surg. 1999;68:244–6.

Huang XH, Wang SY, Xu JP, et al. Surgical outcome and clinical follow-up in patients with symptomatic myocardial bridging. Chin Med J. 2007;120:1563–6.

Huddleston CB, Balzer DT, Mendeloff EN. Repair of anomalous left main coronary artery arising from the pulmonary artery in infants: long-term impact on the mitral valve. Ann Thorac Surg. 2001;71:1985–9.

Hussain T, Fenton M, Peel SA, Wiethoff A, Botnar RM, Burch M, Greil GF. Diagnosis of post-transplant coronary artery disease using contrast-enhanced coronary vessel wall imaging at 3.0 Tesla. J Cardiovasc Magn Reson. 2012;14(Suppl 1):P138.

Ino T, Akimoto K, Ohkubo M, et al. Application of percutaneous transluminal coronary angioplasty to coronary arterial stenosis in Kawasaki disease. Circulation. 1996;93:1709–15.

Isomatsu Y, Imai Y, Shin'oka T, Aoki M, Iwata Y. Surgical intervention for anomalous origin of the left coronary artery from the pulmonary artery: the Tokyo experience. J Thorac Cardiovasc Surg. 2001;121:792–7.

Iwata Y, Takeuchi T, Konuma T, Obase K, Eishi K. Infant coronary artery bypass grafting completely under surgical microscope. JTCVS Tech. 2021;10:441–3.

Jacobs ML. Anomalous aortic origin of a coronary artery: the gaps and the guidelines. J Thorac Cardiovasc Surg. 2017;153:1462–5.

Jaggers J, Lodge AJ. Surgical therapy for anomalous aortic origin of the coronary arteries. Semin Thorac Cardiovasc Surg Pediatr Card Surg Annu. 2005;8:122–7.

Jegatheeswaran A, Devlin PJ, McCrindle BW, et al. Features associated with myocardial ischemia in anomalous aortic origin of a coronary artery: a

Congenital Heart Surgeons' Society study. J Thorac Cardiovasc Surg. 2019;158:822–34.

Jegatheeswaran A, Devlin PJ, Williams WG, et al. Outcomes after anomalous aortic origin of a coronary artery repair: a Congenital Heart Surgeons' Society Study. J Thorac Cardiovasc Surg. 2020;160:757–71.

Jokl E, McClellan CJ, Ross GD. Congenital anomaly of left coronary artery in young athlete. JAMA. 1962;182:572–3.

Kaczorowski DJ, Sathanandam S, Ravishankar C, et al. Coronary ostioplasty for congenital atresia of the left main coronary artery ostium. Ann Thorac Surg. 2012;94:1307–10.

Kamiya H, Yasuda T, Nagamine H, et al. Surgical treatment of congenital coronary artery fistulas: 27 years' experience and a review of the literature. J Card Surg. 2002;17:173–7.

Kardasz I, De Caterina R. Myocardial infarction with normal coronary arteries: a conundrum with multiple aetiologies and variable prognosis: an update. J Intern Med. 2007;261:330–48.

Karl TR, Sano S, Horton S, Mee RB. Centrifugal pump left heart assist in pediatric cardiac operations. Indication, technique, and results. J Thorac Cardiovasc Surg. 1991;102:624–30.

Kato H, Koike S, Yamamoto M, Ito Y, Yano E. Coronary aneurysms in infants and young children with acute febrile mucocutaneous lymph node syndrome. J Pediatr. 1975;86:892–8.

Kato H, Ichinose E, Yoshioka F, et al. Fate of coronary aneurysms in Kawasaki disease: serial coronary angiography and long-term follow-up study. Am J Cardiol. 1982;49:1758–66.

Khan MS, Idris O, Shah J, Sharma R, Singh H. Anomalous origin of left main coronary artery from the right sinus of valsalva: a case series-based review. Cureus. 2020;12(4):e7777.

Kimbiris D. Anomalous origin of the left main coronary artery from the right sinus of Valsalva. Am J Cardiol. 1985;55:765–9.

Kitamura S, Kawachi K, Seki T, et al. Bilateral internal mammary artery grafts for coronary artery bypass operations in children. J Thorac Cardiovasc Surg. 1990;99:708–15.

Kitamura S, Kawachi K, Nishii T, et al. Internal thoracic artery grafting for congenital coronary malformations. Ann Thorac Surg. 1992;53:513–6.

Koh E, Nakagawa M, Hamaoka K, Sawada T, Oga K. Congenital atresia of the left coronary ostium: diagnosis and surgical treatment. Pediatr Cardiol. 1989;10:159–62.

Kosar E, Chandraratna PA. Assessment of coronary artery aneurysms with multiplane transesophageal echocardiography. Am Heart J. 1997;133:526–33.

Kramer JR, Kitazume H, Proudfit WL, Sones FM Jr. Clinical significance of isolated coronary bridges: benign and frequent condition involving the left anterior descending artery. Am Heart J. 1982;103:283–8.

Krause W. Ueber den Ursprung einer accessorischen A. coronaria cordis aus der A. pulmonalis. Z Rat Med. 1865;24:225.

Laks H, Ardehali A, Grant PW, Allada V. Aortic implantation of anomalous left coronary artery. An improved surgical approach. J Thorac Cardiovasc Surg. 1995;109:519–23.

Lambert V, Touchot A, Losay J, et al. Midterm results after surgical repair of the anomalous origin of the coronary artery. Circulation. 1996;94(9 suppl):II38–43.

Le Roy J, Vernhet Kovacsik H, Zarqane H, et al. Submillisievert multiphasic coronary computed tomography angiography for pediatric patients with congenital heart diseases. Circ Cardiovasc Imaging. 2019;12(2):e008348. https://doi.org/10.1161/CIRCIMAGING.118.008348.

Lee MS, Chen CH. Myocardial bridging: an up-to-date review. J Invasive Cardiol. 2015;27:521–8.

Levitas A, Krymko H, Ioffe V, Zalzstein E, Broides A. Anomalous left coronary artery from the pulmonary artery in infants and toddlers misdiagnosed as myocarditis. Pediatr Emerg Care. 2016;32:232–4.

Liberthson RR, Dinsmore RE, Fallon JT. Aberrant coronary artery origin from the aorta. Report of 18 patients, review of literature and delineation of natural history and management. Circulation. 1979a;59:748–54.

Liberthson RR, Sagar K, Berkoben JP, Weintraub RM, Levine FH. Congenital coronary arteriovenous fistula. Report of 13 patients, review of the literature and delineation of management. Circulation. 1979b;59:849–54.

Lipton MJ, Barry WH, Obrez I, Silverman JF, Wexler L. Isolated single coronary artery: diagnosis, angiographic classification, and clinical significance. Radiology. 1979;130:39–47.

Lorber R, Srivastava S, Wilder TJ, et al. AAOCA Working Group of the Congenital Heart Surgeons' Society. Anomalous aortic origin of coronary arteries in the young: echocardiographic evaluation with surgical correlation. JACC Cardiovasc Imaging. 2015;8:1239–49.

Lowe JE, Oldham HN Jr, Sabiston DC Jr. Surgical management of congenital coronary artery fistulas. Ann Surg. 1981;194:373–80.

Lurie PR. Abnormalities and diseases of the coronary vessels. In: Moss AJ, Adams FH, Emmanouilides GC, editors. Heart disease in infants, children, and adolescents. 2nd ed. Baltimore: Williams & Wilkins; 1977. p. 482–96.

Mainwaring RD, Hanley FL. Surgical treatment of anomalous left main coronary artery with an intraconal course. Congenit Heart Dis. 2019;14(4):504–10.

Marey G, Said SM. Unroofing of left main coronary artery with trans-septal course. CTSNet, Inc. Media; 2021. https://doi.org/10.25373/ctsnet.14988588.

Markis JE, Joffe CD, Cohn PF, et al. Clinical significance of coronary arterial ectasia. Am J Cardiol. 1976;37:217–22.

Mavroudis C. Coronary artery anomalies. In: Mavroudis C, Backer CL, editors. Atlas of pediatric cardiac surgery. London: Springer; 2015.

Mavroudis C, Backer CL. Technical tips for three congenital heart operations: modified Ross–Konno procedure, optimal ventricular septal defect exposure by tricuspid valve incision, coronary unroofing and endarterectomy for anomalous aortic origin of the coronary artery. Oper Tech Thorac Cardiovasc Surg. 2010;15:18–40.

Mavroudis C, Dearani JA. Congenital coronary artery anomalies in the adult. In: Mavroudis C, Dearani JA, editors. Atlas of adult congenital heart surgery. Cham: Springer; 2020. p. 383–411.

Mavroudis C, Harrison H, Klein JB, et al. Infant orthotopic cardiac transplantation. J Thorac Cardiovasc Surg. 1988;96:912–24.

Mavroudis C, Backer CL, Muster AJ, et al. Expanding indications for pediatric coronary artery bypass. J Thorac Cardiovasc Surg. 1996;111:181–9.

Mavroudis C, Backer CL, Rocchini AP, Muster AJ, Gevitz M. Coronary artery fistulas in infants and children: a surgical review and discussion of coil embolization. Ann Thorac Surg. 1997;63:1235–42.

Mavroudis C, Dodge-Khatami A, Backer CL. Coronary artery anomalies. In: Mavroudis C, Backer CL, editors. Pediatric cardiac surgery. 3rd ed. Philadelphia: Mosby; 2003. p. 660–88.

Mavroudis C, Mavroudis CD, Jacobs JP. Repair techniques for anomalous aortic origins of the coronary arteries. Cardiol Young. 2015;25:1546–60.

Mavroudis C, Dodge-Khatami A, Backer CL. Coronary artery anomalies. In: Mavroudis C, Backer CL, editors. Pediatric cardiac surgery. 5th ed. West Sussex: Wiley-Blackwell; 2023. p. 835–66.

Mery CM, De León LE, Molossi S, et al. Outcomes of surgical intervention for anomalous aortic origin of a coronary artery: a large contemporary prospective cohort study. J Thorac Cardiovasc Surg. 2018;155(1):305–19.

Meyer BW, Stefanik G, Stiles QR, Lindesmith GG, Jones JC. A method of definitive surgical treatment of anomalous origin of left coronary artery. A case report. J Thorac Cardiovasc Surg. 1968;56:104–7.

Meza JM, Elias MD, Wilder TJ, et al. Congenital Heart Surgeons' Society. Exercise restriction is not associated with increasing body mass index over time in patients with anomalous aortic origin of the coronary arteries. Cardiol Young. 2017;27:1538–44.

Mongé MC, Eltayeb O, Costello JM, et al. Aortic implantation of anomalous origin of the left coronary artery from the pulmonary artery: long-term outcomes. Ann Thorac Surg. 2015;100:154–61.

Moodie DS, Gill C, Loop FD, Sheldon WC. Anomalous left main coronary artery originating from the right sinus of Valsalva: pathophysiology, angiographic definition, and surgical approaches. J Thorac Cardiovasc Surg. 1980;80:198–205.

Moodie DS, Fyfe D, Gill CC, et al. Anomalous origin of the left coronary artery from the pulmonary artery (Bland–White–Garland syndrome) in adult patients: long-term follow-up after surgery. Am Heart J. 1983;106:381–8.

Mookadam F, Green J, Holmes D, Moustafa SE, Rihal C. Clinical relevance of myocardial bridging severity: single center experience. Eur J Clin Investig. 2009;39:110–5.

Mumtaz MA, Lorber RE, Arruda J, Pettersson GB, Mavroudis C. Surgery for anomalous aortic origin of the coronary artery. Ann Thorac Surg. 2011;91:811–5.

Munkner T, Petersen O, Vesterdal J. Congenital aneurysm of the coronary artery with an arteriovenous fistula. Acta Radiol. 1958;50:333–40.

Muriago M, Sheppard MN, Ho SY, Anderson RH. Location of the coronary arterial orifices in the normal heart. Clin Anat. 1997;10(5):297–302.

Musiani A, Cernigliaro C, Sansa M, Maselli D, De Gasperis C. Left main coronary artery atresia: literature review and therapeutical considerations. Eur J Cardiothorac Surg. 1997;11:505–14.

Mustafa I, Gula G, Radley-Smith R, Durrer S, Yacoub M. Anomalous origin of the left coronary artery from the anterior aortic sinus: a potential cause of sudden death. Anatomic characterization and surgical treatment. J Thorac Cardiovasc Surg. 1981;82:297–300.

Mustard WT. Anomalies of the coronary artery. In: Welch KJ, editor. Pediatric surgery. Chicago: Year-Book Medical; 1962. p. 433.

Naimo PS, Fricke TA, d'Udekem Y, et al. Surgical intervention for anomalous origin of left coronary artery from the pulmonary artery in children: a long-term follow-up. Ann Thorac Surg. 2016;101:1842–8.

Najm HK, Ahmad M. Transconal unroofing of anomalous left main coronary artery from the right sinus with trans-septal course. Ann Thorac Surg. 2019;108:e383–6.

Najm HK, Karamlou T, Ahmad M, et al. Early outcomes of transconal repair of transseptal anomalous left coronary artery from right sinus. Ann Thorac Surg. 2021;112:595–602.

Najm HK, Ahmad M, Hammoud MS, Costello JP, Karamlou T. Surgical pearls of the transconal unroofing procedure-modifications and midterm outcomes. Ann Thorac Surg. 2023;115:e29–31.

Nakamura Y, Yanagawa H, Ojima T, Kawasaki T, Kato H. Cardiac sequelae of Kawasaki disease among recurrent cases. Arch Dis Child. 1998;78:163–5.

Neches WH, Mathews RA, Park SC, et al. Anomalous origin of the left coronary artery from the pulmonary artery. A new method of surgical repair. Circulation. 1974;50:582–7.

Newburger JW, Takahashi M, Gerber MA, et al. Committee on Rheumatic Fever, Endocarditis and Kawasaki Disease, Council on Cardiovascular Disease in the Young, American Heart Association, American Academy of Pediatrics. Diagnosis, treatment, and long-term management of Kawasaki disease: a statement for health professionals from the Committee on Rheumatic Fever, Endocarditis and Kawasaki Disease, Council on Cardiovascular Disease in the Young, American Heart Association. Circulation. 2004;110:2747–71.

Newburger JW, Takahashi M, Burns JC. Kawasaki disease. J Am Coll Cardiol. 2016;67:1738–49.

Ogden JA. Congenital anomalies of the coronary arteries. Am J Cardiol. 1970;25:474–9.

Olearchyk AS, Runk DM, Alavi M, Grosso MA. Congenital bilateral coronary-to-pulmonary artery fistulas. Ann Thorac Surg. 1997;64:233–5.

Padalino MA, Franchetti N, Sarris GE, et al. Anomalous aortic origin of coronary arteries: early results on clinical management from an international multicenter study. Int J Cardiol. 2019;291:189–93.

Pahl E. Kawasaki disease: cardiac sequelae and management. Pediatr Ann. 1997;26:112–5.

Paridon SM, Farooki ZQ, Kuhns LR, Arciniegas E, Pinsky WW. Exercise performance after repair of anomalous origin of the left coronary artery from the pulmonary artery. Circulation. 1990;81:1287–92.

Pey J, de Dios RM, Epeldegui A. Myocardial bridging and hypertrophic cardiomyopathy: relief of ischemia by surgery. Int J Cardiol. 1985;8:327–30.

Post JC, van Rossum AC, Bronzwaer JG, et al. Magnetic resonance angiography of anomalous coronary arteries. A new gold standard for delineating the proximal course? Circulation. 1995;92:3163–71.

Potts WJ, quoted by Kittle CF, Diehl AM, Heilbrunn A. Anomalous left coronary artery arising from the pulmonary artery; report of a case and surgical consideration. J Pediatr. 1955;47:198–206.

Poynter JA, Bondarenko I, Austin EH, et al. Congenital Heart Surgeons' Society AAOCA Working Group. Repair of anomalous aortic origin of a coronary artery in 113 patients: a Congenital Heart Surgeons' Society report. World J Pediatr Congenit Heart Surg. 2014a;5:507–14.

Poynter JA, Williams WG, McIntyre S, Brothers JA, Jacobs ML. Congenital Heart Surgeons Society AAOCA Working Group. Anomalous aortic origin of a coronary artery: a report from the Congenital Heart Surgeons' Society Registry. World J Pediatr Congenit Heart Surg. 2014b;5:22–30.

Rab ST, King SB 3rd, Roubin GS, et al. Coronary aneurysms after stent placement: a suggestion of altered vessel wall healing in the presence of anti-inflammatory agents. J Am Coll Cardiol. 1991;18:1524–8.

Reidy JF, Sowton E, Ross DN. Transcatheter occlusion of coronary to bronchial anastomosis by detachable balloon combined with coronary angioplasty at same procedure. Br Heart J. 1983;49:284–7.

Rein AJ, Colan SD, Parness IA, Sanders SP. Regional and global left ventricular function in infants with anomalous origin of the left coronary artery from the pulmonary trunk: preoperative and postoperative assessment. Circulation. 1987;75:115–23.

Roberts WC, Siegel RJ, Zipes DP. Origin of the right coronary artery from the left sinus of Valsalva and its functional consequences: analysis of 10 necropsy patients. Am J Cardiol. 1982;49:863–8.

Romp RL, Herlong JR, Landolfo CK, et al. Outcome of unroofing procedure for repair of anomalous aortic origin of left or right coronary artery. Ann Thorac Surg. 2003;76(2):589–96.

Rosenkranz ER, Murphy DJ Jr, Cosgrove DM 3rd. Surgical management of left coronary artery ostial atresia and supravalvar aortic stenosis. Ann Thorac Surg. 1992;54:779–81.

Sabiston DC Jr, Neill CA, Taussig HB. The direction of blood flow in anomalous left coronary artery arising from the pulmonary artery. Circulation. 1960;22:591–7.

Sakakibara S, Yokoyama M, Takao A, Nogi M, Gomi H. Coronary arteriovenous fistula. Nine operated cases. Am Heart J. 1966;72:307–14.

Satou GM, Giamelli J, Gewitz MH. Kawasaki disease: diagnosis, management, and long-term implications. Cardiol Rev. 2007;15:163–9.

Sauer U, Stern H, Meisner H, Bühlmeyer K, Sebening F. Risk factors for perioperative mortality in children with anomalous origin of the left coronary artery from the pulmonary artery. J Thorac Cardiovasc Surg. 1992;104:696–705.

Sbitli T, Bamousa B, Alburaiki J, Alhussein M, Almasood A. Spontaneous coronary artery dissection in a transplanted heart. JACC Case Rep. 2022;4(21):1439–42.

Schumacher G, Roithmaier A, Lorenz HP, et al. Congenital coronary artery fistula in infancy and childhood: diagnostic and therapeutic aspects. Thorac Cardiovasc Surg. 1997;45:287–94.

Schwartz ML, Jonas RA, Colan SD. Anomalous origin of left coronary artery from pulmonary artery: recovery of left ventricular function after dual coronary repair. J Am Coll Cardiol. 1997;30:547–53.

Schwarz ER, Klues HG, vom Dahl J, et al. Functional, angiographic and intracoronary Doppler flow characteristics in symptomatic patients with myocardial bridging: effect of short-term intravenous beta-blocker medication. J Am Coll Cardiol. 1996;27:1637–45.

Secinaro A, Ntsinjana H, Tann O, et al. Cardiovascular magnetic resonance findings in repaired anomalous left coronary artery to pulmonary artery connection (ALCAPA). J Cardiovasc Magn Reson. 2011;13(1):27.

Sharbaugh AH, White RS. Single coronary artery. Analysis of the anatomic variation, clinical importance, and report of five cases. JAMA. 1974;230:243–6.

Sharma V, Burkhart HM, Dearani JA, Suri RM, Daly RC, Park SJ, Horner JM, Phillips SD, Schaff HV. Surgical unroofing of anomalous aortic origin of a coronary artery: a single-center experience. Ann Thorac Surg. 2014;98(3):941–5.

Singh TP, Di Carli MF, Sullivan NM, Leonen MF, Morrow WR. Myocardial flow reserve in long-term survivors of repair of anomalous left coronary artery from pulmonary artery. J Am Coll Cardiol. 1998;31:437–43.

Smith JC. Review of single coronary artery with report of 2 cases. Circulation. 1950;1:1168–75.

Stephens EH, Dearani JA. Anomalous left coronary artery from the pulmonary artery-Time is of the essence [Commentary]. J Thorac Cardiovasc Surg. 2020;159:1953–4.

Stern H, Sauer U, Locher D, et al. Left ventricular function assessed with echocardiography and myocardial perfusion assessed with scintigraphy under dipyridamole stress in pediatric patients after repair for anomalous origin of the left coronary artery from the pulmonary artery. J Thorac Cardiovasc Surg. 1993;106:723–32.

Suzuki A, Kamiya T, Kuwahara N, et al. Coronary arterial lesions of Kawasaki disease: cardiac catheterization findings of 1100 cases. Pediatr Cardiol. 1986;7:3–9.

Suzuki A, Kamiya T, Ono Y, Okuno M, Yagihara T. Aortocoronary bypass surgery for coronary arterial lesions resulting from Kawasaki disease. J Pediatr. 1990;116:567–73.

Swaye PS, Fisher LD, Litwin P, et al. Aneurysmal coronary artery disease. Circulation. 1983;67:134–8.

Takeuchi S, Imamura H, Katsumoto K, et al. New surgical method for repair of anomalous left coronary artery from pulmonary artery. J Thorac Cardiovasc Surg. 1979;78:7–11.

Tanawuttiwat T, O'Neill BP, Schob AH, Alfonso CE. Left main coronary atresia. J Card Surg. 2013;28:37–46.

Taylor AJ, Rogan KM, Virmani R. Sudden cardiac death associated with isolated congenital coronary artery anomalies. J Am Coll Cardiol. 1992;20:640–7.

Tkebuchava T, Von Segesser LK, Vogt PR, et al. Congenital coronary fistulas in children and adults: diagnosis, surgical technique and results. J Cardiovasc Surg. 1996;37:29–34.

Tunick PA, Slater J, Pasternack P, Kronzon I. Coronary artery aneurysms: a transesophageal echocardiographic study. Am Heart J. 1989;118:176–9.

Turley K, Szarnicki RJ, Flachsbart KD, et al. Aortic implantation is possible in all cases of anomalous origin of the left coronary artery from the pulmonary artery. Ann Thorac Surg. 1995;60:84–9.

Turner II, Turek JW, Jaggers J, et al. Anomalous aortic origin of a coronary artery: preoperative diagnosis and surgical planning. World J Pediatr Congenit Heart Surg. 2011;2:340–5.

Ueyama K, Ramchandani M, Beall AC Jr, Jones JW. Diagnosis and operation for anomalous circumflex coronary artery. Ann Thorac Surg. 1997;63:377–81.

Unzué L, García E, Parra FJ, et al. Congenital atresia of the left main coronary artery in an adult: a rare anomaly with an unfavorable prognosis. Review of the literature. Cardiovasc Revasc Med. 2015;16:498–502.

Urrutia-S CO, Falaschi G, Ott DA, Cooley DA. Surgical management of 56 patients with congenital coronary artery fistulas. Ann Thorac Surg. 1983;35:300–7.

Vasan RS, Bahl VK, Rajani M. Myocardial infarction associated with a myocardial bridge. Int J Cardiol. 1989;25:240–1.

Von Poláček P, Zechmeister A. The occurrence and significance of myocardial bridges and loops on coronary arteries. In: Krutna V, editor. Opuscola Cardiologica. Acta Facultatis Medicae Universitatis Brunensis. Brno: University J.E. Purkinje; 1968. p. 1–99.

Vouhé PR, Baillot-Vernant F, Trinquet F, et al. Anomalous left coronary artery from the pulmonary artery in infants. Which operation? When? J Thorac Cardiovasc Surg. 1987;94:192–9.

Vouhé PR, Tamisier D, Sidi D, et al. Anomalous left coronary artery from the pulmonary artery: results of isolated aortic reimplantation. Ann Thorac Surg. 1992;54:621–7.

Walker TC, Renno MS, Parra DA, Guthrie SO. Neonatal ventricular fibrillation and an elusive ALCAPA: things are not always as they seem. BMJ Case Rep. 2016;2016:bcr2015214239. https://doi.org/10.1136/bcr-2015-214239. PMID: 27033289.

Wilder TJ, Williams WG. Tackling a complex problem via a novel approach: decision analysis may improve quality of life for patients with anomalous aortic origin of a coronary artery. J Thorac Cardiovasc Surg. 2016;152:1376–7.

Williams IA, Gersony WM, Hellenbrand WE. Anomalous right coronary artery arising from the pulmonary artery: a report of 7 cases and a review of the literature. Am Heart J. 2006;152:1004.e9–e17.

Yamanaka O, Hobbs RE. Coronary artery anomalies in 126,595 patients undergoing coronary arteriography. Catheter Cardiovasc Diagn. 1990;21:28–40.

Y-Hassan S. Acute cardiac sympathetic disruption in the pathogenesis of the Takotsubo syndrome: a systematic review of the literature to date. Cardiovasc Revasc Med. 2014;15:35–42.

Zhang W, Hu R, Zhu Y, et al. Surgical outcomes for anomalous left coronary artery from the pulmonary artery: influence of late presentation. J Thorac Cardiovasc Surg. 2020;159:1945–52.

Complications Associated with Pediatric Heart Transplantation

Awais Ashfaq and David L. S. Morales

Abstract

In the current era the majority of programs in the United States use a bicaval-left atrial cuff technique for pediatric heart transplantation. This chapter will review the basic steps of donor cardiectomy and discuss complications related to: (1) implantation, (2) left superior vena cava, (3) bilateral bidirectional Glenn shunts, (4) prior transposition of the great arteries, (5) hybrid interventions, and (6) situs inversus.

Keywords

Congenital heart surgery · Cardiac transplantation · Superior vena cava · Pediatric · Donor · Cardiectomy · Bicaval

A. Ashfaq (✉)
Heart Institute, Department of Cardiothoracic Surgery, Cincinnati Children's Hospital Medical Center, University of Cincinnati College of Medicine, Cincinnati, OH, USA
e-mail: awais.ashfaq@cchmc.org

D. L. S. Morales
Cincinnati Children's Hospital Medical Center, University of Cincinnati College of Medicine, Cincinnati, OH, USA

1 Introduction

According to the International Society for Heart and Lung Transplantation (ISHLT), approximately 600 heart transplants are performed annually in children worldwide (Scientific Registry of Transplant Recipients: Pediatric heart transplant centers 2020). Congenital heart disease is the most common indication for heart transplantation in children, accounting for approximately 40%–50% of cases (Rossano et al. 2016). Dilated cardiomyopathy is the second most common indication, accounting for approximately 25%–30% of cases (Rossano et al. 2016). Hypertrophic cardiomyopathy, restrictive cardiomyopathy, and arrhythmias account for the remaining cases. The survival rate for pediatric heart transplant recipients is generally good, with 1-year survival rates of approximately 85%–90% and 5-year survival rates of approximately 75%–80% (Dipchand et al. 2013). However, long-term survival can be impacted by factors such as graft rejection, infection, and other medical complications.

2 Basic Steps

2.1 Donor Cardiectomy (Fig. 1a)

The method for donor cardiectomy is not illustrated but has not undergone any significant change over the past many decades. A full median

C. L. Backer, C. Mavroudis (eds.), *Complications in Pediatric and Congenital Heart Surgery*,
https://doi.org/10.1007/978-3-032-02661-3_28

a

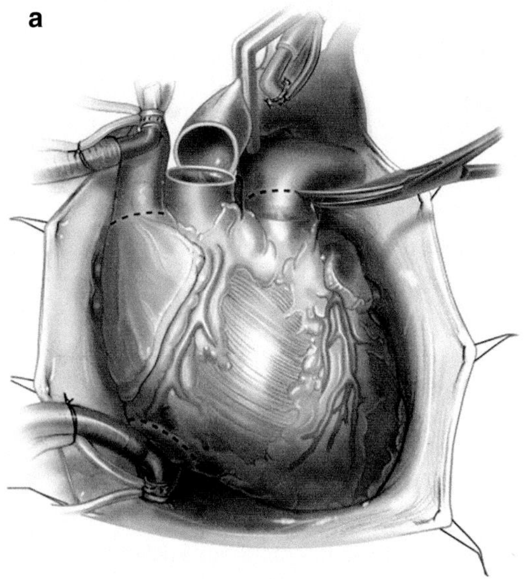

b

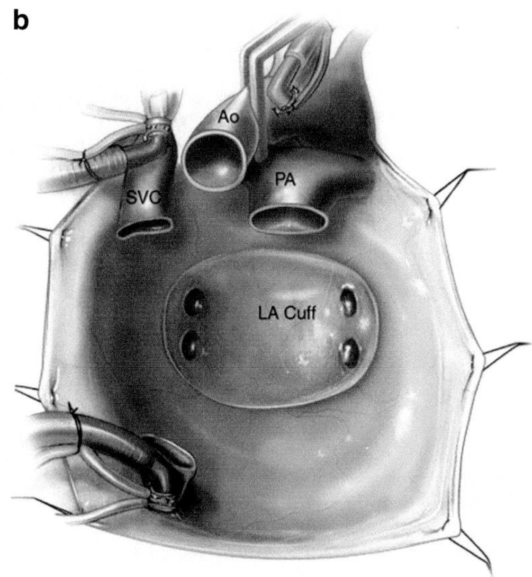

Fig. 1 (**a**) Shows recipient cardiectomy. High cannulation of the aorta and superior vena cava (SVC) is done to ensure there is adequate recipient tissue left. The aorta and the pulmonary artery are separated and the interatrial groove is developed. (**b**) The great vessels are divided just distal to their respective valves. The SVC is transected at the cavo-atrial junction. A large cuff of inferior vena cava (IVC) is prepared by leaving atrial tissue around it. A generous left atrial cuff is left behind around the four pulmonary veins. Hemostasis is achieved by cauterizing the edge of left atrial cuff. *Ao* aorta, *LA* left atrium, *PA* pulmonary artery. (With permission John and Liao 2010)

sternotomy is performed to access the heart and the heart function is evaluated through direct visualization and communicated to the recipient institution. The next step involves creating a space between the ascending aorta and pulmonary artery (PA) to ensure cross-clamp placement. The superior caval vein (SCV) is separated from the pericardial reflections, while the azygos vein is doubly ligated and divided. As much superior caval vein as possible is taken, and in the case of a recipient with a left superior caval vein, the donor innominate vein is also harvested. The pericardial reflection around the inferior caval vein (ICV) is opened to access the vein. Once all teams are ready for cross-clamp, the ascending aorta is cross-clamped, and cold cardioplegia solution is infused. When the cardioplegia is initiated, the right superior pulmonary vein is sharply incised, followed by the inferior caval vein to decompress the heart's right and left sides. Alternatively, the tip of the left atrial appendage is amputated if the lungs are harvested.

The procedure for cardiectomy usually begins by transecting the inferior caval vein while preserving a cava cuff for the liver transplant team. If needed, IVC cuff can be enlarged by cutting into the coronary sinus. Next, the aorta is transected at the site of the aortic cross-clamp, followed by the division of the pulmonary artery just before the branching of the right and left pulmonary arteries. In cases where the lungs are not being harvested, we prefer to transect the pulmonary arteries at the hilum, distal to the branching point of the right and left upper lobe pulmonary branches. This step is particularly crucial for patients who have had previous pulmonary artery repair or a failed Fontan procedure.

We proceed to transect the superior caval vein as close to the innominate vein as possible, sometimes including the innominate vein. Finally, we transect the four pulmonary veins individually before removing the heart from the field after dividing the attachments within the oblique and transverse sinuses (Fig. 1b).

In cases where the lungs are being harvested, we tip the heart anteriorly and select a site on the back of the left atrium, where we perform an encircling left atriotomy, preserving the pulmonary veins with the lungs and using only a small cuff of left atrium for the donor heart. After completing the procedure, the donor heart is placed in a sterile plastic container filled with cold saline, triple bagged, placed it in an ice cooler, and transported to the recipient hospital.

2.2 General Complications Related to Implantation

Although the right atrial technique developed by Lower and Shumway (Shumway et al. 1966) is still used in some medical centers, the majority of programs now employ a bicaval-left atrial cuff technique. This technique was first described by Sievers and his team in 1994 (Sievers et al. 1994).

The bicaval-left atrial cuff technique is performed through a standard median sternotomy with aortic and bicaval cannulation (Fig. 2a, b, c) (John and Liao 2010). High cannulation of the aorta and SVC enables adequate recipient cuffs. Dissecting the diaphragmatic reflection off the IVC allows for low IVC cannulation and an appropriate IVC recipient cuff. After establishing cardiopulmonary bypass, the patient's temperature is lowered to 32 °C. The aorta is then cross-clamped and antegrade cardioplegia is administered until the heart ceases to function.

Next, caval snares are applied, the SVC is transected, and a large right atrial-IVC cuff is created. The aorta is transected, followed by the main pulmonary artery. Once completed, the dome of the left atrium is opened just posterior to the great vessels. The left atrial cuff is created being careful to include all four pulmonary veins but not the left atrial appendage. It is important to ensure hemostasis by cauterizing the left atrial cuff. Once the recipient field is prepared, the donor heart is removed from the transport cooler and prepared for implantation. The aorta and main PA are separated. The left atrium is prepared by opening the pulmonary veins and then making a uniform circular cuff. The atrial septum is then probed from the left atrial side and the right atrial side via the IVC to identify a patent foramen ovale. If present, it can be closed primarily. If lungs were procured, the left atrial appendage was most likely incised for decompression during the procurement procedure; this must be repaired.

Implantation consists of five anastomoses completed with a running polypropylene suture in the following order: left atrial cuff, main PA or aorta and then IVC, SVC (Fig. 2a, b, c) (John and Liao 2010). The right-sided connections can be done with the heart beating on cardiopulmonary bypass. We routinely connect either the main PA and SVC or just SVC as the heart is beating. The left atrial anastomosis is performed first, starting at the base of the left atrial appendage and sewing to the IVC, ensuring that the cuff edges are everted out of the left atrium so that only endocardium is exposed to the blood stream. We believe this to be less thrombogenic. The left atrial anastomosis is not completely finished because a left heart vent is left in place. The aorta is prepared with the idea that it should be the shortest vessel among the SVC and PA so that the donor heart that often is small compared with the pericardial space will "hang" off the aorta. In patients with prior Norwood arch reconstruction, there can be a sizable mismatch with donor aorta. The posterior wall can be sutured primarily with a patch augmentation needed anteriorly after incising into the donor aorta. This will ensure that the SVC and PA are not under tension. As the aortic anastomosis is being completed, the left heart vent is turned off and the heart is de-aired. This anastomosis is completed and an anterior aortic vent is placed. The cross-clamp is removed and, once normal sinus rhythm has been established, the SVC and IVC anastomoses are completed. It is imperative to have the orientation straight while performing the IVC connection as it can be easily twisted and affect venous return (Fig. 2b). It is important, especially with infants, to make the SVC anastomosis tension free, aligned, and free of a purse-string effect. In some instances, anterior patch augmentation may be needed. We also tie the SVC suture line a little loose leaving some room for "distention" as blood fills it. When connecting the main PA, it is important to remember that making it too long is a well described technical error that results in either main PA or branch PA stenosis secondary

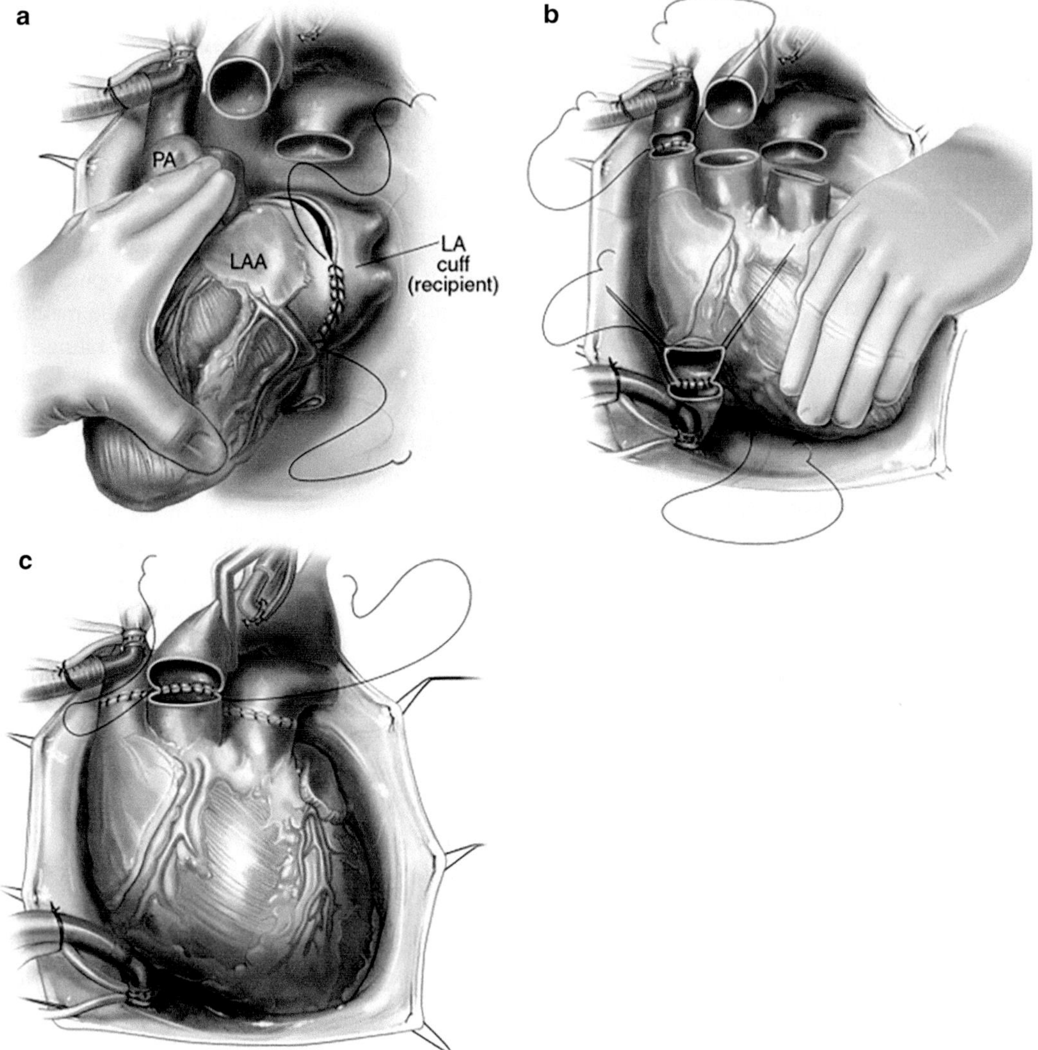

Fig. 2 Bicaval implantation technique. (**a**) Left atrial anastomosis. The left atrial anastomosis is always performed starting at the left atrial cuff adjacent to the left superior pulmonary vein and passing it through the donor left atrial cuff adjacent to the left atrial appendage. The initial few sutures are completed with the donor heart positioned at the level of the sternal edge and the heart is subsequently lowered into the pericardial space. The posterior left atrial suture line is first completed and then subsequently the anterior suture line (as shown). To minimize the risk of left atrial thrombus formation, an everting suture technique should be done to facilitate approximation of the smooth endocardial surfaces of donor and recipient left atrial tissue. A left ventricular vent can be passed through an opening between the 2 untied left atrial sutures that can help with de-airing. (**b**) Inferior vena cava (IVC) anastomosis. During the performance of the IVC anastomosis, care is taken to avoid deep sutures being placed in the region of the donor coronary sinus ostium to avoid potential injury. (**c**) Pulmonary artery and aortic anastomosis. It is important to avoid excess length of pulmonary artery to avoid kinking at the level of the anastomosis. The median raphe on the pulmonary artery may help orient the anastomosis. Next, the aortic anastomosis is completed. Finally, we complete the superior vena cava (SVC) anastomosis. The donor right atrial appendage is medially oriented to facilitate proper orientation of the SVC anastomosis. This is important to avoid the SVC from being kinked or improperly aligned. Further, attention should be closely paid to avoid "purse-stringing" the SVC anastomosis to prevent inadvertent narrowing at the anastomotic level. *LA* left atrium, *LAA* left atrial appendage, *PA* pulmonary artery. (With permission John and Liao 2010)

to buckling of the PA. Therefore, the donor and recipient PAs should be aggressively trimmed, making certain to keep the pulmonary valve and the branch PAs properly aligned (Fig. 2c). In special circumstances for Fontan anatomy, the PA should always be connected, first, after thorough mobilization before performing the aortic anastomosis; otherwise, it becomes very difficult to reach the distal PA adequately. The patient should be completely rewarmed while the PA is anastomosed. Before separating from cardiopulmonary bypass, the heart should be lifted to ensure hemostasis of the left atrial suture line. Separation from bypass is performed under transesophageal echocardiography guidance to ensure excellent de-airing and to assess postbypass ventricular and valvar function.

2.3 Complications Related to Transplantation in Complex Congenital Heart Disease Patients

Planning is paramount for transplantation in complex congenital heart disease patients. There should be a thorough understanding of the anatomy obtained through prior operative reports, imaging studies such as computed tomography scan or magnetic resonance imaging and/or angiography. In some cases, exposure of the femoral vessels may be needed if imaging suggests a high risk of injury to the mediastinal structures. It is imperative to have the cannulation strategy mapped out before for arterial and venous cannulations. Not all patients with bilateral SVCs require both to be cannulated. Most often there are enough collaterals and drainage from the head which is generally adequate. It is also important to remember to use brief periods of circulatory arrest or very low flow, if needed. For Fontan patients, it is important to have bilateral branch pulmonary arteries dissected and controlled. Reconstruction in some cases may be undertaken even prior to the donor heart arriving. In some cases, we have utilized the Organ Care System™ for ex-vivo organ perfusion where patients have a Fontan needing major reconstruction and/or with a ventricular assist device. Virtually all failed Fontan patients have extensive aortopulmonary collateral connections resulting in a large amount of pulmonary venous flow while on bypass flooding the operative field. In addition, it can warm and distend the donor heart once the left atrial anastomosis is completed. A well-functioning left ventricular vent can mitigate this in most instances and also prevent ventricular distention in the new donor heart. For older patients with multiple prior operations, it may be prudent to think about axillary cannulation or dual axillary—femoral arterial cannulation. Alterations in the donor harvest procedure to provide additional tissue for pulmonary artery reconstruction or other anatomic considerations can make for a smoother course of the transplant operation.

2.4 Complications Related to Left Superior Vena Cava

In cases where no bridging vein exists, the systemic venous return from the left SVC needs to be redirected to the donor's right atrium. Typically, the simplest method of reconstruction involves using the donor's innominate vein, either by sewing it end-to-end or end-to-side (Fig. 3) (Chen 2014). If the left SVC is of considerable size (e.g., in heterotaxy with interrupted IVC), an intracardiac baffle can be considered (Fig. 4). If the left SVC drains through a roofed coronary sinus, it may be easier to preserve that whilst creating the left atrial cuff and utilize the enlarged coronary sinus as part of the bicaval anastomosis for easier reconstruction (Fig. 4b) (Chartrand et al. 1990). One could also use the right atrium and create a superior flap where it is anastomosed directly to the left SVC posteriorly and anteriorly a patch is used for augmentation. In cases with hemiazygos continuation a graft/conduit can also be used (Fig. 4c).

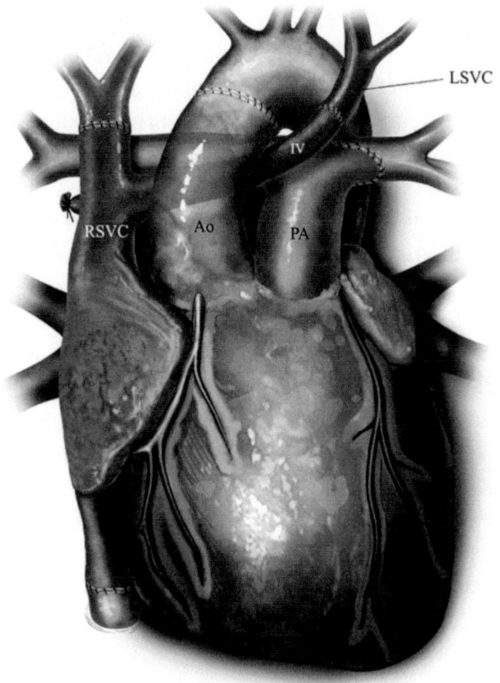

Fig. 3 Drainage from left superior vena cava (L-SVC) without continuation to the coronary sinus can be brought back to the recipient right atrium by utilizing donor innominate vein included at the time of procurement. The anastomosis can be done end-to-end or end-to-side. An additional issue to note is this reconstruction can place the innominate vein posteriorly or anteriorly to the aorta. *Ao* aorta, *LSVC* left superior vena cava, *PA* pulmonary artery, *RSVC* right superior vena cava. (With permission Chen 2014)

2.5 Complications Related to Bilateral Bidirectional Glenn Shunts

Again, the technical difficulty is in attaching the left Glenn to the systemic venous atrium (Huddleston 2014). One strategy is to use the recipient pulmonary artery as the "innominate" vein and leave the Glenn connections intact (Fig. 5a). Branch pulmonary arteries lateral to the Glenn connection can be divided and the medial segment preserved as a conduit (Fig. 5b). Subsequently, the inferior aspect of the right side can then be incised and the donor SVC anastomosed to this. It would also be ideal to harvest the donor pulmonary arteries hilum-to-hilum and use that to reconstruct the branch pulmonary artery segment that was divided earlier. If the lungs are being harvested from the donor, then an extensive patch augmentation almost always does the trick and the donor main pulmonary artery anastomosed into this (Fig. 5c). Alternatively, the technique described above (Fig. 3) of suturing the donor innominate vein to the left SVC as end-to-side can be considered, leaving the recipient pulmonary artery intact. This can prove to be difficult in some situations as the left Glenn is usually very posterior and needs an innominate vein that goes across the mediastinum in an oblique manner.

2.6 Complications in Patients with Prior Transposition of the Great Arteries

The most common scenario involves either congenitally corrected transposition of great arteries where patients have undergone a Mustard or a Senning operation or patients with uncorrected anatomy and heart failure. Because of the anterior-posterior orientation of the great vessels compared with the usual leftward orientation of the donor arteries (Harjula et al. 1988), one has to be mindful of the twist that may occur in using additional donor artery (Fig. 6a). The location of the recipient pulmonary arteriotomy can also be adjusted to counter this discrepancy. However, should the donor or recipient tissue prove inadequate, it is often easier to simply transpose the location of the recipient pulmonary arteriotomy leftward. As shown, this aligns the great vessel connections to more easily match those of the donor heart (Fig. 6b).

2.7 Complications in Patients with Hybrid Interventions

Nowadays, more patients are undergoing hybrid procedures involving ductal stenting, bilateral PA bands, atrial septal stents and flow restrictors as a bridge to transplantation (Fig. 7a) (Huddleston et al. 2019; Sebastian et al. 2010). Waiting times for these patients is usually long and give enough time for the stents to incorporate within the ves-

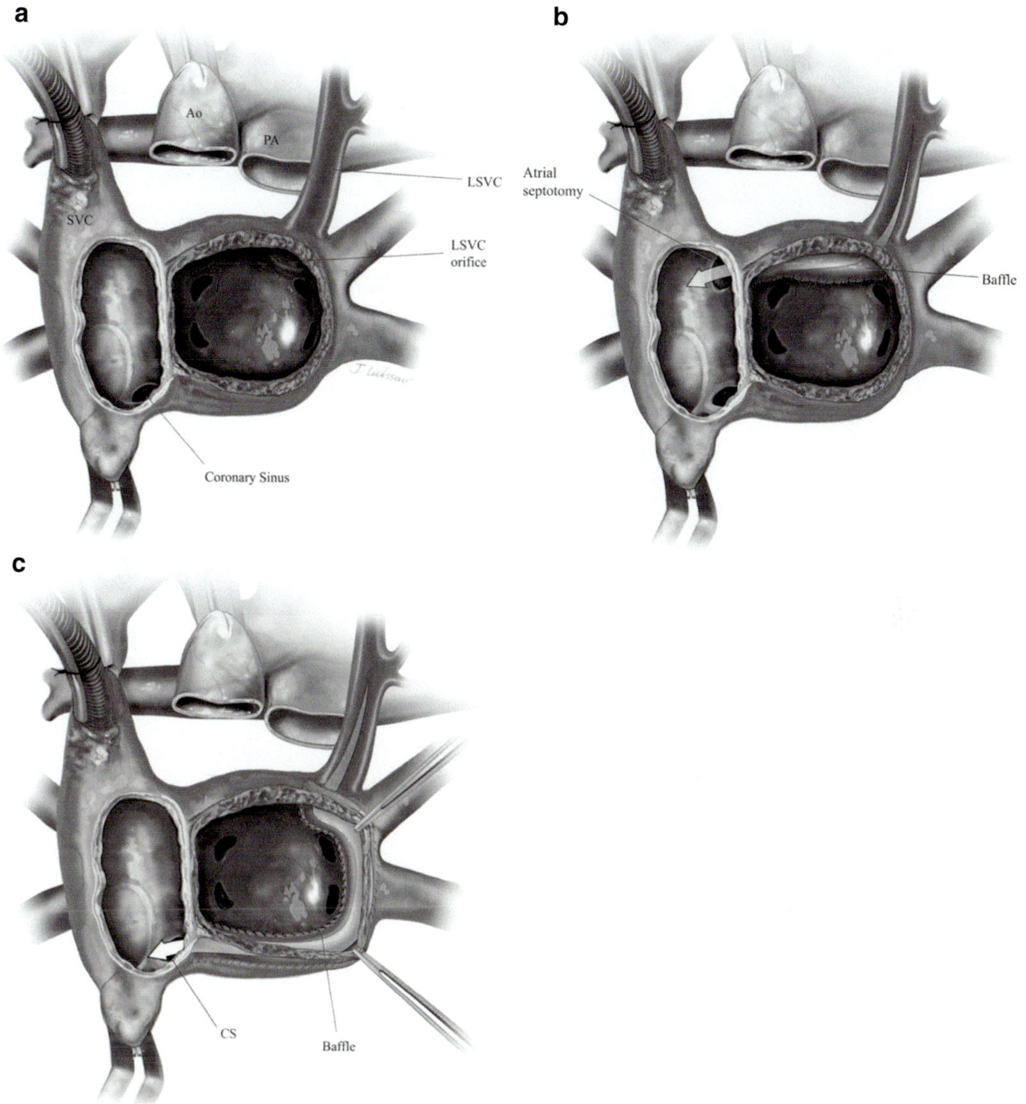

Fig. 4 (**a**) If the donor innominate vein is not sufficient in length, or if the return from the left superior vena cava (L-SVC) is going to exceed the capacity of the donor innominate vein (e.g., heterotaxy and interrupted inferior vena cava with hemiazygos continuation), then other baffles can be created to redirect this systemic venous return. (**b**) The baffle may travel along the roof of the left atrium, above the pulmonary veins to a surgically created atrial septal defect. (**c**) This baffle may also be placed inferiorly to join the right atrium (RA) at the coronary sinus. *Ao* aorta, *CS* coronary sinus, *PA* pulmonary artery, *SVC* superior vena cava. (With permission Chen 2014)

sel walls. As a result, reconstruction following stent and band removal can be challenging and lengthy. Usually, cannulation strategy has to be adjusted by sewing a graft to the innominate artery and cannulating that for arterial cannulation to utilize regional cerebral perfusion and circulatory arrest, if needed. It is also imperative, that during the donor cardiectomy, the entire donor arch distal to the ligamentum arteriosum is harvested so there is sufficient tissue available for reconstruction. Usually, after recipient cardiectomy, one can utilize antegrade cerebral perfusion, remove the ductal stent and carefully examine the remaining quality of the aorta and

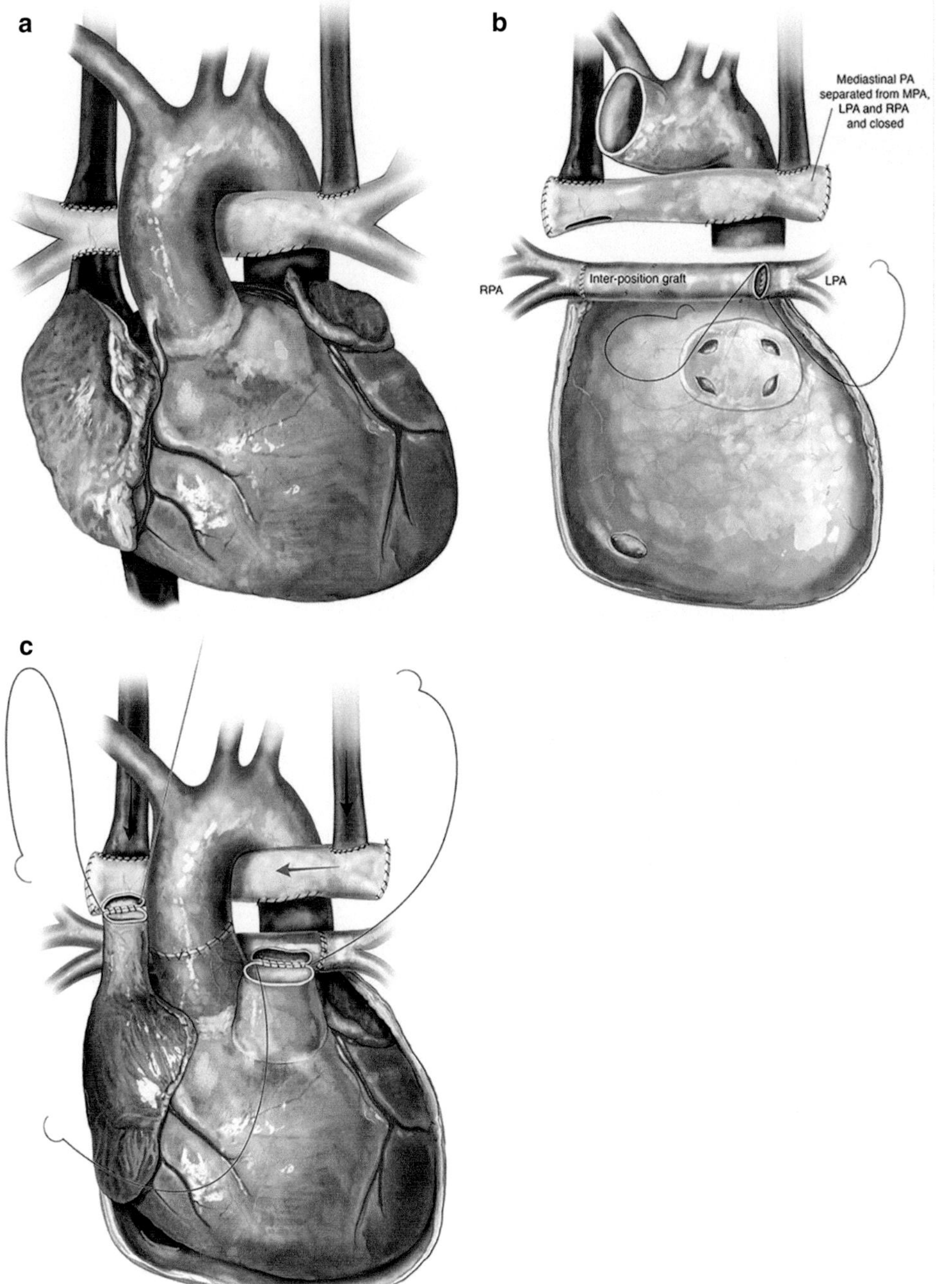

Fig. 5 (**a**) The image here shows a patient with atrial Fontan with bilateral superior venae cavae (SVCs). (**b**) The recipient cardiectomy has been performed leaving the bilateral SVCs attached to the mediastinal pulmonary artery (PA) which is oversewn at each end. The distal branch PAs are connected to one another with an interposition graft; in this case a segment of aortic homograft. An opening is created on the caudad side of the mediastinal PA on the right inferior to the insertion of the right SVC for the superior caval anastomosis. (**c**) The donor heart is sewn in place with the usual left atrium (LA), inferior vena cava (IVC), and aortic anastomoses. The opening for the PA anastomosis is created in the interposition graft. The superior caval anastomosis is to the previously created opening in the right mediastinal PA. *LPA* left pulmonary artery, *MPA* main pulmonary artery, *RPA* right pulmonary artery. (With permission Huddleston et al. 2019)

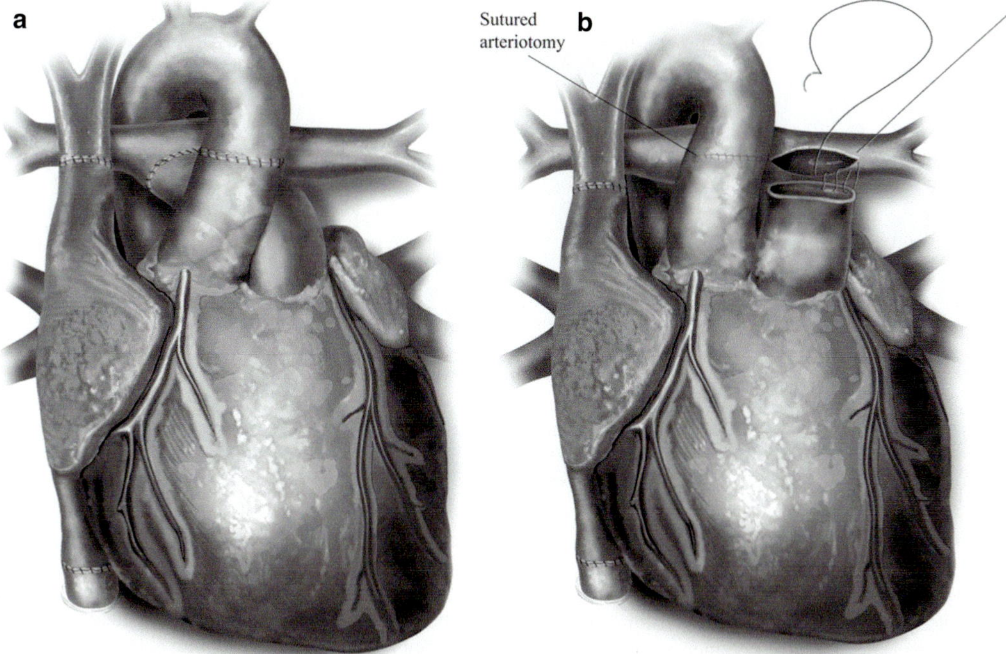

Fig. 6 (**a**) Transposed great arteries may pose little problem for reconstruction. However, often the more anterior-posterior orientation (compared with a more rightward-leftward orientation of the donor heart) can result in a twist. Allowing for extra donor and recipient aorta and pulmonary artery can afford this twist without creating areas of stenosis. (**b**) However, should the donor or recipient tissue prove inadequate, it is often easier to simply transpose the location of the recipient pulmonary arteriotomy leftward. As shown, this aligns the great vessel connections to easily match those of the donor heart. (With permission Chen 2014)

retrograde arch. It is not required to remove the arch/PDA stent in its entirety especially if one plans to reconstruct the arch by replacing the lesser curvature of the arch leaving the arch vessels attached to the descending aorta (Fig. 7b). In cases where there is pulmonary arterial banding, flow restrictors, or stents, it is helpful to do the extensive pulmonary arterial reconstruction prior to donor implant or donor heart arrival to minimize the ischemic time (Fig. 7c).

2.8 Situs Inversus Related Complications

This is perhaps one of the most complex anatomic issues facing congenital heart surgeons for transplantation. Patients may have dilated cardiomyopathy, congenitally corrected transposition of the great arteries, or single ventricle anatomy. The difficulty lies in reconstructing the pulmonary and systemic venous anatomy (Fig. 8a, b, c, d). Recipient cardiectomy should be performed by leaving as much atrial tissue as possible in the chest (Fig. 8b). Pulmonary arterial anastomosis can be "shifted" to the left by suturing the bifurcation closed and incising the pulmonary artery towards the left pulmonary artery. The pulmonary veins return usually more to the "right" of the midline. Some authors have advocated using the atrial septal tissue to baffle the right pulmonary venous drainage as one would do for the Senning procedure (Fig. 8c) (Harjula et al. 1988). We have typically anastomosed the donor left atrium by incising it wide and suturing to the recipient left atrial cuff as the veins would come in. And the remaining anastomosis is then done around this (Fig. 8c). In order for the heart to fit in the mediastinum, the left pericardium is taken down at the diaphragm down to the phrenic nerve. If necessary, the heart is placed outside the pericardium with the phrenic coursing under-

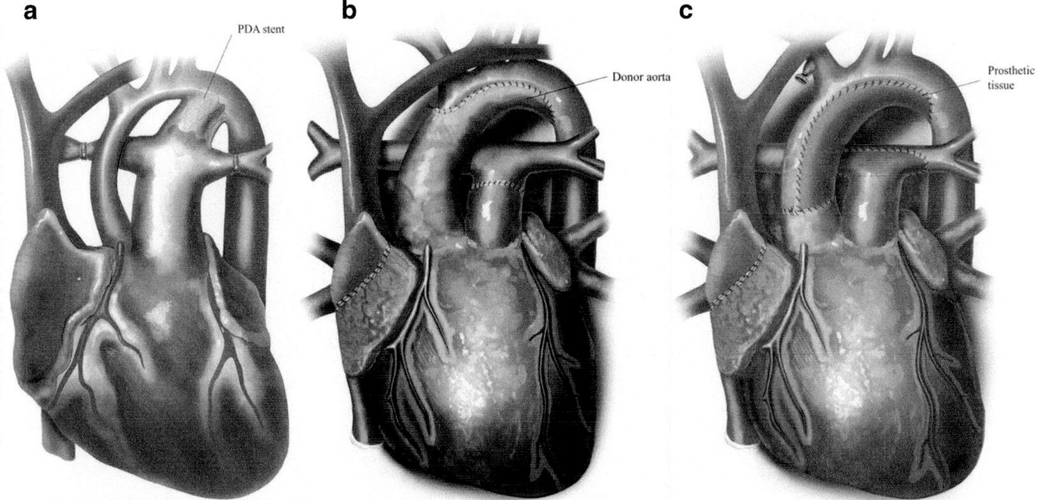

Fig. 7 (**a**) Patients who have undergone prior hybrid procedures, either as a bridge to decision or transplant, or as a primary therapy for hypoplastic left heart syndrome and its variants, present challenges for reconstruction at the time of transplant. The most common scenario is illustrated in (**a**) where bilateral pulmonary artery bands are placed as is a ductal stent (with or without a stent in the atrial septum). (**b**) At the time of transplantation, removal of the pulmonary artery bands often does not result in permanent distortion of the branch pulmonary arteries, and therefore the pulmonary artery anastomosis can proceed without augmentation. Removal of the ductal stent with adjacent descending aorta at its insertion requires reconstruction of the entire arch beyond the ductal insertion. This often is best accomplished with extended donor aortic tissue. (**c**) Alternatively, if removal of the pulmonary artery bands or flow restrictors creates distortion, augmentation of the branch pulmonary arteries is generally effective. *PDA* patent ductus arteriosus. (With permission Chen 2014)

neath the heart. This is done to accommodate the donor heart in a levocardia position. The recipient IVC usually courses to the midline and when enough atrial tissue is left, this can be moved to the right (Fig. 9a, b). In more complicated donor implantation of sinus inversus, hemiazygos continuation of the IVC and dextrocardia, enough of the right atrial wall is left in place to form the tunnel which will direct hepatic venous drainage to the donor right atrium (Fig. 9b). The recipient right atrium is then reconfigured as a composite tunnel from the left-sided hepatic vein ostia, along the diaphragm crossing the midline to connect with the IVC ostium of the donor heart. The recipient left SVC with hemiazygos continuation is connected to the donor right atrium at the transected right atrial appendage with donor descending thoracic aorta as an interposition graft.

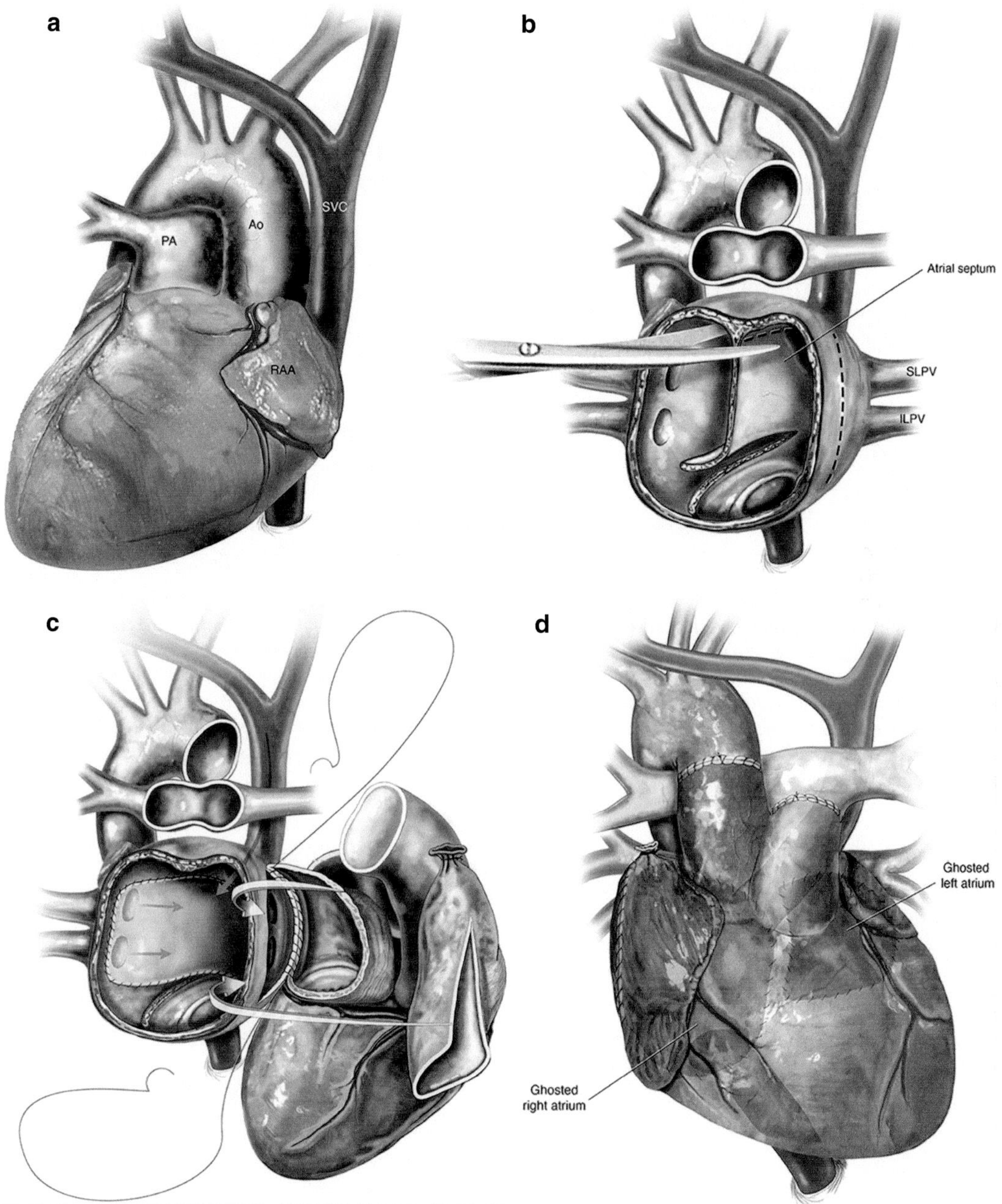

Fig. 8 (**a**) The positioning of the heart with situs inversus totalis. The superior vena cava (SVC) and inferior vena cava (IVC) are on the patient's left. There is right aortic arch and the main pulmonary artery (MPA) is on the patient's right. (**b**) The recipient cardiectomy has been performed leaving as much of the great vessels and atrial tissue as possible. The atrial septal flap is created by incision superiorly and inferiorly. The interatrial groove is developed along the dotted line shown on the patient's left. (**c**) The atrial septal flap has been sewn anterior to the left pulmonary veins. A large opening is created in the previously developed interatrial groove for the left atrial anastomosis. The right atrial anastomosis is performed to the large atrial opening into which the SVC and IVC enter (as well as the coronary sinus). The MPA opening is extended into the left pulmonary artery (LPA) to facilitate the anastomosis to the donor MPA. (**d**) The completed anastomosis, creating levocardia. *Ao* aorta, *PA* pulmonary artery, *RAA* right atrial appendage. (With permission Huddleston et al. 2019)

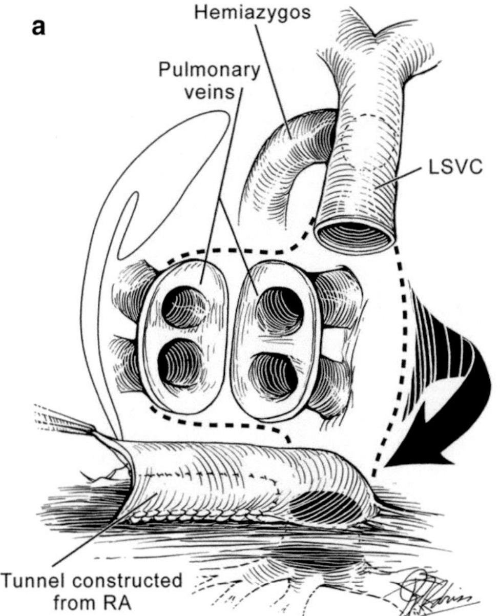

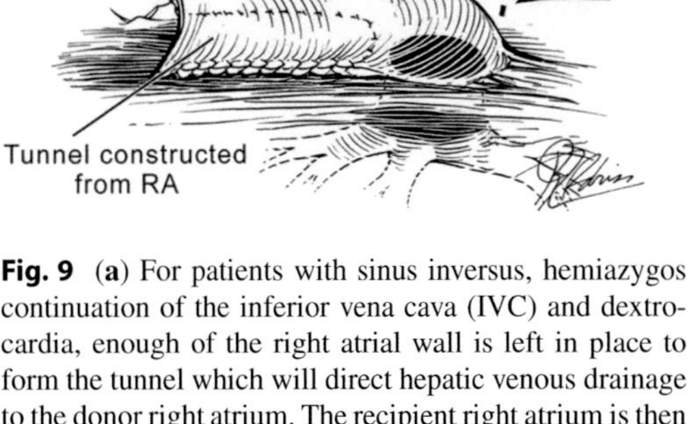

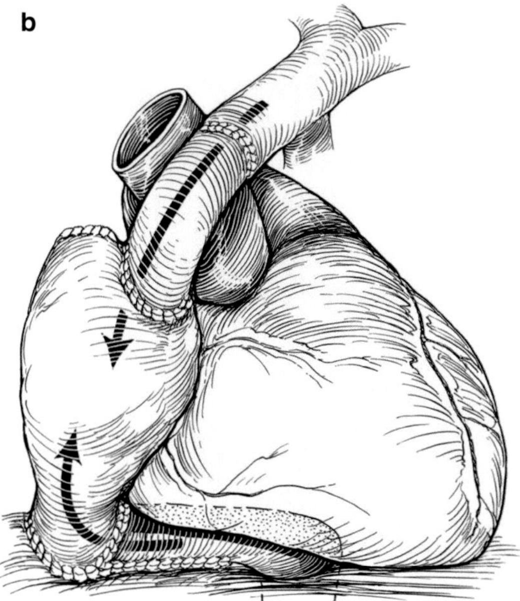

Fig. 9 (**a**) For patients with sinus inversus, hemiazygos continuation of the inferior vena cava (IVC) and dextrocardia, enough of the right atrial wall is left in place to form the tunnel which will direct hepatic venous drainage to the donor right atrium. The recipient right atrium is then reconfigured as a composite tunnel from the left-sided hepatic vein ostia, along the diaphragm crossing the midline to connect with the IVC ostium of the donor heart. (**b**) The recipient left superior vena cava (LSVC) with hemiazygos continuation is connected to the donor right atrium at the transected right atrial appendage with donor descending thoracic aorta as an interposition graft. *RA* right atrium. (With permission Mavroudis and Dearani 2020)

3 Conclusions

There are almost no anatomical contraindications to heart transplantation for congenital heart disease. Surgeons will be challenged in these subgroups of patients but a well-planned strategy will be very helpful for a smooth operation.

References

Chartrand C, Guerin R, Kangah M, Stanley P. Pediatric heart transplantation: surgical considerations for congenital heart diseases. J Heart Transplant. 1990;9(6):608–16.

Chen JM. Heart transplant: transplantation for congenital heart disease. Oper Tech Thorac Cardiovasc Surg. 2014;19(1):30–46.

Dipchand AI, Kirk R, Mahle WT, Tresler MA, Naftel DC, Pahl E, Miyamoto SD, Blume E, Guleserian KJ, White-Williams C, Kirklin JK. Ten years of pediatric heart transplantation: a report from the Pediatric Heart Transplant Study. Pediatr Transplant. 2013;17(2):99–111.

Harjula ALJ, Heikkila LJ, Nieminen MS, et al. Heart transplantation in repaired transposition of the great arteries. Ann Thorac Surg. 1988;46:611–4.

Huddleston CB. Pediatric heart transplantation. In: Kaiser LR, Kron IL, Spray TL, editors. Mastery of cardiothoracic surgery. 3rd ed. Philadelphia: Wolters Kluwer; 2014.

Huddleston CB, Richey S, Fiore AC. Heart transplantation for congenital heart disease. Oper Tech Thorac Cardiovasc Surg. 2019;24(2):103–20.

John R, Liao K. Orthotopic heart transplantation. Oper Tech Thorac Cardiovasc Surg. 2010;15(2):138–46.

Mavroudis C, Dearani JA. Anatomic variation for cardiac transplantation in adults with congenital heart disease. In: Mavroudis C, Dearani JA, editors. Atlas of adult congenital heart surgery. Cham: Springer; 2020. p. 413–22.

Rossano JW, Dipchand AI, Edwards LB, Goldfarb S, Kucheryavaya AY, Levvey BJ, Lund LH, Meiser B, Yusen RD, Stehlik J. The registry of the international society for heart and lung transplantation: nineteenth pediatric heart transplantation report—2016; focus theme: primary diagnostic indications for transplant. J Heart Lung Transplant. 2016;35(10):1185–95.

Scientific Registry of Transplant Recipients: Pediatric heart transplant centers. 2020. https://www.srtr.org/transplant-centers/?query=&distance=50&location=&state=&recipientType=pediatric&organ=heart&sort=transplantRate. Accessed 26 Aug 2020.

Sebastian VA, Guleserian KJ, Leonard SR, et al. Heart transplantation techniques after hybrid single-ventricle palliation. J Card Surg. 2010;25:596–600.

Shumway NE, Lower RR, Stofer RC. Transplantation of the heart. Adv Surg. 1966;2:265–84.

Sievers HH, Leyh R, Jahnke A, Petry A, Kraatz EG, Herrmann G, Simon R, Bernhard A. Bicaval versus atrial anastomoses in cardiac transplantation: right atrial dimension and tricuspid valve function at rest and during exercise up to thirty-six months after transplantation. J Thorac Cardiovasc Surg. 1994;108(4):780–4.

Complications Associated with Right Ventricular Outflow Tract Reconstruction for Congenital Heart Disease in Children and Adults

John W. Brown

Abstract

Repair of numerous complex congenital cardiac anomalies have been made possible utilizing tissue valves and valved conduits for the repair of the right ventricular outflow tract. Most of these patients are now surviving well into adulthood. Intraoperative and postoperative complications following right ventricular outflow (RVOT) tract reconstruction are not rare. Most of these complications are treatable and many, if not most, are preventable. Tissue pulmonary prosthesis durability is limited necessitating the need for multiple reoperations during the patient's lifespan. Percutaneous pulmonary valve replacements have reduced the number of open surgical procedures but will not eliminate the need for repeat surgery. Progress is being made and will continue to be made. This chapter will focus on the management of many of the surgical complications of RVOT reconstruction using several prostheses.

Keywords

Congenital heart disease · Pulmonary-to-artery conduit · Right ventricular outflow tract obstruction · Pulmonary valve · Aortic allograft · Porcine conduits · Mechanical valves · Bovine jugular vein

1 Historical Accounts and Background

Valve pathology at all ages poses numerous challenges to the cardiologist and cardiovascular surgeons. Valve reconstruction is the goal of most pediatric surgical interventions because reconstruction has the potential to restore the anatomy and physiology employing native tissue that has growth potential and resists infection better than prosthetic materials. When repair fails, or is not feasible, valve replacement becomes inevitable. Congenital heart disease with its associated valve pathology, patient age, size, and the requirement for growth all interrelate making valve replacement in neonates, infants, and children more challenging than similar replacements in adults (Husain and Brown 2007).

The pulmonary valve is the most common valve to require replacement in patients with congenital heart disease. Pulmonary valve replacement is 4–5 times more common in our surgical practice than aortic valve replacement. We have

J. W. Brown (✉)
Indiana University School of Medicine, Indianapolis, IN, USA
e-mail: jobrown@iu.edu

C. L. Backer, C. Mavroudis (eds.), *Complications in Pediatric and Congenital Heart Surgery*, https://doi.org/10.1007/978-3-032-02661-3_29

replaced more than 1500 pulmonary valves inside the native right ventricular outflow tract (RVOT) but more commonly inside a conduit in the past 45 years and the prostheses we currently prefer are shown in Figs. 1, 2, 3 and 4 and listed in Table 1. Valve selection has evolved during our experience and has been highly dependent on patient size, age, the congenital anatomy, replacement valve durability, and an obligation to avoid long-term anticoagulation.

In the past (1950s–1970s), infants who had stenotic but patent right ventricular outflow tracts could undergo a transannular outflow tract patch. Transannular patching at that time was thought to be sufficient treatment for a child's lifetime. By the mid-1980s pediatric cardiologists and surgeons learned that many if not most patients who had undergone a transannular RVOT patch in previous decades had developed moderate to severe pulmonary insufficiency, a dilated, sometimes, poorly functioning right ventricle (RV) and evidence of right and left heart failure manifested by fatigue, dyspnea, peripheral edema, and atrial arrhythmias (Husain and Brown 2007; Rastelli et al. 1965; Ross and Somerville 1966; Jonas et al. 1985; Forbess et al. 2001; Dearani et al. 2003; Sinzobahamvya et al. 2001; Tweddell et al. 2000; Chan et al. 1994; Bando et al. 1995; Feier et al. 2005; Wells et al. 2002; Raanani et al. 2000; Discigil et al. 2001; Gundry 1999).

Valveless conduits were introduced in the 1960s (Rastelli et al. 1965; Ross and Somerville 1966; Sinzobahamvya et al. 2001; Tweddell et al. 2000; Chan et al. 1994; Bando et al. 1995; Feier et al. 2005; Wells et al. 2002). Aortic valve allograft conduits (Fig. 5) were introduced in the late1960s–1970s followed by Dacron tube grafts containing glutaraldehyde fixed porcine aortic xenografts (1970s) (Fig. 6). RVOT conduits were introduced to treat complex cardiac lesions without right ventricle-to-pulmonary artery (RV-PA) continuity such as pulmonary atresia, truncus arteriosus, and transposition with ventricular septal defect and pulmonary stenosis/atresia (Rastelli et al. 1965; Ross and Somerville 1966; Sinzobahamvya et al. 2001; Tweddell et al. 2000; Chan et al. 1994; Bando et al. 1995; Feier et al. 2005; Wells et al. 2002; Brown et al. 2005; Askovich et al. 2007; Fiore et al. 2010; Vincent et al. 2009) (Fig. 5). Dacron conduits (Fig. 6) were supplanted by cryopreserved pulmonary allografts (Fig. 4) in the mid-1980s (Forbess et al. 2001; Tweddell et al. 2000; Chan et al. 1994; Bando et al. 1995; Feier et al. 2005; Wells et al. 2002; Raanani et al. 2000; Brown et al. 2005, 2009, 2008, 2011; Askovich et al. 2007; Perron et al. 1999; Hawkins et al. 1992; Yankah et al. 1995; Niwaya et al. 1999; Bielefeld et al. 2001; Gerestein et al. 2001; Boethig et al. 2007; Elkins et al. 2001a; Bibevski et al. 2017; Dave et al. 2003; Schmid et al. 2002; Mery et al. 2016; Ramanan et al. 2015; Dunne et al. 2016; Lee et al. 2011; Jang et al. 2012; Nomoto et al. 2016; Chen et al. 2013; Kwak et al. 2015; Saleeb et al. 2014; Buchholz et al. 2016; Horer et al. 2009; Haas et al. 2005; Rosti et al. 1998; Waterbolk et al. 2006; Ilbawi et al. 1987; Miyamura et al. 1987; Fleming et al. 1989; Kiyota et al. 1992; Yang et al. 2014; Gottlieb et al. 2010; Sacks et al. 2009; Oosterhof et al. 2007; Frigiola et al. 2008;

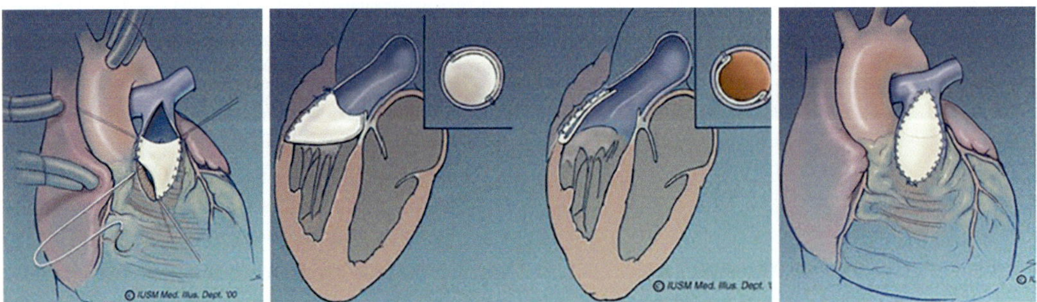

Fig. 1 Drawings illustrating insertion of a 0.1 mm PTFE leaflet and a 0.4 mm RVOT patch for RVOT reconstruction. (With permission Brown and Herrmann 2023). *PTFE* polytetrafluoroethylene, *RVOT* right ventricular outflow tract

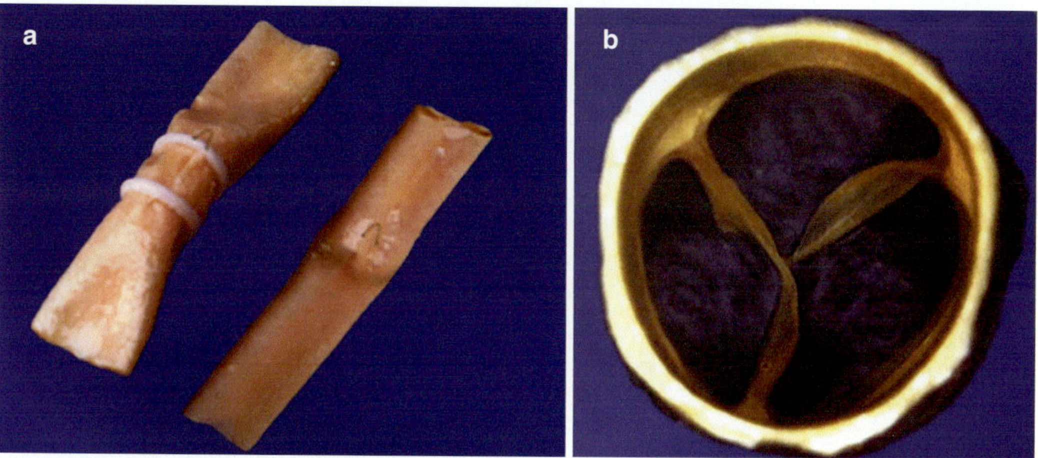

Fig. 2 (**a**) Stented and unstented bovine jugular vein conduit containing an in situ venous valve. (**b**) Trileaflet venous valve of the bovine venous valved conduit. (With permission Carrel et al. 2002)

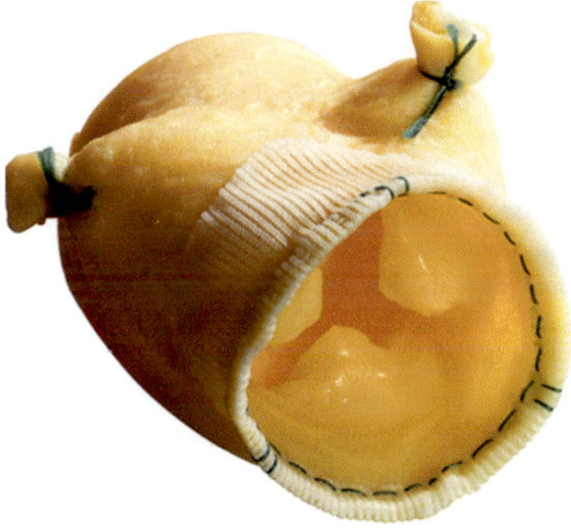

Fig. 3 Porcine aortic xenograft designed for aortic root replacement and used "off label" as a right ventricle-to-pulmonary artery conduit for right ventricular outflow tract reconstruction. (With permission Cohn 2012)

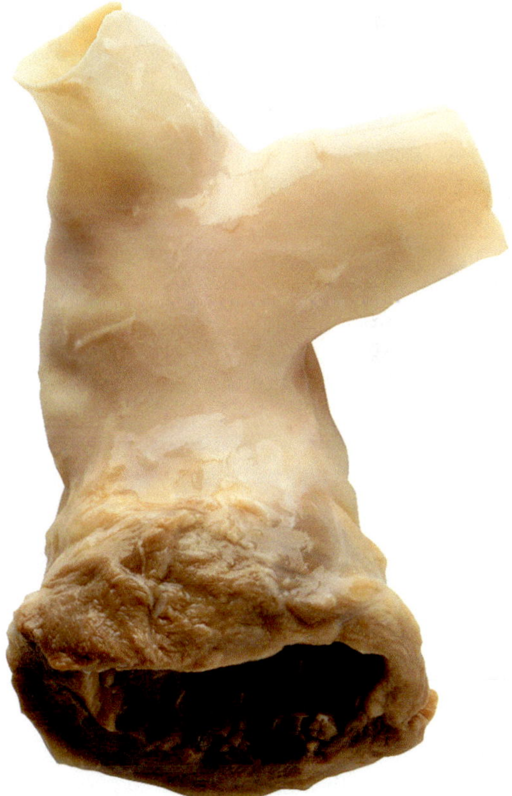

Fig. 4 Decellularized pulmonary allograft for RVOT reconstruction. (Used with the permission of Artivion, Inc. https://artivion.com/)

Table 1 Summary of RV-PA valve/conduits used at Indiana University (IU) from 1980–2024

Type	No. of patients
PTFE monocusps	300
Non-valved conduits	30
Aortic allograft conduits	27
Pulmonary allograft conduits (decellularized)	486 (360)
Stented porcine conduits (Hancock)	47
Stentless porcine valves (freestyle)	170
Mechanical valves	3
Bovine jugular vein conduits (Contegra)	400
Stented bovine pericardial valves	40
Total	1503

RVOT reconstruction currently favored @ IU
Abbreviation: *PTFE* polytetrafluoroethylene, *RVOT* right ventricular outflow reconstruction

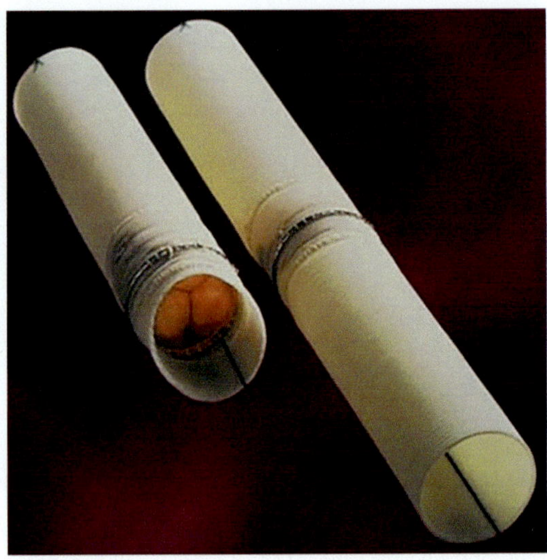

Fig. 6 Dacron conduit with a porcine aortic xenograft (Medtronic conduit). (With permission Vricella et al. 2004)

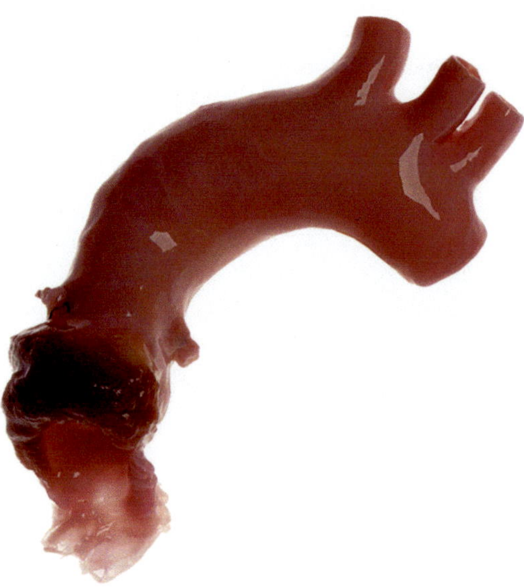

Fig. 5 Cryopreserved aortic homograft used for right ventricular outflow tract reconstruction. (Used with the permission of Artivion, Inc. https://artivion.com/)

Warnes et al. 2008; Anagnostopoulos 2017). Other xenograft conduits like the bovine jugular venous valved conduits (Fig. 2) became available in the early 2000s and decellularized pulmonary allografts starting around 2008.

Poor durability of most tissue RV-PA conduits produced renewed interest in pulmonary valve preservation or valve repair using autologous or xenograft tissue reconstruction.

Our current practice (when a conduit can be avoided) is to preserve as much of the native pulmonary valve as possible and to reconstruct the anterior pulmonary leaflet with a 0.1 mm polytetrafluoroethylene (PTFE) monocusp leaflet and then cover the RVOT with a 0.4 mm PTFE outflow tract patch (Fig. 1). We continue to utilize this technique with our infant tetralogy of Fallot (TOF) patients when a transannular incision is required (25% of our TOF patients). In neonates, infants and children <18 years we have preferred the use of the bovine jugular conduit (Fig. 2) when a Goretex monocusp reconstruction of the pulmonary valve was not possible or when we needed to replace a dysfunctional allograft, xenograft or Goretex monocusp valve. Since 1994 and in adults >18 years we have preferred the stentless porcine xenograft (Medtronic Freestyle valve) (Fig. 3) for RVOT reconstruction because these valves are available in larger sizes (19–29 mm) and have excellent hemodynamics and a lower incidence of infective endocarditis.

When replacing the aortic valve with a pulmonary autograft (Ross Aortic Valve Replacement) we favor the use of the decellularized, cryopreserved, pulmonary allograft (Fig. 4) for pulmonary valve replacement (PVR). We oversize the pulmonary allograft by several millimeters

(3–8 mm) and in children <6 years when we prefer an oversized bovine jugular vein conduit for PVR.

Pulmonary valve replacement usually requires a tissue valve and all the tissue pulmonary valves to date have limited durability (5–15 years) PTFE conduits with PTFE leaflets have been used to a limited degree in recent years and there is currently insufficient follow-up data to know whether they are more durable than tissue pulmonary valves (Oku et al. 1993; Quintessenza et al. 2010; Nunn et al. 2008; Dur et al. 2010; Lee et al. 2016; Miyazaki et al. 2007; Shinkawa et al. 2015).

Due to the life-long potential for the need to surgically replace the pulmonary valve we close the patient's pericardium (since 1994) with a 0.1 mm PTFE membrane to avoid the heart and/or pulmonary valve conduit from adhering to the back of the anterior chest wall.

The purpose of this chapter is to outline some of the surgical complications of RVOT reconstruction during the initial cardiac repair but more commonly during reoperative RVOT repair and how to avoid them or treat them if they occur.

2 Intraoperative Complications During Initial or Re-do Right Ventricular Outflow Tract Reconstruction

2.1 Right Heart Injury on Sternal Reentry

Cardiac injury and bleeding are major causes of mortality and morbidity during redo cardiac surgery. Dilated right heart structures and dense pericardial adhesions produced by prior surgery often cause the heart to be densely adherent to the underside of the sternum and anterior chest wall starting near the diaphragm and extending up to and above the innominate vein. The limited durability (5–15 years) of most currently available tissue valves and conduits used for RVOT reconstruction necessitates multiple redo operations over the course of a patient's life. Five and six time redo operations are not uncommon in our adult/congenital practice and the degree of difficulty tends to increase as the number of redo operations increases. Percutaneous, transcatheter pulmonary valve replaceent (TPVR) is touted to reduce the mortality/morbidity but in a recent series of nearly 2500 TPVRs the cumulative incidence of death was 9% at 8 years (Vincent et al. 2009; McElhinney et al. 2010; Cheatham et al. 2015; Van Dijck et al. 2015; Levi et al. 2016). The number of redo valve-in-valve TPVRs is not limitless (usually 1, at most 2) and surgical PVR after TPVR can be challenging due to stent materials extending outside the RVOT/PA lumen making removal difficult and treacherous.

Since 1994 our group has routinely closed the pericardium with a 0.1-mm sheet of PTFE membrane in all patients with a risk of needing redo cardiac operations. We attach it loosely with interrupted, nonabsorbable, monofilament sutures to the native pericardium laterally and attach it to the diaphragm inferiorly and above the innominate vein superiorly. RVOT reconstruction is one of the largest patient groups needing redo cardiac surgery in our adult/congenital practice. This type of pericardial closure nearly eliminates cardiac adherence to the sternum and anterior chest wall and markedly reduces the risk of cardiac injury on sternal reentry.

3 Techniques Used to Avoid Cardiac Injury During Redo Sternotomy for RVOT Reconstruction (When PTFE Pericardial Closure Was Not Utilized at the Previous Operation)

1. Untwist or cut sternal wires but leave the wires in place. The wires behind the sternum serve as backstop to the oscillating redo sternal saw. Remove wires after oscillating saw use is complete.
2. Begin dissection just below xyphoid process with patient in deep Trendelenburg position.
3. Develop plane posterior and lateral to xyphosternal junction. Enter right pleural space in

order to see and palpate dense attachments of right atrium, right ventricle and/or aorta to posterior sternum and anterior chest wall.

4. Under direct vision with the assistant elevating the xypho-sternal junction and sternal edges with bone hooks or using an internal mammary retractor, sharply dissect cardiac structures from posterior table of sternum and anterior chest wall for a distance of 3–5 cm. before proceeding up the sternum and anterior chest wall.
5. Use bone scissors to divide posterior table of sternum only for that portion of sternum that has been freed from cardiac structures. Move the bone hooks or mammary retractor cephalad to a position just below the next area to be freed.
6. Divide dense lateral cardiac adhesions before inserting/opening sternal retractor to prevent stretching and tearing the right atrium/ventricle as the retractor is opened.
7. In recent years we have been spraying the right atrium, right ventricle, and RVOT with Coseal before positioning the drainage tubes and closing the pericardium primarily or with a PTFE pericardial substitute. We have observed that the pericardial adhesions are much less dense and easier to lyse on subsequent redo cardiac procedures.

4 Air Embolization

Systemic air embolization (SAE) can occur if RVOT reconstruction is attempted on bypass when the heart is beating if there is a known or unknown intracardiac shunt.

Systemic air embolization can also happen if vacuum assisted venous return is used during redo surgery if an intracardiac shunt is present (Brown et al. 1978; Huber et al. 2000).

We often perform RVOT reconstruction or conduit change in a beating heart if our intraoperative ECHO bubble-study is negative. If there is any doubt we cross-clamp the aorta and arrest the heart with cardioplegia or place the patient in a deep Trendelenburg position and vent the ascending aorta with a large bore needle.

If a massive systemic air embolization were to occur while on bypass, we would turn cardiopulmonary bypass off, place the patient in a deep Trendelenburg position, cross-clamp the aorta, give cardioplegia, remove the aortic cannula from the aorta and connect the aortic line to the superior vena cava (SVC) cannula and perfuse the snared SVC cannula at a flow of 500–1000 cc/min. and at a pressure of <40 mmHg. Retrograde cerebral perfusion is continued for 5–10 min while venting the ascending aorta just distal to the aortic cross-clamp to remove the air (Brown et al. 1978; Huber et al. 2000).

5 Other Postoperative Complications of Right Ventricular Outflow Tract Reconstruction

5.1 Coronary Complications

Coronary artery anomalies and/or placement of a rigid pulmonary prosthesis may produce coronary compression during surgical and/or percutaneous pulmonary valve/conduit replacement (Kwon et al. 2023). Eight percent of patients born with TOF have anomalous origin of the left anterior descending (LAD) coronary artery from the right coronary artery (RCA). The anomalous LAD may cross at the pulmonary valve annulus or more commonly 0.5–2 cm below the pulmonary valve annulus. Almost as common, is a dual LAD where there may be a small to moderate LAD branch originating from the right coronary artery and crossing the RVOT and another small to moderate LAD originating from the left coronary artery. Injury, occlusion, division or compression of the LAD or LADs may occur if a transannular incision is required to close the ventricular septal defect and/or relieve RVOT obstruction at the initial repair of tetralogy of Fallot. A rigid prosthetic valve or conduit with a rigid component used to replace the pulmonary valve may compress the left main coronary (LM) or LAD as the sternum is being closed (Kwon et al. 2023). If the anomalous coronary is not recognized visually at operation or preoperatively on the ECHO or catheterization, serious injury or coronary compression may occur. Epicardial scarring from previous surgery or epicardial fat may make visualization of these LAD anomalies difficult. Careful reading of the previous surgeon's operative note can alert the current surgeon of the potential danger that anomalous coronary arteries can pose during redo RVOT reconstruction.

Compression of the normally arising (LM) coronary or the proximal LAD by a rigid prosthesis placed surgically or percutaneously may cause coronary compression and left ventricular ischemia. Balloon distension of the obstructed RVOT is usually done in the catheterization laboratory prior to deployment of a percutaneous pulmonary valve in an attempt to unmask coronary compression and prevent it (Kwon et al. 2023).

Intraoperative treatment of inadvertent LAD division usually requires left internal mammary artery (LIMA) bypass. Left-main and/or LAD compression can often be relieved by opening the left pleural space widely to allow the heart to shift posteriorly. On rare occasions it may be necessary to make a large "trap door" incision in the posterior pericardium medial to the left phrenic nerve starting near the main pulmonary artery and extending down to the diaphragm then transversely to the right and along the diaphragm to the inferior vena cava. The trap door incision is particularly useful in infants where the RV-PA conduit protrudes anteriorly (truncus arteriosus) (Kirk et al. 1995).

6 Right Ventricular Outflow Tract Obstruction and Conduit Length and Diameter Considerations During Initial RVOT Reconstruction

If the RV-PA conduit is left too long it may kink at the distal anastomosis to the native pulmonary arteries that are fixed in place during systole and produce significant obstruction and conduit dilation. This complication is most often seen with the bovine jugular conduit that is provided with several centimeters of venous conduit proximal and distal to the conduit valve. This makes the conduit very distensible. To avoid this complication the surgeon needs to keep the posterior hemicircumference of the conduit as short as possible while leaving the anterior wall just long enough to form an adequate hood over the RVOT incision. The bovine jugular conduit may rarely become aneurysmal if the distal conduit becomes significantly obstructed or native branch pulmonary stenosis is not relieved at the initial correction.

If the RV-PA conduit is of insufficient length anteriorly the conduit may become flattened and compressed at the superior rim of the RVOT incision due to lack of a sufficient hood. This complication is typically seen with aortic and pulmonary allografts and/or stented xenografts. This complication can be avoided by adding a tissue or PTFE hood to the proximal end of the conduit.

Conduit diameter should be as large as can be easily accommodated in the pericardial space because most aortic and pulmonary allograft conduits do not dilate after implantation and typically shrink in diameter by as much as 25% due to an inflammatory response to foreign human tissue. It is easier to oversize the allograft or xenograft RV-PA conduit in the Ross aortic valve repair (AVR) operation due to the fact that the pulmonary replacement is placed orthotopically.

7 Prosthetic Valve/Conduit Dysfunction

Prosthetic pulmonary valve and/or conduit dysfunction continues to occur with all currently available tissue pulmonary prostheses. Mechanical pulmonary valve prostheses are durable but are prone to thrombosis in spite of therapeutic anticoagulation and are rarely used (Haas et al. 2005; Rosti et al. 1998; Waterbolk et al. 2006; Ilbawi et al. 1987; Miyamura et al. 1987; Fleming et al. 1989; Kiyota et al. 1992). Risk factors for early tissue valve dysfunction include young patient age and small valve/conduit size, aortic allografts, and certain glutaraldehyde preserved framed bovine pericardial and porcine valves.

8 Early and Late Postoperative Atrial and Ventricular Arrhythmias

Early and late atrial and ventricular postoperative arrhythmias following RVOT reconstruction are not rare.

Atrial tachyarrhythmias are most commonly observed with right atrial dilation associated with significant residual or recurrent RVOT obstruction and/or regurgitation and/or tricuspid valve regurgitation. If these arrhythmias persist after medical therapy and/or catheterization lab ablative intervention we would strongly consider surgical RVOT revision to include intraoperative cryoablation of aberrant pathways (right-sided maze procedure).

Early ventricular arrhythmias are commonly seen after placement of TPVR prostheses, are usually self-limited, and can be treated medically. These arrhythmias are commonly due to impingement of stent materials on subpulmonary myocardium. Early ventricular arrhythmias are uncommon after surgical RVOT reconstruction but can be associated with myocardial ischemia due to coronary compression by a rigid pulmonary prosthesis after sternal closure. Late ventricular arrhythmias (VT) after RVOT reconstruction are usually associated with subendocardial scarring in the RVOT and are largely responsible for the 5%–8% late mortality over the subsequent 30 years following RVOT reconstruction and particularly when a right ventriculotomy was utilized. Most late ventricular arrhythmias following RVOT reconstruction should be treated, mapped and ablated (Zippenfield et al. 2007).

9 Pulmonary Valve Endocarditis, Thrombosis, and Pulmonary Artery Embolization

Tissue valve thrombosis and pulmonary artery embolization are uncommon occurrences but when they do occur are usually associated with right heart endocarditis on the tricuspid valve, but more commonly, a pulmonary valve prosthesis. Mechanical pulmonary valves are prone to thrombosis despite adequate anticoagulation and in the absence of endocarditis (Haas et al. 2005; Rosti et al. 1998; Waterbolk et al. 2006; Ilbawi et al. 1987; Miyamura et al. 1987; Fleming et al. 1989; Kiyota et al. 1992). The highest incidence of pulmonary valve endocarditis in our clinical series is with the bovine jugular vein conduits (Contegra and Melody) (Fiore et al. 2010; Dave et al. 2003; Schmid et al. 2002; Brown et al. 2006, 2011; Mery et al. 2016; Jang et al. 2012; Elkins et al. 2001b; Ichikawa et al. 1997; Scavo Jr et al. 1999; Herijgers et al. 2002; Breymann et al. 2002, 2009; Bove et al. 2002; Boethig et al. 2005; Corno et al. 2002; Carrel et al. 2002; Chatzis et al. 2003; Rastan et al. 2006; Morales et al. 2006; Sekarski et al. 2007; Dave et al. 2011; Gist et al. 2012; Albanesi et al. 2014). The incidence in nearly 400 Contegra conduits was 6%. One-half of these patients (3%) required surgical replacement and the other 3% were successively treated with antibiotics alone (Mery et al. 2016; Brown et al. 2011). We have observed aortic and pulmonary allograft, bovine pericardial and porcine xenograft endocarditis, thrombosis, and embolization but in less <1% in these patient populations (Mery et al. 2016; Brown et al. 2011). Surprisingly, we have not seen any clinically recognizable episodes of endocarditis, thrombosis, or pulmonary emboli in over 300 children who received a PTFE monocusp RVOT reconstruction (Gundry 1999; Oku et al. 1993; Bogers et al. 1994; Yamagishi and Kurosawa 1993; Turrentine et al. 2002a, b; Gundry et al. 1994; Brown et al. 2007; Kumar et al. 2016).

10 Acquired Right Ventricular Aneurysm

In our experience, an acquired RVOT aneurysm is a rare complication of RVOT reconstruction. However, Seybold-Epting et al. reported that RVOT aneurysms were seen in 6%–25% of patients who underwent repair of TOF that included a right ventriculotomy (Seybold-Epting et al. 1977). In our experience the RVOT aneurysm usually occurs to the left of a transannular RVOT incision and after a conal branch of the right coronary artery has been transected to allow an adequate RVOT incision. These aneurysms develop due to a small area of ischemia or infarction of that portion of the RVOT muscle between the RVOT incision and the left anterior descending coronary artery. They are more commonly seen when pulmonary artery pressure is elevated due to residual, distal PA obstruction. Large aneurysms can produce right ventricular dysfunction, ventricular arrhythmias, thrombus, and potentially pulmonary embolization. Persistent or recurrent RVOT obstruction or progressive enlargement and/or clot within the aneurysm are indications for reoperation to resect the aneurysm and relieve any distal obstruction (Seybold-Epting et al. 1977).

11 Summary

Right ventricular outflow tract reconstruction utilizing tissue valves and valved conduits have made possible the repair of numerous complex congenital cardiac anomalies with most patients surviving well into adulthood. Intraoperative and postoperative complications following RVOT reconstruction are not rare. Most of these complications are treatable and most are preventable. Tissue pulmonary prosthesis durability is limited necessitating the need for multiple reoperations during a patient's lifespan. Percutaneous pulmonary valve replacements have reduced the number of open surgical procedures but will not eliminate the need for repeat surgery. Progress is being made and will continue to be made to produce more durable pulmonary valves and conduits. The "Holy Grail" will be to develop a valve and conduit that is living, will grow and remain competent over the patient's life.

References

Albanesi F, Sekarski N, Lambrou D, et al. Incidence and risk factors for Contegra graft infection following right ventricular outflow tract reconstruction: long-term results. Eur J Cardiothorac Surg. 2014;45:1070–4.

Anagnostopoulos PV. Pseudoaneurysm complicating right ventricle-to-pulmonary artery conduit surgery: why single-center observational studies still matter. J Thorac Cardiovasc Surg. 2017;154(6):2050–1.

Askovich B, Hawkins JA, Sower CT, et al. Right ventricle-to-pulmonary artery conduit longevity: is it related to allograft size? Ann Thorac Surg. 2007;84:907–12.

Bando K, Danielson GK, Schaff HV, et al. Outcome of pulmonary and aortic homografts for right ventricular outflow tract reconstruction. J Thorac Cardiovasc Surg. 1995;109:509–18.

Bibevski S, Ruzmetov M, Fortuna RS, et al. Performance of SynerGraft decellularized pulmonary allografts compared with standard cryopreserved allografts: results from multiinstitutional data. Ann Thorac Surg. 2017;103(3):869–74.

Bielefeld MR, Bishop DA, Campbell DN, et al. Reoperative homograft right ventricular outflow tract reconstruction. Ann Thorac Surg. 2001;71:482–8.

Boethig D, Thies WR, Hecker H, et al. Mid-term course after pediatric right ventricular outflow tract reconstruction: a comparison of homografts, porcine xenografts and Contegras. Eur J Cardiothorac Surg. 2005;27:58–66.

Boethig D, Goerler H, Westhoff-Bleck M, et al. Evaluation of 188 consecutive homografts implanted in pulmonary position after 20 years. Eur J Cardiothorac Surg. 2007;32:133–42.

Bogers AJ, Roofthooft M, Pisters H, et al. Long-term results of the gamma-irradiation-preserved homograft monocusp for transannular reconstruction of the right-ventricular outflow tract in tetralogy of Fallot. Thorac Cardiovasc Surg. 1994;42:337–9.

Bove T, Demanet H, Wauthy P, et al. Early results of valved bovine jugular vein conduit versus bicuspid homograft for right ventricular outflow tract reconstruction. Ann Thorac Surg. 2002;74:536–41.

Breymann T, Thies WR, Boethig D, et al. Bovine valved venous xenografts for RVOT reconstruction: results after 71 implantations. Eur J Cardiothorac Surg. 2002;21:703–10.

Breymann T, Blanz Q, Wojtalik MA, et al. European Contegra Multicentre Study: 7-year results after 165 valved bovine jugular vein graft implantations. Thorac Cardiovasc Surg. 2009;57:257–69.

Brown JW, Herrmann JL. Ventricular to pulmonary artery conduits. In: Mavroudis C, Backer CL, editors. Pediatric cardiac surgery. 5th ed. West Sussex: Wiley Blackwell; 2023. p. 481–97.

Brown JW, Dierdorf SF, Moorthy SS, Halpin M. Veno-arterial Cebral perfusion for treatment of massive arterial air embolism. J Intern'l Anesthesia Res Soc Anest Analg. 1978;66:673–4.

Brown JW, Ruzmetov M, Rodefeld MD, et al. Right ventricular outflow tract reconstruction with an allograft conduit in non-Ross patients: risk factors for allograft dysfunction and failure. Ann Thorac Surg. 2005;80:655–64.

Brown JW, Ruzmetov M, Rodefeld MD, et al. Valved bovine jugular vein conduits for right ventricular outflow tract reconstruction in children: an attractive alternative to pulmonary homograft. Ann Thorac Surg. 2006;82:909–16.

Brown JW, Ruzmetov M, Vijay P, et al. Right ventricular outflow tract reconstruction with a polytetrafluoroethylene monocusp valve: a twelve-year experience. J Thorac Cardiovasc Surg. 2007;133:1336–43.

Brown JW, Ruzmetov M, Rodefeld MD, et al. Right ventricular outflow tract reconstruction in Ross patients: does the homograft fare better? Ann Thorac Surg. 2008;86:1607–12.

Brown JW, Ruzmetov M, Shahriari A, et al. Midterm results of Ross aortic valve replacement: a single-institution experience. Ann Thorac Surg. 2009;88:601–8.

Brown JW, Ruzmetov M, Eltayeb O, et al. Contegra versus pulmonary homografts for right ventricular outflow tract reconstruction: a 10-year single institution comparison. World J Pediatr Congenit Heart Surg. 2011;2:541–9.

Buchholz C, Mayr A, Purbojo A, et al. Performance of stented biological valves for right ventricular outflow tract reconstruction. Interact Cardiovasc Thorac Surg. 2016;23:933–9.

Carrel T, Berdat P, Pavlovic M, et al. The bovine jugular vein: a totally integrated valved conduit to repair the right ventricular outflow. J Heart Valve Dis. 2002;11:552–6.

Chan KC, Fyfe DA, McKay CA, et al. Right ventricular outflow reconstruction with cryopreserved homografts in pediatric patients: intermediate-term follow-up with serial echocardiographic assessment. J Am Coll Cardiol. 1994;24:483–9.

Chatzis AC, Giannopoulos NM, Bobos D, et al. New xenograft valved conduit (Contegra) for right ventricular outflow tract reconstruction. Heart Surg Forum. 2003;6:396–8.

Cheatham JP, Hellenbrand WE, Zahn EM, et al. Clinical and hemodynamic outcomes up to 7 years after transcatheter pulmonary valve replacement in the US Melody Valve Investigational Device Exemption Trial. Circulation. 2015;131:1960–70.

Chen XJ, Smith PB, Jaggers J, et al. Bioprosthetic pulmonary valve replacement: contemporary analysis of a large, single-center series of 170 cases. J Thorac Cardiovasc Surg. 2013;146:1461–6.

Cohn LH, editor. Cardiac surgery in the adult. 4th ed. McGraw-Hill; 2012.

Corno AF, Hurni M, Griffin H, et al. Bovine jugular vein as right ventricle-to-pulmonary artery valved conduit. J Heart Valve Dis. 2002;11:242–8.

Dave H, Kadner A, Bauersfeld U, et al. Early results of using the bovine jugular vein for right ventricular outflow reconstruction during the Ross procedure. Heart Surg Forum. 2003;6:390–2.

Dave H, Mueggler O, Comber M, et al. Risk factor analysis of 170 single-institutional Contegra implantations pulmonary position. Ann Thorac Surg. 2011;91:195–203.

Dearani JA, Danielson GK, Puga FJ, et al. Late follow-up of 1095 patients undergoing operation for complex congenital heart disease utilizing pulmonary ventricle to pulmonary artery conduits. Ann Thorac Surg. 2003;75:399–411.

Discigil B, Dearani JA, Puga FJ, et al. Late pulmonary valve replacement after repair of tetralogy of Fallot. J Thorac Cardiovasc Surg. 2001;121:344–51.

Dunne B, Suthers E, Xiao P, et al. Medium-term outcomes after pulmonary valve replacement with the freestyle valve for congenital heart disease: a case series. Eur J Cardiothorac Surg. 2016;49:e105–11.

Dur O, Yoshida M, Manor P, et al. In vitro evaluation of right ventricular outflow tract reconstruction with bicuspid valved polytetrafluoroethylene conduit. Artif Organs. 2010;34:1010–6.

Elkins RC, Lane MM, Capps SB, et al. Humoral immune response to allograft valve tissue pretreated with an antigen reduction process. Semin Thorac Cardiovasc Surg. 2001a;13(4 Suppl 1):82–6.

Elkins RC, Dawson PE, Goldstein S, et al. Decellularized human valve allografts. Ann Thorac Surg. 2001b;71(5 Suppl):S428–32.

Feier H, Collart F, Ghez O, et al. Risk factors, dynamics, and cutoff values for homograft stenosis after the Ross procedure. Ann Thorac Surg. 2005;79:1669–75.

Fiore AC, Rodefeld M, Turrentine M, et al. Pulmonary valve replacement: a comparison of three biological valves. Ann Thorac Surg. 2010;85:1712–8.

Fleming WH, Sarafian LB, Moulton AL, et al. Valve replacement in the right side of the heart in children: long-term follow-up. Ann Thorac Surg. 1989;48:404–8.

Forbess JM, Shah AS, St Louis JD, et al. Cryopreserved homografts in the pulmonary position: determinants of durability. Ann Thorac Surg. 2001;71:54–60.

Frigiola A, Tsang V, Nordmeyer J, et al. Current approaches to pulmonary regurgitation. Eur J Cardiothorac Surg. 2008;34:576–82.

Gerestein CG, Takkenberg JJ, Oei FB, et al. Right ventricular outflow tract reconstruction with an allograft conduit. Ann Thorac Surg. 2001;71:911–8.

Gist KM, Mitchell MB, Jaggers J, et al. Assessment of the relationship between Contegra conduit size and early valvar insufficiency. Ann Thorac Surg. 2012;93:856–61.

Gottlieb D, Kunal T, Emani S, et al. In vivo monitoring of function of autologous engineered pulmonary valve. J Thorac Cardiovasc Surg. 2010;139:723–31.

Gundry SR. Pericardial and synthetic monocusp valves: indication and results. Semin Thorac Cardiovasc Surg Pediatr Card Surg Annu. 1999;2:77–82.

Gundry SR, Razzouk AJ, Boskind JF, et al. Fate of the pericardial monocusp pulmonary valve for right ventricular outflow tract reconstruction. Early function, late failure without obstruction. J Thorac Cardiovasc Surg. 1994;107:908–13.

Haas F, Schreiber C, Horer J, et al. Is there a role for mechanical valved conduits in the pulmonary position? Ann Thorac Surg. 2005;79:1662–8.

Hawkins JA, Bailey WW, Dillon T, et al. Midterm results with cryopreserved allograft valved conduits from the right ventricle to the pulmonary arteries. J Thorac Cardiovasc Surg. 1992;104:910–6.

Herijgers P, Ozaki S, Verbeken E, et al. Valved jugular vein segments for right ventricular outflow tract reconstruction in young sheep. J Thorac Cardiovasc Surg. 2002;124:798–805.

Horer J, Vogt M, Stierle U, et al. A comparative study of mechanical and homograft prostheses in the pulmonary position. Ann Thorac Surg. 2009;88:1534–9.

Huber S, Rigler B, Machler HE, Metzler H, Smolle-Juttner FM. Successful treatment of massive air embolization during open heart surgery. Ann Thorac Surg. 2000;69:931–3.

Husain SA, Brown JW. When reconstruction fails or is not feasible: valve replacement options in the pediatric population. Semin Thorac Cardiovasc Surg Pediatr Card Surg Annu. 2007;2007:117–24.

Ichikawa Y, Noishiki Y, Kosuge T, et al. Use of a bovine jugular vein graft with natural valve for right ventricular outflow tract reconstruction: a one-year animal study. J Thorac Cardiovasc Surg. 1997;114:224–33.

Ilbawi MN, Lockhart CG, Idriss FS, et al. Experience with St. Jude Medical valve prosthesis in children. A word of caution regarding right-sided placement. J Thorac Cardiovasc Surg. 1987;93:73–9.

Jang WS, Kim YJ, Choi K, et al. Mid-term results of bioprosthetic pulmonary valve replacement in pulmonary regurgitation after tetralogy of Fallot repair. Eur J Cardiothorac Surg. 2012;42:e1–8.

Jonas RA, Freed MD, Mayer JEJ, et al. Long-term follow-up of patients with synthetic right heart conduits. Circulation. 1985;72:II77–83.

Kirk MA, Angelini AJ, Wisheart GD, Hutter JD. Posterior pericardiotomy reduces the incidence of supraventricular arrhythmias following coronary artery bypass. Eur J Cardiothorac Surg. 1995;9:150–2.

Kiyota Y, Shiroyama T, Akamatsu T, et al. In vitro closing behavior of the St. Jude Medical heart valve in the pulmonary position. Valve incompetence originating in the prosthesis itself. J Thorac Cardiovasc Surg. 1992;104:779–85.

Kumar M, Turrentine MW, Rodefeld MD, et al. Right ventricular outflow tract reconstruction with a polytetrafluoroethylene monocusp valve: a 20-year experience. Semin Thoracic Surg. 2016;28:463–70.

Kwak JG, Lee C, Lee M, et al. Does implantation of larger bioprosthetic pulmonary valves in young patients guarantee durability in adults? Durability analysis of stented bioprosthetic valves in the pulmonary position in patients with tetralogy of Fallot. Eur J Cardiothorac Surg. 2015;49:1207–12.

Kwon H, Song MK, Lee SY, Kim GB, Kwak JG, Cho SK, Kim WH. Risk factors for coronary artery complications after prosthetic pulmonary valve implantation in congenital heart diseases. Eur Heart J. 2023;44(Suppl _2):ehad655–2645.

Lee C, Park CS, Lee CH, et al. Durability of bioprosthetic valves in the pulmonary position: long-term follow-up of 181 implants in patients with congenital heart disease. J Thorac Cardiovasc Surg. 2011;142:351–8.

Lee C, Lee CH, Kwak JG. Polytetrafluoroethylene bicuspid pulmonary valve replacement: a 5-year experience in 119 patients with congenital heart disease. Ann Thorac Surg. 2016;102:163–9.

Levi DS, Sinha S, Salem MM, et al. Transcatheter native pulmonary valve and tricuspid valve replacement with the Sapien XT: initial experience and development of a new delivery platform. Catheter Cardiovasc Interv. 2016;88:434–43.

McElhinney DB, Hellenbrand WE, Zahn EM, et al. Short- and medium-term outcomes after transcatheter pulmonary valve placement in the expanded multicenter US Melody Valve Trial. Circulation. 2010;122:507–16.

Mery CM, Guzman-Pruneda FA, De Leon LE, et al. Risk factors for development of endocarditis and reintervention in patients undergoing right ventricle to pulmonary artery valved conduit replacement. J Thorac Cardiovasc Surg. 2016;151:432–41.

Miyamura H, Kanazawa H, Hayashi J, et al. Thrombosed St. Jude Medical valve prosthesis in the right side of the heart in patients with tetralogy of Fallot. J Thorac Cardiovasc Surg. 1987;94:148–50.

Miyazaki T, Yamagishi M, Nakashima A, et al. Expanded polytetrafluoroethylene valved conduit and patch with bulging sinuses in right ventricular outflow tract reconstruction. J Thorac Cardiovasc Surg. 2007;134:327–32.

Morales DL, Braud BE, Gunter KS, et al. Encouraging results for the Contegra conduit in the problematic right ventricle-to-pulmonary artery connection. J Thorac Cardiovasc Surg. 2006;132:665–71.

Niwaya K, Knott-Craig CJ, Lane MM, et al. Cryopreserved homograft valves in the pulmonary position: risk analysis for intermediate-term failure. J Thorac Cardiovasc Surg. 1999;117:141–7.

Nomoto R, Sleeper LA, Borisuk MJ, et al. Outcome and performance of bioprosthetic pulmonary valve replacement in patients with congenital heart disease. J Thorac Cardiovasc Surg. 2016;152:1333–42.

Nunn GR, Bennetts J, Onikul E. Durability of hand-sewn valves in the right ventricular outlet. J Thorac Cardiovasc Surg. 2008;136:290–6.

Oku H, Matsumoto T, Kitayama H, et al. Semilunar valve replacement with a cylindrical valve. J Card Surg. 1993;8:666–70.

Oosterhof T, van Straten A, Vliegen HW, et al. Preoperative thresholds for pulmonary valve replacement in patients with corrected tetralogy of Fallot using cardiovascular magnetic resonance. Circulation. 2007;116:545–51.

Perron J, Moran AM, Gauvreau K, et al. Valved homograft conduit repair of the right heart in early infancy. Ann Thorac Surg. 1999;68:542–8.

Quintessenza JA, Jacobs JP, Chai PJ, et al. Polytetrafluoroethylene bicuspid pulmonary valve implantation: experience with 126 patients. World J Ped Congenital Heart Surg. 2010;1:20–7.

Raanani E, Yau TM, David TE, et al. Risk factors for late pulmonary homograft stenosis after the Ross procedure. Ann Thorac Surg. 2000;70:1953–7.

Ramanan S, Doll N, Boethig D, et al. Pulmonary-valve replacement in adults: results with the medtronic freestyle valve. Ann Thorac Surg. 2015;100:1047–53.

Rastan AJ, Walther T, Daehnert I, et al. Bovine jugular vein conduit for right ventricular outflow tract reconstruction: evaluation of risk factors for mid-term outcome. Ann Thorac Surg. 2006;82:1308–15.

Rastelli GC, Ongley PA, Davis GD, Kirklin JW. Surgical repair for pulmonary valve atresia with coronary- pulmonary artery fistula: report of case. Mayo Clin Proc. 1965;40:521–7.

Ross DN, Somerville J. Correction of pulmonary atresia with a homograft aortic valve. Lancet. 1966;2:1446–7.

Rosti L, Murzi B, Colli AM, et al. Pulmonary valve replacement: a role for mechanical prostheses? Ann Thorac Surg. 1998;65:889–90.

Sacks MS, Schoen FJ, Mayer JE. Bioengineering challenges for heart valve tissue engineering. Annu Rev Biomed Eng. 2009;11:289–313.

Saleeb SF, Newburger JW, Geva T, et al. Accelerated degeneration of a bovine pericardial bioprosthetic aortic valve in children and young adults. Circulation. 2014;130:51–60.

Scavo VA Jr, Turrentine MW, Aufiero TX, et al. Valved bovine jugular venous conduits for right ventricular to pulmonary artery reconstruction. ASAIO J. 1999;45:482–7.

Schmid FX, Keyser A, Wiesenack C, et al. Stentless xenografts and homografts for right ventricular outflow tract reconstruction during the Ross operation. Ann Thorac Surg. 2002;74:684–8.

Sekarski N, van Meir H, Rijlaarsdam ME, et al. Right ventricular outflow tract reconstruction with the bovine jugular vein graft: 5 years' experience with 133 patients. Ann Thorac Surg. 2007;84:599–605.

Seybold-Epting W, Chiariello L, Hallman GL, Cooley DA. Aneurysm of pericardial right ventricular outflow tract patches. Ann Thorac Surg. 1977;24:237–40.

Shinkawa T, Tang X, Gossett JM, et al. Valved polytetrafluoroethylene conduits for right ventricular outflow tract reconstruction. Ann Thorac Surg. 2015;100:129–37.

Sinzobahamvya N, Wetter J, Blaschczok HC, et al. The fate of small-diameter homografts in the pulmonary position. Ann Thorac Surg. 2001;72:2070–6.

Turrentine MW, McCarthy RP, Vijay P, et al. PTFE monocusp valve reconstruction of the right ventricular outflow tract. Ann Thorac Surg. 2002a;73:871–80.

Turrentine MW, McCarthy RP, Vijay P, et al. Polytetrafluoroethylene monocusp valve technique for right ventricular outflow tract reconstruction. Ann Thorac Surg. 2002b;74:2202–5.

Tweddell JS, Pelech AN, Frommelt PC, et al. Factors affecting longevity of homograft valves used in right ventricular outflow tract reconstruction for congenital heart disease. Circulation. 2000;102(Suppl 3):III130–5.

Van Dijck I, Budts W, Cools B, et al. Infective endocarditis of a transcatheter pulmonary valve in comparison with surgical implants. Heart. 2015;101(10):788–93.

Vincent JA, Hellenbrand WE, Zahn EM, et al. Implantation of the medtronic melody transcatheter pulmonary valve for dysfunctional right ventricular outflow conduits: clinical results of initial 99 patients in the US Investigational Device Exemption Trial. Circulation. 2009;120:S930–1.

Vricella LA, Kanani M, Cook AC, Cameron DE, Tsang VT. Problems with the right ventricular outflow tract: a review of morphologic features and current therapeutic options. Cardiol Young. 2004;14(5):533–49.

Warnes CA, Williams RG, Bashore TM, et al. ACC/AHA 2008 guidelines for the management of adults with congenital heart disease. Circulation. 2008;118:e714–833.

Waterbolk TW, Hoendermis ES, den Hamer IJ, et al. Pulmonary valve replacement with a mechanical prosthesis. Promising results of 28 procedures in patients with congenital heart disease. Eur J Cardiothorac Surg. 2006;30:28–32.

Wells WJ, Arroyo H Jr, Bremner RM, et al. Homograft conduit failure in infants is not due to somatic outgrowth. J Thorac Cardiovasc Surg. 2002;124:88–96.

Yamagishi M, Kurosawa H. Outflow reconstruction of tetralogy of Fallot using a Gore-Tex valve. Ann Thorac Surg. 1993;56:1414–7.

Yang CC, Wei HJ, Hsieh SR, et al. Excellent mid-term durability of the On-X mechanical aortic valve in the pulmonary position with a low international normalized ration. J Heart Valve Dis. 2014;23:333–7.

Yankah AC, Alexi-Meskhishvili V, Weng Y, et al. Accelerated degeneration of allografts in the first two years of life. Ann Thorac Surg. 1995;60(2 Suppl):S71–7.

Zippenfield K, Schalij MJ, Bartelings MM, Tedro UB, Koplan BA, Sojima K, Stevenson WG. Catheter ablation of ventricular tachycardia after repair of congenital heart disease. Circulation. 2007;116:2241–52.

Bioethical Complications Associated with Congenital Heart Surgery

Constantine Mavroudis, J. Thomas Cook, and Jeffrey P. Jacobs

Abstract

This chapter discusses ethical complications that are related to congenital heart surgery and offers measures to resolve them. Examples of bioethical controversies such as informed consent, clinical futility, truth telling, conflict of interest, fetal cardiac interventions, the use of bioethical consultation, public reporting, and regionalization of congenital heart surgery care are given. The teachings of ancient philosophers (Aristotle, Plato, Hippocrates) as well as more modern theorists (Kant, Locke) are examined to show how they still cast a profound influence on modern bioethical education.

C. Mavroudis (✉)
Chief of Pediatric Cardiothoracic Surgery (Retired), Peyton Manning Children's Hospital, Indianapolis, IN, USA

Professor Emeritus of Surgery, Johns Hopkins University School of Medicine, Baltimore, MD, USA

J. T. Cook
Rollins College, Winter Park, FL, USA

J. P. Jacobs
Division of Cardiovascular Surgery, Department of Surgery, Congenital Heart Center, University of Florida, Gainesville, FL, USA

Keywords

Congenital heart surgery · Bioethics · Informed consent · Outcomes · Fetal cardiac intervention · Public reporting · Regionalization of care

1 Introduction

This book has considered complications that occur in congenital heart surgery and the associated measures to resolve them. Embedded in this process is the management of bioethical controversies (Mavroudis et al. 2020a) such as: informed consent (Mavroudis et al. 2011, 2014a, b, 2016, 2018; Cook et al. 2020; Mavroudis and Cook 2020), clinical futility (Lantos and Ethical Issues 1994; Sachdeva et al. 1996; Boston Children's Hospital Futility Policy 2013; Truog 2007; Schneiderman et al. 1990; Shepherd 2013; Mavroudis and Siegel 2020), truth telling (Mavroudis et al. 2005) conflict of interest (London et al. 2020), fetal cardiac interventions (Mavroudis 2020), the use of bioethical consultation (Patel et al. 2020), public reporting (Nashif 2020; Jacobs et al. 2009, 2018; Jacobs and Jacobs 2016; Jacobs 2017; Tweddell et al. 2017), and regionalization of congenital heart surgery care (Welke et al. 2019, 2020, 2021; Backer et al. 2020; Karamlou et al. 2020; Backer 2021a, b; 2022a, b, c).

C. L. Backer, C. Mavroudis (eds.), *Complications in Pediatric and Congenital Heart Surgery*,
https://doi.org/10.1007/978-3-032-02661-3_30

The aforementioned list of bioethical controversies are clearly issues that often arise and must be considered in the practice of pediatric cardiac surgery. However, how do they relate to surgical complications? Failure to properly manage these bioethical issues which are often associated with surgical complications can result in lawsuits, loss of professional reputation, and loss of clinical service integrity. We consider how management of surgical complications includes bioethical standards.

2 Autonomy and Informed Consent

Each operation begins with the respect for autonomy and informed consent. No doctor-patient relationship can begin without proper mutual communication, respect for patient autonomy, and the conscientious securing of informed consent. Autonomy is one of the four prime principles of Medical Ethics—which also include, Beneficence, Non-maleficence, and Justice (Cook et al. 2015). It is assumed that these last three principles have been established when the patient is in one's office: namely, that the physician is duty bound to practice Beneficence (to do good), Non-Maleficence (to do no harm) and make sure that Justice is being served in so far as cultural, racial, and gender differences are never negatively considered. Respect for patient autonomy, the fourth cardinal principle, requires that the surgeon secure the informed consent of the patient.

The technique of obtaining consent can best be understood as one of the skills that make up the "Art of Medicine." (Mavroudis 2003, 2005; Mavroudis and Backer 2007) These skills are not to be learned from a textbook, but from observation, practice, and discussion. This generally means that the physician identified a mentor in medical school or training who conducts Informed Consent with practiced proficiency and confident skill. The process is similar to Aristotle's account of how a person attains virtue—by observing and seeking to emulate a virtuous person in one's own practice, thereby acquiring the habit of virtuous behavior which eventually becomes second nature (Aristotle 1954). These lessons and habits become honed and perfected in an Aristotelean sense (Aristotle 1954) over time, allowing the practitioner to form—in a natural and spontaneous way—a proper association with his/her patient.

Recent database studies have approached the practice of Informed Consent based on the incidence of mortality and morbidity for standard operations (Mavroudis et al. 2014a). This information can guide the practitioner as to what is important to discuss in the Informed Consent process. For instance, opinion-based studies in the surgical subspecialty literature (Pleat et al. 2004; McLaren et al. 2001) have determined that complications that occur over 5% of the time should be discussed before any procedure with the patient/parents. While this approach is based on an opinion standard, it may be missing an opportunity for the clinician to bond with the patient/family and avoid the problems of a ruptured relationship and mistrust. For instance, let us consider informed consent for coarctation of the aorta repair. The 5% level of complications, more or less, are recurrent laryngeal injury, chylothorax, residual stenosis at the repair site, wound infection, and bleeding. The incidence of paraplegia after coarctation repair is 4% (Backer et al. 1998; Farag et al. 2019; Serfontein and Kron 2022). Based on the 5% rule, one would not ordinarily discuss the possibility of paraplegia during the informed consent process. So, what is the potential bioethical complication involved herein? Failure to discuss such an important and serious complication will cause much consternation—for both the surgeon and the family—in the event that the complication would occur. The complication is not only paraplegia but also the failure of proper informed consent (Mavroudis et al. 2011, 2014a, b, 2016, 2018; Cook et al. 2020). Court decisions have affirmed this matter (Beauchamp and Childress 2009; Berg et al. 2001; Manson and O'Neill 2007; Salgo v. Leland Stanford Jr University Board of Trustees 1957). In Canterbury v. Spence (Langer 2017), the courts sided with the plaintiff (who wasn't informed of the possibility of paralysis prior to spinal surgery), saying, "The scope of the physician's communications to the patient, then, must be measured by the patient's need, and that need is the information material to the decision [whether to have the surgery]. Thus, the test for determining whether a particular peril must be divulged is its materiality to the patient's decision: all risks potentially affecting the decision must be unmasked." (Murphy 1976). It does not stop there. A failure to show empathy and concern for the affected patient in the postoperative period can develop into further emotional pain, discontent, and in the end, distrust. Distrust often leads to animosity and then comes retribution in the forms of legal suits, the surgeon's loss of reputation, and the hospital's loss of community standing. These are the ultimate results of improper informed consent.

There are many examples of failure to perform proper informed consent based on the procedure and interrelational cultural, racial, and gender issues (Mavroudis et al. 2011, 2014a, b, 2016, 2018; Cook et al. 2020). Does the practitioner omit some potential complications in the Informed Consent process because he/she senses that the patient and family are not capable of understanding the issues? Or does the practitioner omit a more comprehensive discussion because he/she feels that this knowledge might actually be harmful to the patient or family? To be sure, these are sensitive issues and can be mitigated by interpersonal empathy, time spent with the family, and a parting sense of optimism after all the possible but rare adverse complications have been discussed. The basis for communication is Truth Telling (Mavroudis et al. 2005) while creating trust and projecting competence.

There are unfortunate vignettes that have been documented in hospital surgical inquiry proceedings (but not often published) concerning wrong sided surgery, mistaken complicated operations for malignancy when not indicated, and omission of therapeutic standards when clearly indicated. Attempts of the practitioner to avoid inquiry and peer review (after the fact) by lying to the patient and family degrades the practitioner and the patient, violating all four of the basic principles of Respect for Autonomy, Beneficence, Non-Maleficence, and Justice. Of some interest is a study that was performed to assess the implications of practitioners telling the patient who had a complication, "I'm sorry that this complication occurred." (Carmack 2008) Beyond the apology the physician provided an explanation of the conditions that caused the complication including any technical or judgment mistakes as well as the commitment to resolve the complications with transparency and diligence. These authors found (Carmack 2008) that there was a significant decrease in lawsuits with this policy. So, this suggests that when the principles of Medicine are practiced, trust is generally restored.

3 Courage vs. Knowledge: The Moral Imperative to Be Prepared, Competent, and Empathetic

When a practitioner is met with a clinical decision or a surgeon is confronted with a difficult anatomic technical decision, courage will be required to proceed with the clinical course in the absence of supportive data that will facilitate the decision, namely which drug to administer for cancer, or which surgical course to take during an operation (Mavroudis 2003). If, however, there are data to support the proper drug to administer or to guide the surgeon during a difficult case, and if the practitioner/surgeon is unaware of these data, is this a violation of the moral imperative to be prepared? Or is it a situation that could lead to an unwanted complication due to unawareness? Obviously, both questions are related, and the situation can be interpreted as a moral hazard of unpreparedness which can lead to a clinical complication. An example of the relationship between courage and knowledge from my Presidential Address can be drawn from the profession's early experience with the introduction of the heart lung machine and cardiopulmonary bypass. In the early days, much courage was required to apply this technology—courage of both the surgeon and the patient –since there was a paucity of knowledge. As time and research contributed to improved technology and as methods to perform cardiopulmonary bypass reached their present level of expertise, the curve shifted where an abundance of knowledge allowed the practice of cardiopulmonary bypass to be performed safely requiring only a small modicum of courage. While one could invoke the Boy Scout motto of "Be Prepared" (Scout Motto 1908), this principle of preparedness heralds back to ancient times of Hippocrates (2006), Aristotle (1954), Plato (1989), and precursors of modernity such as Locke (1980), and Kant (1993), among many others. Preparation is at the basis of competence and displaying competence will engender trust. And as applied to our discussion, preparation and competence will serve the practitioner well with regard to his/her outcomes and patient satisfaction.

4 Futility

This section on Futility considers medical futility in the settings of philosophical inquiry, spirituality, end of life matters, scientific truths, and societal analysis. Medical/surgical actions or mishaps, accidents, or severe disease entities that have resulted in medical futility are often attended by medical/surgical complications with the potential for heartbreak, distrust, and litigation. There are myriad historical and philosophical issues related to this unfortunate problem. Medical futility is not easily confined to a definition and has been debated throughout the history of thought and medical practice. We quote from a previous publication.

> It was Hippocrates who described the major goals of medical therapy as consisting of cure, relief of suffering, and refusal to treat those who are overcome by their diseases. Plato objected to a cure that results in a life that isn't worth living. He noted that repeated expenditure of energy that is consistently non-productive should not be engaged. (Mavroudis and Siegel 2020)
>
> Futility can be difficult to define. "Schneiderman and associates opined that futile actions are those that cannot achieve the goals of the actions, regardless of how often they are repeated. In addition, they noted that the likelihood of failure can be predictable because it is characteristic of the nature of the action proposed, though futility may become apparent only after many failed attempts. Schneiderman et al offered a useful working definition of futility in the medical field that is centered around the following: when physicians conclude through personal experience, experiences shared with colleagues, or consideration of reported empiric data that in the last one hundred cases, a medical treatment has been useless, they should regard that treatment as futile". (Mavroudis and Siegel 2020)

The practical essence of Medical Futility usually involves parental or family persistence to compel the medical team to continue therapy without regard to the considered medical opinions of attending physicians, nursing staff, and ethics consultants who have determined that the clinical situation is hopeless. In most instances, the recommendation of the medical team in futile conditions is comfort care which generally means terminal care. To define further the issues of Medical Futility and the complications thereto pertaining, Lantos and associates (1994) published an analysis that categorizes the issues that can result in suspicion, confrontation, and disruption of the patient-doctor relationship. Lantos and colleagues offer five categories that can cause complications of medical futility: power, trust, money, hope, and integrity.

4.1 Power

The first category—power—can be discussed in a number of ways, but in this case, the issue is condensed into "Who gets to say no?" (Lantos and Ethical Issues 1994). Historical aspects of this question have roots in discussions during the 1970s and 1980s which considered the rights of patients to refuse medical treatment based on the autonomy principle which recognized that an individual has the legal and moral right to his/her own destiny when it comes to accepting or refusing medical therapy. In particular, the case of Bouvia v. Superior Court (1986) found for Elizabeth Bouvia (The plaintiff) that even if not terminally ill, she has the right to refuse any kind of medical treatment (Langer 2017). This principle has been largely respected except for medical decisions which refer to children who are protected by the moral and legal responsibility of the state. In other words, the state is intensely interested in the wellbeing of her children. For instance, physicians may petition the state to rule on blood transfusions, orphaned subjects, and conflict of interest issues. The law has a way of resolving issues that ordinarily might be mired in unsettled conflict. Opinions in subsequent decades (1990s and 2000s) have evolved in the direction of the rights of patients and their families to demand medical treatment despite futility issues. The issues can be summed up succinctly in the following pair of questions: "Do patients and families have the right to force doctors to squander scarce time and resources on therapies that have no benefit in order to satisfy their potentially irrational wishes?" Conversely, "Do doctors have a right to arbitrarily ignore the values and preferences of patients and families, using only their own value systems to make life and death decisions for others?" Clearly, these debates, stated in confrontational terms for emphasis, require a "Golden Mean" (Aristotle 1954) resolution. Kaplan et al. (1996) introduced the phrase "Odds and Ends" as shorthand for a frame through which this debate can be viewed. Questions that can be asked about a potential futility crisis are: what chance or probability of success is "worth it", what quality of outcome is "worth it" and—equally important—how do we refrain from pursuing long "odds" to achieve bad "ends"? Kaplan further opines that it is hard to choose a position in such a forceful debate. He advises that a theoretical analysis of a bioethical problem should not be expected to bear more weight than can reasonably be sustained. Precision and ambiguity are inherently in tension in such cases and the resolution is not always obvious. Kaplan notes that one reality is secure and unquestionable. The greater the trust that exists between physician and patient, the more willing patients will be to refrain from pursuing long odds to achieve bad ends (Kaplan et al. 1996).

4.2 Trust

When patients trust their doctors, respect their wisdom and agree with their proposed therapeutic options even in the face of futile conditions, the futility debate recedes (Mavroudis and Siegel 2020). Discussions concerning severe complications and futility will be understood amongst family and caregivers and together they will decide to suspend treatment and accept the fatal outcome and associated grieving process. This process can break down however owing to mistrust or misunderstanding of the situation. For instance, one might consider why family members would want to continue a treatment that is futile. The family might not believe that the situation is futile. In addition, there may well be misunderstanding, denial, and psychological stress. Under these circumstances, distrust becomes a challenging situation that will be very difficult to resolve since families are likely to reject doctors' recommendations to withhold life-sustaining treatment and cling to their original thoughts of distrust and misguided hope. The complication associated with this outcome is steeped in the absence or presence of antecedent conscientious informed consent which includes communicating information, shared decision-making, and creating a "connection" with the family. When these "connections" prove to be successful, the chances of a ruptured relationship and resultant distrust fade.

4.3 Money and Precious Resources

There is no getting around the idea that money and precious resources play an active part in medical care—especially when considering futility. The complication is the moral hazard to which physicians are subjected, namely the financial conflicts of interest that are in tension between their loyalty to their patients and their loyalty to the organization that they serve. When futility issues involve inexpensive therapeutic interventions, controversies and moral hazards are not as pronounced as those that require complex technology and avante-garde options. When limited resources are available, one must consider whether it is ethically justified to employ expensive therapeutic interventions that offer minimal benefits, especially when considering futility (Mavroudis et al. 2020b). Bioethical complications come to play when physicians are exposed to financial conflicts of interest regarding their fidelity to their patients, their allegiance to their organizations, and their social obligations. At the heart of it all lies the question of the patients' trust in us. When there is trust, physicians and families have time to deliberate the reality of futility and can come to a rational conclusion about continuing expensive contraindicated care. Distinguishing our obligations in a straightforward and honest manner will become more and more important and will determine whether or not our patients can continue to trust us (Mavroudis et al. 2014b).

4.4 Hope

Hope is a state of mind that is associated with optimistic, religious, and spiritual themes. Physicians are taught never to take hope away from their patients for there is always hope—at least that is what the concept suggests. Hope often implies miracles. A review of selected philosophers can add imprecision to the discussion. David Hume was a famous Scottish philosopher/empiricist and skeptic regarding religion who defined a miracle as a suspension of a law of nature (Hume 1973). His empiricism did not allow for such a suspension, nor for any divine intercession. For him, there is only nature; there are no miracles, and we cannot reasonably hope for one. Alternatively, Reverend William Sloane Coffin, in his interview on National Public Radio in 1994 noted that, "hope is a state of mind independent of the state of the world. If one's heart is full of hope, one can be persistent even though one can't be optimistic. One can keep the faith, despite the evidence, knowing that only in so doing does the evidence have any chance of changing. So, while Reverend Coffin was perhaps not optimistic, he is always very hopeful (Reverend William Sloane Coffin 1994)."

In his book, *The Anatomy of Hope* (Groopman 2003) Jerome Groopman considers the roles of optimism and courage regarding medical therapies when the patient is confronted with severe illness. Another thinker, Viktor Frankl writes about the horrors of his captivity in a Nazi concentration camp which he was able to survive through reflection and perseverance. He developed an analysis that allowed him to endure the hardships that were all around him: that to live is to suffer; to survive is to find meaning in the suffering (Frankl 2006).

This discussion of hope reaches no rational conclusions. The many inquiries pursued by academics, theorists, clergy, and philosophers have resulted in peculiar thoughts about hope. When confronted with futility, our patients and their families are searching for optimistic possibilities in a sea of pessimism and, oftentimes, certain death. Our oath, duty, and empathy require a supportive posture along with and the courage (sensitively but honestly) to tell the truth.

4.5 Attempts to Resolve Futility

Our theme in this chapter is the bioethical complications of congenital heart surgery. There are times when complications relating to surgery or innate disease can lead to futility which will require guidelines to help families to cope with complex decisions (Lantos and Ethical Issues 1994; Sachdeva et al. 1996; Boston Children's Hospital Futility Policy 2013; Truog 2007; Schneiderman et al. 1990; Shepherd 2013; Mavroudis and Siegel 2020; Mavroudis et al. 2005). Judgments of futility will require continued trust and evaluation on a case-by-case basis. Accordingly, ethics committee consultations, hospital policies, and state law have been developed and enacted to make the painful process of recognizing futility and terminating care more tolerable to all concerned. Many hospitals have adopted procedures that require ethics committee consultation, potential patient transfer to another institution, and support for legal representation (Lantos and Ethical Issues 1994; Sachdeva et al. 1996; Boston Children's Hospital Futility Policy 2013; Truog 2007; Schneiderman et al. 1990; Shepherd 2013; Mavroudis and Siegel 2020; Mavroudis et al. 2005).

This process, when conducted in an empathetic manner, rarely results in termination of the patient-physician relationship. In general, families begin to understand the issues and accept them. Furthermore, those families who steadfastly argued for maintenance of life-sustaining treatments, sometimes seem relieved by the process. Comments such as, "If you are asking us to agree with the recommendation to remove life support from our loved one, we cannot. However, we do not wish to fight the recommendation in court and if the law says it is OK to stop life support, then that is what should happen." (London et al. 2020)

The resolution of the complication of futility is stressful and painful for all concerned. As we have noted herein, the events or complications resulting in medical futility can cause regret by the caregivers and resentment by the family. In the end, clinical review will help with the learning process to determine what could have been done better (or not) in the situation of overwhelming complexity and the disease severity. These issues are important to be sure, however, the fact remains that the patient is in a futile condition which requires empathy, understanding, and proper conduct by all parties.

4.6 Regionalization

Regionalization is the process by which pediatric cardiac services are determined by a central center with a large volume of patients and therapeutic experiences. This system puts into tension large volume centers and small volume centers. So, since we are considering complications relating to congenital heart surgery, one asks the question, "Do high volume centers have better clinical results and a lower complication rate than do low volume centers?" The answer to this question is seemingly, "Yes". Many retrospective studies and focused debate have determined unequivocally that patients do better at high volume centers than low volume centers. To solve this problem, authors have determined that low volume centers can partner with other high-volume centers to divide cases based on complexity, the need for cardiac transplantation, and the availability of advanced catheter-based interventions. This system will allow shared educational experiences for all and be a roadmap for improved results and program development (Shepherd 2013).

Nevertheless, there are peculiar situations that are not always solved by interrelational programs. For instance, if a patient presents with a problem to the surgical team at a high-volume center that has some experience but not an abundance of clinical experience that has been accrued by another hospital some five hundred miles away, what does one tell the patient and the family? The clear answer is to be transparent and explain all factors that apply to the situation including the individual surgeon's experience, the expertise of the surgical team, and the postoperative care proficiency. Likely the patient and family will agree to the procedure if the informed consent process is comprehensive and transparent. However, what if there is a complication during the operation that might not have occurred if the patient had traveled to the more experienced location? What if there was a complication that could have happened anywhere? These unanswered questions become problematic and resolution of the same will have required conscientious preoperative consultation and informed consent as well as concern and empathy in the postoperative period. But what about the surgeon and the surgical team? While a complication occurred that will be discussed at the surgical conference, was the surgeon and the surgical team prepared well enough for the operation? Should there have been a trip to the hospital with the larger experience to observe the operation? Introspection and honest self-awareness can help to determine the answers to these troublesome problems.

4.7 Summary

This chapter seeks to remind us that in addition to the many surgical/medical complications that can arise in congenital heart surgery, there are also ethical complications that a conscientious practitioner must consider and be prepared to address. We have mentioned the four cardinal principles of biomedical ethics, while focusing most directly on the complications that can arise with regard to our obligation to respect patient autonomy. We have highlighted clinical examples in which omission of comprehensive informed consent could result in patient dissatisfaction and lawsuits, the practitioner's loss of reputation, and the hospital's loss of public standing. Other examples have been discussed such as truth-telling, shared decision-making, and management of futility.

References

Aristotle. The Nicomachean ethics, book III (Translated by Sir David Ross). London: Oxford University Press; 1954.

Backer CL. Commentary: regionalization = excellence. J Thorac Cardiovasc Surg. 2021a;161(6):2157.

Backer CL. Reply: embracing regionalization worldwide. J Thorac Cardiovasc Surg. 2021b;161(6):e482.

Backer CL. Reply: regionalization: one genotype, multiple phenotypes. J Thorac Cardiovasc Surg. 2022a;163(1):e65.

Backer CL. Invited commentary: regionalization refines surgical dogma regarding trisomy 21 and atrioventricular septal defect. J Thorac Cardiovasc Surg. 2022b;163(4):1445.

Backer CL. Regionalization equals excellence in pediatric tracheal surgery. Ann Thorac Surg. 2022c;113(4):1306.

Backer CL, Mavroudis C, Zias EA, Amin Z, Weigel TJ. Repair of coarctation with resection and extended end-to-end anastomosis. Ann Thorac Surg. 1998;66(4):1365–71.

Backer CL, Pasquali SK, Dearani JA. Improving national outcomes in congenital heart surgery: the time has come for regionalization of care. Circulation. 2020;141(12):943–5.

Beauchamp TL, Childress JF. Principles of biomedical ethics. 6th ed. New York: Oxford University Press; 2009.

Berg JW, Appelbaum PS, Lidz CW, Parker LS. Informed consent: legal theory and clinical practice. 2nd ed. New York: Oxford University Press; 2001.

Boston Children's Hospital Futility Policy. 2013. https://bioethics.hms.harvard.edu/sites/g/files/mcu336/f/CEC-Futility-Report-Jan-2013.pdf. Accessed 13 Apr 2024.

Carmack HJ. How to say I'm sorry: a study of the Veterans Administration Hospital Association's Apology and Disclosure Program, ETH:4614. Ohio University; 2008.

Cook T, Mavroudis CD, Jacobs JP, Mavroudis C. Respect for autonomy as a virtue in clinical medicine. Cardiol Young. 2015;25:1615–20.

Cook T, Mavroudis C, Mavroudis CD. Autonomy and the principles of medical practice. In: Bioethical controversies in pediatric cardiology and cardiac surgery. 1st ed. London: Springer; 2020.

Farag ES, Kluin J, de Heer F, et al. Aortic coarctation repair through left thoracotomy: results in the modern era. Eur J Cardiothorac Surg. 2019;55(2):331–7.

Frankl V. Man's search for meaning introduction to logotherapy. Boston: Beacon Press; 2006. ISBN 978-0-8070-1427-1 (Originally published on 1946).

Groopman J. The anatomy of hope. Random House; 2003.

Hippocrates Microsoft Encarta Online Encyclopedia. Microsoft Corporation 2006. Archived from the original on 2009-10-31.

Hume D. In: Selby-Bigge LA, editor. Enquiries concerning human understanding and concerning the principles of morals reprinted from 1777 edition. 3rd ed. Oxford: Clarendon Press; 1973.

Jacobs JP. The Society of Thoracic Surgeons congenital heart surgery database public reporting initiative. Semin Thorac Cardiovasc Surg Pediatr Card Surg Annu. 2017;20:43–8.

Jacobs JP, Jacobs ML. Transparency and public reporting of pediatric and congenital heart surgery outcomes in North America. World J Pediatr Congenit Heart Surg. 2016;7(1):49–53.

Jacobs JP, Cerfolio RJ, Sade RM. The ethics of transparency: publication of cardiothoracic surgical outcomes in the lay press. Ann Thorac Surg. 2009;87(3):679–86.

Jacobs JP, Shahian DM, Prager RL, Badhwar V, Jacobs ML. Invited commentary. Parents' preferences regarding public reporting of outcomes in congenital heart surgery. Ann Thorac Surg. 2018;105(2):612–4.

Kant I. Grounding for the metaphysics of morals [1785] (Translated by James Wesley Ellington). Indianapolis: Hackett Pub Co; 1993.

Kaplan SH, Greenfield S, Gandek B, Rogers WH, Ware JE Jr. Characteristics of physicians with participatory decision-making styles. Ann Intern Med. 1996;124:497–504.

Karamlou T, Johnston DR, Backer CL, Roselli EE, Welke KF, Caldarone CA, Svensson LG. Access or excess? Examining the argument for regionalized cardiac care. J Thorac Cardiovasc Surg. 2020;160(3):813–9.

Langer E. Court ruling in his case established doctrine of informed medical consent. The Washington Post, 2017, May 21, p. C8.

Lantos J, Ethical issues. Futility assessments and the doctor-patient relationship. J Am Geriatr Soc. 1994;42:868–70.
Locke J. In: MacPherson CB, editor. Second treatise of government. Indianapolis: Hackett Publishing; 1980.
London T, Bautista R-MF Jr, Bhakta AS, Bazan V, Zwischenberger JB. Conflict of interest. In: Bioethical controversies in pediatric cardiology and cardiac surgery. 1st ed. London: Springer; 2020.
Manson NC, O'Neill O. Rethinking informed consent in bioethics. 1st ed. New York: Cambridge University Press; 2007.
Mavroudis C. Presidential address: a partnership in courage. Ann Thorac Surg. 2003;75(5):1366–71.
Mavroudis C. Ethical forces that shape a career in surgery. Am J Surg. 2005;190(2):319–23.
Mavroudis CD. Fetal cardiac interventions. In: Bioethical controversies in pediatric cardiology and cardiac surgery. 1st ed. London: Springer; 2020.
Mavroudis C, Backer CL. The influence of Plato, Aristotle, and the ancient Polis on a programme for congenital cardiac surgery: the virtuous partnership. Cardiol Young. 2007;17(suppl 2):159–63.
Mavroudis C, Cook T. Informed consent. In: Bioethical controversies in pediatric cardiology and cardiac surgery. 1st ed. London: Springer; 2020.
Mavroudis C, Siegel A. Medical futility, when further therapy is hopeless. In: Bioethical controversies in pediatric cardiology and cardiac surgery. 1st ed. London: Springer; 2020.
Mavroudis C, Mavroudis CD, Naunheim KS, Sade RM. Should surgical errors always be disclosed to the patient? Ann Thorac Surg. 2005;80(2):399–408.
Mavroudis C, Mavroudis CD, Farrell RM, Jacobs ML, Jacobs JP, Kodish E. Informed consent, bioethical equipoise, and hypoplastic left heart syndrome. Cardiol Young. 2011;21(Suppl 2):133–40.
Mavroudis C, Mavroudis CD, Jacobs JP, Siegel A, Pasquali SK, Hill KD, Jacobs ML. Informing the informed consent process for congenital heart operations: an analysis from the STS-congenital heart surgery database. Ann Thorac Surg. 2014a;97:1838–49.
Mavroudis CD, Jacobs JP, Siegel A, Mavroudis C. Ethical issues confronting outcomes analysis and quality assurance. In: Barach PR, Jacobs JP, Lipshultz SE, Laussen PC, editors. Pediatric and congenital cardiac disease. London: Springer; 2014b.
Mavroudis CD, Cook T, Jacobs JP, Mavroudis C. Ethical considerations of transparency, informed consent, and nudging in a 9-year-old with aortic stenosis and symptomatic left ventricular endocardial fibroelastosis. Cardiol Young. 2016;26:1573–80.
Mavroudis C, Mavroudis CD, Cook T, Siegel A. Bioethical controversies in pediatric cardiac surgery. In: Mavroudis C, Backer CL, editors. Pediatric cardiac surgery. 5th ed. London: Wiley-Blackwell Inc; 2018.
Mavroudis C, Cook T, Mavroudis CD, editors. Bioethical controversies in pediatric cardiology and cardiac surgery. 1st ed. London: Springer; 2020a.
Mavroudis CD, Lancaster CW, Mavroudis C. Rare diagnoses and allocation of precious resources. In: Bioethical controversies in pediatric cardiology and cardiac surgery. 1st ed. London: Springer; 2020b.
McLaren A, Morris-Stiff G, Casey J. Issues of consent in renal transplantation. Ann R Coll Surg Engl. 2001;83:343–6.
Murphy WJ. Canterbury v. Spence—the case and a few comments The Forum (Section of Insurance, Negligence and Compensation Law, American Bar Association). 1976, Spring;11(3):716–26.
Nashif SAM. The unintended consequences of public reporting. In: Bioethical controversies in pediatric cardiology and cardiac surgery. 1st ed. London: Springer; 2020.
Patel A, Gandhi R, Mavroudis C. Role of ethics consultation in pediatric congenital heart disease. In: Bioethical controversies in pediatric cardiology and cardiac surgery. 1st ed. London: Springer; 2020.
Plato. Republic translated by Paul Shorey. In: Hamilton E, Cairns H, editors. The collected dialogues, Bollingen series LXXI. Princeton: Princeton University Press; 1989.
Pleat JM, Dunkin CSJ, Davies CE, Ripley RM, Tyler MPH. Prospective survey of factors affecting risk discussion during consent in a surgical specialty. Br J Surg. 2004;91:1377–80.
Reverend William Sloane Coffin, as interviewed on NPR radio in 1994.
Sachdeva RC, Jefferson LS, Coss-Bu J, Brody BA. Resource consumption and the extent of futile care among patients in pediatric intensive care setting. J Pediatr. 1996;128:742–7.
Salgo v. Leland Stanford Jr University Board of Trustees (154 Cal. App. 3d 560, 317 P.2d 170 [1957]).
Schneiderman LJ, Kecler NS, Jonsen AR. Medical futility: its meaning and ethical implications. Ann Intern Med. 1990;112:949–54.
Scout Motto. Lieut. Gen. Baden Powell C.B., Scouting for Boys. 1908. "Camp Fire Yarn.—No. 4. Scout Law." (Part I, p. 49).
Serfontein SJ, Kron IL. Complications of coarctation repair. Semin Thorac Cardiovasc Surg Pediatr Card Surg Annu. 2022;5:206–11.
Shepherd D. Bioethics and the law. 3rd ed. Wolters Kluwer Law, and Business; 2013.
Truog RD. Tackling medical futility in Texas. New Engl J Med. 2007;357(1):1–3.
Tweddell JS, Jacobs JP, Austin EH 3rd. Are there negative consequences of public reporting? The hype and the reality. J Thorac Cardiovasc Surg. 2017;153(4):908–11.
Welke KF, Pasquali SK, Lin P, Backer CL, Overman DM, Romano JC, Jacobs JP, Karamlou T. Hospital distri-

bution and patient travel patterns for congenital cardiac surgery in the United States. Ann Thorac Surg. 2019;107(2):574–81.

Welke KF, Pasquali SK, Lin P, Backer CL, Overman D, Romano JC, Karamlou T. Regionalization of congenital heart surgery in the United States. Semin Thorac Cardiovasc Surg. 2020;32(1):128–37.

Welke KF, Pasquali SK, Lin P, Backer CL, Overman DM, Romano JC, Karamlou T. Theoretical model for delivery of congenital heart surgery in the United States. Ann Thorac Surg. 2021;111(5):1628–35.

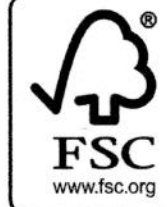

MIX
Papier aus verantwortungsvollen Quellen
Paper from responsible sources
FSC® C105338

If you have any concerns about our products,
you can contact us on
ProductSafety@springernature.com

In case Publisher is established outside the EU,
the EU authorized representative is:
Springer Nature Customer Service Center GmbH
Europaplatz 3, 69115 Heidelberg, Germany

Printed by Libri Plureos GmbH
in Hamburg, Germany